Foundations of Nursing Practice

Your textbook comes with a range of additional online resources

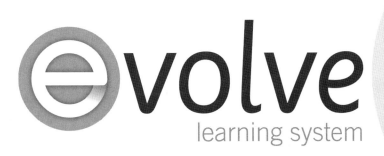

evolve
learning system

**We have created a range of additional online resources
specifically designed to expand the material in your textbook.**

These include:

- 450 self-testing questions with answers
- 100 Multiple Choice Questions
- Illustrations for downloading
- Useful web links
- Learning outcomes

The additional online resources are available on our **Evolve learning system**.

For access, please go to **http://evolve.elsevier.com/Brooker/
foundations/** and follow the on-screen prompts.

Need help? For assistance with accessing your additional online resources, please visit
http://evolvesupport.elsevier.com/

Content Strategist: *Mairi McCubbin*
Content Development Specialist: *Carole McMurray*
Project Manager: *Julie Taylor*
Designer: *Miles Hitchen*
Illustration Manager: *Jennifer Rose*
Illustrator: *Antbits Ltd, Graeme Chambers*

Foundations of Nursing Practice

Fundamentals of Holistic Care

SECOND EDITION

Edited by

Chris Brooker BSc MSc RGN SCM RNT
Author and Editor, Norfolk, UK

Anne Waugh BSc(Hons) MSc CertEd SRN RNT FHEA
Senior Teaching Fellow and School Director of Academic Quality,
School of Nursing, Midwifery & Social Care, Edinburgh Napier University, Edinburgh, UK

Foreword by

Professor Roger Watson BSc PhD RN FRCN FAAN
Editor-in-Chief, Journal of Advanced Nursing, Professor of Nursing,
Faculty of Health and Social Care, University of Hull, Hull, UK

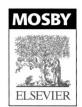

Edinburgh London New York Oxford Philadelphia St Louis Sydney Toronto 2013

MOSBY
ELSEVIER

First edition 2007
Second edition 2013

ISBN 978-0-7234-3661-4

British Library Cataloguing in Publication Data
A catalogue record for this book is available from the British Library

Library of Congress Cataloging in Publication Data
A catalog record for this book is available from the Library of Congress

ELSEVIER your source for books, journals and multimedia in the health sciences

www.elsevierhealth.com

Working together to grow libraries in developing countries

www.elsevier.com | www.bookaid.org | www.sabre.org

ELSEVIER   BOOK AID International   Sabre Foundation

The publisher's policy is to use paper manufactured from sustainable forests

Printed in China

Contents

Contributors

Irene Anderson BSc(Hons) MSc PGCE DPSN RGN FHEA
National Teaching Fellow
Principal Lecturer, Tissue Viability, School of Nursing, Midwifery and Social Work, University of Hertfordshire, Hatfield, UK
25 Wound management

Elaine Ball BA(Hons) MA PhD CertEd PGCHE RN
Senior Lecturer in Nursing, College of Health & Social Care, University of Salford, Salford, Manchester, UK
2 Evolution of contemporary nursing

Emma Briggs BSc(Hons) PhD PGCert(Research)
PGCert(Academic Practice) RN
Lecturer, Department of Adult Nursing, Florence Nightingale School of Nursing and Midwifery, King's College London, London, UK
13 Safety in nursing practice

Chris Brooker BSc MSc RGN SCM RNT
Author and Editor, Norfolk, UK
19 Promoting hydration and nutrition

Carol Chamley BA MA CertEd EdD DipN MSSM RCNT RSCN RNT RGN ONC
Senior Lecturer, Faculty of Health and Life Sciences, Coventry University, Coventry, UK
23 Pain management – minimizing the pain experience

Janis Deane BSc MSc DipLSN RMN RGN RNT
Senior Lecturer, School of Life, Sport and Social Sciences, Edinburgh Napier University, Edinburgh, UK
1 Understanding health and health promotion

Jayne Donaldson BN MN PhD PGCE RN
Head of School, School of Nursing, Midwifery & Social Care, Edinburgh Napier University, Edinburgh, UK
22 Promoting the safe administration of medicines

Christine Donnelly BA PhD DipHV RGN RNT ONC
Senior Lecturer, School of Life, Sport and Social Sciences, Edinburgh Napier University, Edinburgh, UK
18 Mobility and immobility

Jacqui Fletcher BSc(Hons) MSc PGCert Ed RGN
Principal Lecturer, School of Nursing and Midwifery, University of Hertfordshire, Hatfield, UK; Senior Professional Tutor, Department of Dermatology and Wound Healing, Cardiff University, Cardiff, UK
25 Wound management

Maria J. Grant BA(Hons) MSc PGCE
Research Fellow (Information), Salford Centre for Nursing, Midwifery and Collaborative Research (SCNMCR), University of Salford, Manchester, UK
5 Evidence-based practice and research

Morag Gray MN PhD DipCNE CertEd HEAA RGN RCNT RNT FHEA
Emeritus Professor (Nursing and Nursing Education), Edinburgh Napier University, Edinburgh, UK
4 Learning and teaching

Pauline Hamilton MN DipAsthma RNT RCNT RGN RMN
Lecturer, Department of Health and Community Sciences, School of Health and Life Sciences, Glasgow Caledonian University, Glasgow, UK
14 The nursing process, holistic assessment and baseline observations

Annie Holme BSc MSc PGCE[A] RN
Lecturer, Department of Adult Nursing, Florence Nightingale School of Nursing and Midwifery, King's College London, London, UK
3 Health and social care delivery systems

Dorothy Horsburgh BA(Hons) MEd PhD CertEd DipCNE RGN RNT RCNT
Senior Lecturer, Faculty of Health, Life and Social Sciences; Lecturer, School of Nursing, Midwifery and Social Care, Edinburgh Napier University, Edinburgh, UK
7 The NMC Code of conduct and applied ethical principles

Michelle Howarth MSc PhD PGCert RGN
Lecturer, School of Nursing, Midwifery and Social Work, University of Salford, Manchester, UK
5 Evidence-based practice and research

Gay James BSc MSc DipN RGN RCNT RNT
Senior Lecturer, Adult Nursing, Coventry University, Coventry, UK
23 Pain management – minimizing the pain experience

Catriona Kennedy BA(Hons) PhD DipNurs RN DN RNT DNT PWT
Professor of Nursing and Midwifery, Department of Nursing and Midwifery, Univeristy of Limerick, Ireland and School of Nursing, Midwifery and Social Care, Edinburgh Napier University, Edinburgh, UK
12 Loss and bereavement

Rosie Kneafsey BSc PhD MRes PGCE RGN
Senior Lecturer in Nursing, Department of Health Studies, Coventry University, Coventry, UK
5 Evidence-based practice and research

Gill Loughty McCrossan BA MSc PGCert RGN RNT
Lecturer, School of Nursing, Midwifery & Social Care, Edinburgh Napier University, Edinburgh, UK
15 Preventing the spread of infection

Neil Murphy BSc(Hons) MSc RMN
Lecturer in Mental Health, School of Nursing, Mental Health branch, University of Salford, Manchester, UK
11 Stress, anxiety and coping

Sherri Ogston-Tuck BSc MA PGDipHE PGDipLaw RN
Lecturer, Critical Care Nursing, Florence Nightingale School of Nursing, King's College London, London, UK
6 Legal issues that impact on nursing practice

Ah Nya Plant BSc(Hons) MSc DipAA RGN RM RCNT RNT MNIMH
Lecturer/Programme Leader, School of Life, Sport and Social Sciences, Edinburgh Napier University, Edinburgh, UK
10 Sleep, rest and complementary and alternative medicine

Theresa E. Price BSc(Hons) MSc CertEd FE RN RNT FHEA
Senior Lecturer, Department of Health and Community Sciences, School of Health and Life Sciences, Glasgow Caledonian University, Glasgow, UK
14 The nursing process, holistic assessment and baseline observations

Jillian Riley PhD RN RM NFESC
Head of Post-Graduate Education (Nursing) and Harefield NHS Foundation Trust, Royal Brompton Hospital, London, UK
17 Breathing and circulation

Naomi Sharples BSc MBA PGCE Prof Doc RMNH RMN
University Link Lecturer, School of Nursing, Midwifery and Social Work, University of Salford, Manchester, UK
9 Relationship, helping and communication skills

Martin Steggall BSc(Hons) MSc PhD PG Cert AP RN (Adult) FHEA
Associate Dean, Director of Undergraduate Studies, City University, London, UK; Clinical Nurse Specialist (Erectile Dysfunction and Premature Ejaculation), Barts Health NHS Trust, London, UK
20 Elimination of urine: care and promoting continence

Karen Strickland BSc MSc PGCE RGN RNT FHEA
Lecturer & Teaching Fellow in Academic Practice, Office of the Vice Principal (Academic), Edinburgh Napier University, Edinburgh, UK
12 Loss and bereavement

David Tait BSc(Hons) MSc RMN RGN RNT
Lecturer, School of Nursing, Midwifery & Social Care, Edinburgh Napier University, Edinburgh, UK
8 Impact of lifespan on nursing interventions

Susan H. Walker BSc(Hons) MA RGN
Senior Lecturer, School of Nursing, Midwifery and Social Work, University of Salford, Manchester, UK
21 Elimination of faeces: care and promoting continence

Susan Watt BSc MSc PGCertTLHE RN SPQ RNT FHEA
Senior Lecturer for Clinical Skills and Teaching Fellow, School of Nursing, Midwifery & Social Care, Edinburgh Napier University, Edinburgh, UK
24 Caring for the person having surgery

Anne Waugh BSc(Hons) MSc CertEd SRN RNT FHEA
Senior Teaching Fellow and School Director of Academic Quality, School of Nursing, Midwifery & Social Care, Edinbugh Napier University, Edinburgh, UK
16 Personal care, sensory impairment and unconsciousness

My Foreword to the previous edition of this book began with the complaint that the book had appeared too late; my oldest daughter had just qualified as a nurse and would have benefitted from the book. I hoped that the next edition would appear in time if my next daughter decided to study nursing. This one is also too late as my next daughter has, similarly, recently qualified.

This present edition continues in the same vein as the previous volume in terms of relevance and excellence. In fact, this new volume is even more relevant; the previous one was ahead of its time. Nursing in the UK – where the book has most, but not exclusive, relevance – has finally moved to all-graduate entry to the profession. Brooker and Waugh's *Foundations* is precisely what the new curriculum needs; texts of this calibre, if adopted, should enable the new programmes to be substantially different in content and ensure that these degree programmes are not just re-labelled diplomas.

The authorship of chapters has slightly changed, which shows some evolution in and updating of the contents. The division of contents remains more or less the same as the previous volume but 'person-centred care' – an old concept with greater currency than ever before – appears in the title to the fourth section. In the second section, the chapter on Learning and Teaching, which carries over from the previous edition, struck me as demonstrating just how far ahead nursing is in our awareness of educational theories and practice than almost any other subject, including our closest colleagues in medical education and in the allied health professions. My views on complementary and alternative therapies are probably best confined to my Twitter© account (@rwatson1955) but the continued inclusion of these therapies here serves to illustrate their growing influence, with comprehensive coverage of what they purport to do.

I worry about nursing and its continued survival in the face of government cuts, scandals and prejudice from within academia. As I emphasized in my previous Foreword, the order of contents emphasizes that nursing has a history; it has a philosophical and educational basis and it is also profoundly practical…frankly, it is unique. If nursing ever needs to be rebuilt from scratch, then texts like Brooker and Waugh's *Foundations* are there to serve as a template. However, we have not yet reached that extreme situation; nursing survives for the time being and the immediate next generation have an excellent text on which to base their learning and practice. None of my sons has yet expressed an interest in nursing but, if my youngest daughter decides to enter the profession, I hope that the publishers will consult me.

Hull, 2012

Roger Watson

Preface

This book has been written specifically to meet the needs of nursing students in all fields of practice who are working towards the Nursing & Midwifery Council (2010) competencies for the second progression point, hence its title: *Foundations of Nursing Practice: Fundamentals of Holistic Care*. The curriculum and competencies for pre-registration nursing programmes set out by the Nursing & Midwifery Council and which are largely focused on health, health promotion, social and life sciences as they apply to nursing have been used as the basis for this book. It aims to explain how and why sensitive, safe, person-centred and holistic nursing care that is evidence-based is carried out. It includes material that is both common to all and specific to each field of nursing practice. There is an emphasis not only on the theory that underpins nursing practice but also on nursing skills which form an equally important part of nursing programmes. Themes with particular relevance to all stages and fields of nursing practice include safety, infection prevention and control, managing stress, communication, managing wounds and pressure ulcers, and dealing with loss. The authors come from all fields of nursing practice and represent many universities.

The book is organized into four sections:

1. Health, nursing and healthcare systems – the chapters in this section explore theories of health and health promotion (Ch. 1); the evolution of contemporary nursing (Ch. 2) and the health and social care systems within which contemporary healthcare is delivered (Ch. 3).
2. Professional practice – this requires knowledge from other disciplines that are integrated into contemporary nursing practice: learning and teaching (Ch. 4); evidence-based practice and research (Ch. 5) and legal (Ch. 6), moral and ethical (Ch. 7) frameworks.
3. Nursing and lifespan implications – many nursing interventions are specific to patients'/clients' stage of development and/or their stage on the lifespan (Ch. 8). All nursing interventions rely on effective communication, which is discussed in Chapter 9. Sleep, rest, and complementary and alternative medicine are considered in Chapter 10 and stress, anxiety and coping are examined in Chapter 11. Chapter 12 considers loss and bereavement.
4. Developing person-centred nursing skills – this section begins by exploring elements of safe practice (Ch. 13), followed by an introduction to the nursing process, assessment and baseline observations (Ch. 14). Preventing the spread of infection is explained in Chapter 15. A wide range of fundamental nursing interventions and skills needed in a range of care settings are explored in the remaining chapters in this section.

Each chapter contains a range of activities to assist your learning and these are explained on pages xi–xii. Many informative 2-colour illustrations, photographs and tables are used to explain or expand the material in each chapter.

The accompanying website (http://evolve.elsevier.com/Brooker/foundations) contains 450 self-test questions and 100 multiple choice questions and answers to help you further consolidate your learning and to assess your progress.

This textbook therefore provides a comprehensive introduction to nursing, which will meet the needs of a range of students, assistant practitioners, nurses returning to practice, mentors and other registered nurses.

Norfolk and Edinburgh, 2013

Chris Brooker
Anne Waugh

Acknowledgements

Several people at Elsevier have kept us on track in order to ensure the book reached publication, especially Ninette Premdas, Mairi McCubbin, Ailsa Laing, Carole McMurray and Julie Taylor. In addition, we are very grateful to the authors and their families and not least our families, David and Andy, for their patience and support throughout the revision of this book.

CB
AW

This book will help you develop the knowledge base and nursing skills needed to provide holistic patient/client care. Each chapter has the same format and many features to assist your learning. These are outlined below to help you get the best from this book.

Learning outcomes – these provide guidance about what you can expect to learn after reading the chapter and carrying out the activities within it. Reflecting on your clinical experience based on your learning in university after you start undertaking placement learning, will greatly assist consolidation of your learning.

Boxes with information – different types of Boxes have been used to assist learning, break up the text and to highlight information in a concise manner.

Box xx.x | *Plain/text*: these are generally concise lists of relevant information that relate to a topic within the text, e.g. Box 1.15 – UK groups most susceptible to poverty (p. 15); Box 13.19 – When handwashing is carried out (p. 294).

 Nursing skills boxes: these provide the principles of fundamental nursing, e.g. Box 15.7 – Handwashing (p. 347); Box 22.10 – Administration of intramuscular injections (p. 557).

 First Aid: these contain a summary of the principles of first aid for common conditions, which is a Nursing and Midwifery Council requirement, e.g. Box 15.11 – Management of needlestick injuries and exposure to body fluids (p. 351); Box 18.2 – Strains and sprains (p. 432).

Activity boxes – these contain scenarios and related student activities that will help you explore particular topics in more depth. Many are referenced and/or include resources to help you extend your knowledge. The activities are intended to help you consider the following aspects of nursing practice in more detail:

 Reflective practice, e.g. Box 14.4 – Sharing personal information (p. 307); Box 7.2 – Too many patients and too few staff (p. 145); Box 11.16 – Stress associated with pregnancy (p. 257).

 Evidence-based practice, e.g. Box 1.13 – Effects of poverty on children (p. 14); Box 15.15 – Maintaining a clean environment (p. 354).

 Health promotion, e.g. Box 13.10 – Falls prevention (p. 285); Box 19.18 – Reducing hazardous or harmful drinking (p. 478).

 Ethical issues, e.g. Box 7.1 – Maintaining confidentiality? (p. 144); Box 18.10 – Condoning unsafe practice (p. 444).

 Critical thinking, e.g. Box 1.7 – Lay and professional conflict (p. 7); Box 13.2 – Hazards that can cause accidents (p. 282).

Cross-referencing – there are extensive cross-references within the text that signpost links to material and topics from:
* other parts of a chapter – denoted (see p. XXX)
* other chapters – denoted (see Ch. XX).

Summary – this is a list of bullet points summarizing key areas explored within the chapter.

Key words and phrases for literature searching – suggestions are included to help you begin to find out more about key topics within the chapter (see also Ch. 5 – Literature searching).

Useful websites – these direct you to simple and reliable sources of Internet information about relevant topics. They are wide-ranging and include charities and organizations; many provide general information about the topic, although some provide more detailed information about common conditions and illnesses for both lay people and health professionals.

References – extensive use is made of in-text references. The list of references to material used within the text is included at the end of the chapter. These aim to be straightforward and many are easily accessible using the Internet. Learning how these have been incorporated into the text and also how they are listed at the end are essential skills required for nursing students' assignments. Although the method used varies between universities, the principles are always similar.

Further reading – a selection of further reading suggestions is provided at the end of the chapter. These give you the opportunity to access a wider range of related information in order to expand your knowledge base.

Glossary – a selection of commonly used nursing terms and their definitions have been collated into a glossary at the end of the book (p. 631) for easy reference.

Index – an extensive index has been compiled to enable you to locate information quickly and easily.

Website *Evolve* *http://evolve.elsevier.com/Brooker/ foundations*: **Self-test questions and multiple choice questions and answers** – a variety of activities related to each chapter can be found here for you to test your learning. The answers are also found there providing immediate feedback.

Section 1

Health, nursing and healthcare systems

Understanding health and health promotion

1

Janis Deane

LEARNING OUTCOMES

This chapter will help you:

- Reflect on personal and official definitions of health, reviewing your awareness of the factors which influence health
- Discuss common lay health beliefs and their effects on behaviour
- Show awareness of the effects of poverty as the key determinant of health
- Understand the place of health promotion in contemporary nursing
- Describe common methods and approaches to the measurement of health
- Appreciate individual responses to illness.

Introduction

People have close contact with health professionals at key points in their lives – in infancy, during adolescence, pregnancy and childbirth, and in sickness and older age – creating significant opportunities for empowering and health promoting interventions. The importance of this chapter is based within *The Code* (Nursing and Midwifery Council, NMC 2008), which states that nurses and midwives must protect and support the health of individual patients, clients and the wider community (see Ch. 7). One of the NMC (2010) *Essential Skills Clusters* incorporated in all pre-registration nursing programmes is that of promoting health and well-being. In addition, the Government has developed *Essence of Care 2010* benchmarks (Department of Health, DH 2010) for promoting health and well-being which apply to each nurse and midwife (Box 1.1).

To achieve this, it is important for nurses to have an understanding of their own and others' health definitions and beliefs. Nurses also need to take into account the factors that affect health and health beliefs in our increasingly multicultural society. This allows accurate assessment of care needs, the planning of sensitive care and the targeting of relevant

information to help people make positive changes to their health-related behaviour. Furthermore, the increasing focus on evidence-based healthcare means that nurses need to have an understanding of how and why health and illness are measured.

This chapter lays the foundation for the rest of the book by discussing definitions of health, models of health and illness, health beliefs, attitudes and values, factors influencing health, health promotion and health education, measuring health and illness, and illness behaviour. It is important to consider the different terms used to describe people in a variety of health and social care settings. Adult, mental health, children's and learning disability nurses use language that gives clues to their underlying values and assumptions of power and passivity about the person in receipt of care (see Ch. 7):

- *Patient*: A traditional word to describe the recipient of care commonly used by nurses, doctors and other

---

Best practice statements	**Box 1.1**

Promoting health and well-being

- *People*, carers and communities are enabled to find ways to maintain or improve their health and well-being via every appropriate contact
- *People*, carers and communities are enabled to identify their own health and well-being promotion needs
- *People*, carers and communities are involved in planning and actions concerning promotion of health and well-being
- Promotion of health and well-being is undertaken in partnership with others using a variety of expertise and experiences
- *People*, carers and communities have access to information, services and support that meets their health and well-being needs and circumstances
- *People*, carers, communities and agencies influence and create environments that promote people's health and well-being
- *People*, carers and communities have an improved and good quality of health and well-being.

(From DH 2010, p 9).

healthcare workers. It may imply a relative passivity or inequality in the relationship with professionals and is widely used in clinical settings within the NHS.

- *Client*: May imply a more active recipient of care and is sometimes used in situations where a fee is charged, e.g. complementary therapies. The perception is one of greater equality in relationships with professionals, rather than a medical or clinical focus. The term is widely used in community-based settings.
- *Service user*: This is commonly used in mental health and learning disability work but is becoming more widespread in other settings. People with mental health problems may define themselves this way and, by so doing, reject the medicalization of their experience including the mental illness 'label'. They may prefer to use the word 'distress', rather than the diagnosis label given. More radical is the use of the term 'survivor' to describe a person's negative experience of mental health services.
- *Resident or tenant*: Workers in care homes in the community often use these words to describe recipients of their care, whether it is health or social care, often for older people.

Definitions of health

Before reading this section you should undertake the activity in Box 1.2.

The word 'health' is derived from the old English word *hael* meaning whole and, despite being the subject of much research, it cannot be neatly defined. There is no universal definition of health as everyone has their own idea of what it means. When asked to define health, people may highlight the physical functioning of their body, their ability to carry out tasks, feeling content and happy or even respond in terms of relationships with family and friends. In other words, health is multidimensional, composed of different but interrelated dimensions.

Reflective practice · Box 1.2

Your view of health

Student activities

1. Think about your own view of health and write down your own personal definition, or even just some key words.
2. Compare your ideas with those of a friend or co-worker and discuss any similarities or differences.
3. Ask yourself:
   - What attributes might a healthy person have?
   - What would a healthy person look like?
   - Have you always defined health in this way or has it changed since you were a child?
   - Do you think this might change in the future?

Dimensions of health

Six dimensions of health are usually described, five at an individual level surrounded by a further one at the level of society:

- *Physical* – body shape, size or function
- *Mental* – or intellectual health; means the ability to think clearly and coherently, making rational judgements
- *Emotional* – or affective health; means the ability to recognize emotions, adapt to and cope with stress and anxiety
- *Social* – the ability to make and sustain relationships with people
- *Spiritual* – relates to personal beliefs and behaviour, being content or at peace and may include religious beliefs and practices
- *Societal* – relates to everything surrounding a person in their immediate or wider environment, including working and living conditions, employment, income, social norms and the political context.

Being interrelated, problems in one dimension may well affect another. A social dimension issue, e.g. a relationship problem, may cause mental health problems or vice versa. A person with a chronic physical illness may develop an accompanying mood or emotional problem. Societal issues such as poverty and low income determine people's diet and lifestyle, thereby affecting their physical health (Box 1.3).

Reflective practice · Box 1.3

Dimensions of health

Student activities

Look back at the six dimensions of health:

1. From your own life, identify examples of how problems in one dimension may impact on another.
2. Do the same again, but this time thinking about patients/clients you have met in placements.
3. Consider the following situations and suggest the dimensions in which the individual may have problems:
   - A 35-year-old married woman with postnatal depression
   - A 54-year-old man who has been made redundant
   - A 14-year-old boy undergoing treatment for cancer
   - A 78-year-old widow living on minimum benefits.

Holistic health

Nurses applying this multidimensional approach to healthcare need to assess all aspects of health and consider each patient as a whole person rather than as a collection of symptoms or bodily systems. This is called a holistic approach and derives from the Greek word *holos*, meaning whole.

The body as a machine

During assessment interviews, it is common for nurses to hear descriptions related to the physical dimension of health, where anatomy and physiology are described in an oversimplified way, comparing the body to the workings of a machine. This is called 'mechanistic functioning' and descriptive words commonly used include pipes, blockages, tubes, plumbing, waterworks, ticker and pump. This type of comparison is also used by people to describe the workings of the mind or brain, using

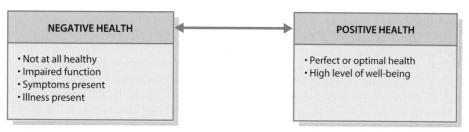

Fig. 1.1 • Health as a continuum.

The continuum of health

Figure 1.1 shows how health can be viewed positively or negatively. Extremes of positive and negative health states are at opposite ends of a health continuum and this reflects the reality that health is much more complex than merely: 'I'm ill' or 'I'm not ill'. The continuum allows for movement along the line, reflecting the dynamic nature of health, which varies over time, with age and stage of development and changing circumstances.

The idea of a single continuum may be seen as unhelpful in mental health. Some people experience high levels of well-being as a symptom of mental illness. For example, a person may experience elation arising from a bipolar mood disorder and would report feeling 'great'.

Positive and negative health

Positive health implies the presence of additional qualities often described as fitness, wellness or well-being. Positive aspects of health are less often used, with a tendency to describe health states in a negative way, focusing on the absence of disease; for example, describing health as being free from the symptoms of illness or not having a medically defined condition – 'I don't have any major illness so that means I'm healthy'. Words suggesting negative health states are more numerous and include: disease, illness, deformity, impairment, abnormality, ill-health, injury, disability, handicap, mental distress or disorder.

The word 'disease' tends to be used as an official label by doctors and nurses for physical conditions with visible signs and symptoms. However, like health, illness cannot be easily defined and is often described as a subjective experience, personally experienced and defined by each individual.

WHO definitions of health

The most well-known definition of health is that of the World Health Organization (WHO 1946): 'Health is a state of complete physical, mental and social well-being and not merely the absence of disease or infirmity'. This definition has many strengths and it:

* Is historically important
* Was written in the post-Second World War optimism of 1946

* Was one of the first authoritative attempts to define health and was proposed by a prestigious international agency
* Promotes a positive view of health by mentioning well-being
* Is a holistic definition, including different dimensions of health
* Can be seen as an idealistic target to aspire for – health as an ideal state.

However, it has been widely criticized because it uses the word 'state', which does not fit well with modern views that health is dynamic, changing with life circumstances. The word 'complete' seems to make this an absolute statement and one which, although idealistic, is unrealistic and unattainable. Lastly, the authority of the WHO to define health has been questioned, as it is acknowledged that everyone has their own definition. Although the original 1946 definition is still commonly quoted, the WHO amended its definition of health in the Ottawa Charter (WHO 1986) to:

> Health is the extent to which an individual or group is able to realize aspirations, to satisfy needs, and to change or cope with the environment. Health is, therefore, seen as a resource for everyday life, not the objective of living. Health is a positive concept emphasizing social and personal resources, as well as physical capacities.

The 1986 definition remains valid today and is considered realistic in comparison to the unattainable 'ideal state' of the earlier definition. This definition focuses on health as enabling adaptation to change and emphasizes the dynamic nature of health, the importance of social aspects of health and the link between health and economic productivity. The WHO definitions of health (1946, 1986) are only two of many, and Seedhouse (2001) summarizes the vast range of health definitions into four major groups (Box 1.4).

Theories of health	Box 1.4

1. Health as an ideal state – the most well-known example is the WHO (1946) definition of health.
2. Health related to physical/mental fitness and role/function – health allows people to carry out normal daily tasks.
3. Health as a commodity – underlying medical practice, health is seen as an external entity, which can be given or even bought.
4. Health as a personal strength or ability – health is seen as related to innate or developed strengths, which can be physical or intellectual. It is possible, in this theory, to be 'healthy' even if disabled or suffering from a disease, illness or social problem.

(Adapted from Seedhouse 2001.)

Defining mental health

Mental health problems are widespread in society (Box 1.5) and are one of the most common reasons for people visiting their GP. Yet mental health remains difficult to define as it is subjective, and something each person defines individually. The WHO (2010) defines mental health as:

> a state of well-being in which an individual realizes his or her own abilities, can cope with the normal stresses of life, can work productively and is able to make a contribution to his or her community. In this positive sense, mental health is the foundation for individual well-being and the effective functioning of a community.

The term mental disorder is often used by medical staff and this implies a clinically recognizable set of symptoms or behaviour associated, in most cases, with considerable distress and substantial interference with personal functioning.

Like the WHO above, other authors have tried describing mental health as one or more of the following:

- Living happily
- Having good self-esteem
- Being able to relate well to other people
- Having a sense of self and identity
- Living productively
- Autonomy
- Maturity
- Coping effectively with stress
- Problem-solving
- Adapting to change.

Many mental health problems and some medical disorders, e.g. cancer or visual impairment, carry an increased risk of suicide.

Although dropping recently, suicide is still the second most common cause of death in men aged 15–44 years, after accidental death (Mind 2011). Nearly 75% of recorded suicides are by people experiencing depression, which is often undiagnosed. The majority of people who commit suicide have had some contact with health professionals shortly before death, so community and hospital staff are very well placed to make a major contribution to suicide prevention (Mind 2011).

In addition to mental health or physical health problems, the causal factors for increased suicide risk are very varied and include social and financial circumstances, biological vulnerability, life events and access to means, e.g. farmers who have shotguns (Box 1.6). This therefore means there can be no single strategy for suicide prevention.

Indicators of suicide risk — **Box 1.6**

Indicators of suicide risk include the following, often occurring in combination:

- Physical or mental illness, accompanied by low mood
- Deliberate self-harm or previous suicide attempts
- History of suicide in the family
- Recent bereavement or other loss such as a close relationship
- A major disappointment (such as failed exams)
- A major change in circumstances (such as retirement)
- Substance misuse
- Changes of behaviour, such as making a will or taking out insurance.

(Adapted from Mind 2011.)

UK Mental health – what are the issues? — **Box 1.5**

- One in six adults will have a mental health problem at any one time but one in three adults of working age in the UK is experiencing some kind of mental distress. This may not be diagnosed as a mental health problem but is affecting their ability to work, e.g. sleep problems
- One in six people in the UK have symptoms recognizable as anxiety/depression
- Over 1 million people in the UK are in contact with specialist psychiatric services, either as out-patients or in-patients
- Over 130 000 people in the UK have a serious mental health condition such as schizophrenia or bipolar disorder
- 10% of children in the UK have a diagnosable mental health condition
- 13–16% of older people in England have severe depression, and up to 50% of older people in residential care
- One in 20 people over 65 in the UK has some form of dementia, rising to one in five people over 80
- One-third of all mental health service activity in England is concerned with the care and treatment of people over 65.

(Adapted from the National Mental Health Development Unit, 2010. Mental Health Factfiles 1–7 Online. Available: www.nmhdu.org.uk August 2012.)

Lay and professional definitions of health

Lay definitions of health refer to the ideas, beliefs and opinions of ordinary members of the public. Lay people may perceive that health can coexist with even serious disease and it is only the last group of theories in Box 1.4 that allows for this, the first three groups must have absence of illness and disease. Professional definitions of health arise from people 'educated in health' such as nurses, doctors, allied health professionals (AHPs) or from official sources, e.g. government experts and agencies. Lay and professional definitions of health vary considerably and may result in differing expectations, lack of understanding or even conflict in issues of relationship, diagnosis, treatment and care. Box 1.7 shows an example of lay and professional conflict.

Models of health and illness

The word 'model' has many meanings but in the study of health and illness, refers to a conceptual framework or a perspective, a way of viewing or thinking about health and illness, which informs research or practice (Seedhouse 2001). The

Critical thinking   Box 1.7

Lay and professional conflict

Jim is 28 years old and has a history of mild asthma going back to childhood. He has had several episodes of bronchitis in the past which have always responded well to treatment with antibiotics. He smokes 30 cigarettes a day.

Jim visits his practice nurse with a heavy cold and a sore throat, and requests a prescription for antibiotics. The practice nurse explains that since his cold is caused by a virus, she will not advise antibiotics. Instead, she starts asking about his smoking habits.

Student activity

After reading the scenario above, identify:

- How Jim might feel about his request being denied and how he may react to this
- What the practice nurse may be thinking
- The differing expectations within the consultation
- The possible effects of any conflict on the future relationship.

---

implication is, therefore, that there may be as many different models in this area as there are different ways of thinking about health and illness. Three common models of health and illness are medical, social and patient-centred.

The medical model

Many health professionals ascribe to the medical model, also known as the biomedical model, which tends to focus on illness rather than health. It has tended to be dominant, although this is now changing. The medical model is underpinned by the growth of scientific thinking, technological progress and research that has developed from the eighteenth century to the present day. The focus is on being objective when identifying physical problems.

Observed symptoms lead to diagnosis, which in turn determines treatment options. Cure and repair are emphasized, with treatment often involving drugs or surgery. The intention is usually to remove the identifiable cause of the problem, returning the patient to a 'normal state'. The medical model assumes that a diagnosis is not valid unless made by expert practitioners. A further assumption is that patients are relatively passive during the process.

Mental health language and the medical model

Foucault (1973) believed that use of language is crucial in determining the way people think and therefore that there could be problems using medical model terminology in the areas of mental distress or mental health problems. The phrase 'mental illness' tends to reflect the medical model, which is neither accurate nor helpful when applied to problems that are often largely social or behavioural. Even use of the adjective 'mental' has been criticized as it relates to the mind rather than to the brain or even to abnormal behaviour where many problems might manifest. It is more accurate to use the term

'mental distress' which fits with modern thinking and is usually preferred by clients.

The social model

The social model considers structural issues within the society in which the individual lives, e.g. social class and poverty, and the barriers which may contribute to ill-health, e.g. difficulties in accessing services. This approach arose in the nineteenth century from the idea that improved health comes from improved environmental and living conditions, e.g. from better housing and improved sanitation. The language of the social model is not of symptoms but instead, uses terms including barriers and enablers, exclusion, distress and disability.

The patient-centred model

This derives from Carl Roger's (1951) work on person-centred therapy and is a dominant model in mental health, learning disability and complementary therapies. The patient's own perception of their physical or psychological health forms the starting point for a more equal, negotiating type of relationship, with the potential for more holistic assessment. The premise is that people have significant and unique knowledge of their own symptoms or problems from which healthcare professionals can learn.

Service user and carer involvement

Service user and carer involvement is crucial to a patient-centred NHS (Box 1.8) and is a feature of national policy recommendations for service planning and change management. This is also required in pre-registration nursing programmes. In mental health and learning disability programmes it is common for service users and carers to have wide-ranging involvement including interviewing and selection of student nurses, curriculum development, classroom input in talks and discussions as well as clinical skills assessment. Service user and carer involvement is becoming much more established in adult and child health nursing.

Evidence-based practice   Box 1.8

User/carer involvement in service design
Student activity

Locate the article below and take short notes to answer the question:

- What are the benefits of engaging people in the planning, delivering and evaluation of cancer care?

Resource

Attree, P., Morris, S., Payne, S., et al., 2010. Exploring the influence of service user involvement on health and social care services for cancer. Health Expectations 14 (1), 48–58.

Health beliefs

Interpersonal relationships are often seen as central to the role of nurses (see Ch. 9). It is therefore essential that nurses are aware of, and understand, the beliefs and perceptions of their patients/clients to facilitate relationship forming. Nurses need to have an informed understanding of the diversity of health beliefs because of their significant position as 'intermediaries' between medical and lay belief systems, acting as translators of patient/client experience to doctors and vice versa. To accomplish this, nurses need sensitivity to people's subjective experience of illness and an open-mindedness regarding the limitations of the medical approach (Jones 1994). Contemporary health beliefs are better understood by briefly considering how they have developed over time.

Early health beliefs

From 3000BC, orthodox Chinese medicine, Ayurvedic medicine and ancient Greek/Roman civilizations used the idea of physical and mental balance or harmony. The approaches were person-centred, holistic and made links between health, illness and the individual's personality, the climate, stage of lifespan and the environment. It is important to note that orthodox Chinese and Ayurvedic medicine are still practised by millions of people throughout the world.

Religion and health

There has been a long and enduring link between religion, moral behaviour and health beliefs. The central idea is that illness may be caused by moral failure; some lapse in good behaviour, or that a person may deserve to become ill because they have brought it on themselves through their own actions (see Box 7.4 (p. 147) for a contemporary example that explores withholding treatment for smokers).

The Latin word for pain, *poena*, comes from the same root as the word for punishment. The idea of illness as punishment for moral failure may seem very old-fashioned, yet it is still a commonly held belief today. This kind of thinking about 'deserving' illness or being punished for bad behaviour by becoming ill is the norm for children of primary school age (see p. 9). It is common to hear phrases like 'you get what you deserve', 'people bring things on themselves' or 'it's in God's hands, everything is for a reason'. Helman (2007) notes that one common image often used in the press is of acquired immune deficiency syndrome (AIDS) as moral punishment, with sufferers divided into two groups: the 'innocent' (children and people with haemophilia) and the 'guilty' (everyone else).

Supernatural ideas and health

Centuries ago, when illness arose for no apparent reason, people sometimes believed that someone had wished them harm by the casting of spells or by giving the evil eye (Helman 2007). Belief in special powers and witchcraft was very common in ancient times but is still held by many people in the UK today, especially as its population becomes more culturally diverse. Large numbers of British people, e.g. those of Afro-Caribbean descent, still hold these beliefs. It is therefore important for all healthcare professionals to be sensitive to cultural aspects of health belief and related behaviour (Box 1.9).

Reflective practice	Box 1.9

Culture and nursing practice

Cultural background has an important influence on many aspects of people's lives, including their beliefs, behaviour, perceptions, emotion, language, religion, rituals, family structure, diet, dress, body image, concepts of space and time, and attitudes to illness, pain and other forms of misfortune – all of which may have important implications for health and healthcare.

Student activities

1. Consider the statement above and reflect on your personal or clinical experience.
2. Try to think of examples of diversity in clients'/patients' beliefs and behaviours which you have encountered in practice, e.g. in relation to:
   * Family roles and involvement
   * Gender roles, clothing and privacy
   * Personal hygiene practices
   * Dietary habits.

(Helman 2007.)

Scientific developments and health

From the eighteenth century onwards, there was rapid development in scientific knowledge accompanied by technological advance with an emphasis on research, evidence and objectivity and the beginnings of the medical model arose.

The miasma model, as espoused by Florence Nightingale in her *Notes on Nursing* of 1859, centred on belief systems which considered that illness was caused by bad air or smells, poor atmospheric conditions, rotting food and sewage. The treatment of illness involved personal and environmental cleanliness, usually involving fresh air, scrubbing, boiling and bleaching. It is still common to hear people voice such concerns about dampness in the air or the importance of cleanliness. Throughout the twentieth century, secularization of beliefs increased so that, for most people, illness tends not to be linked with either moral failure or religious belief. Non-Western notions of health are common, with an increasing interest in, and rise in the use of, complementary therapies (see Ch. 10), which are now embedded in many mainstream NHS settings.

Current lay health beliefs

There is a multitude of common current health beliefs noted in this intensively studied area. Blaxter (1990) studied the health beliefs of lay people and observed that these varied according to age, gender, family responsibilities and cultural background. She found young men tended to emphasize physical fitness and function, whereas older adults described health as linked to social and emotional relationships. Blaxter (1990) summarized lay health beliefs into 10 categories:

1. Health as never thinking about being healthy or ill
2. Health as behaviour, the healthy lifestyle
3. Health as not ill, not going to the doctor
4. Health as social relationships
5. Health as absence of illness
6. Health as ability to function, to carry out tasks
7. Health despite disease
8. Health as energy or vitality
9. Health as a reserve of strength
10. Health as psychosocial well-being.

Box 1.10 provides an activity to help you recognize common, contemporary health beliefs.

 Critical thinking   Box 1.10

Recognizing health beliefs – quotes about health and illness

- 'I think that babies should get aired every day – fresh air in all weathers'
- 'I smoke, have asthma and bronchitis for which I need inhalers, I'm overweight and am partially deaf in one ear but overall I would say that I am healthy'
- 'I really think if you've got to go, you've got to go. It's all mapped out you know'
- 'I can do everything I need to do, earn money, look after my family – to me that's real health'
- 'I'm very healthy, I've got great family and faithful friends'
- 'He lived until he was 89, mind you he was from sturdy stock, they were all long-lived in that family'.

Student activities

- Read the quotes above from lay people expressing their own ideas about health and illness and try to identify what type of belief is being expressed. It may help to look back at Blaxter's 10 categories of health beliefs, the Seedhouse groups of health definitions and the section on history of health beliefs.
- Next time you are on placement, listen for lay health beliefs expressed by patients/clients.

(Adapted from Greig, J., 1995. Men talking about health: a qualitative study. Unpublished MSc thesis, Edinburgh University.)

Lay beliefs about the causes of illness

The study of lay theories of illness causation, also known as 'lay aetiology', refers to people's attempts to make sense of their own or family experience of illness or disease. However, lay people usually have limited scientific understanding of the structure and functioning of the body, the causes of disease and the reasons for body malfunction. They may hold logical but incorrect assumptions about the cause of illness (Helman 2007), e.g. cold (temperature or weather) causes a cold (viral infection).

Like the medical model, lay theories of illness are multifactorial, placing the causes in one of the following four sites: within the individual, in the natural world, in the social world or in the supernatural world (Box 1.11). The first two explanations relate to the Western industrialized world, while the last two usually arise from non-industrialized or rural communities (Helman 2007).

Lay beliefs about the causes of illness   Box 1.11

- *Individual level theories*: Emphasize malfunction within the body. Causes of illness tend to centre on notions of vulnerability, resistance, wear and tear, hereditary predisposition, imbalance and mechanical damage or blockage
- *Natural world theories*: Seek explanation in climatic conditions. Causes of illness typically centre on air quality and seasons, microorganisms which are commonly described as insects (e.g. tummy 'bug'), astrology, accidental injuries, parasites and environmental irritants
- *Social world theories*: Tend to blame other people, emphasizing interpersonal conflict, witchcraft, sorcery, 'evil eye', spells, potions, rituals
- *Supernatural world theories*: Seek explanation in gods, ancestors or spirits. Illness is seen as a reminder for a lapse in behaviour. In industrialized settings, individuals are more likely to blame fate, luck or Acts of God.

(Adapted from Helman 2007).

Children's health and illness beliefs

Children's understanding of health corresponds to their stage of cognitive development, using Piaget's theoretical framework as comparison (see Ch. 8). In a famous study by Hart and Chesson (1998), drawing and writing techniques were used to explore children's health perceptions. Preschool children typically see illness occurring as if by magic and sometimes perceive it as punishment for past misconduct and may even believe that healthcare professionals intentionally set out to hurt them They know the names of some external body parts but internal bodily functions remain largely unknown.

Children aged 6–7 years tend to have a view of health which describes healthy people as being young, sporty, happy, smiling and actively involved in outside activities. In this age group, children may believe that illness is caused by a single factor, often a 'germ' or 'bug'. They are familiar with the names for external body parts and some internal organs and bodily functions. Little is known about children's concepts of mental health, other than feelings related to being happy or sad.

Children aged 9–10 years understand the principles of germ transmission but many believe that all illness is caused this way, even cancer and eczema. Given this, it follows that they sometimes have difficulty in understanding prescribed treatment and medical terms are frequently misinterpreted.

Children aged 11 years have begun to develop a more detailed understanding of health and illness and by 13 years, grasp the complexity of illness with its multiple possible causes. They are able to discuss the complex interplay between biological, lifestyle and environmental factors that influence health and illness (Helman 2007). They can readily identify some health determinants (see Fig. 1.3) and understand health-damaging behaviours such as passive smoking. They can relate, for example, aspects of body functioning to the components of a healthy diet from their studies at school. They are also more likely to appreciate the impact of psychological factors, grasp the notion of drug-related side-effects and the time delay often experienced in response to treatment, e.g. it may take several days before antibiotic medicine is seen to 'work'.

In all age groups, the most common symptoms described as ill-health by children were fever, headache, dizziness or rash (Helman 2007). Thermometers feature strongly in children's descriptions and fever is perceived to be the key symptom used by their parents to determine whether or not they are ill. This reflects children's own experience, which is usually limited to common illnesses such as viral infections.

Unlike adults, positive consequences feature strongly in children's drawings and descriptions of being ill. These include staying off school, being the centre of attention, having visitors, treats and special foods.

Becker's health belief model

There are many health belief models that provide an overview of the factors influencing health beliefs. One is the health belief model (HBM) devised by Becker (1974) to explain how people behave in relation to their health. The HBM (Fig. 1.2) has been shown to be highly predictive of health behaviour. According to the HBM, participation in preventative health behaviour, i.e. behaviour which should decrease the risk of illness, is predicted on the basis of the following:

- How an individual perceives their susceptibility to a given disorder – what is the likelihood of being affected?
- How an individual perceives the seriousness or severity of the disorder – how bad would it be?
- How an individual perceives the benefits of taking action – what will be gained from changing?
- How an individual perceives the barriers to action – how hard is it to change, what will be lost?

- The individual's experience of cues to action – what has been seen or heard which triggers health behaviour action, e.g. GP advice, a health scare or major life event
- Health motivation – how highly a person values health.

Values in health are discussed below and Chapter 7 considers values and ethics in nursing practice. Originally, the HBM had four key beliefs affecting the central concept of health motivation. Later, the HBM was extended to include a fifth key belief: perceived self-efficacy, which refers to a person's confidence in their ability to make/maintain a change in health behaviour. Modifying factors may include sociocultural factors, age and gender. It suggests that people will consider the advantages and disadvantages of engaging in positive health behaviour, even if the existing behaviour is not changed, and relies on a particular cue for action to be taken.

The nurse's role and application of the HBM

Nurses can help people to change their health behaviour in many ways and any contact with health professionals, however brief, can be a 'cue to action' in itself. It is important to use this contact to discuss health behaviours – people expect it and may be surprised if the subject is not broached. Nurses and other health professionals have high credibility with patients/clients and a brief discussion may be all that someone, who has been considering positive health-related change, needs to move forward and actually make a change.

There is a need for nurses to offer factual, balanced health information that clearly indicates individual susceptibility or risk. The language and images used are important considerations, especially in children and people with learning disability.

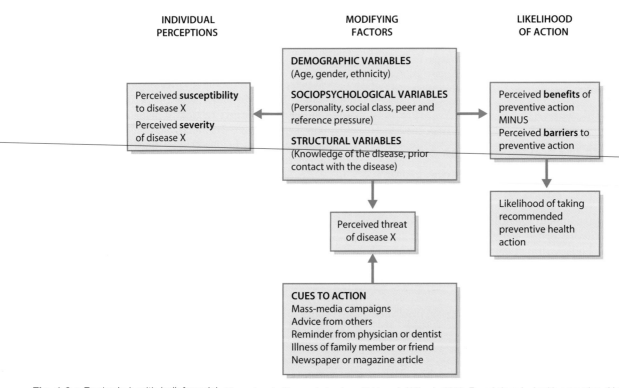

Fig. 1.2 • Becker's health belief model. (Reproduced with permission from Naidoo, J., Wills, J., 2009. Foundations for health promotion, third ed. Baillière Tindall, Edinburgh.)

Shock tactics, moral judgements or emotive language are unhelpful and may alienate patients/clients. Interactions between nurses and patients/clients should stress not only the benefits of preventative health behaviour but also offer encouragement and strategies for dealing with barriers to change.

Attitudes, values and behaviours

This is a complex area of social psychology important in nursing and health promotion since attitudes combine aspects of people's values, feelings and beliefs. An attitude is defined as a relatively stable tendency to respond consistently to particular people, objects or situations. The use of the word 'stable' rather than 'fixed' implies an ability of the attitude to change or be changed. An attitude represents a person's general feelings towards someone or something. It can be negative or positive, strongly held or weak. Attitudes have three components, summarized as ABC:

A – affective component or 'feeling' aspects

B – behavioural aspects

C – cognitive component or knowledge and belief aspects.

Nurses are often involved in assisting patients/clients to change their health-related attitudes with the aim of positively changing behaviour. For example, to explore dietary issues with a person newly diagnosed with diabetes, the nurse needs to:

- Allow time for them to express their feelings about the diagnosis before assessing their understanding of the symptoms and dietary changes needed
- Answer any questions and explore the person's usual eating habits at their own pace
- Provide reinforcement and supplementary reading
- Assess where any practical changes can be made.

To ensure success, all of this must be done sensitively and with the person as participant as possible in the interaction. Care with use of language, visual aids and the opportunity for rehearsal would be of particular benefit to people with a learning disability (see Box 1.28, below).

Public and private attitudes

An attitude openly expressed by a person in public is usually called an opinion. Attitudes may or may not be predictive of people's behaviour. Publicly stated opinions may, or may not, reflect a person's true, privately-held attitude that tends to be divulged only to trusted and close family members and friends. People may express different attitudes to researchers in an attempt to help the interaction, give a more 'textbook' answer or appear more acceptable. An example of this in nursing might be when carrying out an admission assessment, a person who drinks heavily may purposely underestimate their alcohol units consumed per week and describe themselves as a social drinker.

Cognitive dissonance

Festinger's (1964) idea of cognitive dissonance is based on the three components of attitudes mentioned above. It is common for a person who knows and understands the adverse effects of smoking (cognitive component) and who has poor self-esteem because they smoke (affective component), to continue to smoke (the behaviour). This is known as smoking dissonance and is experienced as psychological discomfort or guilt because of the inconsistency that exists among the three components of an attitude.

Festinger (1964) suggested that it is usual for a person feeling this discomfort to have a drive to resolve the conflict between the different components of their attitude and therefore reduce the dissonance experienced. Cognitive dissonance therefore can be viewed as a possible precursor of a positive health-related behaviour change. If nurses or other healthcare professionals perceive a person's cognitive dissonance, then this may be a first step along the road to attitude change and, possibly, behaviour change. Mass media campaigns may purposely seek to induce or increase dissonance for this very reason but it is important to recognize that this approach may not be understood by a large proportion of people with a learning disability.

Values

Attitudes are underpinned by values, which are broad and less specific than attitudes. Values underpin an individual's 'philosophy of life' which are then applied to everyday life. They may relate to moral, ethical or religious issues as well as health, gender roles, family life and the environment. How much a person values their health is a key part of the health motivation section of Becker's health belief model (Fig. 1.2).

A person's value system is composed of broad beliefs developed through early learning, upbringing and socialization within the family and later at school, with peers and through life experiences and work. The cultural context in which this develops is also very important.

Each value may have multiple attitudes associated with it. Although it may be possible to cause attitude change, it is more difficult to change a person's value system as it is an integral part of their early upbringing and life experience. For example, values relating to moral conduct in life may have associated attitudes about crime and punishment, sexual behaviour, marriage and the rearing of children.

Stereotyping

'Stereotypes' are underpinned by direct expressions of beliefs and values and may offer a shorthand way to generalize about a person or a group of people. It may seem natural to try to classify people in society but stereotypes are to be avoided in nursing because they do not acknowledge individual differences and are usually oversimplified and negative. Stereotypes form the basis of prejudice, or unfavourable opinion, formed against a person or group of people, usually based on the following characteristics:

- Age
- Gender
- Mental health problems or physical disability
- Occupation

- Race
- Religion
- Nationality.

Fear of the unknown, e.g. of minority groups, may fuel stereotypes. When people are judged on stereotypes and there is resulting prejudice, this is known as discrimination.

People with mental health problems have historically suffered serious discrimination and can be considered one of the most socially excluded groups in British society. Public fear of mental illness has been fuelled by well-publicized cases in the media where a mentally distressed person has behaved violently. This shows how stereotypes are often untrue because, statistically, people with mental health problems are no more likely than anyone else to engage in violent behaviour and are much more likely to harm themselves than other people. Discriminatory behaviour includes:

- Ignoring or avoiding people
- Abusive language, especially 'jokes'
- Dehumanizing slang
- Name-calling
- Excluding behaviour such as restricted membership of clubs and societies
- Lack of equal access to jobs or promotion.

The result can be segregation and isolation for individuals and, in extreme cases, discrimination is expressed as physical violence.

Discriminatory behaviour which targets children is referred to as 'bullying' and, increasingly, this term is also used by adults in the workplace. Bullying is a common form of discrimination with over 30% of school children reporting some experience of being bullied (National Society for the Prevention of Cruelty to Children, NSPCC 2010). Bullying refers to deliberately hurtful actions, encompassing a broad spectrum of behaviours (Box 1.12). In the case of children, name-calling is the most common type of bullying but other behaviours include teasing, rumour-spreading, theft of possessions or money, abusive text messages, social networking site postings or e-mails (cyberbullying), coercion, being excluded or ignored in play, class, sports and other activities or physical threats and abuse (NSPCC 2010).

Bullying and children	**Box 1.12**

- Vulnerability to bullying often relates to physical and individual characteristics such as body shape, size, physical disability or a learning difficulty such as dyslexia
- More than 30 000 children in the UK call the telephone helpline 'Childline' each year about bullying; up to 20% say that the current 'tormentor' is a former friend
- Bullying causes shame, humiliation and fear. It can also cause feelings of powerlessness and low self-esteem which can last into adulthood
- Concentration problems and increased school avoidance can lead to behavioural problems and deterioration in academic performance
- In some cases, children may attempt self-harm.

(Adapted from NSPCC, 2010. Bullying resources for school and teachers. Online. Available: www.nspcc.org.uk August 2012.)

Lifestyle, health behaviours and locus of control

In relation to health, lifestyle means health-related behaviours over which a person has some choice. These include:

- Sexual health practices
- Tobacco use
- Alcohol use
- Diet
- Exercise

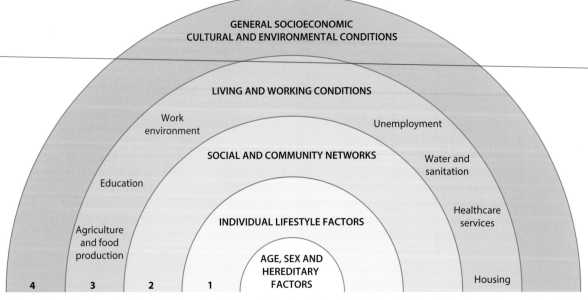

Fig. 1.3 • The main determinants of health. (Reproduced with permission from Naidoo, J., Wills, J., 2009. Foundations for health promotion, third ed. Baillière Tindall, Edinburgh.)

- Keeping healthy during pregnancy (see Box 1.29, below)
- Non-prescribed or recreational drug use
- Stress management
- Use of preventative health services.

The term 'internal locus of control' is used to describe the perception of some people that they have the power to make health-related choices, and that they are ultimately responsible for their own health. Other people demonstrate an 'external locus of control' where they see outside factors controlling their health and health behaviour, with the tendency to blame luck, fate, God, the climate or the environment. You may hear people say things like 'If the bullet's got your name on it …' or 'If you've got to go, you've got to go'. These are examples of fatalism evident in some of the quotes in Box 1.10, above.

It is arguable whether everyone is equally free to make meaningful health-related choices. Some people are severely constrained by issues such as income, education, knowledge and peer group pressure. For example, on a very low income it is hard to afford a healthy wholemeal loaf which may be more than twice the price of the cheaper, and less healthy, white alternative.

Factors influencing health

Factors that influence or determine health are called health determinants. The same factors that determine health also determine ill-health, i.e. they may have either positive or negative effects on health, e.g. housing. Positive health effects related to housing as a health determinant include warmth, space, comfort, well-being and psychological security. Negative aspects of housing as a health determinant are well documented and include overcrowding, noise and safety concerns leading to stress and depression, and dampness and mould resulting in physical illness, e.g. asthma.

Determinants are many, varied, yet interrelated and are described by Dahlgren and Whitehead (1991) as being on five

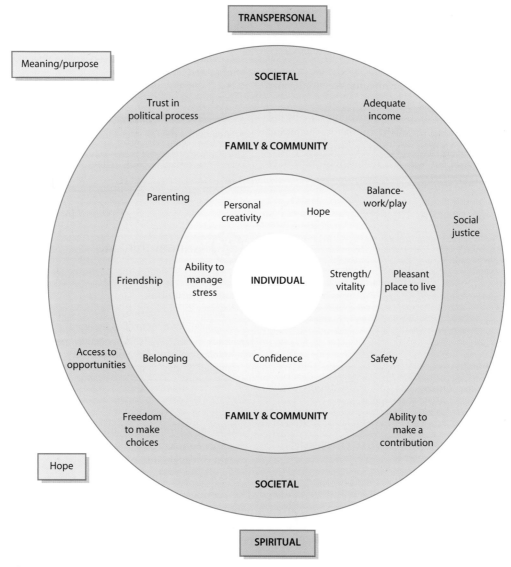

Fig. 1.4 • The confidence spiral: determinants/components of mental health and well-being. (Reproduced with permission from Kennedy, A., 2002. Sorted not screwed up. Report for the Aberdeen Foyer. Online. Available: www.aberdeenfoyer.com/foyer_report.pdf August 2012.)

levels. The multifactorial view shown in Figure 1.3 (see p. 12) illustrates health determinants as layers surrounding a core and allows differentiation between individual and sociopolitical factors. The core factors – gender, ethnicity, age and heredity – are inherited characteristics and largely fixed, while the surrounding layers of influence may be open to some modification. The next layer is individual lifestyle where personal behaviours may not be rationally or voluntarily chosen, but are heavily influenced by family, friends and peer group, and by social and community networks. Wider influences on health include:

- Living and working conditions
- Issues related to housing
- Access to health services
- Clean drinking water and sanitation
- Work environment or unemployment
- Access to education
- Agriculture and food supply.

It is important to note that these wider determinants are not open to action by individuals but need collective action at government level. For example, although individuals can play their part in environmental issues in a small way – by choosing environmentally friendly cleaning products and adopting recycling behaviours – it requires policy, legislation and action at national and international levels to achieve positive changes in some health determinants, e.g. water and air quality.

The outermost layer contains the socioeconomic, cultural and environmental conditions prevalent in society including interest rates, unemployment rates and political stability. Access to health and social services is a major determinant of health.

Determinants of mental health and well-being

Determinants of mental health and well-being are shown in Figure 1.4. Factors influencing mental health are grouped into four spheres:

- Individual
- Family and community
- Societal
- Spiritual.

Each sphere relates to dimensions of self-esteem which together influence mental health and well-being.

Poverty as the key determinant of health

The most important health determinant is poverty but there is no clear consensus on how it is best defined or measured. Poverty can be defined as absolute or relative.

- *Absolute poverty* is the inability to meet basic biological needs such as food, warmth and shelter. This relates to the first level of Maslow's hierarchy of needs (see Ch. 8). Box 1.13 summarizes some of the effects of poverty on children.

 Evidence-based practice | Box 1.13

Effects of poverty on children

Poverty and disadvantage in childhood are key determinants of future mental health for children and young people. A tendency toward adult depression is strongly associated with social deprivation.

- One in 10 children aged 5–16 years has a clinically diagnosable mental health problem, including depression, anxiety or psychosis
- Nearly 80 000 children and young people suffer from severe depression
- It is estimated that 1 in 12 children and young people deliberately self-harm – a behaviour symptomatic of mental distress – and rates of self-harm among girls and young women aged 16–24 have increased dramatically since the year 2000
- It is now widely understood that most adult and adolescent mental illness begins in childhood. Evidence shows that early mental health problems can seriously impact on life chances. In contrast, positive mental health is associated with good educational outcomes, productivity and strong relationships.

Student activity

Search the Office for National Statistics website at www.statistics.gov.uk and find out more about low-income families and any of the following:

- Low birth weight babies
- Teenage pregnancy
- Mental health in children
- Accidental deaths in children.

(Adapted from the Mental Health Foundation, 2010. Children and young people's mental health coalition. Online. Available: www.mentalhealth.org.uk August 2012.)

 Critical thinking | Box 1.14

A satisfactory standard of living?
Student activities

- Reflect on the household items or daily activities you consider essential for a 'normal' standard of modern living.
- Lack of car ownership is one key measure of deprivation and relative poverty. Consider how lack of car ownership might impact on day-to-day life and on health in general today.

- *Relative poverty* is usually defined by a comparison to a country's average living standards, as measured by income level or ownership of certain goods, e.g. a car or access to services, e.g. childcare (Box 1.14).

The European Anti-Poverty Network (EAPN 2010) urges that people's own perceptions of poverty are acknowledged. However, the most commonly used official definition of poverty is living in a household with an income under 60% of the average for the country in which they live. Sometimes, this definition of poverty is further refined by deducting housing costs. Groups susceptible to poverty are shown in Box 1.15.

UK groups most susceptible to poverty   **Box 1.15**

- In mid-2010, almost 2.5 million people in the UK were unemployed. In total, around 6 million were unemployed, 'economically inactive' but seeking work or employed part-time and unable to find full-time work.
- By 2008/2009, 13 million people in the UK were in poverty. Of these, 5.8 million (44% of the total) were in 'deep poverty' where household income was at least one-third below the poverty line, the highest proportion on record.
- By mid-2010, the unemployment rate among people aged 16–24 was at 20%, the highest in 18 years, and three times that for other adults.
- Vulnerable groups include those with in-work poverty, a number of children in the family unit, young adults with few/no qualifications, lack of access of low-income households to essential services, young adult unemployment, those affected by health inequalities and people in social housing.

(Adapted from the Joseph Rowntree Foundation, 2010. Monitoring poverty and social inclusion. Online. Available: www.jrf.org.uk August 2012.)

Classification of social class   **Box 1.16**

Registrar General's Classification of Social Class (used in publications prior to 2001)

Class

1. Professional
2. Semi-professional
3a. Skilled non-manual
3b. Skilled manual
4. Partially skilled
5. Unskilled

National Statistics Socioeconomic Classification (NS-SEC) (used in publications since 2001)

Class

1. Higher managerial and professional
   1.1. Company directors, bank managers, senior civil servants
   1.2. Doctors, barristers, teachers, social workers
2. Lower managerial and professional, e.g. nurses, actors, police, soldiers
3. Intermediate, e.g. secretaries, clerks
4. Small employers and own account workers, e.g. publicans, farmers, taxi drivers
5. Lower supervisory, craft and related occupations, e.g. printers, plumbers, butchers
6. Semi-routine occupations, e.g. shop assistants, traffic wardens, hairdressers
7. Routine occupations, e.g. waiters, road sweepers, cleaners, couriers
8. Never worked and long-term unemployed.

Relative poverty and participation in society

Relative poverty involves more than merely income; it also includes the idea that someone with a low income is unlikely to be able to participate in mainstream society. The European Anti-Poverty Network (EAPN 2010) describe the effects of relative poverty as being unable to or being prevented from meeting one or more needs without outside help. These needs often relate to access to fundamental services such as education, housing and health.

Components of poverty

Poverty is complex and multidimensional. A combination of low pay, inadequate benefits or unemployment can lead to a low household income, which gives rise to separate components of poverty, including poverty of food, fuel, housing, transport, access to recreation/social facilities and, over time, leads to relative powerlessness and possible social exclusion. Ongoing poverty can negatively influence an individual's physical and psychological health, with associated behavioural changes including increased use of alcohol or nicotine, sometimes called 'drugs of comfort'. Box 1.13 highlights the link between childhood poverty and mental health.

Social class and health inequalities

Chadwick's 1842 *General Report on the Sanitary Conditions of the Labouring Population of Great Britain* showed that richer people had a life expectancy more than double that of the poorest in society. Although life expectancy has improved steadily since then, there has not been an equal improvement across social classes; inequalities still remain and have grown.

Social class was previously categorized according to the Registrar General's Classification of Social Class, which was largely unchanged between 1921 and 2000 (Box 1.16). People were allocated to one of five classes on the basis of the occupation of the head of the household. Although suited to men of working age, criticism of this classification centred on the exclusion of people lacking occupation, e.g. students, retired or unemployed people. Women were not included in their own right, their class being derived from that of their husband or father. Publications before 2001 use this classification.

For the 2001 census, classification of social class was revised and the National Statistics Socioeconomic Classification (NS-SEC) has been used since then. Eight categories now take account of changes in the labour market and the role of women, which include categories for the self-employed and those who have never worked or are long-term unemployed. More information is available from the Office for National Statistics website (see Box 1.13).

Research into health inequalities

In 1977, the Labour government appointed Sir Douglas Black to chair a working group to review the information on health inequalities and then identify policy and research that should follow. When published in 1980, it clearly showed that during the first 35 years of the NHS there had been an improvement in health across all social classes. However, there was still a strong relationship between social class and life expectancy, infant mortality and inequalities in the use of health services (Townsend et al 1992).

The Black Committee recommended a comprehensive anti-poverty programme with detailed and costed targets. The two main elements were:

- Fairer distribution of resources
- Provision of the necessary educational and employment opportunities for active social participation.

The *Black Report* advocated that the key approach to tackling health inequalities was preventative work in childhood and in particular the 'first years of life'. This has been borne out by subsequent research and remains the main emphasis in current health promotion targets. The *Black Report's* recommendations were not implemented but, nevertheless, stimulated extensive research and raised the issue of inequalities around the world.

Some 20 years after the *Black Report*, the *Acheson Report* (1998) reviewed inequalities in health in England. The main findings were that poor neighbourhoods are characterized by poor health. Also noted was that health inequalities still affect society and that they are cumulative from before birth to old age and that poverty has a disproportionate effect on children (see Box 1.13). The incidence of premature death was noted to be highest among the poor, and directly linked to inequalities in income. The *Acheson Report* made recommendations in three main areas:

- All policies likely to have an impact on health should be evaluated
- High priority should be given to the health of families with children
- Further improvements should be made to reduce income inequalities and raise the living standards of poor households.

The *Acheson Report* stated that individual lifestyle and personal choice were not responsible for the 'health gap', arguing instead that income levels, changes in society and constraints prevent individuals from choice. For example, changes in transport and shopping contributed to the creation of 'food deserts', areas of social housing with no shops or services, or only one small and expensive corner shop. This makes the purchase of fresh food at reasonable prices almost impossible for some families.

Unlike the *Black Report* which largely led to further research, the *Acheson Report* prompted actual policy change and engendered a climate focusing on health inequalities.

Changing trends in health and illness

Health and illness issues change over time. During the last century there was a shift in the pattern of disease from infectious diseases prevalent in the nineteenth and early twentieth centuries to chronic physical conditions and mental health issues during the twenty-first century. Diabetes is one example of a chronic illness (physical disease) causing premature death and disability. In the UK, it affects 2.6 million of the population and is increasing so rapidly that by 2025 it is estimated that 4 million people will be affected (Diabetes UK 2010).

Diabetes rates in children are increasing and are linked to obesity. Suicide is also increasing in children and young people. The UK also has some of the worst death rates in the world for coronary heart disease (CHD), strokes, cancer and respiratory diseases (British Heart Foundation 2011). These chronic diseases are strongly linked to lifestyle factors such as cigarette smoking, poor diet, physical inactivity and excessive alcohol consumption. Strong links exist between social class and the prevalence of these risk factors, which predominate in the poorest sections of society.

Other health trends related to lifestyle include sexual health and sexually transmitted infections (STIs). Young people aged 16–24 years form 12% of the UK population but account for over 50% of all cases of STIs and, despite dropping throughout the first decade of the twenty-first century, the UK teenage pregnancy rate remains the highest in Western Europe; in England in 2008, the rate was 40.5 per 1000 young women aged 15–17 years (National Children's Bureau 2011). Another contemporary issue is the growing number of children and adults who are overweight and obese (Box 1.17).

? Critical thinking   **Box 1.17**

Obesity trends

- Overweight and obesity rates have grown rapidly in England, doubling over the last 25 years
- Obesity is associated with many health problems some of which are cardiovascular disease, cancer and diabetes
- It is predicted that by the year 2050, 60% of adult males, 50% of adult females and 25% of children will be affected by obesity.

Student activities

Access the National Obesity Observatory website below and locate information on the following:

- Causes of obesity
- Measurement of obesity
- Effects of obesity on health
- Trends and international comparisons.

(Adapted from the National Obesity Observatory, 2010. About obesity. Online. Available: www.noo.org.uk August 2012.)

Apart from the increase in chronic illness and lifestyle-related diseases, another important issue is the emergence of communicable diseases such as Ebola virus, human immunodeficiency virus (HIV) and AIDS, variant Creutzfeldt–Jakob disease (vCJD), severe acute respiratory syndrome (SARS) and avian flu. Longstanding infectious conditions previously thought to be curable are now re-emerging and may be resistant to conventional treatments, e.g. tuberculosis (TB) and methicillin-resistant *Staphylococcus aureus* (MRSA).

Changing issues in health and illness have refocused interest on health promotion and government funding of initiatives. The rationale is based on the largely preventable component of many illnesses, e.g. smoking and lung cancer. There is a huge potential for health gains if morbidity and mortality are reduced, e.g. publicizing the effects of passive smoking on children's health (Box 1.18).

The effects of passive smoking on children's health Box 1.18

The first report on the health impact of passive smoking on children, and the costs to the NHS, concludes that it is responsible for thousands of avoidable hospital and GP visits, as well as for one in five sudden infant deaths.

- More than 22 000 children seek medical help for asthma and wheezing as a result of passive smoking every year
- More than 20 000 chest infections, 120 000 bouts of middle ear disease and 200 cases of meningitis in the young are linked to the effects of second-hand smoke
- Passive smoking results in more than 300 000 GP consultations for children and about 9500 hospital admissions
- Of the £23.3 million spent by the NHS every year treating the effects of passive smoking on the young, £9.7 million is for doctors' visits and asthma treatments
- £13.6 million is spent on hospital admissions; £4 million on asthma drugs for the under 16s.

(From The Royal College of Physicians Tobacco Advisory Group, 2010. Passive smoking and children. Online. Available: www.rcplondon.ac.uk August 2012.)

The 'greying' of the population refers to a growing elderly population with an associated shift from acute to chronic illness. Older adults often have several, concurrent illnesses, known as 'multiple pathology'. This situation has been described as living longer, but not healthier. Chronic illness and multiple illnesses mean a changing emphasis on 'care' rather than 'cure'. Box 1.5 above, shows mental health trends in older adults.

The health needs of people with a learning disability are also changing because of increasing life expectancy and increasing recognition of their more complex health needs.

The huge and growing financial cost of inpatient care, compared with health promotion funding, makes prevention of ill-health and health improvement an attractive strategy for governments.

Health promotion

Health promotion encompasses many activities, some of which are listed below:

- Monitoring children's height, weight and developmental progress
- Encouraging 'flu jab' uptake by TV campaigns
- Organizing access to clean needles for intravenous drug users
- Assessing surgical patients' smoking status
- Encouraging tooth brushing with learning disability residents

- Explaining to parents how their child should use an inhaler
- Teaching stress reduction to people with mental distress
- Helping people access their full benefit entitlements
- Immunizing children
- Supporting people with weight loss programmes
- Undertaking blood pressure checks in workplaces
- Developing anti-bullying programmes in primary schools
- Working with community groups about local traffic issues, e.g. calming measures.

These different activities have a common aim in that they are all positive actions to improve health which, in summary, is what health promotion is all about. It is of note that only some of the activities above relate to physical health and that health promotion encompasses all dimensions of health. Contemporary health promotion often focuses on social and economic issues such as poverty and inequalities in access to healthcare and services.

The focus of health promotion activity could be the whole population but often activities are targeted to meet particular needs, focusing on one or more of the following:

- Key stages of the lifespan – pregnancy and breast-feeding, child development, parenting, retirement
- Particular age groups – e.g. preschool or secondary school children or people over 50 years of age
- High risk groups – homeless people, children and young people looked after by local authorities
- Excluded groups – e.g. minority ethnic groups, travelling people, people with mental distress or learning disability
- Specific physical illnesses – CHD, diabetes, high blood pressure
- Gender-specific issues – testicular cancer, breast or cervical cancer, menopause
- Lifestyle-related issues – smoking, drugs and alcohol, diet, activity levels, sexual health
- Mental and emotional health – awareness raising, suicide prevention, anti-stigma, anti-bullying
- Settings and situation-related – schools, prisons, workplaces, community (Box 1.19).

Health promotion is a useful summary phrase that covers a broad range of activities aimed at improving positive health and preventing ill-health. The most well-known definition is that of the WHO (1984), which defines health promotion as 'the process of enabling people to increase control over, and to improve, their health'.

Mental health promotion is any action to enhance the mental health and well-being of individuals, families, organizations and communities and can be targeted at:

1. Individuals, e.g. promoting life skills, parenting skills, stress management, suicide prevention and improving self-esteem at any stage of the lifespan
2. Communities, e.g. social support, social inclusion, improving neighbourhoods, anti-bullying, workplace health, safety and accident prevention, childcare and self-help networks

Health promotion Box 1.19

Exploring health promotion initiatives
Student activities

1. From the list below, choose a health promotion initiative that interests you:
   - National fruit schemes in school *or* NHS Choices – 5-A-DAY
   - The Drinkaware Trust – reducing alcohol misuse and minimizing alcohol-related harm
   - Paths for All – walking activity for the over 50s
   - SureStart – positive parenting or Healthystart – milk, fruit and vegetable promotion
   - Don't suffer in silence – anti-bullying
   - Baby Friendly Initiative – breast-feeding
   - See Me – reducing stigma for those with mental distress
   - NHS mammography.

2. Using an online search engine, find out more about the specific initiative, noting:
   - Its aim, methods and focus
   - Its target group
   - Whether it is delivered nationally or locally.

3. Thinking back to your recent practice experience, consider which health promotion activities you have been involved with.

3. Structural barriers to mental health, e.g. reducing discrimination and inequalities, combating stigma, promoting equal access to education, housing, services and support (WHO 2010).

Emergence of health promotion

Health promotion grew from the *Declaration of Alma-Ata* (WHO 1978). This was the birth of the 'Health for All' (HFA) movement, the values of which underpin contemporary health promotion, with its aims and principles cascading from international level to inform national legislation. The Alma-Ata declaration states that health for all:

- Involves the population as a whole in the context of their everyday life, rather than focusing on people at risk of specific diseases
- Is directed towards action on the causes or determinants of health to ensure that the total environment which is beyond the control of individuals is conducive to health
- Combines diverse, but complementary, methods or approaches
- Aims particularly at effective public participation, supporting the principle of self-help movements
- Is an activity in the health and social fields but is not a medical service, yet health professionals in primary care have an important role.

The centrality of primary healthcare to health promotion was first acknowledged here and it remains a key feature of all HFA declarations. Primary care is the first tier of health provision,

provided by generalists in the local community 'as close as possible to where people live and work' (WHO 1978). Members of the primary healthcare team include general practitioners (GPs), practice nurses, health visitors, dentists, opticians and pharmacists. Other key aspects of the Alma-Ata declaration are summarized in Box 1.20.

The Declaration of Alma-Ata Box 1.20

This declaration was made in the context of:
- 800 million of the world's population being in absolute poverty
- One-third of all deaths being in the under-5 age group
- Up to 95% of people in developing countries having no access to health services.

It expressed the need for urgent action by all governments, health and development workers and the world community to protect and promote the health of all of the people of the world.

The main foci of the Alma-Ata declaration were:
- State responsibility for health
- Action in social/economic sectors
- Recognizing health inequalities in and between countries
- Sustainable economic and social development leading to increased quality of life
- Participation by individuals and communities to increase their health.

(Based on WHO 1978.)

The Ottawa Charter (WHO 1986) is arguably the most important health promotion document. It described prerequisites of health as peace, education, shelter, food, income, social justice, a stable economy and sustainable resources. Five major types of health action were to:

- Build healthy public policy
- Create supportive environments
- Strengthen community action
- Develop personal skills
- Reorient health services towards primary care.

The Ottawa Charter also highlighted that sustainable health promotion is achieved when working with communities, not just by focusing on individual lifestyle behaviours.

Principles of health promotion

The WHO devised the principles of health promotion (WHO 1984), the key principles of which are shown in Box 1.21.

Health promotion and public health

It may be a source of confusion for students, and indeed health professionals, that there are two similar sounding phrases describing similar types of work – health promotion and public health. Health promotion means different things to different people and there are difficulties in distinguishing between this and public health. The *Acheson Report* (Acheson 1998) described public health as the science and art of preventing

Principles of health promotion   Box 1.21

Health promotion programmes, policies and other organized activities should be planned and implemented so that health promotion can be:

- *Empowering*: Enabling individuals and communities to assume more power over the personal, socioeconomic and environmental factors that affect their health
- *Participatory*: Involving those concerned (the stakeholders) in all stages of planning, implementation and evaluation
- *Holistic*: Fostering physical, mental, social and spiritual dimensions of health
- *Intersectoral*: Involving the collaboration of agencies from relevant sectors
- *Equitable*: Guided by a concern for equity and social justice
- *Sustainable*: Bringing about changes that individuals and communities can maintain once initial funding has ended
- *Multistrategy*: Using a variety of approaches including policy development, organizational change, community development, legislation, advocacy, education and communication, in combination with one another.

(From the WHO 1984.)

---

disease, prolonging life and promoting health through the organized efforts of society.

When comparing health promotion and public health, there are three main views expressed:

- Health promotion and public health are different
- Health promotion and public health are the same
- Health promotion overlaps with, or is part of, a broader concept called public health (Box 1.22).

Health promotion and public health   Box 1.22

1. *Health promotion and public health are different*
Health promotion can be seen as deriving from a more social model of health with a focus on healthy public policy, addressing determinants such as inequalities, using community approaches and advocacy. Public health can be described as an elaboration of the medical model, traditionally involving a focus on communicable disease, environmental health, screening and immunization.

2. *Health promotion and public health are the same*
Increasingly, the two terms are used synonymously in the literature. Many universities have changed their postgraduate programme titles from 'Health Promotion' to 'Public Health' and in primary care, the term public health is more commonly used than health promotion. Other phrases including health improvement and health gain also appear frequently in modern health policies.

3. *Health promotion overlaps with, or is part of, a broader concept called public health*

This may be the most common prevailing view. It is seen as unhelpful to describe health promotion as a separate entity and it should be seen as an integral part of public health. The *Acheson Report* (1998) clearly defines health promotion as part of the broader concept of public health. Health promotion has been described as the implementation arm of public health. The two entities can also be seen as having overlapping spheres of activity such as health education, strategic planning and legislation. Sometimes, the phrase 'new public health' is used to include health promotion.

National health promotion organizations

Each UK country has its own agency or authority for health promotion. Students should explore the relevant links to their own country (see Useful websites, at the end of the chapter). Covering the whole of the UK, the Health Protection Agency (HPA) states on its homepage, that it provides: 'an integrated approach to protecting UK public health through the provision of support and advice to the NHS, local authorities, emergency services, other arms-length bodies, the Department of Health and the devolved administrations' (HPA 2012).

Core public health and health promotion functions in England are undertaken by the Department of Health whose website covers specific topics including alcohol, children and families, drugs, immunization and sexual health.

The Public Health Agency for Northern Ireland supports those working in the areas of health promotion and public health, as well as members of the public.

Public Health Wales coordinates the activities of the public health resources of all health authorities in Wales, including laboratory services and communicable disease surveillance. The Health in Wales website offers a source of information and advice for health professionals and members of the public on health topics and NHS services.

Scotland's agency is NHS Health Scotland, which provides a national focus for collaborative work to improve health and reduce inequalities.

Settings and skills for health promotion

Health promotion covers a wide range of activities which take place in many settings. NHS settings include hospitals and primary care but it also takes place in communities, voluntary organizations, workplaces, schools, in self-help groups and through the media. The skills used in health promotion also vary depending on:

- Type of activity undertaken
- Client group
- Setting (see Chs 3, 9 and 14).

One important client group is children and young people who are commonly the target of health promotion activities because of the scope for prevention. Complex problems like substance abuse, most prevalent in young people aged 16–24 years, need collaborative working and multiple strategies to address them (Box 1.23). This example is specifically designed for the client group of vulnerable and disadvantaged children and young people (National Institute for Health and Clinical Excellence, NICE 2010a).

Health promotion skills vary according to context and may include needs assessment, planning and research, evaluation, communication, a counselling approach, motivational interviewing, management, networking, teaching, marketing, influencing policy and practice change, writing and publication.

Approaches to health promotion

Bottom-up and top-down approaches are the two main views of health promotion. They represent issues of power, control and relationships differently and this underpins their use in health promotion settings.

'Bottom-up' refers to the generation of issues, concerns and expressed needs from clients themselves rather than the experts being in charge. In this approach, clients are encouraged to be participative, taking an active part, or even the lead role, in identifying what information or assistance they need.

'Top-down' is the opposite approach and describes situations where the nurse or health promoter takes the lead and identifies concerns for, or on behalf of, clients. This approach is also described as 'expert-led'. Here, there is less client participation and less equality in the relationship. Sometimes, there is no contact with the client at all as in the case of TV health campaigns. Health advertisements try to market health in the same way as other products and often use celebrity endorsement. Health promotion through the media is also top-down as it has been planned and designed by experts and is one-way and usually impersonal. It is increasingly common for health and illness-related themes to be addressed through TV dramas and soap operas.

There are five ways of thinking about or viewing health promotion: medical, behavioural change, educational, client-centred and societal approaches.

The medical approach

This approach to health promotion is about encouraging people to seek medical help and to comply with prescribed treatment. It employs top-down methods to ensure that patients cooperate and comply. The aim is to reduce risk factors and prevent ill-health. Methods include preventative procedures such as immunization and screening, in addition to information-giving and persuasive advice about lifestyle changes, e.g. giving up smoking. The latter can be carried out in person, by leaflets or through the mass media, e.g. TV advertisements.

The behavioural change approach

Using this approach encourages individuals to make positive health-related changes, however small, e.g. encouraging people in the workplace to increase their exercise levels by using the stairs instead of taking the lift. Other commonly targeted lifestyle behaviours include smoking, alcohol use, diet and nutrition. The aim of this approach remains the prevention of disease by reduction of associated risk factors. It remains a top-down, expert-led approach, although participation may be encouraged.

The educational approach

This approach can be undertaken with individuals but more often involves working in groups. Group work is considered to be essential to explore and challenge people's attitudes, clarify misconceptions and ensure that the knowledge which people need to make informed decisions is available. Communication skills are key to this approach (see Ch. 9).

This approach may also focus on skills development as well as knowledge and attitudes. For example, within the subject of healthy eating, budgeting or cooking skills may be practised. Depending on the design of the session, bottom-up strategies can be used or the approach can be directive and expert-led.

The client-centred approach

This is a wholly bottom-up strategy where clients, either individuals or groups, identify their own concerns or areas where they need more information or assistance. Clients are seen as equals and the aim of this approach is empowerment, i.e. clients are enabled to maintain or increase control over their own lives. This means that the health promoter does not take charge of the situation but acts only as a facilitator. Often this approach is carried out in community groups, e.g. a local mother and toddler group which has concerns about safety and local road crossings.

The societal approach

This approach is large scale and often seen as political. It frequently involves a focus on broader social and environmental determinants of health. It can be bottom-up in approach, e.g. where night-duty nurses organized a petition, lobbied managers and caterers and then successfully negotiated healthier food choices at night in their hospital canteen. It can also be top-down, e.g. when central government legislation made seatbelt-wearing compulsory and enforced no-smoking areas in public places.

Societal change usually requires fundamental and far-reaching political action, which is beyond the scope of individuals. This is especially true when trying to reduce inequalities in health e.g., by addressing minimum wage legislation and levels of state benefits.

Models of health promotion

Models of health promotion are theoretical frameworks giving examples of health promotion activities such as preventative health services, health education, community-based work, public policies and organizational development, and economic and regulatory activities. These activities can be at international, national, regional or local levels.

Tannahill's model of health promotion

The Tannahill model (Fig. 1.5) defines health promotion as comprising efforts to enhance positive health and prevent ill-health, through the three overlapping spheres of:

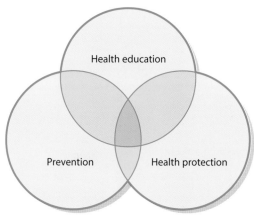

Fig. 1.5 • The Tannahill model. (Reproduced with permission from Naidoo, J., Wills, J., 2009. Foundations for health promotion, third ed. Baillière Tindall, Edinburgh.)

- Health education
- Prevention (of ill-health)
- Health protection.

Health education is defined in Tannahill's model as communication activity aimed at enhancing positive health and preventing or diminishing ill-health. This can be carried out with individuals or groups, through influencing the beliefs, attitudes and behaviour of those with power and of the community at large. This is considered further below.

Prevention of ill-health is described by Tannahill as activities concerned with reducing the risk of occurrence of ill-health, or an unwanted event. Different levels of prevention exist and activities from adult nursing are used as examples:

- Primary prevention of the first occurrence of a given illness or other unwanted phenomena, e.g. immunization
- Secondary prevention of the avoidable consequences of an illness through early detection and treatment, e.g. screening
- Tertiary prevention of the avoidable complications of an established irreversible disease, e.g. rehabilitation.

Box 1.24 shows levels of prevention applied to other nursing settings.

 Health promotion   Box 1.24

Levels of prevention
Learning disability nursing
- Primary prevention – self-care education, e.g. dental hygiene
- Secondary prevention – screening for sensory deficits
- Tertiary prevention – management of epilepsy.

Mental health nursing
- Primary prevention – self-care education, e.g. safe use of prescribed medicines, stress management
- Secondary prevention – screening, using a mental health assessment tool
- Tertiary prevention – rehabilitation techniques for schizophrenia.

Child health nursing
- Primary prevention – positive parenting strategies, accident prevention for toddlers
- Secondary prevention – preschool child development checks
- Tertiary prevention – nebulizer training for parents of children with asthma.

The third sphere of activity in the Tannahill model is health protection, which includes the public policy framework for prevention of ill-health and positive enhancement of well-being. It includes legal, fiscal and political measures, e.g. tobacco tax, or policies, laws and codes of practice, e.g. seatbelt legislation. The Tannahill model is straightforward and easy to use, fitting well with nursing and other healthcare practice in primary care and NHS settings. However, it has been criticized for its medical model approach, its largely individual focus and the lack of emphasis on social determinants of health and illness. It may be less helpful in community settings and when working with disadvantaged or excluded groups. The activities in Box 1.25 will help you apply the Tannahill model of health promotion to nursing practice.

The Tones model

An empowerment model of health promotion was devised by Tones in 1993. It aims to enable people to gain control over their own health and in this way, it sounds very similar to the important WHO (1986) definition of health promotion. A summary of the model (Tones & Tilford 2001) reads like a formula:

Health promotion = health education × healthy public policy.

The full model is more complex than the Tannahill model. Starting at the bottom of Figure 1.6, education is seen as critical to the process of raising awareness so that people can make informed health choices, participate in and influence health policy. This applies to both lay people and health professionals.

In this model, healthy social and environmental factors are emphasized and this view fits better with bottom-up, community-based approaches as in mental health, learning disability and voluntary organizations. It may be harder to envisage this model in relation to working within a traditional NHS setting.

Health education

Although people may use the terms 'health promotion' and 'health education' interchangeably, they are not the same. As seen above, health education is just one part of health promotion and is only one of many methods available to the nurse or health promoter. It has been mentioned above as one of the five approaches to health promotion (see p. 20) and forms one-third of health promotion according to the Tannahill model (see Fig. 1.5). Health education was also described as one half of the summarized Tones Model (Fig. 1.6).

There are many diverse definitions of health education, some of which are listed below. Health education (adapted from Kiger 2004) can be described as:

* A communication activity, e.g. the Tannahill model
* Persuading people to adopt and sustain healthy life practices
* Developing people's skills in decision-making and clarifying beliefs and values about health
* Changing the knowledge, feelings and behaviour of people
* An information-giving activity
* Persuading people to use available health services wisely
* Enabling people to improve their own health
* Enabling people to control their own health, e.g. the Tones model

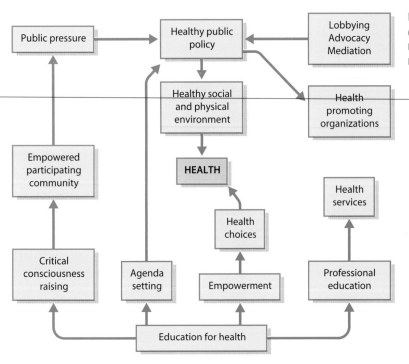

Fig. 1.6 • The Tones model of health promotion. (Reproduced with permission from Naidoo, J., Wills, J., 2009. Foundations for health promotion, third ed. Baillière Tindall, Edinburgh.)

- Assisting communities to engage in conflict with powerful authorities
- Seeking to modify behaviours responsible for disease
- Seeking the roots of health problems and finding them in social, economic and political factors.

Approaches to health education

Kiger (2004) described five approaches to health education: medical, educational, media/propaganda, community development and political action. These can be compared to the five approaches to health promotion explained earlier (p. 20). The approaches to health education are outlined below with examples of the likely methods used:

- *The medical approach* to health education assumes that rational facts will persuade people to change their health-related behaviour. Methods include expert advice, talks, lectures, booklets and leaflets, alone or in combination.
- *The educational approach* to health education does not mean instruction in the same way as the medical model but rather 'leading to learning'. It uses people-centred methods such as discussion groups, problem-solving, values clarification, skills teaching, role play and peer work.
- *The media/propaganda approach* to health education has been described as manipulation for health. Like the medical model it uses the mass media, TV and radio advertisements and markets health as if it were a product.
- *The community development approach* centres on enabling and empowering people. It uses bottom-up methods that include assisting people to organize, change, raise awareness or gain consensus.
- *The political action approach* seeks to promote societal or political change. It uses methods such as providing evidence, lobbying, mobilizing local support and exploring anti-health agencies.

The activities in Box 1.26 will help you think about health education approaches used in your placement.

Health education in the NHS

A medical approach to health education is sometimes known as patient education in NHS settings. Methods such as 1:1

talks/interactions, group work and written information, alone or in combination, have been shown to increase patients' knowledge and understanding of their symptoms, illness, surgery, drugs or other treatments. Effective communication skills are vital to people's understanding of information provided (see Ch. 9).

As long ago as 1975, Hayward's research demonstrated that there are positive effects when patients know what to expect and are prepared by being provided with suitable information prior to clinical procedures (Box 1.27).

Evidence-based practice Box 1.27

The positive effects of health information

A classic study by Hayward (1975) found that the positive effects of preoperative health information and education for patients included:

- Improved informed consent
- Greater patient satisfaction
- Increased compliance with treatment programmes
- Better progress and outcomes
- Reduced levels of distress during invasive procedures
- Reduced anxiety levels
- Reduced pain and need for analgesic drugs (see Ch. 23)
- Faster recovery times
- Shorter hospital stays.

Student activities

- Reflect on the possible benefits of patient education listed above and identify examples from your personal experience, when having information helped you or a family member.
- Identify examples from your placement experience, when having information helped a patient/client or their family.

Levels of health education

As well as having different approaches, health education is also described as having different levels: primary, secondary and tertiary.

Primary health education

Primary health education involves a focus on the structure and function of the body or mind, how bodies or relationships work and how to promote and maintain them. Nurses carry out much primary health education in their everyday practice, e.g. each time information is given before informed consent is sought, lifestyle advice is offered or a procedure or treatment is explained to patients. It is usually undertaken with individuals but can be carried out in groups.

Undertaking health education with learning disability clients can be challenging because they have more complex health needs than the general population and find it more difficult to access health services.

The Government (DH 2009) strategy 'Valuing People Now' outlines four guiding principles which apply to both individuals with learning disability and the services which support them:

- *Rights*: People with learning disabilities and their families have the same human rights as everyone else.

Health promotion Box 1.26

Health education approaches
Student activities

- Look at the list of health education definitions (p. 22) and identify similarities and differences in their approaches.
- Consider the five approaches to health education and the examples of related health education activities and compare them with the health promotion approaches described on page 20. Note the similarities.
- Identify which of the approaches to health education are used in health education activities in your placement.

- *Independent living*: All disabled people should have greater choice and control over the support they need to go about their daily lives; greater access to housing, education, employment, leisure and transport opportunities and to participation in family and community life.
- *Control*: This is about having information and support to understand the different options and their implications and consequences, so people can make informed decisions about their own lives.
- *Inclusion*: This means being able to participate in all the aspects of community – to work, learn, get about, meet people, be part of social networks and access goods and services – and to have the support to do so.

Some people with learning disabilities learn at a slower pace and key considerations for health education are summarized in Box 1.28.

 Health promotion Box 1.28

Health education for people with learning disabilities

Scarborough and Godsell (2011) identify key considerations when planning health education for clients with learning disabilities. Activities should be:

- interactive and designed to meet the needs of particular clients
- conducted in an unhurried fashion, in a supportive and non-judgemental environment
- systematic in planning and delivery so that material is presented in small chunks lasting no more than 30–40 min
- based on everyday life, e.g. healthy eating education being reinforced during shopping trips
- planned so that repetition and opportunities to practise are provided
- provided using the appropriate level of language for each client, with suitable visual aids and other learning materials.

Student activity

Review the principles above and reflect on your placement experience with a client who had learning disabilities.

(From Scarborough, K., Godsell, M., 2011. Enabling good health. In: Atherton, H.L., Crickmore, D.J. (Eds.), Learning disabilities: towards inclusion, sixth ed. Churchill Livingstone, Edinburgh.)

Difficulties in accessing health services is also common among people from black or ethnic minority communities and those for whom English is not their first language. In recognition of this, health promotion materials and NHS information leaflets are often produced in up to 20 languages.

Supporting the health education role of nurses and midwives is NICE. This is an independent organization responsible for producing guidance documents for health professionals, designed to provide national evidence-based guidance on promoting good health and, preventing and treating ill health. NICE guidance is 'based on the best evidence; transparent in its development, consistent, reliable and based on a rigorous development process; good value for money, weighing up the cost and benefits of treatments; and internationally recognised for its excellence' (NICE 2012 Guidance homepage). Box 1.29

provides an example of guidance published by NICE (2010b) for antenatal care during pregnancy. This offers staff detailed guidance on best practice in relation to the content and timing of interventions in relation to information needs or screening activities.

 Critical thinking Box 1.29

Antenatal care

The NICE (2010b) document on antenatal care contains detailed guidance for doctors, nurses and midwives. Following a definition of woman-centred care and principles of antenatal care, three key priority areas are addressed:

- *Antenatal information* – to allow informed decisions about care
- *Lifestyle considerations* – work, medicines and vitamins, infection, exercise, sexual intercourse, smoking, alcohol, diet, cannabis, air and car travel
- *Screening* for clinical conditions and fetal anomalies.

Recommendations are also made about the schedule and timing of appointments and which interventions are not routinely undertaken.

Student activity

Locate the guidance document below and read about the lifestyle considerations section, noting the detailed advice recommended for pregnant women.

Resource

NICE, 2010. Antenatal care: routine care for the healthy pregnant woman. Quick reference guide. Online. Available: www.nice.org.uk/nicemedia/live/11947/40110/40110.pdf August 2012.

Secondary health education

This takes the form of information or advice about services to improve and maintain health, how to get the best out of healthcare and other systems, what is available and how to complain if necessary. Nurses may also carry out secondary health education in their everyday practice, but perhaps less often than primary level health education. In all settings, but especially in community nursing, nurses have to help people to:

- Understand their rights
- Obtain contact details for community-based services
- Be referred to agencies, e.g. housing associations
- Gain access to complaints/suggestions forms.

An empowering resource is the Patient Advice and Liaison Service (PALS). This government initiative in England offers a useful website (p. 30) and ensures that PALS offices provide help, information, advice and support locally and help address any concerns or problems experienced by patients and their families.

Tertiary health education

This is the highest level of health education which focuses on raising awareness of the sociopolitical health determinants such as unemployment, education, pollution, water and food quality, and traffic levels. Another focus is the activities of the anti-health sector of the economy such as advertising and sponsorship by tobacco companies. This is sometimes called consciousness raising, and is common in bottom-up work with community-based groups. In general, it is less common for nurses to carry out this level of health education compared to the other two. Although not often part of mainstream NHS work, tertiary health education features in the education of health professionals and may include study of poverty, inequalities and other health determinants. Box 1.30 will help you consider levels of health education in nursing practice.

 Health promotion **Box 1.30**

Examples of health education

Student activity

Reflect on which level(s) of health education you have seen used in nursing practice and identify examples of:

- Primary health education
- Secondary health education
- Tertiary health education.

UK health policy context

By 1986, the WHO's main target for the following decades was that all citizens of the world should attain a level of health that would permit them to lead socially and economically productive lives by the year 2000. The European region of the WHO later introduced *Health 21*, namely 21 targets for the twenty-first century, to achieve this goal (WHO 1998).

The first UK national targets for health were set in 1992 and each UK country devised its own targets and strategy documents. A further round of revised White Papers on health and healthcare appeared in 1999 following political devolution. *The Jakarta Declaration on Health Promotion into the 21st Century* (WHO 1997) was incorporated into all four national documents with collaborative working as the dominant theme.

While the aims described in the policy documents of all four UK countries are similar in their focus on tackling health inequalities and social exclusion, they are quite different in the use of language, approach and in their organizational development. Despite emphasis on integrated policies and collaborative services, the UK has been described as developing four distinct health services. This is complex for health professionals, so it is recommended that emphasis be placed on the policies relating to the reader's own UK country or that in which they live and work. These policies can be accessed on links from the homepages of each country's national agency for health. Box 1.31 gives examples of some key health policy frameworks from England and Scotland.

Measuring health and illness

Demography refers to the study of populations, with data gathered on the age, gender and size of groups within the

---

Key health policy frameworks **Box 1.31**

England:

The White Paper, *Healthy Lives Healthy People* (DH 2010a) sets out the Government's long-term vision for the future of public health in England. The aim is to create a 'wellness' service (Public Health England) and to strengthen both national and local leadership.

Go to: DH 2010a *Healthy lives healthy people: Our strategy for public health in England*. Online. Available: www.dh.gov.uk/en/Publichealth/Healthyliveshealthypeople/index.htm

The White Paper, *Equity and Excellence: Liberating the NHS* (DH 2010b), sets out the Government's long-term vision for the future of the NHS. The vision builds on the core values and founding principles of the NHS – a comprehensive service, available to all, free at the point of use, based on need and not ability to pay. It seeks to:

- put patients at the heart of everything the NHS does
- focus on continuously improving those things that really matter to patients – the outcome of their healthcare
- empower and liberate clinicians to innovate, with the freedom to focus on improving healthcare services.

Go to: DH 2010b *Equity and excellence: Liberating the NHS*. Online. Available: www.dh.gov.uk/en/Healthcare/LiberatingtheNHS/index.htm

The Health and Social Care Bill 2011 builds on the White Paper *Equity and Excellence: Liberating the NHS* 2010. Its aim is to modernize the NHS and has five themes:

1. Strengthening commissioning of NHS services
2. Increasing democratic accountability and public voice
3. Liberating provision of NHS services
4. Strengthening public health services
5. Reforming health and care – arm's-length bodies (ALBs).

ALBs are a national level network of stand-alone organizations linked to the Department of Health but at 'arm's length'. They help support and manage the health and social care system and are involved in regulation, improving standards and protecting public welfare, e.g. the Health Protection Agency.

Go to: DH 2011 Health and Social Care Bill 2011. Online. Available: www.dh.gov.uk/en/Publicationsandstatistics/Legislation/Actsandbills/HealthandSocialCareBill2011/index.htm

Scotland:

The social policy frameworks below seek to find a common approach to addressing health inequalities across Scotland:

- The Scottish Government 2011 *Child poverty strategy*. Online. Available: www.vhscotland.org.uk/library/executive/child_poverty_strategy.pdf
- The Scottish Government 2009 *The early years framework*. Online. Available: www.scotland.gov.uk/Publications/2009/01/13095148/0
- The Scottish Government 2008 *'Equally well' Report of the Ministerial Task Force on health inequalities*. Online. Available: www.scotland.gov.uk/Resource/Doc/315880/0100454.pdf
- The Scottish Government 2008 *Achieving our potential*. Online. Available: www.scotland.gov.uk/Publications/2008/11/20103815/0

---

population and the geographical spread or migration of those groups. It also covers what are known as vital statistics: births, marriages, divorces, separations and deaths. Box 1.32 shows some examples of UK demographic trends.

Epidemiology is the study of the occurrence, patterns and spread of disease in a population. The data can demonstrate

---

(?) **Critical thinking**   Box 1.32

Demographic trends in the UK

The 2009 data below come from the Office for National Statistics:

- The live birth rate has fallen slightly to 1.96 children per woman in England and Wales after the highest point for 35 years reached in 2008
- Falling death rates means that the population of the UK has slowly increased to over 61.5 million
- In 2009, children under 16 accounted for one in five of the UK population; roughly the same proportion as those of retirement age
- Life expectancy continues to rise and is highest in England, lowest in Scotland
- The average age of the UK population is 39.5 years.

Student activity

Go to: National Statistics online at www.statistics.gov.uk and search the database for information on other health-related topics, e.g. life expectancy, ethnicity, lone-parent families, disability or age on marriage.

---

the scale of a health problem and its trends, showing changes in mortality and morbidity over time. Epidemiological data can highlight the natural history and progression of a disease. Causation can be established when there is evidence that exposure to a particular environmental, lifestyle or socioeconomic factor contributes to ill-health, e.g. use of these methods identified the causal link between tobacco smoking and lung cancer. Epidemiology can also show the severity of a problem and predict the ways in which individuals or communities may be affected. It can assess the likelihood, or probability, of a disease or condition occurring as well as suggesting how it can be tackled or prevented. Later, follow-up studies may show whether changes can be attributed to particular interventions.

Purposes of measuring health and illness

Measuring health and illness in communities provides the opportunity for:

- Assessing a population's health status
- Describing the patterns of disease in populations, in either small groups or whole countries
- Analysing differences between one population and another and, over time, identifying trends
- Directing interventions appropriately, therefore increasing the population's health and maximizing health potential
- Identifying and responding to specific needs of minority groups or sections of the population whose health needs have not been fully met
- Targeting at-risk groups to reduce inequalities in health
- Making resource allocation more equitable
- Influencing policy, research or development of priorities (Pencheon et al 2006).

In addition to measuring ill-health or death, information on the health status of people is also collected, e.g. height, weight and dental health. Such data act as a baseline, allowing comparisons

over time and identification of trends. Another area of study is health behaviour indicators related to individual lifestyle, e.g. smoking status. Environmental indicators are also measured, e.g. air and water quality, housing type and density. Social environment indicators include wealth, income and social class, with one particular focus being the measurement of deprivation. There are many measurements used to identify underprivileged areas with a view to improving or targeting services. Two of the most well-known deprivation measurement tools are the Jarman index and the Townsend index, both of which take into account indicators such as social housing and lack of car ownership.

The advantage of epidemiological and demographic studies is that information is collected regularly, it is relatively consistent and readily available. It is sometimes known as routinely available data and examples are shown in Box 1.33. Both of these quantitative sciences are largely concerned with numerical descriptions relating to groups of people. They do not focus on individuals but instead study the vital statistics or the ill-health of populations within society.

Examples of demographic and epidemiological data   Box 1.33

- Mortality and morbidity rates
- Reasons for primary healthcare consultations
- Immunization rates
- Screening rates
- Accident rates
- HIV, AIDS notifications
- NHS waiting lists
- Children at risk register
- Child developmental health records
- Poverty/inequality measures, e.g. Jarman index of disadvantage
- Sociodemographic statistics.

Common methods of health and illness measurement

The common methods of measurement are counts and rates:

- *Counts* are the simplest numerical description, e.g. 14 people in a nursing home have diarrhoea.
- *Rates* are the number of affected people expressed as a proportion of a total population. Following the example above, if 14 people are affected out of a total nursing home population of 56, then the rate is 14/56 or 25%.

Percentages are the commonest way to express proportions. Sometimes, the numbers per 1000, per 10 000 or per 1 000 000 are used instead of per 100 (percentage).

Incidence

Incidence, or incidence rate, refers to the rate of development, i.e. the new cases, of a disease or problem rather than the total number of people affected in a given period, usually 1 year. The number of people developing a disease in a group of known size over a specific period of time can be expressed in this way. For example, the incidence of depression in men aged 55–59 years in a particular country, was 252 per 100 000 for the year 2002–2003. This means that there were 252 new cases of depression for every 100 000 of the population in this age group during the given year.

Mortality rate is similar to incidence except it refers to the number of deaths from a condition in a particular group during a period of time. SMR refers to standardized mortality ratio and uses the formula below:

$$\text{SMR} = \frac{\text{observed deaths in study population}}{\text{expected deaths in study population}} \times 100$$

The observed death rate in a defined population is compared with the rate expected in a standard population, e.g. the ratio of the rate of lung cancer deaths in smokers compared with that of non-smokers. Therefore, if the SMR is less than 100, the mortality experience of the study population is less than that of the reference population.

Prevalence

Prevalence, or prevalence rate, refers to the total number of people with a disease or condition in a group at a specific time. For example, the prevalence of chickenpox in a preschool nursery on a given day was 10%.

Distribution

Another key term used in epidemiology and demography is 'distribution'. This refers to the spread of a problem or disease by age, gender, race, ethnicity, socioeconomic class, geography or other variable.

Other approaches to measurement of health and illness

Other than epidemiological study, there are three other main approaches commonly used in health and illness measurement: needs assessment, social audit and community profiling. The agency undertaking the measurement exercise and the purpose of the study determine the approach taken. The focus of study may be:

- Using routinely available data or gathering primary data (new research)
- At the individual level or whole populations
- Exploring illness and disease or broader health determinants
- Top-down or bottom-up (see p. 20)
- Primarily using epidemiological data or community participation.

Needs assessment

This is commonly used in health and social care settings, especially in community-based work. It is described as the first phase in health promotion planning, namely identifying what

a client or population group needs to enable them to be more healthy (Naidoo & Wills 2009).

An individual approach to needs assessment focuses on a person's lifestyle and behaviours, such as smoking status. The purpose of this is to gather data directly from individuals in the community under study to inform health promotion planning for behaviour change and risk factor modification. No account is taken of the socioeconomic context or the social and environmental health determinants affecting individuals' lives, leading to criticism that the context of people's lives has been ignored.

Population-based needs assessment, or health needs assessment, is used by statutory bodies to measure health needs in defined populations. In the health arena, statutory bodies are centrally funded agencies, e.g. health authorities, local authorities and health promoting organizations, which undertake health-related work on behalf of the government.

Needs assessment uses an epidemiological approach and tends to be top-down, with limited community involvement. Quantifiable, secondary information is used with heavy reliance on available data such as census and electoral ward information. Electoral wards are the key building blocks of UK administrative geography and data are held by the Office for National Statistics (see Useful websites, at the end of the chapter).

Needs assessment focuses on ill-health and the determinants of disease by measuring the incidence, prevalence and degree of severity of various health problems in a population, although causal links are not always obvious. For example, an increase in the level of youth suicide may be identified in a town but not the reasons behind it.

Social audit

Social audit is a broader approach to health and illness measurement than needs assessment. This is used by a wide variety of voluntary, statutory or community organizations to assess need at local, city or district levels and is wider in scope than lifestyle factors or ill-health rates. Social audit is underpinned by a broad and more social definition of health and health determinants. The interplay of resources, e.g. environment, housing, transport and employment, is a major focus.

Social audit often involves the collection of new primary data and is increasingly called health impact assessment. It tends to be top-down but includes a variable amount of community participation. It has been described as a socioeconomic approach to needs assessment, which uses a wide range of quantitative, secondary data to give a view 'of' a community, rather than 'from' a community. This approach is professionally led and encourages multiagency working because different disciplines need to be involved, e.g. health promoters may be working with local councillors, transport consultants and environmental health specialists to consider the impact of traffic in a community.

Community profiling

Community profiling is the approach commonly used by local health boards, local authorities and councils to measure and evaluate the health and social needs of their populations. Its focus is how local people view their health and social needs in their community. The aim of community profiles is to obtain accurate and appropriate information from local people which is then used to support epidemiological and population data. This is often considered to be the most balanced and helpful approach to measurement of health and illness, as it uses both top-down and bottom-up strategies in the assessment. Community nurses, health visitors and those working in health promotion and public health are often involved in compiling these profiles. Many student nurses undertake a small community profile as part of their coursework.

Community profiling is sometimes known as the community participation approach to needs assessment. It uses client-centred methods and is underpinned by the concept of empowerment. It is described as 'done with' not 'done to' the community. The degree of community involvement is highly variable in this approach but it tends not to be dominated by professionals.

One potential problem in community profiling is trying to encourage meaningful community participation. Any assessment of community needs seeking public involvement requires creative methods of data collection to prevent 'tokenism'. In addition to questionnaires and local surveys, more creative methods of community participation in data collection or evaluation include focus groups, 1:1 interviews, photographs, collage, examples of work from community groups, audiotapes, video work and drama.

Another potential problem is that community involvement can raise unrealistic expectations. Community profiling tends to identify large numbers of needs that cannot all be tackled due to staff, time and financial constraints. Delays or perceived inaction can dishearten participants in the data collection who may have high expectations of change and improvements in their community health and social services.

Priorities

Of the many identified health needs arising from the assessment process, some needs take precedence because they are considered more important than others. They are therefore tackled first and this is called prioritizing, or priority setting. Health economists refer to this as rationing, describing finite resources but infinite needs.

The reasons why one particular issue becomes a priority are many and varied. It may be simply that the local health professional's personal area of interest or expertise is the deciding factor in which need is tackled first or in what order needs are addressed. Usually, however, priorities are set in line with a central or local policy either alone or in combination, e.g.

- National or central government agenda and targets
- Local authority agenda and targets
- Resources and funding availability
- Local people's identified priority.

Illness behaviour

When people are ill their reactions to it are described as illness behaviour, i.e. what they do and how they respond to their changing health state. Illness behaviour is complex and occurs in the context of the family or support system and it is sometimes said that it is not individuals who become ill, but the whole family. The study of illness behaviour focuses on people's experience of illness, their interpretation of, and reactions to, symptoms which may limit their normal function or activities, and how chronically ill individuals cope with the practical and emotional demands of their illness.

Increasingly, instead of illness behaviour, it is called 'illness action' to emphasize the fact that people are active participants in dealing with their own (and others') illness. Each person reacts differently to illness, or the threat of it, in terms of both their behaviour and emotions. Different illness reactions make it crucial that nurses understand and empathize with the experiences of their patients and clients in order to plan suitable, individualized care interventions. The components of Becker's health belief model (p. 10) – including culture, gender, the person's attitude to the illness and their family's reaction to it – are variables which may affect illness behaviour. Another major influence is the nature of the illness itself as patient/client reactions may depend on whether the problem is:

- Short or long term
- Life-threatening or not serious
- Sudden or acute in onset
- Chronic, recurring or progressive in pattern (see Ch. 11)
- Disfiguring or not.

Self-help and self-care

Most symptoms experienced by individuals are dealt with by people themselves without seeking formal medical help. Self-treatment with over-the-counter (OTC) medicines bought from supermarkets, corner shops or community pharmacies is increasingly common, as is the use of homeopathic and other complementary treatments. Community pharmacists are important members of the primary care team (Box 1.34).

Over-the-counter (OTC) medicines and the role of the community pharmacy   Box 1.34

- Community pharmacists play a key role in primary care, having direct patient contact and undertaking health education about prescribed medicines, as well as advising on OTC medicines
- OTC medicines are used to treat minor and short-lived symptoms, which people usually consider not serious enough to visit their GP
- OTC medicines provide the opportunity for people to self-care and manage their own symptoms
- The most common OTC medicines used relate to pain relief or common cold, headache or allergies
- 13 000 community pharmacies in Great Britain are visited by 1.8 million people each day
- The number of prescription items dispensed by community pharmacies in England increased to 886 million in 2009; an increase of 5.2% on the previous year.

(From The Royal Pharmaceutical Society of Great Britain, 2010. What do pharmacists do? Online. Available: www.rpharms.com/ipharmacist/what-do-pharmacists-do-.asp? August 2012.)

It is common for people to use a lay referral system where they ask trusted friends, colleagues or family members for advice about symptoms or treatment. Sometimes it is the lay 'referees' who diagnose and recommend an OTC medicine from the pharmacy. They may also strongly suggest that the person seeks medical help and exert pressure until they comply. This is known as 'sanctioning by significant others'.

The effects of illness

Illness, especially when serious, chronic or life-threatening, can have far-reaching effects on a wide range of issues such as the ability to function physically or mentally, coping with increased stress, family roles and dynamics, caring roles, work roles, finances, body image, self-concept and self-esteem. Reactions to serious illness sometimes resemble loss and bereavement responses such as shock, denial and disbelief (see Chs 11, 12).

Help-seeking behaviour

In the sociology of health and illness, help-seeking behaviour is a major theme for study, which seeks to answer questions such as:

- Why do some people seek medical help for particular symptoms while others do not?
- What factors increase the likelihood of people seeking medical help?

The more visible, frequent and disruptive in day-to-day life a symptom is, the more likely a person is to seek medical help (Box 1.35). This, however, must be set in the context of the

---

Determinants of help-seeking behaviour   Box 1.35

Mechanic (1978) described 10 determinants of help-seeking behaviour, i.e. factors that influence a person's decision to seek medical help:

- How visible a symptom is, e.g. obvious skin rash or limp
- The person's estimate of the seriousness of the symptom, e.g. sleep disturbance
- The person's knowledge and understanding about the symptom
- How much the symptom disrupts usual roles and function, e.g. family, work, social activities
- Frequency or persistence of symptoms, e.g. headache daily for more than 1 week
- How much the symptom is tolerated by family and friends, e.g. smoker's cough
- How much basic needs are affected by the symptom, e.g. dental pain restricting eating
- How much other needs compete with illness responses, e.g. too busy with childcare to rest swollen feet
- How much the person has other reasons for the symptoms, e.g. low mood and tearfulness described as tiredness in the mother of a newborn infant
- How available medical help or treatment is in terms of access, cost and time as well as emotional costs like stigma, e.g. a person with possible symptoms of a sexually transmitted infection delays seeking help because of embarrassment.

(From Mechanic, D., 1978. Medical sociology. Free Press, New York.)

---

person's knowledge, their estimate of the seriousness of the symptoms and the family's tolerance of any restriction of role function caused by it.

There can be a problem with the view that interruption to normal activity is seen as the main trigger for seeking help. For conditions with a slow, insidious onset, e.g. cancer, HIV or Alzheimer's disease, the individual can carry on with normal activities for a lengthy period and there may be a considerable delay in seeking help, allowing symptoms to become more advanced before help is sought.

The sick role

Triggers that strongly influence a person's decision to seek medical help frequently relate to the wider context of their life rather than the symptoms of ill-health directly. For example, someone experiencing interpersonal problems in their wider life may be more likely to notice physical symptoms and then seek help.

In 1952, Talcott Parsons proposed the concept of the sick role, where illness is seen as abnormal and/or disrupting an individual's usual activities. Parsons believed that people learn the sick role through socialization starting in childhood, and change their behaviour when trying to cope with illness. The sick role was described as temporary and conditional on the sick person cooperating to get well again as soon as possible. Parsons (1991) described three main tenets of the sick role:

- *The sick person is not held personally responsible for their illness, meaning that they cannot be blamed for their situation, as the cause of the illness is beyond their control.* Illness is therefore seen as not resulting from personal behaviour or actions. Critique of this first tenet may involve its lack of application to some illnesses or conditions where blame is attributed, e.g. self-harm, STIs or substance misuse, which all have moral overtones.
- *The sick person has certain special rights including the privilege of withdrawing from normal tasks or responsibilities.* The sick person may be expected not to attend work or school and is allowed to withdraw from household tasks. It might be permissible for the sick person to stay in bed and require to be looked after, but this is strictly temporary. Impolite behaviour may well be tolerated or excused because of the illness. Critique of this tenet is that it does not extend to people with disability. Restriction of activity and staying in bed is neither suitable nor required for people with chronic mental or physical illness. Withdrawal from activities, except in the short term, does not fit with modern concepts of rehabilitation (see Ch. 11).
- *The sick person must actively try to get well by seeking expert help and following instructions in the 'patient role'.* Parsons believed that the true sick role can only be conferred by a medical expert whose job it is to legitimize the illness. This removes any doubt that the sick person is malingering and makes the illness official. The patient is expected to cooperate and try to recover as soon as possible by obeying instructions such as adhering to prescribed treatments. Sick role status will not be granted,

and sympathy and special rights quickly evaporate, if the sick person will not seek medical help or cooperate. There has been widespread criticism of the inappropriateness of the sick role concept in relation to people with incurable or terminal illness.

The activities in Box 1.36 will help you think further about the sick role. It is interesting to note how congruent Parson's sick role concept is with the bio-medical view, reinforcing ideas that patients are passive. However, since the sick role was first described in the 1950s, nurses and healthcare workers are much more likely to expect patients to be actively involved in all aspects of their care.

 Critical thinking   **Box 1.36**

The sick role
Student activities

Consider Parson's sick role and think about your experiences, both personal and from your clinical practice.

1. How well does the sick role explain your own experiences of ill-health?
2. Review the following situations and consider how appropriate the sick role is for:
   - A child with chickenpox
   - A teenager with appendicitis
   - A man with longstanding depressive illness
   - A woman with chronic fatigue syndrome/ME
   - A child with a learning disability and cerebral palsy
   - A woman who has recurrent migraine headaches.

SUMMARY

- Personal definitions of health may vary widely from official definitions.
- Health is multidimensional in nature, encompassing physical, mental, emotional, social, spiritual and societal dimensions.
- The medical model is less dominant in contemporary approaches to health promotion.
- Health beliefs vary widely and understanding them is an essential part of nurses' involvement in health promotion activities.
- Changes in health behaviour usually need to be preceded by change in people's attitudes and values but this is often difficult to achieve.
- Many factors influence health and affect life chances; the key determinant is poverty, linked to inequalities in health.
- The 'Health for All' movement and subsequent legislation underpin health promotion activities, which may take place at global, national and local levels.
- Health promotion includes a wide range of activities that are often targeted to particular groups. It takes place in many different settings and forms part of the role of every nurse. The overall aim determines the approach taken and methods used.
- Health education is part of health promotion – it also takes many forms and is carried out in a range of settings.
- Measuring health and illness can involve nurses and provides valuable information for healthcare planning.
- Illness behaviour includes self-help, lay referral systems, help-seeking behaviour and the sick role.
- People today have high expectations of health and healthcare.

KEY WORDS AND PHRASES FOR LITERATURE SEARCHING

Public health
Determinants of health
Dimensions of health
Health beliefs
Health promotion
Health definitions
Inequalities
Poverty

 Useful websites

HSC Public Health Agency Northern Ireland
    www.publichealth.hscni.net
Health in Wales (NHS) www.wales.nhs.uk
NHS Health Scotland www.healthscotland.com
Health Protection Agency UK www.hpa.org.uk
National Institute for Health and Clinical Excellence (NICE)
    www.nice.org.uk
Patient Advice and Liaison Service (PALS) www.pals.nhs.uk
Health topics
   NHS Choices: 'Your health, your choices' has an A to Z list of all
       health topics www.nhs.uk
Health information and advice
   Department of Health: Policy, guidance and publications for NHS
       and Social Care staff www.dh.gov.uk
Office for National Statistics www.statistics.gov.uk
Telephone and Internet support about symptoms, illness and services
   with 24 h coverage
   NHS Direct for England and Wales is a national helpline staffed 24 h
       a day by qualified nursing staff. It offers information on the NHS
       and current health and illness issues Tel: 0845 4647
   NHS Direct is the internet arm of NHS Direct and has links with
       NHS Direct Wales and NHS 24 www.nhsdirect.nhs.uk
   NHS Direct Wales www.nhsdirect.wales.nhs.uk
   NHS 24 provides a similar health information and self-care advice
       service in Scotland. Tel: 08454 24 24 24 www.nhs24.com
All websites accessed September 2012.

References

Acheson, D., 1998. Independent enquiry into inequalities in health. TSO, London.

Becker, M.H. (Ed.), 1974. The health belief model and personal health behaviours. Slack, Thorofare, NJ.

Blaxter, M., 1990. Health and lifestyles. Tavistock Routledge, London.

British Heart Foundation, 2011. British Heart Foundation statistics website. Online. Available: www.heartstats.org September 2012.

Dahlgren, G., Whitehead, M., 1991. Policies and strategies to promote social equity in health. WHO, Copenhagen.

Department of Health, 2009. Valuing people now: a new three year strategy for people with learning disabilities. Online. Available: www.dh.gov.uk/prod_consum_dh/groups/dh_digitalassets/documents/digitalasset/dh_093375.pdf September 2012.

Department of Health, 2010. Essence of care 2010 benchmarks: promoting health and well-being. Online. Available: www.dh.gov.uk/prod_consum_dh/groups/dh_digitalassets/@dh/@en/documents/digitalasset/dh_120394.pdf September 2012.

Diabetes UK, 2010. Diabetes in the UK 2010: key statistics on diabetes. Online. Available: www.diabetes.org.uk September 2012.

EAPN, 2010. European Anti-Poverty Network Resources. Online. Available: www.eapn.eu September 2012.

Festinger, L., 1964. Conflict, decision and dissonance. Tavistock, London.

Foucault, M., 1973. The birth of the clinic. Tavistock, London.

Hart, C., Chesson, R., 1998. Children as consumers. British Medical Journal 316, 1600–1603.

Hayward, J., 1975. Information, a prescription against pain. RCN, London.

Helman, C., 2007. Culture, health and illness, fifth ed. Hodder Arnold, London.

HPA, 2012. Health Protection Agency Homepage. Online. Available: www.hpa.org.uk August 2012.

Jones, L., 1994. The social context of health and health care. Macmillan, Basingstoke.

Kiger, A.M., 2004. Teaching for health, third ed. Churchill Livingstone, Edinburgh.

Mind, 2011. How to help someone who is suicidal. Online. Available: www.mind.org.uk/help/medical_and_alternative_care/how_to_help_someone_who_is_suicidal September 2012.

Naidoo, J., Wills, J., 2009. Foundations for health promotion, third ed. Baillière Tindall/Elsevier, Edinburgh.

National Children's Bureau, 2011. Data and statistics on sexual health. Online. Available: www.ncb.org.uk/ September 2012.

National Institute for Health and Clinical Excellence, 2010a. Community-based interventions to reduce substance misuse among vulnerable and disadvantaged children and young people. Online. Available: http://guidance.nice.org.uk/PH4 September 2012.

National Institute for Health and Clinical Excellence, 2010b. Antenatal care: routine care for the healthy pregnant woman. Quick reference guide. Online. Available: www.nice.org.uk/nicemedia/live/11947/40110/40110.pdf September 2012.

NSPCC, 2010. Bullying resources for school and teachers. Online. Available: www.nspcc.org.uk September 2012.

Nursing and Midwifery Council, 2008. The Code: standards for conduct, performance and ethics for nurses and midwives. NMC, London. Online. Available: http://www.nmc-uk.org/Nurses-and-midwives/Standards-and-guidance1/The-code/The-code-in-full/ September 2012.

Nursing and Midwifery Council, 2010. Standards for preregistration nursing education. Online. Available http://standards.nmc-uk.org/PreRegNursing/statutory/Standards/Pages/Standards.aspx September 2012.

Parsons, T., 1991. The social system. Routledge, London.

Pencheon, D., Guest, C., Melzer, D., et al. (Eds.), 2006. Oxford handbook of public health practice, second ed. Oxford University Press, Oxford.

Rogers, C.R., 1951. On becoming a person. Constable, London.

Seedhouse, D., 2001. Health: the foundations for achievement of potential, second ed. Wiley, Chichester.

Tones, K., Tilford, S., 2001. Health promotion: effectiveness, efficiency and equity. Nelson Thornes, Cheltenham.

Townsend, P., Davidson, N., Whitehead, M., 1992. Inequalities in health: the Black Report and the health divide. Penguin, London.

WHO, 1946. Preamble to the constitution. WHO, Geneva.

WHO, 1978. Alma-Ata 1978: primary health care. WHO, Geneva.

WHO, 1984. Health promotion: a discussion on the concept and principles. WHO, Copenhagen.

WHO, 1986. Ottawa charter for health promotion. WHO, Ottawa.

WHO, 1997. The Jakarta declaration on health promotion into the 21st century. Online. Available: http://www.who.int/healthpromotion/conferences/previous/jakarta/declaration/en/index1.html September 2012.

WHO, 1998. Regional health for all targets: Health21 health for all. WHO, Copenhagen.

WHO, 2010. Mental health: Strengthening our response. Online. Available: www.who.int/mediacentre/factsheets/fs220/en September 2012.

Further reading

Helman, C., 2007. Culture, health and illness, fifth ed. Hodder Arnold, London.

Naidoo, J., Wills, J., 2009. Foundations for health promotion, third ed. Baillière Tindall, Edinburgh.

Naidoo, J., Wills, J., 2004. Public health and health promotion: developing practice. Baillière Tindall, London.

Evolution of contemporary nursing

2

Elaine Ball

LEARNING OUTCOMES

This chapter will help you:

- Appreciate how nursing has evolved since the 1700s
- Explore contemporary nursing and how it is influenced by society
- Outline the different approaches to organizing nursing care
- Describe how to become a nurse in the twenty-first century, showing insight into the four fields of nursing practice
- Develop an awareness of the diverse roles undertaken by nurses in different settings.

Introduction

Nursing has always developed in response to the changing needs of society. As the structure of society alters, new nursing habits, customs, values and knowledge emerge in response to changes in the population and its health issues. Because of the influence of history and its corresponding knowledge-base on nursing, the evolution of contemporary nursing will be considered using a chronological approach from the 1700s to the present day and this chapter will demonstrate how nursing, which does not exist in isolation, has been influenced by society and the sociopolitical agenda of the day. The chapter explores how contemporary nursing and nursing roles have developed in response to the challenges facing healthcare delivery and what it means to become or be a twenty-first century nurse. Approaches to nursing practice are considered along with some key nursing roles in different settings. It is hoped that this chapter will provide a useful introduction for those embarking or enrolled on a pre-registration nursing programme.

Evolution of nursing

To most of us, the term 'evolution' suggests something that changes over time and this is not always easy to map out. This section outlines how early practices provided impetus for subsequent developments. Nursing activities such as understanding, empathy, sensitivity and advocacy, to name but a few, remain steadfast aims in nursing practice. Nursing as a discipline is not defined easily by the many examples located in history, instead it draws its fuller meaning from the women and men who seek to preserve nursing activities in everyday practice such as a caring look, gently holding someone's hand or providing a listening ear.

There is no exact time or place when nursing began. There is, however, a period in history to which we can attribute defining texts that convey the principles of nursing. This section outlines nursing at different periods since the 1700s and some of the main events and contexts that influenced these changes are explored. Florence Nightingale, Mary Seacole and Ethel Fenwick are women who wrote about nursing, and respectively set protocols, policy and shaped nurse registration. Nursing is a responsive ever-evolving profession demanding from those who work within it an ability to translate its developments against the backdrop of historical and political changes. The influence of both World Wars (1914–1918 and 1939–1945), the inception and development of the NHS and the more recent developments in professional regulation and education, are considered together with changes to specialist nursing such as the care of children and people with mental health problems.

Nursing in the eighteenth and nineteenth centuries

In the 1700s, in times of accident or sickness, hospitals, as we know them today, did not exist and being cared for in one's own home was the norm, with lay people largely performing nursing roles in the community. 'Nursing' was also associated with maternity care and the term could be extended to female neighbours who wet-nursed or delivered babies in the local community.

The influence of Florence Nightingale

Florence Nightingale was born in Florence, Italy, in 1820 of wealthy, middle-class parents. After several attempts to receive formalized training in 1850 and 1851, she spent brief periods in Germany at a Protestant institution that trained deaconesses in childcare and nursing. Soon afterwards, Florence Nightingale became Superintendent of Nurses at the Institution for the Care of Sick Gentlewomen in Distressed Circumstances in London. For this she received no pay but was able to display her skills in nursing and nursing administration, which included greatly improved standards of nurses and nursing care, and also the expectation that care should be based on compassion, observation and knowledge. One of her legacies, was the 'Nightingale ward', a ward layout where long rooms have beds spaced out on each side, which can still be found in some areas today. While working in the military hospital during the Crimean War, she established hygienic care and reduced overcrowding; and consequently, reduced the mortality rate of wounded soldiers. In addition, her caring attitude towards the wounded soldiers led to her becoming known as the 'Lady with the Lamp'.

Because Florence Nightingale wrote about nursing, collating information about how nurses worked and recording the nursing activities that produced positive outcomes, an evidence-based structure and philosophy of nursing was established. By observing and testing its rudimentary practices, nursing could become more evidence-based. Florence Nightingale recorded nursing practices and produced statistical outcomes, now known as 'model forms'. As a result of this revolutionary way of working and her model forms – that we would identify today as pie-charts – many now regard her as the first research nurse. Although Nightingale found she was a heroine, she never enjoyed her fame and disliked the sentimental reference that her name inspired. The only testimonial she would accept was a fund, heavily subscribed to by the public and named in her honour, which she used to found training schools for nurses.

The success of the Nightingale reforms led to the rapid expansion of nurse training schools, initially in London voluntary hospitals. This led to the growth of larger provincial voluntary hospitals, and finally to new hospitals being built by local government and poor law authorities (McDonald 2011). Despite this, there was still a lack of hospitals, which led to a need for nursing people at home and Nightingale worked closely with William Rathbone to establish training for district nurses. District nursing started as a voluntary service, run by voluntary committees, until the value of the service was recognized and local authorities gradually began to accept more responsibility for sick people in the community. Professional regulation marginalized those who had previously practiced in often maverick and ungoverned ways, e.g. in the delivery of babies or attempting to cure mental distress through quackery, deception and even rudimentary surgery.

As a result of her work, Nightingale was able to define the role of nursing clearly and how nursing was distinct from, and not subservient to, medicine (Box 2.1). This led to the establishment of nursing as a profession with a sound and specific education base.

 Reflective practice   **Box 2.1**

Florence Nightingale's values

Nursing is a calling

- Religious beliefs in the existence of 'natural laws' could be discovered and used to help people improve their health and existence
- Nursing was all-consuming in terms of time commitment, i.e. more than an occupation
- Nursing work was so important that it should be thought of as a religious vow.

Nursing is an art and a science

- The science of nursing needs formal education
- The art of nursing gave freedom to act, to be creative, proactive and function as an advocate for the patient.

Mankind can achieve perfection

- People can control the outcomes of their lives
- People can pursue perfection by understanding 'nature's laws'. This understanding would enable people to readily use these laws to benefit their existence, so pursuing perfect health
- The role of the nurse was to provide the optimum environment in which perfect health could be achieved.

Nursing requires a specific education

- Education for nurses was revolutionary in the nineteenth century
- The Nightingale approach required a blend of theoretical and clinical experience.

Nursing is distinct and separate from medicine

- Although physician and nurse deal with the same client population, nursing is aimed at discovering the 'natural laws' that will assist in putting the patient in the best possible condition so that nature can affect a cure.

Student activity

- Reflect on the values above and consider the extent to which they influence nursing today.

Mary Seacole

Mary Seacole was another nurse and healer who contributed to the welfare of allied soldiers in the Crimean War. She was of mixed Scottish and Jamaican descent. Although experienced in the treatment of fevers and wound care, the authorities in England rejected her, so working alone she visited battlefields, dispensing comfort and provisions to the wounded. In 1856, she returned bankrupt to England and published a book about her travels, which was one of the few published writings of any black woman before the twentieth century. She was helped financially through funds raised by the soldiers she had nursed and finally received a pension from Queen Victoria. Until the centenary of her death in 1981, Mary Seacole had been forgotten but renewed interest in her achievements resulted in a nursing award being named after her. In 2003, a campaign was launched for a permanent memorial in London and in 2004, in an online poll, she was voted the greatest black Briton.

Health visiting

The first home health visiting began in the mid-1850s as a public health service which focused on problems of sanitation and epidemics; nurses, sanitary engineers or lay visitors were sent into the homes of families with young children to offer advice about health and hygiene (Peckover 2011). At the same time, a 'Sanitary Association' was formed to teach the 'laws of health', followed 10 years later by the 'Ladies Sanitary Association' enabling respectable women, known as 'Health Missioners', to teach health to mothers. From the voluntary work of these health missioners, health visitors (HVs) emerged and the importance of their role in lowering the infant mortality rate ensured that their work became recognized and was brought under the direction of the Medical Officer of Health. The work of early HVs was educative and persuasive; they visited as counsellors to the whole family rather than either inspectors or nurses. The first health visiting course was established in 1892, around the same time as the first social work courses in the United States.

Development of nursing specialties

Specialist nursing services such as children's nursing and mental health nursing have their origins in the 1800s.

Children's nursing

Early accounts of paediatric home visiting started during the mid-1800s (Glasper & Mitchell 2010). Charitable dispensaries were established as the most appropriate means of treating sick children and there was strong opposition to admission of children to hospital (Glasper & Mitchell 2010). Other fears arose because children were often malnourished and susceptible to infection and hospitals were widely viewed as a major source of infection (Jolley 2009). However, in recognition of need for specialist services for sick children, Dr Charles West founded the Hospital for Sick Children in Great Ormond Street, London, in 1852. This was followed by the Edinburgh Sick Children's Hospital in 1860. The aims of the Great Ormond Street Hospital were to teach women the specialist skill of children's nursing and to provide advice for mothers. By 1888, society recognized that sick children required specialized nursing and sick children's nurses required specialist training. A 2-year training programme was introduced almost 10 years before the start of training for adult nurses.

Mental health nursing

During the 1800s, there was also a change in attitude towards the mentally ill. At that time, people with mental distress were labelled as 'insane' and commonly marginalized. Those who could afford treatment were cared for in institutions known as asylums, while many of those who could not were sent to prison.

In the early nineteenth century, there was a desire to tackle poverty, sickness and ignorance; and general acceptance of a common ethical principle, namely, that society had a responsibility for those considered frail or of poor means. It was also recognized that mental health nursing (then known as asylum nursing) should be a skilled profession, needing intellectual and personal skills rather than just strong nerves and powerful muscles.

William Browne, Medical Superintendent at the Royal Edinburgh Asylum in 1838, recognized that the people who were closest to the patients, who spent most of their time with them and who managed them when they became distressed, were untrained attendants (Simmons & Vostanis 2009). In attempting to improve this situation, Browne started a course of lectures, which was a landmark in the history of mental health nursing. The first manual for attendants, working in Mental Hospitals, *The Handbook for the Instruction of the Attendants of the Insane*, was published in 1885. This 'Red Handbook' became the content of training, run by the Medico-psychological Association in the late 1880s, for attendants working with the mentally ill. It included basic anatomy and physiology, principles of general nursing, the mind and its disorders, care of the insane and general duties of the attendant (nurse).

The beginning of education and regulation

By the 1880s, nursing leaders were beginning to question whether nurses should be required to pass a public examination before entry to a register, as medical practitioners had been required to do since 1858. Opposition came from a number of quarters, perhaps most significantly from Florence Nightingale who thought that a central examination might undermine her philosophy of nursing. The matron of the London Hospital was also against registration but the matron at St Bartholomew's Hospital in London, Ethel Gordon Manson, was convinced of the need to raise standards and gain professional status for nursing. In 1887, she married Dr Bedford Fenwick who was active in medical politics and shared his wife's aspirations concerning the registration of nurses. In 1893, Ethel Fenwick took over the publication of the *Nursing Record* and then used this to underpin her campaign for registration. In 1903, the journal title changed to the *British Journal of Nursing* with Fenwick remaining as editor, a position she occupied for nearly 50 years. In 1887, she founded the Royal British Nursing Association (RBNA).

The success of these reforms led to a rapid increase in the number of training schools. Advances in medical science demanded a more conscientious type of nurse. Middle-class women viewed nursing as a worthy career and, at that time, the only real alternatives were teaching or the newly developing civil service.

Nursing in the twentieth century

The Society for the State Registration of Nurses was formed in 1902, with Fenwick as Secretary and Treasurer. She then became President of the National Council of Trained Nurses of Great Britain and Ireland, which was established in 1904. In the same year, the Midwives Act required that all practicing midwives undertook training and registered with the Central Midwives Board.

The Central Committee for the State Registration of Nurses was formed in 1909, with Fenwick as joint honorary secretary. Between 1910 and 1914, the Central Committee introduced annual parliamentary bills on nurse registration but these were blocked. The impact of the First World War (1914–1918) led to unqualified female volunteers, the 'Voluntary Aid Detachment', being sent to assist nurses, which threatened to dilute nursing and led to the establishment of an organization for trained nurses.

In 1916, the College of Nursing (which later became the Royal College of Nursing) was established, and in 1917, there were inconclusive discussions about a merger between the RBNA and the College. The principal objectives of the College sought to:

- Promote better education and training of nurses
- Advance nursing as a profession
- Encourage uniformity of the nursing curriculum.

Other objectives included recognizing approved nursing schools from where a register of persons to whom certificates of training or proficiency could be granted. By promoting a Bill of Parliament in connection with the interests of the nursing profession, education, recognition, and protection of the organization by the State could be made more secure. Shortly afterwards, state lobbying was rewarded when the Nurses Bill received royal assent in 1919.

The General Nursing Council (GNC), chaired by Fenwick, was established in 1920, and sought registration for its practitioners in the way that medical colleagues had done some 60 years earlier, with a syllabus for instruction and examination. The GNC register of qualified nurses included supplementary parts for:

- Male nurses
- Nurses trained in the care of people suffering from mental disease
- Nurses trained in the nursing of sick children.

Later, the register was extended to include parts for nurses trained in the care of people with infectious disease and in the care of 'mental defectives' (people with learning disabilities).

In 1921, the GNC set up a Disciplinary and Penal Committee, which had the power to deal with state registered nurses (SRNs) who were not 'fit and proper persons'. The GNC was able to prosecute those purporting to be registered nurses (RNs) who were not and also to remove from the register those nurses who put patient safety at risk or brought the profession into disrepute. Although standards for competence were tested by examination, the most crucial characteristics of professional status were personal behaviours including obedience, tidiness and unquestioning loyalty. The profession had given much of its control of entry qualifications, and requirements for basic training, to the government who were also responsible for staffing hospitals as cheaply as possible. Although the GNC tried to overcome this tension, statutory control was greatly reduced (Nursing and Midwifery Council, NMC 2010a).

Following the evaluation and refinement of adult and children's nursing, a review of mental health nursing commenced shortly afterwards in 1924. Given the lack of legislation and inadequate working environment in this field, it was recommended that:

- Work would be more attractive if hours were reduced; holiday entitlement and salaries were raised 10% above those of general nurses, plus increased increments for male nurses
- Nurses' accommodation and recreational facilities would be improved
- Mental health nurses would be trained alongside general nurses
- General nurse tutors would be appointed to mental hospitals to raise their standards of general nursing care.

Due to statutory control and prevailing economic conditions at the time, few of these recommendations were realized. Yet, general nursing became increasingly an aspirational career. For women, advantages included the ability to lead an independent life in respectable company, with a recognized education that involved training and the exercise of intelligence. Working class women also flocked into nursing as they could earn more, do less menial work than in domestic service, and move up the social ladder.

The British College of Nurses (BCN) was founded and presided over by Ethel Fenwick in 1926. In 1927, the College of Nursing applied for its Royal Charter. The application, which was opposed by the RBNA, was granted in 1928 and it was renamed the Royal College of Nursing (RCN) in 1939. The RCN remained closed to male nurses until 1960.

The 1930s

The public image of general nursing continued to be that of 'heroine' but the media also recognized that nurses required education, which included development of both skills and knowledge, to practice effectively. Nurses were depicted as brave, rational, decisive, caring and autonomous. It was an era of romance and adventure where the focus of nursing was loyalty to physicians and patients.

The reality was high unemployment and a lack of alternative careers, which made nursing appealing to women who generally commenced adult and children's training, while men undertook mental health nursing. There remained widespread dissatisfaction in the profession over recruitment, pay and conditions, which led the government to set up a committee chaired by Lord Athlone to consider issues of shortages, wastage and training of nurses. This committee made a number of recommendations to improve staff conditions that would encourage nurses to stay in the profession, these included:

- Increasing hospital staff numbers to relieve nurses of non-nursing duties
- Organizing part of nurse training under general education
- Recognizing the role of the nurse assistant who was to be on an official GNC roll.

The impact of the Second World War

The Second World War (1939–1945) changed the situation from an apparently adequate supply of nurses to one of acute shortage. Nurses from all fields were recruited for the armed forces, which resulted in too few nurses to care for civilians. The Ministry of Health set up an Emergency Nursing Committee to organize a Civil Nursing Reserve to assist employing authorities to meet additional staffing needs occasioned by the war. This supplied upwards of 1800 nurses and unwittingly through this, the Ministry of Health played an important part in the development of nursing by:

- Becoming the direct employer of nurses
- Introducing a second grade of assistant nurse, for whom there was no definition or standard of training
- Introducing a third grade called auxiliaries, who had received no training
- Increasing the burden of supervision for trained nurses
- Introducing part-time working
- Paying higher salaries to nurses in the Reserve than those in civilian posts, leading to a rift between the two.

The consequence of this was that in 1941, the Ministry of Health recommended that all hospitals paid salaries equivalent to those in the reserve. In 1943, the Nurses Act came into force with higher pay scales and improved conditions of service (Box 2.2). At this time, a Division of Nursing was created within the Ministry of Health and the first Chief Nursing Officer for England was appointed.

 Reflective practice Box 2.2

Conditions of service in 1943

Proposal of the Nurses Salaries Committee

- Working fortnight to be reduced to 96 hours
- Continuous night duty should not exceed 3 months for student nurses and 6 months for trained nurses
- All nurses entitled to 28 days' holiday a year, taken as stipulated by the hospital, plus 1 day off per week
- Sick pay according to length of service
- Higher salaries according to number of beds.

Student activities

- Reflect on the changes in conditions of service for nurses since the 1940s.
- Try to talk to someone who qualified as a nurse during the 1940s and find out how they felt about their conditions of service.

By the end of the Second World War, many hospital beds had to be closed due to shortages of nursing staff. Through the need to attract sufficient recruits, entry qualifications and the age of entry were lowered. Nursing was to be irrevocably altered – some of the elements of the historical, political and economic shifts alongside post-war displacement and migration meant that every sector of society would be forever altered, including the health sector.

The influence of the National Health Service (NHS) on nursing

The NHS was established in 1948 with the aim of healthcare being free at the point of delivery (see Ch. 3). Nurses were in favour of the NHS and felt part of the service, with Mary Witting commenting in the *Nursing Times* that a great

principle had been met; giving everyone access to a health service, irrespective of their income. However, from the outset, there was a serious shortage of nurses and many hospitals were critically dependent on student nurses. Significantly, during the planned introduction of the NHS, little consideration had been given to how many nurses would be required to staff the NHS. By 1952, training and admission of male nurses to the main nursing register contributed to significant growth with 245 000 full-time equivalent male nurses. During this period, the *Mental Health Act* (1958) abolished the legal separation of psychiatric hospitals, allowing patients to be admitted to any hospital.

This marked a huge change, as large mental hospitals were generally located in the countryside and operated as self-sufficient communities; even having their own graveyards. There was strict regulation with rather impersonal procedures for patients, tight discipline and a much-feared hierarchy for nurses. This level of exclusion from society was justified, to some extent, as the sophisticated combination of pyschotherapeutic and medical therapies we know today had not yet emerged; making psychiatric treatment indiscriminate with unpredictable outcomes. Nevertheless, there was a sense of common purpose in a community that was virtually self-contained and self-maintaining. Increasingly, mental hospitals developed open-door policies, enabling patients to take weekend leave and enjoy a broader range of activities, including art and industrial therapies such as assembling components to provide rehabilitation which occupied their time with meaningful activities. Accommodation and recreational facilities for staff were improved and more effective and professional partnerships were built up between doctors and nurses.

During the 1950s, attitudes to children in hospital also changed. It was suggested that emotional damage might occur if children were separated from their parents for lengthy periods. The Ministry of Health commissioned *The Platt Report* in 1959, into the welfare of children in hospital. At the same time, it was recognized that nurses needed better communication skills and the ability to give patients information prior to admission. There needed to be better signposting within hospitals and other care settings, flexible visiting times and easier access for families to speak to doctors and/or nurses.

In addition, attitudes to people with disabilities, older adults and those with rehabilitation needs also underwent transformation with increased provision and availability of resources such as mobility aids and appliances.

Alongside the growth of technology during the late 1950s, nurses were expected to extend their role to incorporate the impact of this new technical knowledge. However, nursing care was still based on a patient's medical diagnosis rather than on their individual needs. Nursing actions were organized using task allocation (see p. 44) that focussed on familiar ward routines and conformity. This led to patients being depersonalized; they were often categorized according to bed numbers in the ward and their disease. This approach to practice reflected the traditional medical model of care (see Ch. 1).

Emergence of humanism

The values of humanism emerged, from the work of Abraham Maslow and others, during the 1950s and included:

- Valuing humanness and the uniqueness of humans as individuals
- Understanding the meaning and purpose of people's lives from their perspective
- Giving freedom to individuals to make decisions for themselves
- Taking people's physical, psychological, spiritual, emotional and social needs into account.

Since then, these values have been adopted to form the basis of holistic and person-centred care which has increasingly underpinned approaches to healthcare practice and education.

The influence of nursing theory

The 1960s saw the introduction of the first nursing degree by the University of Edinburgh, while the United States established the first nurse practitioner role; both developments signalled the way forward for nurses working more interprofessionally and collegiately with other health and social care practitioners. The changes in practice enabled nurses to accept direct responsibility and accountability for their actions and their consequences, and to understand the decision-making processes that led to those actions.

An influential quote from Henderson (1961, p 42) at that time, stated that:

> The unique function of the nurse is to assist the individual, sick or well, in the performance of those activities contributing to health or its recovery (or to a peaceful death) that he would perform unaided if he had the necessary strength, will or knowledge, and to do this in such a way to help him gain independence as rapidly as possible. This aspect of her work, this part of her function, she initiates and controls; of this she is master.

Nursing was traditionally validated by a set of conceptual terms; indeed dictionary definitions for 'nurse' include 'nurture', 'foster', 'tend' and 'cherish', whereas in today's arena, nursing is validated as much by theory as those early propositions. The levels of abstraction, such as 'assisting the individual' as Henderson describes, has been replaced by an evidence base. The earlier periods of nursing are known for their emphasis on individual moral and principled behaviour, and the importance of rank; the use of non-inclusive language in Henderson's quote is a good example of perceived rank and the positioning of women in nursing.

Since the 1960s, there has been greater focus on developing nursing theory as both a practice and a science. The nursing process (see Ch. 14) emerged bringing a considered and systematic approach to nursing care. At the same time, nurse theorists also began to describe what nursing was about and development of the first nursing models came about. Models are developed to represent and help to mediate abstract ideas either visually or by analogy. So for example, in anatomy and physiology a replica of a healthy heart might show its shape and chambers. In nursing, models are both actual and conceptual. A conceptual model offers a framework from which to guide abstract ideas and thoughts towards evidence-based outcomes. If this is not achieved, then the model would not successfully provide a theoretical process for patient care

based on best evidence. Nursing models are figurative ways of representing theory and practice. They play a central role in signifying collective fields of meaning, bringing points of connection together to see how things work in the bigger picture, especially when the nurse needs to communicate with other health professionals about the care of the patient. For example, a clinical model can outline, through a flowchart, the points of nursing intervention and at what juncture involvement or a rapid response is needed, e.g. early warning scores (EWS, see Ch. 14). This is especially helpful for a student's initial learning that takes place before they become proficient. In this sense, models aim to support the student and facilitator through the processes of learning. Most nursing models are based on beliefs about the following factors:

- *The person* – the individual receiving care
- *Health* – where the patient lies on the health and wellness continuum (see Ch. 1)
- *The care environment* – setting for patient/client/ practitioner interaction
- *Nursing* – the roles of nurses and the knowledge and skills they need to carry out their roles.

There are many models, each reflecting the diverse range and perspectives of nursing roles and care settings (Box 2.3). The nursing process and nursing models are explored in detail in Chapter 14.

Examples of models used in different care settings	Box 2.3
Adult nursing	
• Biomedical	Medical model a traditional form of care planning (see Ch. 1)
• Adaptation	Roy and Andrews (1999) (see Ch. 14)
• Activities of living	Roper, Logan and Tierney (2000) (see Ch. 14)
• Self-care	Orem (1991) (see Ch. 14)
Mental health nursing	
• Developmental	Peplau (1952)
• Tidal model	Barker (1996) (see Ch. 14)
• Recovery Model	Thornton and Lucas (2011)
Learning disability nursing	
• The social model of disability	Grant Carson (2009) Online. Available: http://www.ukdpc.net/site/images/library/Social%20Model%20of%20Disability2.pdf October 2012 Sanderson (2007) (see Ch. 14)
Children's nursing	
• Child as client with family partnership and negotiation	Casey's partnership model (2007) (see Ch. 14)
• Child and family partnership	The Nottingham model (Smith et al 2002) (see Ch. 14)

As nurse education evolved, there has been a move away from traditional didactic (teacher-led) models of teaching to more participative and student-centred learning methods (see Ch. 4). There has been a shift from the traditional apprenticeship training, to university courses that highlight the necessity of critical thinking, giving nurses greater opportunity to reflect and analyse nursing propositions as they evolve. This forms the basis of nursing research.

The early influence of nursing research

In the early 1970s, the Briggs Report (Department of Health and Social Security 1972) set the expectation that nursing courses would incorporate research methods and that their findings would be used in nursing practice. The first nursing research was undertaken around that time. As a profession, nursing has been strengthened and rewarded for its research and evidence-based endeavour and enjoys the research, leadership and scholarly reputation that a collective and discipline-based organization deserves (Northouse 2011). This being so, roles are evolving to include greater responsibilities including prescribing, referring patients to other healthcare professionals and delivery of community services (Department of Health, DH 2009a). The implications for future generations of nurses are, however, obvious and considerable; namely that the more responsibility nurses have, the more robust their knowledge needs to be. Therefore, the profession will be increasingly required to draw upon evidence-based practice as the currency to its future identity if its evolution and developments are to be accredited to nursing.

The late twentieth century

Towards the end of the century, the drive towards evidence-based practice continued, enabled in part by the introduction of university pre-registration qualifications for nurses. Another important development was the introduction of the first code of professional conduct in the 1980s. These are discussed further below.

Code of professional conduct

The United Kingdom Central Council (UKCC) developed the first code of conduct for nurses, midwives and HVs in 1984, which set out for the first time key expectations for professional practice and accountability. Its purpose was to protect the public through providing standards, to inform the public of the standard of professional conduct they could expect, to ensure accountability and to make it clear that RNs, midwives and HVs have a duty of care to their patients and clients. This has been refined and is currently published by the NMC as *The Code: Standards of Conduct, Performance and Ethics for Nurses and Midwives* (NMC 2008a) and is explored in depth in Chapter 7.

University education for student nurses

In the 1980s, it was recognized that, as a result of changing disease patterns and social contexts, and the introduction of reforming modes of care delivery, there would be new healthcare needs that required a different kind of RN. In order to meet this need, a different approach to the education of nurses, commonly known as *Project 2000* (UKCC 1985), was introduced in the late 1990s. The main changes were:

- A common foundation programme for all nursing students before pursuing one of four branch programmes

- Explicit practice-based competencies to be achieved
- The award of a university diploma qualification to all newly registered nurses.

In addition, new parts of the professional register were created for diplomates in each field of practice and supernumerary status for learners was introduced so that student nurses were no longer part of the nursing workforce (Box 2.4). This was made possible, in part, by creating an alternative workforce of healthcare assistants (HCAs). Current nursing courses are discussed on page 50.

? Critical thinking   Box 2.4

Nursing skill mix before the 1990s

Before the 1990s, a typical ward might have had the following staff to cover day-shifts:

- A senior and a junior sister/charge nurse
- Two or three qualified nurses, including enrolled nurses
- Between 6 and 10 student nurses, some from each year of training
- Two or three auxiliary nurses.

Student activities

- Consider the practical issues involved in providing nursing care to patients/clients during the transition from 'learners as workers' to supernumerary students.
- Ask people who were qualified nurses around that time and those who were training as nurses in the old and new systems, about their experiences.
- Discuss your thoughts with your mentor or a peer.

Moving towards evidence-based practice

The development of education and regulation for nurses and midwives failed to bring nursing the autonomy anticipated by early nursing leaders. Over the last two decades, there has been a shift from 'the practitioner knows best' to the belief that one can never take one's own practice for granted. Questioning of nursing practice was encouraged, which saw a move away from nursing actions being based on traditions or rituals and an increasing focus on holistic and evidence-based care. However, nursing had still only developed a limited body of knowledge that could be defined as nursing and which was exclusive of other disciplines. Consequently, the purpose of nursing research is to establish a body of nursing knowledge, which in turn increases the professional status of nursing (see Box 2.5 and Ch. 5).

** Evidence-based practice   Box 2.5**

Professional status: a body of specialist knowledge

Select an area of care that is relevant to your practice.

Student activities

- Identify some evidence that supports the existence of specialist nursing knowledge in your chosen field of practice.
- Discuss the benefit of specialist nursing knowledge to the patients/clients in your placement area, with your mentor.

The attributes of a profession include:

- Having its own body of specialist knowledge
- Having a role in society that is valued
- Employing some means of internal regulation.

There was the expectation that nurses should carry out best practice that was in the interest of their patients and that they would be accountable for their actions. The systematic nursing process gradually evolved into evidence-based decision-making, a process of turning clinical problems into questions and then systematically locating, appraising and using current research findings as the basis for clinical decisions (Box 2.6). By using a structured problem-based approach, practitioners can logically apply the best available evidence to their care, i.e. evidence-based practice (see Ch. 5).

Table 2.1 summarizes the major events influencing the evolution of nursing discussed in this section.

 Evidence-based practice Box 2.6

Nil by mouth

Jenny is a 3rd year student who has just started a new placement on a surgical ward. She has not been in a ward environment for a while, as her last two placements were in theatre and the community. One morning she observes a senior nurse giving a preoperative patient an early morning breakfast. Jenny remembers from an earlier placement witnessing and practising the nil-by-mouth routine on patients having similar surgical procedures.

Student activities

- What is the first course of action Jenny should take?
- What is the mentor's role in this situation?
- What would you do when the same practice appears to be different in different clinical settings?
- Discuss the role of evidence-based practice with your mentor.

Table 2.1 Major events in the evolution of nursing

Date	Context	Influences on nursing practice
1700	Inoculation had been practised in Asia for decades before it became established in Europe. With the outbreak of smallpox in the seventeenth century, inoculation emerged from the discovery that those who became infected and survived became immune to this highly infectious and often fatal disease. Inoculation was first used to protect against smallpox	Nursing has a long association with inoculation and vaccination for the prevention and treatment of disease in both children and adults
1800	Foundation of the Royal College of Surgeons led to a closer relationship between medical education and hospitals	Governors appointed matrons responsible for household affairs, supervision of nurses and other hospital servants. Ordinary nurses were of low status, received some money and a beer allowance, endured appalling working conditions and had little or no education
1834	Poor Law Amendment Act	Workhouses with intolerable conditions for poor, sick and needy people. Sick people nursed by elderly pauper women
1854–1856	Crimean War	Florence Nightingale introduced measures such as sanitary principles, which contributed to a reduction in the mortality rates of wounded soldiers. Mary Seacole visited battlefields, dispensing comfort and provisions to the wounded
1856	Florence Nightingale described as the first research nurse	Using statistics she collected during the Crimean War, she illustrated the need for sanitary reforms in all military hospitals
1858	Improvement of standards	Doctors who passed a public examination were entered on a register. By 1880, nurse leaders were suggesting that nurses should be required to do the same
1860	Florence Nightingale founded the first nursing training school. Attitudes towards the poor changed, poverty implied sickness	The Nightingale Training School and Home for Nurses based at St Thomas' Hospital in London. Poor Law Hospitals and 'probationer' nurses
1914–1918	First World War	Unqualified young women known as Voluntary Aid Detachment (VAD) assisted nurses
1919	Nurses Act	Registration of UK nurses

Table 2.1 Major events in the evolution of nursing—cont'd

Date	Context	Influences on nursing practice
1920	General Nursing Council was established	Prescribed duties and responsibilities for training, examination and registration of nurses and the approval of training schools for the purpose of maintaining a register of nurses for England and Wales, for Scotland and for Ireland
1939–1945	Second World War	Nurses joining military services led to recruitment problems at home. Dissatisfaction over nurses' pay and conditions
1943	Recruitment of nurses remained a problem	Introduction of nursing assistants, later to become enrolled nurses (second level nurses)
1960	More policy decisions for nurses	Salmon Report – formal nursing management structure but no clinical career structure
1979	Nurses, Midwives and Health Visitors Act	Review of registration and education of nurses, midwives and health visitors. United Kingdom Central Council for Nursing, Midwifery and Health Visiting (UKCC) established
1983	Griffiths report	Introduction of general management culture – NHS to be run as a business
1986	Project 2000	Higher education qualifications for nurses, supernumerary status for nursing students
1989	Review of pay scales	Clinical grading structure for nurses introduced
1990	Working for patients; purchaser/provider	Financial performance prominent in healthcare
1997–1999	Nursing programmes to include a 50/50 balance of theory and practice. UK Health Policies	Widening access to nursing education, common foundation programme followed by branch programmes. Expansion of the nursing workforce. Strengthening of nursing leadership. Clinical governance – corporate accountability for the quality of care. Growth in nursing informatics and increased computerization of patient records
2000	The NHS plan (DH 2000)	Healthcare reforms which would lead to extra beds, more hospitals, modernized GP surgeries, more nurses, greater IT support, better food and cleaner wards
2002	UKCC becomes Nursing and Midwifery Council (NMC)	The principal functions of the Council were to protect the public through establishing standards of education, training, conduct and performance for nurses and midwives and to ensure the maintenance of those standards
2004	Agenda for change (DH 2004)	Modernized NHS pay system with the introduction of clinical grading and new pay bandings, job evaluation scheme and knowledge and skills framework (KSF)
2005	Reduction in junior doctors' hours; review of nurses' roles	Nurses increasingly undertaking advanced roles
2006	Reorganization of NHS structures. Some NHS trusts report financial overspends	DH publications *Modernising Nursing Careers* (DH 2006a) and *Towards a Strategy for Research and Development* (DH 2006b) saw a structured and more considered approach to the proliferation of nursing roles
2011–2013		Introduction of all graduate nursing education

Approaches to nursing practice

This section outlines holistic care and patient centredness and then explains the four main approaches to organizing nursing care.

Holistic care

Caring that involves looking after the 'whole person' is truly holistic and healing, and based on the principles of humanism (see above). Holistic care recognizes the uniqueness of each human being, their individuality, personality and human frailty (Watson & Nelson 2011). It can be argued that every nurse knows that the subtle process of caring has physical, psychological, social and spiritual dimensions but that this is often hard to express in words. It involves the integration and coordination of interpersonal, technical and professional skills that results in a complex network of interactions that contribute to successful nurse–patient relationships. Such relationships promote dignity and give the patient confidence in the nurse's ability to listen and help them (Baughan & Smith 2008). Holistic care (see also Ch. 1) therefore requires nurses to think beyond the concept of cure, which is based on scientific facts and technical competence and think more towards person-centred care.

Person-centred care

The promotion of person-centred care in the UK is consistent with the policy direction of person-centredness internationally; the principles of which are concerned with the rights of people to have their values and beliefs as individuals respected, i.e. their personhood (McCormack & McCance 2010). It is said that it is these values that give people their uniqueness and authenticity (Box 2.7). Maintaining person-centredness is central to decision-making and all healthcare practice.

The principles of person-centredness can be applied across health and social care settings and all fields of nursing practice. Everyone experiencing healthcare is on a journey, or pathway of care, that involves new situations, so uncertainty is to be expected. Uncertainty can be challenging but it also provides opportunities for learning and solutions, resolutions and outcomes that, with the appropriate support, can be uniquely created and tailored to meet individual needs.

Involving users and carers

The patient/client/carer (or consumer) is the most important person in the healthcare system. Nurses have an important role in ensuring continuity and maintaining consumer autonomy (the ethical principle that individuals should make their own decisions about their lives) within the maze of the healthcare system, which can be challenging. This may include helping the consumer to:

- Understand what the treatment options are, the benefits and disadvantages of each
- Know who will carry out treatment
- Ensure their rights and views regarding choice are respected.

This helps to reduce feelings of anxiety and isolation. Patient/client/carer involvement has become the norm in contemporary nursing practice as it promotes person-centred decision-making and partnership working, ensuring that services provided meet the service user's specific needs. This approach considers service users as experts in their own lives and promotes patient's/client's rights to be involved in discussions and decisions about their health and the care services they access (DH 2010). People's perceptions of what constitutes quality care are formed by their encounters with an existing care structure and a patient's or carer's experience in the NHS and wider community. This is measured yearly, providing care settings a score for their overall patient experience (DH 2011a).

Contemporary health and social care provision encourages bridging the hospital/community divide through the delivery of more flexible and seamless services, including intermediate care, that is built round patient's care pathways rather than health and social care institutions.

Person-centredness	Box 2.7

Person-centredness involves respecting the rights of each person to make rational decisions, to determine their own goals and to enable them to reach their own decisions. This involves:

- Providing and sharing information
- Recognizing other people's values as being of paramount importance
- Making explicit the aims of nursing actions
- Involving patients/clients in planning and negotiating their care
- Responding to cues that maximize coping resources through the recognition of important things in peoples' daily lives
- Offering personal support and practical expertise, while enabling the person to follow a path of their own choosing in their own way. This may also require the person to be informed about any harmful consequences of their own choices.

(Adapted from McCormack and McCance 2010.)

Effective teamwork

Teamwork is about working together and requires cooperation and understanding to build effective relationships (see Ch. 9). The readiness to develop a collaborative approach is recognized by a group's capacity to experience and manage competition, conflict, risk and stress, and their willingness to achieve a common goal (Northouse 2011). Team members must be aware that their behaviour not only affects others but also the overall performance of the team. The aim should be to adopt the helpful roles outlined in Table 2.2. Moving towards the helpful behaviours involves self-awareness and enhances team working (see Ch. 9).

However, effectiveness is not down to individuals alone. An effective team requires skillful coordination (O'Keefe et al 2011) which involves:

Table 2.2 Helpful and hindering roles in team working

Helpful roles	Hindering roles
Establishing:	**Aggression:**
Helping to start the group along new paths by proposing tasks and goals, defining problems, helping set rules and contributing ideas by: • Getting started • Clarifying purpose • Defining goals • Maintaining direction	Asserting personal dominance and attempting to get own way regardless of others by: • Criticizing • Attacking personality • Dominating • Name-calling
Persuading:	**Manipulation:**
Requesting facts and relevant information on the problem. Seeking out expressions of feelings and values by: • Questioning • Encouraging and guiding responses, advocating • Developing alternatives	Responding to a problem rigidly and using stereotypical responses by: • Topic jumping • Masking statements as questions • Selective interpretation • Gate-keeping
Committing:	**Dependence:**
Helping to ensure that all members are part of the decision-making process by: • Facilitating involvement • Summarizing • Gaining commitment • Problem-solving	Reacting to other people as authority figures, abdicating problem-solving to others, expecting others to lead the solution by: • Agreeing with everything • Avoiding decisions or closure through sarcasm • Seeking sympathy • Expressing futility, resignation or helplessness
Attending:	**Avoidance:**
Demonstrating a willingness to become involved by: • Listening • Showing an interest • Monitoring and observing • Taking notes or recording • Sharing responsibilities • Regular attendance at meetings • Exchanging ideas and suggestions	An emotional retreat in thought or actions by: • Withdrawing psychologically • Withdrawing physically • Reflecting boredom • Escaping the group

• Identifying the right person (or team) to lead or coordinate its activities
• Team referrals and decisions, with consensus of opinion being vital
• Commitment to regular team meetings
• Free flow of information between team members
• Coordinated feedback and team evaluation, rather than a series of unrelated specialist assessments, to give people or patients/clients a sense of clarity and unity, leading to more successful uptake of team recommendations
• A flexible system to meet people's or patients'/clients' differing needs or priorities
• A team commitment to student support to enable engagement in ways that allows students to contribute and learn effectively.

Carrying out the activities in Box 2.8 will help you to understand the characteristics of effective teamwork.

 Reflective practice   **Box 2.8**

Effective teamwork

Think about situations where you have observed members of the multidisciplinary team (MDT) working in your placement.

Student activities

• How is team coordination carried out?
• Who are the team members?
• What are the other team members' responsibilities in the delivery of care?
• To what extent do team members adopt helpful or hindering behaviours (see Table 2.2)?
• How do you think these behaviours may impact on patient/client care?
• Discuss your ideas with your mentor.

Nurses as members of a multidisciplinary team

The multidisciplinary approach is increasingly recognized in healthcare as an essential way of working. Nurses are often part of a multidisciplinary team (MDT) that may include doctors, physiotherapists, pharmacists, dietitians and many other health and social care professionals (see Ch. 3). It is important to understand the roles of all the members and how they interlink to provide 'seamless' healthcare (Box 2.9). Inter-professional learning (see Ch. 4) is an NMC requirement in pre-registration nursing programmes that aims to reflect the reality of the MDT approach to healthcare practice in the twenty-first century.

 Critical thinking Box 2.9

Effective multidisciplinary teamwork

Jane is a 52-year-old married woman recently diagnosed with late onset (Type 2) diabetes. She is overweight with a high body mass index (see Ch. 19). Following a routine appointment to the optician, concern was raised that her shortsightedness (myopia) might be due to diabetes, as she was also developing a cataract in her right eye. The optician notified her GP who called her in for simple tests. From a single fasting blood sugar test, her GP confirmed this diagnosis.

Student activities

- Identify the health issues Jane has and who might help to address them.
- What individuals or teams might be involved in Jane's care?

Approaches to organizing nursing care

There are four approaches that have been used and elements of these underpin nursing practice in most healthcare settings today. Effective teamwork is central to them all.

Task allocation

Task allocation has its historical roots in hierarchical, ecclesiastical and military organizations that value obedience and rank. It was the main method of organization when hospitals were established and still persists to some extent in nursing today (Fig. 2.1). Task allocation dictated ward routines which related to the priority of nursing needs until the early 1980s. For example, wards using task allocation had a dressings book in which wounds were numbered to ensure the nurse allocated to carry out dressings (wound care) progressed from patients with clean wounds to those with infected wounds, thereby minimizing the risk of cross-infection. These practices were not wrong but they have since been superceded by evidence-based holistic care in which the whole person is treated. For wounds, management may be led by a specialist tissue viability nurse, where the whole person and not just their wound is carefully considered. These changes came about not only because of increasing emphasis on evidence-based practice but also due to differences in skill mix and staffing levels in clinical areas.

Patient allocation

Patient allocation was introduced in the 1970s, enabling nurses to focus on the care of individual patients/clients (instead of tasks). Nurses were allocated a group of specific patients to care for, with the aim of providing continuity of care.

Team nursing

In 1956, the RCN developed a theory of team nursing. A number of issues prevented this approach being implemented, largely because hierarchy and rank were so ingrained.

However, during the 1980s, team nursing evolved and allowed care to become more individualized. Team nursing can be associated with task and/or patient allocation and each of these approaches can be permanent or transient. Nurses are allocated to a team who provide care to a specific group of patients/clients (Fig. 2.2). The team leader shares responsibility for patient care, communication and coordination with the ward manager. Ideally, the same team cares for the same group

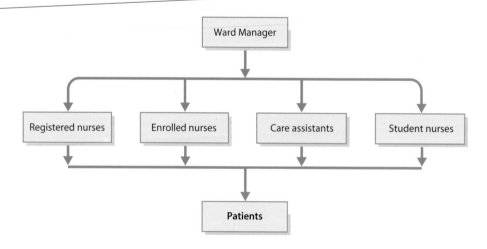

Fig. 2.1 • Channels of communication in task allocation or functional nursing.

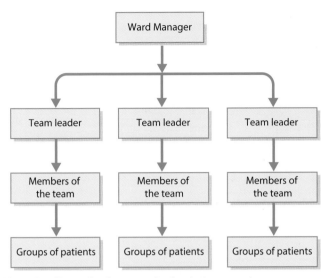

Fig. 2.2 • Channels of communication in team nursing.

of patients for the duration of their stay. This increases continuity of care and provides more meaningful work for nursing teams.

Primary nursing

This approach involves patients/clients being allocated to an individual RN rather than a team of nurses (Fig. 2.3). The focus is on person-centred holistic care, where the participation of patients/clients and relatives is encouraged. The primary nurse has 24-hour responsibility for their group of patients, known as a caseload, throughout their stay. Primary nurses have the knowledge and ability to make decisions, and also the authority to carry them out. In the primary nurse's absence, an associate nurse, another RN or primary nurse carries out the planned care with the involvement of students and HCAs. In settings where primary nursing is practiced, the sister/charge nurse acts as consultant, co-worker, ward manager and in-service educator. In common with other care delivery systems, primary nursing has advantages and disadvantages (Box 2.10).

Care delivery in practice

It has been recognized that when team or primary nursing is used as a method for organizing patient care, less stress is reported by the practitioners involved. Alongside this, there is the belief that patients feel better cared for and their individual needs are met; evidence shows that practice is enhanced, teamwork is more evident and there is greater job satisfaction (Angelini 2011). However, these positives can only be sustained if patient to staff ratio is satisfactory. If not, task allocation returns. An appropriate skill mix is essential, as it ensures effective links between patients' needs and nursing skills.

Figure 2.4 summarizes the key characteristics of the four approaches to organizing care. There is growing evidence that nurses do not work in the four ways described above, but that care settings are organized in more complex ways using attributes from more than one of the different approaches to

Advantages and disadvantages of primary nursing Box 2.10

Advantages

- Patients have the opportunity to develop a therapeutic relationship with one nurse
- Clear documentation by the major caregiver should ensure 24-hour continuity of care
- Primary nurses are accountable for their actions and are encouraged to develop clinical skills, leadership skills and interpersonal skills
- Increased job satisfaction for primary nurses
- Improved communication as relatives and members of the multidisciplinary team (MDT, see p. 44 and Ch. 3) approach the primary nurse to obtain information about patients/clients.

Disadvantages

- Patients may not like their primary nurse
- Nurses may not have the time to develop this relationship
- 24-hour cover is difficult or impossible in many settings
- Requires good education and understanding of the role
- Increased responsibility requires authority and support from the manager
- Can be stressful without adequate support
- Members of the MDT used to a hierarchical system may find it difficult to communicate with primary nurses rather than the charge nurse
- Supervision and normal lines of reporting are different, which – if not agreed – can lead to breakdown in communication.

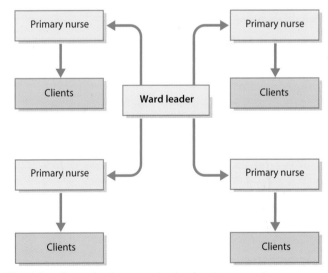

Fig. 2.3 • Channels of communication in primary nursing.

care delivery (Galvin 2010) (Box 2.11). It is interesting to note that patients' perceptions of the quality of care are often dependent on good communication; and that this extends to how good the communication is between the members of the MDT (Doyle et al 2010). Box 2.12 (p. 47) provides an opportunity to consider the importance of clear communication between members of the MDT.

Task orientation	TASK ALLOCATION	PATIENT ALLOCATION	TEAM NURSING	PRIMARY NURSING	Holistic practice
Lack of continuity and fragmentation					24-hour continuity
Professional distance					Premium placed on close nurse–patient relationship
Impersonal routinized care					Individualized care
Shift-by-shift allocation					Fixed allocation from admission to discharge
Centralized responsibility for care invested in charge nurse					Responsibility for care devolved to primary nurse
Hierarchical ward nursing structure					Flat ward nursing structure

Fig. 2.4 • The key characteristics of the four main ways of delivering nursing care.

 Reflective practice Box 2.11

Organization of nursing care

Think back to aspects of care in your last placement.

Student activities

- Which practitioners, including members of the MDT, provided care?
- Were patients/clients/parents involved in decision-making?
- How was care allocated – by tasks or by patients/clients?
- Did patients/clients have the same nurses looking after them every day?
- Did you feel the nurses had time to get to know the patients?
- Who was the coordinator of care?
- What was the role of the charge nurse?
- What was the main system of care delivery used?

Contemporary nursing

This section explores some societal influences on nursing and the roles of nurses in different settings. Characteristics of twenty-first century nursing programmes and nursing in the four fields of practice are outlined.

Nursing today

One feature of nursing today that has not changed over the years is the 24-hour care that is provided; nurses in both hospital and the community function as the MDT linchpin by circulating information across all professional boundaries as required. A main feature of the coordinating role is to maintain the patient's well-being and safety by demonstrating a capacity to observe, listen and think about individual patient's/client's needs in a holistic way. Box 2.13 (p. 47) will help you consider the nurse's role further.

Nurses remain the core of the NHS workforce; they are essential in maintaining continuous patient care and establishing a seamless working relationship across the MDT, with the aim of delivering integrated care. Today's nurses make a significant contribution to patients' treatment and well-being, contributing as members of MDTs. Their roles are often innovative, crossing traditional professional boundaries and also those between hospital and community care. Today's nurses lead in many areas of patient care that may have been traditionally deemed the doctors' role (Box 2.14, p. 47).

Nurse-led clinics and services are just a few examples of the way nurses' roles have developed and offer rewarding career progression and alignment of reputation and status among other allied health professionals (AHPs). Nurses also lead and run clinics in Walk-In Centres that may be entirely nurse-led, where they provide diagnostic services and patient care; many nurses who work in these services are also qualified to prescribe medications. More complex illness or fractures are supported by satellite provision in which patient's reports can be sent remotely to a central diagnostic site managed by senior doctors. Although clinical nurse specialists (CNS) and specialist nurses (SN) hold different titles, they often do equivalent jobs and can be regarded as one group. The CNS and SN may work in

Critical thinking Box 2.12

The importance of good communication

Two new theatre porters have joined the staff at your hospital. They are young, pleasant, good humoured and make the patients chuckle on the way down to theatre. The senior nurse has found that increasingly, they both chat to the staff who accompany the patients to theatre, which means that nurses are not spending this significant time with their patients. Consequently, patients are neither spoken to nor reassured and supported on their way to theatre. Not enough importance is being given to the fact that the patients are being pushed to a potentially life-changing procedure.

Communication is a vital part of nursing care and is outlined in all recent government policy as an essential requisite for best practice. Good and effective communication is a 'tool' that enables structures, people and institutions to develop, evolve and share experiences.

At the monthly staff meeting, the charge nurse takes the opportunity to raise everyone's awareness about the points above, stating that the journey between the ward and the operating theatre is precious time that should be given over entirely to patient communication. Everyone agrees and things do not only return to normal, they are better than before. Staff who had never fully considered the ward-theatre transfer time as an opportunity to be fully spent communicating to their patient start to engage more actively.

Soon afterwards, a new and inexperienced student is asked to escort a patient to theatre and one of the new porters is pushing the bed and begins chatting to the student in his normal friendly manner. Unable to direct the conversation to the patient and deflect the conversation away from him, she tells the porter she is not allowed to talk to him, only to the patient.

At first, the senior nurse thinks it is her imagination when she is ignored by a number of porters, but over the ensuing week, she begins to feel increasingly uncomfortable that some staff are being snubbed by the porters. It now appears that the two new porters are criticized for being pleasant and friendly.

Student activities

- The senior nurse now has a compounded problem, how might he/she go about resolving this?
- Did either the student nurse or senior nurse do anything wrong in the first place?
- Discuss your thoughts about how the situation might be resolved with your mentor.

 Critical thinking Box 2.13

International Council of Nurses (ICN) definition of nursing

Nursing encompasses autonomous and collaborative care of individuals of all ages, families, groups and communities, sick or well and in all settings. Nursing includes the promotion of health, prevention of illness, and the care of ill, disabled and dying people. Advocacy, promotion of a safe environment, research, participation in shaping health policy and in patient and health systems management, and education are also key nursing roles.

Student activities

After reading the ICN Definition of Nursing, look back at Henderson's definition (p. 38) and:

- Compare the two definitions and consider how nursing has changed over the last 40 years.
- Think about your own ideas of what 'nursing' is today.

Resource

International Council of Nurses, 2010. The ICN definition of nursing. Online. Available: www.icn.ch/definition.htm August 2012.

Critical thinking Box 2.14

Identifying nurse-led roles

Nurse-led roles are found in all fields of nursing practice and in both community and hospital settings. Community mental health nurses may provide cognitive behavioural therapy (CBT). In adult nursing, their roles include running clinics for:

- Blood pressure monitoring to identify and manage patients with abnormal blood pressure
- People with long-term conditions
- Medicines adherence
- Smoking cessation using national guidelines
- Promoting healthy lifestyle, e.g. addressing factors such as diet, nutrition and exercise.

Student activities

- List nurse-led clinics and services that might exist in a busy city centre and their benefits to patient well-being and care.
- Identify nurse-led clinics and services that might be found in rural areas and the benefits for patient well-being and care.
- Name and describe two nurse-led services in your area in:
  - The community (primary care)
  - A hospital.
- Discuss the roles of the nurses in these services with your mentor.

similar environments, such as in nurse-led clinics, and undertake almost the same nursing activities. Clinical and nurse specialists (see p. 57) have the added remit of expertise such as those who provide specialist care for patients with congestive cardiac failure under 'home-based' initiatives; nurse-led chest pain clinics, nurse-led delivery of primary mental healthcare and children's cardiac liaison nurses are other examples of these nursing roles. They usually operate and work closely within teams and collaborate with other agencies. However, they also hold a significant degree of autonomy; making referrals and offering specialist advice to patients, carers and other staff.

Influences on nursing today

Nursing will continue to be influenced by factors both inside and outside the profession. The world economy will be one of the most significant factors to shape future healthcare decisions and provision of care. Nursing has become, and will remain, a cost-effective workforce solution to the high cost of doctor's salaries, driving down health service costs while maintaining high quality patient care.

In 1999, the *Fitness to Practice* document introduced greater emphasis on interprofessional partnerships and collaboration; the *Fitness to Practice* white paper looked at trends for the changing disease patterns likely to affect the future health and social care agenda. The influences on nursing today are:

- An ageing population
- New genetic approaches
- New forms of information transfer changing healthcare delivery
- Changing professional roles
- Changing workforce expectations.

On a wider social level, the *Fitness to Practice* document predicted greater information transfer, changing professional roles and expectations. In the 10 years between the publication of the *Fitness to Practice* white paper and *Healthcare Futures 2010*, vast changes have taken place, especially in the area of knowledge transfer and the information available to both patients and healthcare practitioners. Perhaps now, more than at any other time, the need for nurses to document their knowledge and skills is imperative so that they, and other AHPs, can identify the role of the nurse and recognize their contribution to the healthcare arena.

External factors continually influence healthcare and nursing; these include advances in technology, demographic changes, changing patterns of disease, consumerism and increasing recognition of people's rights, e.g. the Human Rights Act 1998 (see Ch. 6).

Technology

Technological advances continue, e.g. in telecommunications and imaging techniques; therefore nurses must be computer literate and be able to embrace new technologies and consequent ways of working. Computerized patient records are increasing and patient data are becoming available via information systems, e.g. laboratory results, prescriptions and integrated care pathways (ICPs, see Ch. 14). ICPs enable members of the MDT to document care against agreed standards to monitor patients' progress.

Consumerism

The users of health services today are more sophisticated, better informed and have high expectations of healthcare. Policy now views patients/clients as consumers whose needs, wishes and expectations will influence the delivery of healthcare.

Diversity and equality

Diversity is about recognizing and valuing human differences for the benefit of patients/clients, carers, staff and the public at large. Diversity goes hand in hand with equity and equality, creating a fairer society in which everyone can participate and has the same opportunity to fulfil their potential. In reality, there is no equity or equality of opportunity if differences cannot be recognized and valued (Aaberge et al 2011).

Human rights

People's rights have become more widely acknowledged since the passing of the Human Rights Act in 1998 (see Ch. 6) and the European Union Social Charter. These have wide-ranging implications for the profession, as they impact on nursing practice and nursing research. Examples include: conscientious objection; age and disability; right to life; patient advocacy; role expansion; healthcare resource allocation; emergency contraception; do-not-attempt-resuscitation (DNAR) orders; rights to privacy and dignity; confidentiality and anonymity; ethics; genetics and informed consent; advance directives (called advance decisions) to refuse treatment in the Mental Capacity Act (2005) and patients'/clients' right to choice (see Chs 6, 7). In practice, diversity should mean that all citizens are treated as equals and can access free healthcare at the point of need. The NHS must challenge discrimination, promote diversity and respect human rights. Given this, it is important to avoid discrimination of individuals, including older adults, drug users, homeless and unemployed people, minority ethnic groups and those with mental health problems who have been recognized as not always receiving equal access to care and treatment in the past (Box 2.15).

(?) Critical thinking — Box 2.15

Avoiding discriminatory practice

Jim has an inner ear condition called Ménière's disease, which causes imbalance, vertigo (dizziness) and noises in his ear (tinnitus). He is a 77-year-old widower who has not looked after himself properly since his wife died a year ago. He fell on the street and was ignored by passers-by who thought that he was under the influence of alcohol and therefore drunk.

When he finally arrived at the emergency department, he was disorientated and dehydrated. Following triage and diagnosis, he arrives on your ward still in a dishevelled state. While chatting to him, Jim tells you that someone called him a vagrant while he was lying on the street.

Student activities

- How do you think Jim felt about being referred to as a vagrant?
- What do you say to Jim when he mentions this?
- Identify community services in your area that may provide support for Jim following his discharge home.

Nursing in different settings

In response to societal influences, new nursing roles have developed in different settings and some of these roles are discussed here. Nurses are increasingly the first point of contact for patients/clients, be it in the community, at home, in hospitals and polyclinics or via NHS direct (England and Wales) or NHS 24 (Scotland).

Community nursing roles

The NHS and Community Care Act (1990) has led to significant changes in the place of care delivery, heralding a move from largely hospital-based provision to care within community settings in which practice nurses work with GPs managing the disease registers and working in prevention of diseases such as measles in children or diabetes in older people (DH 1999). In the ensuing years, the emphasis on community services has further increased as the Government seeks to achieve measurable improvements in community and public health outcomes; creating a shift of resources from hospital-to community-based services (DH 2011c). The modern matron role is central to keeping ill patients at home by using technology.

In addition, nurses are increasingly taking a lead in providing services which often focus on the health of patients/clients and are largely community-based (see Box 2.14, p. 47).

Traditional nursing roles in the community include those of specialist community public health nurses (school health advisors with specialist practice qualifications, HVs and occupational health nurses) and community practitioners such as district nurses, community mental health nurses and community learning disability nurses. Some of these roles are discussed below.

School health advisors

Previously known as school nurses, school health advisors provide an essential link between schools, children's own homes and the community, which helps to safeguard the health and well-being of children and young people. In order to do this, they work with children/young people, parents/carers, teachers and a MDT that includes other health and social care professionals. Their responsibilities include supporting children with complex health needs, organizing immunization and drop-in clinics, assessing the health needs of every 5-year-old and providing health promotion programmes for young people, e.g. on health issues such as safe sex, stress management, discrimination and bullying.

Health visiting

HVs focus on health and social needs, working in collaboration with other healthcare disciplines and other agencies such as the Sure Start initiatives heralded by government initiatives in the late 1990s. Their clients include children and mothers, families, older adults and marginalized groups, including asylum seekers and travelling people.

The HV undertakes health promotion activities to concentrate on the well population from cradle to grave, which may include assessing the health needs of children in the community to provide support and care that will protect and promote health and well-being of other vulnerable groups. HVs work with social workers and others to safeguard children by identifying those who are vulnerable, i.e. whether their safety or welfare is at risk. They also deliver public health programmes that address national and local health priorities such as reducing inequalities, smoking cessation and tackling obesity (see Ch. 1). Other activities include influencing health policy and public health issues. HVs generally have a caseload of clients of one age group, usually children, but some have caseloads of older adults and people with other needs.

Public health nursing

Specialist community public health nurses aim to reduce health inequalities by working with individuals, families and communities to promote health, prevent ill-health and

optimize good health through, e.g. the provision of stress management courses. They also work in secondary prevention (preventative activities that focuses on early diagnosis, use of referral services and rapid initiation of treatment to limit the progress of disease). Public health nurses also undertake culturally sensitive work; e.g. education programmes supporting genetic counselling and the risk management of inherited disease between couples. Such a risk can occur when one or two people carry a gene mutation, increasing the risk of congenital disability in their offspring. Over the last 60 years, services in the UK have grown in response to an increase in the population requiring genetic counselling (Uhlmann et al 2009).

The emphasis is on working in partnership with their clients and other professionals, cutting across disciplinary, professional and organizational boundaries to reach individual and, sometimes culturally sensitive, needs of either individuals or a community. By working at a grass-roots level, the impact of social and political policy to influence the determinants of health (see Ch. 1) can be interpreted positively and implemented effectively to promote the health of whole populations.

Family health nursing

The World Health Organization Europe (Büscher et al 2009), states that greater and more comprehensive workforce planning strategies would provide opportunities to establish and support family-focused community nursing programmes and services, including, where appropriate, the Family Health Nurse (FHN). With initiatives in place, the role of nurses and midwives in public health, health promotion and community development has been enhanced. In little over a decade, Büscher et al (2009) reported considerable improvement in community and FHN provision. The role of the FHN is multifaceted and includes helping individuals, families and communities to cope with illness and to improve their health. The FHN and the family health physician were presented as the key professionals at the hub of a network of primary care services.

District nursing

District nurses (DNs) provide nursing care for people of all ages in a variety of non-hospital settings including patients' homes, GP surgeries and nursing homes. Their work includes health assessments and health promotion, wound management, administering medication and palliative care. Clinics are also provided for people with long-term conditions such as diabetes. DNs often manage a caseload of patients and work with other healthcare professionals in supporting patients and their families and carers.

Hospital nursing

In hospitals, many nurses are expanding their roles to meet demands for increasingly complex care needs, often based on innovative technologies. Many RNs, along with midwives and AHPs, undertake a wide range of clinical activities, including making and receiving referrals, accepting responsibility for admitting and discharging patients, ordering investigations and diagnostic tests, running clinics and prescribing drugs.

Intermediate care

Intermediate care constitutes a range of integrated services that enables people who might previously have been admitted to hospital or community care to remain at home. It helps those with long-term conditions or acute episodes by facilitating a positive transition back into the community following a stay in hospital. Intermediate care provides a range of enabling, rehabilitative and treatment services in community and residential settings. Intermediate care is sometimes required on discharge from an acute hospital for patients who cannot return home immediately as they require some form of rehabilitation. These are often GP beds in a community hospital. Increasingly, nurses work across hospital and community settings, an example being the clinical nurse specialist role (see p. 57).

Becoming a nurse in the twenty-first century

The education of nurses has been influenced by many factors, not least public expectation and scrutiny of what has gone before. Major changes involve the educational outcomes at the point of registration. This section discusses a number of issues including pre-registration nursing programmes, the NMC competencies, the four fields of nursing practice in which nurses may register and the role of the HCA and National Vocational Qualifications (NVQs).

Pre-registration nursing programmes

The NMC requires all pre-registration students to complete a nursing degree programme from 2013 onwards. The NMC (2008b) *Standards to support learning and assessment in practice* and *Standards for pre-registration nursing education* (NMC 2010b) are testimony to a long period of research and reflection within nursing.

The NMC (2010b) introduced changes to pre-registration nursing programmes, where new requirements for teaching, learning and assessment were implemented to address the challenges of meeting new and more flexible ways of working. Services need to be reconfigured and new roles developed to meet the ever-changing needs of patients; such roles and educational routes need to be underpinned by appropriate nursing education.

The NMC (2010b) *Standards for pre-registration nursing education* describe the programme that UK nursing students undertake in order to acquire the competencies needed to meet the criteria for registration. The term 'competencies' replaced the previously used term 'proficiencies', which describe the criteria students must meet in order to complete their programme successfully and apply for registration. The standards identify the knowledge, skills and attitudes students must acquire by the end of their programme and are structured into four domains:

- Professional values
- Communication and interpersonal skills
- Nursing practice and decision-making
- Leadership, management and team working.

The degree level competencies required to meet those standards include both *generic* – skills that all nurses need to learn – and *field-specific* competencies for each of the four nursing fields of practice: adult, child, learning disability and mental health. In addition, the NMC (2010c) *Essential Skills Clusters* set out clinical competencies to be achieved by specified programme progression points within each of the domains above. Furthermore, nursing students must meet the 'Fitness to Practise' requirements of good health and good character (see Ch. 7) during their programmes and confirm these again before applying for registration with the NMC. Professional values, communication and interpersonal skills remain central to the identity of nursing. Although there is clearly a shift from past eras when a small diminution to one's good character could signal dismissal, the prerequisites to good character and professional values remain. Society has evolved to include more liberal views, and so too has nursing, but the high moral standards set generations earlier are still evident in nursing today; albeit in the expression of professional rather than moral conduct.

Students can expect a blended learning approach, which is generally defined as a mixture of classroom teaching, work-based and online learning, with generic and field-specific elements running throughout the programme to provide better understanding of the different fields of practice. These programmes also include interprofessional learning, so that the roles, responsibilities and functions of other nurses and AHPs are better understood and utilized. In order to achieve the required practical skills and competencies, around half of a nursing programme takes place in practice settings where learning is facilitated by and negotiated with mentors (see pp. 55-56). A wide range of placements offer learning opportunities to develop the generic and specific skills needed for registration (Box 2.16).

 Critical thinking Box 2.16

Learning opportunities in placements

Lizzie is on her first placement, and under the supervision of her mentor, has undertaken many fundamental nursing care activities. Towards the end of her placement, Lizzie is asked to carry out oral hygiene on a patient called Jean. Jean's health has deteriorated over the last few days and Lizzie finds when helping with her oral hygiene, that Jean has developed white spots in her mouth. Being observant, Jenny notices this and reports her observations to her mentor who says the likely cause is oral thrush. This is a good learning opportunity for Lizzie, as she has not seen this condition before.

Student activities

- How could Lizzie meet her learning need?
- How might her mentor help in identifying and obtaining relevant resources for Lizzie's learning?
- Consider different ways in which you might get help to meet your learning needs in practice settings.

The rationale for the exercise in Box 2.16 is that from their first placement, students are required to recognize and reflect on learning opportunities to help make links between theory and practice, and to identify any learning needs that could arise. Routinely, students are asked to recall and reflect on their practice so that learning about decision-making takes place (this process also highlights creativity, resourcefulness and ability). Most importantly, it enables development of the science of observing clinical choices in action, tracking the links with appraisal skills and identifying any resultant further learning needs.

While most RNs practice in one of the four fields, patient/client boundaries are not mutually exclusive; there is therefore a need for all RNs to have a clear understanding of all four fields of practice. For example, both adult and children's nurses will encounter clients with learning disabilities when they access primary healthcare through GP surgeries or require admission to hospital, and mental health nurses may have clients with coexisting physical conditions such as diabetes, chronic bronchitis or leg ulcers. The main characteristics of the fields of nursing practice are explored below.

Fields of nursing practice

Although there are four fields of nursing for which registration can be awarded, not all universities provide education in all fields and most students register for adult nursing. The other fields of practice are learning disabilities, mental health and children's nursing. Students in all fields of practice will gain RN status but also require a clear understanding of each field as patients/clients are of all ages, and may have issues which do not occur solely within one field of practice. There are many examples of this: patients who have complex health issues may need to be treated in a general hospital environment but may also have underlying mental health issues. It is not uncommon for children born with a syndrome (e.g. Down's syndrome, which is associated with learning disability), to have underlying congenital heart disease. The heart condition needs to be treated while also being mindful of the individual's capacity to understand, which may require additional nursing understanding and care.

Adult nursing

Adult nurses are primarily responsible for health promotion and providing holistic care for physically ill or injured adults with wide-ranging levels of dependency in both hospital and community settings. The focus is on individual patients, rather than the condition from which they may be suffering; and the needs and anxieties that their condition may generate, including the pressures on their family and friends.

Adult nursing placements include care homes, hospital wards and clinics, and community settings that may involve visiting people at home and/or attachments to health centres. Nurses play an increasingly prominent role in the provision of health-focused care in the community. Many hospital-based nurses are found in specialist areas such as intensive care, cancer care and care of older adults (Table 2.3). Adult nurses work with people over 16 years of age who have acute (short-term) and/or chronic (long-term) conditions.

Despite the wide range of specialties, there are a number of features common to most adult nursing roles (Box 2.17).

Table 2.3 Some adult nursing specialties

Specialty	Focus of care
Palliative care (see Ch. 12)	Holistic relief of symptoms such as pain or breathlessness (rather than effecting a cure), support for patients and their families and friends. This is often, but not necessarily, for people with cancer
Accident and emergency nursing	Any presenting problem that requires urgent intervention
Women's health (gynaecology)	Women requiring health screening, family planning, sexual health advice and interventions involving the reproductive organs
Orthopaedics	Maximizing mobility and independence in people with bone problems such as fractures or congenital bone malformations
Older adults (gerontology)	Holistic approach to problems which are often multiple or specific conditions, which tend to become increasingly common with age
Ophthalmic nursing	Problems affecting the eye and vision
Dermatology nursing	Conditions affecting the skin, which often affect body image (see Ch. 11)
Cancer nursing (oncology)	Helping people to cope with the diagnosis of and treatment for cancer and any related nursing problems
Rehabilitation (see Ch. 11)	Assisting people to achieve, or regain, optimal functioning and reduce the risk of mortality/morbidity through health promotion
Cardiology (see Ch. 17)	Caring for people with heart disorders, supporting families and children with congenital heart disorders; cardiac rehabilitation
Perioperative care (see Ch. 24)	Nursing care required immediately before, during and after surgery

While this often includes physical care, it extends well beyond that, including counselling, advice and education that draws upon interpersonal and communication skills to address psychological, social and spiritual components of holistic care.

Most patients have specific problems but many can eventually look forward to an independent future. The nurse's role is to offer support while it is needed and to give people the skills, strength or knowledge that will help them to regain independence. Box 2.18 provides the opportunity to consider different health-related problems that people may experience as a result of sudden illness and their impact on independence.

Learning disability nursing

Health policy in the UK is explicitly directed at social inclusion and social justice for everyone and is clearly outlined in *Valuing People Now* (DH 2009b) and *Equally Well* (Scottish Executive Health Department 2008). These policy documents aim to ensure that people with learning disabilities are afforded the

Critical thinking Box 2.17

Rehabilitation nursing

As a primary nurse (p. 45), Sandra is the RN responsible for every aspect of nursing care for a group of eight older adults on a rehabilitation ward, who are cared for in two bays of four beds, one male and one female. She directs the work of associate nurses (p. 45), who are less experienced and assist with care delivery. Sandra is accountable for patient care, i.e. she ensures that the care is of good quality and appropriate to patients' needs. Today, Sandra's patients range in age from 69 to 84 and present a variety of nursing problems due to their underlying medical conditions:

- Zayan is unable to move one side and cannot speak coherently following a severe stroke. This means he is very dependent on nurses for all aspects of his care.
- Doris has recently developed swollen legs and becomes very breathless when she exerts herself due to heart failure. She finds it difficult to mobilize.
- Emrys is on the ward for his regular 2-week period of respite care, so that his daughter who normally cares for him at home can have a break. He has slow movements, rigidity and a marked tremor due to Parkinson's disease. This means that he finds it difficult to turn over in bed, feed himself and walk to the lavatory.

Sandra begins her day by reading the notes made by the night staff about her patients' progress and reflecting on the care they have received. Next, she visits each of the patients with the associate nurse, taking the care plans along with her. The purpose of the visit is to discuss the day's care with each patient and to agree the priorities that will meet their needs. Sandra knows from nursing research that it is good practice to involve patients and their families in decisions about their care.

Student activities

- What do you think Sandra will discuss with her patients when she meets them?
- What do you think Sandra will be observing?

Reflective practice Box 2.18

The impact of sudden illness or change in independence

Imagine you wake up one morning to find that you have lost all sensation and power in your dominant hand.

Student activities

- How would you feel?
- What impact would this have on your day?
- Identify some daily activities you would have difficulty in doing by yourself without help.
- Consider the change this would make to your contribution to your family or household situation?
- What assistance could you expect from your family?
- What support could you expect from the university?

same opportunities as everyone else and that they receive the support and services needed to meet their individual needs.

The term 'learning disability' has been adopted in the UK and is the one that users of services prefer. However, the terms 'intellectual disability' and 'developmental disability' are commonly used in other parts of the developed world. In the UK, the term usually refers to a variety of disorders that adversely affects the acquisition, retention and understanding of new or complex information and often also the use of verbal or non-verbal communication. Because learning disability has a lasting effect on development and requires varying degrees of support from others, Mencap launched a 'Getting it Right' campaign to ensure that people with learning disability receive the level of healthcare they have a right to. 'Getting it Right' requests that health professionals commit to a charter to ensure better health, well-being and quality of life for those they support (Mencap 2010).

The role of the nurse is to help people with a learning disability and their families to maintain and improve their lifestyles by promoting health, and to participate fully as equal members of society. Learning disability nurses provide care to vulnerable children and adults. Long-term conditions and end-of-life issues are increasingly part of learning disability nursing, as better ways to treat complex needs related to ageing, cognitive impairment and basic health inequalities are addressed more equitably (Parliamentary and Health Service Ombudsman, PHSO 2010). Approaches to person-centred care in learning disabilities nursing are explored in Chapter 14.

As members of the MDT, nurses may be involved in underpinning people's efforts to enable them to manage daily activities, such as making a pot of tea, or extended activities such as finding a job and bringing up a family. Person-centred care requires considerable sensitivity and skill to offer the best care to people with learning disabilities and their families without being intrusive or offering inappropriate care. 'Reasonable adjustments' were embedded within the Equality Act (2010) to ensure that changes to environment or working practice could be implemented, making reasonable steps to ensure that disabled people are not placed at a substantial disadvantage in comparison with non-disabled people.

It can be more difficult to diagnose health problems and illness in people with learning disabilities, and evidence has shown that hospitalization or regular health checks can be withheld through misunderstanding (Disability Rights Commission 2007). It is important when providing treatment that consent, capacity and advocacy is ensured (see Chs 6, 7). With reasonable adjustments, most individuals should be able to make choices and family carers can feel involved (RCN 2010).

The distinctive contribution of learning disability nurses is their influence on behaviours and lifestyles that promote health and maximize well-being and independence for people with learning disabilities, their families and carers. Care takes place in a wide variety of settings: people's own homes, their family homes, community houses, residential care, schools, workplaces, leisure centres and healthcare facilities. Some nurses maintain this broad spread of activity, whereas others choose a specialist area such as supporting people with interactional challenges and complex needs education, or management of learning disability services.

The main challenge is meeting health needs, since it is apparent that the health needs of people with learning disabilities are greater and more complex, and often present differently from those of the general population. Some conditions occur more frequently in people with learning disabilities, including:

- Vision and hearing impairments (see Ch. 16)
- Mental health problems
- Gastro-oesophageal reflux disorder (GORD) (see Ch. 19)
- Epilepsy (see Ch. 16).

Other health needs are associated with particular groups, e.g. people with Down's syndrome are more prone to depression, thyroid function disorders, hearing impairment and dementia. It is important that learning disability nurses have the ability to recognize these differing health needs but it is also apparent that all nurses require an awareness of them in order to reduce discrimination and enhance access to healthcare services (RCN 2010).

Learning disability nurses coordinate care and work with the whole family and other carers to befriend, teach, support, counsel and carry out therapeutic activities. They also make regular assessments of healthcare needs and ensure the availability of resources to meet them. In this field of practice, it is not only important for nurses to know how to care for the well-being of their clients but also to teach the families, friends and carers who provide regular care to do the same. Often, this entails caring for a person who has seizures or epilepsy, incontinence (see Chs 20, 21), a physical disability that has led to immobility (see Ch. 18) or sensory impairment. Box 2.19 provides the opportunity to consider the impact of this in relation to people with learning disabilities.

 Reflective practice   Box 2.19

The impact of learning disability

John is a 25-year-old man who has complex needs that have affected both his intellectual and physical development. He uses non-verbal communication to convey his needs to his family and carers. John has a specially adapted wheelchair to aid his mobility and his house has specifically designed lifting equipment, including a hoist. On weekdays, he attends a local centre for people with learning disabilities but, when at home, John spends much of his time in the lounge on a special chair, watching television or listening to music. John's physical needs which includes those things we take for granted such as bathing, shaving, using the lavatory, dressing and undressing, are carried out by his parents. He goes out for weekend trips with his parents in a car that has been specially adapted to suit the purpose.

Both parents have taken early retirement to look after John full-time, as his physical needs have increased over the last 2 years. They have had to adapt to their reduced income and becoming full-time carers, which has had an impact on their quality of life.

They have kept in touch with two couples that they have known for many years and meet up once a month for a meal at John's house, with each couple contributing a course. Everyone looks forward to the meal but John's parents always have to leave their guests to help John prepare for bed.

Student activities

Talk to a learning disabilities nurse about:

- The difficulties experienced by families caring for a person such as John who has a profound learning disability.
- The nurse's role in supporting clients like John and his family.
- Facilities available in your area to give people like John's parents a break from 24-hour care.

Using the information in Box 2.19, consider the realities of caring for John. It is frequently physically and psychologically demanding, particularly on parents and other carers. Breaks from physical caring will be few and liable to interruption at any time. Furthermore, there is the need to ensure that John does not become frustrated or depressed by the constraints and demands placed on his life. Since it is difficult for John to travel, the family will hardly ever go away from home together, even to enjoy a meal out. Finally, John's parents may frequently worry about what will happen to John when they grow older and die; most parents of people with a learning disability live in fear of their children going into institutional care when they are no longer there to look after them. The learning disability nurse could help John's parents in a variety of ways, e.g.:

- Their fears could be fully explored
- A plan could be identified for how John may be cared for both now and in the future
- Respite care could be arranged
- Information from support organizations such as Mencap could be provided (see Useful websites, below).

In conclusion, the role of the learning disability nurse is built on developing equal partnerships with the people they work with so that the health needs of people with learning disabilities, their families and carers can be met in an effective, efficient and resourceful manner. Learning disability nurses treat people as unique, whole individuals with specific needs and aspirations. They practise in a sensitive and non-discriminatory manner to enable people with learning disabilities to fully participate within society.

Mental health nursing

Mental health nurses care for people with mental health problems, also known as mental distress, in diverse settings in both hospitals and the community. Mental health nurses distribute work and responsibility among a team so that it is capability- and competence-based with greater shared decision-making than is commonly seen in children's or adult nursing. A major role of mental health nurses is promoting social inclusion, challenging stigma and ensuring a user/carer focus to help individuals develop strategies to enable them to work towards recovery (DH 2007). To facilitate this, mental health nurses must practise in a way that is underpinned by a clear values base which is focused on delivering rights-based care. The publication of reviews of the role of mental health nursing in Scotland and England are set to influence further development of this field of practice (Box 2.20).

Everyone can experience mental distress at some time in their life, e.g. episodes of stress, anxiety or depression (see Ch. 11). At any given time, one adult in six suffers from some form of mental health problem (National Statistics Office 2011); in other words, mental health problems are as common as asthma.

Mental health nurses are at the forefront in providing the support required for people with mental health problems who need to access health services, working as part of MDTs with other professionals such as GPs, psychiatrists, social workers and AHPs to coordinate and provide care. A wide range of

Reflective practice   Box 2.20

The future for mental health nursing

In 2006, the Chief Nursing Officers in both Scotland and England launched reports (see Resources below) of reviews of the future role of mental health nursing. While the reviews were conducted in both countries independently, and used different methods, they share many common messages about the future role of mental health nursing and make several recommendations for the future development of the profession.

Student activities

1. Access both reports and consider the key messages about:
   - The policy that sets out the future direction for mental healthcare and services
   - The role of mental health nursing
   - The future development of the profession.
2. You may also wish to reflect on the differences and similarities between the reports

Resources

The full Scottish Review Report entitled *Rights, Relationships and Recovery*, a summarized version, and a 5-year action plan to support the development of the profession in Scotland. Online. Available: www.scotland.gov.uk/Publications/2006/04/18164814/0

The English Report *From Values to Action*. Online. Available: www.dh.gov.uk/PublicationsAndStatistics/Publications/PublicationsPolicyAndGuidance/PublicationsPolicyAndGuidanceArticle/fs/en?CONTENT_ID=4133839&chk=RJV7mg.

Both websites accessed August 2012.

---

other services, e.g. voluntary organizations, local government and housing agencies, may also be involved. In recent years, there has been a significant shift from hospitals to the community as the main setting for mental healthcare. Nurses work with people in their homes, in small residential units and in local health centres with considerable autonomy in how they plan and deliver care. Community psychiatric nurses (CPNs, increasingly known as community mental health nurses) are key members of the MDT in mental health service provision. The one-to-one therapeutic relationships that mental health nurses form with their clients are at the heart of mental health nursing. Nursing interventions include providing social and physical care, and psychological and psychosocial interventions such as counselling and cognitive behavioural therapy (CBT), as well as working with other professional groups and the voluntary organizations involved in supporting people with mental health problems. Mental health nurses also have a role in assessing and managing individual risk, which requires sophisticated assessment skills. Approaches to care planning used in mental health nursing are explored in Chapter 14.

Mental health nurses work with people of all ages and from a wide range of backgrounds, and mental health nursing provides opportunities to practise in diverse areas including older people's mental health, child and adolescent mental health services (CAMHS), forensic mental health services and acute inpatient care.

Children's nursing

Children and young people's nurses are responsible for teaching families, providing support and helping families to make decisions in the best interest of their child. To do this, nurses frequently develop partnerships with families and acknowledge that family members provide nursing care. Family-centred approaches to care planning in children's and young people's nursing are explored in Chapter 14.

To provide tailored services, the provision of care for children and young people has been divided into four areas (DH 2011b):

- Acute and short-term conditions
- Long-term conditions
- Disabilities and complex conditions, including those requiring continuing care and neonates
- Life-limiting and life-threatening illness, including those requiring palliative and end-of-life care.

Within these four areas, children and young people have very different physical, psychological and social needs; broadened further by different ages and developmental stages (see Ch. 8). Their needs for intervention by health professionals starts before conception and continues through adolescence and transitional care to adult services. The type of intervention required depends upon the particular health needs of the child and family at any given time. Children's nurses learn skills in caring for whole families, including grandparents, siblings, carers and friends. Skills in family-centred care also involve teaching (see Ch. 4) so that the nurse can teach families and empower them with knowledge and skills so that they can carry out almost any nursing care the child requires.

Children's nurses in hospital wards provide care and skilled observation and treatment. They involve parents at all times, helping them to cope with their fears and the trauma of sudden hospital admissions. Parents may be unsure that they have done everything they should have and whether they called the doctor early enough. Children's nurses listen to these worries, explore issues with parents and provide information and health promotion advice, as appropriate. Involving parents helps them to feel included in the nursing care and maintains their relationship with their child.

Children's nurses also work in other settings. They work in special schools for children with learning disabilities or may support children who have long-term health problems such as asthma, cystic fibrosis, diabetes or eczema and those with life-limiting conditions. This can be at home and in the community, as day-care, hospice or hospital settings.

Nurses working with children in any setting must learn to become vigilant, observant and attentive in order to identify vulnerable children, i.e. those at risk or potential risk from physical or emotional injury, abuse or neglect. Although children are generally best looked after by their families, the welfare of children is absolutely paramount and their needs are uppermost if there is conflict between those and carers/parental needs. Nurses have a responsibility to respect and promote children's rights and play an important role in child protection by reporting any suspicion of non-accidental injury, abuse or neglect and following local protocols for safeguarding children (see Chs 3, 6).

Roles of non-registered staff

Non-registered staff such as Health Care Assistants (HCAs), assistant practitioners, clinical support workers (CSWs), therapy assistants or nursing auxiliaries (see Ch. 3) work with RNs and AHPs. They are funded from healthcare budgets and qualified staff retain accountability for them. Traditionally, they helped with fundamental care and treatment, and looking after people's comfort and well-being. However, today, associate practitioners may have complex and technical support roles with skills gained through national vocational qualifications (NVQ). They are employed in many areas in both hospitals and the community. The nature of their role depends on the area in which they work, but it is important to note that registered practitioners are accountable for the work of non-registered staff (including students, see Ch. 7).

A range of unqualified and unregistered practitioners work under the supervision of the RN, and on a hospital ward might make beds, take temperatures and help patients with washing, feeding and toileting. In clinics and high dependency areas, some may undertake more complex procedures, e.g. taking blood samples, undertaking observations, measuring vital signs or managing intravenous infusions. In the community, e.g. health centres, care homes and schools, they might take blood samples, help those with complex needs with eating or going to the toilet or they may have first-aid responsibilities.

National vocational qualifications

NVQs and Scottish vocational qualifications (SVQs) are methods of gaining academic credit through a combination of theory, work-based learning and assessment. Some NHS organizations and other employers have developed work-based training for clinical support workers that lead to the acquisition of NVQs/SVQs levels 2 and 3, which can provide entry into pre-registration nurse education. The main purpose of this development was to widen the skill mix in practice, to ensure clinical support workers are competent in the skills they are expected to carry out and to offer improved career opportunities. NVQs and SVQs are also available in many fields outside the healthcare sector.

Roles of the nurse

This section describes some generic roles of the RN in clinical settings in all fields of nursing practice and then some specialist and advanced roles undertaken by more experienced RNs.

Generic roles of the RN

From your first placement, you will participate in nursing care under the supervision of your mentor. Box 2.21 provides examples of activities RNs may undertake in any clinical setting and the responsibilities they may have.

Reflective practice Box 2.21

RN activities

The nursing activities in the list below include a range of those frequently undertaken by RNs in any setting. From your first placement, you will begin to learn about some of these under the supervision of your mentor while working towards meeting your practice learning outcomes.

- *Caseload management.* If you have worked with nurses who managed a caseload of clients/patients, what particular skills did they use and which members of the MDT did they liaise with?
- *Administering medication* (see Ch. 22). (Some RNs may also prescribe medication after further education)
- Assessing, planning, implementing and evaluating care (see Ch. 14)
- *Documentation of care* (see Ch 14). Reflect on your own experience and identify the documentation you completed during 1 week of your placement (e.g. care plans)
- *Liaison and coordination of care.* This term covers a range of activities. For example in the United States, there are dedicated liaison and coordination of care nurses. In the UK, the term is used to describe ways in which some nurses work, e.g. an RN who links with other members of the MDT to provide a cluster of services and coordination of care for older residents/clients. You will also liaise with other healthcare professionals as a member of the MDT
- *Discharge planning.* This involves planning and arranging the services a patient/client needs to enable transition from one level of care to another or home from a care setting (see Ch. 14)
- *Leading a team.* How an RN manages a team depends on many factors including the environment, the patients/clients there, the team and the philosophy of the care area. Are there any RNs you identified as good team leaders or role models? What type of skills did you learn from them?

Student activities

- Consider each activity above and reflect on your involvement in each one, bearing in mind that your mentor remains responsible and accountable for the care of patients/clients.
- Think about the questions beside some of the nursing activities above.
- Reflect on the your learning to date around each activity above.
- Clarify any questions you may have with your mentor.

Mentoring

It is expected that RNs take on the role of mentoring student nurses about 1 year following registration. RNs must complete a mentorship course that is recorded in a live register within the NHS hospital trust. The role of the mentor is to support and assess student nurses in their practice learning experiences and also to ensure that each student is signed off against NMC competencies for years 1 and 2. The student nurse also has a *sign-off mentor*, from their own field of practice, who signs them off as competent to practice at the end of 3rd year. The NMC (2008b) outlined standards for mentors and mentorship that include:

- Establishing effective communication and working relationships based on mutual trust and respect
- Facilitating learning by understanding students' learning needs and integrating learning from practice and educational settings
- Demonstrating the ability to assess clinical practice
- Demonstrating safe and effective care and good relationships with patients/clients
- Ensuring effective learning experiences by contributing to quality assurance and audit
- Contributing to an environment in which change can be initiated and supported
- Applying research findings to clinical practice (Box 2.22).

This approach is based on a partnership between the student, their mentor and a university lecturer. Promoting this partnership approach encourages student nurses to use the same principles towards the patients/clients for whom they are caring.

Reflective practice   Box 2.22

The role of the mentor

After reading the standards for mentorship above, reflect on your experience and answer the following questions.

Student activities

- What is the role of the mentor?
- What are my responsibilities as a student nurse?
- What is the role of the university when I am on placement?
- Discuss your thoughts with a fellow student.

Roles of experienced RNs

As RNs gain further experience, some may develop their careers by working towards one of the roles below.

Nurse practitioners

A nurse practitioner is an RN who has undertaken a specific course of post-registration study and who takes full clinical responsibility for clinical decisions based on systematic physical assessment, accurate diagnosis and the delivery of a wide range of treatment options. Doctors previously undertook most of these roles, which are diverse and can include pre-assessment to post-discharge follow-up in areas such as dermatology, tissue viability, stoma and breast care, general practice and walk-in centres (Box 2.23).

Teaching

RNs need to provide clinical environments that are conducive to student learning and be able to respond to the individual learning needs of colleagues, students, members of the public, patients/clients or carers. Different roles have evolved to support learning in practice settings; these include mentorship (see above), clinical teacher, practice educator, link lecturer and lecturer practitioner. These roles aim to bridge the

---

? Critical thinking   Box 2.23

Specialist practitioner – tissue viability nurse

The tissue viability nurse (TVN), Louise, has been contacted regarding a patient called Helen who has developed a leg ulcer. Helen was admitted to the ward from a care home and is soon to be discharged from hospital back to her residential home. A leg ulcer is a complex and chronic wound that often requires ongoing management (see Ch. 25). Louise is available to offer support and advice to patients, carers and healthcare professionals on complex wound management and techniques. Aspects of Louise's role include:

- Expert assessment and management of wounds and any related circulatory problems
- Providing appropriate treatments to optimize healing and prevent deterioration in wound conditions
- Having knowledge of the most appropriate wound dressings or pressure bandages that would best treat leg ulcers
- Knowledge of special equipment that may be used to clean infected or heavily discharging wounds
- Providing specialist advice to patients on how to prevent the reoccurrence of wounds or how to prevent and manage circulatory problems, particularly in the lower limbs.

Student activities

- In relation to the specialist nurses you have come into contact with, compare and contrast their different roles.
- Describe the function of the specialist nurse in both the community and hospital
- Discuss the role of the TVN with your mentor.

---

theory–practice gap by closely linking theory and practice, teaching students and staff, assessing competence in practice and contributing to education programmes.

These teaching roles provide an opportunity for student nurses to be supported by experienced mentors and teachers, enabling them to reflect, learn and develop their practice, and improve their level of confidence when interacting with patients/clients.

Lecturers who teach nursing in universities are normally RNs who have undertaken a teaching qualification recognized by the NMC; the learning outcomes of the postgraduate teaching qualification are mapped to the requirements of the NMC teacher qualification (NMC 2008b). In addition to classroom teaching, they facilitate student-centred learning, including reflective groups, provide support to personal students and act as link lecturers in practice placements. Many also undertake nursing research.

Clinical leadership

Clinical leaders are from any discipline within an organization; they are often team leaders but not necessarily line managers. While managers promote organizational structures, leaders promote the achievement of excellence in others. However, in clinical nursing, it is expected that a leader coordinates a team of healthcare professionals whose focus is ensuring that high quality, effective patient-centred care is delivered. The qualities that are central to patient-centred leadership are:

- Learning to manage oneself
- Building and maintaining effective relationships with other staff
- Using person-centred approaches to care of patients/clients
- Internal and external networking to share good practice and to support each other in developing practice
- Increasing political awareness to influence both local and national policy.

Leadership is about setting direction, opening up possibilities, helping people achieve their potential, communicating and delivering; what people do as leaders is even more important than what they say. *The Darzi Report* published in 2009 proposes that every registered clinician has leadership potential, which is about not knowing everything, but about being able to reflect on practice, harness the energy of the clinical team, make continuous improvement part of everyday work and encourage others to lead and improve. Those who lead improvement need to be able to:

- Create a shared vision with their colleagues
- Align improvement with this vision
- Build a more receptive context for improvement
- Engage clinical colleagues
- Support healthcare development through the provision of evidence, data and professional leadership
- Underpin clinical leadership with public health engagement.

Clinical nurse specialists

The clinical nurse specialist (CNS) has acquired extensive specialist knowledge about a specific area of nursing. CNSs often work closely with doctors who specialize in the same area of healthcare and are involved in patient care, family and staff education and support. Many CNSs run clinics where they have a caseload of patients and may have full responsibility for making decisions about care. Some also prescribe and monitor the effects of medication (see Ch. 22). They often work across the hospital and community interface, following the patient pathway.

CNSs share their specialist knowledge with other nurses, help to ensure that national standards are put into practice locally and may contribute to developing care policies, e.g. management of breast cancer, learning disabilities, palliative care and aspects of children's nursing, pain management and mental health.

The CNS role is guided by national standards; programmes of study are delivered by universities and include work-based learning. On completion, RNs have the opportunity to work at a highly specialist level. For example, in critical care, their role may be to enable early identification of patients whose conditions are deteriorating and require more specialist input, provide advice to ward nurses or to transfer seriously ill patients, e.g. to coronary care or intensive care units. Another example is outreach nurses who bridge the gap between community and hospital, providing support for children and/or adults with complex needs and their families/carers.

Nurse consultants

The nurse consultant is an expert practitioner who works with a specific group of patients or clients, improving the quality of care through:

- Demonstrating expert practice
- Demonstrating professional leadership and consultancy skills
- Contributing to education, training and staff development
- Contributing to research and service development.

Expert practice includes both direct and indirect nursing practice, which must make up 50% of the nurse consultant role.

Professional leadership involves a variety of skills and processes that involve facilitating a culture of practice development that allows staff to become leaders themselves. The consultancy role encompasses not only giving advice and guidance but also developing the clinical skills and problem-solving abilities of less experienced RNs. Enhancing outcomes for patient care involves influencing clinical practice in any setting. This encompasses consultancy across traditional boundaries or care settings, interagency working and partnership or community development in addition to the specialist area.

The education, training and staff development roles aim to develop a culture for learning in practice and to maintain links with higher education.

The role of practice and service development, research and evaluation involves establishing a research culture to embed evidence in practice (see Ch. 5). Nurse consultants are required to make a significant contribution to the strategic development of clinical governance (see Ch. 3) and in the promotion of clinical effectiveness in their area of practice. Clinical governance is a monitoring system set up to ensure NHS organizations are accountable for the quality of their services and standards of care. Leaders, such as nurse consultants, work to ensure robust clinical effectiveness mechanisms are in place and to ensure that patient care is as safe as possible. The role is multifaceted and its success is through the promotion of patient-centered practice, development of teamwork and meeting service needs, while demonstrating effective transformational leadership (Stevenson et al 2011).

Lead roles

Charge nurses and hospital and community 'modern matrons' (also known as clinical, ward or nurse managers) have different functions, but share a research and leadership remit with the aim of improving patient experience and providing high quality care. This role was introduced to provide support for ward managers to refocus attention on patient care following the perceived erosion of fundamental nursing care in areas such as infection control, provision of adequate food and drinks for patients/clients, pressure area management, communication, dignity and compassion, as ward managers and clinical leaders were spending more time dealing with management and paperwork. In hospitals, the role of the modern matron has three main functions:

- Providing leadership and ensuring robust care mechanisms are in place within their group of wards in order to secure and assure the highest standards of clinical care

- Ensuring the availability of appropriate administrative and support services within their group of wards
- Providing a visible, accessible and authoritative presence in ward settings to whom patients and their families can turn to for assistance, advice and support.

The role of the 'traditional' matron disappeared in the 1960s when formal management was introduced into the NHS. However, the security, stability and 'care focus' that the role had provided to both staff and patients was overlooked. The old-style matron was often considered to be a formidable character who held considerable authority and commanded respect for their knowledge and expertise from patients and staff alike.

Modern matrons and clinical nurse managers must have credibility and expertise, and present themselves as figures of authority without imposing fear. The role is intermediary; patients can ask to speak to the matron if they have a complaint about their care or the standards of the ward. The matron or manager is ideally placed to resolve complaints at a local level by providing immediate feedback to ward staff.

Their leadership roles include effective communication, mediation, negotiation, understanding and considerable clinical experience within their specialist clinical or community arena. In addition, the role requires the ability to monitor and measure the effectiveness of care, change management skills and the skills to manage interpersonal dynamics that can arise in stressful situations. As a result, ward staff are better supported in their role of caring for patients.

Nurses as researchers

At the heart of the drive to modernize the NHS is a commitment to the development of high quality, person-centred services that are efficient and evidence-based. The vision for nursing in the twenty-first century is for all nurses to be able to both seek out evidence and apply it in their everyday practice, with an increasing number actively participating in research and practice development. All RNs are expected to be able to understand and implement research findings (see Ch. 5) but only a small number will become full-time researchers who will contribute to the development of new nursing knowledge.

Student nurses' contribution to nursing and its evolution

Hospitals, community settings, residential or other clinical surroundings are particular environments that nurses and patients/clients enter into and, either consciously or unconsciously, the environment effects the way they behave; social cues are taken on board, such as when to respect someone's privacy or need for quiet, displays of joyful or sorrowful emotion are assimilated by the environment and understood or contextualized. Employees/patients/clients/residents/carers

all contribute to the environment within care or residential settings. When student nurses enter a practice setting they are quickly assimilated into that environment, which is governed by rules and codes of behaviour (some clear, some less explicit and many that need to be unravelled throughout the pre-registration nursing course). For student nurses, the process of assimilating how more experienced nurses go about their roles, their affiliation with fellow nurses, and developing clinical and caring skills are all important. These lead onto role emergence and the role definition that identifies nursing's future. For nursing to continue to advance, the role of student nurses who will become the RNs of tomorrow is vital.

SUMMARY

- Nursing does not exist in isolation; it changes in response to society and the political agenda of the day. This is what makes nursing an exciting and challenging career.
- Fundamental nursing values include compassion, sensitivity and humanity.
- Nurses practise autonomously and in collaboration with other members of the MDT to ensure that individuals of all ages, groups and communities receive the holistic, person-centred nursing and healthcare that they require.
- Becoming a nurse provides an opportunity to help others, to enable people to cope with difficult and potentially life-changing situations and to provide an environment that allows people to learn about themselves, their health and the impact they have on those close to them.
- Nurses see people at the 'great' times in their lives: great happiness, great sadness and great strength.
- It may be here that we see each other at our most human; for us it is this chance to share with others that which is the essence of nursing.

KEY WORDS AND PHRASES FOR LITERATURE SEARCHING

Accountability

Community nursing

Interprofessional working

Modern matron

Nurse consultant

Nursing theory

Patient allocation

Person-centredness

Practice development

Primary nursing

Professional practice

Nurse specialists

Useful websites

Nursing and Midwifery Council www.nmc-uk.org
Mencap: the voice of learning disability www.mencap.org.uk
Royal College of Nursing Archive www.rcn.org.uk/archives

United Kingdom Centre for the History of Nursing and Midwifery
www.nursing.manchester.ac.uk/ukchnm
All websites accessed September 2012.

References

Aaberge, R., Mogstad, M., Peragine, V., 2011. Measuring long-term inequality of opportunity. Journal of Public Economics 95 (3), 193–204.

Angelini, D., 2011. Interdisciplinary and interprofessional education: what are the key issues and considerations for the future? Journal of Perinatal and Neonatal Nursing 25 (2), 175–179.

Barker, P., 1996. Chaos and the way of Zen: psychiatric nursing and the 'uncertainty principle'. Journal of Psychiatric and Mental Health Nursing 3, 235–243.

Baughan, J., Smith, A., 2008. Caring in nursing practice: a guide for nurses. Blackwell, Oxford.

Büscher, A., Sivertsen, B., White, J., 2009. World Health Organization Europe: Survey on the situation of nursing and midwifery in the Member States of the European Region of the World Health Organization. WHO Regional Office for Europe, Copenhagen.

Casey, A., 2007. Partnership model of nursing. In: Glasper, E., McEwing, G., Richardson, J. (Eds.), Oxford handbook of children's and young people's nursing. Oxford University Press, Oxford.

Department of Health and Social Security, 1972. Report on the Commission for Nursing (Briggs Report). HMSO, London.

Department of Health, 1999. Saving lives: our healthier nation. HMSO, London.

Department of Health, 2000. The NHS plan: a plan for investment, a plan for reform. TSO, London.

Department of Health, 2004. Agenda for change: final agreement. HMSO, London.

Department of Health, 2006a. Modernising nursing careers. HMSO, London.

Department of Health, 2006b. Towards a strategy for research and development. HMSO, London.

Department of Health, 2007. New ways of working for everyone: A best practice implementation guide. HMSO, London.

Department of Health, 2009a. Prime Minister's Commission on the future of nursing and midwifery. HMSO, London.

Department of Health, 2009b. Valuing people now: a new three-year strategy for people with learning disabilities. HMSO, London.

Department of Health, 2010. Healthy lives, healthy people: our strategy for public health in England. HMSO, London. Online. Available: www.dh.gov.uk/en/Publichealth/Healthyliveshealthypeople/index.htm September 2012.

Department of Health, 2011a. Overall patient experience measure updated to include results from the, 2010. inpatient survey. HMSO, London.

Department of Health, 2011b. NHS at home: community children's nursing services. HMSO, London.

Department of Health, 2011c. Healthy lives, healthy people. HMSO, London.

Disability Rights Commission, 2007. Equal treatment: closing the gap one year on. Disability Rights Commission, London.

Doyle, C., Reed, J., Woodcock, T., Bell, D., 2010. Understanding what matters to patients – identifying key patients' perceptions of quality. Journal of the Royal Society of Medicine Short Reports 1: 3.

Equality Act, 2010. Online. Available: www.legislation.gov.uk/ukpga/2010/15/contents September 2012.

Galvin, K.T., 2010. Revisiting caring science: some integrative ideas for the 'head, hand and heart' of critical care nursing practice. Nursing in Critical Care 15, 168–175.

Glasper, E.A., Mitchell, R.M., 2010. Historical perspectives of children's nursing. In: Glasper, E., Richardson, J. (Eds.), A textbook of children's and young people's nursing, second ed. Churchill Livingstone, Edinburgh.

Henderson, V., 1961. Basic principles of nursing care. International Council of Nurses, London.

Jolley, J., 2009. The history of children's perioperative care. In: Shields, L. (Ed.), Perioperative care of the child: a nursing manual. Wiley-Blackwell, Oxford.

Mencap, 2010. Getting it right. Mencap, London. Online. Available: www.mencap.org.uk September 2012.

McCormack, B., McCance, T., 2010. Person-centered nursing: theory, models and methods. Wiley-Blackwell, Oxford.

McDonald, L., 2011. Florence Nightingale at first hand. Journal History of Medicine and Allied Sciences 66 (3), 403–406.

Mental Capacity Act, 2005. Online. Available: Mental health capacity act www.legislation.gov.uk/uksi/2011/2645/contents/made September 2012.

Ministry of Health, 1959. The Platt report: a report on the welfare of children in hospital. HMSO, London.

National Health Service and Community Care Act, 1990. Online. Available: www.legislation.gov.uk/ukpga/1990/19/contents September 2012.

National Statistics Office, 2011. Population estimates. September 2012.

Northouse, P., 2011. Introduction to leadership: concepts and practice, second ed. Sage, London.

Nursing and Midwifery Council, 2008a. The code: standards of conduct, performance and ethics for nurses and midwives. NMC, London. Online. Available: http://www.nmc-uk.org/Nurses-and-midwives/Standards-and-guidance1/The-code/The-code-in-full/ September 2012.

Nursing and Midwifery Council, 2008b. Standards to support learning and assessment in practice. NMC, London. Online. Available: http://www.nmc-uk.org/Documents/NMC-Publications/NMC-Standards-to-support-learning-assessment.pdf September 2012.

Nursing and Midwifery Council, 2010a. Item 8 NMC/10/05 March Council Report of the executive NMC London. Online. Available: http://www.nmc-uk.org/Documents/Council PapersAndDocuments/Council2010/March2010/NMC%2010%2005%20Exec%20Report.pdf September 2012.

Nursing and Midwifery Council, 2010b. Standards for pre-registration nursing education. Online. Available: http://standards.nmc-uk.org/PreRegNursing/statutory/Standards/Pages/Standards.aspx September 2012.

Nursing and Midwifery Council, 2010c. Preregistration nursing education. Annexe 3: Essential skills clusters. Online. Available: http://standards.nmc-uk.org/Documents/Annexe3_%20ESCs_16092010.pdf September 2012.

O'Keefe, M., McAllister, S.M., Stupans, I., 2011. Health-service organization and student clinical workplace learning opportunities. In: Billett, S., Henderson, A. (Eds.), Promoting professional learning. Springer, Dordrecht, The Netherlands.

Orem, D., 1991. Self-care deficit theory. Sage, California.

Parliamentary and Health Service Ombudsman (PHSO), 2010. Improving healthcare for people with learning disabilities. Parliamentary and Health Service Ombudsman and Local Government Ombudsman, London.

Peckover, S., 2011. From 'public health' to 'safeguarding children': British health visiting in policy, practice and research. Children & Society. 27 April 2011, DOI: 10.1111/j.1099-0860.2011.00370.x August 2012.

Peplau, H.E., 1952. Interpersonal relations in nursing: a conceptual framework of reference for psychodynamic nursing. Putman, New York.

Roper, N., Logan, W., Tierney, A.J., 2000. The Roper-Logan-Tierney model of nursing; based on activities of living. Churchill Livingstone, Edinburgh.

Roy, C., Andrews, H.A., 1999. The Roy adaptation model. Appleton & Lange, Stamford.

Royal College of Nursing, 2010. Mental health nursing of adults with learning disabilities. RCN, London.

Sanderson, H., 2007. Person centred planning. In: Gates, B. (Ed.), Learning disabilities, toward inclusion, fifth ed. Churchill Livingstone, Edinburgh.

Scottish Executive Health Department, 2008. Equally well: report of the ministerial task force on health inequalities caring. TSO, Edinburgh.

Simmons, C., Vostanis, P., 2009. Child and adolescent difficulties. In: Newell, R., Gournay, K. (Eds.), Mental health nursing, second ed. Churchill Livingstone, Edinburgh.

Smith, L., Coleman, V., Bradshaw, M. (Eds.), 2002. Family centred care. Palgrave, Basingstoke.

Stevenson, K., Ryan, S., Masterson, A., 2011. Nurse and allied health professional consultants: perceptions and experiences of the role. Journal of Clinical Nursing 20, 537–544.

Thornton, T., Lucas, P., 2011. On the very idea of a recovery model for mental health. Journal of Medical Ethics 37, 24–28.

Uhlmann, W., Schuette, J.L., Yashar, B. (Eds.), 2009. A guide to genetic counselling, second ed. Wiley, Hoboken.

United Kingdom Central Council, 1985. Project 2000: a new preparation for practice. UKCC, London.

Watson, J., Nelson, J., 2011. Measuring caring: international research on caritas as healing. Springer, New York.

Further reading

Benner, P., Tanner, C., Chesla, C., 2009. Expertise in nursing practice, second ed. Springer, New York.

Birchenall, P., Adams, N., 2011. The nursing companion, second ed. Palgrave Macmillan, London.

Gimenez, J., 2011. Writing for nursing and midwifery students, second ed. Palgrave Macmillan, London.

Hand, H., 2006. Promoting effective teaching and learning in the clinical setting. Nursing Standard 20 (39), 55–63.

Mason, D., Stephen, L., Isaacs, D., et al., 2011. The nursing profession: development, challenges, and opportunities. Jossey Bass, San Francisco.

Williamson, G.R., Jenkinson, T., Proctor-Childs, T., 2010. Contexts of contemporary nursing: transforming nursing practice. Learning Matters, Exeter.

Health and social care delivery systems

3

Annie Holme

LEARNING OUTCOMES

This chapter will help you:

- Begin to understand what is meant by health and social care provision and how it is organized
- Outline the structures of the National Health Service (NHS) in the UK and the key developments in the NHS since its inception
- Demonstrate an understanding of the multidisciplinary team (MDT) and multiagency working
- Begin to understand the framework and mechanisms for the provision of high quality health and social care
- Describe how patients/clients and the public can be involved in making decisions about care provision.

Introduction

The health and social care needs of people in the UK are provided by an extensive range of individuals and organizations. The distinction between health or social care needs often determines which organization and the type of caregivers who provide that care. This complex system of care provision is described as multidisciplinary because the individuals providing care are often from a variety of professional disciplines; and multiagency, which refers to the range of organizations involved. To add to this complexity, there are differences in the way that health and social care is delivered between the four countries that make up the UK. These variations have become more marked as a consequence of political devolution that began in the 1990s. This chapter will focus on the structure and function of services in England as the largest and most populous of the four UK countries. Where appropriate, some of the important variations within the other three countries will be highlighted, but readers will need to consider how the services apply to where they live.

Most people in the UK look to the National Health Service (NHS) to meet their health needs. There are many characteristics of the NHS that distinguish it from other countries' healthcare delivery systems; some of which can be traced back to the ideas and values that were behind its creation. The first section considers why the NHS was established, key developments in its history and how these have contributed to the health service that we are familiar with today. Healthcare systems in other comparable countries are also explored.

Social care provision is closely linked to healthcare delivery and for the individuals receiving care, the distinction between their health and social care needs may seem arbitrary. The care itself is often provided by separate organizations with different sources of funding, a range of different professionals and diverse ways of organizing and providing care. This chapter explores the differences between health and social care, how they are organized and funded, and some recent attempts to achieve better integration between the two systems.

The quality of health and social care has become increasingly important and mechanisms in place to maintain and improve care provision are considered in the final section along with ways of involving patients/clients and the public in choices about treatment and other healthcare decisions.

Health and social care provision

The organization of services provided and the delivery of health and social care have undergone numerous changes over past decades in order to meet the changing needs of the UK population. The most recent reforms and new proposals to the way the NHS is organized in England, set out in the *Health and Social Care Act* (HM Government 2012), are outlined.

As well as periodic reforms of NHS structure, governments also seek to address national health and social care issues by on-going development of health and social care policy. Over recent decades, some areas of health policy have emerged as being important to all governments whatever their ideology. These include improving the quality of care, expanding patient choice of care provision and increasing patient and public involvement in decisions about healthcare. These policies have a significant influence on the work currently undertaken by health and social care professionals and will be discussed in more detail below.

Creation and evolution of the NHS

Prior to the Second World War (1939–45), there was little national coordination and no control of health and social care in the UK. A range of private, local government and charitable organizations and individuals provided healthcare and as a consequence, there were disparities in the type, quantity and quality of healthcare available in the UK. For many people, the healthcare they needed was unaffordable or unavailable.

During the Second World War, the Emergency Health Service took control of all hospitals in the UK and for the first time, key components of healthcare provision were coordinated and directed by central government. This persuaded many people including health professionals and politicians that this was a workable, and indeed desirable, model for healthcare delivery. However, the principal impetus for the creation of the NHS was the *Beveridge Report* published in 1942, which identified five 'giants' or problems in UK society, namely:

- Disease
- Idleness (unemployment)
- Ignorance (poor educational standards)
- Squalor (poor housing)
- Want (poverty).

Beveridge (1942) recommended the establishment of a Welfare State to enable central government to address these problems through establishment of the NHS, full employment, state education up to 15 years, public housing and financial benefits for those in need. The welfare state system came into existence after the war with the NHS being established on 5 July 1948.

The founding principles of the NHS have remained constant since its inception with each new government committing itself to upholding them. These principles are that the service should be:

- *Universal* – free at the point of use and available to everyone according to their need and regardless of their ability to pay
- *Equitable* – equal access to high standards of care everywhere in the UK
- *Comprehensive* – quality healthcare provision to meet the needs of all
- *Collective* – centrally and directly funded by government through taxation.

Although the creation of the NHS had met with stiff resistance from some politicians and elements of the medical profession, the 1950s and 1960s were characterized by broad political and societal agreement that the NHS and the welfare state as a whole were beneficial and necessary. NHS costs increased throughout this time not only due to the rapid expansion of new treatments and technologies but also to previously unrecognized, and greatly underestimated, needs and growing public demand for healthcare. This led to an early realization that not all services could be free for all; and from 1952, charges for prescriptions, eye tests and dental services were gradually introduced. There was also recognition that choices would have to be made about which services could be provided (rationing); decisions that every government has faced since (Delamothe 2008). Key developments in the NHS are outlined in Box 3.1.

Changes – 1960s and 1970s

The 1960s saw many new hospitals being built as a consequence of the 1962 Hospital Plan with the aim of providing a district general hospital for every 125 000 people. There was also expansion in primary care services in the community with the development of multidisciplinary primary care teams working from health centres. By the end of the decade there was growing concern about the quality of long-term care provided to older adults, people with mental health problems and those with learning disabilities. Despite initiatives to address these relatively poorly funded services, examples of neglect and inadequate care have continued to come to light up to the present day (Ham 2009).

The 1970s saw a decade of economic and political crises that led to growing criticism of the welfare state for its failure to eradicate the five 'giants' identified in the Beveridge report, which were still very evident in the UK although altered in nature (Alcock et al 2004). The NHS and Social Services experienced major restructuring during this decade against a background of growing industrial conflict and social unrest. Local authority social services departments were established in 1971 following the Seebohm Report taking on responsibility for social care provision, including home helps and residential care. The NHS structure was reorganized with the aim of improving administration and increasing resources for neglected areas (Ham 2009). This period of political and social upheaval culminated in a significant change in the political arena with the election in 1979 of a Conservative government led by Margaret Thatcher.

Changes – 1980s and 1990s

The political and economic beliefs that guided the thinking of the Conservative governments of 1979–1997 aimed to decentralize decision-making and reduce the role of government in society, and focussed instead on 'free markets' and competition to drive the economy. This was in sharp contrast to government policy of the previous decades that had been characterized by state intervention in many industries and a substantial public sector. This change in political ideology led to significant reforms to health and social care provision. Two changes of significance were:

- *The Griffiths Report* (1983) led to the introduction of many more NHS management roles, an imperative to reduce waste and manage budgets more effectively; and contracting out of many services to the private sector, e.g. laundry, catering and cleaning.

| Evolution of the contemporary NHS | Box 3.1 |

The structure of the NHS has been reformed on a number of occasions, with different structures operating in Scotland, Wales and Northern Ireland and increasingly so since political devolution.

- 1948 – NHS inaugurated on 5 July
- 1949 – Patient demand for services outstripped supply pushing costs to worrying levels
- 1952 – Prescription charges introduced
- 1962 – Porrit Report recommended the setting up of primary, secondary and tertiary structures with area boards set up to run the NHS
- 1964 – Salmon Report recommended setting up new grading and pay structure for senior nurses (implemented in 1966)
- 1968 – Seebohm Report on the structure of local authority social services departments
- 1970 – Legislation for local authorities required creation of single Social Service Departments
- 1973 – NHS Reorganization Act set up Area and District Health Authorities to run hospital and community health services with public participation through Community Health Councils; appointment of first Health Service Ombudsman
- 1976 – Publication of the report on the future of child health services; publication of *Priorities for Health and Personal Social Services* in England required that choices would have to be made in healthcare for economic reasons
- 1979 – Publication of *Patients First*, which proposed simplification of the NHS structure for healthcare decisions to be made as near to the point of delivery as possible
- 1980 – *The Black Report:* Inequalities in Health (see Ch. 1)
- 1983 – *The Griffiths Report*; consequences included the introduction of general management which focused on finance and budgets, performance management and management of clinicians
- 1990 – *National Health Service and Community Care Act*; introduced NHS Trusts and competitive internal market which proved very expensive; 'modernization'; clinical governance; emphasis on community care, especially for people with mental illness and learning disabilities, and older adults; introduction of a range of service providers, i.e. NHS, charity, voluntary and informal services
- 1991 – *Citizens' charter* enacted and saw the start of hospital 'league tables'; for health, the Patient's Charter was introduced identifying consumerism, patient's rights and patient choice
- 1992 – White Paper *The Health of the Nation: A Strategy for Health* in England laid down 25 health policy targets; similar documents published in the other three UK countries

- 1997 – White Papers *The New NHS* (England), *Designed to Care* (Scotland) and NHS Wales: *Putting Patients First* published, with Scottish Parliament and Welsh Assembly assuming direct responsibility in these countries; end of internal market and increasing emphasis on cooperation and integrated care
- 1999 – White Paper *The Health Act* describes how the NHS will differ in each of the four nations of the UK and outlines powers to develop more partnerships between the NHS, local authorities and social services
- 1999 – White Paper *Saving Lives: Our Healthier Nation* published in England. Plans policies to improve health and reduce health inequalities
- 2000 – White paper *The NHS Plan: A Plan for Investment, A Plan for Reform* published, saw the introduction of National Service Frameworks (NSFs), associated with setting and monitoring of national standards
- 2000 – Walk-in Centres (now 93 in England)
- 2001 – Commission for Health Improvement (CHI) established
- 2002 – *The Wanless Report: Securing our future health: taking a long-term view*
- 2004 – Healthcare Commission replaces Commission for Health Improvement
- 2004 – White Paper *Choosing Health: Making Healthier Choices Easier* published in England
- 2004 – Foundation Trusts
- 2007 – *The Wanless Report* (A review of NHS funding and performance)
- 2007 – NHS Direct established
- 2008 – Darzi report *High Quality Care for all* – patient-centred care; a focus on primary care, i.e. prevention of ill health rather than treatment and cure; quality improvement, innovation services; nursing to become an all-graduate profession
- 2009 – The NHS Constitution
- 2010 – Care Quality Commission (CQC) replaces Healthcare Commission
- 2010 – White paper *Equity and Excellence: Liberating the NHS* published; more accountable to patients, reducing excessive bureaucracy and top-down control, 'patients will be at the heart of everything we do'
- 2011 – *Health and Social Care Bill* (amended June 2011 following *Future Forum Report*)
- 2012 – *Health and Social Care Act;* the major reorganization of the NHS in England proposed in *Equity and Excellence: Liberating the NHS* becomes law.

- *The National Health Service and Community Care Act* (1990) saw the introduction of an internal market within the NHS which it was believed would further increase efficiency and provide healthcare more relevant to the needs of local populations. This reform introduced a division in organizational roles within the health service with some organizations purchasing (commissioning) health services on behalf of a local population and others providing health services. Some individuals and organizations within primary care, e.g. general practitioners (GPs) became both commissioners and providers, while hospitals became solely providers of

healthcare, largely determined by contracts with commissioners. This division between commissioners and providers of services in the NHS continues today in England, having undergone various developments under both the Labour government of 1997–2010 and the Conservative/Liberal Democrat Coalition government that came into power in 2010. This reform also introduced the term 'Trust' to describe hospitals, a term which is still used in England today, although it also includes other organizations (e.g. Ambulance Service Trusts, p. 70). Acute trusts are those that provide a comprehensive range of emergency and elective (planned) services to adults and children. Mental health trusts provide services to those with mental health problems often on both an in-patient and community basis; while children's NHS trusts provide acute and/or long-term care to children only.

Changes – twenty-first century

The Labour governments of 1997–2010 were responsible for many significant NHS reforms in England. Many government reforms were laid out in *The NHS Plan: a plan for investment a plan for reform* (DH 2000a). Some of the key changes resulting from the *NHS Plan* were:

- Reduced waiting times for treatment (Box 3.2)
- National standards for care and treatment (National Service Frameworks, see p. 76)
- New career and pay structures for NHS staff
- Utilization of the private healthcare sector for NHS patients
- Better use of information technology.

 Critical thinking   Box 3.2

The NHS Plan … Targets: waiting times for surgery

As a consequence of waiting time targets introduced by *The NHS Plan* (DH 2000a), by 2009 most patients in England had their treatment within 18 weeks of being referred by their GP.

Student activities

Alice, who has pain and reduced mobility due to arthritis, has been told that she will be put on the waiting list for a hip replacement but is likely to wait 18 weeks for her surgery.

- Do you think 18 weeks is an appropriate length of time to wait for surgery?
- How would you feel if she was your mother?
- Find out the waiting time for hip replacement and other orthopaedic surgery in your locality.

Many of the ideas behind these reforms have also been reflected in changes in the other UK countries. The split between organizations that commission health services and those that deliver healthcare was maintained but with more emphasis initially on collaboration between providers rather than competition. Primary Care Trusts (PCTs) were established in 2002 to commission health services for their local population controlling 80% of the total NHS budget. They also provided community health services such as district nurses.

Since 2004, hospitals in England have been able to become Foundation Trusts if they meet specific quality and financial management criteria. Foundation Trusts remain within the NHS and are required to work with NHS guidance and standards but have more operational and financial autonomy in how they are run. They also represent an attempt to make the NHS accountable to patients and local populations. Patients, staff and people living in a locality can become members of a Foundation Trust and have an increased say in how care is delivered by attending trust meetings and other activities designed to involve the public.

Other developments included the introduction of the 'modern matron' role, schemes to improve hospital food and mechanisms to improve the joint working of health and social services.

The NHS Plan was followed some years later by the *High Quality Care for All: NHS Next Stage Review Report* (Darzi 2008). Lord Darzi, an NHS surgeon and health minister, produced a report that brought many of the original themes of *The NHS Plan* such as high quality care and patient choice, up-to-date. These two policies could be described as 'policy road maps' that set out the Government vision for health services.

Against a background of global recession, a Conservative/ Liberal Democrat Coalition government was formed in 2010; shortly afterwards, further changes to organization and delivery of the NHS were set out in the White Paper *Equity and Excellence: Liberating the NHS* (DH 2010a) and enacted by the *Health and Social Care Act* (HM Government 2012).

Since 2010, healthcare provision has been separated from the commissioning, with community health services being delivered by a range of organizations including community NHS trusts, non-profit making social enterprise organizations and acute hospital trusts. All NHS trusts are expected to become Foundation Trusts (see above) by 2013–2014. (See Further reading, e.g. Wise 2010 and DH 2012, for more information about the provisions within the *Health and Social Care Act* [HM Government 2012]).

Types of health and social care provision

As described earlier, a range of different organizations provide health and social care. These providers may be:

- Statutory
- Non-statutory
- Voluntary or charitable provision
- Private sector.

Statutory services are those controlled by Acts of Parliament (see Ch. 6). There are some aspects of care provision that are non-statutory, i.e. not governed by Acts of Parliament. Many of these cater for specific client groups, e.g. people with mental health problems or frail older adults. In addition, certain services are provided by voluntary agencies or charitable organizations, e.g. 'Together: for mental wellbeing', a leading UK Mental Health Charity, who provide services (Box 3.3).

Services provided by voluntary and consumer groups tend to be offered by self-help, disease-based or disease-focused groups. Examples of groups that provide support for carers and individuals include:

- Terrence Higgins Trust – HIV and AIDS
- National Osteoporosis Society – osteoporosis
- Scottish Association for Mental Health, MIND – mental health problems
- Marie Curie Cancer Care, Macmillan Cancer Support, Maggie's Cancer Caring Centres – cancer
- Age UK, Alzheimer's Scotland – older people and those with dementia.

Reflective practice   Box 3.3

Voluntary or charitable provision

Many health and social care services are provided by voluntary agencies or charitable organizations, e.g. Together: for mental wellbeing; Macmillan Cancer Support; Mencap, etc.

Student activities

- Choose one of the organizations listed below and find out about the support and services that they offer.
- Reflect with your mentor on the importance of the contribution of the voluntary/charitable sector to health and social care in the UK.

Resources

Age UK – www.ageuk.org.uk.
Macmillan Cancer Support – www.macmillan.org.uk.
Mencap the voice of learning disability – www.mencap.org.uk.
NSPCC – www.nspcc.org.uk.
Together: for mental wellbeing – www.together-uk.org.
All websites accessed August 2012.

Critical thinking   Box 3.4

Meeting Alice's needs

Alice, as you will remember, is on the waiting list for hip replacement surgery (see Box 3.2). Recently, she has fallen at home. Her hip is now very painful and this, in turn, restricts her movement. She is scared of falling again and this has stopped her doing many of the things she would normally do such as having a bath, going to the shops and meeting her friends. Alice tells her family that she is increasingly isolated and this is getting her down and making her feel depressed.

It is important to assess Alice's needs in order to maintain her dignity, improve her quality of life and prevent further deterioration of her mental and physical health.

Student activities

- Think about Alice's needs including:
  - Physical health e.g. arthritis, pain management (which may affect her sleep)
  - Falls
  - Activities of living, e.g. maintaining a safe environment, eating and drinking
  - Mental health, e.g. dealing with feelings of depression and fear of falling
  - Social well-being, e.g. social isolation, shopping.
- Discuss with your mentor how Alice's needs could be met and which service providers would be involved in your area.

As well as providing support and information for professionals, patients/clients and their families, these groups may also work to improve care and assistance provided by statutory services.

Private hospitals, care homes and clinics also provide services to people who in addition to paying taxes, choose to pay directly or indirectly, through private health insurance, for private healthcare services. The demand for private healthcare services is not uniform across the UK. Scotland, Wales and Northern Ireland have fewer private hospital beds per head of population than England.

In reality, the differences between these different types of organizations and the services have become increasingly blurred (Box 3.4). For example, since the 1980s, many acute hospitals have private companies who employ their own staff to provide core services such as cleaning. More recently, private healthcare provision has also been used by the NHS to reduce waiting lists for procedures such as magnetic resonance imaging (MRI) scans or minor, simple surgery such as cataract extraction (removal). NHS patients with mental health problems may be cared for in private hospitals such as The Priory Group.

Older adults requiring support to continue living in their own homes may find that their personal hygiene needs are met by care workers from a private or 'not for profit' company, although their need for this service will have been assessed and determined by their local authority social services department. An older adult requiring residential care will probably live in a home run by a private company, an individual or a 'not for profit' organization such as BUPA. People at the end-of-life may be cared for in a hospice run on a charitable basis but with some funding from the NHS. End-of-life care is increasingly provided in peoples' homes with the support of NHS community nurses or a social enterprise community care provider and specialist palliative care provided by charities such as Macmillan Cancer Support and Marie Curie Cancer Care (see Ch. 12). Social enterprises are those organizations which reinvest surplus funds into the community or business instead of focusing on making the most of profits for owners or shareholders (adapted from the Department of Trade and Industry 2002).

In summary, the NHS has a statutory obligation to look after people's healthcare needs but not their social care needs; these must be met by other organizations and agencies working both independently and together.

Funding of health and social care in the UK

How these services are funded is complex and differs between the four UK countries. Health and social care is funded by taxation collected by the UK government, which is then allocated locally using weighting systems which attempt to reflect the needs of the local population. In England, healthcare providers are reimbursed by Clinical Commissioning Groups through a system called 'Payment by Results' (PbR) with tariffs (prices) determined at a national level (DH 2010b).

The financial contribution that individuals make towards their health and social care depends on where in the UK they live; in England some people pay prescription charges, while in other countries they are free for all. The greatest variations in personal contributions towards care are for personal and social care provided in people's own homes, e.g. washing and dressing, preparing meals and help with cleaning. In Scotland, personal care is centrally funded, while in the other UK countries means-tested contributions are required. In England and Wales, there has been a drive to personalize social care provision; e.g. by giving people direct cash payments or personal budgets

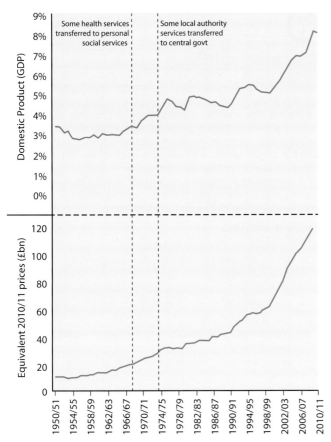

Fig. 3.1 • General government expenditure on UK Health Services: 1948/49–2009/10. (see: www.parliament.uk/briefing-papers/ SN00724 August 2012)

needs. There are many approaches to classifying health systems which use different characteristics for comparison. These include the way the health system is financed and delivered, political and ideological values, the country's economic resources and health outcomes and indicators.

The NHS is probably most usefully compared with its European neighbours not only because of similarities in political systems, economic resources and health needs but also due to having features in common with many European health systems. Germany for example, has a long history of state intervention in healthcare provision dating back to the nineteenth century (Box 3.5). This model of health insurance schemes with a mix of private and public funding is the most common system seen in Europe. A key characteristic in common with the NHS, is universal access to healthcare, regardless of individual income but often with much more choice of healthcare provider than is possible in the UK.

Features of the health system in Germany **Box 3.5**

- Most German citizens are covered by public health insurance providers that are funded through a combination of employer and employee contributions
- Those earning over a certain level can opt for a private health insurance provider
- Healthcare is provided by a range of public, not for profit and private organizations and individuals
- Patients can choose their GP and specialist healthcare providers
- Long-term care insurance is often provided along with health insurance.

---

enabling them to arrange and purchase services suited to their individual needs.

Ongoing increases in healthcare costs (Fig. 3.1) are a challenge for all governments; reflected in policies that aim to improve efficiency and productivity. Although there is evidence that increased health spending does not automatically lead to improved health outcomes (Birn et al 2009); a review of future funding for the NHS produced by Derek Wanless in 2002 led to the conclusion that the NHS needed extra funding to bring about necessary improvements (DH 2002). Consequently, for some years thereafter, NHS funding increased to bring it level with the average amount spent in other European countries. The global economic crisis overshadowing the end of the 2000s meant that NHS spending needed further review. Subsequent governments have all committed to make savings while maintaining and improving quality through innovation, prevention of ill health and increasing productivity collectively known by the umbrella term NHS Improvement, Quality, Innovation, Productivity and Prevention (QIPP) (see Further reading, e.g. NHS Improvement, DH 2009).

Comparisons of the UK funding model with other systems

Birn et al (2009) argue that the healthcare system in each country reflects its political and societal values, and healthcare

The NHS is often contrasted with the healthcare system in the United States (Box 3.6), which Birn et al (2009 p.605) describes as 'one of the world's most fragmented, chaotic and irrational examples of health services organization'. There is no universal health insurance system in the USA but instead, there is a mixture of private and employment-based insurance schemes; and publicly funded schemes for those on low incomes (Medicaid) and those over 65 and long-term disabled (Medicare). Many people are not eligible for these schemes and cannot afford health insurance or have limited coverage, with the consequence that 42% of US citizens are either uninsured or underinsured (Schoen et al 2008). Healthcare provision is mostly private or 'not for profit' and operates in a very competitive market. For those who can afford it, the US

Features of health system in the United States **Box 3.6**

- Mix of private and public funding and delivery
- Significant proportion of the US population uninsured or underinsured for their healthcare needs
- Market-driven private health insurance system with multiple competing providers and a complex system of incentives and disincentives
- Costly system relative to other developed nations.

---

system has the most medically advanced healthcare in the world and spends more *per capita* on health than any other nation. However, because it lacks universal access to care, on some health indicators for the whole population, such as infant mortality, the USA does not perform as well as other high-income countries.

All governments have to make choices about financing healthcare. They also spend more than they would like to and complain of waste and poor control, and all are concerned for the future. Governmental choices are largely determined by their income and resources available, e.g. many Southern African countries are forced to make difficult choices between funding treatment for HIV/AIDS versus treatment for malaria. Low- and middle-income countries have healthcare systems based on different models with some opting for publicly funded and centrally controlled systems and others a mix of private and publicly funded and delivered provision. Many low-income nations struggle with overwhelming health problems and needs due to extreme poverty, difficulties in distributing available health resources as a consequence of poor infrastructure and poor health outcomes such as high infant and child mortality that would be unimaginable in more affluent nations. Yet, there are examples of relatively low-income countries such as Cuba that have developed low-cost healthcare systems with health outcomes and indicators such as life expectancy, infant mortality and number of health professionals *per capita* comparable or better than high-income countries (Birn et al 2009).

The National Health Service

This section of the chapter focuses on how the NHS is structured and the functions of the various bodies within it. It also briefly describes the roles of some of the health and social care disciplines that contribute to MDTs delivering health services.

The original aims of the NHS to provide a comprehensive service to meet the health needs of the entire UK population remain true today and are met by providing services for acute and long-term conditions in a variety of settings, such as hospitals, day hospitals, health centres, home care, walk-in centres, through telemedicine, such as a scan being viewed by an expert who may be many miles away, and through remote sites accessed by telephone or website (e.g. NHS Direct in England, NHS 24 in Scotland). However, the healthcare needs of the population when the NHS was first introduced were very different from the healthcare needs of today's population.

The newly formed NHS was criticized for its focus on cure rather than prevention, perhaps reflecting optimism in the ability of modern medical science to provide 'a pill for every ill'. However, recent decades have seen increasing concern with the growing burden of ill-health on society and the potential economic and social costs. Some of this ill-health reflects changing demographic factors, as the population ages and people live longer; and diseases associated with old age such as cancer, cardiovascular diseases and dementia become more prevalent. The resurgence in infectious diseases such as tuberculosis, emergence of new strains of influenza and *Escherichia*

coli (*E. coli*) food poisoning and, in more recent years, high levels of ill-health associated with lifestyle choices and social behaviours, namely smoking, drinking alcohol, unhealthy diets and lack of exercise, have become a priority in government policy. The increasing emphasis on the prevention of illness and promotion of health within UK healthcare policy is discussed in Chapter 1.

Structure and functions of the NHS

The structure of the NHS in England is the most complex in the UK. This is not only due to its larger population and geographical size but also a consequence of the impact of government reforms that only pertain to England and not to the other UK countries. Information about the differences in structure, health policies and services in Wales, Scotland and Northern Ireland is available from the appropriate government website (see Useful websites, p. 80).

In England, the Department of Health (DH) is charged to ensure that the health of the population is looked after. If necessary, they bring Bills before Parliament to ensure that the appropriate legal framework is in place for meeting their responsibility (see Ch. 6). The Secretary of State and the health ministers within the DH have the responsibility to ensure that the NHS, social care and public health services work together to meet the nation's health and social care needs.

The Secretary of State and health ministers are advised by a group of national clinical directors and key specialists covering the full range of health service provision, e.g. mental health, children, primary care, older people and cancer. These positions are mirrored in the other UK countries.

Central government, in its various forms, is the enacting, funding and driving force for provision of services. The government develops strategies and plans for the health of the nation, legislates how this will be done and provides the funding that enables various professional and non-professional groups to deliver services to the population.

In England, healthcare is commissioned by Clinical Commissioning Groups (CCGs) that replaced PCTs (see p. 64) as part of the reformed NHS structure introduced by the *Health and Social Care Act* (2012) and overseen by the NHS Commissioning Board and locally by Health and Well-being boards within local authorities. CCGs are advised by Clinical Senates and Clinical Networks made up of clinicians from different specialties and disciplines. Hospital and community-based care can be commissioned from private, social enterprise and NHS providers (Box 3.7).

NHS provision is divided into primary, secondary and tertiary care, with various forms of intermediate care used to bridge the gap between primary and secondary care.

Primary healthcare

GPs and other members of the MDT provide a range of primary healthcare services directly to people living in the community. For most people in the UK, their first contact with the health service has, up until relatively recently, been the GP. Traditionally, GPs and other healthcare professionals working

? Critical thinking   Box 3.7

The structure of the NHS varies in each UK country, with organizations having different titles and roles

Student activities

- Ascertain the titles and key functions of NHS organizations in your area.
- How easy was it to find this information?
- Discuss examples with your mentor or a peer.

Resources

See Useful websites, p. 80.

from the same base, such as the GP's premises or a health centre, have provided most community-based primary healthcare services for non-emergency conditions.

The services offered by primary healthcare teams may also include: immunization in schools; sexual health and prevention of teenage pregnancy; the prevention of falls in older people; nurse-led mobile outreach services to rural communities; working with homeless people and cardiac rehabilitation. Community mental health nurses often work in health centres providing nursing interventions for people experiencing mental health problems (Box 3.8).

Reflective practice   Box 3.8

Working with others to improve mental health

Community mental health nurses work with people who are experiencing mental distress and may offer services such as anxiety management and cognitive behaviour therapy (CBT) for people who experience depression as individual or group therapy sessions. They may work with other community mental health nurses, e.g. in group therapy, but they may also work with other professionals such as psychiatrists, occupational therapists, art therapists, complementary and alternative medicine (CAM) practitioners and speech and language therapists.

Student activities

- Reflect on a patient/client you met during a placement who needed help from many different professionals.
- Consider what worked well and the benefits from having different professionals involved in care.
- Identify any problems with team working, e.g. keeping everyone informed; discuss these with your mentor.
- Using the website below, find out more about the roles of key members of the MDT.

Resource

NHS Careers – www.nhscareers.nhs.uk/career.shtml August 2012.

Newer first access routes

People may also access NHS advice and healthcare through walk-in centres (WIC), which are mainly nurse-led, need no appointments and offer advice and treatment for minor

conditions. Telephone and web-based health services, e.g. NHS Direct in England and NHS 24 in Scotland, offer a 24-hour nurse-led telephone health information and advice service, with further information and advice available online; these services provide a single access point to the NHS out-of-hours services (Box 3.9).

Health promotion   Box 3.9

Accessing health information and healthcare

During the last decade there has been a massive increase in ways of accessing health information and healthcare

Student activities

Use the NHS Choices website to find out:
- The location of GPs in your locality and Walk-in Centre (WIC)
- The range of services provided by WICs
- Your rights and responsibilities as an NHS patient
- How to ensure healthcare while on holiday within Europe
- About online health check tools.

Resource

NHS choices – www.nhs.uk August 2012.

Intermediate care

This is designed to blur the boundaries between acute hospital and community care with the aim of preventing unnecessary hospital admissions, providing rehabilitation and recovery for patients discharged from acute care/hospitals. It aims to promote independence at home and prevent or delay long-term admission to residential care. Intermediate care may be provided in nursing homes, community hospitals or in patients' homes by MDTs including nurses and therapists. One example is a dedicated stroke rehabilitation and general rehabilitation unit in Norfolk for patients leaving acute hospital care.

Intermediate care has obvious advantages for both patients and the NHS. Patients can leave acute hospital care sooner or their admission can be prevented by the timely intervention of a fast response specialist team at home.

Secondary and tertiary healthcare

Secondary healthcare is provided by most acute hospitals and usually includes general medicine, surgery (rather than specialist services), orthopaedics and child health, as well as maternity services, some in-patient mental health services and often intensive care and emergency care. Emergency Departments (previously known as Accident and Emergency (A&E) Departments) may also have nurse-led minor injuries units.

Secondary healthcare is usually acute and can be either elective or emergency care and normally takes place in a NHS hospital. Elective care is planned specialist medical or surgical care, which generally follows referral from a community health professional, most often the GP. Examples of elective care include hip replacement operations or a course of chemotherapy for cancer. Elective care can be provided to inpatients, day-patients, or at outpatient clinics. Other examples of secondary care services include services for acute mental health problems and older adults.

Tertiary healthcare services are specialist hospital-based services such as neurosurgery (brain surgery) or cancer care for patients/clients with less common conditions, or needing highly specialized treatments. Tertiary care is usually provided in regional or national large acute teaching hospitals or specialist hospitals which serve large populations. Some of these and also many NHS hospitals where secondary healthcare is delivered, are attached to universities and part of their role is to provide training for health professionals.

Services for specific groups

Specific services such as those for people with mental health problems, children and those needing urgent transport to a healthcare facility are explored in this next section.

Mental healthcare

People who require hospital admission for mental health problems may be treated on a mental health unit of an acute general hospital or in a mental health hospital that will often provide a range of inpatient services including psychiatric intensive care, child and adolescent mental health services (CAMHS) and secure units. Mental health hospitals also often provide community teams to help patients recover from and prevent hospital admissions and also specialist services to support people with drug and alcohol misuse problems. Tertiary (regional) centres, e.g. Broadmoor Hospital in England and The State Hospital in Scotland, provide mental health services, within secure units, for people who pose a high degree of risk to themselves or to others.

Health policies that have shaped and improved mental health services include the *National Service Framework for Mental Health: Modern Standards and Service Models* (DH 1999) and *No Health Without Mental Health: A Cross Government Mental Health Outcomes Strategy for People of all Ages* (DH 2011a). These policies have emphasized the need for clear care planning involving patients and carers whenever possible, well supported and managed community treatment and care, proper attention to physical as well as mental health needs and to optimize each individual's potential for recovery (Box 3.10).

Children's healthcare

It is widely accepted that children are best cared for in their own homes but if they do need hospital treatment, specialist staff and environments are required to ensure their safety and well-being. Action for Sick Children, a UK charity whose purpose is to enable the best quality of care possible for sick children, drew up a document outlining the rights that children should be entitled to should they be admitted to hospital. This has been adopted as the *Charter for Children in Hospital* by the European Association for Children in Hospital (EACH 2001) and sets out good practices when caring for children in hospital. These include ensuring that parents or guardians can

---

| **'No health without mental health'** | **Box 3.10** |

The development of this policy involved a range of different people and organizations including government departments, local government and representatives from patient and carer groups. Six objectives were agreed:

1. More people will have good mental health:
   * More people of all ages and backgrounds will have better well-being and good mental health
   * Fewer people will develop mental health problems – by starting well, developing well, living well and ageing well.
2. More people with mental health problems will recover:
   * More people who develop mental health problems will have good quality of life – greater ability to manage their own lives, stronger social relationships, a greater sense of purpose, the skills they need for living and working, improved chances in education, better employment rates and a suitable and stable place to live.
3. More people with mental health problems will have good physical health:
   * Fewer people with mental health problems will die prematurely, and more people with physical ill health will have better mental health.
4. More people will have a positive experience of care and support:
   * Care and support, wherever it takes place, should offer timely, evidenced-based interventions and approaches that give people the greatest choice over their own lives, in the least restrictive environment, and should ensure that people's human rights are protected.
5. Fewer people will suffer avoidable harm:
   * People receiving care and support should have confidence that the services they use are of the highest quality and at least as safe as any other public service.
6. Fewer people will experience stigma and discrimination:
   * Public understanding of mental health will improve and, as a result, negative attitudes and behaviours to people with mental health problems will decrease.

(From DH 2011a)

---

stay with their child, that children are cared for with other children of a similar developmental age and where appropriate, are involved in making decisions about their care (see Ch. 6).

Children's services have undergone major reforms with the aim of providing every child with the best start in life and protecting them from harm through better integrated health, education and social services. The need for more effective communication between organizations and disciplines and services designed to meet the needs of individuals and populations has been recognized. This led to the establishment of Children's Trusts within each local authority to integrate all children's services provided in that area. Other initiatives include 'Sure Start' Children's Centres, which bring together a range of services to support parents and children from pregnancy to starting school with the aim of giving every child the best possible start in life. The requirement for every local authority in England to have a Children's Trust and to provide Sure Start schemes has been relaxed but integrated and comprehensive children's services remain a priority. See Box 3.11

 Health promotion   **Box 3.11**

'Every Child Matters'

'The five key outcomes that really matter for children and young people's well-being are:

- *Being healthy:* enjoying good physical and mental health and living a healthy lifestyle
- *Staying safe:* being protected from harm and neglect and growing up able to look after themselves
- *Enjoying and achieving:* getting the most out of life and developing broad skills for adulthood
- *Making a positive contribution:* to the community and to society and not engaging in anti-social or offending behaviour
- *Economic well-being:* overcoming socioeconomic disadvantages to achieve their full potential in life'.

(Every Child Matters, p 14 ©Crown Copyright 2003.)

Student activities

- Identify a vulnerable child you have met on placement and consider the interventions in place to enable him or her to reach their potential.
- Think about the contribution of each member of the MDT involved in promoting health and well-being in this situation.
- Discuss your findings with your mentor.

Reference Resources

Children Act, 2004 – www.legislation.gov.uk/ukpga/2004/31/contents.

Department of Health, 2004. National Service Framework for Children, Young People and Maternity Services. Online. Available: www.dh.gov.uk/en/Publicationsandstatistics/Publications/PublicationsPolicyAndGuidance/DH_4089101.

Every Child Matters, 2003 – www.education.gov.uk/consultations/downloadableDocs/EveryChildMatters.pdf.

All websites accessed August 2012.

---

for key government policies that have set these changes in place.

Ambulance Service Trusts

The ambulance service in England provides emergency access to healthcare through paramedic first response vehicles or emergency ambulances staffed by paramedics. Requests (999/112 calls) for attendance of an ambulance are prioritized – the most urgent being for life-threatening situations. If necessary, the patient's condition is stabilized, e.g. intravenous fluid replacement, administration of 'clot busting' drugs (thrombolytics), before onward transport to an Emergency Department or specialist centre; this is usually by road but in urgent cases, might be by air ambulance to regional Major Trauma Centres. Ambulance services are also responsible for transporting many patients to hospital for non-urgent treatment.

Special health authorities

Special health authorities such as the National Institute for Health and Clinical Excellence (NICE) and NHS Blood and

Transplant provide services to the whole of England. They are independent but can be subject to ministerial direction like other NHS bodies.

Multidisciplinary teamwork

Practitioners from a range of professional disciplines provide healthcare within the NHS. To meet peoples' variable and often complex needs, individuals and teams need to work together to coordinate and plan care delivery. In many settings, different disciplines work together as a MDT while in others, individuals and teams have to ensure that there are clear channels of communication between the different professional groups, e.g. by sharing patient records, and holding regular multidisciplinary meetings and case conferences. Within each discipline, there may be many different roles and posts dependent on the area and specialty. Inter-professional learning (IPL) is a feature of preregistration nursing programmes (see Ch. 4), which is designed to ensure that healthcare students become familiar with each others' roles and learn to work together from an early stage in their professional careers.

Nursing is an exceptionally varied and broad health discipline; qualified nurses may work in roles that are scarcely recognizable as the same profession. Some examples are:

- Working as part of an outreach team addressing the mental health needs of homeless rough sleepers
- Providing one-to-one care for very acutely sick babies, children and adults in neonatal, paediatric, adult and psychiatric intensive care units
- Working independently as a nurse practitioner in a health centre or performing diagnostic procedures such as endoscopy in a hospital
- Being part of a rehabilitation team helping patients recover from and learning to live with disability following stroke or other brain injury. (See Ch. 2 for more information about nursing roles and fields of nursing practice.)

Doctors, like nurses, have many different roles and titles. Those who work in hospitals usually specialize in surgery (surgeons) or medicine (physicians), with many specialties within these broad areas. There is also a hierarchy of positions from newly qualified foundation year doctors to consultants. Doctors who choose to work in primary care become GPs and work with a broad base of knowledge although many become specialized in certain areas. They promote health, diagnose and treat patients in the community or refer them for specialist investigations and treatments in hospitals.

Physiotherapists specialize in promoting mobility and helping to rehabilitate people who have suffered loss of physical function due to, e.g. illness, injury or old age. Occupational therapists assess and treat people of all ages who experience physical and mental health problems through the use of physical activities. Dieticians promote health and manage disease by applying the principles of nutritional science to improve people's diet and eating habits. Speech and language therapists (SLT) work with people of all ages assessing and treating speech, language and communication problems and difficulty in swallowing. The roles of social workers are explored below and those of osteopaths, chiropractics and other complementary and alternative medicine therapists are outlined in Chapter 10.

It is important to recognize that individual patient's/client's needs may not reflect fields of practice and professional boundaries; many people will have several members of the MDT providing their care.

Social care provision

Historically, social care has not been a function or a responsibility of the healthcare system but of local government. These authorities organize the provision of social care under the auspices of social services departments (known as social work departments in Scotland). Many of the services offered by the social care sector nowadays are the result of joint ventures between the health service, other statutory services, such as education and the criminal justice system, and non-statutory organizations and the voluntary sector. Multidisciplinary and multiagency working is central to social care provision.

Social care is provided to people of all ages and with a range of social care needs, e.g. older adults (people aged 65 and over), younger adults and children with physical disabilities, adults and children with learning disabilities, 'at risk' children and 'looked after' children. Many social care clients, including the groups above may be particularly vulnerable (see p. 72).

Structure and funding of social care provision

There is some confusion about what 'social care' means because some authors use the terms 'social services', 'social care' and 'social work' interchangeably, but they are, in fact, quite different. Even when there is agreement as to what the different terms mean, the way in which services are delivered and by which organization may vary across the UK.

'Social services' is the broad term used to describe the provision of both social care and social work. It is usually coordinated and managed by a local authority social services department. The social work role is explored below.

Social care refers to the support given to frail, disabled and vulnerable individuals who are unable to fully provide for themselves and may take the form of personal care (help with washing, dressing and feeding) and other services such as domestic cleaning, help with shopping, transport and day centres. A range of organizations including voluntary organizations and unpaid carers provide social care. Although distinct from healthcare, social care is often provided alongside healthcare in people's homes. Think back to Box 3.4 where you considered Alice's needs, e.g. someone may receive the following services to enable them to live in their own home:

- Help with washing and dressing from a social care worker who increasingly have a National Vocational Qualification (NVQ)
- Prepared meals from a 'meals on wheels' service both organized and possibly totally or partially funded by the local authority social services department
- Weekly transport to a day centre or healthcare centre.

Similarly, people who can no longer live independently in their own homes may still receive both social care and nursing care in a residential setting.

Social care is largely funded by central government with further funds from taxation raised by local councils (council tax); however, unlike healthcare, social care services are subject to means-testing and charging. The voluntary sector also provides social care, e.g. through organizations such as Barnardos, Shelter.

Social care provision by the voluntary sector

A growing proportion of social care is provided by voluntary sector organizations. They receive money from both central government and local authorities for specific projects, and services are provided by both paid social care workers and volunteers. For example:

- *SANE*, the mental health charity works to raise awareness of mental health problems and provides emotional support and advice through a telephone helpline, email and an online support forum. It also obtains feedback from service users so health and social care providers can better target their services.
- *Barnardos* runs many projects across the UK dealing with a wide range of issues affecting children and young people; these include homelessness, disability, crime and drug and alcohol misuse.
- *Shelter*, a pressure group, campaigns to end homelessness and poor housing in the UK, and works to support homeless people move into suitable and permanent accommodation. It provides a telephone advice helpline for people with any type of housing problem.
- *Mencap*, 'the voice of learning disability', is a charity for learning disabled people and provides long-term accommodation for those with a learning disability. They also provide support and advice for people with learning disabilities and their families living in their own homes. Mencap also has a National College (two sites in England and one in Wales) where young people with a learning disability can learn the skills they will need for adulthood, developing the personal, social and practical skills required for independence by using local community facilities and engaging in real-life working environments, e.g. shops, cafés, farms.

Social workers

Principles of human rights and social justice are fundamental to social work. Social workers are employed by local authorities and some voluntary agencies, e.g. NSPCC, to identify children or adults who might be in need of individual support or protection as a result of their social or family circumstances. They will either provide this support directly or assist their clients in securing support from other agencies. For their adult clients, social workers generally work in an enabling role. Social workers are professionally accountable for their practice and are not entitled to use the title 'Social Worker' unless they are registered with the Health and Care Professions Council (HCPC) which regulates professional standards.

As with registered nurses, social workers and other professionals are frequently unable to meet all of the needs of their clients. Many social workers work as part of a team that may involve social care workers or support workers in addition to others within the MDT (Box 3.12).

 Reflective practice   **Box 3.12**

Key roles of social workers

All nurses in every setting will have contact with social workers as multidisciplinary and multiagency collaboration increases.

Student activities

- Reflect on your understanding of what social workers do.
- Access the websites below and check your understanding.
- Discuss with your mentor the specific roles that social workers perform in your field of practice.

Resources

Scottish Social Services Council, 2011. A career in social services. Online. Available: www.sssc.uk.com/component/option,com_docman/Itemid,486/format,raw/gid,1712/task,doc_view/tmpl,component August 2012.

NHS Education for Scotland Changing lives – www.knowledge.scot.nhs.uk/changinglives.aspx August 2012.

Safeguarding children and vulnerable adults

In the same way that healthcare staff should prevent those under their care coming to harm, all those who work with children and vulnerable adults have a duty to identify those who may be at risk of abuse and take action to prevent abuse occurring. Abuse can take many forms including:

- Physical
- Chemical, including excessive use of sedating medication in people with dementia
- Psychological
- Sexual
- Financial or material
- Neglect
- Discrimination.

In the past, the role of identifying and dealing with abuse was seen primarily as the responsibility of those in direct contact with children and vulnerable adults such as social workers,

children's nurses, health visitors and teachers. However in recent years, repeated exposures of abuse, particularly of children, has led to this becoming seen as everyone's responsibility. The term 'safeguarding' describes activities that not only protect vulnerable individuals but also work to prevent abuse. For example, there is a legal requirement for all organizations where individuals may have contact with children or vulnerable adults to use the Criminal Records Bureau (CRB) (Protection of Vulnerable Groups, PVG, in Scotland) to check the suitability of their employees and volunteers.

The inquiries that followed high profile cases of abuse such as the tragic death of Victoria Climbie in 2000 produced reports that heavily influenced subsequent government policy and legislation, e.g. the Government Green Paper *Every Child Matters* 2003, the *Every Child Matters: Change for Children* 2004 and the subsequent *Children Act* 2004. However, another child, Peter Connelly (Baby P) died in 2007 within the same London Borough as Victoria Climbie was murdered. Further inquiries and reports have highlighted problems in the way safeguarding and child protection are managed and made recommendations for changes which have been reflected in government policy such as *Working Together to Safeguard Children* (Department for Education 2010). (See Further reading, e.g. Department for Education 2011.)

Other key legislation introduced to protect people who may not be able to make decisions for themselves is *The Mental Capacity Act* 2005 and the *Mental Health Act* 2007 (see Ch. 6).

An equally important problem, is the safeguarding of vulnerable adults. The government paper, *No Secrets: The Protection of Vulnerable Adults* (DH 2000b, p 9) defines a vulnerable adult as someone aged 18 or over 'who is in need of community care services by reason of mental or other disability, age or illness and who is or maybe unable to take care of him or herself or unable to protect him or herself against significant harm or exploitation'. Recommendations for safeguarding vulnerable adults were updated in a series of *Safeguarding Adults: The Role of Health Services* (DH 2011b) papers that emphasized the need for multiagency working, being vigilant for signs of abuse, making decisions and taking appropriate action in response to suspected abuse.

Another area of great concern in recent years has been that of elder abuse which is often hidden, and can take many forms, but does not receive the same media and therefore public attention as child abuse. National and local projects have tried to determine the scale and the nature of elder abuse in the UK, as well as initiatives to address this. Action on Elder Abuse (see Useful websites, p. 80) is a UK charity that works to raise awareness and provide support in this area.

Health and social care staff play key roles in identifying suspected abuse and, more importantly, taking appropriate action and ensuring their concerns are communicated effectively. The role of social workers in dealing with suspected child abuse has been outlined above; however all professional groups have equal responsibilities to work to protect children and vulnerable adults. The Nursing and Midwifery Council (NMC) describe safeguarding as part of everyday nursing practice in all settings (Box 3.13).

Critical thinking   Box 3.13

Safeguarding

The responsibility for safeguarding and protecting children and vulnerable adults belongs equally to all health and social care professionals regardless of their field of practice. It can also be argued that it is a moral responsibility for all members of society to take action if abuse is suspected.

- Tom is 82 years old and a patient on one of your placements; he is regularly visited by his next door neighbour, Jim. On admission, Tom had commented how lucky he is to have Jim next door and how well he looks after him, doing his shopping, paying his bills and managing his affairs for him. One day you notice that Jim is raising his voice with Tom on a visit and that Tom looks quite distressed. After Jim has left, Tom tells you that Jim was asking him for money and that Tom couldn't understand why he needed it as he was in hospital and needed no shopping. This incident has made Tom feel anxious about his relationship with Jim.

- Sarah is a 40-year-old woman with Down's syndrome. She is looked after by her 83-year-old mother who is becoming increasingly frail and is having to share the responsibility of care for Sarah with other members of the family, including an aunt and uncle. You notice that Sarah who is normally very cheerful becomes quiet and withdrawn when she has spent time with her aunt and uncle. You also observe bruising on Sarah's arms and chest – when you ask where they came from, she starts crying and says she is too frightened to tell you.

- One of your neighbours is a young woman who has two pre-school children who often look dirty and poorly clothed. The elder boy occasionally has bruises on his face. You often hear the children crying and their mother shouting at them. One evening, the crying and shouting is worse than usual, and you hear a loud bang and then screaming from one of the children.

Student activities

- After reading each scenario above, consider your responsibilities and possible actions that could be taken.
- Discuss your ideas with your mentor.

Resources

Action on Elder Abuse – www.elderabuse.org.uk
NSPCC – www.nspcc.org.uk.
Nursing and Midwifery Council – www.nmc-uk.org/Nurses-and-midwives/Regulation-in-practice/Safeguarding-New/. All websites accessed August 2012.

Social services for older adults

In England, older adults make up 72% of social care clients (NHS Information Centre 2009). Services offered for older adults generally focus on caring for people in their own homes, promoting independence and reducing time spent in hospital. How independence is promoted and achieved depends upon the context in which people are being cared for, but it is essential that there is close collaboration between health and social care workers when delivering older people's services; especially when these include homecare, meals provision, respite and day-care, and cleaning services.

For most people, being able to look after themselves is fundamental to their independence and self-esteem, and having control and being able to make choices about how people look after themselves is crucial. The promotion of self-care is one way that social care staff and nurses can help people to maintain their independence and dignity. The *Essence of Care 2010 Benchmarks for the Fundamental Aspects of Care* (DH 2010c) (see p. 78, Box 3.19) include one for self-care, acknowledging the importance of this aspect of care planning and delivery (Box 3.14).

Reflective practice   Box 3.14

Benchmarks for best practice in self-care

- '*People* are enabled to make choices about caring for themselves and those choices are respected
- *People's* ability to care for themselves is continuously assessed, planned, implemented, evaluated and reviewed to meet their needs
- *People's* care is continuously assessed for risk of harm to themselves and their carers, and is revised to meet their needs
- *People* and carers have the knowledge and skills to manage relevant aspects of *people's* care
- *People*, carers, staff and/organizations work in partnership to meet care needs
- *People* and carers can access services and resources to enable them to manage relevant aspects of care
- *People's* environment promotes their ability to care responsibly for themselves'.

(DH 2010c, p 8)

Student activities

- Consider the best practice benchmarks above.
- Think about a patient/client you met on placement and reflect on how much choice the person had, and to what extent they participated in planning and evaluating services.

Social services for children

In addition to the social worker roles described earlier, some collaborate with other professionals, within statutory frameworks, to protect and safeguard all children and to identify vulnerable and 'at-risk' children. In England and Wales, Local Safeguarding Children Boards (LSCBs) – comprising local authorities, NHS bodies, the police and others, coordinate the activities of the various agencies to ensure that they work effectively to safeguard children (see Ch. 6).

Following referral and assessment, an interagency child protection conference can make a child subject to a Child Protection Plan if they decide that they are at continuing risk of significant harm such as injury, abuse or neglect. Ideally parents, caregivers and, if they are able, children themselves should be involved in this process. The confidential register of at-risk children is kept by the Social Services Department but is available to professionals involved in safeguarding children, e.g. social workers, health visitors, doctors, teachers, police officers.

In most instances involving children, social workers have lead responsibility for assessment of children's needs as well as assessing their parents' ability to care for them. In the majority of cases, children will remain at home with social services coordinating the plan and interventions to safeguard the child as well as setting out the respective roles and contributions of parents, family members, professionals and other agencies. They will, where necessary, support parents to increase their skills, e.g. through parenting classes.

Sometimes, as a last resort, the child protection team will need to obtain a court order authorizing removal of the child from the family home in order to safeguard their welfare. Where a child has been removed from home as part of a care order, the social worker ensures that appropriate arrangements are in place for their care with their own participation as well as that of other agencies, e.g. the police, school and health services, and the Children's Panel in Scotland. This partnership, wherever possible, will also involve the child's parents.

Social workers may also work with and support families who have a child with a physical disability in order to help minimize the impact of the disability and help them to reach their potential and to lead as full a life as possible. This may involve organizing short-term breaks with foster parents or, where necessary, care in a residential unit or helping with school and leisure activities, e.g. swimming, youth clubs.

Social services for people with a learning disability

There are about 1.5 million people with a learning disability in the UK (Mencap 2011). In 2008, it was estimated that there were 177 000 known users of learning disability services (Emerson & Hatton 2008). Learning disability is defined in *Valuing People: A New Strategy for Learning Disability for the 21st Century* (DH 2001a, p 14) as the presence of:

○ 'A significantly reduced ability to understand new or complex information, to learn new skills (impaired intelligence), with:

○ a reduced ability to cope independently (impaired social functioning);

○ which started before adulthood, with a lasting effect on development'.

There is an equivalent publication in Scotland (see Further reading, Scottish Executive 2000). Services for people with learning disabilities in the UK have since gradually moved from large hospitals into the community. Government policy for people with learning disabilities (DH 2009) is based on four guiding principles, which were reaffirmed in the document cited above:

- *Rights* – People with learning disabilities and their families have the same human rights as everyone else.
- *Independent living* – This means that all disabled people should have greater choice and control over the facilities they need to go about their daily lives; including equal access to housing, education, employment, leisure and transport opportunities and to participate in family and community life.
- *Control* – This is about people being involved in and in control of their life decisions. By having the necessary information and support to understand different options

and their implications and consequences, people are able to make informed decisions about their own lives.

- *Inclusion* – This means enabling people, with support where needed, to be able to participate in all aspects of community life – working, learning, getting about, meeting people – and includes being part of social networks and having equal access to goods and services (adapted from DH 2009).

The overarching aim is to personalize care for each individual, putting the person at the centre of care planning so that they have both choice and control over what they do. These services may include:

- Supported living projects
- Access to training and employment or meaningful daytime activities
- Living at home with supportive or respite care (Box 3.15).

Reflective practice   Box 3.15

Services for people with a learning disability

The Foundation for People with Learning Disabilities (a charity) aims to promote the rights, quality of life and opportunities for people with a learning disability and works with a variety of statutory and non-statutory bodies in order to:

- Conduct research and develop projects that promote social inclusion
- Support local communities and services to include those with a learning disability
- Improve services for people with a learning disability
- Share knowledge and information.

Student activities

- Reflect on how well the services provided by your local authority promote social inclusion.
- Select one area, e.g. day-care, and consider the degree of choice and control the person has over what is provided.
- Access the website below and find out how the organization works with people and local authorities to promote social inclusion.

Resource

The Foundation for People with Learning Disabilities – www.learningdisabilities.org.uk/our-work August 2012.

Providing high quality health and social care

Providing high quality services is a core function of both health and social care organizations. As these publicly funded services are designed to meet the needs of the whole population, there is a potential conflict between improving and maintaining care quality, the need to keep expenditure within allocated budgets and ensuring equality of provision. Successive governments have introduced a variety of mechanisms to ensure that quality of care is prioritized despite other pressures on service provision and several of these are explored below.

At the core of quality care is the patient's experience of receiving care. Being a patient, especially in hospital, can be strange and frightening. Sharing an unfamiliar environment with strangers, experiencing pain, feeling unwell, undergoing medical and nursing procedures and performing toileting and hygiene activities with the help of others and/or in close proximity to strangers can leave people feeling very vulnerable. The importance of ensuring that patients believe that the utmost effort is made to provide care that meets their specific needs is a core aspect of healthcare practice, which has been widely recognized in healthcare policy in recent years, e.g. *Essence of Care 2010* Benchmarks (DH 2010c) and other aspects of health and social care provision discussed above.

This section focuses on how standards of care and quality of health and social care services are promoted and maintained. Some aspects of clinical governance, including benchmarks for best practice, clinical guidelines, National Service Frameworks (NSFs), the Care Quality Commission (CQC) and patient/client involvement in service delivery and evaluation, are outlined below (Fig. 3.2).

Clinical governance and high quality care

Clinical governance is defined as 'the framework through which NHS organizations are accountable for continuously improving the quality of their services and safeguarding high standards of care by creating an environment in which excellence in clinical care will flourish' (DH 1998, Ch. 3, p 2). It describes a range of activities undertaken by healthcare providers to ensure that:

- Care delivery is safe, effective and patient-centred
- Staff are supported, receive appropriate development and have their performance managed
- There are clear lines of accountability for all aspects of clinical governance within organizations.

Clinical governance has been implemented throughout the UK and details of how it works in different regions can be found on local relevant websites. Some of the activities within the clinical governance framework are covered here but others are addressed in more detail in other chapters: evidence-based practice (Ch. 5); continuing professional development (Ch. 7); leadership (Ch. 9); risk management (Ch. 13). Quality care can be hard to define and means different things to different people, however there are some widely held beliefs about the fundamental attributes a quality service should deliver.

Dimensions of high quality care and their implementation

The US Institute of Medicine (2001) has identified six dimensions of quality improvement in healthcare:

- Safety (see below)
- Effectiveness (see below)
- Patient centredness
- Timeliness
- Efficiency (see below)
- Equity.

These dimensions of high quality care reflect the aims of clinical governance above. The importance of the first two dimensions is demonstrated by the many strategies to optimize patient safety (Ch. 13) and promote evidence-based care

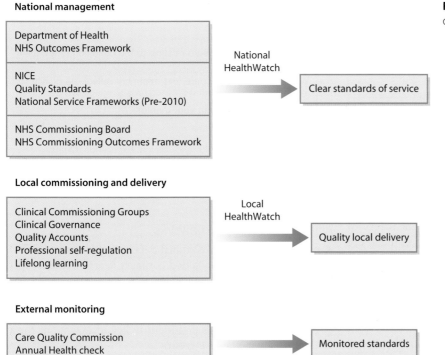

National management

| Department of Health
NHS Outcomes Framework |
| NICE
Quality Standards
National Service Frameworks (Pre-2010) |
| NHS Commissioning Board
NHS Commissioning Outcomes Framework |

National HealthWatch → Clear standards of service

Local commissioning and delivery

| Clinical Commissioning Groups
Clinical Governance
Quality Accounts
Professional self-regulation
Lifelong learning |

Local HealthWatch → Quality local delivery

External monitoring

| Care Quality Commission
Annual Health check |

→ Monitored standards

Fig. 3.2 • NHS Quality management organizations and frameworks.

(see Ch. 5). Most health professionals aim to provide patient-centred care but this has become an explicit objective of government policy by improving systems and processes so they directly involve patients and meet their specific needs. The drive to ensure patients are treated without delay has also been a focus of much recent reform that governs a patient's journey through health and social care. The final two dimensions reflect a view that healthcare provision should use resources prudently and that everyone should have the same access to quality healthcare. It can also be argued that NHS funding and expenditure should be proportionate to that spent on other key economic activities.

Several organizations have been established by government to support quality initiatives in the health services. The principal organizations and quality initiatives in England are considered here, however equivalent organizations perform similar functions in the other three countries, e.g. Healthcare Improvement Scotland (Box 3.16).

Healthcare Improvement Scotland — Box 3.16

Scotland has one main body for supporting the quality of care delivered by healthcare providers and providing public assurance about the quality of services in the NHS and independent sector through a scrutiny process. Healthcare Improvement Scotland was established in 2011 and combined the functions of previous quality improvement and inspectorate bodies.

The organization has four strategic objectives:

- Support innovation and improvement in the delivery of high quality healthcare planned and designed with the patients, their families and the public at the centre of everything we do
- Provide assurance of the safety and quality of healthcare services to the people who use them and to the public in Scotland through risk-based proportionate scrutiny of those services
- Provide authoritative, evidence-based advice and guidance on high quality treatment and care, and best practice in public engagement
- Influence national policies to improve the quality of healthcare.

(Adapted from Supporting Improvement of Healthcare throughout Scotland. Strategic Plan 2011/14 NHS Scotland 2011).

Patient safety

That healthcare should cause no unnecessary harm is fundamental to all healthcare practice. Delivering healthcare is inherently risky and strategies to manage and reduce risk are found in every field of health and social care. Risk management is a core clinical governance activity; all healthcare providers have a statutory duty to maintain and improve the safety of patients in their care. The stages of risk management are explored in more detail in Chapter 13 in relation to patient safety. However, risk management includes many other aspects of care, e.g. surveillance and reporting of hospital-acquired infection (HAI), which is discussed in Chapter 15.

Clinical guidelines

The National Institute for Health and Clinical Excellence (NICE) produces evidence-based clinical guidelines (see Ch. 5) on treatment, care and prevention of ill health; the Scottish Intercollegiate Guidelines Network (SIGN) publish similar information in Scotland. NICE also makes recommendations about the effectiveness of new, and often expensive, treatments including drugs.

As part of the on-going drive to maintain and improve quality in healthcare, NICE produce quality standards for a range of conditions, e.g. stroke and dementia (Box 3.17). These act as guides for commissioners of healthcare as well as care providers in determining the approaches and interventions needed for different patient groups.

? Critical thinking — Box 3.17

NICE quality standards

These are statements written as indicators of high quality, evidence-based and cost-effective care. They cover the treatment and prevention of a range of different conditions and are designed to enable:

- Health and social care professionals to make decisions about care based on the latest evidence and best practice
- Patients to understand what service they can expect from their health and social care providers
- NHS Trusts to quickly and easily examine the clinical performance of their organization and assess the standards of care they provide
- Commissioners to be confident that the services they are providing are of the highest quality and cost-effective.

Examples of quality standards include:

- Dementia
- Depression in adults
- Diabetes in adults
- End-of-life care
- Specialist neonatal care
- Stroke.

Student activities

- Access a quality standard relating to the condition of a patient you have cared for.
- What aspects of their care and treatment reflect the quality standard statements?
- Discuss your ideas with your mentor.

Resource

National Institute for Health and Clinical Excellence. Quality standards. Online. Available: www.nice.org.uk/aboutnice/qualitystandards/qualitystandards.jsp August 2012.

National Service Frameworks

A rolling programme of National Service Frameworks (NSFs), which started in 1988 included coronary heart disease, cancer, mental health, older people, diabetes, long-term conditions, renal services; and children, young people and maternity services. The aim of the NSFs was to:

- Set national standards and identify key interventions for a defined service or care group
- Implement strategies to support the standards

- Establish ways to ensure progress within an agreed timescale
- Identify a range of measures to raise quality and decrease variations in service.

The NSFs have had a significant impact on practice, improving and standardizing care across the country, although there were criticisms of the focus on achieving targets in some NSFs and sometimes the lack of resources to support their implementation. Other disease/health problem focused initiatives were labelled strategies but played a similar role as NSFs in setting standards and outlining key interventions, e.g. one about Sexual Health (DH 2001b), the Alcohol Harm Reduction Strategy for England (Cabinet Office 2004) and the follow-on document (HM Government 2007) and Cancer treatment (DH 2007).

Care Quality Commission (CQC)

The CQC is the independent regulator of all health and social care providers in England, including hospitals, GP practices, residential care homes and formal care provision in people's homes. All health and social care providers, whether run by the NHS, local authorities or the voluntary sector must register with and be licensed by the CQC; this also applies to all private providers that provide care to NHS patients. In order to register with the CQC, providers must demonstrate that they meet essential standards of quality and safety (Box 3.18). The CQC also acts as an inspectorate of care by monitoring the quality of services provided and intervening if problems are identified. The CQC has a specific role in monitoring the care given to people whose rights are restricted under the Mental Health Act.

Essential standards of quality and safety | **Box 3.18**

The Care Quality Commission's (CQC) Essential Standards of Quality and Safety are presented in the form of outcomes grouped together under the following areas of practice:

- Involvement and information
- Personalized care, treatment and support
- Safeguarding and safety
- Suitability of staffing
- Quality and management
- Suitability of management.

Detailed guidance on how organizations should meet these standards and public guides to the same standards for different areas of care provision are available from the CQC website.

Resource

Care Quality Commission. Online. Available: www.cqc.org.uk August 2012.

NHS Commissioning Board (NCB)

Established as part of the health reforms introduced by the *Health and Social Care Act* (HM Government 2012), the NCB oversees commissioning. It guides commissioners in ensuring that quality requirements are built into the commissioning process and is also involved in developing mechanisms for rewarding healthcare providers for quality and innovation through 'Payment by Results' and schemes such as 'Commissioning for Quality and Innovation' (CQUIN) (see Further reading, p. 81).

Effectiveness and efficiency

Although healthcare provision may seem a fairly unique area of activity, it can learn from other industries especially in relation to quality and safety. A good example of this is the 'Productive Series' which, drawing on quality processes from the motor manufacturing and safety approaches from aviation, enables NHS staff to redesign the way they work. The Productive Ward, the Productive Mental Health Ward and the Productive Community Hospital all aim to release nurses and other healthcare professionals from tasks and processes that prevent them spending time giving direct patient care. The programme provides tools and materials that allow staff to change the working environment and the way they work to increase efficiency, productivity and to improve the experience of staff and patients.

Measuring quality and performance

Quality can be hard to define (p. 75) and also challenging to measure. However, it is essential to have some way of assessing whether healthcare meets the needs and expectations of patients/clients and the wider public. It is also essential to examine whether healthcare delivery is achieving its aims in terms of health outcomes for individuals and the population as a whole.

A variety of tools have been developed to endeavour to capture the complex information needed to determine whether quality healthcare is being achieved, maintained and improved. Some of these tools gather data about the process of care delivery, e.g. whether predetermined standards and criteria are being adhered to and targets met; and others consider outcomes of healthcare delivery such as mortality and survival rates. These measures are often objective and results can usually be presented in numerical form, e.g. as league tables. Another approach to assessing quality is to gather information about the patient's lived experience of receiving care. Both types of approach are outlined in this section and patient satisfaction surveys are discussed below.

Benchmarking

Benchmarking is used to compare an organization's care standards against those of an outside, but similar, organization, which is chosen especially for quality excellence. Benchmarking helps organizations to evaluate ongoing improvements. As a quality improvement tool that improves poor practice, this allows organizations and practitioners to learn from each other and contributes to the effective use of resources. The *Essence of Care 2010 Benchmarks* (DH 2010c) provide baseline standards for best practice for health and social care practitioners in a number of areas (Box 3.19, p. 78). While undertaking the activities in Box 3.14, you will have already considered one of these benchmarks, i.e. self-care; others are explored in later chapters.

? Critical thinking   Box 3.19

Essence of Care 2010: Benchmarks for the Fundamental Aspects of Care

- Bladder, bowel and continence care
- Care environment
- Communication
- Food and drink
- Prevention and management of pain
- Personal hygiene
- Prevention and management of pressure ulcers
- Promoting health and well-being
- Record-keeping
- Respect and dignity
- Safety
- Self-care

Student activities

- Access the 'Essence of Care' 2010 benchmarks and select a benchmark relevant to your placement and consider carefully how this is implemented.
- Discuss your ideas with your mentor.

(From Essence of Care 2010; DH 2010c).

Audits

Clinical audit and outcomes measurements are quality improvement tools that can help to close the gap between what is known to be the best care and the care that patients are receiving. They aim to ensure that all patients receive the most effective, up-to-date and appropriate treatments, delivered by healthcare professionals with the right skills and experience. Audits are a commonplace but valuable means of gathering data to assess whether healthcare delivery is meeting required standards or benchmarks and help to answer the question – are patients given the best care? For example, audits are frequently used to monitor staff hand cleansing techniques, correct use of patient documentation and correct cleaning and storage of equipment.

Patient surveys

These are often used by organizations to gather data on patient's views of the service. Traditionally, these are paper-based and given to patients as they are discharged from hospital or leave the GP surgery. Although there is often space provided for free comments, the amount and type of information that can be gathered in this way is limited as patients' views may also be coloured by relief and/or gratitude as their treatment ends. A more accurate means of capturing patients' views on the service is through the use of handheld computer devices that allow patients to enter data in real time as they experience care delivery. These are becoming more popular and increasingly sophisticated in their design, allowing healthcare providers to gain more accurate and useful information.

Patients and relatives can also express their opinions on healthcare provision through websites such as NHS Choices (see Useful websites, p. 80).

Although surveys provide some insight into patient views on the care they received; they often fail to capture important aspects of their experience, e.g. whether the care was delivered with compassion, kindness and respect. However, patient's perception of these qualities is subjective, which makes them hard to quantify and measure and yet there is clear evidence that many patients and relatives are unhappy about the care they receive due to a perceived lack of consideration and kindness from staff (Goodrich & Cornwell 2008, updated 2009). As a result of these concerns there has been a drive to develop accurate measures of patient experiences, an example being the work of the King's Fund *The Point of Care Programme* (see Further reading, p. 81). This topic will be explored further.

User choice and voice

Expanding patient choice of services has been a fundamental component of NHS reforms in recent decades. This has been in the context of the inexorable rise of consumerism in society overall with the public having a better understanding of their rights as consumers of services and also raised expectations of choosing what services are provided in the public sector. It can also be seen as an inevitable consequence of the introduction of market forces into NHS healthcare provision.

Closely linked with patient choice is the concept of 'patient voice' or patient and public involvement in healthcare decision-making, which has also been subject to frequent government policy-making and reform. Organizations and initiatives designed to promote service user/patient/client choice and voice are discussed in this section.

In recent years, more attention has been focused not just on the patient's experience of healthcare but also on their perceptions of the outcomes of their treatment on their health, lifestyle and quality of life. A range of tools has been developed to capture this important patient perspective and is collectively known as Patient Related Outcome Measures (PROMs). Since 2009, all providers of NHS funded care in England have been asked to collect PROM data from patients undergoing a range of procedures including hip replacement, knee replacement, hernia repair and removal of varicose veins.

User choice

Patient choice can be seen as a positive development in the NHS because it promotes competition between providers encouraging them to become more efficient and develop higher quality care. It is also argued that it makes choices about services more equitable, as more affluent patients have always had the choice of private sector services in addition to the NHS. Introducing choice within the NHS ensures everyone is able to choose from a range of services. Choice could also make providers more responsive to patient and public preferences (Dixon et al 2010). However, there are concerns that choice and competition could lead to some services or organizations failing and being closed. It has also been questioned whether health and healthcare can be thought of as commodities or services in the same way as other goods and services: do people have sufficient knowledge and information to make the right choices about their healthcare and how willing are they to do this?

Emergence of 'a market' in publicly funded health services following the *National Health Service and Community Care Act* of 1990 saw GPs and other commissioners making choices on behalf of patients although since then, patients have been offered choices directly. Initially this was for a limited range of procedures with long waiting lists, but gradually the mechanisms to allow choice were expanded and now all patients needing an elective procedure should be offered a choice of providers.

To make choices, people need information to help them choose the option which suits them best. NHS Choices (see Useful websites, p. 80) provides the following types of information:

- Overall quality of service
- Mortality rates
- Other patients' views
- Waiting times
- Infection rates
- Food quality
- Parking facilities and disabled access (Box 3.20).

 Critical thinking Box 3.20

Choice of healthcare provider

Mary is 78 years old and needs to have eye surgery. She is widowed and lives alone. Her son lives close by and her daughter lives about 30 miles away. Until recently, Mary has been fit and healthy and she has not been an in-patient in hospital since her children were born.

Mary has been told by her GP that she can choose the hospital where she would like to have the operation.

Student activities

- What factors do you think would influence Mary's choice of hospital?
- Would you be influenced by the same factors?
- Visit the NHS choices website and find out what choices Mary would have if she lived in your area.
- Identify information that would help Mary to choose a hospital.

Resource

NHS Choices: Find and choose services. Online. Available: www.nhs.uk/servicedirectories/Pages/ServiceSearch.aspx?WT.mc_id=51107 August 2012.

However, research has shown that recommendations from people's GPs, family and friends, as well as their previous experience of a provider are probably more influential than this objective data (Dixon et al 2010).

Having chosen a provider, patients should continue to be offered choices where possible about all aspects of their treatment and care. This commitment to choice in all aspects of NHS care delivery is reflected in the mantra: 'No decision about me without me' (DH 2010a).

User voice

Involving patients and the public in decisions about healthcare is not new and in practice, operates at two levels. At the level of everyday practice, healthcare practitioners should involve patients and, where appropriate, their families and carers in decisions about treatment and care. The role of service users/ patients and the public in making decisions about what and how services should be provided is increasingly viewed as important and examples of how this is achieved are described in more detail below.

Various national and local organizations have been established, abolished, reformed and restructured in recent decades with the aim of improving patient and public involvement in the NHS.

Local HealthWatch

These organizations came into being in England and are funded by local authorities. They are responsible for ensuring the views of patients and local people are shared with commissioners; have the right to enter and view provider services and to be consulted when a change in local services is proposed. If there are concerns about local providers, these can be communicated to the CQC (p. 77) through HealthWatch England. These organizations may also be involved in providing support and advocacy services for people who wish to make complaints about health and social care provision.

HealthWatch England

This body is an independent part of the CQC which investigates concerns raised about services by Local HealthWatch and can ask the CQC to intervene when necessary.

Patient Advice and Liaison Services

Patient Advice and Liaison Services (PALs), as the name suggests have, as a major part of their role, the responsibility to provide information and advice that patients/clients need when they use hospital NHS services. For example, when problems arise, the PALs team liaises and works with NHS staff, organizations and support groups and, if there is no resolution to the identified problem, patients/clients will be supported to make formal complaints to appropriate service managers (see Useful websites, below for information about the core functions of PALs).

Complaints

Inevitably, due to the complex and often very personal nature of healthcare delivery, there will be occasions when patients and relatives are unhappy with the service provided. In 2008/2009, 89139 people made complaints about their hospital or community care (NHS Information Centre 2011). These complaints may have arisen either because the service did not meet their needs or expectations at that time and/or because the care provided was of poor quality and did not meet the standards and requirements of the organization or the NHS overall.

Recent reforms in the NHS complaints procedure have not only aimed to simplify the process and assist with effective local resolution but also to set organizational targets for

Reflective practice Box 3.21

Complaints

In 2008/2009, over 89 000 people were unhappy with the care provided by the NHS in hospitals and the community.

Student activities

- Discuss with your mentor the procedure for dealing with a complaint in your placement.
- Access The NHS Constitution and reflect on the patient's rights outlined there on page 8.
- Using the NHS choices resource, consider the NHS complaints procedures and other options.

Resources

Department of Health, 2009. The NHS Constitution for England (see p 8). Online. Available: www.dh.gov.uk/en/Publicationsandstatistics/Publications/PublicationsPolicyAndGuidance/DH_093419 August 2012.
NHS Choices: Complaints. About NHS complaints. Online. Available: www.nhs.uk/choiceintheNHS/Rightsandpledges/complaints/Pages/AboutNHScomplaints.aspx August 2012.

SUMMARY

- ◆ Knowledge of the history, policies and legislation underpinning the NHS and health and social care provision, and how they are organized is crucial for practitioners to understand how important it is for both the NHS and social care provision to be dynamic in order to meet changing needs.
- ◆ An understanding of the evolving professional roles within health and social care allows nurses to work collaboratively and effectively with other professionals in the MDT and in multiagency working (statutory and non-statutory agencies).
- ◆ Nurses also need a good understanding of the complexity of the current systems of organization and funding arrangements in order to have flexible working relationships with other professionals, volunteers and service users.
- ◆ Holistic care depends on nurses having a greater awareness of the complex needs of patients/clients, families and other carers.
- ◆ Holistic care depends on the commitment of nurses to plan and deliver services by working together in MDTs and with many agencies. Multiagency working is vital for holistic care of all the population but especially so for vulnerable groups that include children, people with mental health problems or learning disabilities and older people.
- ◆ The frameworks and mechanisms for ensuring high quality care are important in guaranteeing improvements in the patient's/client's or carer's experience. Experience of a quality healthcare system is dependent upon all those involved having a voice in how, where and when care is delivered and developed and by whom.

responses to complaints. Healthcare providers are encouraged to view complaints as a rich source of data to help maintain and improve the quality of the care they provide. Box 3.21 provides an opportunity for you to reflect on complaints about care and the process for dealing with them.

KEY WORDS AND PHRASES FOR LITERATURE SEARCHING

Audit
Clinical guidelines
Commissioning
Frameworks
Funding
Governance
Multiagency working
Multidisciplinary teams
National Health Service
NHS Trusts
NHS Policy
Private sector
Quality
Social care
Social work
Statutory services

Useful websites

Action for Sick Children www.actionforsickchildren.org
Action on Elder Abuse www.elderabuse.org.uk
Care Quality Commission www.cqc.org.uk
Department of Health www.dh.gov.uk
History of the NHS www.nhshistory.net/shorthistory.htm
King's Fund www.kingsfund.org.uk
NHS choices www.nhs.uk
NHS Information Centre www.ic.nhs.uk
National Institute for Health and Clinical Excellence www.nice.org.uk
Devolved NHS structure:
  Northern Ireland www.n-i.nhs.uk
  Scotland www.show.scot.nhs.uk
  Wales www.wales.nhs.uk
NHS Surveys www.nhssurveys.org
Patient Advice and Liaison Services (PALS) www.pals.nhs.uk
All websites accessed September 2012.

References

Alcock, C., Payne, S., Sullivan, M., 2004. Introducing social policy, revised edition. Pearson Prentice Hall, Harlow.
Beveridge, W., 1942. Report on social insurance and allied services, Cm 6404. HMSO, London.
Birn, A.E., Pillay, Y., Holtz, T., 2009. Textbook of international health: global health in a dynamic world. Oxford University Press, New York.
Cabinet Office: Prime Minister's Strategy Unit 2004 Alcohol harm reduction strategy. TSO, London.
Darzi, A., 2008. High quality care for all: Next Stage Review final report. Online. Available: www.dh.gov.uk/en/Publicationsandstatistics/Publications/PublicationsPolicyAndGuidance/DH_085825 September 2012.

Delamothe, T., 2008. NHS at 60. A comprehensive service. British Medical Journal 336, 1344–1345.

Department for Education, 2010. Working together to safeguard children: a guide to inter-agency working to safeguard and promote the welfare of children. Online. Available: https://www.education.gov.uk/publications/standard/publicationdetail/page1/DCSF-00305-2010 October 2012.

Department of Health, 1998. A first class service: quality in the new NHS. Online. Available: www.dh.gov.uk/prod_consum_dh/groups/dh_digitalassets/@dh/@en/documents/digitalasset/dh_4045152.pdf September 2012.

Department of Health, 1999. National service framework for mental health: Modern standards and service models. Online. Available: www.dh.gov.uk/en/Publicationsandstatistics/Lettersandcirculars/LocalAuthorityCirculars/AllLocalAuthority/DH_4004760 September 2012.

Department of Health, 2000a. The NHS plan: a plan for investment, a plan for reform. Online. Available: www.dh.gov.uk/en/Publicationsandstatistics/Publications/PublicationsPolicyAndGuidance/DH_4002960 September 2012.

Department of Health, 2000b. No Secrets: Guidance on developing and implementing multi-agency policies and procedures to protect vulnerable adults from abuse. Online. Available: www.dh.gov.uk/en/Publicationsandstatistics/Publications/PublicationsPolicyAndGuidance/DH_4008486 September 2012.

Department of Health, 2001a. Valuing people: a new strategy for learning disability for the 21st century. Online. Available: www.archive.official-documents.co.uk/document/cm50/5086/5086.pdf September 2012.

Department of Health, 2001b. Better prevention, better services, better sexual health – The national strategy for sexual health and HIV. Online. Available: www.dh.gov.uk/en/Publicationsandstatistics/Publications/PublicationsPolicyAndGuidance/DH_4003133 September 2012.

Department of Health, 2002. Securing our future health: taking a long-term view – the Wanless Report. Online. Available: www.dh.gov.uk/en/Publicationsandstatistics/

Publications/PublicationsPolicyAndGuidance/DH_4009293 September 2012.

Department of Health, 2007. Cancer Reform Strategy. Online. Available: www.dh.gov.uk/en/Publicationsandstatistics/Publications/PublicationsPolicyAndGuidance/DH_081006 September 2012.

Department of Health, 2009. Valuing people now: a three-year strategy for people with learning disabilities. Online. Available: www.dh.gov.uk/prod_consum_dh/groups/dh_digitalassets/documents/digitalasset/dh_093375.pdf September 2012.

Department of Health, 2010a. Equity and excellence: liberating the NHS. Online. Available: www.dh.gov.uk/en/Publicationsandstatistics/Publications/PublicationsPolicyAndGuidance/DH_117353 September 2012.

Department of Health, 2010b. A simple guide to payment by results. Online. Available: www.dh.gov.uk/en/Publicationsandstatistics/Publications/PublicationsPolicyAndGuidance/DH_119985 September 2012.

Department of Health, 2010c. Essence of care 2010: Benchmarks for the fundamental aspects of care. Online. Available: www.dh.gov.uk/prod_consum_dh/groups/dh_digitalassets/@dh/@en/@ps/documents/digitalasset/dh_119978.pdf September 2012.

Department of Health, 2011a. No health without mental health: a cross-governmental mental health outcomes strategy for people of all ages. Online. Available: www.dh.gov.uk/en/Publicationsandstatistics/Publications/PublicationsPolicyAndGuidance/DH_123766 September 2012.

Department of Health, 2011b. Safeguarding adults: the role of health services. Online. Available: www.dh.gov.uk/en/Publicationsandstatistics/Publications/PublicationsPolicyAndGuidance/DH_124882 September 2012.

Department of Health, 2012. Health and Social Care Act explained. Online. Available: http://www.dh.gov.uk/health/2012/06/act-explained/ August 2012.

Department of Trade and Industry, 2002. Social enterprise: a strategy for success. DTI, London.

Dixon, A., Robertson, R., Appleby, J., et al., 2010. Patient choice. How patients choose and how providers respond. The King's Fund. Online. Available: www.kingsfund.org.uk/publications/patient_choice.html September 2012.

European Association for Children in Hospital (EACH), 2001. EACH charter. Online. Available: www.each-for-sick-children.org/each-charter September 2012.

Emerson, E., Hatton, C., 2008. People with learning disabilities in England. Centre for Disability Research, Lancaster.

Goodrich, J., Cornwell, J., 2008 (updated 2009). Seeing the person in the patient. The Point of Care Review Paper. The King's Fund. Online. Available: www.kingsfund.org.uk/publications/the_point_of_care.html September 2012.

Griffiths, R., 1983. NHS management inquiry. DHSS, London.

Ham, C., 2009. Health Policy in Britain, sixth ed. Palgrave Macmillan, Basingstoke.

HM Government, 2007. Safe. Sensible. Social. The next steps in the National Alcohol Strategy. Online. Available: www.dh.gov.uk/en/Publicationsandstatistics/Publications/PublicationsPolicyAndGuidance/DH_075218 September 2012.

HM Government, 2012. Heath and Social Care Act. Online. Available: http://www.legislation.gov.uk/ukpga/2012/7/enacted August 2012.

Institute of Medicine, 2001. Crossing the quality chasm: a new health system for the 21st century. National Academic Press, Washington.

Mencap, 2011. About learning disability. Online. Available: www.mencap.org.uk/all-about-learning-disability/ September 2012.

National Health Service and Community Care Act, 1990 HMSO, London. Online. Available: www.legislation.gov.uk/ukpga/1990/19/contents September 2012.

NHS Information Centre, 2009. Personal social services home care users in England aged 65 and over. 2008–2009 survey. Online. Available: www.ic.nhs.uk/webfiles/publications/Social%20Care/socialcarepubs/Personal_Social_Services_Home_Care_Users_aged_65_and_over_England_2008_09_Survey.pdf September 2012.

NHS Information Centre, 2011. Data on written complaints in the NHS, 2008–2009. Online. Available: www.ic.nhs.uk September 2012.

Schoen, C., Collins, S.R., Kriss, J.L., et al., 2008. How many are underinsured? Trends among U.S. adults 2003 and 2007. Health Affairs 27 (4), w298–w309.

Further reading

Baggott, R., 2007. Understanding health policy. The Policy Press, Bristol.

Baggott, R., 2010. Public health: policy and politics. Palgrave, Basingstoke.

Buse, K., Mays, N., Walt, G., 2007. Making health policy. Open University Press, Maidenhead.

Department for Education and Skills (DfES), 2004. Every child matters: change for children. Online. Available: www.education.gov.uk/publications/standard/publicationDetail/Page1/DfES/1081/2004 September 2012.

Department for Education, 2011. The Munro review of child protection: final report: A child-centred system. Online. Available: www.education.gov.uk/publications/standard/publicationDetail/Page1/CM%208062 September 2012.

Department of Health, 2008 (updated 2010). Using the Commissioning for Quality and Innovation (CQUIN) payment framework. Online. Available: www.dh.gov.uk/en/Publicationsandstatistics/Publications/PublicationsPolicyAndGuidance/DH_091443 September 2012.

Department of Health, 2009. NHS 2010–2015: from good to great. Preventative, people-centred, productive. Online. Available: www.dh.gov.uk/en/Publicationsandstatistics/Publications/PublicationsPolicyAndGuidance/DH_109876 September 2012.

King's Fund, 2009 (updated 2012). The Point of Care Programme. Online. Available: www.kingsfund.org.uk/current_projects/the_point_of_care/ September 2012.

NHS Improvement EQIPP Delivering quality efficiently. Online. Available: www.improvement.nhs.uk/Default.

aspx?alias=www.improvement.nhs.uk/qipp September 2012.

McMurray, A., Clendon, J., 2010. Community health and wellness: primary healthcare in practice, fourth ed. Churchill Livingstone, Oxford.

McSherry, R., Pearce, P., 2011. Clinical governance. A guide to implementation for healthcare professionals, third ed. Wiley Blackwell, Chichester.

Peckham, S., Meerabeau, L., 2007. Social policy for nurses and the helping professions, second ed. Open University Press, Maidenhead.

Scottish Executive, 2000. The same as you? A review of services for people with learning disabilities. Online. Available: www.scotland. gov.uk/Resource/Doc/1095/0078271.pdf September 2012.

Wise, J., 2010. GPs are handed sweeping powers in major shake up of NHS. (See box 'Key proposals in the government's white paper'). British Medical Journal 341:c3796 Online. Available: www.bmj.com/content/341/bmj.c3796 September 2012.

Section 2

Professional practice

Learning and teaching

4

Morag Gray

LEARNING OUTCOMES

This chapter will help you:
- Outline the major theories of learning
- Describe the factors associated with effective learning
- Recall three different reflective models
- Write aims and SMART learning outcomes
- Summarize the key components of successful teaching.

Introduction

> Success is a journey ... not a destination
> Your greatest asset for the journey is your mind
> Learning how to use it is the secret.
>
> (Egle 2009)

Nursing programmes aim to provide safe, knowledgeable, skillful and caring practitioners who are able to provide effective evidence-based care (see Ch. 5). Nursing students take on the role of learner at both university and in placements. In placements, mentors are involved in formal and informal teaching and learning experiences with students and patients/clients. From an early stage, you will be involved in informal and simple patient/client teaching activities, assuming the role of teacher while the patient/client becomes the learner. It is therefore important to understand the processes of teaching and learning from both learner and teacher perspectives to maximize both your own learning and that of the people in your care.

'Learning is the process whereby knowledge is created through the transformation of experience' (Kolb 1984, p 38). Learning is all about educating oneself to think, as well as appreciating the importance of reflecting on that thinking in order to learn. Individuals learn and behave in different ways as a result of their educational experiences. The result of learning is commonly seen as a relatively permanent change in behaviour.

Theories of learning

There are different theories of learning, none of which has gained universal acceptance, and these are discussed in this section.

Behaviourism

Behaviourism as a theory of learning was dominant in the 1960s. Its origins lie with the Russian psychologist, Pavlov and the American behavioural psychologist, Skinner. Classic conditioning is the type of learning made famous by Pavlov's experiments with dogs, where Pavlov found that if he rang a bell and at the same time fed the dogs, the dogs began to associate the sound of the bell with food. Eventually, the dogs would salivate when they heard the bell despite not receiving food. This is called a 'conditioned response'.

Skinner's experimental work involved rats, pigeons and latterly, humans. Skinner found that rats or pigeons placed within a cage-like box containing a food tray and a lever to release food would demonstrate trial and error behaviour until the lever was pressed. Over time, the animal learned the connection between pressing the lever and the release of food. Skinner's work led to what is known as 'operant conditioning', by which a new behaviour can be taught assuming that rewards are related to the learner producing successive approximations to the desired behaviours.

Behaviourists assert that memory is the result of strengthening of associations between a stimulus and a response. Therefore, according to behaviourists, almost all kinds of learning can be described and explained in terms of the gradual learning of stimulus and response. A stimulus is equivalent to an event, person or thing in an environment, whereas a response is something that the learner does. The theory of stimulus–response in learning is most useful in providing advice regarding how to teach simple knowledge and skills, and has also made a valuable contribution to training programmes for people who have a learning disability (Bastable 2008).

Any event that increases the probability of a piece of behaviour being displayed by the learner is called a 'reinforcer'. Skinner proposed that by providing reinforcement to an individual in a particular situation displaying certain behaviour, they would be more likely to display this behaviour again when a similar set of stimulus conditions prevailed. For example, when training an animal to perform particular tasks, the teacher looks for behaviour consistent with what is desired and positively reinforces that until the animal displays the desired behaviour. This technique is called 'shaping'. Following shaping, prompting or guiding, or 'chaining' can be commenced.

Once each component of a task has been learned, the steps have to be joined together into a sequence so that completion of the first step becomes a stimulus signalling the second step, and so on. Backward chaining can also be useful, particularly when teaching children and people with a learning disability (Box 4.1).

Using backward chaining in teaching   Box 4.1

Goal: John will put his trousers on.

The technique involves breaking down the task or skill to be learned into small manageable steps. For example, teaching John how to put on trousers with an elasticated waist could be broken down as follows:

1. Pick up trousers by waistband
2. Lower trousers and lift up leg
3. Put left leg into left trouser hole
4. Put right leg into right trouser hole
5. Pull trousers up to knees
6. Stand and pull trousers to waist.

To use backward chaining, the teaching sequences would start with step 6. The teacher would carry out steps 1–5 for John and then get him to do step 6 himself.

On completion of step 5, John would be asked to put his hands on the sides of his trousers with his thumbs inside the waistband. Then, while guiding John's hands, the teacher asks him to pull his trousers up. On completion of the task, praise is given by saying, e.g. 'That's great, you pulled your trousers up!'

Once John has learned step 6, he would then start at step 5 and so on until he is able to complete all six steps by himself.

The learner is presented with a task with all the steps completed except the last one, which they must complete and the process of completion then reinforces the behaviour. In this way, the individual gains instant satisfaction of completing the task and is more likely to have a positive learning experience. In this type of learning, it is important to use social reinforcement along with praise for completing the task because social approval is very powerful. Social reinforcers include non-verbal communication such as smiling, eye contact, winking, physical contact such as a hug or pat on the back, nodding or clapping (see Ch. 9). Social reinforcement can be particularly effective with children and young people and to some adults when given by people whose opinions are valued or respected. It is vital that any form of social reinforcement is:

- Sincere and non-ambiguous
- Clear about the specific behaviour being praised.

These Skinnerian techniques are reputed to be most effective in teaching social skills. They can also be used to decrease the occurrence of undesirable behaviours. To summarize, behaviour which is rewarded is likely to be repeated; conversely, behaviour which is ignored is likely to fade.

Another strategy used to reduce behavioural problems is positive programming. LaVigna and Donnellan (1986) suggest this is the preferred strategy and provide an example of an individual who hits staff. First, this behaviour needs to be seen within the context of the setting so that a judgement can be made as to whether it is inappropriate. Assuming it is, the reason for such behaviour needs to be identified. In this case, the individual hits out at staff when he is engaged in an activity that he does not enjoy and hits out to signal that he wants a break. Using the positive programming strategy, the individual is provided with a card that says 'Break' and is told that when he shows this to staff, they will allow him a 5-minute break before resuming the activity.

Cognitive theories of learning

Cognition relates to the mental processes involved in thinking, perceiving, problem-solving and remembering. The mainstay of cognitive theory is that thinking and reasoning play a major part in how people learn. Reinforcement is not an automatic process but rather the learner realizes the benefits of adopting certain behaviours. Through paying attention, the learner selectively observes and extracts what they perceive as valuable components of behaviour. Proponents of cognitive theory argue that people learn from experience, by 'doing', and that this learning is then inserted into their framework of existing knowledge. The act of doing involves repeated practice and the provision of reinforcement or rewards encourages further learning.

Gestalt learning theory is an example of cognitive theory which emphasizes that it is important to view the whole when learning rather than taking a reductionist approach which involves looking at small parts that make up the whole. For example, when teaching a skill, it is best to demonstrate the whole procedure at normal speed, so that the learner gains a holistic view of what is expected. Thereafter, the skill is usually broken down into its component parts in order to learn. The aim is that, with practice, the learner will be able to perform the whole skill competently.

Humanistic theories of learning

These emerged in the 1950s and 1960s from individuals such as Abraham Maslow and Carl Rogers. Both Maslow and Rogers rejected the behaviourist theory that human beings were unthinking and could be shaped and programmed by patterns of rewards and punishments. Instead, they focused on people's potential, believing that humans strive to reach the highest possible level of achievement.

Maslow (1954) is best known for developing the hierarchy of needs which is important in respect to learning, as these needs play an important role in motivation. The hierarchy is usually presented as a pyramid with the most basic needs (physiological) at the base. The key aspect of Maslow's work is that, before someone can learn effectively, their most basic needs must be met. For example, if people are hungry, thirsty or in pain, they are unlikely to be able to concentrate in order to learn. The next layer in the pyramid relates to safety needs. If learners' physiological needs are met but they fear for their physical or psychological safety, then their learning will be impeded.

The third layer relates to the need to belong and be loved. Even if the previous two levels are met, if a learner feels excluded from a group, this will affect their learning because their belonging and love needs will not be met. The fourth layer relates to esteem. Despite having their belonging and love needs met, if they perhaps ask a question and someone ridicules them for asking a silly question, then that too will affect their learning, as their self-esteem needs would not be met. Individual self-esteem needs can be met through recognition, acceptance, praise and a belief that others acknowledge their worth. The final layer in the pyramid is called self-actualization. This, according to Maslow, is the highest form of achievement where the learner achieves their full potential.

Rogers (1994) argues that human beings have a natural potential for learning, which is most significant when what is to be learned is perceived as relevant and the learner is active in the process. Furthermore, Rogers argues that self-concept and self-esteem are necessary during any learning experience. The most lasting form of learning, according to Rogers, is that which involves the learner being self-directed. In other words, the self-directed learner is motivated to explore a topic at their own pace and in their own time and relishes the experience of being independent and creative. If, however, learning involves a change in someone's behaviour or is viewed as a threat to how they organize themselves or to the way they live, it is often resisted. That is why, for example, attempts to change one's eating habits or sedentary behaviour can be very difficult to achieve.

Rogers (1994) developed 'client-centred therapy' in which he aimed to provide his clients with the knowledge and skills necessary to find their own solutions to their problems, rather than being told what they should do. Roger's work led to what we know today as student-centred learning. This involves the teacher being the facilitator of learning: guiding students on how to learn, fostering their enthusiasm, initiative and responsibility, and providing them with a variety of learning experiences through which they can discover and learn. It also encourages the use of group learning so that, as well as having peer support, students also learn about working in teams (Bastable 2008). Learning how to work effectively as a team member is a fundamental skill for all healthcare professionals.

Andragogy

Malcolm Knowles (1990) coined the term 'andragogy' at the end of the 1980s to differentiate it from 'pedagogy'. Pedagogy, in its strictest sense, relates to how children learn. The word pedagogy is derived from the Greek words *paid*, meaning child, and *agogus*, meaning leader of, and therefore pedagogy

literally means the art and science of teaching children. Pedagogy involves:

- The teacher as the expert
- Learners being dependent on the teacher for the transmission of knowledge
- Learners being ready when they are told what they have to learn
- External motivation for learning led by the teacher (Knowles et al 1998).

Andragogy is about how adults learn. Knowles et al (1998) argue that adults learn best when they are involved in doing something or are active in the process. In short, andragogy reflects a student-centred approach to learning. Being active in the learning process facilitates the formation of meaning and provides depth to understanding. Knowles identified certain characteristics of adult learning. Adults need to know why they should be learning something and how it will be beneficial to their work or other facets of their lives. Adults' approach to learning is more problem-solving in nature as opposed to subject-centred. Adults prefer to take charge of their own learning, that is, to be self-directive and responsible. Adults use their varied life experience as a rich resource for learning and connect any new learning to their existing knowledge and experience. When planning any educational activity involving adults, it should be underpinned by adult learning principles (Box 4.2).

Summary of adult learning principles   **Box 4.2**

- Allow adult learners to exercise autonomy and self-direction in the learning process
- Help adult learners achieve the personal learning goals they have identified
- Ensure that all learning experiences designed for adults are relevant
- Encourage adult learners to solve practical problems
- Develop learning experiences that build on the life experiences of adult learners
- Help adult learners fulfill their potential
- Involve learners in making judgements on their own learning – this can develop their skills of critical reflection.

(Adapted from Cannon and Boswell 2012, p 65).

In relation to the principles of adult learning, or andragogy, the models of experiential learning by Kolb (1984) and Race (2011) are now explored.

Kolb's experiential learning cycle

Kolb (1984) presented a model of learning consisting of four phases, known as Kolb's experiential learning cycle (Fig. 4.1). The cycle is based on the premise that people learn much more effectively when they are encouraged to be active in the process. Kolb suggests that learning results from two things: the way an individual perceives and the way the individual processes what they perceive. Kolb (1984) suggested that learning styles are composed of a combination of the four

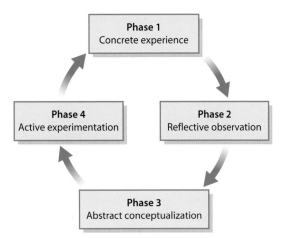

Fig. 4.1 • Kolb's experiential learning cycle. (Reproduced with permission from Kolb, D.A. 1984. Experiential learning: experience as the source of learning and development. Prentice Hall, Englewood Cliffs.)

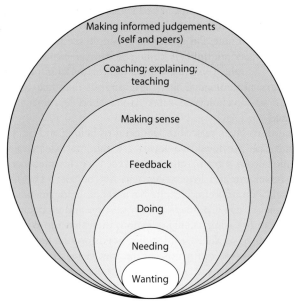

Fig. 4.2 • Representation of Race's (2012) seven factors underpinning successful learning. (Adapted from http://phil-race.co.uk).

phases in his experiential learning cycle. He stated that individuals perceive either through concrete experience or through more abstract concepts and that they process information in one of two ways: through active experimentation or through reflective observation.

Concrete experience

A concrete experience starts when the individual begins by doing something. During the concrete experience, learners are actively involved and tend to rely on their feelings rather than using a systematic approach to problems or situations. According to Mills (undated) during concrete experience, individuals use all five senses: sight, smell, touch, taste and hearing in order to deal with the obvious, i.e. the here and now.

Reflective observation

During this phase, the learner requires to take time out to consider, or reflect, on what has happened during the concrete (or doing) phase. The learner relies on objectivity and careful consideration to search for meaning by studying things from a variety of different perspectives and asking questions (Bastable 2008).

Abstract conceptualization

This phase involves trying to make sense of what has happened. It involves visualization, use of imagination and conceiving ideas to move beyond the obvious to uncover the more subtle implications (Mills undated). The learner makes comparisons between what they have done and what they have reflected upon, and draws on their existing knowledge. During abstract conceptualization, learners tend to rely more on logic and ideas in regard to problems or situations rather than on their feelings (Bastable 2008).

Active experimentation

This is the final phase of the cycle where the learner considers what they have learned and how they are going to implement it into practice. In other words, they place what they have learned into context so that it is both meaningful and useful to them (Bastable 2008).

Summary

The above way of thinking about learning follows the principle that learning is continuous, as people continually test out new ideas in practice and adjust their ideas and behaviour in light of their experience. Kolb highlighted two particular aspects:

- The use of 'here and now' experiences to test ideas
- The use of 'feedback' to change practices and theories.

Race's ripples model

Race, a British educationalist, first presented his alternative experiential model of learning in 1993 and since then it has been further developed and refined (Race 1993, 2005, 2012). This model is also based on experiential learning – or 'learning by doing'– and reflects Kolb's view that by receiving feedback from others and reflecting on one's learning is of paramount importance to the learning experience. Race's model consists of seven elements or processes (Fig. 4.2), which together constitute successful learning. Race's model differs from Kolb's because, rather than using a cycle, Race's model involves processes that interact with one another rather like ripples on a pond.

Wanting to learn

This is the central process and lies at the heart of the model. Race believes that wanting to learn is crucial to the internal motivation that drives the learner in the first place. Motivation ripples out from the heart of the model into the surrounding layers.

Needing to learn

Here, the learner takes charge or ownership of their need to learn stimulated by their intrinsic motivation of wanting and needing to learn.

Learning by doing

From wanting and needing to learn the next ripple in the process is doing, which reflects the belief that adults learn best by doing, and being active in the process.

Learning through feedback

Receiving timely feedback is viewed as essential since it is important to the quality of the learning experience to see both the results of one's learning and to obtain feedback from others regarding how effective it has been. According to Race's model, feedback is as crucial as the central process of wanting to learn, needing to learn and learning by doing.

Making sense of things

Race asserts that making sense of what has been learnt is the most important part of the ripple on the pond. This is where learners realize that they have solved something and how they did it successfully so it can be tested out again in the future. It can be experience of 'oh now I get it!' or 'that explains why …'.

Coaching, explaining and teaching

Race explains that the next ripple invoves learners' coaching, teaching and explaining things to their peers. In this role, students further develop their understanding of the topic area through the process of coaching, explaining and teaching.

Making informed judgements

In this last of the seven ripples, Race asserts that students should develop their self-assessment skills to make informed judgements about their own progress. They should also provide informed judgements as part of a peer-assessment process with the provision of appropriate feedback.

Summary

Figure 4.2 suggests that motivation ripples outwards in successive layers, with positive feedback sending the ripples back towards the centre; this in turn has a positive effect on needing and wanting. The position of feedback in the model symbolizes the fact that feedback is gained from a variety of sources (teachers, peers, self-assessment) and needing and wanting are derived internally. In between these two are 'doing' and 'making sense of things', both of which are influenced by internally generated needing and wanting as well as by externally generated feedback. The outer two ripples reflect growing student autonomy whereby learners expand their repertoire to include coaching and teaching others as well as the ability to make informed judgements of their own and other's progress.

Interprofessional learning

Interprofessional learning (IPL) has been defined as 'occasions when 2 or more professions learn with, from, and about each other to improve collaboration and the quality of care' (Centre for the Advancement of Interprofessional Education, CAIPE 2011). The NMC (2010 p 148) defined interprofessional learning as: 'An interactive process of learning which is undertaken with students or registered professionals from a range of health and social care professions who learn with and from each other'.

IPL has become increasingly important for all health and social care professionals as a result of tragedies such as the cases of Victoria Climbie and Beverley Allitt, which demonstrated a lack of joint working across professional boundaries (Darbyshire & Machin 2011). It is a means of learning about, promoting and facilitating interprofessional team working (Mitchell et al 2010). IPL is based on the fundamental principle of being able to understand the variety of professional roles involved in providing holistic patient/client centred-care. The NMC (2010) requires students to be involved in IPL and to provide evidence of being able to understand and coordinate interprofessional care as part of the standards for leadership, management and teamworking.

The learning process

People have a tendency to adopt ways of learning with which they feel most comfortable. These are known as learning styles, which are now explored. Thereafter approaches to learning and reflection and critical thinking are considered.

Learning styles

The term 'learning styles' refers to the way in which individuals choose to learn. Different people have different learning needs and bring their own individual knowledge, experience and resources to the learning process and learn in different ways. It is important to be aware of the differing learning styles because it is recognized that people learn better and more quickly when teaching methods match their preferred learning style. When someone learns successfully, their self-esteem increases, which in turn has a positive effect on their learning. Honey and Mumford (1992, 2006) built on Kolb's work and identified four learning styles/preferences that individuals naturally prefer to use: activists, reflectors, theorists and pragmatists.

Activists

People who prefer doing things and involving themselves fully in new experiences are referred to as activists. They have the following characteristics:

- Open-mindedness
- 'Try anything once', usually without any planning
- Learn best when being 'thrown into things' and enjoy working alongside others in order to solve a problem
- Learn least well from passive activities such as reading, watching or listening
- Prefer activities that have a short timespan
- Get bored with repetition and resist replaying past events in their minds, preferring instead to live in the present.

Reflectors

Reflectors prefer to reflect and observe. They tend to collect information, sift through it thoroughly, look at the issues from a range of perspectives and, not surprisingly, can be slow to make decisions or come to any conclusions. They have the following characteristics:

- Learn best when they are able to stand back, listen and observe
- Learn least well when rushed into things with insufficient information or time to plan
- Cautiousness, postponing making decisions or definitive conclusions as long as possible; however, when they do so, their decisions are usually soundly based on what they have learned.

Theorists

People who prefer to focus on trying to understand reasons, ideas and relationships are called theorists and ask the question: 'Why?' They enjoy using their logic and ideas (rather than their feelings) in order to understand situations and problems and have the following characteristics:

- Tendency not be to happy until they have an understanding of what underpins their observations
- Tendency to be perfectionists and need to know the underlying principles and theories to ensure that any actions are based on logic rather than subjectivity or ambiguity
- Learn best when they can use a theory, model, framework or other system
- Learn least well when they are asked to engage in activities which are unstructured, ambiguous and/or lack depth.

Pragmatists

Those who are receptive to new ideas and like to try things out to see if they work are called pragmatists. They have the following characteristics:

- Enjoyment of experimentation and problem-solving
- Very practical
- Prefer to work quickly, avoid delays and progress things that interest them
- Respond well to problems and challenges

- Learn best when there is an obvious link between the subject matter and their current job
- Learn least well when there are no immediate benefits or rewards from the activity.

Deep, strategic and surface learning

Another facet to learning styles is the depth of effort to which learners exert themselves. Different intentions lead to contrasting study strategies and learning experiences. People do not usually just adopt one approach but rather, based on the circumstances, choose the approach that most suits a particular set of circumstances. Using deep or strategic approaches is associated with a better quality of learning (Table 4.1).

Deep approach to learning

This approach is generally expected of learners studying at university. Students who adopt a deep approach to their learning study with the aim of deriving meaning from what they learn, and then compare that meaning to previous experiences and ideas. Such students are intrinsically motivated to learn successfully about the subject area and, as a result, the deep approach to learning is associated with long-term success (Baeten et al 2010). The same applies to patients or clients who learn about their illnesses or conditions, as those who adopt a deep approach are likely to access the Internet to obtain information and question healthcare professionals in order to clarify their understanding.

Strategic approach to learning

The intention of learners using this approach is to achieve the highest possible grades. Learners take a strategic approach to maximize their marks or grades by systematically managing the time and effort they put into their study. These learners, often motivated by competition, are alert to assessment criteria and other requirements and often gear their work towards the perceived preferences of lecturers.

Table 4.1 Characteristics of surface, deep and strategic approaches to learning

Characteristics of students adopting a surface approach	Characteristics of students adopting a deep approach	Characteristics of students adopting a strategic approach
• Most likely to have poor study skills and worry excessively about their assessments. • Tendency to focus on memorising facts and rote learning. • Focus of their study is to acquire sufficient knowledge in order to recall it when needed. • No attempt to actively engage with the learning material. • No desire to reflect or make connections so their learning is fragmented and disconnected.	• Usually have well-developed study and time management skills. • Have a genuine desire to learn and enjoy the process. • As they study, they are very much active in the process. • There is a conscious deliberation to seek out and make links with what they already know so that they gain a more holistic understanding of the material.	• Usually have well-developed study and time management skills. • Tendency to focus on the requirements of the assessment as opposed to focusing on learning for learnings sake. • Will adopt deep or surface approaches depending on how they view what they are being asked to do in their assessment. • Tendency to question, spot and pick up tutor cues and preferences.

Surface approach to learning

The intention in this approach is to cope with course requirements. Learners adopting this approach are primarily motivated by a fear of failing and study without reflecting on what they are doing or why they are doing it. Each aspect of learning is treated as an unrelated bit of knowledge, which in turn makes it difficult to make sense of new ideas. Learners try to 'suss out' what the teacher wants and aim to provide this by concentrating solely on assessment requirements and routinely memorizing facts and procedures. Learners using a surface approach rarely achieve understanding and, unsurprisingly, this approach is associated with poor academic performance.

Summary

Before reading on, you should carry out the activities in Box 4.3. When overloaded with coursework it is likely that a strategic approach will be taken. If the subject matter is compulsory but boring, a surface approach may be taken in order to meet minimum requirements. Where there is an intrinsic interest in the subject matter, such as when a client or patient wishes to learn about a health problem, then a deep approach is more likely to be taken.

 Reflective practice Box 4.3

Your approaches to learning

Student activities

- Think of your own experiences as a student. Identify examples of when you engaged in deep, strategic and surface learning
- How useful was each type of learning for your understanding of the subject?
- What were the reasons for engaging in each type of learning? (See Table 4.1.)

Reflection

Essentially, reflection is an active, conscious process in which an individual examines their experiences, beliefs, values, behaviour and knowledge that leads to a new understanding and appreciation of the situation which prompted the reflective process (Boud et al 1985). This process involves looking beyond the immediate situation and delving below the surface in order to provide care relevant to the particular context of the patient or client. Stepping back in this way informs practice, creates learning and brings new meaning. From that understanding, judgements can be made on how to ensure one's practice is based firmly on evidence. Reflection is a key requirement in nursing programmes (NMC 2010, Essential Skills Clusters 12.3, 14.1).

Dewey (1933) initially brought the idea of reflection to nurses' attention. In the 1980s, Schon's work highlighted the central role of reflection in professional practice, predominantly in teaching and nursing (Johns 2009). Schon (1995) described reflection as having two constituents:

- Reflection-*in*-action, which is generated from an experience and involves thinking about what one is doing while actually doing it
- Reflection-*on*-action that occurs when the practitioner considers aspects of their practice afterwards.

Greenwood (1993) added a third dimension to reflective practice – 'reflection-before-action'. Greenwood argued that reflection-before-action was important as it related to practitioners reflecting about what they intended to do before they actually did it and in this way, minimize the risk of making errors.

Reflection is therefore the process of examining and thinking about what we do within the context of the world around us. Reflection is more than just describing what we do or an event that has occurred. It goes beyond that to thinking about why we do things, whether they have gone as intended, why they did or did not go well and/or why and how we might do things differently the next time.

Purpose of reflection

Becoming a reflective practitioner is essential to becoming a nurse. Reflection facilitates understanding of both oneself and others within the context of practice and encourages thinking about practice. Nursing students must learn about the importance of reflection as a way of linking theory to practice. There are several ways to facilitate the use and development of these skills, which include regular reflective group sessions with peers and academic staff, keeping a reflective journal, log or diary, and incorporating reflection within written assessments.

Models of reflection

There are several models of reflection and three are considered below. They all contain the same principles but are differentiated by the level of detail they provide.

Gibbs' reflective cycle

Gibbs (1988) presented a reflective cycle as a way of providing structure for practitioners to follow when reflecting. It consists of six sequential steps, beginning with the description of an event through to producing an action plan for future practice (Fig. 4.3A).

Atkins and Murphy's framework for reflection

Atkins and Murphy presented the framework for their reflective model in 1993 (Fig. 4.3B) and is more detailed than Gibbs' model. This model emphasizes the skills used in the reflective process, namely:

- Self-awareness (see Ch. 9)
- Description
- Critical analysis
- Synthesis
- Evaluation (see p. 94).

When using Atkins and Murphy's model, it is important to recognize that the first step of awareness of uncomfortable feelings and thoughts can be stimulated by positive as well as

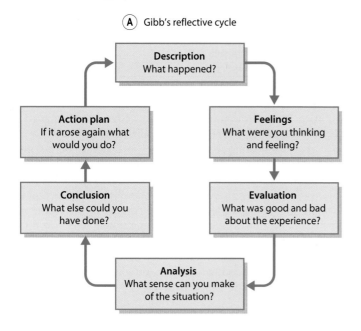

Ⓐ Gibb's reflective cycle

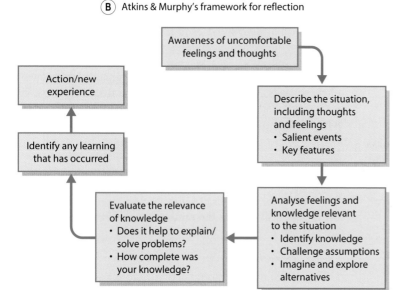

Ⓑ Atkins & Murphy's framework for reflection

Fig. 4.3 • Models of reflection. (A) Gibbs' reflective cycle. (Reproduced with permission from Gibbs, G., 1988. Learning by doing. Further Education Unit, Sheffield.) (B) Atkins and Murphy's framework for reflection. (Reproduced with permission from Atkins, S., Murphy, K., 1993. Reflection: a review of the literature. Journal of Advanced Nursing 18 (8), 1188–1192.)

negative experiences. For example, during a teaching session you realize that there is now new evidence which demonstrates that an aspect of care you have been performing in practice is no longer appropriate. The experience is positive in that the teaching session involved disseminating up-to-date good practice, but it also produced uncomfortable feelings as the evidence supporting the new practice was more than 6 months old and in that time, you have been practising unaware of the new evidence.

The final step in Atkins and Murphy's model involves action as in all reflective models. Finishing a reflective account with an action plan is essential because, as a practice-based profession, nursing is about seeking to learn from experience in order to improve practice.

LEARN framework for reflection

The College of Nurses of Ontario, Canada (1996) developed this framework. It is presented as a cyclical process containing the five steps that should occur during the process of reflection. LEARN is an acronym for these five steps (Box 4.4).

The process of reflection

There are a number of triggers or stimuli for reflection. Petersson and Springett (2009) suggest the following:

• A successful event
• A problematic event
• A problematic event that ended successfully.

Reflective practice   Box 4.4

Using the LEARN framework

Step 1 – **L**ook back at an experience or event that has happened in your practice recently. Review it in your mind as if you were watching a video.

Step 2 – **E**laborate and describe, verbally or in writing, what happened during the event. How did you feel and how do you think others felt? What were the outcomes? Were you surprised by what happened during the event or did it turn out as you expected?

Step 3 – **A**nalyse the outcomes. Review why the event turned out the way it did. Why did you feel or react the way you did and why did others feel/react the way they did? If the event or outcomes were not what you expected, consider how you could improve on them next time. This is an opportunity to really question your beliefs and assumptions, and ask yourself what the experience reveals about what you value. It is also a good time to ask for feedback from others.

Step 4 – **R**evise your approach based on your review of the event and decide how, or if, you will change your approach. This might involve asking others for ideas for dealing with the situation next time or how to work on a learning need. With your new learning, you may decide to try a new approach, learn more about the subject, or decide that you handled the situation very well.

Step 5 – **N**ew trial. Put your new approach into action. This may require anticipating or creating a situation in which you can then try out your new approach.

Student activity

Think of a scenario or an incident which you have either observed or been involved in while on practice placement and work through it using the five steps of the LEARN framework.

(Reproduced with permission from the College of Nurses of Ontario.)

The trigger or stimulus for reflection is often referred to as a critical incident. A critical incident is an event that has an impact or significant effect on your learning or practice. Analysing critical incidents is a useful way of gaining an understanding of the dimensions of your role and better understanding interactions with patients/clients and other healthcare professionals.

Reflection begins with choosing an incident which represents an issue that warrants further exploration for any of the reasons listed above. The first step involves the nurse becoming self-aware, accepting that there may be other ways of thinking about or practising nursing, and being honest about how a significant event affected them as an individual and the impact that this had within the practice setting. This is important for linking theory to practice.

The next step is a comprehensive verbal or written description, of all components of the significant event, constantly bearing in mind the importance of maintaining confidentiality (NMC 2008a, see also Ch. 7). The incident should be described by including where and when it happened, what actually happened in detail (who did what, said what, etc.) and your own thoughts and feelings during and after the incident.

This is followed by broadening and deepening your understanding by exploring existing knowledge and theories that influenced what happened in the significant event, and exploring and challenging your assumptions. Probe the incident by answering the following questions:

- Why was the incident significant to me?
- Why do I view the incident in that way?
- Why was this incident particularly effective/ineffective?
- What assumptions have I made about the problem, patient(s)/client(s) or colleagues?
- How else could I interpret the incident?
- What other action(s) could have been taken that may have been more helpful?
- What have I learned from this process?
- What can I do to improve my own or others' practice in light of this process?

New knowledge is integrated with existing knowledge to solve problems creatively and predict consequences. It is usually at this stage that the process identified in the above steps is written up using relevant literature to support assertions, judgements and conclusions.

When writing up a critical incident analysis or a reflective account, the first person voice (I) is used rather than the third person, which is normally used in academic writing. Use of the third person provides distance from both the incident and the reflective process, which is inappropriate when the focus should be on the individual's journey. It is essential that written reflective accounts abide by *The Code: Standards of Conduct, Performance and Ethics for Nurses and Midwives* (NMC 2008a) and protect the anonymity and confidentiality of those involved in any incidents or events (Box 4.5).

Maintaining confidentiality in reflective accounts   Box 4.5

On an early shift in the third week of my surgical placement I watched Staff Nurse Robin Hood (pseudonym) teaching a patient called John Smith (pseudonym) how to change his colostomy bag. The way that Robin explained the procedure to John was very clear and as John had been encouraged to watch how his bag was changed since his operation, the whole teaching process seemed to go well. Robin was very careful to explain each step to John, emphasizing particular points such as the importance of cleaning and drying the skin surrounding the stoma, making sure that there were no wrinkles in the adhesive dressing around the stoma and ensuring that the bag was securely fastened. I really thought the way that Robin stressed the importance of listening for the bag clicking into place was especially useful as that is one of the points that I always find reassuring when I change a colostomy bag.

In longer reflective accounts or coursework, this may be achieved by inserting the following near the beginning: 'In order to maintain confidentiality (NMC 2010, Essential Skills Clusters 7.1) all the names of those involved have been replaced with pseudonyms'.

Once written, it is useful to share your reflective analysis with others as this facilitates learning from others' perspectives, allowing further exploration to be undertaken as appropriate. It is also good practice to further reflect on the process of sharing your analysis with others.

The final step in the reflective cycle is evaluation, where a judgement takes place in order to develop a new perspective on the critical incident or significant event. The new perspective is developed from the broadening and deepening of understanding and the acknowledgement of how the individual would adopt different practices in the future. The cycle ends with the development of an action plan including specific learning outcomes (see Box 4.14, p. 103) for future development. Bulman and Schutz (2008) suggest practical tips to assist in the process of reflection (Box 4.6).

Practical tips for reflection   Box 4.6

1. Use a reflective model – stick it on your notice board above your desk where you study; refer to it as you work on your first jottings.

2. Get something down on paper as soon as possible, not necessarily something academic or part of assessed work, but something you can check out with your mentor in the first instance.

3. Keeping a reflective diary is helpful for some people – write down what happened and why, then ask yourself what did I learn and what would I do next time?

4. Look back over your diary – use it to inform your academic work.

5. Make sure you fix up an early meeting with your mentor and keep it! Check your mentor knows what is expected of both of you.

6. Develop a repertoire of practice to draw on, store up experiences that you could use later in your reflective work, e.g. by making notes, jotting things down, so that important experiences are not lost.

7. Get to know your mentor, and use learning opportunities and experiences for writing reflective accounts.

8. Make the most of any individual or group opportunities to get feedback.

9. Write some notes on your reflection(s), then leave them for a while (about 2 days). When you re-read your reflective notes you may find it easier to engage in more critical reflection. Ensure that your writing does not reveal any confidential details.

10. Refer to your reflective model/framework and ensure all stages are covered in order to complete your analysis.

11. Go deep, not wide, in your analysis.

12. Live with the lack of perfection – realize you won't always achieve the ideal, just do what you can to the best of your ability.

(Adapted from Bulman and Schutz 2008, p 35).

Critical thinking

Critical thinking is an important part of your learning and is closely aligned with reflection. In order to be an autonomous reflective practitioner you need to develop critical thinking. This is recognized in the NMC (2010) Essential Skills Clusters (10.4, 10.9, 14.9). Jasper (2006, p 75) defines critical thinking

as: '… one of the ways in which practitioners make decisions about their practice'. Cox and Hill (2010) provide the following characteristics of critical thinkers: being open-minded; being inquisitive; being courageous about asking difficult questions; using critical analysis; being systematic in problem-solving; questioning and, challenging and trusting their own reasoning, skills, insights and judgements. Gopee (2002) provides a useful framework to illustrate the processes involved in critical analysis (Fig. 4.4).

Factors influencing learning

There are a number of factors that influence learning. These include motivation, feedback and readiness to learn, difficulties people may have in the process of learning and the environment in which learning takes place.

Motivation

Motivation influences what people do (if there is a choice), how long they do something and how well they do it. Motivation is a key factor in successful learning and a central feature in most theories of learning. Without motivation, learning does not take place, as we need to be motivated enough to pay attention while learning. There are two sources of motivation:

- Internal
- External.

Internal, or intrinsic, motivation arises from within the individual and is made up of personal factors that make them want to learn. Internal motivation is longer lasting and more self-directive than external motivation. This is because praise, reward or incentive must be provided repeatedly to reinforce external motivation (see Behaviourism, above). For individuals who are externally motivated, the desire to learn is secondary to the reward gained from learning. According to Knowles et al (1998), adults' motivation to learn is largely internally generated through self-esteem, quality of life and job satisfaction. Adults who are motivated to seek out learning experiences do so primarily because they have a use for the knowledge or skill being sought.

Since motivation is essential to learning, it is important to be aware of the factors that enhance and diminish it. Factors that enhance and sustain motivation include a warm and accepting learning environment, incentives such as praise, feedback and knowledge of one's progress, and the way in which learning materials are organized. As can be seen from Box 4.7 (p. 96), the factors associated with diminishing motivation are more numerous than those which enhance it. The best way, therefore, to motivate adult learners is to enhance their reasons for learning and decrease the barriers.

When thinking of motivation related to patient/client education, additional barriers must also be considered. The individual's perception of their state of health can shape their motivation to learn as can their stage of development (Ch. 8) and ability to understand (Ch. 9). Confusion, pain, lack of sleep, noise, interruptions or lack of privacy can interfere with

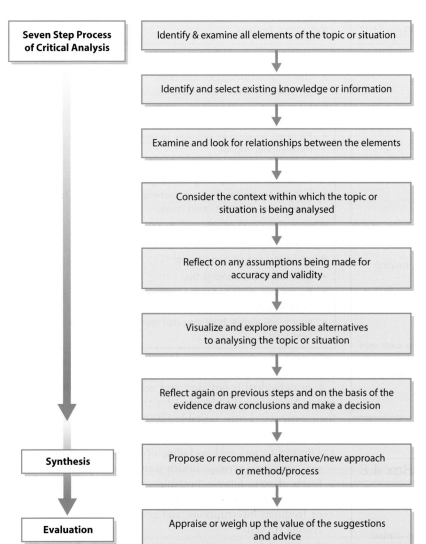

Seven Step Process of Critical Analysis	
	Identify & examine all elements of the topic or situation
	Identify and select existing knowledge or information
	Examine and look for relationships between the elements
	Consider the context within which the topic or situation is being analysed
	Reflect on any assumptions being made for accuracy and validity
	Visualize and explore possible alternatives to analysing the topic or situation
	Reflect again on previous steps and on the basis of the evidence draw conclusions and make a decision
Synthesis	Propose or recommend alternative/new approach or method/process
Evaluation	Appraise or weigh up the value of the suggestions and advice

Fig. 4.4 • Seven factor framework for critically analysing a health topic or issue. (After Gopee, N., 2002. Demonstrating critical analysis in academic assignments. Nursing Standard 16 (35), 45–52.)

a patient's/client's ability to concentrate and therefore learn. The nurse as teacher who is insensitive to people's cultural, ethnic, spiritual and/or social needs can also diminish their motivation to learn (Box 4.8).

The place of feedback in learning

Learning is an active process which requires feedback so the learner knows how effective their learning has been. In addition to providing information about how well a learner has performed, feedback should also identify areas for further personal and professional improvement. (Using and responding to feedback are highlighted in the NMC (2010) Essential Skills Clusters 12.4, 12.6, 12.8; and 14.4.) As a nursing student, it is important to understand the purpose of feedback and to learn to respond positively to constructive feedback on both your written and practical performance.

Feedback should be specific rather than general, it should be immediate and contain details of what was good about your performance and why. In addition, it should highlight which elements require further practice and attention with an explanation of how this can be achieved. It is also a good idea for you to assess your own performance so that you develop the ability to make judgements about your own performance. The quality of the feedback is important, as praise is motivating and can encourage you to try to do better next time. Although receiving and giving feedback on both positive and negative aspects of a performance is important, the manner in which this is done is even more important. The key factors are listed in Box 4.9.

How do you learn?

As a nursing student you should be thinking about how you yourself learn as a life-long reflective learner. Successful learners have specific characteristics – take a few minutes to look at Figure 4.5 and see how many of these you have. Do not worry if you are missing some of these characteristics, as they can be learned. That is why successful learners are often not the most intelligent in the class, but the ones who have learned and used strategies to help them become successful.

Reflective practice Box 4.7

Motivators: your study habits

Barriers to motivation

- High levels of anxiety
- Sensory deficits
- Low literacy
- Fatigue
- Inability to concentrate
- Poor past learning experiences
- Stress
- Lack of time
- Lack of money
- Lack of child-care facilities
- Low self-confidence
- Poor learning environment, e.g. inadequate lighting, heating and acoustics
- Being told that the subject matter is difficult and/or hard to understand.

Student activities

1. Think about an occasion when a learning experience went well and identify factors that may have led to this.
2. Thinking about your usual study habits and routines, identify:
   - Barriers that may impede your learning
   - Strategies you could employ to reduce them.

 Reflective practice Box 4.8

Motivators: patients and clients

Student activities

1. Reflect on patient/client teaching that you have seen carried out in your placement and:
   - Identify factors used to motivate patients/clients
   - Identify potential barriers to their motivation
   - Identify the extent to which learning activities integrate people's cultural, spiritual and social needs
   - Discuss your findings with your mentor.
2. Think about how the following scenarios could affect the individual's motivation to learn about their health problem.
   - Ian Fraser, who is in pain and remains anxious following his recent myocardial infarction (heart attack)
   - Harriet Harrison, who is suffering from postnatal depression following the birth of her second baby
   - Jennifer King (aged 8), who has recently been diagnosed with diabetes and is frightened about learning how to give herself injections
   - Sam Donaldson, who has a learning disability and needs to learn how and when to wash his hands.

Readiness to learn

'Readiness to learn' means that a learner is receptive and wants to engage in the learning process. In other words, they are motivated and able to learn. This is usually signalled by the learner asking a question and is crucial to the learning process

Effective feedback Box 4.9

Feedback should:

- Use clear unambiguous language
- Be specific, honest and personalized
- Be given in a way that respects the individuality and worth of learners
- Be given as soon as possible to provide the highest motivational impact
- Be delivered in a quiet and private setting
- Comment positively on good things
- Use the feedback sandwich technique: good news, not so good news and then good news.

When giving good news:

- Tell the learner what was good/right and why.

When giving not so good news:

- Be honest and constructive
- Be specific, kind and non-judgemental
- Tell the learner what was poor/wrong and why
- Inform the learner how they can improve their performance next time.

– if an individual is not alert and motivated, learning will not occur. Nurses need to be alert for these signals, or cues, from their patients/clients. Bastable (2008) presents four groups of factors affecting readiness to learn:

- *Physical factors* such as failing eyesight, e.g. seeing the markings on a syringe; health status and in particular levels of pain, fatigue, breathlessness; unfavourable surrounding conditions such as high levels of noise or frequent interruptions; and generally 'not feeling rushed'
- *Emotional factors* such as motivation, levels of anxiety (that impairs the ability to concentrate and retain information) and generally one's 'frame of mind'
- *Experiential factors* relating to past experiences with learning including the level of aspiration, past coping mechanisms (e.g. support structures); cultural background and language (including ethnicity, religious and health beliefs, see Ch. 1); and locus of control when one is internally motivated
- *Knowledge-related factors* including current knowledge base, cognitive ability and learning and reading problems (see p. 98).

Readiness to learn influences the timing of useful teaching. Patients/clients are generally more receptive to information about their illness shortly after diagnosis or prior to treatment and want information that is immediate and personally relevant (Bastable 2008). There are a number of ways in which relevant information can be imparted and at a time when readiness to learn is often at its highest. For example:

- Patients attending a pre-admission clinic before planned surgery (see Ch. 24)
- Children having nutritional support at home
- People with a learning disability attending the GP or accessing screening procedures (see Ch. 1).

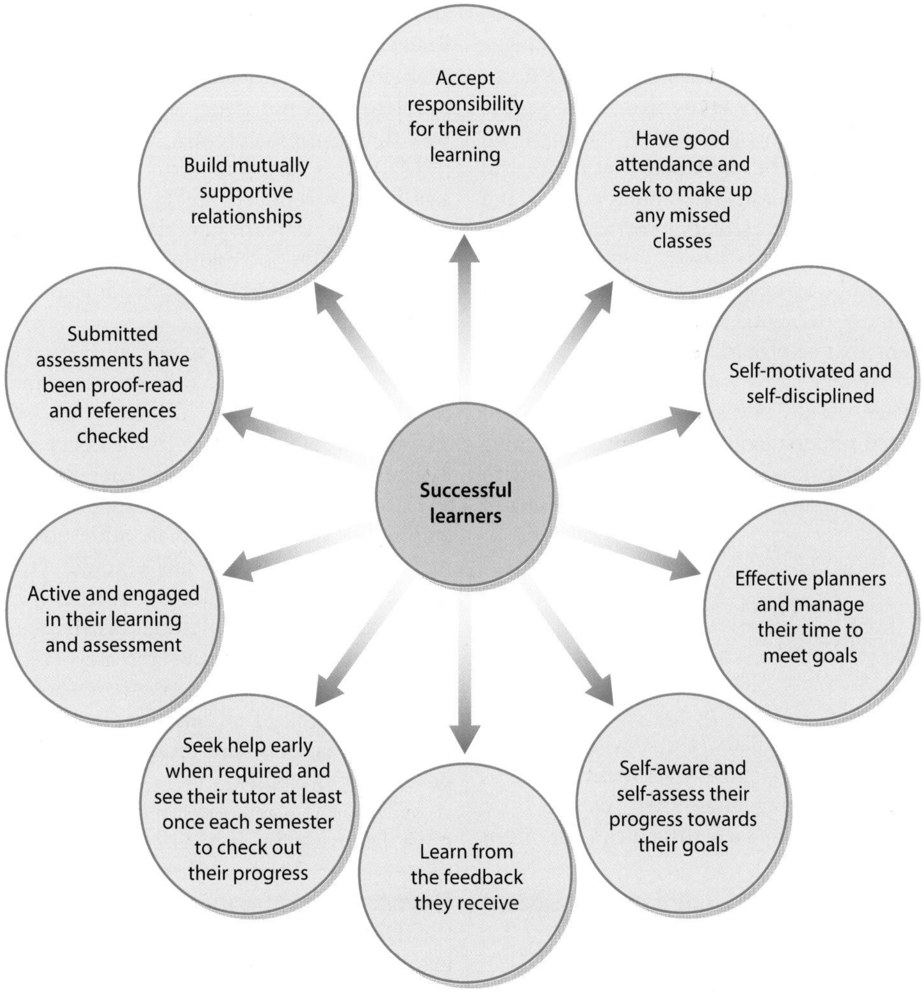

Fig. 4.5 • Characteristics of successful learners. (Based on Rowles, J., 2011. Learning is not easy: How can we help our students to learn? Currents in Pharmacy Teaching and Learning 3 (2), 159–162 and Cottrell, S., 2008. The study skills handbook, third ed. Palgrave Macmillan, London.)

Bastable (2008) presents four types of readiness to learn and uses the acronym PEEK to describe these:

- **P**hysical readiness
- **E**motional readiness
- **E**xperiential readiness
- **K**nowledge readiness.

All of these should be considered as they can have an adverse effect on the degree to which learning will take place.

Assessment of physical readiness is important, especially when the proposed learning requires physical strength or capability. For example, learning to walk with crutches requires physical strength and coordination, learning to inject a drug requires fine motor skills and good vision. Children or people with a learning disability who are learning to fasten buttons also need fine motor coordination. Learning also requires the individual to be alert and have enough energy to concentrate (Bastable 2008).

Emotional readiness relates to a number of areas. For example, a little anxiety can motivate learning but undue levels are counterproductive. If patients/clients are scared or anxious about something they have to learn, this must be managed before learning can begin. For example, learning to self-administer injections may produce fear because of the necessity to inflict pain on oneself. Furthermore, fear and/or anxiety may cause patients or clients to deny the existence of their illness, which severely limits their readiness to learn. Emotional readiness also extends to students and 'fear of the unknown' often causes them anxiety. Despite mentors orientating nursing students into a new placement, students' high anxiety levels may mean that although they are hearing what is being said, they may be unable to take in what is actually being said.

Experiential readiness is related to individuals' past learning experiences and whether these have been positive or negative. Someone who has had previous poor learning experiences is unlikely to be motivated or willing to risk trying to acquire new knowledge or skills. According to Bastable (2008), experiential readiness involves the level of aspiration, past coping skills, cultural background and motivation.

Knowledge readiness relates to the individual's current knowledge, their level of learning capability and their learning style. It is important to establish the individual's knowledge base, as teaching what is already known is boring, demotivating and can be construed as insulting. Teaching should move from the known to the unknown. For example, when teaching a patient about their diabetes and the need for insulin, the nurse could ask them whether they already know that many people with diabetes require insulin. If this is the case, moving from the known to the unknown could be explaining that the reason why insulin must be injected is because it is broken down and digested if taken orally and therefore would not work if given in tablet form.

Cognitive ability should be assessed because factors such as developmental stage, illness, dementia or learning disability can impair this to an extent that explanations need to be broken down into simple and smaller steps with frequent repetition built in. Simple language should be used. Including pictorial information can enhance understanding and convey meaning more readily. Nurses must seek ways to help individuals with a learning disability overcome any problems with processing of information (see below).

Individuals disadvantaged when considering information needs

Consideration requires to be given to people with particular needs, e.g. those who use wheelchairs, those with visual or hearing impairments (see Ch. 16), those with mental distress or illness, and those with learning disabilities. With a little thought, the needs of people with such difficulties can often be easily met. For example:

- For wheelchair users, having leaflets and posters at an accessible height may be sufficient
- People with a visual impairment may benefit from audiotapes or Braille sheets
- Access to videos or written information for those with hearing impairment.

Computers are another learning tool that can be used by many people, particularly since technology permits accessibility, i.e. the ability to access material regardless of peoples' needs. They can be used in various ways such as accessing the Internet to find information and sending e-mail messages to experts so that individual questions can be answered.

People who have problems in learning

There are a variety of problems that may impinge on how individuals learn. These include people with visual and/or hearing impairment, with mobility problems and those with mental health problems, e.g. dementia. Others may be those with:

- Dyslexia, which involves a range of abilities and/or a variety of problems that may affect several aspects of learning including reading, spelling, writing and numbers
- Autism, a lifelong condition that impinges on how an individual communicates with and relates to others
- Asperger syndrome, which is a form of autism.

Chapter 2 describes what learning disability nursing involves. In relation to teaching and learning, it is important to realize that many individuals with learning difficulties have average or above average intelligence. In fact, Albert Einstein, Richard Branson and Tom Cruise are among those known to have had problems with learning. So, having a learning difficulty or problem does not mean a person cannot learn, it just means that they learn differently. The Department of Health (2001, p 14) states that the term 'learning disability' includes: 'A significantly reduced ability to understand new or complex information, to learn new skills (impaired intelligence), with a reduced ability to cope independently (impaired social functioning) which started before adulthood, with a lasting effect on development'.

It is also important to recognize that people with learning disabilities form a very diverse group and can have a number of problems such as difficulty in solving practical and abstract problems, difficulty in conceptualizing patterns and difficulty in communication generally. Having one or more of these difficulties means that such people acquire knowledge and skills more slowly than other people. Not surprisingly, feelings of frustration can emerge. However, being taught different learning strategies can help people learn more effectively, e.g. using pictorial instructions on cards or a computer screen to illustrate the key steps in the task to be learned. Good teaching practices should meet most of the disparate needs of all learners, including those with disabilities, whether these are caused by physical problems, dyslexia or learning disability.

Within the university and practice settings, adjustments must be made by law, as set out in the Equality Act (HM Government 2010) and the Disability Equality Duty in the Disability Discrimination Act 1995, sometimes referred to as the 'DDA', (HM Government 1995) that will help those with learning and/or physical disabilities. The changes that require to be made are known as 'reasonable adjustments' and identified on an individual basis. Now read the information in Box 4.10 and carry out the activity at the bottom.

The learning environment

Regardless of where learning takes place – at university, at home, in placements, clinics or day centres – creating a supportive environment is essential to successful learning. A supportive or conducive learning environment:

- Is free from physical or psychological harm
- Encourages mutual trust, respect and helpfulness
- Allows active participation and a questioning approach
- Is free from intimidation or rejection
- Is high in acceptable challenge
- Takes differing learning styles and cultural and ethnic origins into account.

Anxiety has a direct bearing on an individual's ability to learn as, physiologically, the stress response limits the individual's thinking capacity and inhibits attention. A conducive learning environment includes acquaintance of group members and this is why many courses start with ice-breaking exercises. Over time, the peer group develops cohesion in which each member begins to feel secure and knows that their contributions will be valued.

Critical thinking Box 4.10

Language and reading difficulties

Language difficulty

Sheena has an expressive language difficulty. She has difficulty with expressing herself clearly and precisely because she finds it difficult to know which words are appropriate and how sentences should be structured. She also has problems copying from whiteboards, overheads and PowerPoint slides, and with note-taking, handwriting and spelling. To help, Sheena should be:

- Allowed to use a word processor with a spelling checker
- Encouraged to use specialist advice and guidance
- Given both written and verbal instructions
- Allowed to tape-record lectures or let someone take notes for her (a scribe).

Reading difficulty

Fred has dyslexia. This causes him difficulty with decoding unfamiliar words, understanding what he reads, knowing the meaning of words read, and maintaining an efficient rate of reading. To help Fred, he should be encouraged to:

- Skim-read the chapter before actually reading it to get an idea of its structure and content
- Use different coloured pens to highlight main points or definitions
- Stop at the end of each page to check his understanding of what he has just read
- Read aloud parts that he finds particularly difficult and ask when he needs help or advice about meaning.

Student activities

- There is a client with dyslexia in your placement. Using the Internet, find out what services are available to help.
- Find out about the support available for students with learning difficulties at your university.

Resource

Guildford Technical Community College – www.gtcc.edu/students/student-services/disability-access-services/student-resources/tips-for-success.aspx October 2012.

In applying Maslow's hierarchy of needs (see pp. 86-87) to the educational environment, Freitas and Leonard (2011) explain that an individual's physical needs must be met first. Being in a cold or overheated room, sitting for long periods without adequate breaks or struggling to hear because of background noise all impinge on the ability to relax and pay attention. In terms of safety, Freitas and Leonard (2011) point out that those involved in teaching need to ensure that the learning environment is safe enough for learners to feel able to voice concerns or ask questions. Fostering mutual respect and acknowledging that learners' self-esteem and pride can be injured through humiliation and lack of sensitivity can enhance the latter. Mutual respect also falls into Maslow's belonging level by ensuring that all learners have their voice heard and their presence acknowledged. Self-esteem needs are met by providing feedback to make learners feel valued. Careful use of positive and constructive feedback nurtures the development of self-esteem, while negative or destructive comments speedily reverses it (Freitas & Leonard 2011).

Stuart (2007) identifies four categories that make up a learning environment, namely:

- People
- Learning opportunities and experiences
- Staff commitment to teaching and learning
- Material resources.

At university, academic staff are responsible for creating a good learning environment and many institutions use a personal tutor system, where a named lecturer guides and supports learners through their programme by providing feedback on draft assignments and one-to-one discussions regarding their personal and professional development.

In practice settings, ward managers, members of the multidisciplinary team and mentors are responsible for creating and fostering a supportive learning environment. Mentors play a pivotal role in supervising, supporting, facilitating and assessing students' learning. In addition, healthcare assistants, patients/clients and their carers and families are sources from which to learn. An effective mentor is a good role model who has the ability to enhance students' learning experiences by being approachable, planning a variety of different learning experiences and maximizing learning opportunities. They appreciate the need to provide detailed feedback on how their mentee is progressing and offer guidance and support to improve their practice (Gray 2011; Kragelund 2011). The same characteristics apply to any teaching, including that involving patients and clients.

Role models

Children are eager to find role models to copy or imitate, usually their parents. They watch them closely and follow their example. The NMC Standards for Education (2010, Domain 2) recognize that role models are important to nursing and other healthcare students and that it is from them that students learn how to socialize into their profession. Nurses and other healthcare workers tend to choose professional role models on the basis of their clinical skills, personality and teaching ability. From role models, nursing students learn both appropriate and inappropriate behaviours, as role models can be good or poor. A good role model is someone students can look up to, value and admire what they do and say, and may wish to emulate. They demonstrate professionalism in all aspects of their practice, whereas poor role models do not. Nurses may think that they will only learn from good role models but by reflecting on what makes someone a good or poor role model means that students can learn from both. However, inexperienced nursing students may not be knowledgeable enough to discriminate between safe and unsafe practice and therefore inadvertently learn poor practice (Box 4.11).

It is important to note that individuals do not deliberately choose to be role models. Healthcare professionals are role models, good or bad, at all times because others are constantly watching them and forming opinions. Not only are students observed by qualified healthcare professionals but also by other students, patients/clients, carers and their relatives. Nurses are also expected to be role models in pursuing healthy lifestyles, promoting health and, in time, implementing health promotion

---

Reflective practice   Box 4.11

Role models

Student activities

Think of three people who you would identify as either good or less effective role models:

- What characteristics do they have?
- What makes them a good role model?
- If they are a less effective role model, why did you identify them in this way?

---

strategies. Nurses can also learn from patients/clients and carers as role models, as they can inspire them in many different ways. Learning from people with longstanding health problems can be very valuable, as they often know more about their conditions than many healthcare professionals.

Summary

In terms of the learning environment, learning opportunities and experiences are paramount in achieving learning outcomes. As well as academic and placement staff ensuring that there are appropriate learning opportunities and experiences available, learners also have a responsibility to take maximum advantage of the opportunities afforded to them.

Teaching and learning methods

There are different teaching and learning methods that include mass instruction, individualized and group methods. The method used impacts on the effectiveness of learning and retention of information. The more active people are in the learning process, the better their learning, which means that experiential learning is the most effective method. A variety of teaching and learning methods are discussed in this section, including action learning, problem-based learning and the use of portfolios.

Mass instruction methods

These include lectures using a variety of learning technologies such as PowerPoint, videos, patient information leaflets and posters. These methods do not encourage an active approach from participants. Lectures are only 5% effective as a teaching method, while reading is 10% effective and a video or poster is 20% effective (National Training Laboratories, NTL undated).

Individualized methods

These include directed study such as online or computer-assisted learning, reflection, portfolios, workbooks, demonstrations and flexible learning materials. These methods encourage a more active approach from participants and are therefore more effective. Demonstrations are about 30% effective, while practice by doing is around 75% effective (NTL undated).

Group methods

These include reflective group sessions, group work, self-help groups, action learning (see below), problem-based learning (see below), tutorials and seminars. Again, these methods require active participation. NTL (undated) states that discussion groups are about 50% effective in terms of the learning process.

Role of teacher

Student nurses will be involved in using these methods both to teach others (peers and patients) and as active participants. The teaching role is the most active of all and this is reflected in the effectiveness of teaching others (90% effective) as a way of improving one's own learning (NTL undated). In summary, teaching using methods where the learner is passive are much less effective than those where the learner is active during the learning process.

Action learning

Action learning involves learning in small cooperative groups, usually referred to as action learning sets. The fundamental premise of action learning sets is working on solving real-life issues and/or problems by learning from others and reflecting on the process. The emphasis on 'real-life' problems means that adult learners bring their own problems to the action learning set and work together on how these can be solved. There is no one correct answer or solution, so the task is to develop a workable solution for a particular context. Action learning is based on a number of educational beliefs:

- Adults normally work better in groups
- The experience of working together in a supportive and constructive environment is beneficial
- Adults are capable of solving their own problems.

Through team working, individuals learn from each other by respecting different perceptions, perspectives, experiences and knowledge bases, all of which are harnessed in developing a solution to a problem or critical incident. Action learning is used to encourage team working in solving practice-based problems, finding resources, preparing presentations and placement-related activities (Box 4.12).

Principles of action learning   Box 4.12

- An action learning set is normally composed of between four and six members who remain together as a supportive group and meet regularly until the end of the action learning set
- Every member takes their turn in presenting their work related to the problem and being questioned by the others. The nature of the questioning should be open-ended and inquisitorial, and intended to encourage reflection. An action plan is then prepared for the next meeting
- The action learning set has an experienced advisor who establishes the ground rules about how members work together, with particular emphasis on confidentiality and the importance of building trust.

Problem-based learning

Problem-based learning (PBL) has its origins in medical education at McMaster University School of Medicine in Canada. Its use is widespread in a variety of disciplines, including nursing (McAllister 2007). PBL is a student-centred learning and teaching strategy that promotes learning by encouraging learners to actively engage with others to analyse and solve problems – a fundamental skill required of all healthcare professionals. The key principle of PBL is that students take control of their own learning. PBL is 'a strategy that promotes the development of critical thinking, analysis and reflection, alongside teamworking and collaboration' (Mannix & McIntosh 2011, p 138).

The teacher, acting as a facilitator, introduces a problem-based scenario to learners without any previous teaching input or study. Working in groups of 5–10, learners attempt to solve the problem(s) by suggesting a number of possible hypotheses and in doing so realize that their knowledge base is insufficient to solve the problem or explain how it can be solved. This leads to learners identifying areas for further learning and collecting material to build the necessary knowledge and evidence base in order to solve the problem. Learners work through the problem in a systematic way and then reflect on both the content and the process so that they can meet the learning outcomes associated with the scenario (McAllister 2007). Box 4.13 contains seven steps to solving a problem that can be used in any context, not just in PBL.

Seven steps to problem-solving	Box 4.13
1. Identify and define the problem 2. Obtain all the facts 3. Determine a number of workable solutions 4. Evaluate each solution for workability 5. Select the action that appears to be the most practical 6. Implement the selected solution 7. Evaluate the results.	
(*Source*: Mannix & McIntosh 2011.)	

Portfolios

Jasper (2006, p 155) states that 'a portfolio, when used in a professional context, is simply a collection of documents that present a picture of the practitioner'. A portfolio can be used for a variety of purposes such as to:

- Value practical experience as a source of learning
- Encourage reflective practice
- Provide a storehouse for information about and evidence of experience, learning and achievements
- Encourage personal and professional development (Buckley et al 2010).

Portfolios are a means by which learners accumulate evidence to demonstrate achievement of learning outcomes and/or competencies. As evidence is collected, a portfolio represents an individual's learning, progress and achievement over a period of time. Portfolios encourage personal and professional development by the use of reflection, self-assessment, evidence of attainment of specific learning outcomes and competencies, and action plans for future learning. Reflection (see above) is central to the learning processes involved in constructing and maintaining portfolios.

Completing a portfolio encourages deep learning, as the learner is required to actively engage in understanding the learning outcome and then compile evidence that demonstrates its achievement. Since portfolios are situated within practice, they encourage learners to make links between practice and its underpinning theory (Timmins & Dunne 2009; Buckley et al 2010).

Portfolios provide a vehicle for discussion between learners and their mentor/tutor and, as such, are useful for monitoring progression. Learners should keep copies of all feedback from coursework and practice placements in their portfolio. This should be read through carefully before meetings with personal tutors and/or mentors so that they can discuss the positive aspects of feedback and also those highlighted as requiring further development. Reflecting on feedback, as well as discussions with your tutor and/or mentor, should underpin your action plan to meet your personal learning needs. Portfolios are also the basis of Post-registration Education and Practice (PREP, NMC 2008b) and provide evidence of achieving both personal and specific professional learning outcomes.

The process of teaching

The information in this section is common to all teaching methods/activities explored below and it is also important to bear in mind that the information relates to readers in the roles of both student and teacher of others.

Nursing students are often required to give presentations to their peers as part of their coursework. The rationale for this is that when preparing to teach others, teachers engage with the material very effectively and consequently, their own learning becomes more in-depth and longer lasting. Similarly, when students are involved in teaching patients, clients and/or carers they find that through the preparation required for the teaching session they also develop their knowledge of the subject matter.

Teaching is about passing on information, communicating, informing and instructing. Telling is not teaching. Teaching is usually perceived as a planned structured activity based on aims and learning outcomes (see p. 103), designed to increase or improve a person's knowledge, skill or attitude on the subject.

Patient/client education 'is a process of assisting people to learn health-related behaviours that can be incorporated into everyday life with the goal of optimal health and independence in self-care' (Bastable 2008, p 12). Patients or clients often need to be taught skills and/or knowledge to help them maintain optimum health (see Ch. 1), prevent disease, manage illness and/or facilitate their independence. According to Bastable (2008), patient/client education has the potential to:

- Increase patient/client satisfaction with the nursing care delivered
- Improve quality of life
- Ensure continuity of care
- Reduce anxiety so that patients/clients know what to expect
- Reduce the incidence and onset of complications associated with illness
- Promote agreement with treatment plans and help people make informed choices about treatment
- Maximize independence in performing everyday activities
- Energize and empower patients/clients as they become actively engaged in planning their own care, which in turn provides them with a sense of control.

The last bullet point above relates to information giving, so that patients/clients can make informed decisions or give informed consent (see Chs 6, 7). Consent is normally prefixed by the word 'informed' and it is this which ensures that an individual who, before giving their informed consent, must:

- Have the relevant information
- Understand the information
- Be able to understand the probabilities and/or complications with any procedures and treatments being explained/suggested
- Be able to understand alternative choices to treatments/ therapies being suggested
- Be mentally competent (see Ch. 6)
- Consent voluntarily.

Conflicts and challenges in giving information can arise for a number of reasons. Timing of information giving is important. Giving it too early can mean that key messages are forgotten and giving it too late can lead to individuals not having enough opportunity to reflect upon the information given and ask further questions for clarification. The Department of Health has key documents on the topic of consent (see Useful websites, p. 104).

Just as nurses assess, plan, implement and evaluate their care using the nursing process (see Ch. 14), the same stages apply to teaching. Bastable (2008) draws parallels between the process of education and the nursing process. The headings used in Table 4.2 are used to underpin discussion of the teaching process below.

Assessment

Before setting out to 'teach' someone, it is essential to identify what the person/patient/client or groups of peers/patients/clients (hereafter referred to as learners):

- Need to know
- What they already know
- Their readiness to learn (p. 96)
- Their preferred learning style (p. 89).

Assessment of learners' needs prevents unnecessary repetition of known material, which saves time and energy for all parties. In order to teach, it is essential to read around the topic area including all the up-to-date literature and evidence (see Ch. 5 for literature searching and sources of evidence). Once what the learners already know has been established, assessment of what should be taught can begin.

Planning

The purpose of this phase is to plan what, how and when the intended teaching will take place. Following assessment, it will be evident what is already known and what remains to be taught. Knowing what to teach is not enough. Planning identifies which particular elements of the topic are essential to teach and those that are interesting, but not essential. Writing aims and learning outcomes helps in deciding what is essential and what is not. The nature of the learning outcomes provides the basis of deciding which teaching methods are most appropriate to use.

Consideration needs to be given to creating a motivating learning environment (see p. 98). To achieve this, it is important to involve learners in setting their own learning outcomes when possible and to ensure that the outcomes are at the appropriate level so they move learners to a higher level of understanding.

Table 4.2 Nursing process and education process in parallel

Nursing process		Education process
Appraise physical and psychological needs	Assessment	Ascertain learning needs, readiness to learn and learning styles
Develop care plan based on mutual goal setting to meet individual needs	Planning	Develop teaching plan based on mutually predetermined behavioural outcomes to meet individual needs
Carry out nursing care interventions using standard procedures	Implementation	Carry out teaching using specific instructional methods and tools
Determine physical and psychological outcomes and compare with intended plan	Evaluation	Determine behavioural changes (outcomes) in terms of knowledge, attitudes and skills, and compare with intended plan

(From Bastable, S.B., 2008. Nurse as educator, third ed. Jones and Bartlett, Boston.)

Table 4.3 Examples of levels within the cognitive domain

Domain level	Verbs associated with domain level	Example used in practice: On completion of the placement students should be able to:
Knowledge	Define, recall, identify, list, describe, draw, record	Recall knowledge and skills of assessment and its relation to planning, implementing and evaluating care
Comprehension	Describe, rephrase, explain, recognize, discuss, sort, rearrange, differentiate, estimate, conclude	Discuss barriers to communication within the assessment process
Application	Apply, generalize, demonstrate, illustrate, practise, relate, choose, develop, organize, use, transfer	Demonstrate a holistic approach to the assessment of patients and clients
Analysis	Analyse, distinguish, calculate, detect, deduce, classify, discriminate, categorize, test, inspect	Analyse the psychological and development needs of the sick child
Synthesis	Relate, produce, construct, organize, document, design, plan, propose, specify, derive, synthesize	Document the outcomes of nursing and other interventions relating to a patient or client with complex needs
Evaluation (see p. 94)	Judge, argue, justify, evaluate, assess, decide, compare, appraise, validate, select	Evaluate the role of the nurse within the multidisciplinary team context when caring for patients/clients with complex needs

Aims and learning outcomes

If there are no aims or learning outcomes, it is very difficult to focus one's learning or indeed provide evidence that any learning has actually occurred. In other words:

If you don't know where you are going, any road will get you there.

(Lewis Carrol 1831–1898)

Aims attempt to provide shape and direction to teaching and learning. They are general statements representing an ideal, or aspiration, and illustrate the overall purpose of a course. Learning outcomes should be clear, specific and contained within one sentence. Their purposes are to:

- Allow the learner to know what is expected of them
- Help the teacher define what has to be taught
- Assist the assessor by providing a means of deciding if the learner has met them.

Bloom (1964) proposed three main areas, also called domains, which are helpful in writing learning outcomes:

- The cognitive domain, concerned with knowledge and thinking
- The affective domain, which is concerned with feelings and attitudes
- The psychomotor domain that refers to manual, manipulative or practical skills.

Each of these domains is further broken down into a hierarchy with the simplest ones at the bottom. For example, the cognitive domain begins with knowledge and then moves upward to comprehension, application, analysis and ends with synthesis. This means that once knowledge of a topic is acquired, that knowledge can be applied by examining the relationship between elements and functions. Analysis is the next level that involves considering the context in which the topic area is being analysed, identifying and challenging assumptions by exploring alternatives and then making a judgement. Synthesis occurs when the findings from analysis are used to make suggestions or recommendations (Gopee 2011). An example of each level is given in Table 4.3.

Effectively written learning outcomes must be unambiguous and should be SMART (Box 4.14). Chapter 14 identifies the need to be able to write SMART goals as part of the nursing process. Once SMART learning outcomes have been written, the next step is to devise a teaching (or lesson) plan.

SMART learning outcomes   Box 4.14

S – **S**pecific
M – **M**easurable – so that there is evidence that they have been achieved
A – **A**ction-orientated – verbs should lead or drive them
R – **R**elevant – in both nature and reason
T – **T**ime-restricted – so that there is a target date for successful completion.

Example

By the end of this module you should be able to:

- Collaborate with others in the multidisciplinary team to ensure continuity of care.

SUMMARY

◆ There are three major theories of learning: behaviourism, cognitive theory and humanism.

◆ Andragogy and experiential learning are the preferred ways of learning for adults.

◆ Pedagogy describes how children learn.

◆ The learning process is associated with four main learning styles and deep, strategic and surface approaches.

◆ Reflective models provide a basis for learning the skills of reflection.

◆ Learning outcomes must be unambiguous and should be specific, measurable, action-orientated, relevant and time-restricted.

◆ The key components of successful learning and teaching are that:
  ◆ We learn best by doing
  ◆ Without readiness, learning is inefficient and may be harmful
  ◆ Motivation is essential
  ◆ Responses need immediate reinforcement
  ◆ Meaningful content is learned most easily and retained for longer
  ◆ A conducive environment is necessary
  ◆ Deep learning is most successful.

KEY WORDS AND PHRASES FOR LITERATURE SEARCHING

Critical thinking

Interprofessional learning

Learning

Learning outcomes

Learning styles

Learning theories

Patient/client education

Reflection

 Useful websites

British Dyslexia Association www.bdadyslexia.org.uk

Informed consent http://webarchive.nationalarchives.gov.uk/+/www.dh.gov.uk/en/Publichealth/Scientificdevelopmentgeneticsandbioethics/Consent/Consentgeneralinformation/index.htm

Learning styles www.xmarks.com/site/www.support4learning.org.uk/education/learning_styles.cfm

Sense UK (charity that provides services to support individuals with sensory impairment) www.sense.org.uk

Race's ripples – model of learning http://phil-race.co.uk/downloads

All websites accessed September 2012.

References

Atkins, S., Murphy, K., 1993. Reflection: a review of the literature. Journal of Advanced Nursing 18 (8), 1188–1192.

Baeten, M., Kyndt, E., Stryven, K., et al, 2010. Using student centred learning environments to stimulate deep approaches to learning: Factors encouraging or discouraging their effectiveness. Educational Research Review 5 (3), 243–260.

Bastable, S.B., 2008. Nurse as educator, third ed. Jones & Bartlett, Boston.

Bloom, B.S., 1964. Taxonomy of educational objectives. McKay, New York.

Boud, D., Keogh, T., Walker, D., 1985. Reflection, turning experience into learning. Billing, Worcester.

Buckley, S., Coleman, J., Khan, K., 2010. Best evidence on the educational effects of undergraduate portfolios. The Clinical Teacher 7 (3), 187–191.

Bulman, C., Schutz, S. (Eds.), 2008. An exploration of the student and mentor journey into reflective practice. In: Reflective practice in nursing, fourth ed. Blackwell Science, Oxford.

Cannon, S., Boswell, C., 2012. Evidence-based teaching in nursing. Jones & Bartlett, Sudbury.

Centre for the Advancement of Interprofessional Education, 2011. Definition of Interprofessional learning. CAIPE, London. Online. Available: www.caipe.org.uk/resources/principles-of-interprofessional-education September 2012.

College of Nurses of Ontario, 1996. The LEARN model of reflection. College of Nurses, Ontario.

Cox, C.L., Hill, M.C., 2010. Professional issues in primary care nursing. John Wiley, Oxford.

Department of Health, 2001. Valuing people: a new strategy for learning disability for the 21st Century. Cm5086. TSO, London. Online. Available: www.dh.gov.uk/en/Publicationsandstatistics/Publications/PublicationsPolicyAndGuidance/DH_4009153 August 2011.

Darbyshire, J.A., Machin, A.I. 2011. Learning to work collaboratively: nurses views of their pre-registration interprofessional education and its impact on practice. Nurse Education in Practice 11 (4), 239–244.

Dewey, J., 1933. How we think. Heath & Co., Lexington, DC.

Egle, C., 2009. Rural Health Education Foundation, Australia.

Freitas, F.A., Leonard, L.J., 2011. Maslow's hierarchy of needs and student academic success. Teaching and Learning in Nursing 6 (1), 9–13.

Gibbs, G., 1988. Learning by doing. Further Education Unit, Sheffield.

Gopee, N., 2002. Demonstrating critical analysis in academic assignments. Nursing Standard 16 (35), 45–52.

Gopee, N., 2011. Mentoring and supervision in healthcare. Sage, London.

Gray, M., 2011. Mentorship. In: McIntosh, A., Gidman, J., Mason-Whitehead, E. (Eds.), Key concepts in healthcare education. Sage, London, Ch. 22.

Greenwood, J., 1993. The apparent desensitisation of student nurses during their professional socialisation: a cognitive perspective. Journal of Advanced Nursing 18 (9), 1471–1479.

HM Government, 1995. Disability Discrimination Act. TSO, London. Online. Available: www.legislation.gov.uk/ukpga/1995/50/contents September 2012.

HM Government, 2010. Equality Act. TSO, London. Online. Available: www.equalities.gov.uk/equality_act_2010.aspx September 2012.

Honey, P., Mumford, A., 1992. The manual of learning styles, third ed. Peter Honey, Maidenhead.

Honey, P., Mumford, A., 2006. Learning styles helper's guide. Peter Honey, Maidenhead.

Jasper, M., 2006. Professional development, reflection and decision-making. Blackwell, Oxford.

Johns, C., 2009. Becoming a reflective practitioner, third ed. Wiley-Blackwell, Chichester.

Knowles, M.S., 1990. The adult learner: a neglected species, fourth ed. Gulf, Australia.

Knowles, M.S., Holton, E.F., Swanson, R.A., 1998. The adult learner: the definitive classic in adult education and human resource development. Gulf, Houston.

Kragelund, L., 2011. The windmill of learning processes: A learning and teaching tool for student nurses and mentors. Nurse Education Today 31 (1), 54–58.

Kolb, D.A., 1984. Experiential learning: experience as the source of learning and development. Prentice Hall, Englewood Cliffs.

LaVigna, G.W., Donnellan, A.M., 1986. Alternatives to punishment: solving behavior problems with non-aversive strategies. Irvington, New York.

Mannix, J., McIntosh, A., 2011. Problem-based learning. In: McIntosh, A., Gidman, J., Mason-Whitehead, E. (Eds.), Key concepts in healthcare education. Sage, London.

Maslow, A., 1954. Motivation and personality. Harper and Row, New York.

McAllister, M., 2007. Solution-focused nursing: rethinking practice. Palgrave Macmillan, Houndmills.

Mills, D.W. Undated Applying what we know: student learning styles. Online: Available: www.ldpride.net/learningstyles. MI.htm#Learning%20Styles%20Explained September 2012.

Mitchell, M., Groves, M., Mitchell, C., et al, 2010. Innovation in learning – An inter-professional approach to improving communication. Nurse Education in Practice 10 (6), 379–384.

National Training Laboratories. Undated. Learning pyramid – average learning retention rates. Online. Available: http://lwvbae.org/civ_pyramid.pdf September 2012.

Nursing and Midwifery Council, 2008a. The Code: standards of conduct, performance and ethics for nurses and midwives. NMC, London. Online. Available: http://www.nmc-uk.org/Nurses-and-midwives/Standards-and-guidance1/The-code/The-code-in-full/ September 2012.

Nursing and Midwifery Council, 2008b. The PREP Handbook. NMC, London.

Nursing and Midwifery Council, 2010. Preregistration nursing education. Annexe 3: Essential skills clusters. Online. Available: http://standards.nmc-uk.org/Documents/Annexe3_%20ESCs_16092010.pdf September 2012.

Petersson, P., Springett, J., 2009. Telling stories from everyday practice, an opportunity to see a bigger picture: a participatory action research project about developing discharge planning. Health and Social Care in the Community 17 (6), 548–556.

Race, P., 1993. Never mind the teaching feel the learning. SEDA Paper 80. Online. Available: www.londonmet.ac.uk/deliberations/seda-publications/race.cfm September 2012.

Race, P., 2005. Making learning happen. Sage, London.

Race, P., 2012. Race's ripples model of learning. Online. Available: http://phil-race.co.uk/?s=model+of+learning August 2012.

Rogers, C.R., 1994. Freedom to learn, third ed. Merrill, New York.

Schon, D., 1995. The reflective practitioner: how professionals think in action. Arena, Aldershot.

Stuart, C.C., 2007. Assessment, supervision and support in clinical practice, second ed. Churchill Livingstone/Elsevier, Edinburgh.

Timmins, F., Dunne, P.J., 2009. An exploration of the current use and benefit of nursing students' portfolios. Nurse Education Today 29 (3), 330–341.

Further reading

Braungart, M.M., Braungart, R.G., 2008. Applying learning theories to healthcare practice. In: Bastable, S.B. (Ed.), Nurse as educator, third ed. Jones and Bartlett, Boston.

Grainger, A., 2010. What if …? Reflective practice: Treating non-cooperative patients. British Journal of Healthcare Assistants 4 (12), 610–611.

Irvine, F.E., Roberts, G.W., Tranter, S., et al, 2008. Using critical incident technique to explore student nurses' perception of language awareness. Nurse Education Today 28 (1), 39–47.

Levett-Jones, T., Gerbach, J., Arthur, C., et al, 2011. Implementing a clinical competency assessment model that promotes critical reflection and ensures nursing graduates' readiness for professional practice. Nurse Education in Practice 11 (1), 64–69.

Luiselli, J., 2011. Teaching and behaviour support for children and adults with autism spectrum disorder. Oxford University Press, Oxford.

Miola, J., 2009. Informed consent and the rise of autonomy. British Journal of Nursing 18 (8), 504–506.

Evidence-based practice and research

5

Maria J. Grant   Michelle Howarth   Rosie Kneafsey

LEARNING OUTCOMES

This chapter will help you:

- Understand the concept of evidence-based practice
- Discuss how evidence is used in practice
- Use information technology (IT) skills to perform a basic search for evidence using bibliographic databases
- Evaluate research evidence
- Reflect on own practice and identify evidence gaps
- Use problem-solving skills to work with peers/colleagues to identify how evidence could be used in your own area of practice.

Introduction

The term 'evidence-based practice' (EBP) has been used synonymously with 'evidence-based medicine' or 'evidence-based healthcare' or 'evidence-based care' in the National Health Service (NHS) since the early 1990s. While many practitioners may have heard about EBP, it has been defined in many ways and some practitioners may be uncertain about its meaning. Despite this ambiguity, EBP plays a pivotal role in health and social care and is reflected in the Nursing and Midwifery Council (NMC) *Standards for pre-registration nursing education* (NMC 2010) and the *The Code: Standards of conduct, performance and ethics for nurses and midwives* (NMC 2008).

At a national level, EBP is promoted through the National Institute for Health and Clinical Excellence (NICE), National Service Frameworks (NSFs) and Scottish Intercollegiate Guidelines Network (SIGN). But what does the practitioner think about EBP? Can all practitioners really claim that their practice is evidence-based? On what evidence are clinical decisions based?

These questions will be explored in this chapter through the use of themed activity boxes and issues for reflection that will guide you through the maze of EBP, what it means and how it is used in healthcare practice.

This chapter covers the main components of EBP and encourages you to reflect on your own practice and clinical decision-making. EBP is an idea that is used in all fields of practice. You will be encouraged to relate the chapter text to your own clinical experience. You will be supported and directed to locate and appraise evidence relating to a chosen topic area and to develop your understanding of EBP.

What is evidence-based practice?

Evidence-based practice (EBP) encourages practitioners in health and social care to ensure that their practice is underpinned by the best available evidence. EBP was first introduced into health policy in the early 1990s with the emergence of 'Clinical Governance'. As an overall approach, it encourages practitioners to be 'clinically effective' by providing a framework within which evidence used in practice is constantly appraised for its effectiveness, relevance and trustworthiness.

EBP is now promoted in many Department of Health (DH) documents and through the Clinical Governance agenda. The *Making a Difference* document (DH 1999a) emphasized the need for reliable and robust evidence to underpin nursing, midwifery and health visiting. A similar strategy is promoted within *Saving Lives: Our Healthier Nation* (DH 1999b), which clearly advocates the need to implement EBP to improve services that promote public health. The significance of EBP is echoed in the current NHS health reforms through which the Government encourages evidence-based policy-making within a culture of evaluation and learning (DH 2010a, p 11). The importance of EBP is also reflected in many professional regulatory standards. For example, the Nursing and Midwifery Council (NMC 2008) statements 35–37 clearly states the need for nurses to deliver care based on the best available evidence or practice. Cox and Reyes-Hughes (2001) consider that EBP has a pivotal role in clinical effectiveness and argue that it is the main driver for clinically effective practitioners. If practitioners are unaware of the effectiveness of an intervention, how then can they claim to be clinically effective?

Defining EBP

Several definitions of EBP exist and, initially, the concept of EBP was applied to medicine in the early 1990s. Practitioners may find that they prefer one definition over another, or may find that they do not have a preference. In each case, the important issue is that practitioners develop an understanding of evidence-based care and are able to question their own practice and the types of evidence used to underpin this. Barker (2010) provides a useful overview of the key components of EBP. These include using the best available evidence, combining it with clinical expertise, taking into account the patient's preferences and considering the context within which care and treatment is being provided.

All of the definitions of EBP suggest that research evidence is the 'best' evidence, although this view is hotly debated. Others, however, have broadened this to include additional types of evidence. For example, the Royal College of Nursing (RCN 1996) identifies audit, client feedback and expertise as valuable sources of evidence. While all of the definitions advocate the use of evidence to support decision-making, there is an assumption that evidence is easily used in everyday practice. However, this is not always the case. To help practitioners underpin their practice with evidence, a series of steps have been developed. These steps include:

- Questioning practice and acknowledging areas of uncertainty about practice
- Developing clear questions about clinical practice for which answers are needed
- Searching for and retrieving the evidence
- Judging the quality of the evidence
- Using knowledge gained from the evidence to make improvements to practice
- Evaluating or auditing practice to assess the impact of changes.

Each of these steps will be explored throughout this chapter.

The EBP cycle

EBP has become an important mechanism for improving the quality of clinical practice, for reducing risk to patients/clients and ensuring the most effective allocation of resources.

The steps described earlier can be viewed as a cycle, whereby evaluation or audit always leads back to further questioning of practice. This cycle of events ensures that up-to-date practices are carried out and good standards of clinical practice are maintained.

Questioning practice

The first step towards EBP is the ability of practitioners to question their own practice. To do this, practitioners will need to identify *why* they make decisions in a particular way and acknowledge what or who has informed the decision. Often, practitioners may not take the time to think about *why* and *how* they made a decision and, all too often, these are based on ritual and custom rather than a reliable evidence base. All

practitioners need to consider what decisions they are making and what evidence is being used to support such decisions.

Now consider the material in Box 5.1. Here we can see that Staff Nurse Dyer now questions the type of dressings she applies. By questioning her practice, Staff Nurse Dyer is influencing the care she gives and clinical decisions she makes as a result. Questioning practice involves thinking about the appropriateness of the care being provided, e.g. is it the right treatment? How do practitioners know that treatment works? How do different treatments compare? Is the treatment cost-effective?

◯ Evidence-based practice   Box 5.1

Effective decision-making and questioning practice

Sister Robbins asks Staff Nurse Dyer to redress a person's wound using Brand A as a dressing. Staff Nurse Dyer does not question the Sister as to her choice of dressings. She follows Sister Robbins' instructions and applies Brand A to the person's wound.

Later on that week, Staff Nurse Dyer observes Staff Nurse Flynn applying a different dressing to the same person's wound. Staff Nurse Dyer wonders which dressing is best for the person and questions her own practice.

Student activity

Think about a recent decision you have made in practice:

- What was the decision?
- How did you make the decision?
- What/who influenced your decision? For example, was your decision based on any of the following types of evidence: research; guidelines; tradition; intuition; experience; advice from your mentor, colleagues, peers, qualified staff; ritual practice?

Refining the question into a workable search question

If decisions are based on tradition or ritual, then there is a need to find out if more reliable evidence to support decisions about practice is available. To accomplish this, it is useful to formulate a structured question to guide the search for evidence. Formulating workable questions is discussed in the searching for evidence section (see p. 110).

Finding the evidence

Once the question has been formulated, the next step is to find the evidence. This will involve using electronic databases such as MEDLINE and CINAHL, as well as Government websites, national guideline databases, professional organizations and service user forums. Finding evidence can be difficult and there is a need to practise in order to develop the skills required to search effectively on databases.

Appraising the evidence

When the evidence has been located, practitioners then need to make sense of it. A range of guidelines has been designed to help practitioners make sense of the evidence and decide whether it is robust and believable. Guidelines for appraising evidence are explained later in the chapter.

Implementing the evidence

Following appraisal of the evidence, and once the practitioner is satisfied that the evidence is reliable and trustworthy, it is important to plan how to use this evidence in practice. Implementing evidence-based findings is not easy, but with support from others and through reading this chapter, students and clinicians should be able to make comprehensive plans to help them use evidence to guide practice.

Evaluating or auditing practice

Finally, once practitioners have introduced the evidence into practice, there is a need to reflect on and audit practice to assess whether it is safe and effective for the patient/client in their care. This may involve other colleagues and professionals who observed their actions.

Practitioners may find that they need to continually audit their practice to ensure that it is based on 'best' evidence. For example, practitioners may need to return to the original practice question and refine it, or they may discover that there is a gap in evidence. Whatever the situation, the important message is to be able to improve practice by questioning the decisions that practitioners make about a patient's or client's care needs.

Literature searching

A crucial way of finding out what is the best practice for a clinical situation is to discover what has been written about it in the literature. This means that practitioners need to be able to carry out a search of the literature and a review of the evidence (NHS Executive 1996).

There are numerous reasons for conducting a literature search. Searching and reviewing the literature identifies whether previous studies or audits have been carried out in relation to the topic of interest or whether practice guidelines exist. This might be important if practitioners wish to make changes in practice, as it may be possible to read about how other practitioners improved their practice – both what they did and how they did it. It may also help to highlight potential problems or difficulties that might be encountered during the process of practice innovation (NHS Executive 1996). Determining what the literature identifies provides an opportunity for practitioners to incorporate new knowledge into their decision-making.

A dramatic rise in the amount of scientific literature published has resulted in the need to ensure that practitioners have the skills to find the literature they need. Typically, practitioners lack the required skills and find it hard to search the literature efficiently. This has implications for practice as it means that it may not be based on current evidence despite it being available.

This section will provide an introduction to the basic principles and practice of searching for literature and evidence for practice. This will include exploring:

- Sources of literature
- Developing a search question
- Searching databases.

Sources of literature

There are many different sources of information available including books, the Internet, journals and professional organizations. Some will provide examples of original research, while others – often referred to as evidence-based sources – will provide an up-to-date review of the evidence available. In both cases, it is necessary to undertake an appraisal of the quality of the information presented (see p. 119).

The reason for choosing to use one source over another will depend on the type of information the practitioner wants to find. The following gives a brief overview of some of the key resources that can be used in a search for literature.

Bibliographic/electronic databases

Databases gather together and index large numbers of articles within specific subject areas, (e.g. nursing, social sciences), so choosing the right database(s) to search will depend on the topic area. Some databases also distinguish between including examples of primary research projects and literature reviews (reviews of research). A list of some useful databases is presented in Box 5.2.

By searching a database systematically, practitioners can retrieve a list of references of relevant articles. Normally, the full text of the article is not provided and a trip to the library is needed to look up the article in a printed journal. Although databases often look different, they can usually be searched in the same way, and use similar formats to provide information, e.g. the author, title, journal source and often an abstract (a clear and concise summary of the study design, results and implications for practice) of the article. This information enables practitioners to find the full version of the article in the library. If the local library does not stock the required journal, it is usually possible to request the article using the interlibrary loan system. You will probably need to pay a fee and the library will then request a photocopy of the article from another library.

Books

This group of resources includes textbooks, specialist dictionaries and encyclopaedias. They are useful for obtaining background information and will generally provide a standard account of a specific subject area. Books are good for obtaining a distinct piece of information, but because it can take a considerable length of time to get into print, the information they contain may not always be up-to-date.

The Internet

The Internet provides a way of accessing information and resources in a variety of formats. These can include web pages that provide information, and web pages that provide access to resources such as bibliographic databases. The quality of websites is sometimes difficult to assess, so a good place to start is to use a gateway service. A gateway service is

---

Useful databases	Box 5.2

AMED – Allied and Complementary Medicine indexes physiotherapy, occupational therapy, rehabilitation, speech and language therapy, podiatry and complementary medicine and palliative care articles from 1985 onwards.

BNI – British Nursing Index covers over 240 UK journals and other English language titles, including core international nursing/midwifery titles and selective content from medical, allied health and management from 1985 onwards. It has a strong UK focus.

CINAHL – Cumulative Index of Nursing and Allied Health Literature indexes all English-language nursing journals and publications from the National League for Nursing and the American Nurses' Association including nursing and allied health disciplines, biomedicine, health sciences librarianship and consumer health from 1982 onwards. It has a strong US focus.

The Cochrane Library – A 'virtual library' or collection of six databases that provide a starting point for accessing systematic reviews. These reviews are primarily concerned with the effectiveness of interventions and therefore concentrate on using randomized controlled trials (RCTs) as their foundation. A seventh database provides information about groups in The Cochrane Collaboration. The Cochrane Library includes:

- Cochrane Database of Systematic Reviews (CDSR)
- Cochrane Central Register for Controlled Trials (CENTRAL)
- Cochrane Methodology Database
- Database of Abstracts of Reviews of Effects (DARE), a collection of systematic reviews which include studies other than randomized clinical trials (RCTs)
- Health Technology Assessment Database
- NHS Economic Evaluation Database
- About The Cochrane Collaboration.

MEDLINE – A general biomedical database which covers international literature on medicine, allied health, biological and physical sciences, humanities and information science as they relate to medicine and healthcare, communication disorders, population biology, and reproductive biology. It indexes articles from 1948 onwards with an additional archive of non-indexed items from 1946. It has a strong US focus. Research has suggested that for the majority of nursing queries, MEDLINE is likely to retrieve a higher number of relevant (and often unique) references (Okuma 1994; Brazier & Begley 1996; Brand-de Heer 2001).

---

usually subject specific and provides access to quality-assessed websites. An example of a gateway service is the Health Information Resources (formerly National Library for Health) which provides access to a wide range of health-related services including an index of UK national clinical guidelines. (Other examples are included in the Useful websites on pp. 123-124.)

Journals and newsletters

Published at regular intervals, journals are a useful resource in obtaining the full text versions of primary research projects and articles on practice development, e.g. *Nursing Times*, *Nursing Standard*. More recently, journals have also begun to summarize or make evaluations of original pieces of research. Some adopt quite a formal or structured approach to providing information, e.g. Evidence-Based Nursing, Clinical Knowledge Summaries, NHS Evidence, whereas others are more informal, e.g. Bandolier (see Useful websites, below).

Some journal sources are more reputable than others because they publish articles that have been peer reviewed. Peer review means that the articles have been sent for evaluation and comment by experts in the area before being accepted for publication, e.g. *Journal of Advanced Nursing*, *Journal of Learning Disabilities*. Journals are becoming increasingly available online either via a local library or information service, or via commercial ventures such as PubMed Central (see Useful websites, below). PubMed Central represents one of a growing number of services which provide free and unrestricted access to a full-text digital archive of life sciences journal literature, in this instance, provided by the US National Library for Medicine.

Reports

Like books, reports can be good for obtaining an overview of a subject area. They are often produced by government departments, e.g. Department of Health; professional organizations, e.g. Royal College of Nursing; universities and other statutory and voluntary organizations, e.g. Joseph Rowntree Foundation.

Developing a search question

Before beginning a literature search it is important to think through what information is needed. Developing a focused search question helps to ensure that the search for literature is structured and time is used efficiently. If the search question is vague, too many references are likely to be retrieved from a database search and the question will not be answered. Conversely, if the search question is too focused it may mistakenly appear that nothing has been published in that area.

A useful framework to help in structuring a search question is the PICO acronym (Richardson et al 1995) (Box 5.3). PICO helps the practitioner to identify key elements of the search question with each letter representing a different element:

P – the patient or problem under consideration

I – the intervention or treatment under consideration

C – the comparison intervention or treatment under consideration

O – the clinical outcome(s) of interest.

Once the key elements of the search question have been identified, the next step is to organize these elements in order of importance. When starting a literature search, it is probable that only two search areas will be needed. However, by having a clear idea of the whole topic area before starting to search, it will be easier to add a third or even a fourth element to the search strategy, and narrow down the type of information being retrieved, without getting sidetracked.

Critical thinking Box 5.3

Structuring a search question using PICO

You are on placement with a practice nurse running a 'well man' clinic. John is 72 years of age and is waiting to go into hospital for prostate surgery. He has been suffering from recurrent urinary tract infections (UTIs) and has read that cranberry juice is good at preventing UTIs. He asks about the effectiveness of cranberry juice. The nurse tells John that she is unsure but will make enquiries and discuss the findings with him.

Student activity

Use the PICO acronym to plan the ideas you would use to search for information to answer John's question.

PICO acronym	Search idea identified using PICO
P – *Patient or population*	
I – *Intervention*	
C – *Comparison*	
O – *Outcome*	

You will probably have identified search ideas similar to the following:

- Patient/population – urinary tract infections
- Intervention – cranberry juice
- Comparison – water
- Outcome – reduced levels of infection.

Once the search question has been clearly defined, it is then necessary to decide on the most appropriate place to look for the information. Depending on the type of information needed, this might include some or all of the following:

- Reading books
- Contacting subject specialists
- Visiting recommended websites via gateway services (pp. 123 and 124)
- Searching electronic/bibliographic databases.

Searching databases

Searching a database can seem daunting but there are a number of steps that, if followed, will make this process easier and more successful. It is sensible to ask the librarian for help in getting started.

The way databases present information can often look quite different, but there are some basic ways of searching which are common to all. The examples used here are from the MEDLINE database via the OVID search interface, but a typical database record will include the name of the author, the title of the article, the source of the article, i.e. which journal is it published in, and a list of indexing terms or subject headings (Fig. 5.1).

The reason for the search will determine how comprehensive or complete the coverage of the database search will be. For those undertaking a thorough review of the literature for a dissertation or, once qualified, looking to change practice, it is necessary to find as much information on a topic as possible.

However, when searching for a couple of references to support an argument in an assignment, it probably will not matter if you miss a few papers. In both instances, the best place to start is by searching using the database's list of indexing terms.

Indexing terms

Indexing terms are also called Medical Subject Headings (MeSH), subject headings, thesaurus terms or descriptors, but they all mean basically the same thing. These indexing terms are split into subject areas and are organized within a hierarchy (Fig. 5.2).

The most precise indexing terms – which are assigned by the database producer – are given to describe the content of each article. Using John's request for information on the effectiveness of cranberry juice in preventing urinary tract infections as an example, every article that mentions urinary tract infections would be given the indexing term 'Urinary Tract Infections'. It does not matter which specific words have been used to describe the idea/topic because if they were discussing infections of the urinary tract, they will be indexed using 'Urinary Tract Infections'. However, if the search is for bacteriuria (bacteria in the urine), then the specific indexing term 'Bacteriuria' is used because the broader indexing term of 'Urinary Tract Infections' would not retrieve articles discussing this specific area of interest within the category of urinary tract infections.

Although it may initially take some time to identify the most appropriate indexing terms to use, searching using indexing terms can retrieve more accurate search results. Most databases will have an option which will suggest the most likely indexing term in the subject area. This feature is sometimes called mapping, when the database makes a 'best guess' at suggesting which term(s) will be helpful. If available, it is a good idea to check the description of the indexing term to make sure it means what you think it does (Box 5.4).

Although a database will often provide an opportunity to search for more than one term at a time, it is usually a good idea to search for each term separately. In this way, if an indexing term is not working as expected, e.g. it is retrieving irrelevant information, it is much quicker to exclude it from the search than having to retype the terms that are to be kept.

It is important to bear in mind that each database will have a slightly different set of indexing terms, so it is necessary to check the list of terms each time a search is started on a new database.

Free text terms

If it is necessary to undertake a more thorough literature search, e.g. for a final year project, this will probably need to use a combination of indexing terms searching with free text searching.

Free text searching is the development of a list of words, or free text search terms, that describe each component of the search question in more detail. For example, this might be a list that includes alternative spellings (including Americanisms), plurals, synonyms and abbreviations (Box 5.4).

Free text searching will help ensure the retrieval of the maximum possible literature on a topic area, and will compensate for any mistakes by the database producers in missing or

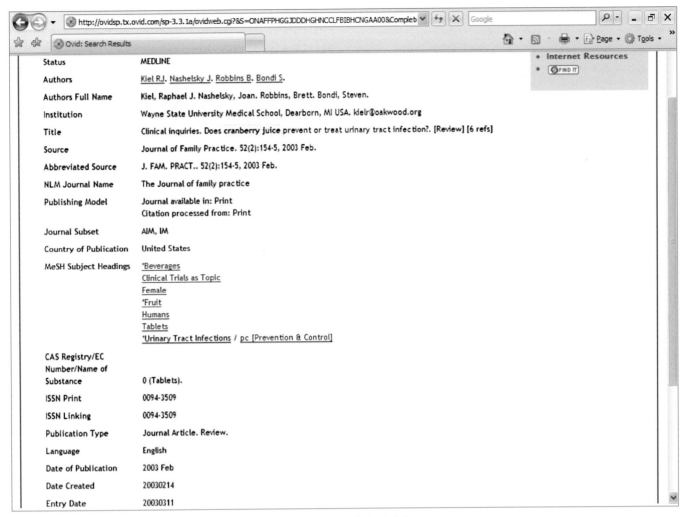

Fig. 5.1 • A typical database record. (Reproduced by kind permission of OVID Technologies).

misapplied indexing terms. It is important to remember that as well as increasing the number of potentially relevant articles retrieved, there is also the possibility that it will increase the number of potentially irrelevant references too. In both instances, there is a need to allow extra time to read through the retrieved abstracts.

Combining your search terms

Once the indexing terms for the subject area (and any free text terms for an extended search) have been identified, it is necessary to link the words together using the 'AND' and 'OR' functions of the database. These are known as the 'Boolean Operators'.

When searching within a single element of the search question, it is necessary to use the 'OR' Boolean operator. 'OR' enables the user to search for a range of alternative ways of describing an idea/topic, so that any one of a number of indexing or free text terms may appear. Using the urinary tract infection as an example, the 'OR' Boolean operator will enable a search for any combination of indexing or free text search terms, e.g. 'Urinary Tract Infections' or 'UTI' (Fig. 5.3A). An

easy way to remember how to use the 'OR' Boolean operator is the mnemonic 'OR is more' (Palmer & Brice 1999).

Users may worry if, at this stage, they seem to be retrieving too much information. However, once the indexing terms have been combined for each individual element of the search question, users then need to search for articles where both ideas appear, e.g. where cranberry juice is mentioned in the same article as urinary tract infection, and the numbers will quickly decrease. In order to do this, the 'AND' Boolean operator is used (Fig. 5.3B).

A third Boolean operator – the 'NOT' Boolean operator – enables users to exclude papers that mention a particular topic/ word (Fig. 5.3C). While this may initially appear to be a good thing, there is a distinct possibility that users could inadvertently exclude potentially relevant papers. You are advised to use the 'NOT' Boolean operator with extreme caution – if at all.

A more effective way of reducing the number of papers retrieved is to add a further element to the search strategy (remember four elements were identified using PICO, but searching began by using only the two most important ones)

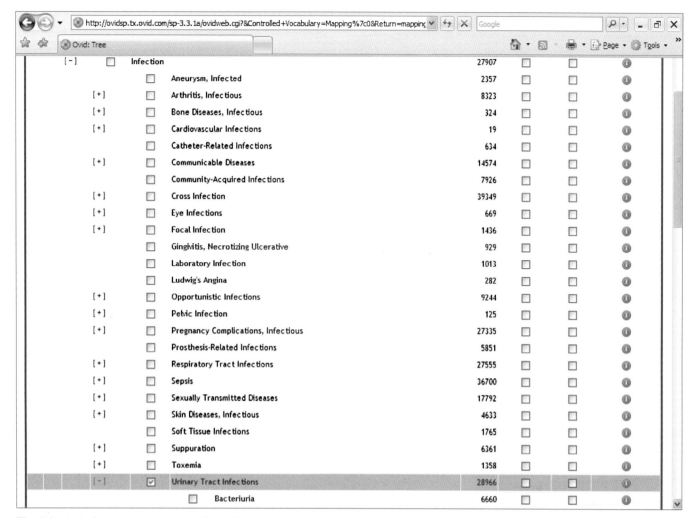

Fig. 5.2 • Indexing terms are organized in a hierarchy. (Reproduced by kind permission of OVID Technologies).

(?) Critical thinking   Box 5.4

Identifying indexing terms on a database

Access a database of your choice and identify the indexing terms for the four main elements of the PICO acronym (you might want to have another look at Box 5.3).

PICO acronym	Search idea identified using PICO	Indexing term identified on database
P: *Patient or population*	Urinary tract infection	
I: *Intervention*	Cranberry juice	
C: *Comparison*	Water	
O: *Outcome*	Reduced levels of infection	

If you searched on the MEDLINE database, you will probably have identified the following indexing terms:

- Patient/population – urinary tract infections
- Intervention – beverages
- Outcome – randomized controlled trial

Although the indexing term 'Review Literature as Topic' is potentially available as an 'Outcome' search term, there are many types of review (Grant & Booth 2009). The MEDLINE scope note does not make specific reference to systematic reviews and notes that reviews cover 'subject matter at various levels of completeness and comprehensiveness …'. When searching for examples of systematic reviews, it is therefore more appropriate to limit your search by 'Publication Type' for 'Review'.

There does not appear to be a suitable indexing term for water, so you may wish to consider using free text searching.

Developing a list of free text search terms

Add as many synonyms, alternative spellings, Americanisms, plurals or abbreviations to each of the elements of the PICO acronym (you might want to have another look at Box 5.3).

You will probably have identified a range of free text search terms similar to the following:

- *Patient/population* – urinary tract infection, urinary tract infections, UTI, UTIs
- *Intervention* – cranberries, cranberry, cranberry juices
- *Comparison* – drinking water, H_2O, water
- *Outcome* – randomised controlled trial, randomized controlled trial, randomised controlled trials, randomized controlled trials, RCT, RCTs, systematic review, systematic reviews

Note: When free text searching, the database will search for the precise match of the terms typed in, so be sure that the spelling is correct.

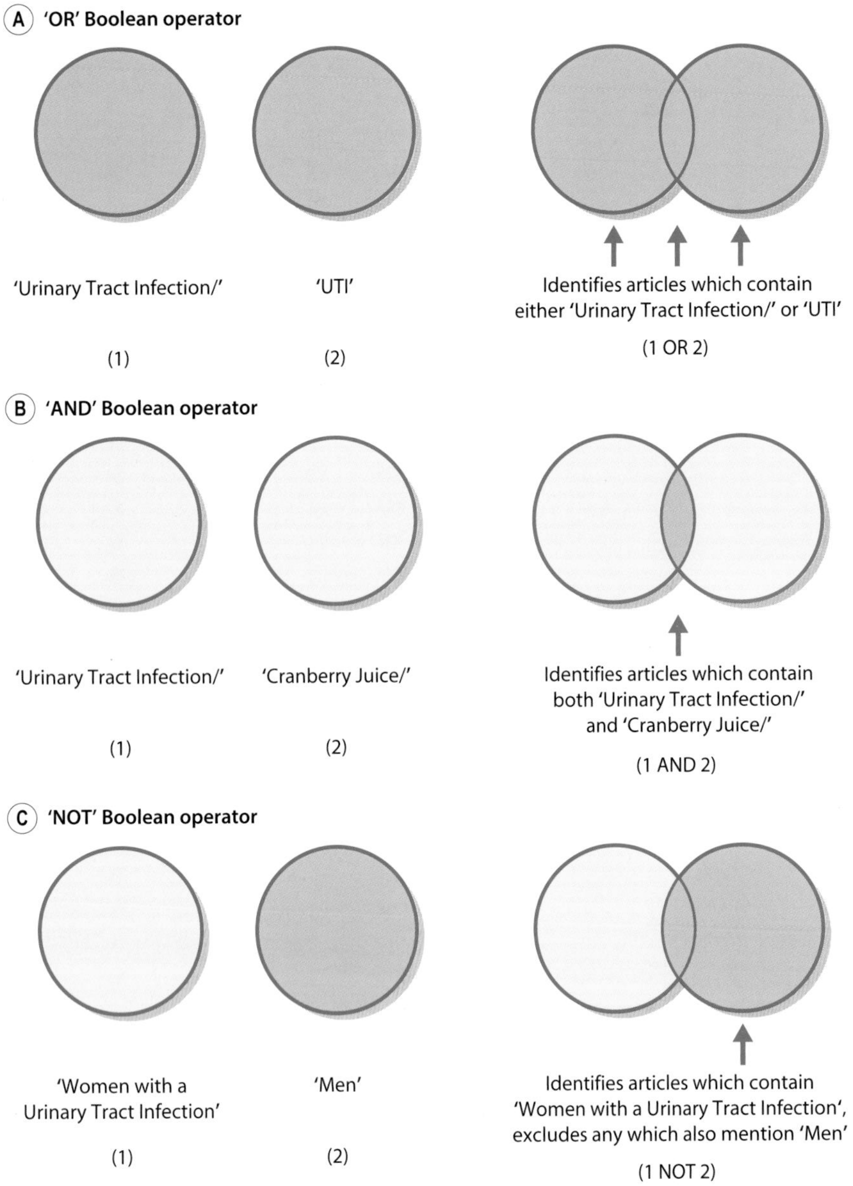

A 'OR' Boolean operator

'Urinary Tract Infection/'

(1)

'UTI'

(2)

Identifies articles which contain
either 'Urinary Tract Infection/' or 'UTI'

(1 OR 2)

B 'AND' Boolean operator

'Urinary Tract Infection/'

(1)

'Cranberry Juice/'

(2)

Identifies articles which contain
both 'Urinary Tract Infection/'
and 'Cranberry Juice/'

(1 AND 2)

C 'NOT' Boolean operator

'Women with a
Urinary Tract Infection'

(1)

'Men'

(2)

Identifies articles which contain
'Women with a Urinary Tract Infection',
excludes any which also mention 'Men'

(1 NOT 2)

Fig. 5.3 • Boolean operators. (A) 'OR' Boolean operator. (B) 'AND' Boolean operator. (C) 'NOT' Boolean operator.

or by adding limits such as date range, publication type, e.g. review/systematic review, or language, e.g. English.

The aim of searching is to start off with a selection of references, sometimes called a 'sensitive' search, and then narrow the search down until the number of references is reduced to those that will be useful, sometimes called a 'precise' or 'specific' search.

Once the search is completed, it is important to make a note of the search strategy. It is good practice to include this in any assignment or report. If it is necessary to return to the search at a later date, it will also mean that there is no need to try to remember which search terms were used.

Sources of knowledge to support evidence-based practice

During the process of providing care, nurses and others must make a wide range of decisions. These decisions have important effects on the person's and family's experience of care, and the outcomes of healthcare interventions. Nurses may also be involved in assisting people to make decisions about their own care, such as whether to consent to a particular treatment or not.

For nurses to be able to make safe and effective clinical decisions, they must draw on a range of different sources of knowledge and information. For example, past experiences, guidance from a colleague or a practice protocol. These different sources of knowledge can be defined as types of 'evidence' underpinning practice.

The provision of safe, evidence-based nursing care depends on how health information is managed and used (Box 5.5).

What is meant by 'evidence'?

Everyone uses evidence from a variety of sources, both in daily life and in professional practice. However, what constitutes 'evidence' has been debated for many years. Different types

---

Health informatics   Box 5.5

Many of the problems associated with patient care can be linked to poor information management. Therefore, by improving the management of health information, the delivery of healthcare can also be improved. This is the goal of health informatics (HI).

Predominantly associated with the application of information technology in healthcare provision, computer systems represents just one tool of what might be defined as HI. HI extends to all types of information systems including oral, printed and electronic and embraces 'the knowledge, skills and tools which enable information to be collected, managed, used and shared safely'. (UK Council for Health Informatics Professions 2011.)

Originally established in 1967, the International Medical Informatics Association (IMIA) acts as a coordinating organization, seeking to bring together multidisciplinary interests to facilitate an improvement in the health of the world population. (International Medical Informatics Association 2011.)

Many branches of informatics exist including nursing informatics, the safe use of information in the provision of healthcare by nurses.

Resources

International Medical Informatics Association, 2011. The IMIA vision. Online. Available: www.imia-medinfo.org September 2012.

UK Council for Health Informatics Professions, 2011. The UKCHIP vision. Online. Available: www.ukchip.org/ Oct 2012.

Reflective practice   Box 5.6

Questioning your practice

Think about and reflect on a recent example of ritualistic care, which has caused you to question the nursing care provided.

Student activities

- Try to identify the aspect of nursing care that was different from that given elsewhere or contradicted what you have learnt during your course.
- Discuss this with a fellow student or your mentor.

---

of evidence include the information gained from tradition and ritual, experience, intuition, authorities and experts, patients and families, research, audit and guidelines.

Tradition and ritual

Large parts of daily life are based on trusted traditions and rituals learnt from others during childhood (see Ch. 8). Traditions and rituals allow people to undertake activities with little thought or consideration as to the reasons why – they provide structure to everyday life (Walsh & Ford 1989). The process of learning traditions and rituals by observing the actions and activities of peers continues from childhood into adulthood and into the world of employment.

Learning traditions and rituals is a central means of transmitting knowledge and is an important mechanism through which nursing students learn to 'become' nurses (Parahoo 2006). Students learn from effective colleagues who practise safely and on the basis of best evidence. This can be a useful means of sharing knowledge and good practice. However, relying on traditional knowledge may also lead to the transmission of outdated information and practice, putting both nurses and clients at risk (Box 5.6).

Experience

Practitioners use their own or the experiences of others to inform decisions they make about nursing practice. After experiencing an event, the memory of this is stored and is ready to draw upon in similar circumstance in the future. Practitioners may also discuss experiences with colleagues, thus passing their experiential knowledge on to others. However, while experience brings confidence, experiential knowledge is based on a limited range of events or practice situations to which practitioners have been exposed. As such, practitioners may be unaware of new or different practices or treatments, or recommendations from research (Parahoo 2006).

Intuition

Intuition is defined as a way of knowing and behaving that is not based on rational or conscious reasoning (Parahoo 2006). While many nurses explain the importance of intuition in their nursing care, it is difficult to define exactly what it is. In addition, it is also easy to dismiss another person's intuition. For example, Polgar and Thomas (1995) describe the activities of the nineteenth century physician, Ignaz Semmelweis, who noted the high levels of maternal deaths at his hospital and suspected that medical students attending the mortuary were spreading infection via their hands. Unfortunately, while handwashing is now recognized as the cornerstone of effective infection prevention and control, at that time, Semmelweis and his intuition was ignored and dismissed.

Authorities and experts

Often, practices in healthcare and nursing are determined by the knowledge and opinions of those members of the healthcare team in positions of authority. Knowledge is considered true because the person who states it has authority or is considered an expert. While experts may well possess high levels of knowledge, conflict may arise when one expert or person in authority holds differing opinions from another. It is also possible for experts to hold misplaced views or be biased in some way, as demonstrated in the example of the now discredited 'evidence' regarding the safety of the MMR vaccination.

Service users and their families

During the process of providing individualized care, it is important to ascertain the views of people and their families. In this way, it is possible to work in partnership with them to tailor care and treatment to individual needs. This is an important aspect of evidence-based healthcare because it recognizes that people can be, and often are, the experts in their own care. As such, they should be able to make choices and decisions about what happens to them. Although this is a very important source of knowledge upon which to base nursing care, people often feel that they are not involved enough in their own care and are not asked about what services they think should be offered by the NHS. The Department of Health now recognize that service users should have more say in the care that they receive and the types of health service research carried out. In order to ensure that patients' views are listened to, NHS Trusts have expert patient groups and Patient Advice Liaison Services (PALS).

Research studies

While other sources of knowledge constitute important aspects of the evidence base, knowledge derived from research is crucial to evidence-based practice. This is because, unlike other forms of knowing, research is a systematic approach to generating knowledge using well-established methods. While there are many different types and ways of carrying out research, the main aim of nursing research is to improve the quality of care and to enable effective clinical decision-making (Parahoo 2006). For example, research can tell practitioners which treatments work best or why they may not be so effective. Research can also help practitioners to find out about how people feel and experience things. For example, research can tell practitioners which drugs are effective in treating high blood pressure and also how people may feel about having a chronic condition or a learning disability.

Audit

Many aspects of nursing care are influenced by the results of audit, which students may come across during their clinical placements, e.g. audits of the incidence of pressure ulcers or the occurrence of violent behaviour. The *Essence of Care* 2010 document (DH 2010b) is an important nursing audit tool currently being used in many NHS Trusts (Box 5.7).

 Evidence-based practice | Box 5.7

Benchmarking

Student activities

Locate information about the ***Essence of Care 2010 Benchmarks for the Fundamental Aspects of Care*** (DH 2010b).

- What are the key objectives of *Essence of Care 2010*?
- How many benchmarks are included?
- Are there any benchmarking groups/activities in your organization?

Essentially, clinical audit involves measuring an aspect of practice (such as how often nutritional assessments are carried out, see Ch. 19, or risk assessments for pressure ulcer formation, see Ch. 25) and comparing it to agreed standards for best practice. Clinical audit can provide knowledge about nursing care and highlight where improvements are needed. Audit is an important link within the evidence-based practice cycle as, without it, it is not possible to state whether the right practice is actually occurring.

Guidelines

Practitioners may also use guidelines as a source of knowledge from which to base care that they provide. Guidelines are written after the best available evidence, research and/or clinical expertise (where research evidence is lacking), and client views have been gathered and scrutinized. This evidence is then used to set a standard for best practice for a particular

treatment or aspect of care. For example, a guideline for pressure ulcer management has been produced by NICE and the RCN (2005). In Scotland, the Scottish Intercollegiate Guidelines Network (SIGN) and NHS Quality Improvement Scotland (NHSQIS) produce guidelines (Box 5.8). Guidelines can also be used as the standard against which to assess the quality of care during the audit process and may be a way of eliminating variations in clinical practice that exist in different parts of the country.

 Evidence-based practice | Box 5.8

Guidelines

Student activity

Locate *one* local practice guideline from the following examples which you have come across during your clinical placements:

- The management of schizophrenia
- The management of obesity
- Pressure ulcer management
- Management of attention deficit and hyperkinetic disorders.

Resources

- Visit the SIGN website (*www.sign.ac.uk*) and locate the guideline about the management of obesity (A national clinical guideline No. 115), or the management of attention deficit and hyperkinetic disorders in children and young people (A national clinical guideline No. 112). Compare and contrast the published guidelines with those produced locally for any similarities or differences.
- Visit the NICE website (*www.nice.org.uk*) and locate the latest guideline about pressure ulcer management (Clinical guideline No. CG29), or schizophrenia (National Clinical Guideline No. 82). Compare and contrast the published guidelines with those produced locally for any similarities or differences.

Best evidence

Knowledge is thus derived from many different sources and, used in combination, can ensure that the care and treatment provided is as effective as possible (Box 5.9).

The notion of 'best' evidence is controversial. Some argue that experimental research that demonstrates the effectiveness of an intervention is the best evidence; however, others disagree, viewing other types of evidence as more informative for certain clinical situations (Cox & Reyes-Hughes 2001).

A number of hierarchies now exist, enabling different types of research and evidence to be graded or ranked according to their ability to predict effectiveness, remove bias and control confounders and provide more confidence in the reliability of the findings (see pp. 120-122 for further information). One such hierarchy is described by Thompson and Cullum (1999) where the highest level of evidence is a systematic review of several high-quality randomized controlled trials (RCTs), through various grades to expert opinion, which is the lowest level in the hierarchy.

Experimental research such as RCTs is seen by many as the 'highest standard' of evidence because the findings are thought to be more valid and reliable than that of non-experimental descriptive research and other evidence.

Types of evidence

Mrs Kaur is a 73-year-old woman who has an infected venous leg ulcer and is due to have her dressings changed today by Staff Nurse Smith. After removing the dressing, Staff Nurse Smith observes that the ulcer has worsened. She asks Mrs Kaur what she thinks about the ulcer who agrees that it does look worse. Mrs Kaur also states that she has been in more pain. Staff Nurse Smith begins to plan a course of action. She remembers that she has used another type of dressing on a venous ulcer in similar circumstances. She decides to discuss this with her colleague and, with Mrs Kaur's consent, invites her colleague to review the ulcer. Staff Nurse Smith and her colleague look at the tissue viability guidelines and hospital protocol for the management of venous leg ulcers. After some discussion with Mrs Kaur, and her colleague, Staff Nurse Smith makes a decision to contact the tissue viability nurse for an opinion.

Student activity

- Reflect on the different types of evidence used by Staff Nurse Smith. You can include the following types of evidence:
  - Mrs Kaur's opinion
  - Colleague's opinion
  - Expert opinion (tissue viability nurse)
  - Her own experience
  - Guidelines
  - Hospital protocols.
- Through your reflection, you may have thought of other types of 'evidence'. For example, you may have attended a lecture, spoken with your personal tutor or attended a conference. What is important is that you develop the skills needed to differentiate between good or 'best' evidence and bad evidence.

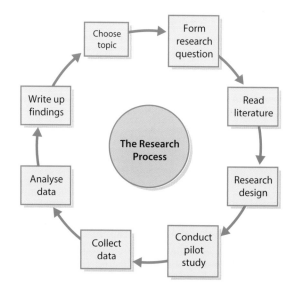

Fig. 5.4 • The research process.

In general, research is viewed by many as the most important source of knowledge for practice. It is a large topic area and the next section provides an introduction to some of the key aspects.

Overview of the research process

In order to carry out research correctly, certain rules and logical steps need to be followed. This is known as the 'research process' and is often viewed as cyclical in nature, rather than linear (Fig. 5.4).

When research projects are reported in academic journals and reports, they will often describe the research process followed. For the reader, this is important as it makes it clear how the research was carried out. It should also provide enough detail for readers to decide whether the project followed the proper rules or research process.

There are many different forms of research evidence and although there are exceptions, research can be defined broadly as quantitative or qualitative in nature.

Quantitative research

Quantitative research is described as the logical collection of numerical data under controlled conditions that uses statistics to analyse the data. This type of research is based on the belief that the world, events and phenomena are governed by laws that can be uncovered by measuring and counting, and searching for correlations between different phenomena (Parahoo 2006). For example, this type of research might try to find out about 'cause and effect' – i.e. does A+B=C? It often (but not always) involves the testing of hypotheses through objective measurements and observations to see whether the hypothesis is supported or rejected.

Qualitative research

Qualitative research focuses on understanding human behaviour, experiences of life and the social processes we participate in (Gerrish & Lacey 2010). It can be defined as the logical collection of subjective data that often include narrative or observational materials without additional researcher control. This type of research assumes that the complexity of everyday life cannot be reduced to numbers, as much meaning could be lost. It is also accepted that there is never simply one reality – that there will always be different experiences, perspectives and interpretations. There is no attempt to control the environment in which data are being collected, as the aim is to understand events and interactions, as they unfold, from the perspective of those people experiencing them (Craig & Smyth 2007).

Quantitative and qualitative research in nursing

Both approaches to research are needed within nursing, as many research questions require the measurement of objective facts to inform the development of clinical practice. However, much nursing work cannot be broken down into measurable parts without the meaning of that phenomenon being lost.

Often, a particular research topic or research question will require a combination of quantitative and qualitative research.

This allows for a more complete understanding of the particular phenomenon to be gained. For example, back injuries in nurses and the links between patient handling activities have been explored using both quantitative surveys and qualitative interview studies. Surveys have allowed researchers to find out how many nurses suffer from back injury while interview studies have helped to shed light on the factors that influence nurses' manual handling practices.

Different types of research design

In order to begin collecting data to answer a research question, a plan or research design must be decided upon. The research design sets out whether the research approach will be quantitative or qualitative, how data will be collected (data collection tools), where/who data will be collected from (the sampling strategy or sample) and how data will be analysed. Different research questions require that different research designs be used. For example, if the researcher was trying to find out about the effectiveness of a treatment (e.g. does drug A work better than drug B?), it would be most appropriate to use an experimental design such as a randomized controlled trial. Alternatively, if the researcher were seeking to understand people's thoughts and feelings, a qualitative approach would be used. It is important that the researcher chooses the best research design to answer the research question. There are many different research designs, including:

- Systematic review
- Randomized controlled trial
- Survey
- Qualitative (ethnography, grounded theory and phenomenology; see Glossary).

For a fuller explanation of the many different research designs, data collection tools and sampling strategies, it is important to consult a more in-depth research text (see Further reading, p. 124).

Sampling strategy

When a study is conducted, it is not usually possible to collect information from every single person because the total target population is too large. For example, in a study on the factors causing heart disease, it would not be possible (due to costs and time constraints) to contact every single person in the UK with heart disease to complete a lifestyle survey. It is therefore necessary to target a smaller number of people from within this total population. This is known as the sample (defined as a subset of the target population).

- In quantitative research, the goal of sampling is to gain access to a representative sample of the target population. This makes it possible to then make generalizations from the sample population to the population as a whole.
- In qualitative research, the goals of sampling are different. The purpose is to recruit people who are most likely to be able to contribute to an understanding of the phenomenon being studied. Although the emphasis on qualitative

research is not on generalizability, if the respondents within the sample are known to be 'typical' or 'atypical', then the findings from the sample may be used to throw light on other similar phenomena.

Like the large number of research designs that may be selected, there are also different ways of sampling that will depend on the nature of the research design. Readers may come across a range of sampling approaches but further reading will be required to explore these aspects further.

Types of data collection

In the same way that there is a range of research designs and approaches to sampling, there are also a variety of ways of collecting data. These include techniques such as observation, questionnaires, documentary analysis and interviews.

Observation

Observation focuses on the researcher 'seeing' and perhaps experiencing what happens in a particular context by watching, documenting and then analysing events of interest. The researcher may either take part in the activities being observed (participant observation) or may 'sit at the sidelines' at a distance (non-participant observation).

Questionnaires

Questionnaires are a common way of collecting data and consist of a pre-set list of written questions to be answered, either in writing or verbally, by the respondent.

Documents

Documents may also be a useful source of data. Examples of documents include patient care records, policy documents, historical documents archived in a library, census statistics and reports, and institutional documents.

Interviews

Interviews involve talking with and listening to people, asking questions and discussing issues with them. Interviews may be structured or unstructured and can be undertaken face-to-face or over the telephone. They may occur on a one-to-one basis or may be conducted as a focus group with up to eight people.

Ethical issues and research

All research projects raise ethical issues whether they involve direct contact with people or the use of documentary evidence. To ensure that ethical issues are fully addressed, the plans for all research projects in health and social care must be submitted to Research Ethics and Governance Committees for review prior to the project being carried out. In addition, nurses conducting their own research, assisting other researchers or caring for people involved in research studies, need to do all that they can to ensure that the research they are involved with is of the highest standards.

A number of key ethical principles must be considered in relation to research. The first is the principle of 'respect for persons' (see Ch. 7). This means that researchers must protect individuals from harm and protect their autonomy. Research participants must be able to make informed choices and decisions about what happens to them, such as whether or not to take part in the research. Thus, researchers must ensure that informed consent is gained prior to including anyone in a study (Box 5.10) (see Chs 6, 7).

Ethical issues   Box 5.10

Informed consent in research

Imagine you are a research nurse responsible for recruiting people into a study.

Student activities

- What information would people need in order to give informed consent to their inclusion in the research study?
- How would you ensure that people understood what they were agreeing to do?
- How would you take account of a research participant who is unable to consent due to age, mental distress, learning disability, dementia or who is unconscious?

In some situations, individuals may be unable to make an informed decision to take part in a study, due to illness, age, cognitive impairment or consciousness level or any other feature that increases their vulnerability, such as an inadequate understanding of English, poor literacy, etc. Special measures must be taken in this situation. Confidentiality must also be ensured in order to protect the dignity of people taking part in research. This means that, e.g. personal information, or views expressed by respondents, or photographic images must be stored safely to comply with the 1998 Data Protection Act (DH 1998). Similarly, this is reflected in the Essential Skills Clusters (ESC), No. 7, 1–4 (NMC 2007; now incorporated into NMC 2010 *Standards for pre-registration nursing education*), which states that nurses are obliged to treat any information, including that which is collected through research, as confidential. In particular, all fields of nursing are required to adhere to the principles of data protection. Effective ways of protecting and disguising the identity of participants must also be devised, as respondents should be assured of anonymity (Royal College of Nursing Research Society 2003).

Appraisal of the evidence

The ability to identify good quality evidence requires the development of critical appraisal skills, in order to differentiate weaker evidence from stronger (Box 5.11). Appraising evidence is not just about identifying a paper's flaws, but determining the value or otherwise of the paper to an area of practice. This involves developing a critical awareness that will enable practitioners to read, digest and understand the evidence.

This section provides an introduction to the process of critical appraisal and an example of an appraised article. Once practitioners become familiar with the appraisal process, they find that their skills will advance and develop over time.

Evidence-based practice   Box 5.11

Evidence on the effectiveness of cranberry juice

Refer to Boxes 5.3 and 5.4 based on 'John' and the use of cranberry juice. You need to think about this scenario and the idea of clinical effectiveness and the EBP cycle.

Student activities

- Read the evidence you previously located on cranberry juice.
- Identify two 'types' of evidence, e.g. an RCT, a qualitative study or a guideline, which you think may help you to provide evidence-based care for John. Discuss your two 'types' of evidence with your mentor.

Critical awareness

While many practitioners are able to read the findings from a research paper, most may have problems evaluating the relevance of the findings for their own practice (Avis 1994). Often, people will read the abstract, introduction, findings and conclusions of a research paper, while ignoring the section on research methods. Unfortunately, by ignoring the methods section of the article, it is possible that vital details that provide insight into the strengths or weaknesses of a paper will be missed. This is important when considering the application of findings to practice.

Critical thinking   Box 5.12

The challenges of critically appraising research

Read the example below.

Staff Nurse Brown: 'I read an article yesterday which said that eating soya products is good for you.'

Staff Nurse Sanchez: 'Yeah… Really, what did it say?'

Staff Nurse Brown: 'Well, it said that something found in soya can help to prevent breast cancer.'

Staff Nurse Sanchez: 'So how did they come up with that conclusion?'

Staff Nurse Brown: 'Oh easy really, they compared the diet of a group of women who had breast cancer with the diet of a group of women who didn't have breast cancer and the findings showed that the women who didn't have breast cancer ate more soya products.'

Staff Nurse Sanchez: 'But how many women did they look at?'

Staff Nurse Brown: 'Erm… I think about 100.'

Staff Nurse Sanchez: 'Well, did any of the women smoke?'

Staff Nurse Brown: 'Oh, I'm not sure, I think I missed that bit out – it was a lengthy article.'

Student activities

- What problems does this example highlight?
- Why did Staff Nurse Sanchez ask how many women were in the study and whether any of the women smoked?
- What other details about the paper would you need to know before deciding whether you can trust the findings?
- Discuss with another student what other confounding variables could be associated with breast cancer.

Box 5.12 provides an overview of how important details could be missed. This example highlighted the need for Staff Nurse Brown to read the article in full. Because she did not read the research methods section, she was unable to answer Staff Nurse Sanchez's questions about the sample size and variables which may have significantly influenced the findings of the study. For example, it is known that smoking increases the risk of breast cancer. If any of the women smoked in either group, then this could have influenced the findings. For example, in this case, soya acts as the control variable: women in the non-soya diet group may have smoked more than the women in the soya group which would have led to an increased risk in developing breast cancer, irrespective of whether they consumed soya in their diet. Smoking is therefore a confounding variable that should have been taken into account.

Strategies to develop critical appraisal skills

The development of an evidence-based culture within the NHS is being supported by the government's modernization agenda. This has involved the introduction of clinical governance, NSFs, NICE and other guidelines used to help standardize care. As part of this, it is also recognized that NHS staff such as nurses, midwives and health visitors need better critical appraisal skills (DH 1997) to enable them to use evidence in practice. One way of developing practitioners' appraisal skills is through the use of journal clubs. Journal clubs are an ideal way to develop appraisal skills in a friendly and supportive atmosphere. Journal clubs have expanded and there are now online journal clubs as well as local clubs (see Useful websites, p. 123).

Critical appraisal skills are essential to the delivery of EBP and a variety of critical appraisal tools have been designed to help the reader decide on the quality of research papers (Box 5.13). These appraisal tools usually take the form of a series of questions that the reader needs to ask of the paper. A

number of other tools/guidelines have been developed to help with the process of critical appraisal. Some of these are available online and can be downloaded free of charge (see Useful websites, p. 123).

Questions to ask when critically appraising a research paper

The first and perhaps most crucial stage in the process of critical appraisal is that of identifying a clear research question. If the question is not clear at the outset, then the rest of the research process may be confusing to the reader.

There needs to be a good reason for undertaking a study and it needs to be transparent to the reader. The reader needs to know what type of study has been done and whether the research design was appropriate to meet the study aims. The stages of the research process should be transparent throughout the paper, to enable the reader to understand and make full use of the findings. If the design used was inappropriate, then this may lead to confusing findings that do not address the aims of the study.

There are also other questions that the practitioner needs to consider (Box 5.14).

Questions to consider when reading a research paper   **Box 5.14**

Is the study of interest? – Read the title and abstract.

Why was the study done? – Look into the introduction.

How was the study done? – The methods section will explain the methodological approach to the study and rationale for the approach.

What were the results of the study? – Look into the results or findings section.

What are the implications of the study? – These are normally outlined in the discussion section. The discussion may draw on previous literature to highlight similarities or differences between the study findings and existing literature.

What else was of interest? – As healthcare practitioners are constantly developing their skills and knowledge they may learn something unexpected from the study that could inform their practice.

 Evidence-based practice   **Box 5.13**

What evidence and how to appraise it?

Look at the evidence on cranberry juice you have already located (see Box 5.11).

Student activities

- What type of evidence have you located (e.g. a systematic review, RCT, guideline)?
- How are you going to make sense of the evidence?
- What tools or guidelines will you use to appraise the evidence?
- Obtain copies of some critical appraisal guidelines and, using one of the research papers you located on cranberry juice, compare and contrast the critical appraisal guidelines. Make a list of any similarities or differences.
- Discuss your findings with your mentor.

Appraising different research designs

When appraising different research designs, it is important to identify the stages of the research process carried out by the researcher. Without this, it will not be possible to make sense of the paper, which could limit the application of the findings to practice. In all cases, the paper must be relevant to the practice issue. Readers need to look for evidence that the author has considered the methodology chosen and the rigour the researcher has applied to the methodology. The next section explores four different research designs and highlights key points that should be considered when appraising these designs.

Appraising qualitative research

Qualitative research (Box 5.15) attempts to explore the meanings and experiences of individuals or groups about a particular topic. For example, practitioners may have read about mood disorders and understand the effects and treatment. But what is it like to have depression? Only those who have suffered the condition will be able to describe their experiences. Qualitative research provides a method to explore these thoughts and feelings to gain insight into the experiences of people with depression. In order to obtain the rich, in-depth data required to explore perceptions and feelings, the researcher becomes the data collection tool. Hence, the role of the researcher is important and should be clearly described, as their role is pivotal in the collection of data and analysis of the findings. Qualitative research should demonstrate a clear purpose, an appropriate methodology, and a rationale for the sampling strategy adopted.

Points to look out for in qualitative research   **Box 5.15**

- Is there a description of the researchers' relationship and role with the research participants?
- Was the methodology used appropriate for the study?
- Did the authors provide any extracts from the interviews/focus groups/observation data to support their analysis?
- Is there any evidence of other literature used to support the researchers' findings?
- How were the data analysed?

Appraising systematic reviews

Systematic reviews (Box 5.16) use a series of logical steps that bring together the results of several studies on a single topic in a reliable way to provide an overall conclusion.

Points to look out for in systematic reviews   **Box 5.16**

- How many reviewers were involved? (There should be at least two.)
- How comprehensive was the search strategy?
- Were all the relevant databases searched?
- What were the inclusion and exclusion criteria?
- Were all the studies incorporated in the review similar?
- Were English and non-English articles included?
- How did the reviewers assess the quality of the research studies included in the review?

In a systematic review, research evidence about a specific topic is located through a comprehensive search strategy. The evidence located is then appraised using validated appraisal tools to provide a summary for the reader. Strict inclusion and exclusion criteria are normally used to help the reviewers decide on the best type of papers to be included in the review. Systematic reviews embrace international literature, including published and non-published work, and may take up to 2 years to complete. They are, therefore, considered to be a valuable form of evidence. Systematic reviews of quantitative research (RCTs in particular) are designated as the 'gold standard' of evidence within the hierarchy of evidence. This is reflected in many guidelines currently in use, e.g. the National Service Framework for Older People (DH 2001, pp 14–15).

Appraising randomized controlled trials

Randomized controlled trials (RCTs) (Box 5.17) are an important quantitative method and are another valuable type of evidence. They attempt to manipulate variables within a control and an experimental group to establish treatment cause and effects. As a result, they reduce researcher bias, introduce control and limit confounding variables. Many believe that RCTs are a good type of evidence because they are reliable and it is often possible to generalize from the findings if the study is well designed.

Points to look out for in randomized controlled trials (RCTs)   **Box 5.17**

- Was there a robust randomization procedure?
- Were the researchers and subjects 'blind'? (meaning that neither the researcher nor the research subject knew whether they were in the experimental group or the control group). This helps to reduce bias, e.g. preventing the researcher from entering healthier subjects into the experimental group.
- Was everyone who entered the trial followed up and accounted for? It may be that some subjects left the trial for a variety of reasons. It is important to know what happened to the subjects.
- Were the groups treated equally? Unequal treatment may have a significant impact on the findings.

Appraising survey designs

Surveys (quantitative method) (Box 5.18) are large-scale questionnaires of a selected population. They can provide details about the demographic make-up of a population or trends in lifestyles. For example, they may be used to provide data about how many people smoked in a geographical area.

Points to look for in survey designs   **Box 5.18**

- What was the length of the questionnaire? Was it too long?
- What types of question were included in the questionnaire?
- How was the questionnaire analysed?
- What was the response rate? (Questionnaires are notorious for their poor response rates; sometimes less than 10% are returned.)
- What was the sample population?

An example of a survey that you may have been involved in is the Census. In the UK, this is undertaken every 10 years by the government to find out about the population's lifestyle status. Surveys use questionnaires to elicit details about a

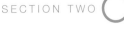

population. Short, closed-ended questions are used to uncover a variety of details from the respondent.

Box 5.19 provides an opportunity for you to reflect on your experiences of completing a survey.

 Reflective practice   Box 5.19

Experiences of completing a survey

Reflect on an experience where you were asked to complete a questionnaire, e.g. as part of market research or a satisfaction questionnaire about a service.

- What type of questions did the questionnaire use?
- How were they structured?
- Did you complete and return the questionnaire?
- What factors helped you to decide to complete the questionnaire or not?

Discuss with your mentor how you could use your personal experiences positively when designing a questionnaire.

Appraising guidelines

Clinical guidelines and integrated care pathways (ICPs) pull together evidence and set out what services and treatments people should receive (see Chs 3, 14). By providing service users with access to information, it is hoped that they will be more empowered and knowledgeable regarding their own care. However, it is also important to remember that not all guidelines/ICPs are reliable and evidence based. The following key points should be considered before using one:

- Are the statements referenced?
- Are the references current?
- When was the guideline/ICP written?
- When is it due for review?
- Who wrote the guideline/ICP?
- Is it clear and free of jargon?

All of these points should be present in a guideline so that practitioners can be reassured of the guideline's evidence base and reliability (Box 5.20).

 Critical thinking   Box 5.20

Integrated care pathways (ICPs)

- Find an ICP used in your clinical placement.
- Locate the care pathways database (see Resource, below – this provides up-to-date information and contact details for ICPs that have been developed and those being piloted).
- Identify an ICP that covers the same condition as the ICP from your clinical placement.
- Compare and contrast the two ICPs and discuss your findings with your mentor/personal tutor.

Resource

Health Information Resources, (formerly the National Library for Health, NLH). Online. Available: www.library.nhs.uk.

Putting evidence into practice

There are important reasons for ensuring that the best evidence is used in practice. First, it is a crucial way of ensuring that people get the treatments and services that are most effective and will have the best health outcomes. EBP ensures that the public funding that supports the NHS is used wisely and that the treatments and services offered are cost-effective. Together, these factors lead to the provision of clinically effective care.

Practitioners, managers, researchers and educators are responsible for ensuring evidence is used in practice. For practitioners, there is a professional responsibility for using the best evidence in practice and to ensure accountability in their practice (NMC 2008) (see Ch. 7). As such, nurses must attempt to keep up-to-date with developments within their field in order to fulfil the continuing professional development requirements for periodic re-registration (see Ch. 7). Practitioners must provide evidence-based advice and keep abreast of contemporary developments (NMC 2008). Equally, nurse managers must support practitioners in using evidence in practice, by developing environments in which EBP can flourish. They must base decisions, e.g. about services, staffing and treatments, on the best available evidence.

Researchers have an important role in generating new knowledge and evidence for practice. However, they must be able to share this information with the practitioners who need to use it. This is dissemination and is usually done by publishing research findings within professional journals. Educators may work with both practitioners and researchers and can help to teach the principles of EBP and support practice development. They may also be involved in research projects.

Finally, but importantly, service users also have a role in ensuring that evidence is used in practice to support a patient-centred approach to care. It is important that service users do ask about the best treatment or care options that are available and are able to challenge practices that they are concerned about.

Challenges to the use of evidence in practice

Unfortunately, despite the vast amount of evidence now available, there are many challenges to using it in practice. In many areas of the NHS, decisions are made on the basis of custom and practice that can lead to outdated or ineffective treatment and care being offered. For example, despite evidence to suggest a shorter fasting time for some types of surgery, people are still fasted preoperatively for too long. This type of practice does not use research to support or change practice. This is often described as the 'research-practice gap'.

There are many reasons for the failure to use research in practice. These often relate to the attitudes of practitioners who may be satisfied with routine practices and are reluctant to change. Barriers to using evidence in practice include lack of time, poor communication and limited research skills (Barker 2010). In other cases, there is a lack of high quality research to guide practice. This means that practitioners have no option but to follow their own experience. Research studies may be small scale, methodologically flawed or produce findings that are difficult to implement. It is also a problem when research seems irrelevant to practitioners who would have asked different research questions had they been involved in the design of the research. Different studies on the same topic can also produce conflicting results, making it problematic to use the information. Systematic reviews of particular topics collate evidence into a more usable form. By combining the results of multiple studies, clearer implications can be indentified and put into practice.

Overcoming the challenges is essential to improving care and service delivery. The most important approach is to improve the communication or dissemination of research findings. Unfortunately, while publication in academic and professional journals is the usual approach to sharing research information, this type of dissemination remains relatively ineffective and does not necessarily lead to changes in practice.

Implementing evidence

The process if incorporating research findings and other good sources of evidence into practice is complex. Generally, the publication of evidence on its own will not lead to changes and improvements in clinical practice. Specific change management strategies will be required to overcome the numerous barriers to change and EBP that have been documented. One important way of translating evidence and research into practice is through the production of clinical practice guidelines. There are also numerous models for knowledge translation (see Gerrish & Lacey 2010, p 508). Bucknall et al (2010) suggest that there are five key attributes to successful change. These include:

- Consideration of the evidence in relation to the type, compatibility, trustworthiness and relevance
- The clinicians involved and their personalities, the meaning of the clinical issue and the clinicians' ability to change practice
- The organizational context and the structural determinants. This involves ascertaining the type of organizational structure and whether it is receptive to change
- Communication and facilitation, particularly in relation to the organization's demographics, boundaries, leaders and those who are likely to support change
- The patient, and determining at what level they should be involved and their competence to be an active participant in change.

Thus, preparation to effect change in practice is complex and requires considerable input from all those involved, including the professionals, patients and their carers, to be truly clinically effective.

SUMMARY

- EBP acts as a bridge between different types of evidence and nursing practice.
- By promoting the uptake and implementation of research and other types of evidence, high standards of effective practice in

healthcare are supported. Models and guidance have been developed to sustain the use of research.

- EBP is viewed as a means to challenge outdated, ritualistic practices by encouraging practitioners to be more questioning of their work and care delivery.
- Research is a valuable form of evidence that can be used to support, improve and develop practice. There are a number of steps to the research process including locating the evidence. At first, the prospect of conducting a literature search can be quite daunting. However, it is a skill that develops over time and, with practice, your abilities to search for literature will improve.
- Once practitioners have located relevant research they should then appraise the evidence critically. When reading a research paper, each step should be made transparent so that it is possible to judge the value of the study. EBP relies on the availability of good quality evidence to improve practice. To ensure the implementation of good evidence in practice, practitioners need critical appraisal skills that help the reader to make sense of research evidence. By using a validated tool or guide, the reader can work through a research paper in a systematic way to judge the credibility and value of research papers.
- While practitioners may question their practice, find and appraise evidence, practice will not change unless evidence is effectively implemented. This requires the involvement of the individual practitioner, the nursing team and the organization.

KEY WORDS AND PHRASES FOR LITERATURE SEARCHING

Evidence-based practice

Health informatics

Literature review

Qualitative

Quantitative

 Useful websites

Action for Sick Children http://actionforsickchildren.org

Bandolier www.medicine.ox.ac.uk/bandolier

Centre for Reviews and Dissemination www.york.ac.uk/inst/crd

Clinical Knowledge Summaries www.cks.nhs.uk/home

Cochrane Library www.thecochranelibrary.com

Evidence-based Nursing http://ebn.bmj.com

Health Information Resources (formerly the National Library for Health, NLH) – provides access to a wide range of health related services including an index of UK national clinical guidelines www.evidence.nhs.uk

Mental Health Foundation www.mentalhealth.org.uk

National Institute for Health and Clinical Excellence (NICE) – develops clinical guidelines, undertakes appraisals and provides other clinical guidance for the NHS for England and Wales www.nice.org.uk

NHS Evidence www.evidence.nhs.uk/topics

NHS Quality Improvement Scotland (NHSQIS) – sets standards, monitors performance, provides advice, best practice statements, guidance and support on clinical effectiveness and improvement for the NHS in Scotland www.nhshealthquality.org

NHS Solutions for Public Health Critical Appraisal Skills Programme – appraisal tools/guidelines available for free download www.sph.nhs.uk/what-we-do/public-health-workforce/resources/critical-appraisals-skills-programme

PubMed Central www.ncbi.nlm.nih.gov/pmc

Scottish Intercollegiate Guidelines Network (SIGN) – appraisal tools/guidelines available for free download www.sign.ac.uk/methodology/checklists.html

US National Library of Medicine www.nlm.nih.gov

All websites accessed September 2012.

References

Avis, M., 1994. Reading research critically I. An introduction to appraisal: designs and objectives. Journal of Clinical Nursing 3, 227–234.

Barker, J., 2010. Evidence based practice for nurses. Sage, London.

Brand-de Heer, D.L., 2001. A comparison of the coverage of clinical medicine provided by PASCAL, BIOMED and MEDLINE. Health Information and Libraries Journal 18 (2), 110–116.

Brazier, H., Begley, C.M., 1996. Selecting a database for literature searches in nursing: MEDLINE or CINAHL? Journal of Advanced Nursing 24, 868–875.

Bucknall, T., Rycroft-Malone, J. (Eds.), 2010. Evidence-based practice doing the right thing for the right patients. In: Models and frameworks for implementing evidence-based practice: linking evidence to action. Wiley Blackwell, Chichester.

Cox, C.L., Reyes-Hughes, A., 2001. Clinical effectiveness in practice. Palgrave, Basingstoke.

Craig, J.V., Smyth, R.L. (Eds.), 2007. The evidence based practice manual for nurses, second ed. Churchill Livingstone, Edinburgh.

Department of Health, 1997. The new NHS: modern and dependable. TSO, London.

Department of Health, 1998. Data protection act. Department of Health, London.

Department of Health, 1999a. Making a difference: strengthening the nursing, midwifery and health visiting contribution to health and healthcare. Department of Health, London.

Department of Health, 1999b. Saving lives: our healthier nation. A contract for health. TSO, London.

Department of Health, 2001. National service framework for older people. Department of Health, London.

Department of Health, 2010a. Equity and excellence. Liberating the NHS. Online. Available: www.dh.gov.uk/en/Publicationsandstatistics/Publications/PublicationsPolicyAndGuidance/DH_117353 September 2012.

Department of Health, 2010b. Essence of care 2010. Benchmarks for the fundamental aspects of care. Online. Available: www.dh.gov.uk/prod_consum_dh/groups/dh_digitalassets/@dh/@en/@ps/documents/digitalasset/dh_119978.pdf September 2012.

Gerrish, K., Lacey, A., 2010. The research process in nursing, sixth ed. Wiley Blackwell, Oxford.

Grant, M.J., Booth, A., 2009. A typology of reviews: an analysis of 14 review types and associated methodologies. Health Information and Libraries Journal 26 (2), 91–108.

National Institute for Health and Clinical Excellence and the Royal College of Nursing, 2005. The management of pressure ulcers in primary and secondary care. A Clinical Practice guide. Clinical Guideline CG 29 Online. Available: www.nice.org.uk/nicemedia/live/10972/29885/29885.pdf September 2012.

NHS Executive, 1996. Achieving effective practice: a clinical effectiveness and research information pack for nurses, midwives and health visitors. NHS Executive, Leeds.

Nursing and Midwifery Council, 2007. Introduction of essential skills clusters for pre-registration nursing programmes. Online. Available: www.nmc-uk.org/Documents/Circulars/2007circulars/NMCcircular07_2007.pdf September 2012.

Nursing and Midwifery Council, 2008. The Code: Standards of conduct, performance and ethics for nurses and midwives. Online. Available: http://www.nmc-uk.org/Publications/Standards/The-code/Introduction/ September 2012.

Nursing and Midwifery Council, 2010. Standards for pre-registration nursing education. Online. Available: www.nmc-uk.org September 2012.

Okuma, E., 1994. Selecting CD-ROM databases for nursing students: a comparison of MEDLINE and the Cumulative Index to Nursing and Allied Health Literature (CINAHL). Bulletin of the Medical Library Association 82 (1), 25–29.

Palmer, J., Brice, A., 1999. Information sourcing. In: Hamer, S., Collinson, G. (Eds.), Achieving evidence-based practice: a handbook for practitioners. Baillière Tindall, London.

Parahoo, K., 2006. Nursing research: principles, processes and issues, second ed. Palgrave Macmillan, Basingstoke.

Polgar, S., Thomas, S., 1995. Introduction to research in the health sciences. Churchill Livingstone, London.

Richardson, W.S., Wilson, M.C., Nishikawa, J., et al., 1995. The well built clinical question: a key to evidence based decisions. ACP Journal Club 123 (2), A12–A13.

Royal College of Nursing, 1996. Clinical effectiveness: a Royal College of Nursing guide. Royal College of Nursing. In: Cox, C.L., Reyes-Hughes, A. (Eds.), 2001 Clinical effectiveness in practice. Palgrave Macmillan, Basingstoke.

Royal College of Nursing Research Society, 2003. The Royal College of Nursing Research Society: nurses and research ethics. Nurse Researcher 11 (1), 7–19.

Thompson, C., Cullum, N., 1999. Examining evidence: an overview. Nursing Times Learning Curve 3 (1), 7–9.

Walsh, M., Ford, P., 1989. Nursing rituals: research and rational actions. Butterworth Heinemann, Oxford.

Further reading

Bowling, A., 2009. Research methods in health: investigating health and health services, third ed. Open University Press (McGraw-Hill Education), Maidenhead.

Brettle, A., Grant, M.J., 2004. Finding the evidence for practice: a workbook for health professionals. Churchill Livingstone, Edinburgh.

Evans, D., 2003. Hierarchy of evidence: a framework for ranking evidence evaluating healthcare interventions. Journal of Clinical Nursing 12, 77–84.

Polit, D.F., Beck, C., 2011. Nursing research: Generating and assessing evidence for nursing practice, ninth revised international ed. Lippincott Williams & Wilkins, Philadelphia.

Legal issues that impact on nursing practice

6

Sherri Ogston-Tuck

LEARNING OUTCOMES

This chapter will help you:
- Have an overview of the English legal system
- Develop an understanding of relevant law and legislation
- Understand the legal and professional responsibilities and obligations integral to nursing
- Understand the important legal issues that apply to nursing practice.

Introduction

This chapter provides an overview of the legal system as it pertains to nursing. The law varies across the UK, but the emphasis here is the law in England and Wales. Practitioners should be aware that there are different systems in Scotland and Northern Ireland. The law is a specialist area with its own language but highly relevant to nursing practice. The law is outlined with the aim of providing a better understanding of relevant terminology and legislation relevant to all fields of nursing.

It is necessary to have an understanding of the legal system for those working in healthcare. The law is not static; it is constantly changing, as is healthcare and nursing practice. Changes affecting nursing practice result from research and changes in technology and society; giving rise to evidence-based practice (see Ch. 5) and change in practice. Nurses need to be aware that statutes affecting their practice may be amended or repealed.

Nurses must think how the law affects their role and to always consider it in their day-to-day practice. Often it is only when something 'goes wrong' that nurses consider the law. All practitioners should maintain knowledge of and adherence to the law as it is important to standards of care and expectations of practice, patient/client outcomes and public well-being. Professional and ethical issues pertain to this and it is therefore important for nurses to think about influences on practice and decision-making. There have been significant changes in policy

and practice that reflect patient rights, changes within the NHS and government initiatives – all of which must also be considered in relation to the law, to the practitioner and to the patient/client. Having an understanding of this will provide you with the necessary foundations to reflect on your practice and how the law impacts upon this.

Legal frameworks

A country's system of justice reflects its morals, history and politics. UK law and the structures within it have developed over hundreds of years. Thus, terminology, legislation and systems of law, all stem from the past and from tradition. The UK is unique in that it has an unwritten constitution, which is unlike the majority of the civilized world (Boylan-Kemp 2011). This gives rise to our understanding of governance; which encompasses the distinctive structure, power and duties of government in relation to the rights of citizens of the state. By not having a written constitution, the law can reflect society and be modified; avoiding a rigid and inflexible codified constitution. The rules and principles of law can be found within statute and case law, custom and conventions. The UK's constitution is entrenched in its historical development which is primarily parliamentary supremacy.

The law can be conceived as a set of rules which govern society and create a structure of authority of government to run the social order (Stychin & Mulcahy 2010).

Structure of law

Our legal system is referred to as a common law system, where legislation created by Parliament, is at the centre. Notwithstanding the role of parliament, it is the judiciary's function to interpret the law.

A fundamental doctrine of English law is the 'rule of law' which is characteristic of the English constitution and supremacy. It is the principle of legality, where the rule is that no person is above the law (Boylan-Kemp 2011).

Sources and types of law

The law is derived from three major sources:

- Legislation
    Acts of Parliament (statute or written law)
    Secondary legislation (statutory instruments)
- The Courts (judicial decisions)
- The European Community and Human Rights law

Note: Case law or judge-made law predates statute; however, common law rules may be regarded as secondary because of the many statutes that now exist. The rules in case law are derived from legal principles laid down by judges over many years, hence the historical development of English law. Nevertheless, case law still remains an important source of law, particularly in negligence cases (see pp. 133 and 134). Case law is subject to a system of precedent where the earlier decisions made by a higher court mean that a lower court must follow their decision. Rulings of the Supreme Court (the highest court) are binding on all lower courts, whereas those rulings of the Court of Appeal are generally binding on the lower courts.

The legal system is divided into two divisions: public and private law. Public law concerns itself with preserving the order of society, whereas private law is concerned with disputes between individuals. The law is further divided into criminal law and civil law:

- *Criminal law* – deals with actions/behaviour regarded as wrong. Criminal offences relate to people and property and result in a prosecution, and if the defendant is convicted, usually results in punishment (discharge, fine, community penalty or a custodial sentence). The burden of proof in criminal cases means that the prosecution must prove the facts 'beyond reasonable doubt'. Most (95-96%) criminal cases are heard in the Magistrates' court and more serious or complex cases or appeals are heard in the Crown court. The Crown Prosecution Service or another prosecuting body brings the case against the defendant.
- *Civil law* – deals with the conduct and conflicts between people. A person (the claimant) who has suffered a perceived wrong can seek redress by bringing an action or claim in the civil courts. The claim may be settled with an award of financial compensation or damages, or an order (injunction) banning an unlawful act or an order that requires some action. The burden of proof in civil cases is lower; the claimant must prove the facts 'on a balance of probabilities'. Civil cases are between the claimant and another person or organization and are heard in the County court or the High court depending on the amount of damages or degree of harm.

Acts of Parliament

Most English law is in the form of Acts of Parliament (statutes). Codification is a means of putting a rule of the common

law into a written statute (Griffith & Tengnah 2010). An example of primary legislation is the Disability Discrimination Act 2005; secondary legislation may be in the form of Regulations: Lifting Operations and Lifting Equipment Regulations 1998 (LOLER); or Orders: Medicines for Human use (Prescribing) (Miscellaneous Amendments) Order 2006, which introduced independent and supplementary prescribing by nurses and other healthcare professionals (Griffith & Tengnah 2010).

An Act results from a Bill (a draft proposal). Proposals for legislative changes may be contained in government White Papers. Consultation papers, sometimes called Green Papers, which set out government proposals and seek comments from interested parties, including the public, may precede these. Figure 6.1 illustrates the procedure of how a Bill becomes an Act.

The law undergoes constant reform in the courts as established principles are interpreted, clarified or reapplied to meet new circumstances; laws become outdated, new policies require new laws, or new laws are needed to ensure that the

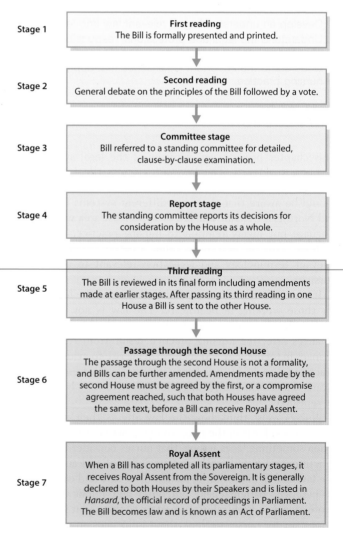

Fig. 6.1 • How a Bill becomes law.

UK complies with international or European Law, e.g. The Convention of Human Rights Act 1998.

Court system (England and Wales)

The courts are entirely independent of parliament and government, and can act as a control mechanism to these powers (Boylan-Kemp 2011). The use of precedent binds a court in decision-making, giving certainty and meaning to law and in maintaining equality (see above). The hierarchy of the court system (criminal and civil proceedings) in England and Wales is outlined in Figure 6.2.

Important legislation for nursing

Many Acts of Parliament are relevant to nursing. Although a detailed discussion of every Act is beyond the scope of this book, Table 6.1 outlines some important Acts and sources of information for nursing and healthcare. Some of these have far-reaching effects for nursing and are discussed in the chapter.

UK Supreme Court
The most senior domestic court. Deals with appeals from the Court of Appeal and some cases with exceptional circumstances from the High Court.

Court of Appeal
Criminal and Civil division - deal with appeals from the crown court, tribunals and some county court cases.

High court
Divided into three divisions: Queen's bench – contract, tort and administrative cases, supervisory of lower courts, tribunals and local authorities; Family – deals with appeals from the magistrates' courts; Chancery – deals with appeals from county courts on bankruptcy and land law.

Crown court
Deals with serious and complex cases committed by magistrates for trial or sentence. Hears appeals against conviction and or sentence, etc. from the Magistrates' court.

County court
Civil litigation and disputes between individuals and some family matters.

Magistrates' court
Deals mostly with criminal cases and with some civil cases. These courts deal with around 95-96% of all criminal cases to completion. Magistrates with specific training deal with family proceedings in the family court and young offenders in the youth court.

Tribunals
Deals with cases on immigration, social security, child support, pensions, tax and land, etc.

European Court of Human Rights (ECtHR)
Located in Strasbourg. Enforces the Convention on Human Rights and deals with human rights complaints from countries belonging to the Council of Europe. It hears appeals against the UK Supreme Court judgements that relate to the Convention and is subject to relevant precedents set by the ECJ.

The European Court of Justice (ECJ)
The highest court of the European communities (European Union (EU)) located in Luxembourg. It adjudicates on all matters of European law relating to trade and civil matters.

Fig. 6.2 • The court system (England and Wales).

Table 6.1 Important legislation for nursing (England and Wales)

Act of Parliament	Where to access the Act or explanatory notes
Access to Health Records Act 1990	www.legislation.gov.uk/ukpga/1990/23/contents
Children Act 1989	www.legislation.gov.uk/ukpga/1989/41/contents
Children Act 2004	www.legislation.gov.uk/ukpga/2004/31/contents
Data Protection Act 1998 (DPA)	www.legislation.gov.uk/ukpga/1998/29/contents
Disability Discrimination Act 2005	www.legislation.gov.uk/ukpga/2005/13/contents
Freedom of Information Act (FoIA) 2000	www.legislation.gov.uk/ukpga/2000/36/contents
Health and Safety at Work Act 1974 (see Ch. 13)	www.legislation.gov.uk/ukpga/1974/37/contents www.hse.gov.uk/legislation/
Health and Social Care Act 2001	www.legislation.gov.uk/ukpga/2001/15/contents
Human Rights Act 1998 (HRA)	www.legislation.gov.uk/ukpga/1998/42/contents
Human Tissue Act 2004	www.legislation.gov.uk/ukpga/2004/30/contents http://www.organdonation.nhs.uk:8001/ukt/default.asp
Medicinal Products: Prescription by Nurse Act 1992 (see Ch. 22)	www.legislation.gov.uk/ukpga/1992/28/contents
Mental Capacity Act 2005	www.legislation.gov.uk/ukpga/2005/9/contents www.legislation.gov.uk/all?title=mental%20capacity%20act%202005 www.dh.gov.uk/en/SocialCare/Deliveringsocialcare/MentalCapacity/MentalCapacityAct2005/index.htm
Mental Health Act 2007 (MHA)	www.legislation.gov.uk/ukpga/2007/12/contents
Public Interest Disclosure Act 1998	www.legislation.gov.uk/ukpga/1998/23/contents

All websites accessed September 2012.

The Human Rights Act

The Human Rights Act (HRA 1998) is wide ranging and promises that the state will respect the rights and freedoms of individuals. Human rights are very much a part of everyday life and aim to protect the public, professionals and patients/clients. Nurses need to be aware of the potential implications of this Act in their practice and care provision. The HRA 1998 applies to children (a person under the age of 18) as well as adults. It became law in 2000 and incorporates the rights and freedoms guaranteed under the European Convention on Human Rights (the Convention, ECHR). The Convention was drafted following the Second World War and the UK was one of the first countries to sign up to be a member in 1953. At present, 47 states have signed the ECHR (Boylan-Kemp 2011).

The ECHR contains a number of basic human rights and is divided into schedules, which are further divided into articles. These are:

- Article 2 – Right to life
- Article 3 – Prohibition of torture
- Article 4 – Prohibition of slavery and forced labour
- Article 5 – Right to liberty and security
- Article 6 – Right to a fair trial
- Article 7 – No punishment without lawful authority
- Article 8 – Right to respect for private and family life
- Article 9 – Freedom of thought, conscience and religion
- Article 10 – Right to freedom of expression
- Article 11 – Freedom of assembly and association
- Article 12 – Right to marry and found a family
- Article 14 – Prohibition of discrimination

as well as

- Article 1 of the First Protocol – Protection of property
- Article 2 of the First Protocol – Right to education
- Article 3 of the First Protocol – Right to free elections (right to vote).

Since coming into effect in 2000, English courts deciding on a matter connected with one of the Rights must, as far as applicable, regard those decisions made by the European Court of Human Rights (ECtHR) previously and any new legislation must also comply. All public bodies must act in accordance with the Convention, including health services and healthcare professionals. Indeed some articles impact on nursing practice such as effective pain management, clinical decision-making, palliative care and end-of-life choices (Box 6.1). Examples impacting on practice include:

- Article 2 impacts on decisions regarding withholding and/or withdrawing of life-preserving or life-saving treatment. It is clear, however, that there will always be challenges with regard to non-resuscitation orders and demands for

Reflective practice   Box 6.1

The Human Rights Act and nursing practice

- Bob, aged 82, has advanced brain cancer, and has been unconscious for 24 hours. Following consultation with Bob's family and the care team, it is decided that he will not be resuscitated
- Shelagh is 5 years old and has a learning disability. She screams and kicks when the nurses try to give her oral antiseizure drugs. One nurse usually holds Shelagh on her lap while another nurse administers the drug
- John has liver cirrhosis after many years of alcohol misuse; he refuses to stop drinking and is denied a liver transplant
- Francis has severe dementia and lives in a care home. His niece visits and finds him dressed in clothes that are not his and that he has outdoor shoes on, but no socks.

Student activities

- Reflect on the scenarios above and consider which Articles are relevant.
- Discuss with your mentor situations in placements where an Article(s) of the HRA was pertinent to patient/client outcomes.

Resource

Department for Constitutional Affairs, 2006. A Guide to the Human Rights Act, 1998, third ed. Online. Available: http://webarchive.nationalarchives.gov.uk/+/www.dca.gov.uk/peoples-rights/human-rights/pdf/act-studyguide.pdf September 2012.

Reflective practice   Box 6.2

Mental distress

Sam is wandering in and out of the pub and the takeaway. It is Saturday evening and he is increasingly agitated and distressed by the noise and unfamiliar people. The pub landlord calls the police when Sam starts shouting at people having a meal. The police officer, who knows Sam well, is worried about his distressed state and, also noticing that he has a head wound, summons an ambulance. When Sam arrives at the Emergency Department accompanied by the police officer, he is very distressed and will not allow the staff near him. The charge nurse fears for Sam's safety. The duty psychiatrist is asked to come to assess Sam.

Student activities

- How would you have felt sitting in the pub when Sam came in?
- Speak to a mental health nurse and ask which provisions of the mental health legislation in your part of the UK can be used to both help and protect Sam in the short term.

---

more aggressive treatments for serious illness. This is of particular relevance with an ageing population, technological advances and other challenges concerning dying with dignity and end-of-life choices

- Article 3 states that no-one shall be subject to torture or inhumane, degrading treatment or punishment. Inhumane treatment is deemed to be any treatment that causes intense physical and mental suffering.

Nurses act as advocates for their patients/clients, to safeguard standards of care and to speak out where the patient/client may be at risk. Moreover, the Nursing and Midwifery Council (NMC) (2008) *The Code: Standards of conduct, performance and ethics for nurses and midwives* requires registrants to bring any circumstances that may compromise patient/client care and safety to the attention of an appropriate authority.

Mental health legislation

The Mental Health (MH) Act 2007 made a number of amendments to the MH Act 1983; introduced 'Bournewood' safeguards; and amended the Mental Capacity Act (MCA) (2005) introducing new *Deprivation of Liberty Safeguards* (Box 6.2). The 1983 Act is largely concerned with the circumstances in which a person with a mental disorder can be detained for treatment for that disorder, without his or her consent. The main purpose of the legislation was to ensure that people with serious mental disorders which threaten their health or safety or the safety of the public can be treated irrespective of their

consent where it is necessary to prevent them from harming themselves or others.

The safeguards came about in response to the Bournewood judgement from the ECtHR case *HL v UK [2004]* involving a man with autism who was kept at Bournewood Hospital by doctors against the wishes of his carers. The ECtHR found that admission to and retention in hospital of HL under the common law of necessity amounted to a breach of Article 5(1) ECHR (deprivation of liberty) and of Article 5(4) (right to have lawfulness of detention reviewed by a court).

The 'safeguards apply to anyone:

- aged 18 and over
- who suffers from a mental disorder or disability of the mind – such as dementia or a profound learning disability
- who lacks the capacity to give informed consent to the arrangements made for their care and/or treatment and
- for whom deprivation of liberty (within the meaning of Article 5 of the ECHR) is considered after an independent assessment to be necessary in their best interests to protect them from harm …'

(DH 2011)

The MCA (2005) which came into force in 2007 replaces the common law provisions and provides a statutory definition of capacity and sets out clear steps in determining the best interests for a person who lacks capacity. Situations of necessity are now covered under this Act; which recognizes the duty of a healthcare professional to take action that is in the 'best interests' of the patient. The basic principles (Dimond 2011; NMC 2008) of the MCA are:

1. A person must be assumed to have capacity unless it is established that he lacks capacity
2. A person is not to be treated as unable to make a decision unless all practicable steps to help him to do so have been taken without success
3. A person is not to be treated as unable to make a decision merely because he makes an unwise decision

4. An act done or decision made under this Act or on behalf of a person who lacks capacity must be done or made in their best interest

5. Before the act is done or the decision made, regard must be had as to whether the purpose for which it is needed can be effectively achieved in a way that is less restrictive of the person's rights and freedom of action.

The MCA sets out steps which must be taken in determining what the 'best interests' are for the patient. The guidance is that where healthcare professionals are involved in the care of those lacking capacity, they must exercise a professional duty of care in regard to the NMC Code. The MCA also addresses advocacy and lasting powers of attorney (LPA), for health and financial interests.

Rights for children and child protection

There is growing recognition that children have rights (McHale & Fox 2007) with much of the impetus of this from the following:

- The leading case of *Gillick v West Norfolk and Wisbech AHA [1986] AC 112 (HL)* (see p. 136)
- Children Act (2004) and safeguarding children
- *Keeping Children Safe* published by the DH following the inquiry into the death of Victoria Climbié
- The Green Paper published in 2003 'Every Child Matters'
- National Service Frameworks (NSFs) for Children, Young People and Maternity Services (2004) (www.dh.gov.uk/).

The Children Act 2004 provides the legal underpinning for safeguarding children and sets out those provisions that address the duties and arrangements for the protection and welfare of children and young people. It is the responsibility and duty of local authorities, NHS organizations, etc. that child protection policies are in place and must be followed by healthcare professionals and others working with children (Box 6.3). Regarding confidentiality and disclosure, the NMC reminds registrants with an extract from *The Code* 'You must disclose information if you believe someone may be at risk of harm, in line with the law of the country in which you are practising' (NMC 2009a).

Data Protection Act

The Data Protection Act (DPA) 1998 is designed to balance the right of individuals to privacy and the rights of those people/organizations who have valid reasons for holding and using personal data, such as healthcare professionals. It sets out the principles with which users of personal information must comply, and also gives individuals the right to gain access to information held about them and provides for a supervisory authority the right to oversee and enforce the law (Dimond 2011).

The DPA applies to electronic records as well and sets out terminology of such data. The Act should be read in conjunction with the Human Rights Act (HRA) 1998 and the Freedom of Information Act 2000 as the DPA gives rise to our duty of confidentiality; all three Acts are interlinked (see Table 6.1, p. 128).

 Reflective practice Box 6.3

Safeguarding children: Baby P

Peter Connelly was a 17-month old boy who died in London after suffering many injuries over an 8-month period, during which he was repeatedly seen by Haringey Children's services and NHS health professionals.

The case caused shock and concern among the public and in parliament, partly because of the magnitude of Peter's injuries, and partly because Peter had lived in the London Borough of Haringey, under the same child care authorities that had failed 10 years earlier in the case of Victoria Climbié. This had led to a public enquiry which resulted in measures being put in place in an effort to prevent similar cases happening.

The child protection services of Haringey and other agencies were widely criticized. Following the conviction of Peter's mother, his step-father and the step-father's brother, three inquiries and a nationwide review of social service care were launched. Another nationwide review was conducted by Lord Laming into his own recommendations concerning Victoria Climbié's killing in 2000.

(Victoria Climbié was abused, neglected and tortured to death by her great-aunt and the woman's boyfriend. Both were convicted of murder and sentenced to life imprisonment. The police, health professionals and social services all had contact with Victoria while she was being abused. A public inquiry chaired by Lord Laming exposed a picture of incompetence and error at every level. Lord Laming promised to make recommendations to ensure such a tragedy would never happen again.)

Student activities

- Access the reports on the failings that allowed the abuse of both Peter and Victoria and ultimately their deaths and discuss the findings with your mentor.
- Find out what services/protocols are in place in your area for safeguarding children.

Resources

Care Quality Commission (CQC) Report 2009 Inspection of progress made in the provision of safeguarding services in the London Borough of Haringey.

Communitycare.co.uk 2010 Baby Peter case in Haringey. Online. Available: www.communitycare.co.uk/Articles/2010/12/09/109961/baby-peter-case-in-haringey.htm.

Department of Health, 2009. Safeguarding children and primary medical care. Online. Available: www.dh.gov.uk/en/Publicationsandstatistics/Lettersandcirculars/Dearcolleagueletters/DH_109407.

The Victoria Climbié inquiry, Chairman Lord Laming, 2003. Online. Available: www.dh.gov.uk/prod_consum_dh/groups/dh_digitalassets/documents/digitalasset/dh_110711.pdf.

All websites accessed September 2012.

Nurses have a responsibility to protect data as most manage, or will manage, personal information about people (see Documentation and record-keeping, and Confidentiality, below). It is also important to be aware of the patient's/client's rights in relation to personal information held about them, how it is managed and how they can request access to it (see Access to Health Records Act 1990, Table 6.1).

Legal concepts integral to nursing

This section considers legal concepts that are important for nurses: accountability, safeguarding practice, duty of care, clinical negligence, consent, professional and legal obligation and responsibility.

Nurses are accountable for their actions and omissions (NMC 2008) (see Ch. 7). Registered nurses remain accountable even when acting on the instructions of another practitioner such as when administering drugs prescribed by a doctor. Nurses have a professional duty of care not to harm patients and to act in a way that minimizes risk of harm at all times. Therefore, even where the prescribing doctor, for example, has made the original mistake, the nurse has responsibilities and is accountable. This is illustrated in the case of *Prendergast v Sam and Dee [1989] 1 MED LR 36*, where both the prescribing doctor and the pharmacist were held to account for causing harm to the patient who was given the wrong drug as a result of poor handwriting.

Furthermore, nurses (including students) will not generally be able to argue that they are unaccountable because they lack experience (Griffith & Tengnah 2010) where failing to refer a matter to a more senior nurse may fall below an acceptable standard of care (*Nettleship v Weston [1971] QB 691 (CA)*). It is therefore essential that nurses work within their limitations and be aware of their capabilities. It is also crucial that they take responsibility for checking and where necessary, challenging lack of clarity, errors or discrepancy in drug prescriptions or other treatment.

The four arenas of accountability relating to the nurse's duty of care, negligence and patient harm are:

- Employer
- NMC
- Civil law
- Criminal law.

All four arenas are discussed in this section.

Safeguards for practice

There are various safeguards that protect both patients/clients and nurses accountable for planning and providing care. These include statutory regulation, professional indemnity insurance, documentation and record-keeping, etc.

Statutory regulation

Health, psychological and social work professionals are subject to statutory regulation, e.g. the NMC regulates nurses and midwives (see Ch. 7), the General Medical Council (GMC) regulates doctors, and the Health and Care Professions Council (HCPC) currently regulates 16 professions, e.g. physiotherapists, paramedics, etc. The purpose of statutory regulation is to ensure standards of care and practice and to provide public protection.

The NMC regulates the profession and maintains a register of practitioners (Box 6.4). When a practitioner seeks employment, the employer would ensure the practitioner is registered

---

> ### Reflective practice Box 6.4
>
> **Fitness to practise**
>
> Registered practitioners must be 'fit to practise', i.e. meet standards for safe practice and work within guidelines of professional and safe practice.
>
> **Case history**
>
> The NMC Conduct and Competence committee removed a registered nurse from the register for failing to administer insulin to a patient, reporting and documenting that it had been given when it had not. The Committee found the nurse's fitness to practise impaired by reason of misconduct and dishonesty.
>
> **Student activities**
>
> - Discuss with your mentor the circumstances of the case and consider other reasons why a practitioner may be considered 'unfit to practise'.
>
> **Resource**
>
> NMC – www.nmc-uk.org/

---

with the NMC as well as requiring a satisfactory Criminal Records Bureau check.

The law protects the title of registered nurse/midwife and it is a criminal offence to use the title without NMC registration.

The Code: Standards of conduct, performance and ethics for nurses and midwives (NMC 2008) has two key functions: to inform the nurses/midwives of the standard of professional conduct of registrants, and to inform the public, other professionals and employers of those standards and conduct expected of professionals.

Nursing students must achieve the mandatory theory hours, practice learning hours and competencies and be of good character prior to registration. Following registration, the NMC continues to monitor professional development and education as a requirement for periodic re-registration.

The NMC provides guidance for clinical experience for nursing students. For example, nursing students must always introduce and identify themselves as students, as some patients/clients may refuse care provided by a nursing student. If the patient/client asks the student to leave they must do so (NMC 2010). Although nursing students are not accountable professionally to the NMC until they become registered, they can be called to account by the law or to their college or university for any actions or omissions (NMC 2010).

Contracts of employment

Employees are protected by a contract of employment but have responsibilities to the employer to fulfil their contractual obligations. Thus, the nurse's employer would have the expectation that the nurse acts in accordance with that contract, e.g. keeping confidential information secure. In an employment contract, boundaries or limitations of practice are clearly stated and responsibilities identified. It is important to be aware of how the employer and the practitioner interpret it. A job description should provide clear expectations of the practitioner and identify functions expected within that role. Contracts also protect the employer. For example, if a nurse were to practise outside their job description or contract, their employer may not accept liability for any negligent acts or omissions (see p. 133).

Direct liability is where the employer is at fault; indirect or vicarious liability is when the practitioner is at fault. Some employers accept the liability (see below) but others may not.

When disputes arise between employee and employer they may be referred to a tribunal. These hear unfair dismissal, discrimination and other cases in relation to statutory employment rights as well as some breach of contract actions.

Professional indemnity insurance

The NMC recommends that registrants have professional indemnity in the event of a claim for negligence: 'Some employers accept vicarious liability for negligent acts and/or omissions of their employees' (NMC 2008, p 8). However, this cover does not include actions outside work. Registrants working independently will need to obtain their own insurance cover. As some agency work may not be covered by insurance, registrants should check their insurance status and if necessary, obtain cover through a professional organization or trade union.

The situation is set to change following the response to an independent review to have insurance or indemnity as a condition of registration as a healthcare professional (DH 2010).

Conscientious objection

Healthcare professionals, patients or their family may have a conscientious objection to a particular procedure, such as termination of pregnancy. Although nurses may object to their participation in abortion on religious or cultural grounds, there is no statutory definition of conscientious objection and the law does not give an interpretation of 'participation in treatment'.

There are only two areas of care in law where nurses and midwives have the right to conscientiously object:

- The Human Fertilization and Embryology Act 1990 – technological procedures to accomplish conception and pregnancy
- The Abortion Act 1967 – direct involvement in abortion procedures. However, the statutory right of conscientious objection does not include persons more remotely associated to abortion processes.

The NMC standard relating to conscientious objection is contained within *The Code*; practitioners must inform someone in authority if they experience problems that prevent them from working within this code or other nationally agreed standards (NMC 2008). It is important to reiterate that nurses and midwives have no right of refusal to take part in emergency treatment. In any emergency, they would be expected to provide care and this is explicit in *The Code* (NMC 2008).

The NMC expects all nurses and midwives to be non-judgemental when providing care, treat people kindly and considerately, as individuals, respect their dignity and not discriminate (NMC 2008). Nurses must act as an advocate for their patients, which may require helping patients in their care to access relevant health and social care, information and support.

Policies, procedures and guidelines

In addition to NMC guidance, nurses have access to national guidelines and local policies, procedures and practice guidelines (see Ch. 5). Nurses must consider how the law affects professional guidelines, practice and patient/client outcomes.

Documentation and record-keeping

Proper documentation is a fundamental aspect of recording what nurses do and how they decide on a particular course of action. Nursing records can be used as evidence in professional conduct hearings and courts, therefore documentation must meet both the NMC standards and policies (Box 6.5). If nothing is documented, then nothing was done, or it was not noted or acted upon – this could have detrimental effects and it could jeopardize 'fitness for practice'. Full and accurate records can protect nurses if allegations of poor or negligent care are made.

 Reflective practice   Box 6.5

Documentation and record-keeping

Proper documentation is a fundamental aspect of recording what nurses do and how they decide on a particular action.

Case history

A nurse was required to answer allegations of inappropriate documentation; failure to create and/or maintain the appropriate care documentation for a patient along with other numerous counts of neglect and unacceptable practice to the NMC Conduct and Competence committee.

Student activities

- Discuss with your mentor a situation during a clinical placement where documentation was not completed or was inadequate.

Resource

NMC – www.nmc-uk.org/

The NMC *Guidelines for records and record keeping* offers guidance for both paper and electronic records – stating 'good record keeping is an integral part of nursing and midwifery practice, and is essential to the provision of safe and effective care' (NMC 2009b, p 1). All nurses should consider its contents along with relevant legislation; DPA and FoIA and also the Access to Health Records Act, 1990, which ensures that records are accurate and used appropriately by those to whom they relate and others, such as nurses and the interprofessional team.

The interpretation of what is written may be quite different from its intended meaning; thus viewed as uncaring or judgemental, or seen as unprofessional. Sparse detail and abbreviations can make the meaning unclear and open to misinterpretation if used in a court of law. Information needs to be accurate, measurable, quantifiable and qualitative. For example, '++' on a chart portrays none of these. Documentation is a means of recording data about a patient/client, which is shared with other healthcare professionals. If words lack clarity or meaning, this can be dangerous, fails to achieve what it is intended to do and could lead to patient harm.

Reporting incidents/accidents

Following any clinical incident – whether it is a drug error, verbal abuse or violence, or accident or injury to a patient/client, staff, visitor or member of the public – it is essential that this be reported and documented (Box 6.6). Importantly, 'near misses' should also be reported and documented (see Ch. 13).

 Reflective practice Box 6.6

Reporting incidents/accidents

Reflect on an incident or accident that occurred while on placement. Who completed the incident form, when and what information was recorded?

Student activities

- Access the incident form used in your clinical area.
- Consider what information is recorded on the form and the questions asked.
- Discuss with your mentor what other documentation is required following a clinical incident – where else are details of the incident recorded?

A statement is a formal account of an incident or sequence of events that must be recorded by those who witness or are involved in a clinical incident or event. All NHS organizations have a protocol and documentation for the reporting of clinical incidents (see Ch. 13), most of which are electronic with limited space to record the event, therefore facts should be accurate and concise. In the case of litigation, records of this nature are used when presenting the facts in court and referred to in an investigation. As this process could take months, it is crucial that accurate documentation is completed at the time of an incident.

Some incidents, e.g. an injury lasting more than three consecutive days or a work-related disease, must be reported to the Health and Safety Executive under Reporting of Incidents, Diseases and Dangerous Occurrences Regulations (RIDDOR) (see Ch. 13).

Duty of care and negligence

In law, we are not generally required to owe a duty to be careful to *just* anyone (Griffith & Tengnah 2010), however in certain situations, the nature of the relationship gives rise to a duty of care (*Kent v Griffiths and Others [2000]3 CLL Rep 98)*. Nurses have a duty of care to patients/clients and visitors – this is the legal obligation to take reasonable care, to be careful and not to be careless to patients (*Bolitho v City and Hackney HA [1998] AC 232)*. Duty of care extends to off-duty times; the

NMC (2008) indicates that nurses have a professional duty to provide care in an emergency, in or outside the work setting. However, the care provided would be judged against what is reasonably expected from someone with your knowledge, skills and abilities when placed in those particular circumstances (*Bolam v Friern [1957] 1 WLR 582)*. This is a general rule, as applied in the courts, however, what is logical and a reasonable standard (*Bolitho v City and Hackney HA [1998] AC 232)* is determined by the courts. The standard set by the NMC is, however, higher (where protection of the public is their highest concern) than those of the courts.

Once nurses volunteer to help in an emergency, a duty of care is established. If nurses then act in-keeping with professional standards and have not fallen below that standard in law, there will be no liability in negligence (Griffith & Tengnah 2010).

Negligence

Negligence is an act with *any* element of carelessness or lack of regard resulting in injury, harm or loss. It is any act or omission that falls short of a standard to be expected from 'the reasonable man' (*Bolam v Friern HMC [1957] 1 WLR 582)*. Negligence can result in a civil claim for compensation or in a criminal prosecution – duty of care is an essential element in negligence claims (Box 6.7). Failure to communicate effectively or within a team may be grounds for negligence (*Wilsher v Essex HA [1998] AC 1074 (HL))*.

 Critical thinking Box 6.7

Negligence

Renata has been returned to a surgical ward following abdominal surgery. During the night, Renata becomes disorientated with her surroundings. She attempts to get out of bed in search of the lavatory. There is a crash and a nurse nearby rushes to the bedside to find her on the floor.

Student activities

- Discuss with another student whether the nurse is liable for negligence.
- Does the nurse have a duty of care to Renata? Has there been a breach in her duty of care? Then consider if this breach of care led to reasonable foreseeable harm (*Wilsher v Essex HA [1998] AC 1074 (HL))* and to what degree of harm did the patient suffer?

Note: It would have to be shown that the nurse failed in the approved and acceptable standard of practice that resulted in the harm suffered by the patient (Dimond 2011).

There are three civil wrongs or torts, which must be proven for a successful claim of negligence. These are:

- A duty of care is owed
- The duty of care is breached
- The breach must have caused damage.

Over 1 million patient safety incidents were reported in 2009/2010 (National Patient Safety Agency, NPSA 2010).

'In 2009/2010, 6652 claims of clinical negligence and 4074 claims of non-clinical negligence against NHS bodies were received by the Authority, up from 6088 claims of clinical negligence and 3743 claims of non-clinical negligence in 2008/09' (NHS Litigation Agency, NHSLA 2010a). Interestingly, few cases (<2%) handled by the NHSLA reach court; most are settled out of court or discontinued by the claimant (NHSLA 2010b).

If a nurse has been negligent, generally it is the employer, i.e. the NHS Trust, that would be sued. However, a claim may also be brought against the nurse. Self-employed practitioners require personal indemnity insurance, as they are personally liable for their actions and omissions (see p. 132).

It is therefore essential that nurses recognize their accountability; being accountable for acts, omissions and outcomes means that nurses must consider the consequences of everything they do in relation to patient/client care.

Where an official complaint by the patient or family results from a clinical incident, the employer would initiate a full and thorough investigation. A negligence claim is a lengthy process, and all witnesses and anyone else involved are questioned and investigated. Statements given represent oral testimony of the events that occurred and legal advice would be sought. All four arenas of accountability may be considered and in the event of a patient's death, criminal courts would be involved.

Accountability to employer

Where negligence has occurred and harm caused because the nurse failed to follow reasonable instruction, guidelines or protocols, the employer has the right to take disciplinary action against the employee.

For example, *a staff nurse fails to assess the patency of a peripheral access device prior to injecting intravenous medication. The patient reports pain and burning at the site. The staff nurse says that this sometimes happens and not to worry. However, on further assessment the site appears blistered and discoloured. The incident is later reported by a senior nurse claiming the patient suffered extravasation. Following an investigation, it was found that the staff nurse had not followed local guidelines for the administration of intravenous antibiotics.*

This incident could lead to litigation (Dougherty 2010). In this scenario, an official complaint from the patient's family could amount to professional misconduct and suspension from practice. The employer would insist the staff nurse undertake further training and work under direct supervision until deemed competent. The employer has a duty to report this to the NMC. The patient and their family would receive an apology, however this may not prevent them from pursuing legal action for negligence.

Professional accountability to the NMC

Nurses and midwives accused of misconduct, such as an action/ omission that is found to be negligent, or are convicted of certain criminal offences, will be reported to the NMC. The NMC has a responsibility to review the information surrounding the allegation and inform the individual. An Investigating Committee decides whether there is a case to answer and also decides if interim suspension or interim conditions of practice are justified. If the Investigating Committee decides there is no case to answer, the case is closed. Where there is a case to answer it will be referred to the Conduct and Competence Committee (CCC) or to the Health Committee if the nurse is considered unfit to practise by virtue of their physical or mental health.

The standard of proof required by the CCC is the civil standard, however if the CCC finds the facts proven, they may, depending on the degree of unfitness to practice and risk to the public, decide to:

- Take no further action
- Remove or suspend the nurse from the register
- Impose conditions of practice or a caution.

Misconduct cases are published by the NMC and hearings are open to the public.

Civil accountability

Nurses may encounter the civil courts in claims of negligence or trespass against a person – any interference with the person's bodily integrity and liberty, touching a person without consent, including assault and battery. Assault is an attempt or offer of unlawful contact wherein the person is put in fear of violence or unlawful force. Battery is defined as unlawful contact or touching.

The scenario (intravenous injection) above demonstrates how an action (claim) for negligence and compensation for the harm can involve the civil courts. What has been emphasized is the elements of tort that must be satisfied, based on reasonableness, foreseeability and a balance of probability. Judges use the 'Bolam test' when determining whether a nurse has been negligent. This test is not only a rule of substantive law to determine what amounts to adequate care, but also to determine standards of care. In determining the 'legal standard', advice would be sought by lawyers acting for the nurse/NHS Trust, etc. and the claimant. If the case goes to court, an 'expert opinion' is obtained. The judge would draw conclusions based on this standard of professional practice. It is important to note that the courts are more testing of expert evidence than in 1957 and the case of Bolam, where the legal principles stem from. The judge's comments in this case later became known as the 'Bolam test', which applies equally to nurses and other health professionals.

Criminal accountability

Criminal law is concerned with intent, i.e. the person intended to commit the crime, or was reckless or negligent about the consequences of their actions. Nurses are answerable to a criminal court when there is an allegation that a crime has been committed, e.g. a grossly negligent act (injecting intravenously an oral medication) by a nurse results in a patient's death. In such a case, the nurse could be charged with manslaughter and if convicted, face imprisonment. In this situation the nurse is answerable in all four arenas of accountability, i.e. dismissal, action by the NMC, a civil claim and criminal charge.

Confidentiality

Confidential information is limited to those who use it and access it, and their use must be legitimate. Nurses are responsible for protecting the confidentiality and security of the patient's/client's personal and health information (see Ch. 7). However, nurses may be required to provide information, e.g. if required by law, order of the court or if it is in the public interest.

All written and electronic information about patients/clients must be stored securely and access limited, e.g. by password, to the care team. Confidentiality applies to written and electronic records and verbal information (Box 6.8).

 Reflective practice   Box 6.8

Idle chatter

Two nurses are discussing a patient/client in the canteen. At surrounding tables there are other members of staff, visitors, patients and outside contractors.

The nurses' conversation, which is loud enough for others to hear, centres on a patient's history of mental health problems.

Student activities

* What might be the consequences of other people overhearing the conversation?
* Reflect on how you would feel if you were a relative or patient/client overhearing the conversation.

Patient/client records contain a great deal of information including: name and hospital identification, date of birth, address, marital status, next of kin, etc. In addition, records contain details of the person's health, lifestyle, current and past medical conditions and other confidential information. Therefore, nurses should always 'seek patients' and clients' wishes regarding the sharing of information with their family and others' (NMC 2008, p 3). When it is not possible to obtain permission, such as with children, some people with mental health problems or learning disabilities, the nurse must seek advice from colleagues.

Breaches in confidentiality are potentially very harmful to patients/clients and families. Unauthorized or inadvertent disclosure can lead to disciplinary action by the employer or action by the regulatory body for professional misconduct (see p. 134).

Consent

Consent has a legal and clinical purpose (Griffith & Tengnah 2010). It is a state of mind in which a person agrees to the touching of their body as part of an examination/treatment (*Sidaway v Bethlem RHG [1985] 1 ALL E.R 643*)..It is the *absolute right* of an adult, competent patient to give or withhold consent and in doing this, prevent physical contact becoming a civil or criminal actionable wrong; namely trespass against the person (see p. 134).

Very often, a patient/client may give 'implied' consent, e.g. by rolling up their sleeve for blood pressure recording. However, patients still require information and an explanation, such as the reason for carrying out the task. The implications of the procedure should be made clear to the patient/client. In some instances, e.g. prior to an injection, verbal consent is appropriate and in other instances, written consent will be necessary, e.g. prior to an examination, invasive procedure or surgery. There are three criteria to satisfy validity of consent:

* Capacity
* Voluntarily
* Informed.

A person must be able to understand the information to make a decision; they must be able to weigh up the information given; and consider the consequence of having the procedure or not.

However, sometimes further information or explanation may be needed and it must be acknowledged that a person may be competent to make some decisions, even if they are not competent to make others. It is also important to remember that obtaining consent is a 'continuing process' and not a one-off event (DH 2001) and it may be withdrawn at any time.

The NMC clearly states your professional responsibility with regard to consent in *The Code* – 'Ensure you gain consent …' (NMC 2008, p 3).

In order that consent is legally binding and compelling (or valid), the patient/client has to be given the information they require to make a *conscientious decision*, whereby they may accept or refuse treatment. Thus, patients/clients must not be forced, coerced or tricked into making the decision, nor should other professionals or institutional pressures or family or friends influence them.

What is sufficient information? The patient/client must always be informed of the risks involved in the proposed procedure (*Sidaway v Bethlem RHG [1985] 1 ALL E.R 643*), so that they have an opportunity to avoid or reduce these risks. Thus, the patient/client needs to understand in broad terms, in a language they can understand, the nature and purpose of the procedure. The person who will be carrying out the procedure usually obtains consent but registered nurses who have had special training may obtain consent in certain circumstances.

In all cases, patients/clients should be provided with sufficient information in order to make a decision (*Chester v Afshar [2004] EWCA 724*) and this should include the benefits and the risks, and alternative treatments or therapies. If the patient/client is not offered as much information as they need to make a decision, and in a form they can understand, then their consent may not be valid (DH 2001).

The Mental Capacity Act (MCA) 2005 identifies those elements of the consensual process for adults with capacity, and sets clear principles for patients who lack capacity. It is important for nurses to understand that *capacity* is based upon a test of understanding and it is not a professional or status test – one cannot assume lack of capacity simply because of a person's age, physical appearance, condition or behaviour (Griffith & Tengnah 2010). Importantly, the MCA requires healthcare professionals to assume those who are 16 years of age or older have the capacity to make decisions, even if considered unwise. The need to assess capacity would arise where circumstances or behaviour places doubt in one's mind. The MCA identifies practicable steps to help make a decision: using simple language or their own language, using pictures or objects rather than words if appropriate, seeking advice from someone who knows the patient well about the best methods of communication, choosing an appropriate time and location, and waiting until a person's capacity improves before requiring a decision.

Consent in children

Children should always be consulted (subject to age and understanding) and kept informed about what is planned. The Children Act (2004) provides guidance.

There are three key points in relation to age of children that need to be emphasized:

* At 16, a young person can be treated as an adult and can be presumed to have capacity to decide
* Under the age of 16, children *may have* capacity to decide, depending on their ability to understand what is involved
* Where a competent child refuses treatment, a person with parental responsibility or the court may authorize investigation or treatment which is in the child's best interests.

Maturity is a key factor and older children can have the maturity and capacity to make important decisions about their own medical treatment, whereas others may not have reached that level of maturity at the same age. It is imperative that professionals assess maturity and the individual's capacity to understand issues surrounding the proposed treatment and risks.

An important ruling regarding the competence of a child to consent to treatment is the 'Gillick competence' (*Gillick v West Norfolk and Wisbech Area Health Authority [1986] AC 112 (HL)*) (Box 6.9).

In caring for children, the main priority for the nurse is to obtain valid consent from the appropriate person, i.e. the child or the person with parental responsibility. Usually, this is the mother or father of very young children. However, parental consent does not cover whatever treatment the parents believe to be in their child's best interests and any treatment is ultimately dependent upon the healthcare professional's assessment of what is appropriate for the child. While parents do have the power to give consent – this is not an absolute power (Dimond 2011).

The law makes a distinction between a child's right to consent to treatment and to refuse treatment. Where the parents refuse to give consent to treatment, decisions by healthcare professionals that are made in the child's 'best interests' often override. No child should die because the parents have unreasonably refused their consent to a necessary treatment (Dimond 2011). In this instance, healthcare professionals should hesitate before giving treatment and consider the potential outcomes of giving the treatment or of withholding treatment. Often, it is the urgency of the child's condition that dictates justification for treatment without parental consent. In cases of an emergency, essential action is taken in the best interests of the child. The Children Act 1989

? Critical thinking   Box 6.9

Gillick competence: Fraser guidelines

'... it is considered good practice for doctors and other health professionals to follow the criteria outlined by Lord Fraser in 1985, in the House of Lords' ruling in the case of *Victoria Gillick v West Norfolk and Wisbech Health Authority and Department of Health and Social Security*. These are commonly known as the Fraser Guidelines:

* 'the young person understands the health professional's advice;
* the health professional cannot persuade the young person to inform his or her parents or allow the doctor to inform the parents that he or she is seeking contraceptive advice;
* the young person is very likely to begin or continue having intercourse with or without contraceptive treatment;
* unless he or she receives contraceptive advice or treatment, the young person's physical or mental health or both are likely to suffer;
* the young person's best interests require the health professional to give contraceptive advice, treatment or both without parental consent ...' (DH 2004, p 4)

Student activity

* Discuss with your mentor how a school nurse might assess a young person's competence before supplying/prescribing emergency contraception.

---

emphasizes the principle where children can give consent if it is not possible to contact the parent, and the child is mature and capable of understanding the situation. This is where the Gillick case would be considered, however there are exceptional circumstances set out from this case.

The refusal may be from both the parent and child, e.g. where the child and family are refusing a blood transfusion according to the teaching of their religion (Jehovah's Witness). In such a situation, the outcomes and consequence of refusal must be made clear to both the child and parents. The dilemma for health professionals is if that refusal could lead to the death of that child. Authorization for treatment would be dependent upon the court's decision.

Consent – people with learning disability or fluctuating mental capacity

There are situations where capacity may be in doubt – a patient/client may not understand what they have been told or they may appear confused. The nurse may need to assess if the patient/client is capable of making a particular decision. This can be especially difficult in some patients/clients who have a learning disability or suffer from fluctuating mental capacity (Box 6.10). There is legislation to guide decision-making on behalf of people lacking in capacity and the Mental Capacity Act (MCA) 2005 sets out principles for testing capacity and decision-making, thereby providing a statutory framework for decision-making on behalf of adults, thus protecting vulnerable adults and their carers, and professionals. In Scotland, the Adults with Incapacity (Scotland) Act 2000 fulfils a similar function.

Reflective practice — Box 6.10

The 'Bournewood' case

A man, aged 40 years, was unable to speak and had limited understanding. He had a history of self-harming behaviour and frequent outbursts of agitation. For over 30 years, the man was cared for in an NHS hospital.

He was discharged on a trial basis but after an incident where he became agitated with self-harming behaviour he was detained in hospital under the MHA. Because the man was compliant and did not resist admission, he was admitted as an informal patient in his own best interests under the common law principle of necessity.

Legal action was commenced to secure his discharge from hospital. This was unsuccessful in the High Court but later the Court of Appeal held that the man had been unlawfully detained, and that because of the MHA 1983 the common law principle of necessity could not be used to detain someone for treatment for a mental health disorder. The man was formally detained under the MHA 1983 and later discharged.

The House of Lords overturned the Court of Appeal's judgement and the case was taken to the European Court of Human Rights. This Court found that there had been a violation of Articles 5(1) Right to Liberty and 5(4) Right to Security.

Student activity

- Discuss with your mentor how this judgement affects your area of practice.

Resource

Department of Health, 2006. Protecting the vulnerable: the 'Bournewood' consultation. Online. Available: www.dh.gov.uk/prod_consum_dh/groups/dh_digitalassets/@dh/@en/documents/digitalasset/dh_4137959.pdf September 2012.

The Act applies to adults who lose mental capacity, e.g. due to dementia, and to people who lack mental capacity due to conditions present at birth, e.g. some forms of learning disability, and governs decisions about welfare, health, financial matters and participation in research. It also includes a new scheme for LPA, which can include health-related decisions, making it clear who can take decisions in which situations and how they should go about this.

Adult refusal to treatment

A competent adult patient has an absolute right to refuse or withdraw from treatment or change their mind about treatment. Their decision must be respected, even if it results in death, e.g. the case of *Ms B v An NHS Trust [2002] 2 All ER 449*, in which the judgement was that Ms B had the necessary mental capacity to refuse treatment, which in this case meant switching off the ventilator and allowing her to die (Box 6.11).

Advance decisions and advance statements

People can maintain control or choice in decisions about their health or life or circumstance (when their mental capacity is altered) through the use of advance decisions (referred to as an *advance decision to refuse treatment* in the MCA). Advance

---

 Reflective practice — Box 6.11

Refusal of medical treatment/Right to die

The debate continues: who has the right to die and at what point should one be able to refuse treatment?

In the case of *Ms B v An NHS Trust* it was clear to all concerned that she would die once treatment ceased. The implications for other refusals of treatment are not always so clear-cut.

Student activities

- Discuss the case of Ms B with your mentor.
- Access the resource and reflect on the feelings of the people involved.

Resource

BBC 29 June, 2009. Radio play questions right to die. Online. Available: http://news.bbc.co.uk/1/hi/northern_ireland/8125507.stm September 2012.

---

decisions (AD) to refuse treatment can be made, where the wishes of the patient must be respected and treatment withheld. For example, *Re: AK (Adult Patient) (Medical Treatment: Consent) [2001] 2 FLR 35*, where a man with motor neurone disease had made a long-established AD refusing treatment that was explicit as to when and under what circumstances artificial hydration and nutrition would be withheld. It was confirmed in the courts that these decisions were expressed by the patient when he had capacity and it was lawful to therefore withhold the treatment. There are clear guidelines for AD in the MCA. Although an AD can be verbal, the guidance is that they are written; these are legally binding providing they are prepared in advance by a competent adult before they lose the mental capacity to make decisions (see Box 6.12).

 Critical thinking — Box 6.12

Advance decisions and advance statements

There is sometimes confusion about what advance decisions and advance statements cover and the criteria that must be met for them to be valid.

Student activities

Visit the Age UK website and find answers to the following questions:

- What are the differences between advance decisions and advance statements?
- Can a person refuse basic nursing care in either?
- Who should know that the advance decision exists?

Resource

Age UK Advance decisions, advance statements, and living wills. Fact Sheet. Online. Available: www.ageuk.org.uk/documents/en-gb/factsheets/fs72_advance_decisions_advance_statements_and_living_wills_fcs.pdf?dtrk=true September 2012.

End-of-life issues, information sources	Box 6.13

Specific sources

1. Withholding or withdrawing treatment:
   - *Airedale NHS Trust v Bland [1993] AC 789* – the landmark case concerning Anthony Bland who was left in a permanent vegetative state (PVS) following the Hillsborough disaster. Artificial feeding was not in the best interests of the patient and could be withdrawn.

2. Maintaining artificial nutrition and hydration (ANH)
   - Court of Protection judgement – *W v M and S and A NHS Primary Care Trust* 28 September 2011. Concerning the withdrawal of artificial nutrition and hydration (ANH) for 'M' who is in a minimally conscious state (MCS). His Hon. Mr Justice Baker ruled that withdrawing ANH would not be in the best interests of 'M'. Online. Available: www.judiciary.gov.uk

3. Assisted dying and euthanasia:
   - Assisted Dying for the Terminally Ill Bill (HL), reintroduced into parliament in October 2005
   - RCN moves to a neutral position on assisted suicide. July 2009. Online. Available: www.rcn.org.uk/newsevents/news/article/uk/royal_college_of_nursing_moves_to_neutral_position_on_assisted_suicide
   - Judgements – *The Queen on the Application of Mrs Dianne Pretty (Appellant) v Director of Public Prosecutions (Respondent) and Secretary of State for the Home Department (Interested Party)* 29 November 2001. Online. Available: www.publications.parliament.uk/pa/ld200102/ldjudgmt/jd011129/pretty-1.htm

4. Organ donation and transplant:
   - Human Tissue Act. Online. Available: www.legislation.gov.uk/ukpga/2004/30/contents

5. Do not attempt resuscitation orders
   (see above, *W v M and S and A NHS Primary Care Trust*)
   - Decisions relating to cardiopulmonary resuscitation: A joint statement from the British Medical Association, the Resuscitation Council (UK) and the Royal College of Nursing. November 2007.

General sources

Johnstone, M.J., 2009. Bioethics. A nursing perspective, fifth ed. Churchill Livingstone, Edinburgh.

Mason, J.K., Laurie, G.T. (Eds.), 2011. Mason & McCall Smith's law and medical ethics, eighth ed. Oxford University Press, Oxford.

Royal College of Physicians (RCP)/British Society of Gastroenterology, 2010. Oral feeding difficulties and dilemmas. Online. Available: http://bookshop.rcplondon.ac.uk/contents/pub295-ca2ff0c8-85f7-48ee-b857-8fed6ccb2ad7.pdf.

UK Clinical Ethics Network Access. Online. Available: www.ethics-network.org.uk.

All websites accessed September 2012.

End-of-life issues

Prior to the Suicide Act 1961, English law did not recognize a right to suicide and for a person to take their own life was a criminal offence (McHale & Fox 2007). However, it remains a criminal offence to assist in ending a life. The prohibition on assisted suicide was first challenged in the case of *Pretty v DPP [2001] UKHL 61; Pretty v UK [2002] 2 FLR 45ECHR*, a woman with motor neuron disease, who failed in her attempt to see section 2 of the Suicide Act incompatible with her right to a dignified death (and a breach of human rights Article 2, 3, 8 and 14) and failed at the ECHR. Pretty wanted a pardon for her husband if he assisted her to take her own life; the HL held that Article 3 gave rise to a right to life, not to die, and that her sanctity of life could not allow the state to sanction an intentional intervention to end life (Griffith & Tengnah 2010).

The law has not been supportive to proposals to change the law on euthanasia, however several attempts have been made to pass an Assisted Suicide law but have failed.

Following the loss of Debbie Purdy's attempt to have the law clarified, the law is being revisited and at the time of writing, the Bill being proposed to parliament is to allow terminally ill people to end their lives with the help of loved ones in their home country lawfully. Euthanasia is currently lawful in the Netherlands and Switzerland, however it is unlawful for persons to assist in their passage abroad. The Crown Prosecution Service recently issued new guidelines regarding the prosecution of family members who assist, but the debate continues.

Healthcare professionals are presented with many dilemmas for end-of-life issues: withholding/withdrawing treatment; 'do not attempt resuscitation' (DNAR)/'do not resuscitate' (DNR) orders. The legal, ethical and professional issues are difficult to resolve and currently require consultation and clear communication that considers the best interests of the patient, while respecting their autonomy and human rights. Detailed discussion of this controversial topic is beyond the scope of this chapter, however it is important that nurses are aware of these issues (see Chs 7, 12 and 17).

While it is likely that nursing students will encounter some of these situations, they will not be directly involved in the decision-making but should take the opportunity to observe and discuss the issues with their mentor (Box 6.13).

SUMMARY

- The law is constantly evolving, therefore practitioners must be aware of new developments.
- Duty of care and accountability for practice are central responsibilities for all nurses.
- Nurses are accountable to their employer, the NMC and the civil and criminal courts.
- Issues that include consent to treatment, refusal or withdrawal of treatment and mental capacity affect all nurses.

KEY WORDS AND PHRASES FOR LITERATURE SEARCHING

Civil law

Confidentiality

Consent

Criminal law

Duty of care

Legislation

Liability

Negligence

Useful websites

Age UK http://ageuk.org.uk

Court of Protection www.justice.gov.uk/guidance/courts-and-tribunals/courts/court-of-protection/

Health and Safety Executive www.hse.gov.uk

Law Commission www.justice.gov.uk/lawcommission/publications.htm

Office of Public Sector Information *(source for UK legislation)* www.opsi.gov.uk

The children's legal centre www.childrenslegalcentre.com

All websites accessed September 2012.

References

Boylan-Kemp, J., 2011. The English legal system: the fundamentals, second ed. Sweet & Maxwell, London.

Department of Health, 2001. 12 Key points on consent: the law in England. Online. Available: www.dh.gov.uk/en/Publicationsandstatistics/Publications/PublicationsPolicyAndGuidance/DH_4006131 September 2012.

Department of Health, 2004. Best practice guidance for doctors and other health professionals on the provision of advice and treatment to young people under 16 on contraception, sexual and reproductive health. Online. Available: www.dh.gov.uk/en/Publicationsandstatistics/Publications/PublicationsPolicyAndGuidance/DH_4086960 September 2012.

Department of Health, 2010. Response to the Independent Review of the requirement to have insurance or indemnity as a condition of registration as a healthcare professional. Online. Available: www.dh.gov.uk/prod_consum_dh/groups/dh_digitalassets/@dh/@en/@ps/documents/digitalasset/dh_122610.pdf September 2012.

Department of Health, 2011. The Mental Capacity Act Deprivation of Liberty Safeguards. Online. Available: www.dh.gov.uk/en/SocialCare/Deliveringsocialcare/MentalCapacity/MentalCapacityActDeprivationofLibertySafeguards/index.htm September 2012.

Dimond, B., 2011. Legal aspects of nursing, sixth ed. Pearson, Harlow.

Dougherty, L., 2010. Extravasation: prevention, recognition and management. Nursing Standard 24 (52), 48–55.

Griffith, R., Tengnah, C., 2010. Law and professional issues in nursing, second ed. Learning Matters, Exeter.

McHale, J., Fox, M., 2007. Healthcare law, second ed. Sweet & Maxwell, London.

NHS Litigation Agency, 2010a. Key facts about our work. Online. Available: www.nhsla.com/ September 2012.

NHS Litigation Agency, 2010b. Claims. Online. Available: www.nhsla.com/ Claims September 2012.

NHS National Patient Safety Agency, 2010. NPSA Annual Report & Accounts 2009/10. Online. Available: www.npsa.nhs.uk/corporate/corporate-publications September 2012.

Nursing and Midwifery Council, 2008. The Code Standards of conduct, performance and ethics for nurses and midwives. Online. Available: http://www.nmc-uk.org/Publications/Standards/The-code/Introduction/ September 2012.

Nursing and Midwifery Council, 2009a. Confidentiality. Online. Available: www.nmc-uk.org/Nurses-and-midwives/Advice-by-topic/A/Advice/Confidentiality September 2012.

Nursing and Midwifery Council, 2009b. Guidelines for records and record keeping. NMC, London. Online. Available: www.nmc-uk.org/Documents/Guidance/nmcGuidanceRecordKeepingGuidanceforNursesandMidwives.pdf September 2012.

Nursing and Midwifery Council, 2010. Guidance on professional conduct: For nursing and midwifery students. Online. Available: www.nmc-uk.org/Documents/Guidance/NMC-Guidance-on-professional-conduct-for-nursing-and-midwifery-students.pdf September 2012.

Stychin, C.F., Mulcahy, L., 2010. Legal methods and systems, fourth ed. Sweet & Maxwell, London.

Further reading

Carvalho, S., Reeves, M., Orford, J., 2011. Fundamental aspects of legal, ethical and professional issues, second ed. Quay Books, London.

Department of Health, 2010. Confidentiality: NHS code of practice. Supplementary Guidance: Public Interest Disclosures. Online. Available: www.dh.gov.uk/prod_consum_dh/groups/dh_digitalassets/@dh/@en/@ps/documents/digitalasset/dh_122031.pdf September 2012.

Hodgson, J., 2010. The UK's Supreme Court: how it works and why it exists. British Journal of Nursing 19 (3), 194–195.

Information Commissioner's Office, 2005. Data Protection Act Factsheet. Online. Available: www.ico.gov.uk/for_organisations/data_protection.aspx September 2012.

McInroy, A., 2005. Blood transfusions and Jehovah's Witnesses: the legal and ethical issues. British Journal of Nursing 14 (5), 270–274.

McHale, J.V., 2009. Conscientious objection and the nurse: a right or a privilege? British Journal of Nursing 18 (20), 1262–1263.

Walters, T.P., 2009. The Mental Capacity Act – a balance between protection and liberty. British Journal of Nursing 18 (9), 555–558.

The *NMC Code of conduct* and applied ethical principles

7

Dorothy Horsburgh

LEARNING OUTCOMES

This chapter will help you:

- Outline the role of the Nursing and Midwifery Council (NMC) in protecting the public within the UK
- Demonstrate a knowledge of the NMC's (2008a) *Code: standards of conduct, performance and ethics for nurses and midwives*
- Understand the NMC's (2010a) *Guidance on professional conduct: For nursing and midwifery students*
- Discuss implications of the NMC's (2010b) *Essential skills clusters for your practice as a nursing student*
- Demonstrate an awareness of, and apply, ethical principles and theories to nursing practice
- Identify, and reflect upon, ethical issues in everyday nursing practice (NMC 2010b).

Introduction

Registered nurses (RNs) practise in a variety of care settings and provide care for individuals with a wide range of needs. Nursing students receive theory- and practice-based education, by the end of which they must have achieved specified competencies (Nursing and Midwifery Council, NMC 2010b) in order to register with the Nursing and Midwifery Council as a nurse in one of the following fields of practice: Adult, Mental Health, Child Health, Learning Disability.

People who require nursing care are vulnerable by virtue of the problems for which they require assistance. This chapter will describe and discuss ways in which protection is provided for patients and clients, and some of the challenges that student nurses and registered practitioners may encounter in everyday practice. This chapter should be read in conjunction with Chapter 6, which deals specifically with legal issues and nursing. The focus of this chapter is the requirements that the statutory regulatory body (NMC) has of RNs and nursing students, and it addresses some ethical and moral issues integral to nursing practice.

The role of the Nursing and Midwifery Council (NMC)

Protection of the public

Since 1919, when the Nurses' Registration Act was passed, public protection has been provided by a statutory body, originally the General Nursing Council (GNC). Changes in policy and in the statutory regulatory body's remit over time resulted in replacement of the General Nursing Council by the United Kingdom Central Council (UKCC) and, later, by the Nursing and Midwifery Council.

Quality assurance of educational programmes

The NMC has a UK-wide remit for quality assurance of educational programmes that lead to registration as a nurse or midwife and all other recordable NMC qualifications, e.g. specialist practitioner. While there are national differences in UK health and education policy and provision, the NMC uses a management and development consultancy to approve and assure the quality of all its programmes.

Registration of students as qualified practitioners

Protection of the public is a constant feature of the NMC and this includes regulating theory- and practice-based components of educational programmes and the criteria for students' registration as qualified practitioners (NMC 2010b). There are five essential skills clusters for which students' competency is assessed at the end of years 1, 2 and 3:

- Care, compassion and communication
- Organizational aspects of care
- Infection prevention and control
- Nutrition and fluid management
- Medicines management.

Students are required, at intervals during and on successful completion of their pre-registration programme, to provide a self-declaration of good health and good character (NMC 2010c). This declaration must be supported by the RN accountable for students' educational programmes at the approved educational institution. This person must also verify students' attainment of the theoretical and practical competencies required for registration (NMC 2010b).

Register of practitioners

The NMC maintains a register of practitioners and supervision of their subsequent practice. Periodic re-registration of practitioners requires evidence of the individual's continuing fitness to practise, including ongoing professional development. The NMC's requirements in relation to post-registration education and practice (PREP) are set out in *The PREP Handbook* (NMC 2008b).

Post-registration education and practice

PREP's purpose is to provide optimum care for patients by ensuring that registered practitioners update and develop their practice. PREP requirements are professional standards, set by the NMC and required by law for renewal of registration. There are two separate PREP standards, one of which relates to continuing professional development (CPD), which the NMC identifies as a key component of clinical governance. Clinical governance essentially means that the quality of nursing care people receive should be of an equally acceptable standard, in all care settings in the UK, rather than varying from one area to another. The second PREP standard relates to the minimum number of hours for which practitioners must have worked, by virtue of their registration, during the previous 5 years.

To fulfil PREP requirements, practitioners identify their own learning needs and activities by which these can be met. They document these activities and must produce this record if required to do so by the NMC.

Fitness to practise

Allegations made against practitioners of misconduct or unfitness to practise (e.g. due to ill health or drug misuse) are investigated by the NMC and, if these are upheld, action is taken. Depending on the nature of the offence the practitioner may be reprimanded, or their name removed from the register, thus removing their right to practise as a nurse. If unfitness to practise due to ill health is found, treatment may be necessary before the person can continue to practise. Students must provide annual confirmation of their health and good character, as defined by the NMC (2010c). Allegations of misconduct or unfitness to practise against student nurses or midwives are investigated by their university and referred to the university's Fitness to Practise Committee when appropriate.

NMC expectations of nursing students

Nursing students are not professionally accountable during their preparation for practice: the individual accountable for the consequences of their actions and omissions is the registered practitioner with whom they work. This person is usually referred to as a mentor and will have undergone preparation for this role. Expectations of nursing students are set out in *Guidance on professional conduct: For nursing and midwifery students* (NMC 2010a). An outline of *The code: standards of conduct, performance and ethics for nurses and midwives* (NMC 2008a) with which RNs must comply will place in context subsequent discussion of the NMC's (2010a) guidance to students. Implications for students in practice placements will be discussed using practical examples to highlight relevant points. *The code* (NMC 2008a) is not intended to provide practitioners with specific answers to each and every situation, but to set overall standards with which their practice must comply.

NMC documentation

The NMC publishes online documents, which cover all aspects of professional practice. These are reviewed and updated on a regular basis, following consultation with practitioners and other stakeholders.

This provides the UK public (including practitioners, employers and clients) with information about standards expected of all registered nurses and midwives. The aim is to ensure that public safety is maintained by provision of a satisfactory standard of care.

The code of professional conduct

While *The code* (NMC 2008a) applies to RNs and not students, you should obtain a copy now (if you have not already done so), as it is important that by the point of registration, you have understood and internalized the elements of *The code* and their relevance to your future practice. A copy may be obtained online or in paper format from the NMC. The NMC's (2010b) Essential Skill Cluster 1.1 requires you to be able to articulate the underpinning values of *The code* and Essential Skill Cluster 14.1 and expects you to work within the NMC *code* (2008a) and adhere to the NMC's (2010a) *Guidance on professional conduct: For nursing and midwifery students*.

The purpose of *The code* (NMC 2008a) is to:

- Inform the professions (nursing and midwifery) of the standard of professional conduct required of them in exercise of their professional accountability and practice
- Inform the public, other professions and employers of the standard of professional conduct that they can expect of a registered practitioner.

RNs are expected to:

- Make care of people their first concern, treating them as individuals and respecting their dignity
- Work with others to protect and promote the health and well-being of those in their care, their families and carers, and the wider community
- Provide a high standard of practice and care at all times
- Be open and honest, act with integrity and uphold their profession's reputation.

As professionals, nurses are personally accountable for actions and omissions in their practice, and must always be able to justify decisions. They must always act lawfully, whether in relation to their professional practice or personal life (NMC 2008a). In addition to professional accountability, RNs are legally accountable for their practice (see Ch. 6).

At government level, increasing emphasis has been placed on care provision with compassion and dignity; and national initiatives have developed policies, procedures and cultural change to enhance healthcare delivery (Scottish Government 2010; Department of Health, DH 2010; RCN 2008a; RCN 2009).

Implications of *The code* for nursing students

The *Guidance on professional conduct: For nursing and midwifery students* (NMC 2010a) emphasizes the need for students to have good health and good character in order to have fitness to practise. (While good health means that a person must be able to practise safely and effectively without supervision, it does not mean absence of any health condition for which reasonable adjustment may be required.) Good character involves a person's conduct, behaviour and attitude, while fitness to practise adds demonstration of the skills and knowledge necessary to be a safe practitioner. Cheating, plagiarism, criminal convictions, dishonesty and drug or alcohol misuse would bring into question a student's fitness to practice and the NMC (2010a) emphasizes that nurses' conduct in their personal lives is important in addition to their professional practice. The core principles for student conduct are:

- Making care of people your first concern, treating them as individuals and respecting their dignity. This includes being polite and compassionate and ensuring that you recognize and respect diversity and do not discriminate against anyone in any way. You should be able to demonstrate understanding of how individuals' culture, religion, spiritual beliefs, gender and sexuality can impact on their illness and disability. In doing so, you respect people's rights and adopt a principled approach to care.

You need to respect confidentiality, collaborate with those in your care, gain consent before providing care and maintain professional boundaries. Confidentiality extends beyond placements, e.g. if writing about a person's care for an assignment, their identity should be protected by use of a pseudonym and by omitting details of the area within which care took place.

- Working with others to protect and promote the health and well-being of those in your care, their families and carers, and the wider community.
- Providing a high standard of practice and care at all times, including awareness of the limits of your competence (NMC 2010b Essential Skill Cluster 15.1 and 18.1). You must work at all times under the supervision of an RN and request assistance when appropriate.
- Be open and honest, act with integrity and uphold the reputation of your profession.

(NMC 2010a)

One element of *The code* reminds RNs that they 'must facilitate students and others to develop their competence' (NMC 2008a, p 5). RNs have an obligation to teach and supervise students, while students have a responsibility to develop stipulated competencies prior to registration (NMC 2010b, Annexe 3). This includes ensuring that care students do not exceed their current level of understanding and competence. While students are not professionally accountable to the NMC, they are accountable to their university (whose recommendation to the NMC is a prerequisite for registration) and the law.

Patients and clients are at the centre of healthcare and their wishes must be respected at all times. Students should identify their status, if the client does not already know this, in order that the latter may indicate acceptance or refusal of care provision. (Indeed, it is a criminal offence for individuals to represent themselves falsely and knowingly as RNs.) If a patient or client refuses care from students, or asks them to leave while care is being carried out, students must comply. While the majority of patients and clients accept that students' participation in nursing care is an integral component of preparation for practice as RNs, respect for the rights of patients/clients overrides students' rights to knowledge and experience (NMC 2010a). Similarly, if a patient, client or their friends or family voice disquiet at any aspect of care, students should refer this immediately to their mentor or RN in charge of the placement at the time. Students should be familiar with the local policy for documenting concerns or complaints and work within clinical governance frameworks (NMC 2010b). Similarly, when involved in administration of medicines, the student must demonstrate understanding of the relevant legal and ethical frameworks (NMC 2010a). (See also Ch. 22.)

Confidentiality

Patients and clients provide information that is frequently of 'a sensitive nature', as defined by the Data Protection Act (HM Government 1998a). Patients and clients therefore need to be assured that information provided is not divulged, other than for the purpose for which it was supplied, i.e. their healthcare. Students must avoid talking about patients/clients when their conversation may be overheard and, if discussing patient/client care in, e.g. a reflective session in their university, then they need to take measures to protect confidentiality. This ensures that students apply principles of confidentiality and data protection (NMC 2010b).

Access to patient and client records

Access to patient/client records should relate only to the need to implement effective care; local policies and practices on handling and storage of records must be adhered to (Ch. 6). Documentation by students of care that they have provided should be carried out under supervision of an RN who should countersign the student's signature. The NMC has advice within *The code* (NMC 2008a) specific to confidentiality and guidelines for records and record-keeping (NMC 2009a), with which students should familiarize themselves. Failure to maintain accurate records of care has contributed to RNs' removal from the Register.

Confidentiality in practice

Maintaining confidentiality of information provided by patients/clients is not always clear-cut, as the following situation illustrates.

The situation outlined in Box 7.1 illustrates a number of points, one of which is the importance of ensuring that patients and clients are made aware of a student's status. Students are frequently involved in direct, and often intimate, care provision and may be viewed by patients/clients as approachable and as someone in whom they may confide information that they might be more hesitant to reveal to qualified staff. As can be seen in the situation described in Box 7.1, this degree of intimacy may place students in a difficult position. On the one hand, there is a requirement to maintain confidentiality and accede to individual wishes (NMC 2010a); on the other hand, there is the need to ensure that qualified staff have access to all information relevant to a patient's/client's care.

 Ethical issues   Box 7.1

Maintaining confidentiality?

You are undertaking a placement in a surgical ward. It is suspected by the qualified staff that Katie, a 37-year-old patient who has been admitted to the ward via the Accident and Emergency Unit, has sustained injuries that are non-accidental and the nature of which preclude self-infliction. While you are assisting Katie to carry out personal hygiene, she tells you that her partner was the perpetrator. She emphasizes that this information should not be passed on to anyone else.

Student activities

• What should you, as a student, do in this situation?
• Write down the reasons for your answer.

It is not clear, in the scenario, whether Katie was told in advance that information might be shared among the care team. In situations in which information may need to be disclosed outwith the immediate care team, the person's consent should be obtained. If consent is withheld, disclosure is only justifiable when:

• It is required by law or court order
• It is believed by those involved in the patient's/client's care that divulging information is in the wider public interest, i.e. to prevent harm to the patient/client or a third party
• There is an issue of child protection, in which case action must be taken in accordance with national and local policies.

For students, the answer is that they should explain to Katie that the information provided cannot be kept confidential. Students are not in a position in which non-disclosure of the information is justifiable, as it is the responsibility of students to ensure that information relevant to patients'/clients' current and future care is passed to their mentor or the RN in charge of the placement at the time. When an assurance of confidentiality cannot be provided to a patient or client, they should be informed of this and of the rationale for the decision.

For the RN to whom this information is divulged, there is an obligation to discuss its implications with other members of the care team, as it may impact upon the patient's/client's current and future care requirements. It is also important to document the information in their notes (NMC 2009a). In relation to divulgence of information beyond the immediate care team responsible for the patient's/client's welfare, the position is less clear. It might be argued that information should be passed to the police, e.g. in order to investigate allegations made and provide protection for the patient/client from further harm. However, Katie is an adult and there is no indication within the scenario that she lacks the mental capacity (Ch. 6) to make her own decisions.

Qualified staff might discuss the situation and the potential consequences for Katie of reporting, or not reporting, the matter to the police, but if she refuses to make a statement, then there is little staff can do. Respecting Katie's wishes may cause disquiet among staff as to the possibility that future harm may result, but this may not be a justification for interference. Indeed, it is difficult to predict outcomes of actions and omissions and reporting of the incident could, at least in Katie's view, have the potential to create further problems.

It would probably be the case that staff would discuss with Katie the possibility that she could, at a future date, bring a charge against her partner and that documentation of her current condition and care would be available, should she wish to call upon it. Staff might also provide Katie with information about sources of support, formal and informal (e.g. family, workplace colleagues, Samaritans, Women's refuge, police), which she could draw on if she chose to do so.

Katie's situation presents a dilemma to staff, i.e. it is a problem that does not have a clear-cut solution. Whichever action, or inaction, staff consider most appropriate, is likely to cause them disquiet at the time and on subsequent reflection.

If a child is involved, there is no room for debate. If Katie had divulged that her partner was abusing her 12-year-old child, then the situation would be quite different, as is made clear by *The code* (NMC 2008a), and the law (see Ch. 6). In such circumstances, it would be explained to the woman that, as the welfare of a child was in question, the information would have to be reported to Social Services in order that they could investigate the situation.

Ethical principles

Having discussed the situation in Box 7.1 in general terms, it is useful to examine it further, to identify the principles underpinning decisions that might be made. These ethical principles are sometimes referred to as being *prima facie*. The phrase means 'at first sight', i.e. each principle should be respected 'at first sight' but, in light of the situation, another principle might need to take precedence. For example, autonomy (the right to make one's own decisions) appears, at first sight, to be one that should be respected, but there may be circumstances in which another principle would override it. This will be identified in the discussion that follows.

Autonomy and justice

Within Western societies, great importance is placed on autonomy. The word autonomy literally means to be 'self-governing', but clearly within society, there are limits upon the degree to which one may exercise autonomy. For example, it is usually accepted that the right of one individual to exercise autonomy should not interfere with the rights of other individuals to exercise their autonomy. The right of one person to hold regular noisy parties would interfere with the rights of others to have a peaceful night's sleep. The right of one person to drive recklessly interferes with the rights of other individuals to use the roads in safety. In situations such as reckless driving and breach of the peace, society usually places legal penalties upon those who infringe or threaten the rights of others. So, autonomy may be exercised, provided that harm is not caused to others in the process.

In Katie's situation, exercise of autonomy in refusing to report the injuries to the police does not directly appear to interfere with the rights of others. (Indeed, were staff to ignore the patient's wishes and report the matter to the police, a prosecution would be unlikely, in the absence of the victim's cooperation.) Were the welfare of a child involved, the patient's 'autonomy' could, and should, be overruled, as the patient is not able to make a decision that would place a child at risk of continuing abuse.

Non-maleficence and beneficence

One reason that staff wishing to intervene on the woman's behalf might give would be the desire to prevent harm to the patient (an idea known as 'non-maleficence') and to act in the patient's best interest (known as 'beneficence'). There is also the problem that consequences of actions or omissions are difficult to predict: anticipated harms or benefits may not materialize in reality. Identification of 'best interests' can also be problematic, as the attitudes, values and beliefs that individuals bring to any situation will influence the decisions that they make (Ch. 1). Actions that nursing staff consider to be in patients' best interests are not necessarily ones with which patients would agree. A respect for patients, the importance of which is emphasized by *The code* (NMC 2008a), indicates that staff should comply with patients' wishes when these are clearly expressed and when the patient has the legal capacity to make decisions (Ch. 6).

Client autonomy in healthcare is not always straightforward, as the right to autonomy is usually based on a person having insight into the consequences of their actions or omissions. (One would not consider a small child to be autonomous, e.g. in their desire to run across a busy road to reach the park. Interference would be considered not only justifiable, but mandatory.) In order to be autonomous therefore, patients need to be provided with information upon which to base their decisions and be able to understand, retain and act upon it. In Katie's situation, if the available options were discussed with her along with the possible outcomes of each, this would facilitate an autonomous decision.

In summary, the four principles that were used in the discussion above are:

- *Autonomy* (the ability to make one's own decisions): This is linked to another principle – respect for persons, which means that even in the absence of the ability to make an informed decision, the individual is at the centre of the decision-making process
- *Justice*: A person has the right to refuse to take the matter further, but equally a right to protection from the law, should they wish to avail themselves of it
- *Non-maleficence* (prevention of harm)
- *Beneficence* (creation of benefit).

While Katie's situation created a problem unlikely to be encountered on a daily basis, there are many problems that nurses can encounter on a regular, if not everyday, basis (Box 7.2). While this is not a 'life and death' issue, decisions made by staff impact on patients' quality of life.

 Reflective practice Box 7.2

Too many patients and too few staff

In a busy placement several patients need assistance to eat and drink, but few staff are on duty. Some patients therefore have to wait longer than others and their meal may be cold by the time they receive it.

Student activities

Identify a practice placement in which several patients or clients required help with an activity of living, e.g. washing, dressing, eating, bathing:

- Identify how staff decided which patient or client should be cared for first.
- Consider whether decisions were based on needs of individual patients or clients, or on the number of staff available.

The ethical and moral dimensions of nursing practice

The nature of healthcare provision is such that decisions made and the treatment and care provided, or withheld, may alter the duration and quality of the lives of the individuals who experience it. The relationship of nursing to health and well-being (Ch. 1) provides it with a moral dimension such that it is usually impossible to identify some elements of its practice as morally significant and others as morally neutral. It might be thought, for example, that measuring a patient's blood pressure is a psychomotor skill that is morally neutral, but the nurse's ability to measure and record the blood pressure accurately has the potential to affect the patient's health and well-being and this is morally significant. All decisions and actions taken (or omitted) in relation to client care are closely connected to their beneficial, or harmful, effects. While some aspects of nursing are technical, competence or lack of it affects clients' welfare. If nursing practice is accepted as having a highly significant moral dimension, then evaluation of nursing care quality involves moral reasoning processes in order to arrive at moral judgements. In Box 7.2, where staff shortages prevented all patients being provided with the help needed to eat and drink simultaneously, decisions made about whom to assist, and when, were not only technical, but also moral in nature. It is now useful to examine concepts of ethics and morals and their implications for nurses.

Ethics and morals

Ethics and morals are terms frequently used interchangeably. When differentiating between the two, the term ethics is usually taken to refer to the study of morals, whereas morality relates to people's behaviour.

Ethics and morals are sometimes viewed as something to which we resort in time of crisis, but it is arguable that morality is not one single dimension of life within society but is essential for society to function successfully. Thompson et al (2006) stress that not all moral decision-making is associated with drama and crisis, but that moral choice is an integral, and inescapable, part of everyday life and a focus on life and death dilemmas clouds the fact that most moral issues faced by nurses are encountered in daily practice.

The notion that it is impossible to demarcate clearly between the work and private life of an RN is one that is made clear in *The code* (NMC 2008a) and in the *Guidance on professional conduct: For nursing and midwifery students* (NMC 2010a), which emphasize that nurses have a professional duty to provide care and uphold the standing of their profession within and outwith their work setting.

Having said that, ethics and morals are central to nursing practice, it is the case that problems or dilemmas can, and do, occur. A dilemma is, by definition, a situation with no solution and any action taken will be with the purpose of creating the least harm. More common than dilemmas are problems, to which solutions may be found, although these may not be without complexity.

Ethical theories

Ethical theories are sometimes used within UK healthcare provision and these will now be described and discussed in the light of a particular situation. In the situation outlined earlier, Katie, who had been abused, was central to the discussion illustrating the application of ethical principles. Now carry out the activities in Box 7.3 that relate to decisions that may be made in relation to allocation of healthcare resources.

⚖ **Ethical issues** Box 7.3

Allocation of resources

It is sometimes argued that individuals whose health problems can be perceived as 'self-inflicted' should not have the same entitlement to treatment as others. One example is that of cigarette smokers.

Student activities

Do you consider that smokers should have the same rights to treatment as non-smokers?

- Take 5–10 minutes to explain your answer.
- Then, take another 5–10 minutes to provide counter arguments to those you put forward.

You can do this on your own or in discussion with others.

Responses and reasons that people provide to activities in Box 7.3 will vary, but it is useful to identify and discuss the most commonly used arguments in favour of, and against, equal entitlement of cigarette smokers to treatment.

In your own discussion, you may have arguments additional to those listed in Box 7.4, although those in the box are often used. It can be seen that the issue of whether or not cigarette smokers should enjoy equal access to treatment as non-smokers is not a clear-cut and straightforward issue.

It is important, in nursing practice, to be able to identify arguments for, and against, a particular course of action and to analyse which arguments appear most compelling and why. The activity in Box 7.3 was useful in relation to the *process* of identifying arguments for, and against, a particular viewpoint, as well as in relation to the *product*, in this case compiling a list of arguments. Reflection *on* practice (Ch. 4) also involves this type of activity. Over time, and with experience, reflection *in* practice enables practitioners to analyse and evaluate situations at the time they occur, thus enabling the practitioner to be reflexive, in addition to reflective. This is a skill that develops throughout a student's educational programme and further development continues following registration. Events that facilitate reflective and reflexive practice are those in which practitioners explicitly identify *why* a particular situation proceeded well or badly in relation to its component parts.

Practitioners also need to acknowledge their own attitudes, beliefs and values. In arguments for and against equal access to treatment for cigarette smokers, it is likely that personal attitudes, beliefs and values, rather than a notion of 'objective' judgements, may come into play initially. These may be clearly

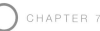

Arguments for, and against, equal entitlement of smokers to treatment | Box 7.4

Arguments *for* equal entitlement of smokers to treatment

- Treatment decisions should depend on individuals' needs
- Healthcare workers should provide care for people who require it, not make value judgements about lifestyle or behaviours
- Each individual is equally important – one cannot deem some people more 'deserving' of treatment than others
- Cigarettes are addictive; smokers should receive help, not be censured
- If an individual stops smoking they may have many years of life ahead
- Outcomes are unpredictable: a person who smokes may outlive a non-smoker
- Cigarette smokers, over their lifetime, generate significant government revenue (excise duty and VAT in the UK comprise approximately 76% of the cost of 20 cigarettes; ASH 2011)
- Cigarette smokers claim less state benefits in the UK, in the long term, than non-smokers. Some 50% of smokers die prematurely, losing an average 8 years of life (Edwards 2004), and therefore receive less pension benefit and are less likely to require long-term care in old age
- Cigarette smoking is a legal activity
- Criteria for designating ill-health as 'self-inflicted' are problematic, e.g. sports injuries may be 'self-inflicted' and many people's lifestyle has, to some extent, contributed to their health problems

Arguments *against* equal entitlement of smokers to treatment

- Healthcare resources are limited, therefore allocation decisions must be made
- Scarce resources should be allocated where they can provide greatest healthcare benefit for the greatest number of individuals: cigarette smokers are less likely to benefit from many treatments than non-smokers and may be at greater risk of development of complications of treatment, e.g. a greater likelihood of chest infection following anaesthesia
- If cigarette smokers are treated, but continue to smoke, benefits of specialized treatment may be minimal or of short duration
- Cigarette smoking is an individual choice, therefore healthcare problems that arise as a result of smoking are self-inflicted
- Cigarette smoking has been recognized for many years as being harmful: individuals who smoke are aware of the risks
- It is unjust to those who care for their health if cigarette smokers have equal or preferential access to treatment
- Treating cigarette smokers equally to non-smokers provides official endorsement of cigarette smoking or at least no incentive for individuals to stop smoking

ASH (Action on Smoking and Health) 2011 Basic facts: Economics. Online. Available: www.ash.org.uk/information/facts-and-stats/fact-sheets September 2011.

---

evident in your replies, or may have been implicit in reasons provided for the response.

Some arguments outlined in Box 7.4 will now be examined to identify ethical theories that underpin them.

Consequentialist ethics

One argument put forward in Box 7.4 was that, when health resources are finite, they should be allocated to create the greatest health benefit for the greatest number of people. This type of thinking is 'consequentialist' and one form of consequentialism, called 'utilitarianism', was proposed by Jeremy Bentham (1748–1832). His theory was further developed and refined by John Stuart Mill (1806–1873). Bentham used the term 'happiness', but this was later re-defined by Mill as 'benefit', and, whereas Bentham's focus was clearly upon the good of the majority, Mill also advocated tolerance for minority beliefs and lifestyles.

The utilitarian theory of deploying resources to provide the greatest benefit for the greatest number of individuals frequently underpins UK government policy, both at central and local levels (Box 7.5). It is a consequentialist theory because the focus is on the consequences of action or inaction: methods taken to achieve desired consequences (i.e. greatest benefit for the greatest number of individuals) are deemed morally right or wrong insofar as they facilitate, or inhibit, attainment of benefits. (This type of theory is sometimes also referred to as 'teleological', i.e. derived from the Greek *teleos*, meaning 'end'.) For example, if cigarette smokers are less likely than non-smokers to benefit from a particular treatment, and resources to provide that treatment are limited, then the treatment should be available to those who will benefit most, i.e. non-smokers.

 Ethical issues | Box 7.5

Utilitarian approaches

Student activity

Identify what you consider to be the strengths and limitations of allocating scarce health resources where they will create the greatest benefit for the greatest number of individuals.

Strengths and limitations of a utilitarian approach

Some arguments in favour of a utilitarian approach are that it is the only feasible way in which to cater for the healthcare needs of a large, and fairly diverse, population. The impossibility of addressing the needs of every individual within a country means that policy makers have to adopt a 'broad brush' approach and aim to create the greatest benefits for the greatest number. This strategy is intended to ensure that health needs of the majority of the population are addressed.

Unpredictability of outcomes

One problem with a utilitarian approach is that it is based on the ability to identify the actions, or inactions, that ensure beneficial outcomes. (It is important to recognize that 'inactions' as well as 'actions' have consequences, e.g. if a decision is made *not* to treat a patient – 'inaction'– then this will have consequences, as will providing treatment – 'action'.) In reality it is often difficult to predict outcomes of actions and/or inactions. If the intended action is treatment so that an individual will have many more years of a healthy life, then not only may the action itself fail to achieve this end, but the unpredictability of life may result in an individual dying of another, possibly unrelated, cause. For example, if a non-smoker is treated in preference to a smoker, on the grounds that they are likely to achieve a greater long-term health benefit, it is possible that the non-smoker may die from another cause within a year of treatment, whereas the smoker may survive for many years. Unpredictability of outcomes is one factor used to criticize a utilitarian approach to resource allocation.

What counts as 'benefit'?

Another concern about implications of consequentialist theories is that they may encourage a simplified view of 'benefits' as equating neatly with 'years of life'. This is a quantitative approach (see Ch. 5), in which numbers of survivors and length of survival are important. It may be argued that quality of life can be of equal importance as length of life. For example, treating non-smokers who have certain forms of heart disease may provide them with many years of health, whereas treating smokers with similar problems may enable them to mobilize outdoors as opposed to being housebound and this may improve their quality of life, if only for a relatively short time.

Are numbers all that count?

Another limitation of consequentialist theories is that individuals who suffer from relatively rare health problems, or those not considered to be healthcare priorities, may be unable to access treatment if resources are geared towards provision of treatment for the majority. For example, relatively few individuals require a liver transplant, whereas many people have heart disease or cancer, or know of someone with these problems.

Does the end result justify the means?

Consequentialist theories focus on results and not actions and inactions that create these may be deemed unacceptable, at least in some instances. It may be considered that actions and inactions are, in themselves, of moral importance. For example, it may be anticipated that telling a patient the truth about an unfavourable diagnosis and prognosis will create distress for that patient, for their friends and relatives and for the care team. A consequentialist might argue that, if creation of the greatest benefit for the greatest number of people will be achieved by telling a lie, then that is the morally correct thing to do. It is the end result, or consequence, that is of moral importance and not the means used to achieve it. An alternative viewpoint is that telling the truth, or telling a lie, is morally right or wrong in itself, independent of the consequences.

Taking consequentialism to extremes might (at least in theory) entail that for a person who was in need of healthcare, but without friends or relatives and who wished to die, it would not only be acceptable, but desirable, for that person to

die. This would free up resources that would be used in the care of others and thus maximize benefits for the greatest number of people.

Rule utilitarianism

One way to circumvent the potential problem outlined in the previous paragraph is to refine the theory. Rule utilitarianism states that, rather than deciding in individual instances what will create the greatest benefit for the greatest number, the 'rule' should be implementation of actions (or inactions) that will, if adopted by society as a whole, create the greatest benefit for the majority. It might then be argued that it would not create the greatest benefit for society as a whole if a culture was promoted in which lives of individuals were held in low regard.

Consequentialist ethics: summary

There are strengths and limitations in a consequentialist approach to ethics, some of which have been identified here. Overall, its charm may lie in its relative simplicity. It contains no spiritual or religious elements and relies on identification of factors that will create the largest net benefit for the greatest number of individuals. However, the relative simplicity may be a shortcoming when it encounters the complexity of individuals' needs for care and debate about what comprises a 'benefit'. The difficulty in predicting outcomes is also problematic, as is the idea that actions and inactions are, in themselves, neutral and morally relevant only in respect of their results. For further reading about utilitarianism, see Thompson et al (2006).

Deontological ethics

Some arguments for, and against, smokers' equal access to treatment use justifications that are not dependent upon intended consequences. One example is the idea that treatment decisions should be made on the basis of individual need and that healthcare workers have a duty to provide care regardless of individuals' lifestyles or behaviours. This argument is evident in *The code* (NMC 2008a), which emphasizes the importance of respecting patients and clients as individuals. Deontological argument proposes that actions and/or inactions are morally acceptable or unacceptable in themselves, independent of their anticipated or actual consequences.

Deontology derives from the Greek words *deon*, meaning 'duty' and *logos*, meaning 'science' or 'study of'. A deontological theory specifies moral requirements and moral prohibitions. *The code* (NMC 2008a) is an example of a deontological code. *The code* does not refer at any point to maximization of benefits for the greatest number of patients, nor does it refer to the end result justifying the means by which it was attained. Rather, *The code* specifies duties of RNs, including their duty of care to all patients as individuals.

Kant (1724–1804) developed deontological theory, including the concept of the categorical imperative. Basically, this involves asking oneself whether, if one's proposed action (or inaction) was to be implemented by people universally, it would be morally acceptable? For example, if a person considered telling a lie, they should first consider whether, if this practice were universal, the result would be acceptable. It is likely that, while an individual might consider that their own action (in this instance telling a lie) might be acceptable, they might also realize that, if lying was adopted universally, chaos would ensue, as individuals would be unable to trust one another. If individuals behave in a manner that would be acceptable if universally practised, then they are acting in accordance with a categorical imperative. A deontological approach to truth telling would be that telling the truth, or a lie, is of moral importance, *in itself*, rather than solely in terms of its consequence. The individual's intentions are also important, e.g. that the intention of an individual in carrying out a particular action was fulfilment of a duty.

While *The code* (NMC 2008a) is a secular, or non-religious, document, and while a deontologist may be agnostic or atheist, the majority of religions can be classed as deontological, i.e. a religion usually requires adherents to behave in specific ways, which are deemed to be right or wrong *in themselves*, as opposed to right or wrong in relation to beneficial or deleterious consequences.

Areas of potential conflict

One area of potential conflict is that deontologists may have a variety of backgrounds: their commonality lies in the requirement, duty or obligation to behave in particular ways. One person's idea of duty may vary considerably from, and indeed may be diametrically opposed to, that of another individual, if they have a different set of deontological beliefs. In relation to termination of pregnancy, for example, individuals who believe strongly in the right of women to decide whether to continue with, or terminate, a pregnancy, may express a deontological belief that healthcare workers have a duty to provide termination of pregnancy on demand. On the other hand, individuals strongly against termination of pregnancy may base their belief on a perceived duty to preserve human life, or potential human life, at all costs. This example shows that deontologists may hold diametrically opposed views, although they share in common the belief that individuals have certain obligations or duties, with which they must comply.

Virtue ethics

A theory of ethical behaviour, originally expounded by Aristotle in the fourth century BC and developed more recently by Macintyre (1981), concerns the role of the virtues. A virtue is a character trait perceived as socially valuable and a moral virtue is one which is morally valuable (Beauchamp & Childress 2009). Virtue theorists consider that morality, rather than being the domain of ivory-tower academics, is a practical skill exercised on a daily basis. If children are socialized into behaving in a morally acceptable manner in relation to others, then this should become habitual practice over time. Within this theory, humans are perceived as social in nature, but they must practise certain behaviours or virtues on a regular basis to maintain them. It is insufficient only to know what is right: it is necessary to put that knowledge into practice (Ch. 1). The concept of moderation in behaviour is important and individuals must take responsibility for their voluntary actions.

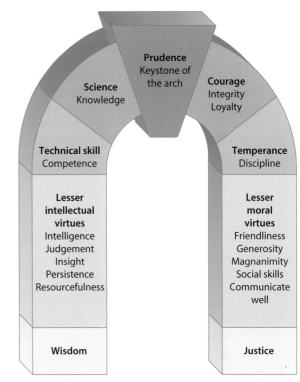

Fig. 7.1 • Symbolic representation of Aristotle's view of the relationship between prudence and the intellectual and moral values. (Reproduced with permission from Thompson, I.E., Melia, K.M., Boyd, K.M., et al, 2006. Nursing ethics, fifth ed. Churchill Livingstone, Edinburgh.)

Thompson et al (2006, p 302) explain that Aristotle's system of ethics requires both intellectual and moral virtues (Fig. 7.1).

Intellectual and moral virtues

Intellectual virtues relate to skill in decision-making and problem-solving, while moral virtues are character traits (or habits) that are prerequisites for an individual to be reliable, effective and efficient in action. The keystone (Fig. 7.1) that links and binds intellectual and moral virtues together is prudence, also referred to as practical wisdom. Thompson et al (2006, p 308–309) argue that 'situation ethics' is needed, as this actively acknowledges the importance of the 'specifics' of particular situations, rather than, as some ethical theories require, attempting to develop principles that are universal in application and applicable to any situation. Consequentialist and duty-based approaches to ethics are viewed as attempting to force unique events to comply with inappropriate general frameworks. Neo (i.e. modern versions of) Aristotelianism, or virtue ethics, requires consideration of each situation as unique, comprised as it is, of individuals. Individuals are not identical to one another and all have needs that should be addressed in an understanding, individualized and caring manner.

Concerns about virtue ethics

Concerns are raised in relation to the idea of virtue ethics. It is arguable that the idea that virtues can be cultivated in all individuals is impossible. Qualities deemed to be virtues might lack consensus among the population at large. For example, for some people, intellectual endeavour may be perceived as a virtue, while for others this is not valued. It can be argued that, even if practice of the identified virtues becomes habitual over time, situations may arise in which individuals abandon virtuous behaviour, at least temporarily. For example, in response to continuing severe staff shortages, which complaints to management have failed to rectify, a normally thoughtful and caring practitioner may find that their capacity, or motivation, to be virtuous has diminished or is absent. For virtues to flourish, it is important to recognize that responsibility is not solely that of the individual: the environment must be one in which qualities deemed to be virtues are promoted and may flourish.

Constraints on ethical behaviour

It may be argued in relation to any ethical theory that, while some behaviours are those for which individuals (sometimes referred to as 'agents') are directly responsible, the structures (physical and cultural) within which individuals work and live may inhibit, or facilitate, moral conduct. This interaction between an individual (the agent) and the structures within which they live and work may be a powerful determinant of people's ability to behave morally.

Ethical theories: summary

The previous section outlined three ethical theories of relevance to UK healthcare provision. Detailed explanation and discussion of ethical theories is provided by Thompson et al (2006).

Power: its use and abuse

Power has a variety of definitions, but most include notions of command, authority, control and ability to influence events and produce effects. Individuals who seek healthcare are usually, due to their need for assistance, in a situation in which their ability to exert power is limited. Students may not consider themselves powerful players within the healthcare team, but patients or clients are to some degree vulnerable. Abuses of power reported by the media tend to be extreme in nature, e.g. the case of Harold Shipman, an English GP, convicted in 2000 for the murder of over 200 of his patients. It is important to remember that many decisions in everyday nursing practice are not those of life and death, but of care quality, and relate to treating patients and clients as individuals who are entitled to compassion, dignity and respect. Now consider the scenario outlined in Box 7.6.

An abuse of power?

Individual reactions to the scenario in Box 7.6 will vary, but some relevant points are identified below:

- It is not a 'life or death' situation
- Alex is not subjected to physical abuse
- Healthcare workers may exert considerable influence and control (power) over clients
- Alex is subjected to misuse of power

? Critical thinking Box 7.6

An abuse of power?

John is a student undertaking his first practice placement in a community house for adults who have learning disabilities. He had no experience of care settings before starting his university programme 4 months ago. One of the residents, Alex, who has a moderately severe learning disability and is overweight, asks John for sugar in his tea. John is about to comply when one of the healthcare assistants shouts across the dining room that Alex is 'not allowed sugar' as he is on a diet. Alex protests loudly and swears at the healthcare assistant, who replies that, unless Alex 'behaves', he will have to return to his room.

Student activities

- Take a few minutes to discuss the above situation with others, or to jot down your own thoughts about what should be done in this situation. In particular, identify what action, if any, John should take.
- Write down a rationale for your ideas, including reference to bioethical principles or ethical theory.

- Alex's autonomy is disregarded, i.e. his right to make his own decisions
- Alex's 'capacity' (Ch. 6) to make his own decisions is unknown,
 but
- The healthcare worker's action (shouting, rather than speaking discreetly with Alex) is abusive.

In this short scenario, and with no direct knowledge of the people concerned, it is impossible to place the situation in context and to understand individuals' motivations for actions. However, the fact that Alex is in a position of vulnerability as he needs care does not justify decisions being made on his behalf, without prior consultation and agreement. It also does not mean that he should be subjected to a form of emotional abuse, i.e. humiliation in front of other residents and threats of removal to his room.

On reflection then, while it may be that the healthcare assistant acted in what she perceived to be the resident's best interest, and it is the case that beneficence is a *prima facie* ethical principle (i.e. a principle that, at 'first sight', should be respected), it remains arguable that it was unacceptable to take action as she did, as her actions interfered with John's autonomy, which is another *prima facie* ethical principle. An individual's autonomy in relation to health issues usually overrides beneficence by others (for exceptions to this, see Ch. 6). It may also be argued that the resident's 'best interest' was not served by the way that the healthcare assistant handled the situation.

What should John do in this situation? While students are not professionally accountable to the NMC, John should, as a future RN, have residents' interests as his main concern and take action to protect these. There are several options available to John:

- Confront the healthcare assistant (within or outwith the dining room) and tell her that he found her action unacceptable

- Discuss the situation with his mentor, or person in charge of the placement, at the time
- Contact the university to express his concerns
- Do nothing because, as a new student, John might be uncertain as to what constitutes acceptable or unacceptable practice. Even if John did feel that this was poor practice, he might feel unable to complain, for fear of repercussions during the remainder of his placement. He could reassure himself that the resident had not suffered physical abuse and that, as a student, he was not in a position to alter practice or have a complaint upheld
- Do nothing because John is aware that he has to work closely with the healthcare assistant and her colleagues for the remainder of his placement and does not wish to make himself unpopular. Additionally, John knows that he has to achieve a satisfactory placement assessment and does not wish to jeopardize this.

Of the above, while John does not perhaps have a legal or professional obligation to report the incident, it is arguable that he has a moral obligation to do so. Alex is a vulnerable individual who has received treatment that appears detrimental to his emotional, although not physical, well-being. If there are valid reasons for the healthcare assistant's response to the resident these should be made clear. John could perhaps approach the healthcare assistant and ask why she had spoken to Alex in the way that she did. An alternative would be for John to request clarification from his mentor or person in charge of the placement. Formalized care policies, guidelines and procedures provide benchmarks for staff, clients and other interested parties against which quality of care delivery may be measured. Benchmarks clarify acceptable and unacceptable staff behaviours and would have been a helpful resource for John.

If John failed to receive a satisfactory explanation from staff, or from policies, guidelines or procedures, he could contact his university to explore the incident with the Link Lecturer or his Personal Tutor. John could make a written complaint about the healthcare assistant's behaviour, which would then be the subject of official investigation (Ch. 3).

Such action may be termed 'whistleblowing' by the media. The Public Disclosure at Work Act (HM Government 1998b) provides legal protection for employees who divulge unacceptable work practices (Ch. 6, Further reading). Students are not employees within placement areas and are not subject to their disciplinary processes and procedures, but they are subject to those of their university. RNs are provided with legal protection by the Act (HM Government 1998b) if they disclose unacceptable practice(s), although this does not prevent potential censure by colleagues for having divulged unacceptable practice(s).

John, as a student, may feel that it is difficult to raise concerns about poor, or unacceptable, practice within a placement area for fear of intimidation by staff (this concern may also be experienced by registered practitioners). The Royal College of Nursing (RCN 2002) provides guidance for students in relation to bullying and harassment at work and the NMC (2010d) identifies ways in which raising and escalating concerns may be achieved.

The situation above showed that power does not reside solely in managers within healthcare settings. People who provide direct care for patients and clients wield considerable power over their well-being and abuse of this power is often not the sort that makes news headlines. Additionally, this situation identifies different staff with whom students work as part of a multidisciplinary team. The NMC (2010e) and Scottish Government (2011) propose that healthcare assistants should be regulated and that this would enhance healthcare and protection of the public. The example also illustrated that students who witness what they consider unacceptable practice may be uncertain about how to proceed in making a formal complaint. Advice should, in those instances, be sought from the sources identified in the previous section.

Vulnerable groups

The most vulnerable members of society are likely to become the victims of abuse, both in institutional and domestic settings. These include:

- Children
- Women
- Individuals who have a learning disability
- Individuals who have limited ability to speak or express themselves
- Individuals who have a mental health problem
- Older adults, especially those who are physically and/or psychologically frail
- Non-English speakers
- Asylum seekers
- Individuals without legal authority to be in the UK.

Some client groups are more vulnerable to abuse than others, including individuals who receive ongoing (as opposed to short-term) care and those with limited ability to articulate or whose reports of abuse are unlikely to be heeded, e.g. if they receive few visitors in whom they could confide. The NMC (2008c) provides advice for nurses working with children and young people and guidance for the care of older people (NMC 2009b) to ensure that the care of potentially vulnerable individuals is emphasized and RNs' responsibilities clarified.

Vulnerable adults and children

Abuse within healthcare settings may be classified in a number of ways (Box 7.7) and is more likely to occur in certain circumstances. Care settings and management styles that may result in poor, or unacceptable, practice include the following:

- Minimal preparation of staff for practice
- Minimal ongoing support and supervision of staff
- Failure of management to value staff's work.

In these circumstances, clients may be perceived as units of work, rather than individuals. Care areas without clear lines of accountability or policies and procedures that do not state acceptable (and unacceptable) staff behaviours facilitate, or at least do not inhibit, care that is of poor quality or could be categorized as abuse.

Categories of abuse	Box 7.7

- *Physical*: Restriction of a person's movement; misuse of medication, e.g. sedation
- *Sexual*: Acts to which an individual is unable to consent; was not in a position to give consent, e.g. below the age of consent, due to incapacity, under pressure to consent
- *Psychological/Emotional*: Threats, humiliation, isolation
- *Financial*: Exploitation
- *Neglect*: Failure to provide appropriate care and attention or access to services
- *Discriminatory*: Race, sex, disability, sexual orientation, religious or cultural beliefs.

Restrictive physical intervention and therapeutic holding

Forcible restraint of individuals within care settings is controversial. The scenario in Box 7.8 describes a situation that relates to care of a child, but the principles can be generalized to care of patients and clients of varying ages and diverse needs.

? Critical thinking	Box 7.8

Restrictive physical intervention/therapeutic holding of a child

Anna is a student undertaking a placement within a children's hospital. She is involved, under supervision of her mentor, in carrying out a variety of procedures for young children, but is uneasy about the use of restraining measures to ensure that children remain still and by the distress that this causes some children. Anna wonders whether these measures are justifiable.

Student activity

Identify the grounds on which you would consider restrictive physical intervention or therapeutic holding of a child to be ethically justifiable.

The United Nations *Convention on the Rights of the Child* was based on the premise that children have an active contribution to make within society (United Nations, UN 1989). Therapeutic holding is used frequently by parents or carers during procedures such as immunization by injection, venepuncture and lumbar puncture. The Royal College of Nursing (RCN 2008b) provides general guidelines about use of restraint, and also guidelines specific to care of children (RCN 2010). The latter places emphasis upon prior explanations to the child about procedures, use of alternatives to restrictive physical intervention and therapeutic holding, e.g. distraction, wherever possible. They emphasize the need to obtain the child's consent wherever possible and the importance of documenting measures used, their rationale and duration.

It may be seen from the above that the disquiet that Anna experienced in the situation outlined in Box 7.8 was justified. Perhaps the situations where Anna witnessed (and perhaps participated in) therapeutic holding of children were those in which actions of staff were justified, but it is important that such measures are not carried out without reflection on, and in, practice and that an evidence base is used to support the rationale for their use (see Chs 4, 5). If practices that may cause patients or clients distress are implemented, it is of particular importance that the rationale for these is explained and potential alternatives explored.

The situation in Box 7.8 related to children but, as identified earlier, many individuals who require healthcare are vulnerable. Guidance is available for individuals with different care needs, e.g. the NMC (2009b) provides guidance for care of older people.

Ethical frameworks and models

Reflecting on, and in, practice can be structured (Ch. 4). In relation to ethical problems or dilemmas, frameworks or models may also be used to reach decisions in specific situations, e.g. the DECIDE model (Thompson et al 2006).

The DECIDE model

The authors of the DECIDE model (Thompson et al 2006) (Fig. 7.2) advocate that, in a crisis situation (originally defined in Greek as a 'decision time'), structured questions can assist ethical problem-solving. These are shown in Box 7.9. The first step is to verify the facts, then identify 'stakeholders' (i.e. parties involved in the situation). Stakeholders' rights are then established, as are the duties of other parties in fulfilment of these.

Following this initial process, it is important to define the problem and identify relevant ethical issue(s). Once this has been established, a review to identify ethically relevant principles is carried out and available options are considered. Investigation of the options explores their potential outcomes and the costs and benefits attached to each. The action deemed most appropriate is decided upon, implemented and subsequently evaluated for its effectiveness or otherwise in solving, or at least alleviating, the problem.

The DECIDE model in practice

The following discussion illustrates issues that may arise from the activities in Box 7.10 and, because the scenario is brief, there is limited information on which to base a discussion. It is not intended to provide the 'ideal' answer. The steps of the DECIDE model are each considered in turn using the framework in Box 7.9.

Defining the problem(s)

The first step is to verify the facts, which are:

- Tom has a mental health problem
- Tom lives in a community house with support

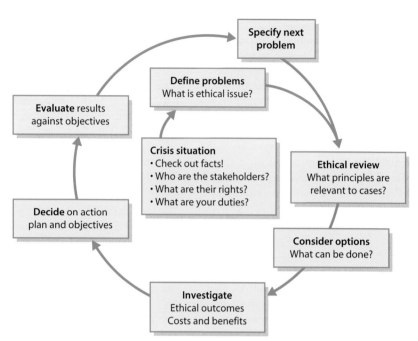

Fig. 7.2 • The DECIDE model for ethical decision-making. (Reproduced with permission from Thompson, I.E., Melia, K.M., Boyd, K.M., et al, 2006. Nursing ethics, fifth ed. Churchill Livingstone, Edinburgh.)

The DECIDE model	Box 7.9

D – Define the problem(s)

What are the key facts of the case? Who is involved? What are their rights, your duties? What is the main ethical problem to be addressed?

E – Ethical review

What ethical principles have a bearing on the case and which principle or principles should be given priority in making your decision?

C – Consider the options

What options do you have in the situation? What alternative courses of action? What help, means and methods do you need to use?

I – Investigate outcomes

Given each available option, what consequences are likely to follow from each course of action open to you? Which is the most ethical thing to do?

D – Decide on action

Having chosen the best available option, determine a specific action plan, set clear objectives and then act decisively and effectively

E – Evaluate results

Having initiated a course of action, monitor how things progress, and when concluded, assess carefully whether or not you achieved your goals.

(From Thompson et al 2006, p 324)

⚖ Ethical issues	Box 7.10

Whose rights?

Tom is a young man who has schizophrenia. He has been in hospital on two occasions and now lives in a community house with support from a residential care worker and community mental health nurse. Tom takes medication as prescribed which alleviates, but does not eradicate, some of his distressing thoughts, experiences and feelings. These include hearing voices (auditory hallucinations) that mock and frighten him, and consequent feelings of suspicion and uneasiness cause him considerable distress.

Some of the residents in the neighbourhood raised objections when the proposal for the community house was put forward 2 years ago under the misapprehension that people who had mental health problems might display antisocial behaviour. Tom has, on several occasions, shouted in the street in response to distress caused by his auditory hallucinations. Tom's feelings of mistrust understandably worsen when people stare at and talk about him. Neighbours are worried about his shouting, believing it is directed at them, and complain that it has become unsafe for their children to walk, or play, outdoors because of Tom's behaviour.

Student activities

- Write down, or discuss with others, your perspective on the above scenario.
- Explain the reasons that support your views.

- Tom takes medication as prescribed
- The medication controls Tom's symptoms, but does not eradicate them
- Tom's symptoms include auditory hallucinations and feelings of paranoia, which he finds distressing

- Tom is sometimes verbally aggressive to people who stare at him or talk about him
- Some of the people who live near the community house objected to its existence at the planning stage
- Some of the neighbours find Tom's behaviour threatening.

The stakeholders are Tom, the neighbours who complained that Tom's behaviour was threatening, Tom's support workers (including yourself as the RN), his psychiatrist and, in a wider sense, possibly other individuals who have mental health problems, and all other members of society.

The rights of all the stakeholders appear to be those of freedom (autonomy) to live their lives within society. Your duty, as the RN responsible for Tom's care, is to act to ensure that Tom's best interests are served (NMC 2008a). You do, however, also have a duty to take action if you consider that Tom's behaviour presents an actual threat to others. You have a duty to comply with your contract of employment.

The next step is to define the problem and, as the problem is not only practical (e.g. accompanying Tom to the shops) but also has implications for Tom's future health, freedom and well-being (and also has implications for the perceived freedom of some of the neighbours and their children), it appears to be an ethical problem.

Ethical review

The next stage of the model is to review the ethical elements. These appear to be those of competing rights, i.e. Tom's right to move around freely and not be prescribed medication to the point where side-effects (including lethargy and drowsiness) impede this right. The principles involved are:

- Preventing harm to Tom: non-maleficence
- Acting to preserve his best interests: beneficence
- Preserving his autonomy as much as is possible without it interfering with the autonomy of others
- Justice.

Unless Tom is being held under an appropriate section of the Mental Health Act (see Ch. 6), he is entitled to freedom of movement. Ethical review would include acknowledgement of your duty as the RN responsible for Tom's care to uphold his best interests and act as his advocate if required to do so.

The rights of the neighbours to be free from harassment are also important within the ethical review, but it is not clear that there is an *actual* threat to their well-being. Their negative perception of Tom's behaviour may be based on lack of knowledge about the nature of his illness.

Consider and investigate options

The next two stages in the DECIDE model (Fig. 7.2) are identification of options available and investigation of ethically acceptable outcomes, including the costs and benefits of each. The options in this case appear to be:

- Do nothing and hope that, over time, the neighbours will accept that Tom's behaviour does not constitute a threat. This does not, however, seem ethically acceptable, as the neighbours will remain uneasy and Tom's feelings of worry and isolation will probably be reinforced by the neighbours' behaviour
- Request that the psychiatrist increase Tom's medication in an attempt to reduce his symptoms to a 'socially acceptable' level. However, as this might increase deleterious side-effects and constitute chemical restraint, it does not seem an ethically justifiable solution
- Encourage Tom to remain indoors. This also seems ethically unjustifiable, as it attempts to restrict Tom's freedom of movement

- Arrange to discuss the situation with concerned neighbours to allow them to express their concerns and allow you to explain Tom's behaviour. This seems ethically justifiable, but there is the problem of ensuring that your duty of patient confidentiality is maintained (NMC 2008a). It might be possible to carry out such a discussion so long as no specific details about Tom or his particular mental health problem were divulged. It might be possible to seek Tom's permission to divulge information, but dependent upon the severity of his problems there might be the issue of whether he is in a position to provide informed consent (Ch. 6) to this request.

Your duty, as the RN responsible for Tom's care, is to act to ensure that Tom's best interests are served (NMC 2008a) and to act as his advocate if required to do so. The term advocacy has its origins in the judicial system and retains rather a confrontational association. An advocate is an individual who speaks on behalf of another, either in response to a request from that person or because their position in relation to the other person may require them to do so. The position of RNs in relation to their clients, so far as *The code* (NMC 2008a) is concerned, is that nurses should support clients' best interests and this may be assumed to include advocacy, if required. There are arguments for, and against, RNs adopting advocacy roles in relation to their clients (see Ch. 6). It may be argued, for example, that independent advocates (i.e. those who have no other formal input into the client's care) are better placed to act purely in accordance with the client's known, or assumed, wishes.

Decide on action

The next stage is to decide on action, in conjunction with Tom, and to compile a plan and identify objectives. The investigation indicated that the best action might be to speak with Tom in an attempt to explore how he understands and feels about the situation and to speak with the neighbours, ensuring that specific details of Tom's condition were not discussed, thus maintaining client confidentiality. Reassuring neighbours that Tom did not present a risk to their safety would be important and they might wish advice as to how best to interact with Tom when they meet. With Tom's permission, it might be useful for him to meet with the neighbours, accompanied by an independent advocate. The intended objectives or outcomes, would be:

- That Tom's symptoms would not be exacerbated by the neighbours' negative reactions towards him
- That the neighbours' anxieties would be alleviated and that their attitude towards Tom (and the community house) would be more positive.

Evaluate results

The final stage of the DECIDE model (Fig. 7.2) is an evaluation of the effectiveness of the action taken. This may be measured against the objectives that were identified during the decision stage, so those who worked with Tom, Tom himself and the neighbours would be able to provide feedback as to whether the intended objectives had been fully, or partially, met. (There is a further step in the DECIDE model, which is to specify the next problem; whether another problem would arise would remain to be seen.)

The framework provided by the DECIDE model is relevant across a wide range of healthcare settings and for individuals with varying needs. Box 7.11 provides an opportunity for you to reflect on a situation within your own practice experience.

> **? Critical thinking**   **Box 7.11**
>
> ### The DECIDE model in practice
>
> **Student activities**
>
> - Identify and reflect on a situation from your own practice placement experience in which an ethical problem was present.
> - Use the DECIDE model to work through the actions that either were, or might have been, carried out in that situation.

SUMMARY

- An introduction to the role of the NMC and the guidance it provides for nursing students and registered practitioners to enable it to meet its primary duty: protecting the public.
- An overview of fundamental ethical principles, theories and frameworks.
- Discussions of some everyday ethical issues that may arise in nursing practice using scenarios. The underpinning themes can be generalized to a variety of care settings and to clients with diverse needs.
- A basis for further understanding of professional and ethical issues that may arise during nursing programmes and following registration.

KEY WORDS AND PHRASES FOR LITERATURE SEARCHING

Nursing and Midwifery Council

Ethics

Morals

Nursing students

 Useful websites

Nursing and Midwifery Council www.nmc-uk.org
Royal College of Nursing www.rcn.org.uk
All websites accessed September 2012.

References

Beauchamp, T.L., Childress, J.F., 2009. Principles of biomedical ethics, sixth ed. Oxford University Press, Oxford.

Department of Health, 2010. Dignity in care. Department of Health, London. Online. Available: www.dh.gov.uk/en/SocialCare/Deliveringsocialcare/DH_121415 September 2012.

Edwards, R., 2004. The problem of tobacco smoking. British Medical Journal 328, 217–219.

HM Government, 1998a. Data Protection Act. TSO, London.

HM Government, 1998b. Public Disclosure at Work Act. TSO, London.

Macintyre, A., 1981. After virtue, second ed. Notre Dame University Press, Notre Dame.

Nursing and Midwifery Council, 2008a. The code: standards of conduct, performance and ethics for nurses and midwives. NMC, London.

Nursing and Midwifery Council, 2008b. The PREP handbook. NMC, London.

Nursing and Midwifery Council, 2008c. Advice for nurses working with children and young people. NMC, London.

Nursing and Midwifery Council, 2009a. Record keeping: Guidance for nurses and midwives. NMC, London.

Nursing and Midwifery Council, 2009b. Guidance for the care of older people. NMC, London.

Nursing and Midwifery Council, 2010a. Guidance on professional conduct: For nursing and midwifery students. NMC, London.

Nursing and Midwifery Council, 2010b. Standards for pre-registration nursing education. NMC, London.

Nursing and Midwifery Council, 2010c. Good health and good character: guidance for approved education institutions. NMC, London.

Nursing and Midwifery Council, 2010d. Raising and escalating concerns: Guidance for nurses and midwives. NMC, London.

Nursing and Midwifery Council, 2010e. Regulation of healthcare support workers. NMC, London. Online. Available: www.nmc-uk.org/About-us/Policy-and-public-affairs/Politics-and-parliament/PMs-Commission-on-the-future-of-nursing-and-midwifery/Regulation-of-healthcare-support-workers-/ September 2012.

Royal College of Nursing, 2002. Dealing with bullying and harassment: a guide for nursing students. RCN, London.

Royal College of Nursing, 2008a. Dignity: a pocket guide. RCN, London.

Royal College of Nursing, 2008b. Let's talk about restraint: rights, risks and responsibility. RCN, London.

Royal College of Nursing, 2009. Dignity in healthcare for people with learning disabilities. RCN, London.

Royal College of Nursing, 2010. Restrictive physical intervention and therapeutic holding for children and young people: guidance for nursing staff. RCN, London.

Scottish Government, 2010. NHS Scotland Quality Strategy – putting people at the heart of our NHS. Edinburgh, Scottish Government. Online. Available: www.scotland.gov.uk/Publications/2010/05/10102307/0 September 2012.

Scottish Government, 2011. Regulation of Health Care Support Staff and Social Care Support Staff in Scotland: Consultation. Scottish Government, Edinburgh.

Thompson, I.E., Melia, K.M., Boyd, K.M., et al., 2006. Nursing ethics, fifth ed. Churchill Livingstone, Edinburgh.

United Nations, 1989. The United Nations convention on the rights of the child. CRDU, London.

Further reading

Beauchamp, T.L., Childress, J.F., 2009. Principles of biomedical ethics, sixth ed. Oxford University Press, Oxford.

Thompson, I.E., Melia, K.M., Boyd, K.M., et al., 2006. Nursing ethics, fifth ed. Churchill Livingstone, Edinburgh.

Section 3

Nursing and lifespan implications

Impact of lifespan on nursing interventions

8

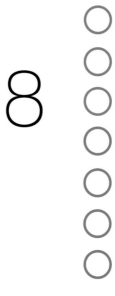

David Tait

LEARNING OUTCOMES

This chapter will help you:

- Develop an awareness of psychological and sociological aspects of development
- Describe the main stages and processes of human development through the lifespan in relation to theoretical frameworks
- Outline the main stages of physical development and milestones
- Describe psychosocial development
- Describe some common mental health problems across the lifespan
- Discuss the emergence of self and self-concept, cognitive and moral development and emotional attachment
- Discuss the main points of psychosexual development, personality and social integration
- Begin to appreciate the relevance of these events and frameworks for nursing practice.

Introduction

This chapter provides an overview of the multifaceted process of development that occurs throughout a person's life. It begins with an outline of two social sciences, psychology and sociology, with explanations of contrasting approaches to both. Key topics from each subject are explored, namely motivation, culture, socialization and family. Physical development is described from conception through infancy and childhood milestones, adolescence and adulthood to old age. Psychosocial development covers the emergence of the self-concept, cognition and morality, emotional attachment and separation, aspects of sexuality and personality, and social integration. Implications of this subject matter for student nurses and nursing practice are highlighted as they arise, i.e. its importance for nurses when planning and implementing patient care.

Psychology and sociology related to development and nursing

This section outlines the psychological and sociological theories, approaches, frameworks and important topics such as motivation and culture, required for understanding developmental processes.

What is psychology?

The word psychology derives from the Greek terms *psyche*, relating to the mind, and *logos*, meaning investigative discussion. In modern terms, it can be taken to mean 'the study of the mind' or of mental processes. It is clearly useful for nurses to understand what is happening in a patient's/client's mind and the resulting consequences, i.e. behaviour.

In 1879, Wilhelm Wundt initiated scientific research into the mind. Wundt aimed to study perceptual discrimination of sensory input under controlled conditions, and so understand what he termed the 'elements of consciousness' – building blocks of the mind. He described differences in intensity and quality of stimuli, inferring structural aspects of the mind – the 'Structuralist' approach to psychology.

William James likened Wundt's method to comprehending a house by contemplating its individual bricks, and considered the 'whole' mind as an integrated entity of more significance than the sum of its parts (inspiring the 'Gestalt' viewpoint, which gained currency from the 1920s). James was more interested in what the mind could *do* and its purpose, the 'Functionalist' approach. This focuses on thoughts and emotions, and how they help people to survive their environment. From these early origins, psychology branched into at least three distinct schools or approaches: Psychodynamic, Behaviourist and Humanistic.

Psychodynamic approach

This stemmed from Sigmund Freud (1890s onwards). Essentially, he emphasized the importance of unconscious processes in emotions and behaviour. Freud developed a therapeutic approach called 'psychoanalysis', designed to gain access to the unconscious mind, using means such as hypnosis, sedation and dream analysis.

Behaviourist approach

By the early 1900s, psychologists such as J.B. Watson increasingly criticized the subjective methods of Freud and Wundt, arguing that mental events were inaccessible to and thus inappropriate for scientific investigation; psychologists should concentrate on accurately observing outward behaviour, e.g. responses to experimental stimuli. Much of the behaviourists' focus was on animal learning, taking two forms:

- *Classical conditioning* – passively associating things that seem linked in time and place, e.g. Pavlov's dogs relating a ringing bell to imminent food
- *Operant conditioning* – noting the consequences of one's actions, e.g. behaviour 'reinforced' or strengthened, by gaining rewards, or weakened by ensuing punishment.

This approach assumed the validity of comparisons between humans and animals, and that environmental factors determine or 'shape' an individual's behaviour, including training animals to perform 'unnatural' skills. Psychologists could thus devise methods of 'engineering' people's behaviour in 'desirable' directions via 'conditioning' programmes. Behaviourism held sway until the 1950s, when its approach began to be seriously questioned.

Humanistic approach

A new school of psychologists, including Abraham Maslow and Carl Rogers, then emerged as a 'third force'. Humanists focused purely on human experience, including personal will and fulfilment. Their methods were subjective and person-centred, such as interview and self-report. Offshoots included therapeutic self-help groups and learner-directed education. Humanism emphasizes each person's positive potential and fostering appropriate choices to maximize their well-being and life satisfaction.

Applying psychology to health

The three approaches can be used to understand a health issue such as smoking.

- The psychodynamic approach would propose unconscious processes prompting smoking, e.g. troubling thoughts generating nervous tension, which tobacco alleviates. Smoking might also be an 'oral' pleasure or by-product of self-destructive instinct (see p. 161). To discontinue smoking, underlying concerns must be brought to awareness, so they can be consciously addressed and resolved. 'Orality' might be satisfied by other means, e.g. chewing (nicotine) gum.

- Behaviourists would view smoking as a learned behaviour, a habit created by associations, including routine and reward. This might include automatic 'lighting up' at certain times or under particular circumstances, e.g. after meals or when stressed or bored, gaining 'escape' from a hospital environment or to feel 'grown-up' or sophisticated. It occupies smoker's fingers from fidgeting. The aim would be to 'unlearn' these associations, e.g. suggesting changes of routine and using non-smoking facilities. UK health campaigns have emphasized tobacco odorizing of clothes and hair and quitters regaining 'a mind of their own'. Inconveniencing smokers, e.g. restricting smoking to outside premises, or delaying surgery until they stop are examples of 'punishment' within operant conditioning.

- Humanists would presume that smokers derive positive benefits from tobacco – often ignored by health promoters. For example, relaxed reading or drinking may be enhanced by tobacco smoking, a relatively affordable pleasure for the socioeconomically disadvantaged. The client would be encouraged to review their choice to smoke, comparing the benefits gained from smoking with those from stopping, e.g. improved fitness, longevity, disposable income and 'odour'. Humanists might also harness smokers' respectfulness by highlighting adverse effects imposed on others, e.g. fumes, coughing or harm from secondary smoke – especially in children.

Motivation

Motivation is the cause underlying actions. Without it, people would be inert and non-functional. It provides individuals with stamina and focus to perform activities.

Motivation explains behaviour; inexplicable behaviour appears fruitless, perplexing or threateningly unpredictable. Nurses need to understand the actions of others in their environment, in order to predict eventualities and plan appropriate interventions. Box 8.1 considers motivation to become a nurse.

 Reflective practice Box 8.1

Motivation to become a nurse

Think about your reasons for becoming a nurse; perhaps compare your reasons with those of colleagues, and note any that are different from your own.

Student activities

- Try to compile a list with several distinct 'motives'. These might include wanting to care for others, to work with and help people, or professional/career aspirations.
- Consider why people have different reasons for becoming a nurse.
- Read the theories/approaches relating to motivation (pp. 160-162). Then return to your original motives for becoming a nurse and discuss with a fellow student how they relate to the theories outlined.

The 'instinct' theory of motivation

Animal behaviour has been studied and compared with that of humans, deemed the most evolved and complex members of that kingdom.

Considering 'what makes cats hunt, birds sing and monkeys climb?', the usual response is respective 'instincts'. This poses 'what is meant by the term instinct?' One answer might be an unlearned behaviour pattern, more than a single reflex, specific to a species, elicited by a specific stimulus or 'releasor', e.g. a mouse appearing before a cat. The word derives from the Greek to 'impel'/'instigate'.

'Acting on instinct' is often used to describe automatic behaviour, such as using touch to comfort a distressed patient. However, the notion of human instincts remains questionable, as even characteristics like associating with others, sexual desire, aggression, parenting and intuition all involve learning and are not ever-present.

Early attempts by William McDougall to explain all human behaviour via instincts foundered; because of the complexity and variability of human behaviour, his approach identified innumerable instincts to explain why humans differ so widely in preferences and responses, e.g. only some humans hunt, sing and climb, and very few enjoy all three. This approach was also criticized for lack of explanatory value and circular argument. Asking 'what makes humans act in certain ways?' would be answered 'instincts'. To the follow-up 'what are instincts?', MacDougall's response might be 'things we naturally possess that make us act so'.

Freud proposed that just two instincts motivated behaviour:

- Eros – the 'life-force' promoting survival, sexuality and creativity, e.g. individuals' desire to live 'carrying them through' illness against medical predictions; patients persisting with unpleasant and expensive fertility treatment; and individuals damaging their health in pursuing their work or 'art'.

- Thanatos –the polar opposite, generating destructive impulses, its most extreme expression a 'death wish' (e.g. risk-taking behaviours like dangerous sports or unsafe sexual practices, recreational drug-use, deliberate self-harm, attempted suicide, the vicarious appeal of action movies).

Behaviourist theories of motivation

Lorenz demonstrated that newly hatched goslings follow the first large moving object they encounter in this early 'critical period' (experimentally either human or inanimate figures) – thought to be an instinctive releasor enabling them to be led to the safety of water. Subsequently, they seemed attached to or 'imprinted on' this initial figure, their particular 'Mother Goose'.

Critical periods in human development may include language acquisition (Ch. 9) and 'healthy' personality development – socialization (p. 167) and attachment (p. 185) – each dependent on exposure to normal human society in the first 4 years of life. Parental feelings and caring skills may be 'released' for the first time after having one's own child and

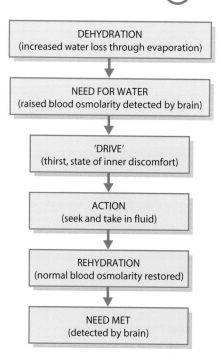

Fig. 8.1 • An example of a drive.

perhaps following a parent into the nursing profession may be an example of imprinting.

Drive theory

Clark Hull argued that all behaviour was impelled by 'drives', hypothetical internal states arising from 'needs'. Figure 8.1 shows how this approach can be used to explain increased fluid intake on a hot day, a homeostatic process (Ch. 19).

Hull's theory explains biological or 'primary' needs, such as hunger, thirst and sleep, but seems less convincing when proposing 'secondary' drives to explain wider human pursuits, e.g. intellectual or social activities.

Nonetheless, the terms 'drive' or 'driven' are often used regarding motivation, and Hull's framework reflects that it is sometimes better to want or pursue something than attain it.

Humanistic motivation

Humanists view people as uniquely possessing a rich mental life, including free choice of action, dreams and personal goals, rendering comparison with other species futile.

Maslow proposed a 'hierarchy of needs', explaining human behaviour. Although originally comprising five levels of need, two more levels were added (Box 8.2). Some descriptions omit levels 5 and 6. The goal at the highest tier is individual fulfilment (self-actualization), which can normally only be attained following satisfaction of lower needs. The hierarchy can be represented as a pyramid with self-actualization at the apex and the physiological needs at its base (Nolen-Hoeksema et al 2009), as shown in Box 8.2. Examples of how nurses may help patients/clients include:

- *Physiological needs*: Assistance in relation to nutritional and fluid intake (Ch. 19), breathing (Ch. 17), temperature regulation (Ch. 14), rest and sleep (Ch. 10)

Maslow's hierarchy of human needs	Box 8.2

7 – Self-actualization

Achieving one's personal aspirations and potential

6* – Aesthetic needs

Beauty in one's surroundings; an ordered environment

5* – Cognitive needs

Knowledge and understanding, curiosity and exploration; search for meaning

4 – Esteem needs

Being valued by others and oneself; a sense of personal worth and competence

3 – Love and belongingness (affiliation) needs

Giving and receiving affection; trust and acceptance of others, being part of a group

2 – Safety needs

Both physical preservation and psychological composure

1 – Physiological needs

Homeostatic necessities required for bodily survival

*Omitted in some descriptions.

and elimination (Chs 20, 21). This may extend to other nursing activities such as advising on sexual matters, e.g. family planning, as reproduction is another basic need.

- *Safety needs*: Include maintaining physical safety, e.g. against environmental hazards, protecting people from falls, traffic during outings or scalding liquids (Ch. 13), and infection (Ch. 15). Psychological aspects include offering explanation or reassurance before investigations/ treatments to increase patient cooperation and reduce fear of the unknown (Chs 9, 11), providing a consistent routine and minimizing pain (Ch. 23).
- *Affiliation or belongingness needs*: Enabling people to feel loved and not alone, e.g. by encouraging visitors, conveying telephone messages, displaying greetings cards, celebrating birthdays, organizing appropriate social activities and establishing a sound nurse–patient/client relationship (Ch. 9).
- *Esteem needs*: Nurses should be respectful towards patients/clients, recognize their achievements, e.g. progress in rehabilitation (Ch. 11), counter self-deprecation, e.g. in depression, reinforce positive aspects of their self-image (Chs 9, 11) and help them to feel/look 'their best' (Ch. 16).
- *Cognitive needs*: Provide patients/clients with the prerequisite knowledge/skills to optimize self-care (Chs 3, 11) and prevent relapse, keep them informed and facilitate active mental occupation, e.g. via reading materials, crosswords, television/radio, liaising with occupational therapists or employment trainers (see Ch. 4).
- *Aesthetic needs*: May relate to the patient's/client's appearance, e.g. help in selecting well-matched clothes,

organizing a hairdresser or beautician. Nurses may improve the attractiveness of care surroundings, e.g. tidying bedding, minimizing unpleasant odours, arranging flowers and recognizing important festivals for patients/clients, e.g. putting up Christmas decorations or helping clients to observe Diwali (Deepavali), the Hindu festival of light, in exchanging presents and managing illuminations.

- *Self-actualization*: Individual goals and possibilities may be heavily constrained by ill-health or disability. For some, being able to walk after an accident, or return to home or work after treatment, may be a major aspiration. A person with a learning (intellectual) disability or with mental health problems might aspire to a relatively independent existence in the community. Rehabilitation or recovery is not simply the absence of symptoms. It is based on hope, involvement, participation, inclusion, meaning, purpose, control and self-management, meaningful activity, employment, maintaining social networks and activities when distressed and having the chance to contribute, or give back, in some way. Nurses are part of the therapeutic relationship, skills provision and support network required, enabling the client to attain their individual aims.

Maslow's concept of self-actualization is embodied in *peak experiences*, moments of ecstatic happiness when everything seems to 'feel right', and a person's ambition is fulfilled. He considered that all humans were capable of these, although infrequently, some perhaps 'once in a lifetime'.

There are, however, exceptions to lower needs always preceding higher needs in the hierarchical structure. Reverse instances include:

- Fasting before anaesthesia places safety (level 2) before eating and drinking (level 1)
- People may pursue higher needs such as social, sporting, career and creative activities (levels 3–5) at the expense of their physical health or safety (levels 1–2)
- A terminally ill patient may waive analgesia (level 2) in order to keep their mind clear for crucial decisions, e.g. testamentary amendments (levels 5–7).

What is sociology?

Definitions vary, reflecting the author's standpoint. Macrosociology studies society overall, while microsociology focuses on individual interactions within it. All degrees of magnification between these extremes are possible, e.g. studying groups within society. Health applications can consider one-to-one dealings between individual nurses and patients/clients, the functioning of ward teams, types/grades of nurses, the profession as a whole, or the entire NHS workforce.

The focus could widen to cover people in Britain, Westerners or all of mankind. Sociology can therefore be defined as the study of societies, their component groups and individual interactions.

However, all sociologists would agree that people cannot be understood as individuals in a vacuum; humans are social beings. People arise from groups and from within society, and are part of its fabric during their lifespan; they comprise society, i.e. each person is equivalent to a brick in the building and society is 'within' everyone, as contact with others shapes each person. Consequently, appreciating this common social dimension enables nurses to understand others and themselves.

Several sociologists' views have been particularly influential over the past two centuries (Box 8.3).

Conflict approaches

These view society as riven by competition between antagonistic groups, each pursuing opposing interests, including:

- Marxists stressing economic disparity in Western societies
- Feminists protesting against male domination of wealth and social institutions, e.g. family life, politics or senior healthcare posts.

Conflict perspectives argue the need for radical revision or overthrow of society's attitudes, institutions and way of life.

Microsociological approach

This examines individuals and groups whose daily interactions comprise societal life, e.g. how nurses behave towards patients/clients and colleagues, experiences of student nurses in practice or whether nursing is a 'profession'. It views people as entering social situations with pre-existing ideas about themselves, others and the situation, e.g. their relative status and expected actions, and this subjective perspective largely determines interpersonal behaviour. Members of a society possess shared meanings conveyed by symbols such as language, gestures and other non-verbal behaviour, including dress (see Ch. 9).

Why is sociology relevant to nursing?

> No man is an island, entire of itself … any man's death diminishes me because I am involved in mankind; and therefore never send to know for whom the bell tolls, it tolls for thee.
>
> (John Donne 1624)

Donne observes how each person is bound up inextricably with other members of society, even if the person is not conscious of this communality in their individual day-to-day concerns. It is reminiscent of one explanation of why people are inclined to help others – the cardinal function of nursing. Due to a common evolutionary ancestry, sociobiology argues that as all humans are genetically related to each other, assisting others to survive helps preserve some of our own genes.

Knowledge of sociology helps nurses to understand the behaviours of patients/clients, families and colleagues. For example, a patient's/client's distress is automatically attributed to pain, or fear regarding the experience or findings of surgery (Box 8.4), i.e. physical or psychological factors specific to the individual tend to be the initial assumption.

However, patients'/clients' concerns often arise from a wider social context, involving worries about family members, employment or care of pets. A patient/client might be more concerned about inability to move heavy items at work after

---

Influential sociologists   Box 8.3

Auguste Comte

During the nineteenth century, the 'Father of Sociology' was positive that his 'Queen of Sciences' would establish truths about recently urbanized, industrial society and so be able to prescribe remedies for its social problems. He confidently dubbed himself 'Great Priest of Humanity' and his optimism has been shared by many of his sociological successors.

Karl Marx

Marx was particularly conscious of the extreme economic inequalities within newly industrialized nineteenth century society. He predicted that the masses of employed workers (the Proletariat) would come to realize their exploitation and the need to wrest ownership of factories and land, the source of societal wealth, from their employers (the Capitalist minority). The post-revolutionary sharing of society's 'means of production' would inaugurate an era of classless, socialist utopia.

Max Weber

Weber modified Marx's 'conflict' interpretation of society by focusing more narrowly and deeply on the perspectives and interactions of individuals and groups within society. For example, he noted the diverse skills, status and aspirations within the working class, which Marx had tended to treat as a homogeneous mass. Weber also advocated greater subjectivity within sociology, empathy being required to understanding the shared meanings in human interactions – Verstehen. An example would be to consider the many possible factors contributing to anxiety experienced by a patient newly admitted to hospital.

Emile Durkheim

Comparative study between societies was Durkheim's hallmark. He used newly accumulated population data, such as census information, to make deductions about the actions, thoughts and feelings of individuals. He came to view suicide as a reflection of the circumstances, expectations and laws of the groups, organizations and society to which one belongs, rather than a purely private, individual act. It is possible to comprehend phenomena like 'suicide bombings', only by taking their social context into account.

Park, Cooley and Mead

The nineteenth and early twentieth centuries saw huge expansion of industrial cities in the United States. Together with mass immigration, this led to many social problems such as crime, ghetto squalor and inter-group hostility. Robert Park and his colleagues used the city of Chicago as a laboratory for research 'in the field', while Charles Cooley and G.H. Mead worked on the social interactions of key significance in childhood development (see the 'self', pp. 177, 179-181).

Talcott Parsons

During the twentieth century, Parsons envisaged society as a functioning entity, with each individual, group and organization playing its part or 'role' to make the system work and deriving benefits in return for their contribution. This represents an alternative macrosociological ('big picture') structuralist viewpoint to that of Marx, both looking at society as a single, whole entity. Parson's 'structural functionalist' or 'consensus' approach views society as a harmonious arrangement wherein people basically agree on fundamental operational principles, making society function effectively. Each member works to benefit society, and in return society benefits each member, e.g. nurses provide healthcare, while potential patients transport them to work and staff the canteen.

Critical thinking Box 8.4

Michael

Michael is recovering from technically successful surgery. Despite receiving appropriate information and nursing care to maximize his physical comfort, he remains restless, tearful and frequently demands nursing attention.

Student activities

- Consider why Michael might be reacting in this way.
- Discuss the scenario with your mentor.

back surgery and the effects on their livelihood and self-worth than about transient postoperative pain or discomfort. Health professionals rarely gain such insights from case notes or superficial encounters with the patient/client; they often emerge only through gradual development of a trusting relationship with the patient/client (see Ch. 9).

Sociology provides insights into the nurse's own culture and other cultures, particularly significant with the increasing diversity of British society. Examples include social practices specific to members of minority groups. A patient/client or their relatives may feel offended if an otherwise caring environment fails to accommodate their cultural norms such as food preferences, consultation of their spouse or prayer requirements.

This awareness can also enhance the nurse's self-understanding, for instance by analysis of their own social experience, e.g. of an unfamiliar setting (Box 8.5).

 Reflective practice Box 8.5

Adjusting to new nursing environments

All student nurses encounter the unfamiliar in new placements, which can initially provoke anxiety.

Student activities

- What is involved, e.g. in settling into a new clinical environment?
- What social rules have to be learned, and why?
- Discuss the required adjustments with your mentor.

The environmental layout and respective roles of new colleagues, in addition to the names and needs of the patients/clients, must all be learned. The management style of the nurse in charge is important, e.g. whether using first name terms is acceptable and the time constraints for completing tasks or meal breaks. Appropriate use of initiative has to be gauged through experience, and may be different for a nurse in a student role compared with their concurrent part-time or former auxiliary role. Understanding this may help to diminish the stress of a new placement.

Sociological research can also investigate and suggest remedial strategies to wider social issues (see Ch. 5). This may include compiling and analysing quantitative data, e.g. the incidence of teenage pregnancy, and qualitative measures such as surveying attitudes, e.g. to binge drinking.

Whatever their theoretical standpoint/focus, social scientists provide insightful appraisal of social realities to complement or refute those of religious belief and secular assumption.

Common sense and sociology

Nurses need to consider whether sociology can enhance common-sense thinking (Box 8.6).

 Critical thinking Box 8.6

Is common sense all we need?

Read the statements below and decide whether they are true or false.

- A long and healthy life results from inheriting a sound constitution.
- Older people are repositories of wisdom and are consequently viewed with universal respect.
- The provision of a high quality, effective educational system that is accessible to all would diminish social inequalities.

Student activities

- Discuss these statements with your mentor or a fellow student and decide why your true/false decision was made.
- Consider the sociological aspects of each statement and their relevance to nursing.

Perhaps the best way to ensure a long life is to pick healthy parents, as longevity tends to run in families. However, although genes play a role in determining susceptibility to many diseases, environmental factors appear to contribute equally. This explains the close association between health and wealth, apparent in the significantly raised incidence of nearly all serious diseases in the poorest sections of society (Graham 2009). (See Ch. 1 and Further reading, Dowler & Spencer 2007.) Relevant factors include quality of housing, diet, occupation, leisure activities and, more controversially, healthcare provision. Thus a person's environment may have more significance to health than their genes.

Regarding the second statement in Box 8.6, most older adults retain their mental vigour, with around 1.5% of those aged 65–69 years, and 20% of those over 85 years of age exhibiting dementia (NHS Clinical Knowledge Summaries 2010). Older people undoubtedly represent stores of accumulated knowledge and skills, distilled into wisdom by a lifetime's reflected-on experience. Despite this, older adults in Western society have been typically viewed as redundant and an economic burden on the productive section of society. They tend to be functionally marginalized – excluded from the social mainstream – in, e.g. occupation and leisure, rationed in resources such as facilities and benefits, and viewed not with respect but in a derogatory manner, ranging from well-meaning pity to outright contempt, the many expressions of ageism.

Although education is often regarded as the key to universal achievement and equality, there is much to suggest that the Western system perpetuates and cements inequalities. Middle-class children tend to achieve more and better qualifications than their working class counterparts, perhaps in part because their parents provide better preparation, encouragement and opportunities, but also because they seem to relate more easily to teachers and their style of communication. This disparity is accentuated by other social factors that predominate in the working class, e.g. early pressure to earn, widely varying facilities even within the state system and peer group distractions. Thus, children from affluent backgrounds are more likely to progress directly to higher education and from there to better paid jobs, often in their parents' own professions.

Culture

Consider what the term 'culture' means to you. Common responses include normal patterns of behaviour within one's country, including eating, drinking and speech patterns, plus 'lofty' forms of social expression such as art, music and literature.

Culture can be defined as the way of life of a society – people who share a distinct identity, often within a circumscribed locality. Components of a culture include beliefs, values and norms.

It is important to remember that the components of culture may change within a society over time, allowing it to gradually adapt to changing circumstances and evolve. An example of this is the insistence in Victorian times that student ('probationer') nurses were female and would attend Christian services each Sunday, stay within the nurses' home when off duty and leave the profession once married – quite different to experiences of students of nursing in the twenty-first century.

Beliefs

Beliefs are specific ideas held to be factual such as faith in one God (or more, or none). Some beliefs may involve lifestyle issues, e.g. what is appropriate to eat, or how it should be prepared, varying hugely between societies, as does the acceptability of alcohol. Traditional cultures may revere people experiencing visions and divine voices, whereas in Western cultures, mental health services often intervene.

Values

Values mean broad guidelines, conveying what principles a society deems valuable and worth preserving. In the West, freedom of speech, occupation and choice of partner are highly prized, perhaps conflicting with values such as patriotism, equality of wealth and respect for older people, which may take precedence in other societies. Values tend to be more absolute than beliefs, i.e. subscribed to whole-heartedly or not at all, so that optimizing 'health' may either govern one's lifestyle fully or be ignored. The sanctity of life, i.e. that life is precious and should be prolonged where possible, is another value central to healthcare but not all human situations.

Norms

These are more specific behavioural expectations in particular circumstances, equivalent to everyday 'do's' and 'don'ts'. Tongue protrusion and bare torsos are expected from hosts at Maori welcoming ceremonies, but not at a wedding in the UK. Conformity increases the likelihood of social acceptance and success, often mirroring the underpinning value, e.g. paying for goods reflects honesty or adhering to nursing advice suggests a patient/client valuing health. Norms are often subdivided into folkways, customs, mores and rules (Box 8.7).

Types of norm — **Box 8.7**

- *Folkways*: Common conventions whose original rationale is obscure, e.g. throwing rice at newly-weds (symbolizing fertility), buying and decorating a Christmas tree, or referring to mundane events such as time of rising from and going to bed. Non-adherence tends to be condoned or viewed as harmless eccentricity.
- *Customs*: More universal traditions, whose original sense is apparent, e.g. shaking hands, singing national anthems, giving presents at weddings and birthdays. Non-adherence may cause offence.
- *Mores*: Strict regulations governing conduct, or 'thou shalt nots', which may be formalized in legislation (see Ch. 6), with punitive sanctions for transgression. Mores range from minor offences such as driving just over the speed limit, which may result in a fixed penalty fine, through more severe disapproval of theft – in some cultures punishable by limb amputation – to *taboos*, which are totally prohibited activities such as cannibalism, incest and paedophilia.
- *Rules*: Specific guidelines that vary from informal local instructions to written policies or codes of professional conduct, such as that published by the NMC (2008).

Cultural universals

As well as the foregoing components, certain elements of culture are common to all societies, e.g. language, both verbal and non-verbal, enables interpersonal communication (see Ch. 9). Mutual understanding of the spoken and written word gives members of a society a communal currency, unique where restricted to small populations, e.g. Celtic tongues in the UK.

Facial expressions conveying universal emotions like joy, sorrow, fear and surprise are recognized across cultural groups, but conventions governing meanings of gestures and acceptable degrees of interpersonal touch and distance vary widely. Other aspects common to all cultures, past and present, include:

- Religious ceremonies
- Communal buildings and housing
- Money and property
- Art forms including graphics, music and dance
- Humour
- Jewellery and attire
- Exchange of gifts
- Courtship and marriage
- Specific dietary and hygiene-related practices (Chs 16, 19).

Cultural bias and relativism

On comparing practices and underpinning belief systems across cultures, people tend to favour those of their own society. There are many possible reasons for this bias, including respect for those who have nurtured them, greater familiarity with their own ways and boosting self-esteem through criticizing foreign behaviours. However, in a culturally diverse society, this may lead to intergroup hostility and discrimination, then unequal treatment, e.g. in healthcare settings. It is important to remain aware of this tendency, and to try to accept cultural differences as indicating the distinctiveness of a particular group rather than their perceived comparative shortcomings. Indeed, aspects of Western culture might seem odd to an outsider (Box 8.8).

Reflective practice — Box 8.8

Some characteristics of Western culture

- Preoccupation with material goods
- Working hours leaving little time for family life or requiring delegation of child care to non-family members
- Pursuit of individual success
- Contraception and abortion practices
- Consumption of convenience food and alcohol
- Ideal of thin women
- Interest in spectator sports
- Pampering of companion animals .
- Overt sexuality
- Media portrayal of violence
- Pressure to observe seasonal customs, e.g. buying chocolate eggs, although not attending an Easter church service
- Varied political opinions and their free expression.

Student activities

- Think about your views on the ideas above.
- Discuss your views with a fellow student or a friend from a different background.

Subcultures

Individuals within a society form groups with distinctive views and practices. These variations inside a culture give rise to subcultures ('cultures within a culture'). One example is 'youth culture'; young people have independent values, beliefs and norms, e.g. in relation to dress, speech and musical taste. These may vary markedly from those of societally powerful older adults, who provide the cultural yardstick. Other variant subcultures include those of minority ethnic groups, students and healthcare professionals. Some subcultures openly defy existing laws in a society, and are termed 'deviant' subcultures, e.g. criminal gangs. 'Counter-cultures' are antagonistic towards the prevailing dominant culture, although may not break any laws, e.g. travelling people, self-sufficient smallholders and pacifist campaigners in the UK (Giddens 2009).

Culture shock

This term describes the disorientation experienced when exposed to an unaccustomed culture or subculture. Varying degrees of this occur when on holiday abroad, or when entering a new workplace or setting (Box 8.9). Admission

---

Reflective practice — Box 8.9

Culture shock

Think about when you started a new school, met your partner's family or commenced your nursing course, i.e. joined a new subculture.

Student activities

- Feeling anxious is inevitable – why?
- Were there any similarities to the stressors associated with admission to a care setting (see below)?
- What helped reduce your anxiety (e.g. preparatory information sent about your course)?
- Reflect on the extent to which nurses can help people to overcome aspects of 'culture shock' and discuss it with your mentor.

---

to a care setting may provoke anxiety. The possible stressors (see Ch. 11) associated with the healthcare subculture might include:

- Strange language, e.g. technical terms used by staff
- Changes in norms, e.g. regarding what and when to eat and drink, bed/rising times, taking medication, undergoing investigations, wearing nightclothes during the day, undressing in front of strangers, restrictions on where one may go
- Questioning values/reappraising priorities, e.g. health over pleasure, one's occupation and its pressures
- Threats to composure, e.g. facing one's own mortality, religious practices being compromised
- Tolerating other's behaviour, e.g. noisy staff, visitors and patients
- Challenged preferences, e.g. communal television channels, self-disclosure between residents.

Culture and healthcare (see Ch. 1)

A profound interconnection exists between these. People from different cultures may conceptualize health and illness differently, e.g. diagnostic criteria for mental health problems such as schizophrenia are dissimilar between Western and Eastern perspectives, while studies show wide cultural variations regarding pain tolerance (see Ch. 23), recreational drug use, e.g. of cannabis by Rastafarians, and sexual behaviours (e.g. involving the spread of the human immunodeficiency virus (HIV) in sub-Saharan Africa).

To deliver holistic care, nurses must be sensitive to the cultural expectations of individual patients/clients and families, without making stereotypical assumptions (Box 8.10). This may involve aspects including:

- *Health beliefs* (see Ch. 1)
- *Naming systems*: e.g. Sikh names comprise a personal name, a gender designation (Singh for males and Kaur for females) and a last/family name. Preferable terms are 'first name' rather than 'Christian name' and 'last/family name' instead of 'surname'

Critical thinking   Box 8.10

Cultural awareness in nursing practice

You are helping the registered nurse (RN) to admit an obviously tense client. The RN asks the client for his Christian name and is surprised when he challenges her, saying that he is Muslim.

Student activities

- Find out about Muslim naming systems.
- Ascertain the policy for name enquiries on your next placement.
- Choose a religion/culture that you are unfamiliar with and identify its usual practices related to activities described in this section.

Resource

BBC (Religion and Ethics) – www.bbc.co.uk/religion/religions September 2012.

- *Assessment interview* (see Ch. 14): In patriarchal cultures, a man may expect to answer questions and make decisions, or be present at interviews, concerning his wife or children. Nurses in the UK must be guided by The Nursing & Midwifery Council (NMC) *The code: Standards of conduct, performance and ethics for nurses and midwives* (2008), which covers consent to treatment or care (see Ch. 7).
- *Dietary considerations* (see Ch. 19): Proscriptions include avoidance of pork by Jews and Muslims, and beef by Sikhs and Hindus; many sects are vegetarian; vegans eat no animal derivatives, including eggs and dairy products; Mormons avoid caffeine and alcohol. Foods may be prescribed, e.g. Muslims require Halal meat from animals slaughtered in accordance with Islamic law; Jews require Kosher food prepared according to Judaism. Religious fasting may be observed, e.g. by Muslims during Ramadan. However, extremes of age or illness may be exempt from fasting restrictions and not all followers adhere to orthodox practices.
- *Dignity*: Members of several cultural/religious groups prize modesty and would be unhappy wearing revealing hospital gowns, or sharing sleeping, bathing and lavatory facilities with/being nursed by the opposite sex.
- *Personal hygiene/elimination* (see Chs 16, 20, 21): Hindus and Muslims prefer to wash using running water, and do this after elimination rather than use toilet tissue. Strict Muslims must wash before prayers. The left hand is used for 'dirtier' areas and the right hand for handling food. Women may wash their whole bodies at each personal hygiene intervention during menstruation.
- *Medical interventions*: Blood transfusions and tissue transplants are not permitted by Jehovah's Witnesses; Christian Scientists may refuse any treatment beyond prayer, even for sick children; Hindu women may refuse vaginal examinations; Chinese patients/clients may prefer traditional

options, e.g. herbal remedies and acupuncture (see Ch. 10) to those of Western medicine.
- *Family planning*: Many religions, including Buddhism and Roman Catholicism, disapprove of artificial birth control and termination of pregnancy. Many cultures such as Chinese and Indian prefer male babies.
- *Palliative care* (see Ch. 12).

Socialization

A society transmits its culture (or a group its subculture) to future members by this process. Thus, individuals acquire the knowledge and skills that allow them to function socially, leading to personal and communal success. Two phases of socialization are usually distinguished: primary and secondary (Box 8.11).

Reflective practice   Box 8.11

Personal experience of socialization

Think back to when you learned something from a parent or person close to you, from the mass media and from an RN while on placement.

Student activities

- Reflect on the agents of socialization in each case, your relationship with them and any feelings experienced.
- Did your feelings differ between the three examples and did this affect your learning? Discuss your feelings with your mentor

Note: You may find that emotions colour such recollections. As socialization is an interpersonal process, it often imparts learning in a profound and affective (emotional) manner.

Primary socialization

This occurs in early childhood, its main 'agents' usually close family members. The preschool child acquires fundamental social skills including speech, gesture and appropriate behaviour, and self-care, e.g. continence, dressing, feeding. Additionally, attitudes including moral and religious beliefs are transmitted. Sometimes teaching can be formal, or deliberate, e.g. tying shoelaces, but may be unconscious, or informal, e.g. a child overhearing their parent's private opinion about something. Due to its initial and personal nature, primary socialization carries long-term emotional undertones.

Secondary socialization

This refers to cultural transmission after entering school, continuing throughout life. It equips the growing person to survive and prosper outwith the family environment. Agents include teachers, peers (equals, e.g. friends and fellow students), work supervisors and colleagues, and the mass media, e.g. authors, journalists and broadcasters.

The term tertiary or 'professional' socialization (see p. 181) relates to the acquisition of knowledge, skills and attitudes required in high-level occupations such as nursing.

Socialization is a two-way process, the novice challenging the 'mentor' by asking questions and proposing alternatives, so that parenting involves learning from interactions with one's children, the same give-and-take occurring during grandparenting.

Roles

Functionalist sociology pictures socialization as gearing individuals to fulfil roles, social positions involving expected behaviours. Typically, everyone performs several roles, focusing on one at a time, including:

- Familial, e.g. mother, daughter, grandmother, sister, aunt
- Occupational, e.g. nurse, doctor, cleaner
- Miscellaneous, transient ones such as patient, client or customer.

Many roles have reciprocal partners, one to some extent defining the other, e.g. it is hard to imagine the role of nurse without someone filling the role of patient/client.

Each role can be viewed as benefitting other members of society but also the performer; although every role carries duties or obligations, it also confers rights and privileges if fulfilled adequately (Box 8.12).

Rights and responsibilities related to the role of student nurses (UK)　　Box 8.12

Possible rights
- Paid a bursary/salary, no tuition fees (currently)
- To be educated
- To receive free uniforms where appropriate
- A safe and healthy environment in which to work and study
- Supernumerary status in placements

Possible responsibilities
- Attend classes and placements
- Apply oneself to study
- Meet assignment deadlines
- Be presentable when on duty
- Conduct oneself professionally

Society can therefore be viewed as a symbiotic community, each role-bearer contributing to its smooth running, in turn receiving rewards such as healthcare, when sick. Parsons extended this to formulate the 'sick role', which people could legitimately adopt when unfit to perform their normal roles (see Ch. 1). Domestic inactivity and sick pay are granted if the person 'cooperates' in recovering swiftly (i.e. follows medical advice).

Role conflict

Fulfilling multiple roles can be a tricky balancing act. Conflict occurs where fulfilling one role impairs performance of another,

e.g. family commitments undermining study or nursing duties (Box 8.13).

 Reflective practice　　Box 8.13

Potential role conflict

Student Nurse Sarah has two children of school age. Her husband works full-time, and Sarah works as a care assistant 2 days a week to supplement the family income.

Student activities
- What roles does Sarah fulfil?
- What competing pressures is she likely to experience?
- Consider with your mentor how Sarah might minimize role conflicts.

Domestic commitments often reduce energy and time for relationships, study and work. Caring for older relatives can also significantly affect a person's own parenting, employment and personal life.

The family

The term 'family' pervades our world, evident in terms such as 'Father Time' and 'Mother Earth'. Political parties vie to be 'the party of the family' and espouse 'family values'; the family is regarded as the basic unit, or even microcosm of society (Box 8.14).

 Reflective practice　　Box 8.14

What 'family' means

Although used in everyday speech, it is not easy to agree on a concise, universally acceptable definition of 'family'.

Student activities
- What does the term 'family' mean to you?
- Reflect on the ways in which the family in Western society has changed over the past 100 years; perhaps seek the views of people from previous generations. Discuss with your mentor how changes in family structure influence healthcare.

'Family' means different things to different people, but is commonly associated with emotions such as love and affection (or mixed/negative feelings), 'togetherness', intimacy, shared experiences, communal housing, financial support, advice, the roles mentioned earlier and caring for one another.

Although people have different familial experiences, a general definition is 'a group of people, bound by kinship ties, who live together, share resources and look after each other in times of need'. All societies have some form of family unit that performs – some would say *controls* – essential functions including the reproduction, economics and socialization of its members.

Family structures

Family structures vary widely between and within cultures. Variants include:

- *Nuclear family*: Two adults, a man and a woman living just with their biological children.
- *Extended family*: Three or more related generations living in close proximity, including indirect relatives such as cousins, aunts and uncles.
- *Reconstituted family*: Two adults who regroup with children from their current and previous relationships.
- *One-, single-or lone-parent family*: One parent living with her/his biological children.
- *Gay-parent family*: Where a gay or lesbian person, often with their partner, brings up a child.
- *Polygamy*: A man or woman with several concurrent spouses. Generally illegal in Western societies, it usually refers to a man living with more than one 'wife'. It is sometimes culturally sanctioned to facilitate procreation.
- *Commune/Kibbutzim*: An arrangement common in Israel where unrelated people share living facilities and cooperate to produce food/income and provide mutual care, e.g. of offspring (Haralambos & Holborn 2008).

With its universal and pivotal position in society, the family has received much consideration as an integral part of healthcare provision or a contributing factor to many physical and mental health problems.

There are many ways in which the family may influence an individual's health and healthcare, both positively and negatively. These include transmitting 'healthy' genes or those producing abnormal conditions; providing the emotional climate surrounding child-rearing and adult interactions, e.g. loving care or forms of abuse. Communication patterns may be supportive or disruptive to mental health, and family income is usually crucial in determining material comfort. Links between wealth and health are well documented (Ch. 1); lifestyle choices such as diet, smoking and exercise are often influenced by domestic attitudes. Close relatives may be understanding of, or intolerant of, certain conditions, e.g. intellectual disabilities, mental health problems, substance misuse or HIV infection. Family dynamics may involve mutual devotion (or discord at refusing) to shoulder the burden of a family member's care needs. Relatives may also disagree with care decisions, e.g. prolonging active treatment or disclosing poor prognosis, and place great value on customs in a loved one's care or treatment (Denny & Earle 2009).

As with individuals and cultures, the family does not remain static but continuously evolves, adapting to changing pressures and circumstances. It represents a mirror of society at any given time, reflecting its development, limitations and current challenges, its successes and its shortcomings.

Trends in family structures

Considerable changes in family structure have taken place over the last few decades.

Examples of these trends suggested by Abercrombie and Warde (2005), which do not necessarily apply to all social groups or countries, include:

- Divorce has become more common, and death before retirement age is now a less common cause of family disruption
- Cohabitation of unmarried adults is widely accepted, extending to children being born out of wedlock
- Choice of partner is now less subject to constraint
- The extended and, more recently, nuclear arrangements have become less common, with increasing reconstituted, one-parent, and gay-parent families
- The average number of children per family has generally fallen in the UK, but survival rate has improved
- The importance of wider kinship groups, e.g. 'clans' and mothers' networks, has diminished and the family unit is more home-centred or 'privatized'
- Male status and power ('patriarchy') has been eroded, with more legal rights, work opportunities and economic independence for women; domestic roles are more symmetrical, with both genders contributing to housework, childcare and decision-making
- Families tend to be more geographically mobile, often prompted by employment opportunities. This potentially removes them from supportive networks, such as grandparents for childcare
- More people are following a single lifestyle for longer; women tend to have children later in life, an increasing proportion choosing to remain childless.

Development across the lifespan

Until Victorian times, children were considered miniature adults, pre-programmed for adult knowledge and behaviour to emerge. This view, implying the importance of growth in physical size and strength, changed with publicization of child exploitation and misery, e.g. in the novels of Charles Dickens. Protective legislation began conferring rights on children, such as education. Prior to 1833, under 9s could work up to 12 hours a day in factories. Only after the Education Act of 1870 did school attendance become compulsory for most British children until age 13; the leaving age became 15 after the Second World War and 16, in 1972. Another factor in reappraising childhood was increasing scientific interest in the process of adaptation following Darwin's publications on evolution. From the early 1900s, enquiry focused on how the concept of 'self' was formed, in parallel with Freud's ideas about unconscious processes being formative in adult sexuality and personality. The latter would inspire Erikson's model of each individual integrating socially through resolution of a series of 'personal crises'. The mid-twentieth century saw much investigation of how cognitive, moral and emotional maturity is acquired, e.g. the work of Piaget, Kohlberg and Bowlby.

This section outlines stages of physical and psychosocial development throughout the lifespan, plus factors affecting development and their potential significance to health. Developmental milestones from birth to school age are introduced, alongside the Denver II (Frankenburg et al 1990) screening test (pp. 174-175). (Readers requiring more information should consult the Further reading, e.g. Hockenberry & Wilson 2010.)

Physical development

This section outlines how the body grows and develops before birth and then through the stages of infancy, childhood, adolescence, adulthood, middle and old age. Chapters 14 and 19 discuss monitoring children's progress in height/length and weight.

Various hormones influence growth and development throughout the lifespan, including those that stimulate growth during infancy and initiate the events of puberty. Some examples are offered in Table 8.1.

Conception to birth

Every month following the establishment of menstrual cycles during puberty until the menopause (cessation of menstruation) approaches, a non-pregnant woman ovulates or releases (usually) a single oocyte (egg), from one of two ovaries. The frequency of ovulation decreases some years before the menopause. The oocyte enters a uterine tube, where it may be fertilized by one of the millions of spermatozoa deposited into the vagina by a sexual partner. The nuclei of the oocyte and spermatozoon (the gametes) each have 23 chromosomes (the genetic material), so that when they merge forming a zygote at fertilization or conception, the normal human complement of 46 chromosomes per cell is restored. Thus an individual receives half of their genes from each parent.

After 24–36 hours, the first cell division occurs, and mitosis rapidly recurs. Within 3 days, a cluster of cells about the size of a pinhead is formed. During the 2nd week, the cluster of developing cells implants into the specially prepared lining of the uterus known as the decidua, which provides nourishment until the placenta develops. The term 'embryo' is used from earliest developments until the 8th week of pregnancy/gestation. Thereafter, until birth it is known as a fetus.

The cell-mass continues to develop, eventually differentiating into all the specialized cells of the human body. Concurrent processes result in formation of two protective membranes, the chorion and amnion, that enclose the embryo/fetus, umbilical cord and placenta. The amnion contains (amniotic) fluid in which the developing fetus floats throughout pregnancy. The placenta, which has close contact with maternal blood vessels in the uterus, delivers oxygen and nutrients to and removes waste from the fetus through blood vessels in the umbilical cord. The fetal circulation of vessels and shunts mostly bypasses the developing lungs and gastrointestinal tract; these adaptations are normally reversed after birth.

Soon after implantation, the organ systems start to develop, so that a heartbeat, lungs and limbs are detectable within 4 weeks; rudimentary digits, eyes, ears, nose and mouth can be visualized after 8 weeks' gestation. At this stage, the embryo is particularly vulnerable to harmful agents such as toxins and microorganisms, which may have major effects on developing

Table 8.1 Hormones affecting growth and development

Hormone	Source	Effects
Growth hormone (GH)	Anterior pituitary gland	Stimulates growth in many tissues, e.g. bone and skeletal muscle Stimulates protein synthesis Cell growth and repair
Thyroid hormones	Thyroid gland	Needed for normal development of central nervous system Deficiency during early childhood results in small stature, impaired mental development and learning disability
Parathyroid hormone (PTH) with vitamin D and the hormone calcitonin (CT) secreted by the thyroid gland	Parathyroid glands (PTH); C-cells of thyroid (CT)	Bone formation, growth and repair
Insulin	Pancreas	Glucose uptake and storage; fall in blood glucose level
Glucagon	Pancreas	Glucose release and usage; rise in blood glucose level
Glucocorticoids, e.g. cortisol (see also Ch. 11)	Adrenal glands (cortex)	Regulates tissue growth, electrolyte and glucose levels Excess during periods of growth inhibits growth in height
Oestrogen	Ovaries	Female secondary sexual characteristics Female body fat distribution Bone density enhanced
Testosterone	Testes	Male secondary sexual characteristics Widespread anabolic effects on many body (somatic) tissues to produce male physique

(Adapted with permission from Hinchliff, S.M., Montague, S.E., Watson, R., 1996. Physiology for nursing practice, Second ed. Baillière Tindall, London.)

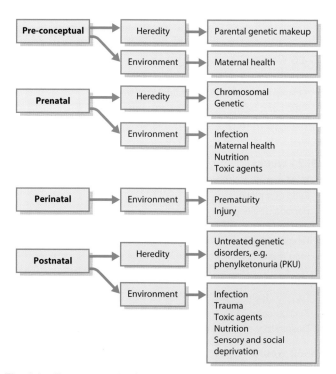

Fig. 8.2 • Factors causing learning disabilities by timing. (Adapted with permission from Watson, D. 2011. Causes of learning disability. In: Atherton, H.L., Crickmore, D.J. (Eds.), Learning disabilities: toward inclusion, sixth ed. Churchill Livingstone, Edinburgh.)

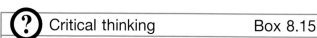

? Critical thinking   **Box 8.15**

Down's syndrome

A friend and her partner are planning to have a baby and she asks you what causes Down's syndrome and her risk of having a baby with this. She also asks what diagnostic tests are available during pregnancy.

Student activities

- Use the websites below to find answers to your friend's questions.
- Talk with a learning disability nurse about the ways in which Down's syndrome may affect individual people.

Resources

Down's Syndrome Association – www.downs-syndrome.org.uk
Down's Syndrome Scotland – www.dsscotland.org.uk
UK NHS Screening information – http://
    fetalanomaly.screening.nhs.uk
All websites accessed September 2012.

---

organs, e.g. the rubella virus may cause heart defects and deafness.

There are many possible causes of learning disabilities, either genetic (hereditary) or environmental (Fig. 8.2), which can occur during various stages of development, i.e.:

- Preconceptually, e.g. adverse parental genes
- Prenatally, e.g. Down's syndrome (Box 8.15), exposure to microorganisms such as cytomegalovirus (CMV) or maternal alcohol misuse
- Perinatally, e.g. insufficient oxygen or brain trauma during birth
- Postnatally, e.g. meningitis, brain injury and social deprivation (Watson 2011).

From the end of the 2nd month to the completion of pregnancy (usually 40 weeks) the fetus grows from 2.5 cm in length and 7 g in weight to around 50 cm and over 3500 g. Gender is distinguishable between 12–16 weeks (Serci 2009), while development of the brain, lungs and heart make viability possible from about 24 weeks' gestation (Bee & Boyd 2009). Box 8.16 provides further detail of embryonic and fetal development.

Infancy (0–12 months)

Although infants lose some weight in the days immediately following birth, once feeding and digestion are established, growth is extremely rapid, with up to 0.5 kg being gained per week, so that birth weight is usually doubled by 18 weeks.

Similarly, an infant can increase in length by 1 cm per week during this stage (see also Developmental milestones, below).

The first teeth erupt around 6 months of age (see Ch. 16); a delay in the eruption of teeth may indicate other developmental problems.

Motor strength and coordination also steadily advance during infancy. The head is disproportionately large, and requires support in the neonatal period (first 28 days). However, by 8–12 weeks, the infant's neck muscles can prevent the head lolling backwards, and by 9–12 months the infant will sit and latterly stand unaided.

Mobility also increases; by 3–6 months, the typical infant can roll over, crawl by 6–9 months and some walk well by 12 months.

Childhood (1–10 years)

The rate of growth slows, but by 2–3 years, children attain half their adult height, although less than one-fifth of a healthy adult weight.

From 3–5 years of age, size and strength continually increase, accompanied by apparently boundless energy, punctuated by the appearance of skilled behaviours, e.g. doing up buttons (see Developmental milestones, below). (For further details of childhood growth, see Further reading, e.g. Hockenberry & Wilson 2010.)

Adolescence (11–18 years)

During adolescence, the period between the onset of puberty and adulthood, further growth spurts are stimulated by the sex hormones oestrogen and testosterone (Table 8.1). This episodic sudden growth may pose challenges regarding coordination of a typically gangling frame. Self-consciousness is further increased by the appearance of secondary sexual characteristics (Box 8.17) with inherent, unavoidable challenges to self-image (see p. 173).

Summary of embryological and fetal development   Box 8.16

0–4 weeks

- Primitive streak appears
- Some body systems laid down in primitive form
- Primitive central nervous system forms
- Heart develops and begins to beat
- Covered with a layer of skin
- Limb buds form
- Sex determined

4–8 weeks

- Very rapid cell division
- More body systems laid down in primitive form
- Blood is pumped around the vessels
- Lower respiratory system begins
- Head and facial features develop
- Early movements
- Visible on ultrasound from 6 weeks

8–12 weeks

- Rapid weight gain
- Eyelids fuse
- Urine passed
- Swallowing begins
- External genitalia present but sex not distinguishable
- Fingernails develop
- Lanugo (see Glossary) appears
- Some primitive reflexes present

12–16 weeks

- Rapid skeletal development – visible on X-ray
- Meconium present in gut
- Nasal septum and palate fuse
- Gender distinguishable

16–20 weeks

- Constant weight gain
- 'Quickening' – mother feels fetal movements
- Fetal heart heard on auscultation
- Vernix caseosa (see Glossary) appears
- Skin cells begin to be renewed

20–24 weeks

- Most organs functioning well
- Eyes complete
- Periods of sleep and activity
- Ear apparatus developing
- Responds to sound
- Skin red and wrinkled

24–28 weeks

- Legally viable and survival may be expected if born
- Eyelids open
- Respiratory movements

28–32 weeks

- Begins to store fat and iron
- Testes descend into scrotum
- Lanugo disappears from face
- Skin becomes paler and less wrinkled

32–36 weeks

- Weight gain 25 g/day
- Increased fat makes the body more rounded
- Lanugo disappears from body
- Head hair lengthens
- Nails reach tips of fingers
- Ear cartilage soft
- Plantar creases visible

36 weeks–Birth

- Birth is expected
- Shape rounded
- Skull formed but soft and pliable.

(Reproduced with permission from Serci 2009).

Younger adulthood (18–40 years)

Early in this stage, most people reach their maximum height, because the epiphyseal plates (cartilage) of long bones ossify (become bone), preventing further growth in stature. However, growth in height may cease earlier in young women. It is important to maximize bone density during the teens and 20s (Box 8.18). Bone mass peaks during the late 20s but after 35–40 years of age, it starts to decline. Individuals are now at their peak of skeletal muscle bulk and physical strength, speed and athleticism, the cardiovascular system possesses its maximum oxygen-carrying capacity and immune responses are at their peak, so young adults recover quickly from exercise, injury and illness. Brain mass and sensory powers are also maximal, optimizing stimulus discrimination.

The middle years (40–65 years)

Most adults in Western society can anticipate living into their 70s or 80s, owing to reduced mortality from disease, occupational accidents, etc. compared with past generations (see Ch. 1). By the mid-40s there is detectable, but not serious, deterioration in all body systems (Box 8.19).

Even into their 50s, however, many consider themselves healthy and if no longer at their physical zenith, functioning at their best intellectually and socially – their 'prime of life'.

Older adulthood

Beyond the relative physical and functional plateau between young adulthood and middle-age, individuals must

Secondary sexual characteristics Box 8.17

Both sexes

- Growth and development of external genitalia
- Maturation of gametes (oocytes or spermatozoa)
- Larynx enlarges, deepening voice, especially of males
- Appearance of body hair, e.g. axillary, leg and pubic areas
- Sebaceous glands become active, perhaps causing greasy skin and acne
- 'Musky' body odour as sex hormones stimulate apocrine sweat glands

Females

- Breasts develop and pelvis widens
- Subcutaneous fat redistributed
- Onset of menstruation: the first period (menarche) occurs between 10 and 14 years, dependent on reaching a critical body mass

Males

- Increased muscle bulk and shoulder girth
- Facial hair
- Penile erections
- Nocturnal emission of semen.

 ## Health promotion Box 8.18

Eating disorders and bone density

Eating disorders such as anorexia and bulimia nervosa can have far-reaching consequences for bone health. Apart from inadequate intake of nutrients needed for bone growth and density (e.g. calcium, vitamin D, protein), there are other issues for young women with eating disorders. Those with a very low body weight may stop having periods and consequent lack of oestrogen risks further loss of bone density, which may never be rectified even if they gain weight and their periods return. This may also occur when young women exercise excessively without an eating disorder. Loss of bone density or a failure to reach peak density increases the risk of osteoporosis (see Ch. 18).

Resource

National Osteoporosis Society. Online. Available: www.nos.org.uk September 2012

Changes in body systems in middle years Box 8.19

The integumentary system

- Skin may sag; wrinkles ('crow's feet') develop around eyes and mouth
- Pigmentation becomes patchy and there is an increased risk of skin cancer through the cumulative effects of sun damage over many years
- Hair may become grey and thin in both sexes. In men, there may be typical male pattern baldness, although this can happen much earlier.

The senses

- Thickening and reduced elasticity of the lens of the eye results in problems with near vision (presbyopia), where the person eventually needs to hold a book at arm's length. It is corrected by wearing reading or bifocal spectacles
- Slow adjustment to changes in light intensity
- Hearing changes with an inability to hear sounds at the extremes of pitch. This may be apparent only on audiometric testing
- Sensitivity to touch and pain diminishes, although tolerance of discomfort may be lowered.

Cardiovascular and respiratory systems

- The power of cardiac muscle contraction is reduced
- Arterial walls lose elasticity
- The lumen of arteries may be reduced by hard fatty deposits (atherosclerosis), which raises blood pressure and significantly increases the risk of heart attacks and strokes (see Ch. 17) – the commonest serious health problem in this age group
- Elasticity in the lungs and lower air passages also diminishes, although resultant breathlessness is only usually noticed during unaccustomed exercise.

Body weight in middle years

- Individuals tend to gain weight steadily from as early as their late 20s until their mid-50s, a result of reduced physical activity in tandem with the same or increased kilocalorie intake. Women have a greater tendency to increase weight at this time, with fat accumulating over the hips and lower abdomen – 'middle-age spread' – whereas men tend to accumulate fat over the abdomen above the waist.
- For both sexes in Western society, obesity is of special concern for those in middle adulthood, being linked to type 2 diabetes mellitus, hypertension, cardiovascular complications and some cancers (see Ch. 19).

The reproductive system

- While sexual appetite (libido) usually persists, alterations in function become evident
- Between 45 and 55 years, most women experience the climacteric, including the menopause (cessation of menstruation), ending natural fertility. This can cause variable psycho-physical symptoms including mood fluctuations, headaches, insomnia and 'hot flushes'. The vagina becomes smaller and its lining becomes thinner. This can make intercourse uncomfortable, although sexual interest may increase at this time.
- Men tend to find penile erection slower and less reliable from middle-age onwards, with delayed and less forceful attainment of orgasm.

---

progressively adapt to the changes that accompany ageing, often advances of those which appear in the middle years. As indicated by Mader (2009), anatomical aspects include:

- Skin changes, e.g. wrinkles, dryness, reduced tone, widespread pigmentation including 'age spots' and slower healing
- Hair loss in both sexes
- Loss of height (1.2 cm per 20 adult years) due to vertebral curvature and intervertebral disc compression/erosion
- Reduced bone mass with increased risk of fracture, especially in women due to postmenopausal reduction in oestrogen; men exhibit this at a later age
- Usually inconsequential, but progressive loss of neurones.

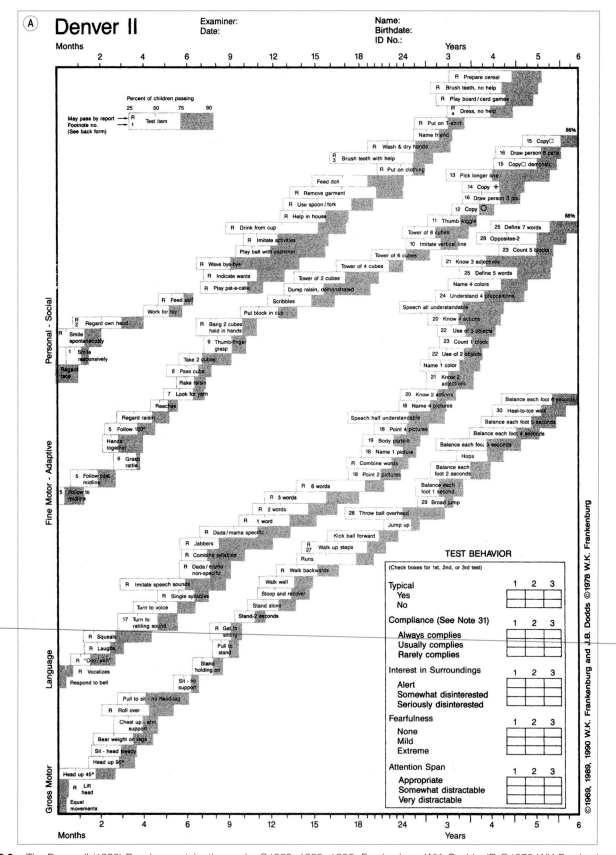

Fig. 8.3 • The Denver II (1990) Developmental rating scale. ©1969, 1989, 1990. Frankenburg WK, Dodds JB ©1978 WK Frankenburg.
(Reproduced by kind permission of Denver Developmental Materials Inc.)

Continued

B DIRECTIONS FOR ADMINISTRATION

1. Try to get child to smile by smiling, talking or waving. Do not touch him/her.
2. Child must stare at hand several seconds.
3. Parent may help guide toothbrush and put toothpaste on brush.
4. Child does not have to be able to tie shoes or button/zip in the back.
5. Move yarn slowly in an arc from one side to the other, about 8" above child's face.
6. Pass if child grasps rattle when it is touched to the backs or tips of fingers.
7. Pass if child tries to see where yarn went. Yarn should be dropped quickly from sight from tester's hand without arm movement.
8. Child must transfer cube from hand to hand without help of body, mouth, or table.
9. Pass if child picks up raisin with any part of thumb and finger.
10. Line can vary only 30 degrees or less from tester's line.
11. Make a fist with thumb pointing upward and wiggle only the thumb. Pass if child imitates and does not move any fingers other than the thumb.

12. Pass any enclosed form. Fail continuous round motions.
13. Which line is longer? (Not bigger.) Turn paper upside down and repeat. (pass 3 of 3 or 5 of 6)
14. Pass any lines crossing near midpoint.
15. Have child copy first. If failed, demonstrate.

When giving items 12, 14, and 15, do not name the forms. Do not demonstrate 12 and 14.

16. When scoring, each pair (2 arms, 2 legs, etc.) counts as one part.
17. Place one cube in cup and shake gently near child's ear, but out of sight. Repeat for other ear.
18. Point to picture and have child name it. (No credit is given for sounds only.) If less than 4 pictures are named correctly, have child point to picture as each is named by tester.

19. Using doll, tell child: Show me the nose, eyes, ears, mouth, hands, feet, tummy, hair. Pass 6 of 8.
20. Using pictures, ask child: Which one flies?... says meow?... talks?... barks?... gallops? Pass 2 of 5, 4 of 5.
21. Ask child: What do you do when you are cold?... tired?... hungry? Pass 2 of 3, 3 of 3.
22. Ask child: What do you do with a cup? What is a chair used for? What is a pencil used for? Action words must be included in answers.
23. Pass if child correctly places and says how many blocks are on paper. (1, 5).
24. Tell child: Put block on table; under table; in front of me, behind me. Pass 4 of 4. (Do not help child by pointing, moving head or eyes.)
25. Ask child: What is a ball?... lake?... desk?... house?... banana?... curtain?... fence?... ceiling? Pass if defined in terms of use, shape, what it is made of, or general category (such as banana is fruit, not just yellow). Pass 5 of 8, 7 of 8.
26. Ask child: If a horse is big, a mouse is __? If fire is hot, ice is __? If the sun shines during the day, the moon shines during the __? Pass 2 of 3.
27. Child may use wall or rail only, not person. May not crawl.
28. Child must throw ball overhand 3 feet to within arm's reach of tester.
29. Child must perform standing broad jump over width of test sheet (8 1/2 inches).
30. Tell child to walk forward, heel within 1 inch of toe. Tester may demonstrate. Child must walk 4 consecutive steps.
31. In the second year, half of normal children are non-compliant.

OBSERVATIONS:

Fig. 8.3 • The Denver II (1990) Developmental rating scale (cont'd). ©1969, 1989, 1990. Frankenburg WK, Dodds JB ©1978 WK Frankenburg. (Reproduced by kind permission of Denver Developmental Materials Inc.)

Functional aspects typically include troublesome reductions in:

- Sensory acuity, with obvious visual and hearing loss (Ch. 16)
- Muscle strength, speed of movement, joint flexibility (Ch. 18)
- Organ efficiency, e.g. kidney function reduced by 50% at 75 years of age.

Despite the increasing incidence of illness and disability with age, most older people, especially under 75 years, are healthy and independent. They retain their mental faculties and continue to enjoy life, especially if reconciled to adapting to their limitations. Although the proportion of older people in Western society is increasing, health-related factors such as diet, housing, technological and medical advances suggests their prospects to be brighter than for previous generations.

Developmental milestones

Human development is often considered a process of achieving competencies or 'milestones', i.e. the ability to perform tasks that society expects of its members. These competencies are acquired during physical maturation (increasing age, size, strength and coordination) and through opportunities for practice. Development is viewed as a complex interplay of biological, environmental and social factors.

The usual way of assessing an infant's/child's developmental progress is to compare their behaviours with those of the majority of their contemporaries. Following detailed studies, abilities have been organized into comparative grids, e.g. the Denver II (1990) (Fig. 8.3), which divides infant's/children's milestones into four categories:

- Personal/social – relating to other people and self-care
- Fine motor – adaptive: concerning vision and use of the hands
- Language – responding to and using speech
- Gross motor – maintaining posture and moving head/limbs/whole body.

Cross-comparison establishes whether a particular infant/child has attained a series of milestones established as typical for their age. This will concern parents, but compiling 'average' scores involves rating some children as showing behaviour relatively early or late. It is only significant if all related behaviours and overall progress are slow. Additionally, it is common for children to be advanced in some abilities and delayed in others, and for boys and girls to develop at slightly different rates (Box 8.20).

 Reflective practice   Box 8.20

Developmental assessment

In order to detect problems promptly, it is important to assess the progress of infants and children in attaining certain milestones, such as smiling or building a tower of bricks.

Student activities

- Think about infants/children you have met on placement or within your own family and reflect on their progress using the four categories of Denver II.
- Ask your mentor or a Health Visitor what physical criteria are assessed in infants/children aged 0–5 years, starting with the Apgar scoring system (heart rate, respiratory effort, muscle tone, reflex irritability and colour) performed immediately after birth.

Psychosocial development

This refers to psychological and sociological aspects of development. Stages are considered by age group.

Infancy and childhood

The main issues relating to infancy are considered under self-concept and attachment, below.

Early in childhood, preschool milestones must be attained, a process that may occur naturally, but may be awaited anxiously and require facilitation. By age 5, children are required to attend school, mix with peers and accept direction from unrelated adults (see Socialization, below), which can prove traumatic.

Young children possess enormous energy (expended in a shorter day than their parents'/carers' reserves), as well as increasing bodily strength and frame size. Awareness of this growing power, constraints from adults and intense emotions all promote behavioural problems. These range from tantrums of the 'terrible twos' to destructive rages, scuffles and vandalism in school years. Such features can be pronounced in the behaviour of young people with learning disabilities, whose psychological resources may be overstretched by the demands of normalization, i.e. the myriad stresses of life lived within mainstream society. In these situations, it is important that parents/carers consider communication strategies and useful environment modifications.

Adolescence

Physical changes during puberty generate psychosocial challenges for the adolescent coming to terms with new experiences, including:

- Sexual desires, fantasies and decision-making regarding sexual orientation (see also p. 190)
- Intensification of peer relationships
- Impending autonomy from parents
- Establishing personal identity
- Feelings of ambivalence towards the preceding.

All this is accompanied by cognitive, e.g. scholastic, and ethical developments that will be considered later. Teenagers are acutely aware of their bodily appearance and hygiene (taking much time over self-care), and concerned about issues of modesty and privacy, relevant to those nursing them. By the late teenage years, many have reached their highpoint in terms of physical suppleness, speed and reproductive ability, but outlets for these may be limited and restrictions resented.

Younger adulthood

This phase begins around 20 years of age, although attainment of adulthood may be culturally defined in various ways, e.g.:

- Reaching an age milestone, e.g. 18 or 21 years
- Related legal entitlements, e.g. being allowed to purchase alcohol, enter certain occupations such as nursing or have sexual intercourse
- Social events such as leaving home, attending university or getting married.

The nervous system functions at its peak, resulting in optimal ability to detect and memorize information, and solve problems. Physical attractiveness is often most prized at this time. Consequently, self-confidence may simultaneously expand. While such attributes may gradually diminish from the age of 26 onwards, factors such as experience, reasoning ability and motivation may more than compensate.

The middle years

A common psychological challenge for women in their mid-40s to 50s is the 'empty nest syndrome', their children entering young adulthood and leaving home. This can prompt women to re-enter the labour market or restart their career, which may coincide with marital separation or divorce. Career opportunities can, however, be offset by the need to care for older relatives. Childless women also come to realize that they are now unlikely to conceive.

Male awareness of sexual difficulties, occupational and relationship stagnation – perhaps contrasting with their spouse's new lease of life – and of approaching mortality can combine to precipitate the 'male menopause', expressed in introverted self-doubt or the purchase of a Harley-Davidson motorcycle!

Older adulthood

Psychological aspects of old age are well documented (Gross 2010), including diminished ability to solve new problems, memorize and retrieve information. As these changes seem negative and relate to loss, it is unsurprising that depression is common in older adults, and the prospect of ageing may be dreaded or defused through humour.

Retirement can be a rewarding period where the person has more time to devote to relationships (e.g. with partners, children, grandchildren and friends), hobbies and part-time or voluntary work. Lifestyles advocated for contentment in old age vary between authorities, for instance 'disengagement' versus 'activity' models (Gross 2010).

Mental health problems across the lifespan

The stages of the lifespan are associated with a range of potential mental health issues. Table 8.2 outlines some common problems, their presentations and treatment options.

The 'self' and 'self-concept'

These terms are used interchangeably when appraising how people think about themselves, their nature and actions, a process also referred to as 'self-awareness' or 'self-consciousness'. Generally viewed as a straightforward, natural part of a person's existence, the 'self' is a complex notion, unique to human beings, that is developed and modified throughout our lives. It involves forming the ability to simultaneously take the role of subject and object, observer and observed. Self-consciousness is particularly intense when a person is aware of being viewed as an object, e.g. suddenly finding oneself before a group of 'spectators', as when arriving late for class (Box 8.21).

| | Reflective practice | Box 8.21 |

Self-consciousness and nursing

Feeling self-conscious is an uncomfortable but universal experience.

Student activities

- Think of instances of self-consciousness during a nursing placement.
- Discuss with a colleague how this might be alleviated.

Possible instances might include:

- You are starting a placement in an unfamiliar nursing environment. Try to arrange a prior orientation visit at a 'quiet' time or with another student.
- Patients/clients often feel like objects when being examined or having nursing procedures performed. Try to maximize their privacy and dignity, and facilitate natural conversation when appropriate.

The self comprises three interrelated elements: self-image, self-esteem and ideal self.

Self-image

The first of these is the impression people hold of themselves, how they think they appear to others and the kind of person that they believe they are (Box 8.22).

| ? Critical thinking | Box 8.22 |

The TST

One way of investigating a person's self-image is to ask people to describe themselves. Kuhn and McPartland used this approach in their 'twenty statements test' (TST) of 1954.

Student activity

- Write down 20 different responses to the question, 'Who am I?', i.e. 'I am …' etc.

Note: There are **no** right or wrong answers.

Kuhn, M. H., McPartland, T. S., 1954. An empirical investigation of self-attributes. American Sociological Review 19, 68–76.

'Twenty statements test' (TST) answers may fall into three main categories: personality traits, roles and factual.

Personality traits

These are adjectives that allow people to describe their mental processes such as thoughts and feelings, or their behaviour. Examples might include: 'I am … *kind, caring, practical, hardworking*' (all good characteristics for a nurse) *outgoing* or *shy*. These can be grouped to form a personality 'type', e.g. traits such as 'shy and retiring', 'thoughtful', 'serious' and 'cautious' may characterize an *introvert*, contrasting descriptions such as 'sociable', 'lively', 'fun-loving' and 'impulsive' relating to the opposite *extrovert* type (Eysenck 2008). Hans Eysenck also distinguished between:

- '*neurotic*' (anxious, moody) versus '*stable*' (calm, consistent) and
- '*tough-minded*' – hard-headed, ruthless, versus '*tender-minded*', sensitive, empathetic types.

Trait and type self-descriptions are commonly used in everyday language and psychological research, and imply that aspects of the self are fixed once established, and can be compared/contrasted between individuals.

Roles

Related answers may include familial roles (see p. 168) such as 'parent' or 'sibling', or occupational ones such as 'student' or 'nurse'. There may be statements of religious identity, e.g. 'I am an 'atheist' or 'Muslim'.'

Table 8.2 Common mental health problems across the lifespan

Initial stage	Mental health problem	Presentation (signs and symptoms)	Treatment options/Recovery approach
Childhood	Autistic spectrum disorders	Impaired communication skills, restricted/stereotyped behaviour patterns	Specialized education, language/artistic therapies, dietary modification, varied psychoactive medications
	Attention deficit hyperactivity disorder (ADHD)	Hyperactivity, distractibility, difficulty following instructions, impaired educational performance, strained relationships	Supervision, ensuring safety; energetic outlets; minimize distractions; establish routine; encourage positive behaviours; dietary appraisal; medication, e.g. methylphenidate
	Separation anxiety/Reactive attachment disorders	Fear of parental absence/loss; insomnia and somatic complaints; shyness. Lack of/indiscriminate response to social interaction/physical closeness	Understanding support; facilitate coping strategies. Parental/carer education; family therapy (common strategy for all childhood disorders)
Adolescence	Conduct disorders	Aggression/cruelty, truancy, vandalism, theft	Social skills input; behavioural/family therapy, specific, e.g. 'anger management', challenging substance abuse
	Eating disorders	Range from self-starvation (anorexia nervosa) through chaotic extremes (bulimia nervosa) to obesity from excessive intake; preoccupation with food/weight, distorted body-image, purgative abuse, feelings of guilt/self-deprecation	Nutritional stabilization (may be emergency); psychotherapeutic approaches (individual, e.g. cognitive–behavioural or family/group); supervisory regimens
	Self-injury; Parasuicide	Repeated superficial incisions (scarring on wrists/legs); ingestion of harmful items (razor blade fragments, chemicals); 'suicidal' gestures without serious intention to die (e.g. summoning help after overdose)	Monitor for recurrence; provide opportunity to express/understand emotions and resolve underlying issues (counselling/group therapy); Family education; Supportive, consistent carer relationship
Young adults	Schizophrenia	Varied; may include deficient self-care/motivation, over-/under-activity, bizarre behaviour, incongruent affect, psychosis (delusions, hallucinations)	Antipsychotic medication, e.g. chlorpromazine, haloperidol; supportive nursing; family education; community-based rehabilitation
	Mental health disorders postpartum, e.g. puerperal psychosis, postnatal depression	Puerperal psychosis results in 2/1000 women requiring admission to a psychiatric unit (Raynor & Oates 2009). Low mood (plus anxieties about coping/baby's health) in around 10% of mothers postpartum	Admission to hospital with baby (prevents neglect/harm/disrupted bonding); gentle support; antidepressant medication; refer for counselling/group psychotherapy
	Personality disorder	Many forms; features include emotional immaturity, impulsiveness, dysfunctional relationships/role-fulfilment, dependent and antisocial behaviour	May be lifelong pattern, yet ameliorates with age; calm, consistent response; set behavioural limits; promote self-awareness; group therapy insightful; interprofessional support and communication vital
Middle years	Bipolar disorder	Extreme mood swings/activity variations, possible psychotic symptoms	Mood-stabilizing medication, e.g. lithium salts, behavioural supervision, prevention of self-damage
	Anxiety states	Feeling of dread, inability to relax, adrenaline 'rushes'; may have obsessive thoughts or specific fears (phobias)	Short-term/acute minor tranquillizing medication (e.g. benzodiazepines); psychological support; clinical psychology referral
	Abnormal grieving	Prolonged, ruminative misery following loss; delayed acceptance of reality	Individual or group psychotherapy (e.g. referral to CRUSE)

Continued

Table 8.2 Common mental health problems across the lifespan—cont'd

Initial stage	Mental health problem	Presentation (signs and symptoms)	Treatment options/Recovery approach
Older adults	Depression	Persistent unhappiness/joylessness; slowed movement and speech; lethargy, insomnia, poor appetite, hypochondriasis	Antidepressant medication, e.g. amitriptyline; monitor for self-harm; supportive nurse–patient relationship; psychotherapy
	Dementia *Note*: dementia is a syndrome caused by a number of disorders (Bridges & Wilkinson 2011)	Accelerated death of brain cells causes forgetfulness, disorientation, reduced awareness, decline in communication skills and personality changes; consequent loss of independent living skills	Terminal illness, though medication (e.g. anti-cholinergic) may slow its progress. Reminiscence, reality orientation and validation are among therapies that supplement increasing physical care provision; support family, e.g. refer to Alzheimer Society

Factual

Factual matters include gender, marital status and age (commoner if the respondent is towards the extremes of lifespan). Literal answers characterize younger age groups: children under 8 years often answer the TST in terms of activities, e.g. 'I am *playing*', '… *at school*', or even '… *talking to you!*' Between 8 years and adolescence, answers usually revolve around facts such as:

- Names, e.g. '*I am Sandra*'
- Sex, e.g. '*I am a girl*'
- Size, e.g. '*I am tall*'
- Nationality
- Age
- Preferences, e.g. '*I am keen on music*', or '*I am going to be a nurse*'
- Performance, e.g. '*I am good at football/sums/playing the piano*'

(From Miell 1990).

The relative significance of a person's TST answers can be gauged by asking them to be ranked in importance. This enables construction of a concentric model of self-image (Fig. 8.4), with the central part representing the most important self-descriptor and true 'core-self', compared with the progressively less important 'peripheral-selves' outside.

Physical characteristics, e.g. size and appearance, partially form the 'bodily self', or 'body image', and may be elicited by the TST if perceived to be particularly significant. The bodily self also includes sensations such as hunger, thirst, warmth, cold, pleasure and pain – common preoccupations during ill-health, and help to direct consciousness towards survival-related actions. It also covers anatomical components (body structures), which might be regarded as *the* essential part of people's living selves, although aspects are lost without concern, as when cutting hair and nails. Possession of body parts or even fluids can be an ambivalent matter, e.g. when considering donating or receiving organs or blood.

However, there will be circumstances where an adolescent or adult patient/client particularly fixate on the bodily self in response to the TST. For example, chronic pain, preoccupation with weight in anorexia nervosa or obesity, burn injuries, paralysis, loss of continence, breast removal or stoma-forming surgery; depression may also engender self-deprecation.

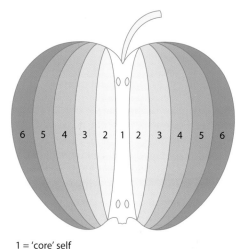

1 = 'core' self
2–6 = increasingly 'peripheral' selves

Fig. 8.4 • A concentric representation of the self.

Self-esteem

The ability to evaluate our self-image leads to the second component of the self – 'self-esteem'. This is how people *feel* about their self-perception, the degree to which it pleases or displeases, whether it is a source of pride or shame. People can vary in emotion when appraising themselves, from conceit to despair including all points in-between, and these judgements vary with time, behaviour and circumstances. Self-evaluation may be directed at specific aspects of the self, e.g. appearance, thoughts about issues or other people, emotions like desires or past actions. Alternatively, a 'global' amalgamation of such detailed appraisals may generate overall estimation of self-value at a given moment.

Self-esteem is enormously influenced by culture, which in the West values material wealth and individual attainment. An individual member of such society will have their self-esteem bolstered by financial security, ownership of impressive clothes, house and car, academic qualifications and a high-status job, often mutually contingent. Absence of such indicators of personal success is liable to lower a person's self-esteem, unless in non-materialistic subcultures, e.g. religious organizations or anti-capitalist protesters, which may prize quite different yardsticks of personal worth.

Self-esteem has a major bearing on emotional well-being and so is integral to personal happiness. If people aim for personal fulfilment and happiness, this implies an aspirational element to the self-concept. If self-image represents the 'person' that people consider themselves to be, the 'actual self', it may not be all they would like to, or could be. The wished-for improvement was termed the 'ideal self' by Rogers (see p. 160). Another way of tackling low self-esteem is to avoid exacerbating factors. People evaluate their self-image by comparing themselves with others. If inappropriately successful figures are chosen for reference purposes, disappointment will ensue, e.g. comparing one's physical attractiveness with a supermodel's or one's material success with a billionaire's. Similarly, a student nurse will feel inferior in poise and skills to an experienced registered nurse.

William James suggested a formula:

$$\text{Self-esteem} = \frac{\text{success}}{\text{ambitions}}$$

In other words, the higher one's expectations, the likelier they are to exceed our achievements, increasing probability of disappointment. This indicates the need for realistic personal targets, e.g. goals negotiated with a patient/client for rehabilitation. It could be equally argued that without aspirations, people are unlikely to improve or achieve anything significant in life. Rearranging James' formula gives:

$$\text{Success} = \text{self-esteem} \times \text{ambitions}$$

Therefore, nurturing high self-regard and goals is likely to enhance success, a positive view of the present and future self being conducive to generating advancement, e.g. in a student/nursing career.

Development of the self

If the self-concept is not innate, how is it formed? Piaget (p. 181) proposed that infants younger than 6 months are egocentric or self-centred, unaware that a world separate from themselves actually exists. It takes at least a further year before they develop realistic understanding of their surrounding environment and people within it. Studies of object permanence suggest that young children only have consistent interest in/concept of absent things and people, i.e. the 'not self', by about 18 months (see p. 182). Furthermore, Lewis and Brooks-Gunn in the late 1970s determined that only above this age do children recognize their own image, for instance in photographs or mirrored reflection, distinct from images of other similarly aged children.

This echoed Gallup's findings in primates, that only higher apes seemed able to develop self-recognition, dependent on previous early exposure to other members of their species. Naturally, this usually occurs, and seems essential to future social functioning such as mating and parenting (see Development of interpersonal bonds (attachment), below). From his results, Gallup asserted that the self is 'a social structure, and arises through social experience'. So, infants begin to form their self-image through being reared by other humans, and gradually recognize their form as similar to the children and adults around them, until they conceive their own physical boundaries and appearance towards the end of their 2nd year.

From infancy, children spontaneously interact with those around them, exchanging gaze and facial expressions like smiling with their mother, then during their 2nd year uttering recognizable words of their 'mother tongue'. Such symbols, along with gestures such as waving, allow shared meaning during interpersonal interactions, the basis for the 'social interactionist' perspective, originated by George Herbert Mead in the 1930s. Mead developed observations made in the 1890s by William James on the linguistic distinction between the terms 'I' and 'me' – both in this context given the prefix 'the'. The first-person pronoun 'I' is used to denote the self as subject of the act of thought, speech or behaviour. James likened this to a knowing but hidden observer, almost like an ever-active camera, operating within what he termed a person's 'stream of consciousness'. The 'I' might be equivalent to the essential 'core-self', a secret entity, unattainable even to its owner.

On the other hand, the pronoun 'me' refers to the self viewed or treated as an object, amounting to what is outwardly observable about someone, such as their physical appearance, clothes (e.g. when you ask another whether a new garment is 'me' or 'not me'), overt behaviour, even reputation. This evaluation is much affected by social influences such as perceived or anticipated opinions of others. Thus the 'me' may be modified to maximize one's self-esteem, and the 'I' in this framework makes these judgements and decisions.

Although the social interactionist model and its linguistic peculiarities/interrelations is complex, it suggests that consistent use of the terms 'I' and 'me' demonstrates the child's awareness of parallel existence of both 'self' and other people, and how their standpoints interact.

As well as through acquiring language skills, Mead contended that the self-concept developed by assuming roles, which occurs in the three stages of his own 'primary socialization' process. In the initial preparatory stage, the young child closely imitates parental actions, e.g. housework tasks. The child is very sensitive here to parental feedback, whether encouraging or disapproving, and internalizes implicit judgements (Miell 1990).

In the second stage, play often involves re-enactment of adult behaviour when the child is alone, accompanied by a commentary conveying previous parental attitudes, e.g. via praise or criticism of what a toy is being made to do.

Finally, participating in relatively formal games, the older child must adhere to rules established by others. To be successful, the child must learn to take the viewpoint of others, both on their side and in opposition, e.g. in ball games, in order to anticipate what others are likely to do. Thus, through each stage, the child engages with the viewpoints of other people, developing empathy. Eventually, they are able to imagine typical perspectives of those within their culture, e.g. what the average person might think of their thoughts, behaviour and appearance – Cooley's 'looking-glass self'. Mead termed this adoption of the 'role of the generalized other', providing a yardstick to evaluate one's 'self', a virtual mirror reflecting it as viewed by others. This limitless source of socially grounded feedback enables a person to subtly modify and refine their 'selves' throughout life, both in interactions with the agents of socialization (p. 167) and in moments of solitary 'self-reflection'.

Refinement of self in adulthood occurs during 'professional' or 'tertiary' socialization, whereby people acquire the knowledge, skills and attitudes peculiar to an occupational role. Goffman (1971) described the process of assuming behavioural elements of such roles in terms of participating in a drama. Initially, an actor may feel unnatural in a part, and uncertain about how convincingly they can fulfil a well-established role, just as a student might about performing that of 'nurse'. A professional 'mask' is self-consciously adopted to begin with, and feedback gained from observers, e.g. mentors. Aspects can be modified until the performer feels confident about fulfilling the role's requirements and can routinely 'play' it naturally.

To summarize, the 'self' is a vague, elusive concept. It comprises psychological and physical components that interrelate. People develop their self-concept in the course of continuing social experience, through their interactions with others. Their view of themselves is much influenced by their cultural milieu, and the reactions to them of people they encounter, both real and imagined. The self-concept is fluid; 'selves' can be adapted to varying situations, e.g. behaving quite differently in professional and domestic roles. Lastly, because the self-image is constantly evaluated, and generates one's self-esteem, the self-concept is crucial in determining a person's emotional well-being, intrinsic to inner contentment.

Cognitive (intellectual) development

The most influential researcher in this field was Jean Piaget (1896–1980), who helped develop early intelligence tests. These implicitly assume that intelligence is determined at birth/early in life, and that it can be estimated through standardized questions/puzzles. Piaget however, became fascinated with children's incorrect answers to questions beyond their chronological ability. He felt that these offered insights by reflecting the characteristic, if immature, ways in which children think. Consequently, he devised a series of tests specifically to investigate intellectual processes at different ages.

Piaget believed that human understanding of reality was not inborn, but had to be actively 'discovered' through interactions with the world, the child learning as a scientist would. Hence, intelligence 'evolves', like the characteristics of species responding to environmental challenges, promoting survival and success. Initially, reflexes ('automatic' responses) suffice, so the infant can derive nourishment from its mother's breast or a bottle's teat and investigate objects such as toys through sucking and licking. A comforting state of 'equilibrium' follows being able to 'assimilate' or successfully respond to encountered challenges by existing strategies – 'schemata' (singular 'schema'), the building blocks of Piagetian intelligence. However, the growing infant comes to find sucking and licking

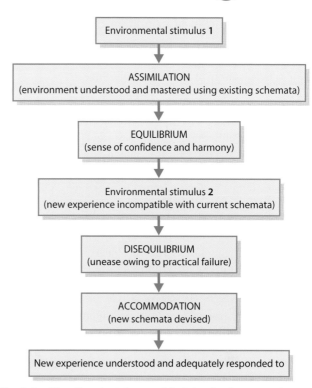

Fig. 8.5 • Piaget's adaptation model of the development of intelligence.

unsatisfactory for dealing with solid food or unpleasant-tasting objects, producing inner dissatisfaction or 'disequilibrium'. This necessitates formation of new strategies, e.g. biting and chewing food, scrutinizing and fingering objects, better suited to new challenges – the process of 'accommodation'. According to Piaget, this process – 'equilibration' – of employing old schemata until they fail and then replacing them with more suitable ones characterizes adaptation/intellectual development throughout life (Fig. 8.5).

Assimilation allows practice of recently acquired skills, e.g. in nursing, until we achieve routine competence in them. Accommodation enables formulation of innovative solutions to new problems. Both processes are complementary and integral to lifelong learning and development of the mastery of expert nurses.

An everyday example might be using chopsticks for the first time in a Chinese restaurant, which you might try if others do. Assimilation would involve using the sticks as a blunt spoon to scoop the food up with. Much rice and sauce will drop before reaching the mouth, creating embarrassment and frustration (*disequilibrium*). With practice, each chopstick moves separately, the tips grasping food securely (*accommodation*), the diner feeling competent and well-fed (*equilibrium*). Feeding dependent patients similarly involves new strategies, e.g. prior consideration of comfort, hygiene and dignity, discerning the desired sequence or mixtures, offering drinks and pausing until the mouth is empty (Ch. 19). All this occurs automatically when we feed ourselves (adapted from a Napier University Module booklet, 1997, 2001).

Piaget's four stages of cognitive development

Piaget contended that children progress through four consecutive stages to acquire adult intellect. Each stage has its characteristic schemata/way of thinking/intelligence.

Piaget envisaged intellectual development proceeding continuously, driven but limited by accumulating experience and biological maturation. His ideas have received considerable cross-cultural confirmation, although studies have since suggested the need for revision of details. Criticisms have been directed at:

- The questioning method adopted in his studies, perhaps influencing children's answers
- The age parameters accorded to the stages, now thought to underestimate children's abilities
- An adolescent end-goal of cognitive development, as this may continue developing throughout life.

Sensorimotor stage (0–2 years)

The title derives from infant 'thought' appearing limited to sensing events and objects, and reacting by muscular movements, e.g. reaching for rattles, crying if wet. Consequently, sensorimotor intelligence is 'practical', as infants react only to circumstances and objects that appear evident to them. It takes some months for them to show awareness of absent things, e.g. searching for objects that are hidden, even if they witness their disappearance. This convinced Piaget that 'object permanence' – objects and people accepted as having an independent and permanent existence of their own – has to be developed through experience. Piaget described the infant before acquiring this notion as experiencing pure 'egocentrism'.

By about 18 months, the child starts using symbols to represent absent people and objects, e.g. words, imitative behaviour and toys. They will ask for 'Mum' or a favourite soft toy by name, re-enact behaviour previously exhibited by others ('deferred imitation') and use a building brick as if it were a car (representational or 'make-believe' play).

Preoperational stage (2–7 years)

The child continues to develop use of language and other symbols, but tends to be convinced, and confused, by how things outwardly appear rather than operate on a logical basis, i.e. logical 'operations' do not yet characterize thought. During the first 2 years of this stage, the 'preconceptual' substage, the child focuses ('centres') on one striking aspect of an object, ignoring other relevancies. So adult males of similar age and appearance may be indiscriminately called 'Daddy', and four-legged animals ranging in size from cats to ponies are called 'doggies'. Moving inanimate objects, like the sun and moon, cars or footballs are deemed 'alive'.

By 4 years of age, the child progresses to the 'intuitive' substage, where some logic is present but intuitive thought, relying on what 'feels right', makes cross-classification ('class-inclusion') tasks difficult, e.g. comparison of toy cows, either white or black in colour. Identifying the more numerous colour is easy, but this sub-group are also thought to outnumber the total number of toy cows. However, this might be due to the task's lack of practical relevance to a small child. In the 1970s, Donaldson showed children the cows, some standing and others laid on their side, which she said were 'sleeping'; 4–5 year-olds easily judged that 'all' cows outnumbered 'sleeping' cows.

Before 7 years of age, the child still displays egocentrism, but a lesser form than in the sensorimotor stage, equivalent to relative inability to see a situation from another's standpoint. For instance, the child will know if they have a brother, name him, yet insist this brother does not have a brother or sister of his own. However, children expected by age to be egocentric can perform empathetic skills such as 'talking down' to and selecting suitable toys for 2 year olds, which inexperienced adults find difficult (Box 8.23), and understand that keeping a secret means that others are excluded from it.

Concrete operational stage (7–11 years)

After entering this stage, children become able to solve previously tricky logical operations such as 'conservation tasks', e.g. confronted with two identical short, broad tumblers, and asked when both are filled with milk to the same level. The milk from one of these is then poured into a taller glass as the child watches. The child is then asked if there is the same in it as in the original broad tumbler, or whether there is less or more. Piaget thought the essential indicator of attaining this stage was to agree that they were the same. Focusing on more than one feature simultaneously, 'decentring', allows understanding that height compensates for breadth so that milk transferred to a different-shaped container 'conserves' its volume and physical identity, despite its changed appearance. Preoperational children insist that the tall glass has more, even if agreeing that none was spilled in transfer. Other measures of conservation ability relate to substance and number.

One criticism of this research focuses on the word *more*; for a child below 7 years, perhaps the term simply means a higher level of milk or juice in a glass, so that the preoperational immaturity may be linguistic rather than logical. Another questions the method of enquiry and the power relationship between experimenter and respondent. How might a child interpret an adult repeating the question, 'Are both the same or does one have more?' after rearranging the test items? A child might feel that they should ignore what is logically correct, suspecting some magical trickery, or that they should change their answer to the question second time around, as a grown-up presumably expects this if asking twice.

Finally, relative terms such as *big*, *bigger* and *biggest*, previously used interchangeably, are employed appropriately now,

Health promotion   Box 8.24

Health promotion for different stages of cognitive development

Nurses in all fields of practice have an important health-promoting role. However, effective health-promoting initiatives require careful planning, considering the person's/group's stage of cognitive development.

Student activities

- Think about an area of health promotion relevant to your field of nursing, e.g. healthy eating, relaxation/stress reduction, dental care, hand hygiene, etc.
- Plan a series of health-promoting activities appropriate for each of Piaget's stages.
- How would you modify your approach for an adult with a learning disability?

Resource

Department of Health, 2010. Essence of care 2010 benchmarks for the fundamental aspects of care. Online. Available: www.dh.gov.uk/prod_consum_dh/groups/dh_digitalassets/@dh/@en/@ps/documents/digitalasset/dh_119978.pdf September 2012

 Critical thinking   Box 8.25

What can children do?

A series of practical, age-related activities are provided here for you to use.

3–15 months

Hide a toy behind a cushion. Observe if the child tries to search behind it. If they do, move it behind an adjacent cushion. Usually 'seeking' occurs from about 8 months, but the child is easily 'fooled' if the hiding place is discreetly changed, and until into their 2nd year, will not persist in searching.

2–3 years

Find out whether the child can consistently distinguish between different animals, perhaps using a picture book or visiting a zoo.

4–5 years

See if the child can play hide-and-seek, a game requiring participants to imagine where others would conceal themselves to avoid detection.

6–8 years

Try out the liquid conservation test; can the child 'conserve' or not?

9–14 years

Ask the young person, 'What would happen if people could fly?' In the concrete operational phase, this is either considered seriously or answered in a literal manner, e.g. 'That would be fun'; 'Where would our wings be attached' or 'Don't be silly'. Those at the formal operations stage are likely to be flippant, and suggest 'You could sleep longer before school' or 'It might save fossil fuels'. These answers reflect the differences between the literal reaction of children to science fiction and fantasy, viewing supernatural powers as something to emulate, and adults' intrigue about the interesting notions involved and their possible ethical ramifications.

Student activities

- Observe the abilities of children that you know (e.g. in a nursery placement or within your family) in relation to the practical activities.
- Consider their abilities in relation to Piaget's stages and discuss these with your mentor.

allowing accurate verbal comparison between two or more objects. The stage is named from the observation that the new logical strategies are reliably used only when the components of the problem can be seen or touched, i.e. they have a *concrete* presence.

Formal operational stage (11–15+ years)

This refers to the ability to follow the *form* or theoretical outline of a problem remote from its physical reality or lacking a concrete context. Examples include following verbal or written instructions rather than observing then imitating someone demonstrating how to do something, or being able to delay implementation of new learning. Comparing two absent objects, e.g. people described independently of one another becomes straightforward, e.g. 'if John is taller than Mary, and Jim is smaller than Mary, who is tallest?' – a transitivity test, requiring correct use of relative terms.

Logic can now be applied in an abstract way, making future practical applications easier, since general principles can be applied to many different situations, as in linking nursing theory to practice settings. The contrast between formal and concrete operational thinking is akin to that between insight and behavioural or social learning (Ch. 4). However, there is some doubt if all or even most adults function consistently at this level, as adults may persist in using trial and error or observational approaches to tasks solvable through creative, abstract thinking, sometimes with frustrating results. For example, when setting up unfamiliar equipment, one can push buttons randomly or ask another's opinion, rather than consulting written instructions.

Hypothetical thinking enables consideration of (im)possibilities, e.g. science fiction, surreal humour and alternative courses of action, leading to some of the conflicts that typify adolescence, e.g. friction with elders, personal identity crises and vacillation over career choice.

Formal operational thought represents the highest level of thinking in Piaget's model. People with learning disabilities may have particular difficulty with formal operational thinking, as it requires intellectual ability at the level of secondary school age. They may benefit from practical demonstrations and supervised experience, e.g. in living skills and health promotion, rather than more abstract methods of verbal or written explanation (Box 8.24).

Box 8.25 provides an opportunity to consider what children can do, and relates practical observations to Piaget's four stages.

Alternative theories of intellectual development

Jerome Bruner studied the changing ways in which the child represents the world. In the initial 'enactive' stage this is through actions, i.e. motor responses, akin to Piaget's sensori-motor stage. In the following 'iconic' stage, formation of mental images becomes paramount, roughly equivalent to preoccupation with appearances in Piaget's preoperational stage. Finally, around 7 years of age, the 'symbolic' stage commences, in which use of increasingly sophisticated language directs thought and its development. Piaget preferred to regard changes in language usage as reflecting rather than engineering cognitive advances. Research tends to support his opinion, e.g. deaf children's language skills are typically delayed more than their thinking abilities.

In the 1930s, Vygotsky also argued the importance of inner speech or verbal thought in development. He considered this and other forms of social activity as instrumental in encouraging problem-solving and self-sufficiency. For example, an adult may tutor a child in tasks such as dressing through general advice or specific prompts, providing the 'apprentice' with the 'scaffolding' of another's experience, accelerating mastery. Student nurses can similarly benefit from practical expertise passed on by mentors. Cultural learning is similarly imparted by interpersonal means between generations (p. 167), and people's most highly developed cognitive skills tend to be those most valued by the society to which they belong (Gross 2010).

Cognitive approaches to moral development

Cognitive approaches also regard morality as developing through childhood and adolescence via a predictable succession of distinctive stages.

In Piaget's view, 5–9-year-olds conceive morality as an absolute system of rules and sanctions directed by higher/adult authorities ('external' morality), demanding one-sided respect, with obedience a virtue in itself ('moral realism'). The over-10s increasingly feel reliant on their own principles of right and wrong ('internal' morality), which evolve through mutual negotiation. Lying to an adult is now viewed as no worse than to a peer. Understanding and respecting the viewpoints of others becomes a prerequisite of trusting social relationships ('moral relativism'). Piaget considered that these qualitative ethical changes result from, therefore lag behind, the cognitive transformations (e.g. reduced egocentrism and ability to decentre) which typify attainment of operational thought.

Kohlberg's work

In the mid-1950s, Kohlberg designed nine scenarios with moral dilemmas, i.e. problems juxtaposing two or more ethical principles, impossible to resolve entirely satisfactorily (see Ch. 7).

What interested Kohlberg was the rationale given for favouring one course of action over another. Analysis of participant responses led him to formulate a theory that individuals can progress through three levels of moral development, each comprising two substages and, like Piaget's types of morality, contingent on preceding intellectual advances (Box 8.26).

Kohlberg's stages of moral development	Box 8.26

I – Pre-conventional morality

Stage 1 – Moral behaviour is what goes unpunished by authority

Stage 2 – Moral acts are those that are rewarded

II – Conventional morality

Stage 3 – Moral behaviour is that which would please most other people

Stage 4 – Moral acts constitute performing one's public duty

III – Post-conventional morality

Stage 5 – Moral behaviour must adhere to applicable democratic laws

Stage 6 – Moral behaviour is purely a matter of individual conscience

---

Kohlberg reported that only 20% of adults are governed by 'post-conventional' morality and just 10–15% operate on the most advanced sub-level. This finding may relate to the limited proportion of adults who consistently demonstrate Piaget's formal operational thought. As well as advancing through cumulative reasoning ability, Kohlberg thought that morality developed alongside biological maturation and practical challenges within new social experiences. His work has received criticism on the basis of his research methods (seen as both subjective and abstract) and his implicit assumptions, e.g. that 'Western liberal' morality is superior to a 'traditional conservative' standpoint. However, it may be the best explanation of how a child's pragmatic sense of right and wrong may progress to generalized ethical codes in adulthood.

Alternative theories of moral development

The cognitive approach of Piaget and Kohlberg may downplay the emotional aspect of moral development, integral to the alternative approaches to moral development discussed below.

Freudian psychodynamic theory and moral development

Freud proposed that innate, amoral ('id') impulses from infancy until around 4 years of age are tempered by the ('ego') assessing 'what can be got away with'. At around 5 years of age, the conscience ('superego') emerges through identification with the words and deeds of one's same-sex parent and 'internalizing' his or her values. The self is punished for the 'should-nots' it commits, engendering guilt, while fulfilling moral obligations generates self-satisfaction and pride. Conscience thus comes to replace parental authority as an internal moral watchdog. Freud contended that sexual and aggressive impulses that cannot be expressed are forced out of conscious awareness (see Defence mechanisms, pp. 187, 188, and Ch. 11).

Behaviourism (conditioning)

Eysenck suggested that people learn from childhood to connect wrongdoing with punishment through recollecting past associations; thereafter even anticipating misdeeds may arouse negative emotions like fear and guilt. Similarly, good deeds are associated with rewards e.g. praise and ensuing pleasant feelings like self-congratulation. Moral behaviour is usually thus 'reinforced' and predominant.

Social observational learning theory

In the 1960s, Bandura emphasized the significance of other individuals, known as 'models', that people observe from childhood onwards and whose behaviour they come to emulate. These include relatives, acquaintances, sporting champions, celebrities and fictional characters in various entertainment media. Factors influencing the likelihood of 'modelling' include perceived similarities between observer and model (e.g. gender, age, ethnicity, culture, status and personal qualities), and whether the model's behaviour has positive consequences.

Development of interpersonal bonds (attachment)

This process occurs with particular intensity during preschool childhood, the nature of the experience being of lifelong significance. Formation of these bonds is referred to as 'attachment', their severance, whether temporary or permanent, as 'separation'.

Infants tend to receive adult attention due to their natural attractiveness and the curiosity they arouse, as well as any parenting instinct they evoke. By 6 weeks of age, infants smile at human faces, then after 3 months seem able to distinguish familiar ones from those of strangers, showing increasing discomfiture at the latter. They actively engage in exchanges of expression, like mutual gazing for up to 20 seconds and reciprocal smiling, and seem able to detect differing moods through facial scrutiny, e.g. appearing perplexed if mother maintains a blank expression.

By 6 or 7 months of age, children should start to form a lasting emotional bond or attachment to one specific adult, usually the natural mother. Attachment will further develop until the child is around 3 years old (Bowlby 2005). This is inferred from the child attending to and seeking attention from this 'figure', and craving physical closeness to them. The toddler typically shows distress on separation and relief when reunited. Accordingly, Bowlby described attachment behaviour as the child's 'first love affair'.

It was initially suggested that infants become attached to the person who feeds them, i.e. essentially motivated by the need to secure nourishment. As the child relies on its mother to satisfy primary drives (see p. 161) such as hunger and thirst, it develops a secondary drive for this service supplier.

However, Harlow's work with infant Rhesus monkeys separated from their mothers and all such monkeys at birth, suggested otherwise. They preferred to cling to a cloth-covered contraption which rocked soothingly rather than a wire 'mother' containing their milk-feeding bottle, suggesting warmth and comforting physical contact to be the more powerful attraction.

Later, it was argued that the attachment figure is the person who usually responds to the human infant's behaviour in general and is the main provider of stimulation. Sometimes this might be father, who perhaps returning from outside work, having had little to do with feeding or comforting, becomes the child's preferred playmate, his stimulating intermittent interactions, e.g. energetic games or bedtime story-reading, proving important in attaching his child to him. As the child ages, it may develop multiple attachments, e.g. to grandparents, aunts and uncles, older siblings, neighbours and nursery carers, who substitute for maternal absences with minimal emotional upset.

The significance of attachment

Fear of strangers, some of whom might be ill-intentioned, and of isolation from the dependable adult that provides care has significant survival value to vulnerable youngsters. The attachment figure also acts as a safe base from which to explore things, places and people, so paving the way for future 'detachment' and self-sufficiency.

Bowlby believed that continuous loving care in early childhood was a prerequisite for developing interpersonal trust and fulfilling emotional relationships in adulthood. It is therefore crucial to a person's future social competence, happiness and mental health, 'as important to the latter as vitamins to physical health' (Bowlby 2005).

Reactions to separation from attachment figures

In the 1950s, evidence filmed by James and Joyce Robertson on the distressed behaviour of hospitalized children startled many childcare professionals (Box 8.27).

 Reflective practice Box 8.27

Separation anxiety

You may observe this occurring with your own children or during a nursery placement. Think of occasions when parents leave their children in the care of unrelated adults, e.g. at nurseries or in hospital.

Student activities

- Did you witness any signs of separation anxiety?
- Do children react any differently to separation from their fathers, compared with their mothers?
- Does it make a difference if the 'replacement' carers are familiar to the child?
- Reflect on your observations and discuss them with a fellow student.

Subsequently, Bowlby described three behavioural stages typifying children in these circumstances:

- *Protest*: The child cries and fights to cling onto the departing mother/person. After separation, intermittent distress is evident.
- *Despair*: After a week's separation, the child becomes apathetic and inconsolably sad, possibly blaming himself for his mother's absence; her future return seemingly no longer anticipated.
- *Detachment*: Later, the child begins to respond again to others, e.g. nurses. When reunited with his mother, he may rebuff her and take time to 'relearn' their original loving, trusting bond.

These stages recall those described in various models of loss and bereavement (see Ch. 12) and suggest that separation from the mother can be emotionally traumatic for a preschool child. Bowlby used the term 'maternal deprivation' to convey the effects of such separation when prolonged, although this is criticized for implying that only the mother is important in childhood attachment. Some specific situations where attachment is likely to be significant are discussed below.

Looked-after children, fostering and adoption

There have been concerns about effects of institutional care on orphans and whether children really need to attach to replacement parents early in life. In 1978, Tizard and Hodges observed that 4-year-olds domiciled in institutions were over-friendly towards strangers and 'clingy' towards carers. These children seemed unselective and superficial in their attachments, displaying little emotion when staff members left (possibly a self-protectory response following repeated separation/loss experiences) and quarrelsome with their peers (Hayes 2000). Adopted children reportedly fared better scholastically and emotionally than those returned to their biological parents, although socioeconomic factors may partially account for this (Meggitt 2006). Other studies suggest that adopted adolescents display significant adjustment and behavioural problems, unless adoption had occurred in infancy (Santrock 2009), and offer support for Bowlby's theory.

Working mothers

Dr Benjamin Spock expressed influential concerns in the 1950s that children might be damaged if denied continuous mothering. However, many children may benefit from the stimulation of substitute carers and unrelated children in nurseries. Moreover, their mothers' psychological (plus financial) well-being may be significantly enhanced through working outside the home, through adult social contact and occupational stimulation. Preschool children may form multiple attachments, including with regular carers at nursery or child-minders, but still show obvious emotional preference for their returning parent.

Hospitalization

Separation due to hospitalization is stressful for both child and parents, whichever is the patient/client. Separation can occur in widely varying circumstances and hospitals now have a range of measures to minimize its impact (Box 8.28).

Parental loss by death or divorce

Bowlby's theory would predict no differences in children's emotional reaction to loss of a parent through death, parental break-up or abandonment, all being permanent separations from an attachment figure (see Ch. 12).

Evidence has suggested that divorce increases the likelihood of antisocial behaviour, particularly in boys, as does separation from both parents, but only if preceded by prolonged and severe marital disharmony. This leads to the conclusion that amicable parting of parents is preferable to continuing marital strife for their children's mental well-being (Hayes 2000). There are also well-established links between parental loss in childhood and depression (and increased risk of divorce) in adulthood (McLeod 1991).

? Critical thinking Box 8.28

Reducing the effects of separation for parent and child in hospital

It is accepted that separation due to hospitalization causes distress to children and their parents.

Student activities

1. Choose circumstances relevant to your field of nursing, e.g.:
   - Full-term neonates
   - Pre-term babies requiring special or intensive care
   - Young children under 5 years
   - Mothers who have been admitted for treatment
   - Palliative care.
2. Find out what strategies are in place within your particular field of practice to reduce the effects of parent–child separation.

Resources

Action for Sick Children – http://actionforsickchildren.org/ October 2012.

Variations in the attachment process

Ainsworth et al (1978) distinguished between:

- *Secure attachment* (characterizing about two-thirds of children): The child uses the mother as a base for exploring or playing, returning periodically for comforting contact. Brief separations are tolerated, reunions joyful.
- *Insecure avoidant attachment*: Mother is avoided or ignored on returning, comfort from others being accepted.
- *Insecure ambivalent attachment*: Maternal departure distresses the child, who rejects physical contact with his reappearing mother.

Secure attachment has been linked to social assurance and emotional balance, regarded as a kind of psychological 'immune system' for future mental resilience (Holmes 2001). Other factors such as later life experiences and family stressors are, however, likely to be significant, and insecure attachment does not invariably foreshadow future psychological problems.

The nature of the attachment relationship appears to stem partly from parental approach. If consistently loving, sensitive and responsive, the secure pattern usually follows. If neglectful, critical or abusive, the insecure forms seem likelier. The child itself may also be influential, e.g. an unwell child may demand more parental interventions, and the youngster's personality may also be significant. Thomas and Chess (1977) described three types of infant temperament/natural predisposition:

- *Easy* (the most common) – the child is typically predictable, cheery and unfussy
- *Difficult* – the opposite of easy, above
- *Slow to warm up* – the child is wary of new situations, but usually contented once 'familiarized'

These early characteristics seem not to indicate a child's future personality. Parents may also vary in preference regarding their child's temperament. A mother lacking confidence might be reassured about her competence by an 'easy' infant, while one domineered as a child herself may welcome the assertive behaviour of a 'difficult' baby.

Culture and genetics may also be of significance. Chinese infants appear more restrained, calm and easily soothed than Caucasian ones. This could reflect inherited characteristics or the value placed by Chinese culture on self-control. Chinese-American parents are reported as less likely than other North American racial groups to encourage their infants' smiling and vocalizing, or independent play (Bernstein et al 2007). Such factors may in turn influence the attachment process.

Freud's psychodynamic theory

Sigmund Freud (1856–1939) published numerous works to explain his medical treatment, psychoanalysis. Its underpinning psychodynamic theory conceives mental processes as heavily influenced by interplay between three active and largely unconscious structures, namely the:

- Id
- Ego
- Superego.

The id constitutes the inborn source of mental energy, generated by two antagonistic instincts, Eros and Thanatos (p. 161). Eros represents the positive life-drive, whose energy, the libido, impels behaviour conducive to survival (including feeding and reproduction). Meeting such needs involves self-gratification, so the id is described as operating via the 'pleasure principle'. The opposing instinct Thanatos initiates negative impulses such as aggression and self-destructive behaviour. Infants are regarded as functioning via pure id.

The ego develops in response to 'real world' constraints, as the child finds its demands increasingly unmet by reflex activity or the intervention of others. Practical strategies have to be devised to satisfy id impulses in accordance with parental expectations and social rules. As it seeks compromise to gain an individual's goals, the ego operates on the 'reality principle', i.e. what actions a person can get away with.

Growing exposure to and identification with the values of parents and significant others promotes their adoption or internalization, creating the ethical principles known as the superego, effectively one's conscience (p. 184). The ego is compelled to obey the dictates of conscience and comply with the newly governing 'morality principle'.

A person's basic wants (id), practical options (ego) and moral considerations (superego) often conflict, causing a build-up of tension in the 'pressure cooker' of the unconscious (mind). Squeezed between the incessant demands of the id below and the inhibitions of the superego above (Fig. 8.6), the ego has to formulate on-going behavioural compromises. Freud suggested that the outcome determines each person's personality and mental health.

Safety valves

In order to protect the ego from being overwhelmed, Freud suggested that two principal methods of pressure/steam release develop: dreaming and defence mechanisms.

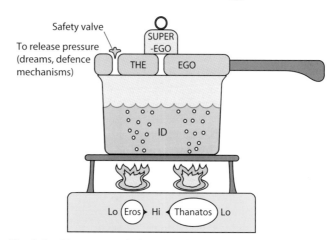

Fig. 8.6 • 'Pressure-cooker' model of unconscious mental structures.

Dreaming is deemed a disguised method of expressing unacceptable desires, or wish-fulfilment. Intense fears can also be enacted during sleep, although the true meaning of the experience is concealed from the dreamer by rich symbolism as well as loss of recall on awakening. Interpretation of dreams became a major tool of psychoanalysis.

Defence mechanisms (DMs) are a range of unconscious tactics by which the ego can prevent unpleasant thoughts and emotions from troubling the conscious mind. Each involves self-deception and distortion of reality, and can at best provide temporary respite rather than a true solution to the underlying problem (see Ch. 11 for more information about defence mechanisms in stress and coping). The main defence mechanisms are:

- Repression – unpalatable memories or emotions are prevented from entering consciousness, but still leave an uncomfortable tinge, a state of 'unblissful unawareness'. Repression is the basis for all other DMs, so each carries discomfiting emotional undertones
- Denial – unpleasant realities are driven out of awareness and ignored, allowing the person to function normally within a 'fool's paradise'
- Reaction formation – attitudes are expressed completely opposite to those unconsciously held, reminiscent of Shakespeare's 'methinks thou dost protest too much'
- Displacement – emotions are redirected from their actual target towards a safer, innocent recipient, e.g. 'slaying the messenger' of bad news
- Rationalization – constructing a logical explanation to justify dubious actions, then believing one's own argument, claiming 'I have my reasons'
- Intellectualization – minimizing anxiety in a situation by appraising it in abstract, objective terms, focusing on 'logic in adversity'
- Projection – perceiving undesirable qualities or motives that you possess yourself in others, a case of 'the pot calling the kettle black'
- Identification – characteristics, even if unpleasant or threatening, of other acquaintances are incorporated into

one's own behaviour, a case of 'if you can't beat them, join them'

- Sublimation – unacceptable impulses energetically channelled into socially approved pursuits.

Even if repressed out of conscious awareness, covert thoughts and impulses may occasionally surface in the form of slips of the tongue ('Freudian slips'), memory lapses, e.g. of unwanted events or responsibilities or physical mishaps (e.g. damaging disliked objects), which suggest to Freudians that there is no such thing as an innocent accident.

However, if the lid is kept too firmly on unconscious turmoil, the energy of suppressed anxieties may be converted into emotional and physical ailments ('psychosomatic disorders'). Box 8.29 provides an opportunity to identify the defence mechanism operating in a series of scenarios.

 Critical thinking Box 8.29

Which defence mechanism?

Scenarios

- The consultant made critical remarks to the Ward Sister about inaccuracies on patients' charts. Shortly afterwards, the sister shouted at a student nurse for being a few minutes late on duty
- The staff nurse said that she didn't mind that someone else had been chosen for promotion, as she had just wanted the interview experience
- On failing his assessment, Moses told his parents that they should accept it philosophically, and view it as an educational experience for their son
- Karen had been told that the two charge nurses loathed each other, but they always seemed very polite to each other
- The student took a long time to feel at ease in her ward placement. Later she discovered that she had been a patient there as a small child
- Dr Njuguna was terminally ill with breast cancer. She had ignored a suspicious lump for a year
- During the coffee-break with her fellow nurses, Julia denounced their absent colleagues as terrible gossips
- Joanna worked as a theatre nurse and had two main hobbies: gardening and pottery
- Eric knew that he worked with insensitive colleagues. He was taken aback when his girlfriend complained that she found him increasingly brusque.

Student activities

- Consider the scenarios and identify the likely defence mechanism.
- Discuss your findings with a fellow student and decide which mechanisms might be used to explain events in your own practice.

Psychosexual personality development

Freud believed that personality developed through a series of consecutive stages, each distinguished by the part of the body affording most contemporary stimulation and resultant pleasure. Particularly controversial was his contention that this

gratification was sexual in nature, even in infants. Either insufficient or excessive enjoyment within a stage could result in fixation there – remaining preoccupied with or continuing to indulge pursuits characterizing that period. This could be manifest in connected traits and activities during adulthood. These primitive vestiges could become particularly pronounced during stressful episodes, when the individual might dramatically revert, or regress, to strikingly immature behaviour. Freud identified five psychosexual stages: oral, anal, phallic, latent and genital.

Oral stage (0–24 months)

This reflects Piaget's sensorimotor intelligence (see p. 182) and is subdivided into two phases:

- An initial *passive* phase, when the mouth's principal activity is sucking, either to feed at the breast or bottle, or to investigate objects
- A later *active* phase, coinciding with the emergence of the first teeth from around 6 months, enabling the infant to bite as well as chew. Attempts at speaking now become increasingly distinct.

Freud regarded weaning as the main goal by the end of the oral stage, and common problems as resulting from prematurely stopped or protracted breast-feeding.

Effects of fixation in the 'passive oral' personality may be behaviours redolent of infant-like dependence: incessant demands ('wailing' for attention), greed/gluttony, breast-obsession and 'sucking' behaviours, e.g. smoking, excessive alcohol intake, pen- or thumb-sucking, with marked regression to this when stressed.

The 'active oral' personality is talkative, prone to sarcasm or abusive outbursts (the mouth is used as a weapon), as well as chewing gum, pencil nibbling or nail biting if anxious.

Anal stage (2–3 years)

The focus changes to the structures and processes of elimination, particularly of faeces. This stage also comprises two substages:

- An initial *expulsive* phase, when satisfaction and parental praise is derived from expelling excrement
- Later, parents try to encourage continence, with praise and the child's pleasure becoming related to retaining excrement until appropriate opportunities for voiding, the *retentive* phase.

Reliable continence is the goal by the end of the anal stage. Toilet training can be a frustrating and ambivalent process for all concerned, with difficulties resulting from both prolonged incontinence and rigid, authoritarian supervision (see Chs 20, 21).

The effects of fixation early on, an 'expulsive anal' personality, may be characterized by a person who is untidy, messy, wasteful, over-generous, unpunctual, prone to coarseness and vulgarity in speech and humour.

Fixation later results in a 'retentive anal' personality, the person being fastidious, hygiene-obsessed, methodical, perfectionist, obsessive, restrained, miserly and obstinate.

Phallic stage (4–5 years)

The child now becomes fascinated with genitalia, their own and those of other people, provoking genital self-fondling and curiosity about the mechanism of reproduction. Adult disapproval often follows, complicated by the child's increasing attraction to the opposite sex parent and hostility to that of the same sex. Freud termed this gravitation the 'Oedipus complex' in boys and 'Electra complex' in girls.

The stage's goal is that the 'mummy's boy' and 'daddy's girl' complexes resolve naturally through gradual acceptance of and identification with the same-sex parent. Sexual inwardness and parental preoccupation should not persist.

Effects of fixation here may include lifelong worship of one's opposite sex parent and choosing love partners by their resemblance to that figure, or a competitive, ambitious and boastful nature, expressing an unconscious need to surpass the same sex parent. Narcissism (preoccupation with one's own attractiveness) and teasing flirtatiousness may reflect the self-directed and abstract nature of sexual impulses inherited from this stage, while another vestige may be difficulties relating to authority figures.

Latent stage (6–11 years)

This involves temporary submersion of preceding sexual awareness into unconscious undercurrents. The child appears immersed in their hobbies and school activities. Playmates are typically of the same sex, revulsion being commonly expressed at any exhibitions of affection, nudity or sexual passion that they may encounter, e.g. on television or between parents.

The focus switches to scholastic and sporting prowess (see stage 4 of Erikson's model, Table 8.3, below).

Fixation is apparent in adulthood with immersion in work, study or pastimes, sexual coldness or indifference to the opposite sex.

Genital stage (12 years and above)

At puberty, sexual impulses reappear in a more conscious and urgent form, requiring satisfaction in intimate relationships and ultimately through physical intercourse. This need persists throughout adult life, Freud envisaging its ultimate fulfilment in enduring monogamous love. Equally conventional was Freud's view of males as naturally aggressive, adventurous and dominant compared with females' passivity, maternalism and domesticity.

The main goal is physical love and reproduction; fixation in this stage is desirable. However, earlier fixations can interfere with its accomplishment.

Criticisms and benefits of the psychodynamic approach

Criticisms of Freud's approach include its lack of scientific basis, and subjectivity. Some lament its pessimism about human nature (as at core irrational, hedonistic and destructive), and its 'irresponsible' focus on childhood sexuality, a charge which surprised Freud. Additionally, it may offend modern sensibilities as sexist, e.g. viewing males as behaviourally and anatomically superior.

However, the benefits of Freud's approach may include:

- Greater tolerance of sexuality, e.g. of its open discussion and idiosyncratic expressions
- Increased understanding and acceptance of people suffering from mental dysfunction; anxiety, Freud's clinical focus, is a universal experience
- The emergence of gentler, 'talking' treatments for mental disorders; psychoanalysis is the forerunner of modern psychotherapy
- Enrichment of Western language and thought, as many of its terms and notions are now part of wider cultural heritage.

Table 8.3 Erikson's stages of psychosocial development

Stage	Approximate age range	Significant others
1. Basic trust versus mistrust	0–1 year	Mother-figure, main care providers
Infants develop awareness of how sensitively and consistently their needs (e.g. nourishment, comfort and stimulation) are met, and so whether or not the world seems to be a safe, predictable and welcoming place		
2. Autonomy versus shame and doubt	2–3 years	Parents, child-minders, nursery staff
Toddlers develop a sense of individual 'self' and increasing muscular power, and often wish to exercise choice and do things for themselves. Adults may feel obliged to intervene at times, e.g. for reasons of safety or efficiency, and children may feel ashamed at failed initiatives or doubt their abilities, e.g. when struggling with toilet training		
3. Initiative versus guilt	4–6 years	As in previous stage, teachers latterly
Preschool children ask probing questions of adults to deepen their own understanding, participate imaginatively in games and are boldly energetic. Such independent actions bolster self-confidence, but this may be shaken if adults show disapproval of the enquiries, or criticize play as 'silly' or dangerous, resulting in self-censure and guilt		

Continued

Table 8.3 Erikson's stages of psychosocial development—cont'd

Stage	Approximate age range	Significant others
4. Industry versus inferiority	7–12 years	Teachers, friends, parents
Primary school children are keen to learn, to make things and see how they work. Their self-esteem depends largely on their ability to fulfil set tasks in comparison with their peers' performance. Opportunities, guidance and encouragement are crucial, as a sense of failure results from perceived underachievement		
5. Identity versus role confusion	13–19 years	School 'chums', boyfriend, girlfriend, mentors
Adolescents begin to formulate a concept of who they are in relation to society, including their intended occupational and sexual preferences – their cultural, work and sexual identities. They engage with and either commit to or reject ideologies, e.g. political and moral. Inability to emerge with clear roles and values can result in anger or apathy, and lack of future direction		Ambivalent towards parents
6. Intimacy versus isolation	20–30 years	Colleagues, employers, lovers, spouse/partner
Young adults build on their new identity to seek proximity and share interests and feelings with others, in the workplace and through committed sexual relationships. Isolation may result from fear of self-revelation or inability to select or obtain rewarding employment or partners		
7. Generativity versus stagnation	31–50s	Children and partner, customers or clients, mentees/pupils/students
In middle adulthood, the main concern is to care for and raise children, benefit others with your experience and/or be productive in rewarding work or art and craft, so making a contribution to society. If denied these outlets, middle-age can feel empty and wasted		
8. Ego integrity versus despair	50s onwards	Oneself and all humanity
Mature adulthood is seen as a phase for reflection on one's life cycle, which should be seen as having had a meaningful pattern and having been useful, despite inevitable adverse experiences. This allows the person to anticipate death with dignified acceptance and composure. An unsatisfactory life review focuses on failures and missed opportunities, fear of dying and a futile wish for sufficient time to start anew		

(After Gross, R.D., 2010. Psychology: the science of mind and behaviour, sixth ed. Hodder and Stoughton, London.)

Erikson's stage theory of psychosocial development

In the 1950s, Erik Erikson explored the relationship between psychological and social development. He produced a framework in which personal development naturally occurs via eight stages, each dominated by a major issue or crisis presented by the social environment (Table 8.3). If the child, adolescent or adult positively resolves the contemporary challenge, a sound foundation is established for progression to later stages, and a healthy personality and functioning are more likely. However, a maladaptive response will result in poor resolution of the issue, psychological problems and diminished ability to cope with later crises. Erikson suggested that it is possible to retrospectively rectify inadequate confrontation of an issue, even if an earlier stage's time parameters are the ideal point at which to resolve it. Conversely, previously gained ground can be lost once chronologically beyond a stage, e.g. possible disappointment or regaining of trust in life during adulthood.

SUMMARY

- An understanding of the major psychological and sociological concepts related to the human lifespan is important for nurses wherever they work.
- The contrasting approaches of psychology and sociology each yield useful insights into individual and social behaviour.
- Considering motivation assists nurses to understand the behaviour of others and to meet their needs.
- Culture, socialization and family are significant factors in health.
- Physical development relates not only to increasing size/strength over the lifespan, but also to changing function of body systems. This affects a person's ability to function in a social context.
- Both genetic and environmental (including social) factors are important in development.

- A variety of mental health problems may occur across the lifespan.
- Psychosocial development encompasses advances in self-perception, thought, morality and personality.

- Both conscious and unconscious processes may be significant in development and health.
- Aspects of development may be envisaged as a necessary progression through a series of age-related stages.

KEY WORDS AND PHRASES FOR LITERATURE SEARCHING

Adaptation	Developmental milestone	Psychology
Ageing/aging	Family	Psychosexual
Attachment	Growth	Psychosocial
Behaviourism	Intelligence	Role
Cognitive	Motivation	Self
Conditioning	Normalization	Socialization
Culture	Norms	Sociology
Development	Psychodynamic	Values

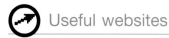 Useful websites

NHS Evidence www.evidence.nhs.uk/topics
Public Health Genomics Foundation www.phgfoundation.org
Scottish Recovery Network www.scottishrecovery.net
US National Library of Health MedlinePlus Medical Encyclopedia – provides information of developmental milestones at different ages www.nlm.nih.gov/medlineplus
All websites accessed September 2012.

References

Abercrombie, N., Warde, A., 2005. Contemporary British society, third ed. Polity, Cambridge.

Ainsworth, M.D., Blehar, M., Waters, E., et al., 1978. Patterns of attachment: a psychological study of the strange situation. Erlbaum, Hillsdale, NJ.

Bee, H., Boyd, D., 2009. The developing child, twelfth ed. Pearson International, Boston.

Bernstein, D., Penner, L.A., Clarke-Stewart, A., et al., 2007. Psychology, eighth ed. Houghton Mifflin, Boston.

Bowlby, J., 2005. A secure base: clinical applications of attachment theory. Routledge, London.

Bridges, J., Wilkinson, C., 2011. Achieving dignity for older people with dementia in hospital. Nursing Standard 25 (29), 42–47.

Denny, E., Earle, S., 2009. Sociology for nurses, second ed. Polity, Cambridge.

Denver Developmental Materials Inc, 1990. The Denver scale II. Denver Developmental Materials, Denver.

Eysenck, M.W., 2008. Fundamentals of psychology, third ed. Psychology Press, Hove.

Frankenburg, W.K., Dodds, J.B., Archer, P., et al., 1990. The Denver II (developmental rating scale). Denver Developmental Materials, Denver.

Giddens, A., 2009. Sociology, sixth ed. Polity, Cambridge.

Goffman, E., 1971. The presentation of self in everyday life. Penguin, London.

Graham, H. (Ed.), 2009. Understanding health inequalities, second ed. OUP, Oxford.

Gross, R.D., 2010. Psychology: the science of mind and behaviour, sixth ed. Hodder and Stoughton, London.

Hayes, N., 2000. Foundations of psychology, third ed. Thomson, London.

Haralambos, M., Holborn, M., 2008. Sociology: themes and perspectives, seventh ed. Collins, London.

Hinchliff, S.M., Montague, S.E., Watson, R., 1996. Physiology for nursing practice, second ed. Baillière Tindall, London.

Holmes, J., 2001. The search for the secure base. Brunner-Routlege, Hove.

Mader, S.S., 2009. Human biology, tenth ed. McGraw-Hill, Boston.

McLeod, J.D., 1991. Childhood parental loss and adult depression. Journal of Health and Social Behaviour 32 (3), 205–220.

Meggitt, C., 2006. Child development: an illustrated guide, second ed. Heinemann, London.

Miell, D., 1990. The self and the social world. In: Roth, I. (Ed.) Introduction to psychology, Vol. 1. Open University Press, Milton Keynes.

Napier University 1997, 2001. The individual, family and society: Module booklet 2. Faculty of Health and Life Sciences, Edinburgh.

NHS Clinical Knowledge Summaries, 2010. Dementia – Background information. Online. Available: www.cks.nhs.uk/dementia/background_information/

epidemiology_and_societal_burden September 2012.

Nolen-Hoeksema, S.N., Fredrickson, B., Loftus, G., et al., 2009. Atkinson & Hilgard's introduction to psychology, fifteenth ed. Cengage Learning, Florence, KY.

Nursing and Midwifery Council, 2008. The code: Standards of conduct, performance and ethics for nurses and midwives. Online. Available: http://www.nmc-uk.org/Publications/Standards/The-code/Introduction/ September 2012.

Raynor, M.D., Oates, M.R., 2009. Perinatal mental health. In: Fraser, D.M., Cooper, M.A. (Eds.), Myles textbook for midwives, fifteenth ed. Churchill Livingstone, Edinburgh.

Santrock, J.W., 2009. Life-span development, twelfth ed. McGraw-Hill, New York.

Serci, I.G., 2009. The fetus. In: Fraser, D.M., Cooper, M.A. 2009 (Eds.), Myles textbook for midwives, fifteenth ed. Churchill Livingstone, Edinburgh.

Thomas, A., Chess, S., 1977. Temperament and development. Brunner and Mazel, New York.

Tizard, B., Hodges, J., 1978. The effect of early institutional rearing on the development of 8-year-old children. Journal of Child Psychology and Psychiatry 19, 99–118.

Watson, D., 2011. Causes of learning disability. In: Atherton, H.L., Crickmore, D.J. (Eds.), Learning disabilities: toward inclusion, sixth ed. Churchill Livingstone, Edinburgh.

Further reading

Barker, P., 2009. Psychiatric and mental health nursing: the craft of caring, second ed. Hodder Arnold, London.

Colbert, G., Ankey, J., Lee, K., et al., 2009. Anatomy & physiology for nurses and health professionals. Pearson, London.

Dowler, E., Spencer, L.J., 2007. Challenging health inequalities: from Acheson to choosing health. Policy Press, Bristol.

Durkin, K., 2007. Developmental social psychology. In: Hewstone, M., Strobe, W., Jonas, K. (Eds.), Introduction to social psychology: a European perspective, fourth ed. Wiley, Hoboken NJ.

Gerhardt, S., 2004. Why love matters; how affection shapes a baby's brain. Routledge, London.

Hockenberry, M.J., Wilson, D., 2010. Wong's nursing care of infants and children, ninth ed. Mosby, St Louis.

Light, P., Oates, J., 1990. The development of children's understanding. In: Roth, I. (Ed.) Introduction to psychology, Vol. 1. Open University Press, Milton Keynes.

National Institute for Health and Clinical Excellence, 2007. Antenatal and postnatal mental health. Clinical guideline CG 45. Online. Available: www.nice.org.uk/nicemedia/live/11004/30431/30431.pdf September 2012.

National Institute for Health and Clinical Excellence, 2008. Attention deficit hyperactivity disorder. Clinical guideline CG 72. Online. Available: www.nice.org.uk/nicemedia/live/12061/42059/42059.pdf September 2012.

National Institute for Health and Clinical Excellence, 2009. Depression. Clinical guideline CG 90. Online. Available: www.nice.org.uk/nicemedia/

live/12329/45888/45888.pdf September 2012.

National Institute for Health and Clinical Excellence, 2009. Schizophrenia. Clinical guideline CG 82. Online. Available: www.nice.org.uk/nicemedia/live/11786/43608/43608.pdf September 2012.

National Institute for Health and Clinical Excellence, 2011. Common mental health disorders. Identification and pathways to care. National clinical guideline CG 123. Online. Available: www.nice.org.uk/nicemedia/live/13476/54604/54604.pdf September 2012.

Videbeck, S.L., 2009. Mental health nursing, UK edn. Wolters Kluwer, London.

Relationship, helping and communication skills

Naomi Sharples

LEARNING OUTCOMES

This chapter will help you:

- Discuss aspects of communication
- Outline the development of language
- Describe the use of language
- Outline interpersonal communication skills
- Describe communication in nursing relationships, therapeutic and professional
- Recognize, minimize or overcome communication barriers
- Start to develop the skill of communicating significant information
- Discuss the importance of leadership skills and team working.

Introduction

This chapter explores how knowledge of communication, language and interpersonal skills can enhance professional nursing practice and nursing relationships; and considers how people understand language and communication. The reader is offered various frameworks and activities to practise with the aim of developing their interpersonal skills and so developing the quality of the care and positive relationships and interactions they are able to engage in.

Well-developed interpersonal and communication skills are considered essential for all nurses, regardless of where they work. This is promoted by the Nursing and Midwifery Council (NMC) *Competency Framework Domain 2: Communication and interpersonal skills; Essential skills cluster: Care, compassion and communication* from the *Standards for pre-registration nursing education* (NMC 2010) and *Essence of Care 2010* (Department of Health, DH 2010) (Box 9.1). Good interpersonal skills positively affect people, enhancing emotional and physical well-being (West & Turner 2009).The information, skills and techniques offered will enhance the nurse's ability to deliver care within the context of a positive and empowering communication environment.

The primary aim is to enable the reader to recognize good communication, barriers to communication and also how to improve communication and interpersonal skills. It is of paramount importance for nurses to consider exactly what they say to people, how they say it and how this affects the person.

When nurses start to focus attention on their own communication skills, they may feel a little anxious, unsure if they are saying the right thing. Feeling unsure is good because it indicates that nurses are starting to think carefully and more critically about what they say to people, how they relate to them and how this affects the person's experience of health professionals.

The chapter will bring readers out of their 'unconscious competence' zone, to work within the 'conscious competence' and 'conscious incompetence' areas. This model represents our zones of learning and experience:

- *Unconscious competence*: People do not think about what they are saying – they just open their mouth and speak and *generally* get it right
- *Conscious competence*: People know what they are going to say, why they are going to say it and what result they want

- *Conscious incompetence*: People will be aware of what they do not know about communication and interpersonal skills – 'they know what they don't know'
- *Unconscious incompetence*: People do not know what they do not know, e.g. meeting someone who speaks a different language, a language they have no knowledge of or the skills to understand or express ideas.

(This model can be found at: www.businessballs.com.)

The model helps you to think about what you do know and search for things you need to know; the skills you need to possess. Gibbs' (1988) reflective model (see Ch. 4) will also encourage nurses to consider more deeply their thoughts, feelings and behaviours; it will bring communication to the forefront of the mind and help move understanding from an innate level – an unconscious competence level – to a more critically considered consciously competent level.

Good communication offers pathways into relationships between individuals and the ability to effectively care for people. Caring for someone entails looking after their needs on many different levels – from physical needs to emotional support, from information giving to working in partnership. Caring is a fundamental nursing value and to communicate care nurses must show concern, attention, empathy and respect.

Communication theory

People's brains are 'wired' to communicate, to develop language, reason, empathy and even storytelling skills. Parents and carers are innately skilled in developing the language ability of their children; people have the capability and importantly the motivation to match the communication needs of other people in various situations and from diverse cultures, social strata and backgrounds. We are born with the ability and the language faculty to understand any natural language (Pinker 2007). This ability is like no other learning experience: it does not require conscious effort and exceeds all other notions of learning theory – all the child needs is to be stimulated by a language environment.

Despite these innate abilities, people still make errors when communicating; some errors are small, such as 'pacifically speaking' rather than 'specifically speaking', but others are more serious. Practitioners who do not communicate effectively with the patient/client/child may cause anxiety or fear, which can in turn negatively affect the patient's health.

Models for communication

Various models for communication exist and two models are outlined here: the Blueprint of Behaviour model and another derived from Shannon and Weaver's (1949) model.

Blueprint of Behaviour model

The neurolinguistic programming (NLP) model showing the 'blueprint of behaviour' is a tool to help understand how people comprehend the world around them, how this influences the person's communication and therefore how others may respond to them (Fig. 9.1).

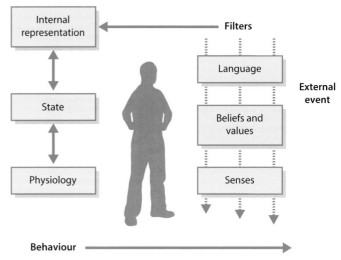

Fig. 9.1 • Blueprint of Behaviour model.

Everyone has unique life experiences that affect the way they understand the world. Our senses are also unique: people see, hear, smell, touch and taste in ways that are particular to them. The language used and understood is also unique to and influenced by background, social class, education, family, spirituality and cultural heritage. Given so many individual distinctions, it is our capacity to communicate that enables people to create such effective connections with others.

Language, senses, experiences, beliefs and values act as filters influencing the way people interpret and internalize external stimuli and this determines the way people communicate and behave. The term 'filter' represents the environmental, physiological and neurological processes that act on information as it comes through the senses and into our language, values and belief systems. Filtered external stimuli are internally represented and understood by each individual in a different way. These representations influence emotions, which in turn influence the language used and person's subsequent behaviour.

Understanding how these filters create accessible or inaccessible pathways between individuals and groups enables nurses to be clear and creative in communicating often vital information to patients/clients, carers and colleagues (Box 9.2).

 Reflective practice   Box 9.2

What influences the effectiveness of communication?

Consider a typical communication in a familiar placement and look at it using the Blueprint of Behaviour model.

Student activities

- Reflect on how the people involved will be influenced by their view of the world – how will this affect the communication?
- Discuss with your mentor how you can ensure that the information you provide is clear.

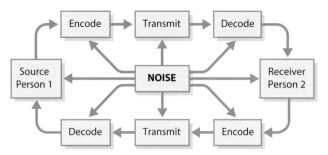

Fig. 9.2 • Communication model derived from Shannon and Weaver's model.

A model derived from Shannon and Weaver's model

A communication framework, derived from Shannon and Weaver's model (Fiske 2010), provides a description of the communication process between two people (Fig. 9.2): person 1 encodes, creates their message and transmits it to person 2 who decodes the message for meaning, and encodes or creates a response, which is transmitted to person 1 to decode and understand.

It would be useful to consider this model while at the same time keeping the Blueprint of Behaviour model in mind. It helps to build a picture of the factors that affect:

• People individually
• The communication process between people
• The communication process between people and their environment.

Communication process – getting the message across

Most people have a preference for either the auditory or the visual channel for sending and receiving messages (see p. 194), choosing the most appropriate channel is vital for effective communication.

For example, the sender thinks of an idea that will have been triggered by an internal or external event. The thought/message is encoded into words in the brain; the message is transmitted from the brain to the structures involved in voice production (e.g. larynx, tongue, palate and lips), then to the outside world and the listener. The listener picks up the sound through their ears and the sound is transmitted along the vestibulocochlear (auditory) nerves to the brain. There it is decoded and understood by the listener who will react to the message and respond to the sender.

At any point in this sequence, 'noise' can influence the quality of the message. A noise could be environmental interference, such as a noisy classroom where people are competing to be heard, or clinical equipment beeping and buzzing. The person may be experiencing pain and is concentrating on this rather than on the person speaking.

Other factors that impact on the communication process in care settings are language differences, anxiety, fear and anger. People who are experiencing extremes of emotions are not in a position to fully understand a message, e.g. a distressed

relative in the Emergency Department, a person with psychosis experiencing hallucinations. People who are distressed find their ability to comprehend others can be limited.

'Noise' changes the message. To understand how it has been changed, the sender relies on the listener's feedback or a change in behaviour to check if the message has been understood. In a situation where the message is clear and understood, the sender has been successful. If the message was not understood, the sender is responsible for adjusting the message and possibly the channel chosen to transmit the message to communicate their idea again (Box 9.3).

Reflective practice   **Box 9.3**

Getting the message across

They tap their ear, shake their head and shrug their shoulders. The nurse may think that they have not heard the message:

• By quickly analysing the message – the sender feels it was clear
• The situation – the message was in context
• Possible noise factors – these were at an acceptable level.

By ruling out many possibilities, the nurse may conclude that the person is deaf or hard of hearing. If the nurse has sign language skills and encodes the message in sign, the visual channel can be used to transmit the message. The patient/client receives and understands the message via the visual channel. Feedback could be a smile and thumbs up.

Student activities

Reflect on a situation from clinical practice, where the listener did not hear your spoken message:

• How did you know the listener had not heard?
• What other communication channels did you consider?
• Discuss with your mentor how might you have communicated with the person.

Acknowledging potential noise in communication helps the nurse to change the message to suit the situation. The nurse is 'accommodating' the communication to the needs of the person rather than 'diverging' from their needs (see p. 200).

More considered strategies are needed in some situations. For example, when a nurse communicates with a person with a learning disability, the communication is determined by the nurse's knowledge of the person and their linguistic and cognitive ability. The person, their carers, friends, family and speech and language therapists (SLTs) can inform this knowledge and help the nurse (Box 9.4).

Language is a transactional process influenced by what has been said before, what is happening between the speakers in the present and what could follow. Good communicators attend to the whole transaction, rather than only one aspect (West & Turner 2009).

Language

Earlier sections have emphasized that each person has a different blueprint of behaviour. We all have the ability to change,

Children and adults with a learning disability may face greater challenges in acquiring language. These difficulties not only relate to their cognitive development but also to the physical problems that coincide with some developmental differences. They may have problems with articulation, expressive language or receptive language (see pp. 197-198).

Structured assessments by the multidisciplinary team (MDT); comprising audiologist, SLT, ophthalmologist and physiotherapist, are therefore vital to this client group. The assessments focus on:

- Hearing and communication skills – hearing loss is more common for people with learning disabilities (see Ch. 16)
- Assessment of oral cavity, larynx, pharynx and nasal cavity to ascertain if there are any anomalies that would preclude speech development, or the ability to produce sound or factors affecting the quality of the sound
- Vision is crucial to language learning and should be assessed regularly
- Gross and fine motor movement ability will also have impact on their ability to use gesture, sign language or to vocalize
- Cognitive impairments are also assessed by the SLT to discover if there is a neurological basis for any problems the client has.

Following the assessments, the MDT plans interventions with the client, family and carers to facilitate the client's move towards communicative competence. These are evaluated and the plan reviewed on a regular basis. Examples of interventions could include:

- Naming games, completing the sentence games
- Mouth/tongue exercises
- Voice practice and breathing exercises
- Listening games, rhythm games, sound identification games
- Social skill development to enhance interpersonal communication skills
- Advice to family/carers about the best method of communication, e.g. signing, or some other aid.

Language development in children

Language development is vital for a child to progress from a point where they express thoughts or feelings through behaviours; to one where they can express abstract thoughts, complex emotions, describe intricate behaviours and develop engaging relationships with others (Box 9.5).

Normal early language development   Box 9.5

- *Newborns* cry, scream, coo and whimper, alerting parents/carers that they are hungry, cold, want contact or are content. This is the pre-linguistic phase.
- *At 3 months* the palate and pharynx begin to develop; before this age they are unable to create speech sounds.
- *Around 6 months* babies start to 'babble'. This is where they learn to differentiate true language sounds from those that will not be needed. Deaf babies 'babble' with their hands forming the hand shapes that are some of the finite set of shapes they will use. Babies start to practise the articulation of words later in this stage. Although babies cannot use words, they listen intently, watch people's faces and imitate mouth movements, shapes and voice intonation. This communication and language stimulation is imperative for the child's development (Boysson-Bardies 1999).
- *Between 7 and 12 months* babies babble with more clarity, particularly certain sounds that move easily into fundamental words, e.g. 'Mama', 'Dada'. Such words and sounds help to develop the speech muscles. Babies develop one-word skills, focusing this development on the things/people around them, e.g. 'Mama', 'no', 'up'. Mostly the words have a naming function, show an emotion or give a command (Fromkin et al 2010).
- *In their 2nd year* children begin to form two-word sentences. These often contain more information than people may at first think. For example, 'cat dirty' could be describing the cat's fur or that the cat has done something dirty. The child can put two concepts together that when 'translated' mean more than the words alone. This reinforces the fact that babies and young children can understand and conceptualize at a level beyond their ability to articulate. As the child develops, so their ability to form sentences increases and they begin to develop the rules of language.
- *From 3 to 7 years* children continue to develop skills in the complex rules of grammar and word usage. By the age of 7 most children have developed understanding and skill in most of the language rules that they will need for their future.

to develop and, in the case of our senses, to deteriorate. Our choices of communication strategies depend on many factors, one of the most important being language.

All human languages comprise words or signs, sounds, visual movement, rules, grammar and vocabulary to express desire, knowledge and creativity. All languages are complex and based on a finite number of sounds or, in the case of sign language, hand shapes. All languages provide the users with the ability to produce an infinite number of sentences (Crystal 2010).

Some people feel that language is a complicated and difficult subject with hidden depth and complex rules making the idea of learning a new language daunting. Babies and children learning their first language do not share these anxieties; they usually have a natural curiosity that supports language acquisition. Play is an important component in the processes involved in language development. Depending on a child's age and stage of development, one of the main sources of communication with children is through play (see below).

Box 9.6 provides an opportunity to reflect on communication with a child. Children who are denied access to a language environment have problems acquiring language. Feral children or children who experience severe neglect are confounded by the complexity of language rules and social relationships, particularly if the child misses the formative language development years.

Play as a communication tool

In all societies, people can recollect the games they played with other children and adults as they grew up. Remembering imaginary stories that were re-enacted, games with rules or songs

Reflective practice   Box 9.6

Communicating with children

Think of a child that you have met in a caring capacity.

Student activities

Using Gibbs' (1988) model of reflection, consider the following questions:

• What were you doing? What was the child doing? How old were they? Who was present? What were they doing? What were you saying? What was the child communicating?

• What did you do to ensure the child understood you? How did you speak to the child? How did you know that the child understood you, on what evidence? What effect did the communication have on the child's behaviour? What effect did their communication have on your behaviour? What would you do differently next time to enhance the communication?

• What do you need to know to enhance your communication with children? How will you obtain that information? How will you know that accessing and understanding the information has changed your behaviour?

and deep attachments to favourite toys can give a sense of happiness. Play is crucial to language development, understanding relationships and developing an understanding of 'self' and how the 'self' relates to the outside world. Play enables the child to make sense of the world and develop strategies to enable them take their place in society.

Play is of vital importance for children who are either in receipt of healthcare or for children who are trying to understand and come to terms with illness, disability and death (see Ch. 12). Nurses can provide support for children by utilizing play in the child–nurse therapeutic relationship.

Babies use 'practice' play to understand their movements and sensations. Play is vital in developing control over gross and fine motor movements and to start interacting with the world. This involves: grasping, taking objects to the mouth, pulling, hitting, clapping, pushing, grabbing and moving objects, fitting one object inside another, delighting in the movement of the objects and the interaction and responses of parental figures. Babies continue with the trial and error approach to affecting change on objects in their environment, e.g. rolling balls away by pushing or discovering that hard objects make louder noises than soft objects.

During the 2nd year, children continue to develop by using play to explore more complex ideas, e.g. learning to feed themselves by pretend feeding of adults or toys. Adults actively encourage pretend play but their interactions are often triggered and controlled by the child who leads the play. This person-to-person interaction encourages the child to modify behaviour according to the reactions of others. It also enables the child to practise social skills such as turn taking, waiting, requesting, constructing and destructing scenarios.

Preschool children delight in 'rough and tumble' using large pieces of furniture or nursery props to design sets for play. This play is vital for the development of coordination, muscle development, playing with others and fighting battles against good and evil. This helps children understand a wider range of emotions and strategies for life.

From the age of about 4 years children start to understand games with rules; these games support the development of the person in a number of ways. All games for two or more players require communication and language skills. They develop the child's understanding of competition, fair play, choosing a team, working together and developing a defensive or offensive tactic to win. The child develops a sense of what it means to belong to a group, and how to form and work in a team. Games with rules can play a major part in developing a child's self-esteem and self-awareness, and understanding their own skills and limitations.

Pretend play allows the child to develop and practise life skills. Children use the scenarios around them to develop their meaning of the world. Children will role-play scenes from family interactions, taking on the role of carer or healer, and developing skills in looking after others. They will also use information from wider cultural roles, from the media and current characters such as 'Postman Pat' or an action hero/heroine. Objects are used to trigger play, e.g. dressing-up boxes can provide an infinite range of possibilities. Children can use pretend play to work through conflict situations, negotiate results and stage the scenarios so that they can understand or impose their views and wishes on the events.

Nurses and play specialists utilize play with children in a number of ways, such as in relation to painful or invasive interventions. Play becomes the communication vehicle for identified aims of the child's care (Table 9.1).

Adults also play, and many care settings, e.g. mental health units, provide facilities for play such as board games, pool or table tennis. Play with adults has a number of benefits:

• Alleviates boredom
• Motivates activity to help people to stay mobile and fit
• Provides distractions
• Develops teamwork between clients and staff
• Develops rapport
• Shows people aspects of their life other than illness or distress
• Provides a sense of achievement
• Develops the concepts of sharing and empowerment.

Developmental problems – receptive and expressive language

Language development problems may affect reception and/or expression of language.

Children who have hearing loss may have problems developing language because of the quality of sound information. It is crucial to provide access to language for the child in a mode that is accessible. Children with a useful residual level of hearing may be helped by hearing aids or a cochlear implant, depending on the cause of the hearing loss. These children develop speech, comprehension and expression by relying on aids and lipreading. For children from signing families, or for children whose residual hearing is not at a level that would facilitate understanding, sign language is preferable. Children who learn to sign from an early age follow the same developmental process as children learning speech.

Table 9.1 Therapeutic play – uses in healthcare	
Aim	**Process**
Distraction from a procedure they may find upsetting or painful	Identifying the type of play appropriate to the age of the child, the nurse will use play to focus the child's concentration away from the procedure
Information giving	The nurse will use toys and other media such as paints, modelling materials, online games and specifically designed dolls to inform the child about their health
Play as a 'normal' child function, promoting physical and psychological development	Nurses and play therapists will use play to create a sense of normality for children in situations that are not normal Play can be a valuable coping strategy for children to use
Assessing child's development	Specialist practitioners use play as an assessment tool to ascertain the child's stage of development, thus identifying any deficits in cognitive, linguistic, emotional or physical development All nurses should be able to identify any obvious differences in the age of a child and their level of play, language and social interactions
Encouraging the child to express their fears and wishes	Provide toys and creative materials to assist a child in expressing their thoughts without the child having to resort to language Children need space and time to develop their understanding and the language of new or emotionally difficult issues and toys provide this opportunity
Assisting parents in their appreciation of how their child understands the situation	Involve parents in the child's play and help parents to understand the concepts the child is working on Help parents link the play themes to the child's situation so that they can support the child in this process

Children who are deafblind face immense challenges in learning language. SLTs, parents/carers, educators and support groups such as Sense (www.sense.org.uk) facilitate their language development.

Children with cerebral palsy may have difficulties in speech production (expression) due to muscle control issues. Nurses need to be aware that people with cerebral palsy may take longer to express themselves; people who are familiar with their speech may help the nurse in understanding the person. However, it is important to be aware that family members acting as interpreter may not be appropriate (see pp. 215, 217).

Children with a cleft palate and/or cleft lip (an opening in the palate connecting the nasal and oral cavities; may also involve the upper lip) may also experience difficulty in speech production. Most cleft palate problems are swiftly and effectively rectified by early surgery but input from specialist dental/orthodontic services and an SLT may be needed.

Language styles and influences

The way people communicate with others depends on a number of influences that are usually subconscious. Nurses will find it useful to understand why they speak to people the way they do and how this is dependent on the situation, the people they are communicating with and the background of everyone involved.

Formality

Consider the following statements:

- 'Wow, work was hard today, one man was really ill, but he's on the mend now.'

- 'It has been a busy day. Mr Clark has been taken off the ventilator and is breathing independently.'
- 'On the thirteenth of May between 10.00 and 10.45 hours, Staff Nurse Elliot and I worked with Mr Clark ensuring he could breathe independently of the ventilator. I then proceeded to input the account of the intervention in Mr Clark's notes.'

The same person spoke each sentence but in different situations, at home with his partner, during shift handover and in a court of law. It is obvious which statement was used in each situation, but what is it about the sentence that fits the context in which it is spoken? The level of formality in each situation determines the level of formality in the language used.

The first sentence suggests an informal setting, a friendship or relationship with a person not involved in the speaker's work life. Not a great deal of factual information is given because of confidentiality (see Ch. 6). Social information is provided to inform the listener of the speaker's feelings.

The second sentence is more formal, the context supports increased information about the patient rather than the member of staff. The sentence does suggest some informality initially, which can have a positive effect on team and individual connections, though it moves quickly on to deal with the pertinent issue of care.

The final sentence is very formal, there is a high degree of clarity, and more words are used to provide detailed information. There are no feelings expressed at all. People would certainly find it odd if people spoke in this way on a daily basis; it is highly structured and by the absence of emotional information it lacks any social use and could distance the listener. In a court situation, however, the facts of the matter are of ultimate importance and feelings are less relevant. In each example, the situation determines the language style used.

The people within the situation also determine the language used. For example:

- 'Pick those up … clever girl … That's it. Ah, good girl.'
- 'Please could you pick those books up, thanks.'
- 'I need all those books picked up and put away, immediately.'

One person is speaking to a small child of about 2 years old, another is speaking to a colleague and the third is speaking to an adult who has annoyed them considerably. How do people know?

- When speaking to young children people adjust the number of words and the amount of information given in each sentence. They also give words of encouragement.
- The second sentence is quite neutral, clear information prefixed and ended by pleasantries. The formality is reduced by the use of 'thanks' rather than 'thank you'.
- The final sentence is very different in tone. It is one sentence containing three commands. There are no pleasantries and suggests either that the speaker is annoyed or is in a position of authority.

Clearly, reading the statements above requires some degree of guesswork because it is not possible to hear or see the speaker. Different tones, emphasis, facial expressions and gestures could change the meanings completely.

Age

Age has an interesting influence on language; people may speak to older people in the same 'singsong' style as for children, using short encouraging sentences with emphasis on intonation and emotion. This can be a useful strategy only if the language used reflects and respects the life experience of the individual. When people are caring for individuals who have difficulties responding, the carer may inappropriately resort to language that reinforces a care relationship and a power dynamic that favours the carer. This tendency is neither appropriate nor useful to the client. Caring in a way that is respectful and dignified for older people is a high level accomplishment that requires nurses who are skilled in communication (Box 9.7).

People with learning and physical disabilities, and mental distress

People with learning and physical disabilities also face similar situations. Again, carers must cope with a complex communication situation and sometimes, rather than adjust their language to suit a person with cognitive difficulties in an age-appropriate way, they resort to speaking to the individual as if the person was a child. These limitations in carers' communication skills must be addressed, because this disempowers the individual. Understanding the transactional nature of communication and each person's blueprint of behaviour will help the nurse develop their skills.

Nurses who work with people with learning disabilities or with children, or nurses who work in more than one language, show skills in 'convergence' (see below). They develop skills

? Critical thinking   Box 9.7

Stefan

Stefan, who is 79 years old and has dementia, lives in a care home. It is nearly lunchtime and Stefan is very agitated about his house keys. Stefan's carer is keen to take him to the lavatory before lunch. Stefan is frantically searching the drawers in his bedroom. The carer says: 'Come on Stefan, don't be silly. The house was sold years ago. Your lunch is getting cold. Come on, there's a good boy.'

Student activities

- Using the *Essence of Care 2010 benchmarks for communication* (DH 2010), think about the scenario involving Stefan, or a similar experience in a placement.
- Compare the carer's communication against the benchmark and identify areas for change.

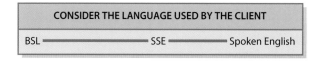

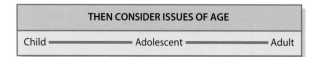

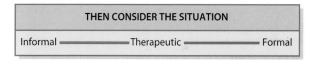

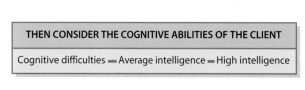

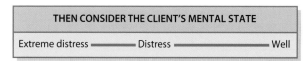

Fig. 9.3 • Considerations in communications to meet clients' needs.

in talking to each individual in a way that meets the person's communication and cognitive ability.

Another example of this can be found in services for deaf people with mental health problems. Some specialist mental health nurses work with deaf people in services where clients may use British Sign Language (BSL), Sign-Supported English (SSE; a variation of BSL) and speech. Figure 9.3 models these languages and language variations and other considerations such as distress.

Nurses move up and down each cline depending on the communication needs of the person with whom they are engaging. By doing this, they match the needs of the clients to provide access to communication while considering the skills and limitations of the nurse and the client. The nurse and the client accommodate to the needs of each other in this fluid situation – remember that clients also have the innate skill to match the needs of the nurse. Typically in settings where more than one language is used, clients do assist nurses and other professionals in understanding their (the client's) language. This puts the client in an empowered position, thus giving respect to and acknowledgement of their language skills.

In addition to the considerations on the cline, nurses consider issues of gender, social background, education experience, family connections, spirituality and culture. This creates a very complex communication situation where skilled communicators are essential.

Accommodating and diverging in communication

People usually accommodate other people's communication style quite naturally (Fromkin et al 2010). When travelling abroad with little or no knowledge of the language, people reduce conversation to more simple sentences, use clear pronunciation, and increase the use of gesture to assist the message. As already discussed, when talking to small children, people adjust language to suit their needs, speaking in simpler terms, using fewer key ideas per sentence, and breaking down sentences into chunks that the child can more readily access. When speaking to a person they relate well to, people 'converge'; they use similar vocabulary, pronunciation, conversation tempo and may change their accent or dialect to accommodate the other person.

Nurses accommodate the needs of patients/clients/carers when they explain complex therapies. They speak in non-technical terms using less jargon to enable the other party to understand. Where the nurse speaks Hindi and Punjabi and the client speaks Gujarati and Punjabi, the client and the nurse will accommodate each other by using Punjabi, even though it may not be either person's first language.

Occasionally, people do not accommodate the listener's needs – they 'diverge'; this occurs when the:

- Speaker is not skilled at understanding the needs of others
- Other person has upset them
- Person is making a political statement by distancing the listener
- Person aspires to a higher social class or intellectual status
- Person wants to show a difference in backgrounds (Holmes 2001).

There are numerous examples of speech divergence in healthcare. For instance, a healthcare professional provides technical information to the patient/client very quickly, without eye contact; disempowering the patient/client. It requires confidence to challenge the speaker, something that people in hospital may lack due to their illness, anxiety or because they may feel in a subordinate position (see Ch. 7).

Table 9.2 Representational word systems		
Representational system	**Examples of words used**	**Possible responses**
Visual	'I see the idea'	'Does that give you a clearer view of things?'
Auditory	'That rings a bell'	'I heard that you wanted to sound out the options'
Kinaesthetic	'I have a bad feeling about this drug'	'How would you feel about taking a similar drug?'

It is clear that converging often creates effective communication, whereas diverging creates difference. However, people can use divergence to assist people to change their level of formality or informality to help them to adjust to the needs of the situation. When people converge too much it can sound patronizing. Where a patient/client is relying on the nurse to make them feel confident in the therapeutic process, it is useful to use technical terms and to support the client with an explanation of the meaning of each term.

Interpersonal communication skills

Interpersonal communication can be divided into verbal/signed, non-verbal and listening skills. In addition, we consider how, for nurses, courtesy is crucial to interpersonal communication.

People represent their world in different ways and have different preferences in the way they access information about their world. People tend to use a visual system, an auditory system or a kinaesthetic system. Some people like to 'see' what people are saying, some like to 'hear' a good idea and some like to 'feel' a sense of what is happening.

When communicating with patients/clients it is useful to be able to use their preferred representational system because this will enable them to access the information with less effort and develop rapport quickly. Initially, this may seem rather complicated, but by looking at the words that may suit people it will be easier to understand and practise.

In order to recognize someone's representational system, it is necessary to listen to the words they use to describe their world, perhaps by asking them to talk about something that they have enjoyed, e.g. their favourite place. Listening for the 'describing' words the client uses, will provide clues about their preference for one or two systems or all three (Table 9.2).

Courtesy

Most patients/clients and carers rightly expect nurses to be civil, courteous and polite. People are more likely to complain when they feel others are being rude to them. The number of such complaints is increasing. The signs of courtesy include:

- Paying attention to people when the nurse is with them or when they request the nurse's attention

- Being civil to a person, treating them with respect, behaving towards them as a valued person
- Being polite, which is essential to developing rapport, e.g. saying please and thank you, not rushing people, smiling and using the person's preferred name, all help to ensure the person feels they are important and valued.

Consideration for others also depicts courtesy. Considering the other person in all dealings with them sounds obvious, but unfortunately people feel that nurses do not always show consideration. This could be not listening to requests, rushing care or not considering individual preferences, e.g. in food, cosmetics, clothing, etc. This all shows a lack of consideration for the person.

The signs of courtesy are clear, although it may feel they are sometimes difficult to achieve due to resource (time, people, money) allocation, the emotional context in which nurses work and the barriers to communication that must be overcome (see p. 214). Developing sensitive skills in courtesy and customer care allows nurses to meet the needs of all stakeholders in the healthcare system.

Verbal communication

Spoken words are arbitrary representations of ideas that have been agreed over time by those using a language. In other words, they are an agreed sound or group of sounds that we know represent a thing or an action. Without such agreement on meaning, words would be nonsensical or idiosyncratic – understood only by the person who produced them. Verbal communication usually has written equivalents to the words produced, although some languages do not.

Nurses employ various verbal communication strategies to develop relationships, seek and understand information, provide feedback to others and to demonstrate professional compassion and self-awareness. Some strategies are outlined below. It is useful for nurses to recognize when they use these strategies naturally, before developing their skills further.

Strategies – questioning with good intentions

People use positive intentions when questioning others. This helps them to show courtesy and respect and this develops trust; therefore they get the correct information in a short space of time with 'ecology', i.e. without damaging the relationship environment.

Open questions

Open questions are used to gain information about people, their feelings, their beliefs and values, their perceptions and wishes. Open questions usually begin with a 'What …? Who …? How …? When …? Where …?'. To help people accept these questions, nurses can also use a 'softener' such as 'It would be good to know how …'. Open questions 'open up' the listener's mind to answers that they can give; information that they hold. Softeners, however, may be so gentle that it becomes a closed question, e.g. 'Please could you tell me when …'. It is so easy to respond 'no' to this very polite request.

Closed questions

Closed questions are used when specific information is needed quickly or if there are other limitations causing barriers, e.g. the client is distressed. Closed questions are those to which a person can answer 'yes' or 'no', e.g. 'Do you like soap on your face?'; 'Are you unhappy?'. It may be the nurse's intention to gather more information than purely a 'yes' or 'no'. It can be very frustrating trying to get beyond the yes/no responses. Closed questions can be opened by leaving the end of the sentence unfinished, e.g. 'Are you unhappy … or …?'. This is a useful strategy when the client/child/carer really does not want a lengthy conversation but the nurse needs to open a way for further discussion.

Funnelling

Funnelling is a strategy used first to obtain general information and then to narrow the information down to an agreement, specific point or clear conclusion.

Summarizing

A summary is a strategy whereby the listener summarizes information given by the speaker, in the speaker's own words. The purpose of summarizing is to check the listener's understanding at the same time as acknowledging what has been said.

Paraphrasing

This strategy is similar to summarizing but with more use of the listener's own words. This often helps the listener get the information straight in their own mind.

Clarifying

This enables the listener to present the information back to the speaker, then to question if this is what they heard. It is also useful for the speaker to identify with their own thoughts coming from another source; sometimes it sounds or feels different, thus providing another perspective.

Feedback

Feedback provides the listener with acknowledgement of their performance. It can reinforce the behaviour so that it is more likely to happen again and it helps to motivate people through the knowledge that their behaviour was appropriate.

Box 9.8 provides an example of some of these strategies.

Assertive communication

The skill of assertiveness is important to nurses. Assertiveness enables people to be honest with themselves and in their relationships with others. Assertiveness helps to enhance relationships, avoid power games and is a vehicle for clear outcomes. Hargie (2006) details four elements of assertive communication:

- *Content* – where the rights of the people involved are embedded gently in the statement. This could be done using an explanation, empathy for the listener, praise for the listener, an apology for the consequence for

Nursing skills 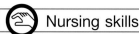 Box 9.8

Verbal communication strategies

Occupational therapist (OT) – 'Ghedi has been out with the student to the sports centre. He relaxed once he knew that he could choose a time that was set aside for people new to the gym. He said that he was happy to attend twice a week, so he bought a 6-month off-peak pass. It was really reasonable; I have one, they really are worth the money. Anyway, he went to his first session, Tai Chi, then back for lunch. He says he feels confident and relaxed and he really does look it too.'

Summarizing

Keyworker – 'Oh, thanks for that information, so [*in summary*], he's got his membership, will be attending at off-peak times, he had his first session of Tai Chi and he is feeling confident and relaxed. Great.'

Paraphrasing

Keyworker – 'OK, so Ghedi has been out, joined the sports centre, paid for 6 months off-peak and has already started to use the facilities. He's fine with this and feeling confident.'

Clarifying

Keyworker – 'OK [*let me get this clear*], Ghedi has been out this morning to the sports centre, got an off-peak membership, he is feeling better because he knows this is a quieter time and he has already been to his first Tai Chi class and feels fine about the arrangements?'

Feedback

Keyworker – 'That's great news. I hope the student will be going with Ghedi again soon as this is so important to him.'

the listener or a compromise that is favourable to both people
- *Covert elements* – where the speaker is able to recognize their rights and the rights of the listener in the communication process. These include respect, expressing feelings, having your own priorities, being able to say 'no', being able to make mistakes and choosing to say nothing (see Further reading, e.g. Holland & Ward 1997)
- *Process* – concerned with how a person expresses themselves assertively. Is their body language (see Non-verbal communication, below), intonation (see p. 216) and choice of language reflective of a confident assertive person? Are the processes that make up communication congruent, in keeping with what is being said? The process also involves managing the setting so that people are not embarrassed, or the 'noise' levels are kept to a minimum (see pp. 214-215). Increasing the likelihood of assertive communication happening again involves feedback to the listener to show that their accomplishment is appreciated
- *The non-verbal cues* – gesture, touch, proxemics and posture – also need to reflect confidence, regard and respect for self and others (see below and pp. 203-204).

Negotiation and delegation

These are areas that depend on assertive communication. Negotiation is the process where people come together with their own ideas, discuss their ideas and agree on an outcome that is acceptable to both parties. It could be as simple as negotiating an off duty change, e.g.

> Nurse A asks Nurse B to change a duty on Wednesday because she needs the morning off. Nurse B agrees if Nurse A will do the same for her next Sunday. They agree and the plan is negotiated.

Delegation is another way of getting things done. Delegation often occurs between people of different authority, e.g.:

> Staff Nurse A: 'Andrew, Ms Wilkinson's medicines are ready to be picked up and her lift home will be here soon. Please could you go over for them?'

Staff Nurse A has delegated the task of collecting the prescription from pharmacy to Andrew, a 1st year student nurse. When delegating to another person it is imperative to be polite, assertive and clear. Offering information to support the request allows the other person to understand why they are being asked to perform a task. Delegation is reliant on a number of issues:

- Can the person accept the delegated task? Do they have the right level of knowledge, experience, skills, responsibility or status?
- Is it the right time to delegate this task to this individual?
- Are you delegating because you have left something too late? If so, how will the timeframe for completion affect this person?
- Does the situation allow for the task to be delegated?

Non-verbal communication

Non-verbal communication is that part of communication that is not reliant on words. As approximately 60% of communication is non-verbal, non-verbal skills are essential for effective communication. It is clear that people determine a great deal of meaning from aspects of communication other than words. People who are blind or partially sighted generally place more emphasis on the intonation of a person's voice to pick up the non-verbal messages (see Ch. 16). Argyle (1994) suggested that non-verbal communication was made up of:

- Accent
- Bodily contact
- Direction of gaze
- Emotive tone in speech
- Facial and gestural movements
- Physical appearance
- Posture
- Proximity
- Speech errors
- Timing of speech.

This section focuses on gesture, touch, proxemics and posture. Paralinguistic issues, i.e. the voiced aspects of non-verbal behaviour, for instance 'guggles', are discussed later.

Gesture

Gesture is a crucial aspect of non-verbal communication. Some psychologists and linguists suggest that early humans used gesture before they used spoken or signed language (Armstrong et al 1995). Gestures can be classified into categories of increasing complexity.

Universal gestures that are understood by most people include opening arms and eyes wide to suggest bigness; furrowed brows, pursed lips, drawing body inwards and moving index fingers together would suggest smallness. Subtler gestures include a cupped hand to the mouth to indicate a drink, or a single upwards gesture of the hand with palm facing upwards suggests that someone stand up.

Certain gestures are recognized as specific to a language community, such as the 'OK' gesture with thumb and index finger touching to make a circle with the other fingers raised. However, it is important to be aware that some gestures that are acceptable in one community are possibly offensive in another.

Touch

This is a complex communication subject and often difficult to tackle. Children tend to be touched more than adults. Interestingly, babies and young children who do not experience touch do not thrive as well as those who do (Hargie 2006).

Touch for many people is an essential aspect of their working lives. Nurses in particular must learn how to touch people in a professional context without causing embarrassment or concern to the patient/client. In addition, nurses must ensure their own safety. Nurses use two clear types of touch: first and often the most intimate type is the necessary touch nurses use when attending to people's physical needs and during other nursing interventions; the second type is the touch that communicates a feeling or a meaning, such as, 'I am here for you'. Everyone has a personal view about touch, when it is appropriate and when not. People from different cultures will touch each other according to their accepted norms.

It is suggested that a well-timed touch on the shoulder or hand can help a person in distress to feel comforted, which in turn creates a sense of trust. Touch in this scenario is thought to encourage the person's cathartic release by communicating that you are with them in the moment, supporting them and sharing their feelings. This affirms their sense of self, respects their distress and shows the nurse's commitment to their needs.

Touch is more appropriate in some clinical settings than in others. Understanding what is acceptable in each area is important and nurses can learn much from each other (Box 9.9). As a student new to a client group, it is useful to know how people deal with clients' emotions. Also crucial is an understanding of common courtesy (see pp. 200-201) and the social norms of the patients/clients and carers who are most likely to attend the clinical setting. Nurses should attend to their developing professional boundaries at all times and question the actions of others that are discourteous or abusive.

It is vital that nurses also recognize their own feelings around touch (Box 9.10).

Reflective practice   Box 9.9

Appropriate touch – learning from others

Nurses who are consciously competent in respecting a client's dignity will more readily engage their trust, and therefore be more likely to be able to work therapeutically and less likely to cause offence. Think about occasions when you worked with registered nurses who perform the most intimate of procedures while maintaining the dignity of the patient/client.

Student activities

- How did the nurse behave in relation to touch?
- What did they say to the patient/client?
- Reflect on how the patient/client may have felt

Reflective practice   Box 9.10

Feelings about touch

Think about your feelings about being touched and touching others.

Student activities

- What is your norm?
- How does that fit in with the clinical environment?
- Could you leave yourself or others open to the risk of inappropriate touch or at risk of feeling alone and isolated when in distress?

Proxemics

Proxemics is a fascinating area of communication – people have very different views about their own personal space – how close people like to be to others and how close they like others to be to them, can be very complex and bound by personal rules.

Boundaries enable people to feel comfortable in their environment. Some boundaries are fixed, such as walls and rooms within buildings; others are semi-fixed, such as the seating in the clinic or seating arrangements in a dining room and the location of the television. These arrangements are an indication of where to sit, where to eat and which way to face. Fixed and semi-fixed boundaries can help or hinder communication.

Another boundary is the informal space between people. This space is fluid and utilized in different ways for different messages and in different settings.

The person listening will be aware of the distance between themselves and the speaker and vice versa. There are clear cultural differences in the distance people accept between each other.

Knowingly intruding into someone's personal space can be very intimidating for the listener. This approach is used to interrogate or bully people, resulting in their disempowerment. It may be necessary to gently remind colleagues or children or clients that their comfort zone may be smaller than that of other people.

Posture

How a person holds their body in relation to other people and in relation to the fixed and semi-fixed boundaries communicates a great deal about what they are feeling and thinking. Posture sends a very clear message, e.g. leaning forward indicates interest and respect for the other person. On the other hand, despite looking at the other person, a lack of interest is portrayed if the listener's body is orientated towards the door, or sitting back in the chair arms folded and head down.

How a person filters the information provided by the external event will affect their thoughts, feelings and behaviours; therefore their posture is a mirror of their inner beliefs (see below).

When a nurse wants to create a sense of confidence, they walk into the situation with their head held high, at a moderate pace. People will look at the nurse's posture and decide very quickly whether they like them or not and whether they can be trusted or not. Once people have made a judgement, it is difficult to convince them otherwise. This may seem a little harsh but it is a survival technique that has helped people to function socially for thousands of years.

Listening skills

How do people know that they are really listening to someone, or that someone is really listening to them? Many nurses claim to be good listeners, because in the clinical environment to suggest otherwise is as bad as saying they are poor nurses.

People often know when someone is not listening to them; they feel ignored, undervalued, frustrated and disempowered. Not listening to the other person can seriously affect the relationship. In a nurse–patient/client relationship the outcome of not listening to a client can result in their choices being reduced, e.g. not eating their choice of food, the nurse not understanding their fears/anxieties, the potential for misdiagnosis and ultimately ineffective or even harmful treatment. If nurses fail to listen to colleagues, not only is vital information missed but it can also affect the colleagues' motivation, trust, self-esteem and skills.

There are a number of reasons for listening and different types of listening skills are needed. Wolvin and Coakley (1996) identified four types of listening:

- *To comprehend in order to understand information*: When listening for understanding the focus is on main topics, ideas and data. In the clinical setting it is used during ward rounds and handovers, for receiving information from patients/clients, etc.
- *To appreciate sound, to feel relaxed or at ease*: This includes listening to music on headphones or in a Snoezelen room (see Ch. 11); listening to a meditation tape or to recordings of 'sounds of nature' in order to relax – all for pleasure, meditation or well-being
- *To evaluate information, when the speaker wants to persuade or to influence behaviour*: This may include evaluating information from a drug company representative, wound care advisors and continence nurses, and to weigh up points in team meetings

- *To empathize where the focus is on the speaker rather than the listener*: In this situation, the aim is to listen to patients/clients, etc. who need to talk/express themselves in order to alleviate stress, to problem-solve or to release tensions. This type of listening is a therapeutic skill that practitioners must acquire.

Characteristics of good listening

Good listening skills are vital to rapport and empathy (see pp. 207-208). The following characteristics of good listening are based on English-speaking Western cultural norms. People from different linguistic and cultural groups have different norms of communicative behaviour (see pp. 216-217).

Appropriate eye contact

Appropriate eye contact is where the listener looks at the speaker. They blink just after the speaker blinks or when they are ending a sentence. The listener's blink rate matches that of the speaker and corresponds with their head nods of encouragement. The eye gaze is generally soft, as opposed to staring and hard (eyes slightly wider than usual denotes some muscular tension). However, the listener's gaze also mirrors the verbal and non-verbal expressions of the speaker.

Mirroring

When engaged in listening, people naturally find themselves 'mirroring' the speaker's posture. This does not mean copying their every movement as if playing a game; instead the listener may be leaning slightly in the same direction, tapping their pen at the same time the speaker is tapping their foot, folding one arm across the body as the speaker folds both arms (Box 9.11).

 Critical thinking   Box 9.11

Mirroring

Watch an experienced nurse and patient/client or a couple who are getting on well.

Student activity

Observe their posture, their mannerisms, their tempo or timing of their movements. See if you can notice how much the listener is mirroring the speaker. For example, do they have similar facial expressions, gestures, posture and movements?

This behaviour is a natural sign for the speaker to show that the listener is with them, acknowledging their mood, recognizing their feelings and trying to understand them. This behaviour increases rapport between them and encourages the process to continue.

Nurses and other healthcare professionals often need to develop trust and rapport quickly in order to work effectively with people. Being aware of their skills in mirroring another person is vital in enhancing the therapeutic or professional relationship (see pp. 205-214).

Guggles

Guggles are the sounds (non-words) uttered when listening, e.g. 'mmmms', 'ahs', 'hmm'. These affirm the speaker's point, agree with them and confirm their view or idea. To do this, guggles rely heavily on intonation and tunes (see p. 216). The use of guggles by the listener encourages the speaker to continue by providing evidence that the listener is listening (Box 9.12).

(see p. 216)

Reflective practice   Box 9.12

Skills that encourage and discourage conversation

Next time you are listening to a friend telling you a story (one that is not too sensitive), listen to your own guggles.

Student activities

- Gently increase the number of guggles you use. What difference does it make to your friend's storytelling?
- If you gently reduce the number of guggles so that you hardly express any, how does this affect the storytelling?
- If you increase them a little more, does this make any difference?
- How many guggles become too many and stop your friend telling the story because they feel uncomfortable?
- Tell your friend what you having been doing, apologize and ask them how it made them feel.
- Reflect on the experience with your friend and consider how you will use it to improve your listening skills.

Active listening

Nurses and others often highlight active listening as an essential skill; as the term implies there is a need for energy and concentration on the part of the nurse when they actively listen. The aim is to enhance the quality of the therapeutic relationship and to facilitate problem-solving by being with the speaker on a social, psychological and emotional level (Egan 1998). In active listening, the listener:

- Listens to the speaker, bearing in mind the context of the speaker's message with regard to their background, life experience and current situation, i.e. their 'blueprint of behaviour'
- Attends to the speaker's non-verbal behaviours
- Listens and understands the speaker's message
- Listens for inconsistencies in the message and incongruence between what is being said and the speaker's non-verbal behaviour.

Active listening requires the practitioner to understand:

- How and why people communicate the way they do
- What language they are likely to use
- How a person's non-verbal communication provides information about the message.

Nursing relationships

So far, this chapter has provided the knowledge and encouragement needed to develop skills in a variety of ways to create a good communicator. This section draws upon this learning for enhancing communication in a range of relationships with different outcomes.

The types of relationship that people connect with on a day-to-day basis are intimate, social, professional and therapeutic. The focus here is on the therapeutic and professional relationships that nurses experience and how these relate to care and health outcomes.

Therapeutic relationships

Nurses have therapeutic relationships with the patients/clients/children, families and carers they work with. The therapies they offer cover a wide range of interventions from an adult nurse providing education about insulin therapy to mental health nurses providing cognitive behavioural therapy. Interventions also include assisting adults and children with the activities in ways that maintain the individual's independence, dignity and health, e.g. eating and drinking, bathing. An essential component that underpins all nursing interventions, from daily living needs, to sophisticated procedures, is the 'therapeutic relationship' (Box 9.13).

The therapeutic relationship   Box 9.13

Who
- Nurses and other health professionals.

Who may
- Provide a specific health-related service.

Who will
- Have skills to maximize the personal exploration and health of the patient/client
- Use strategies to underpin these skills
- Focus on the patient's/client's needs
- Be led by the patient's/client's issues
- Develop problem-solving capacity in the patient/client
- Evaluate the change in the patient/client to identify progress towards optimum health.

Who don't
- Work outside contractual boundaries
- Relate on an intimate or social level with the client
- Need the client to like them
- Expect mutual appreciation to occur.

This relationship is the foundation on which the nurse and patient/client can work in alliance to identify issues that are affecting them and that require change. The therapeutic relationship facilitates the patient/client to move from their current state of ill health, distress or need to their desired state of maximum attainable health, well-being and strength. Where patients/clients are unlikely to achieve full health, the therapeutic relationship is used to assist reconciliation, alleviate stress and provide solace and support.

The therapeutic relationship relies on specific components being in place, including rapport, empathy, trust, genuineness, warmth and positive regard (see pp. 207-209). The therapeutic relationship requires the nurse to have active listening

(see pp. 207-209)

skills and proficient interpersonal skills (see pp. 204-205). It is also vital for the practitioner to know their own values and beliefs and how these can trigger filters that may affect their resourcefulness.

Skills that develop 'connectedness', the emotional connection between two people, are great; however, the nurse also needs to develop a range of communication strategies. This may sound quite manipulative and in the wrong hands, good communication skills can be devastating if the aim of the strategy is to gain at the expense of another person. When developing relationships and communication strategies, it is necessary to reflect on the desired outcome and decide whether it is ethically and morally correct; to do this, first and foremost nurses require self-awareness.

Self-awareness skills

Self-awareness involves exploration of thoughts, feelings and behaviours. It includes an understanding of how internal and external events influence people and how they behave. The more nurses search within themselves for meaning and understanding, the better they understand their skills and limitations and how their responses can affect others. The concept of self-awareness suggests that people are always able to learn, develop and improve. Some people are very self-aware; they clearly understand how they are affected by internal and external stimuli and know how their response may affect other people. Others lack this level of understanding of self and, as a result, they do not know the likely effects on others and this can be a barrier to effective communication.

Nurses are strongly encouraged to work within their limitations. When people work beyond their competence through lack of self-awareness, mistakes occur and people can suffer. Most nurses can recall an occasion where communication was impeded by lack of self-awareness, e.g. by people not listening properly or by only looking at a problem from their point of view.

What influences people's knowledge about themselves to make them more self-aware? People are influenced by their beliefs and values: those who are internally motivated will only accept feedback on their behaviour from people whom they hold in high regard; others do not rely on their own internal beliefs but instead like to know other people's opinions about their thoughts and behaviours. People who are either entirely internally motivated or entirely externally motivated will limit their own development. A mixture of both approaches is the most reasonable way to develop knowledge about self and others.

There are life experiences that provide feedback to deepen self-awareness by seeing how others see you, e.g.:

- Social links and friendships
- Emotional lives
- Close relationships
- Spiritual and ethical beliefs
- Financial concerns/control
- Current job role and career aspirations
- What meanings they place on words of value such as love, life, happiness, honour, care, professionalism, etc.

People are shaped by information that enables an increasing self-awareness and ability to empathize and develop rapport with others. The knowledge people gain through reflection and meaningful self-questioning allows them to develop a wider perspective of life (Box 9.14). Limited knowledge of themselves and others means that they are unable to contribute effectively.

⟳ **Reflective practice**   **Box 9.14**

Self-questioning skills

In order to develop self-questioning skills, you can try layering your questions around the themes known to influence people's lives. To begin the layering process, ask yourself simple questions around the meaning of the words you chose to use and 'listen' to the answers. You will find a natural focus for your next question, as part of your answer leads to another meaningful question. For example:

- *What does my career mean to me?* My career means that I am part of a profession.
- *What does being in a profession mean to me?* It means that I have a responsibility to enact my roles and responsibilities in a way that respects nursing as an art.
- *What does the term 'the art of nursing' mean to me?* The art of nursing is about the relationship nurses have with patients/clients and families that promote care giving.

Student activities

- What does the relationship nurses have with their patients and families mean to you?

When questioning yourself, get used to asking the question using the words you have just 'heard' from the last answer. This strategy of reflection will help you develop your reflective skills when dealing with patients/clients and carers, as reflection enhances the therapeutic relationship.

Attributes of a nurse–patient/client relationship

Not all nurse–patient/client relationships are the in-depth type utilized by nurses working in learning disability or mental health settings. The focus of nursing relationships is to bring about change in a person's health or facilitate an optimum quality of life. Sometimes this involves empowering the person to do this independently; on other occasions the nurse will undertake a nursing intervention for a client. There are some attributes common to all nurse–patient/client relationships and in nurse–family/carer relationships.

Being there

O'Brien (2000) suggests that patients/clients like the nurse to 'be there' for them. This appears a simple job but it is an intense and emotionally powerful task to do for someone. Being there is being present for the patient/client when needed. This can provide a sense of achievement for the nurse and will sometimes leave the nurse feeling exhausted having worked hard emotionally (see Ch. 11).

Self-disclosure

O'Brien (2000) also found that, in developing and sustaining a nurse–patient/client relationship, the nurse needed to disclose some information about him/herself. This was to show humanity and put the two people on an equal footing. The more people share with another person, the closer they can feel to them, thus increasing rapport.

Patients/clients sometimes think that they are the only ones who are having difficulties; by some self-disclosure, the patient/client is able to see that others share their difficulties. This also validates their feelings and provides perspective for the problem.

It is also easy to disclose too much information, particularly when nurses have developed a good rapport with the patient/client or carer. Having good rapport (see p. 208) enables nurses to feel comfortable with the other person and to discuss things not usually discussed. This can be damaging to both nurse and the patient/client if the information shared can be used to make the other person feel vulnerable or limit the therapeutic value of the relationship (West & Turner 2009).

Being concerned

Being concerned enhances the nurse–patient/client relationship (O'Brien 2000). Nurses develop a protective feeling towards the people they work with, while recognizing the need for the patient/client to make their own decisions about their lives and health. Nurses were clear that their role was to offer choice and alternatives to facilitate the patient/client in problem-solving and this helps develop a confirming relationship (West & Turner 2009).

Trust

Trusting another person is sometimes hard and at other times, easy. Some people automatically trust medical professionals because they believe they are in a position of expert knowledge and power, and are caring. In trusting someone, people tend to expect certain behaviours. For example, they want the person to be:

- Honest and not to lie
- Kindly and not to be cruel
- Consistent in their behaviour towards them so that they 'know where they stand'
- True to their word – if they say they are going to do something and they do, then people will trust them to be true to them again.

Trust is hard won and very easy to lose, and regaining lost trust is very difficult. Losing trust is best avoided by giving time, energy, concern and regard to everyone involved.

Being 'as if' – emotional labour

It would be naive to assume that nurses will never be challenged by wanting to ignore a person, to snap at a patient/client who appears overly demanding, to wish that the patient's/client's family would realize that the nurse has other people to look after, or that they feel like crying too. At the most challenging times, nurses who manage to maintain their professionalism tend to use clear strategies for dealing with such situations. Some strategies to maintain a professional profile include:

- Wearing a uniform or clearly defined work clothes helps to give some identity to the task – 'in these clothes I am

first and foremost a nurse'. A uniform/work clothes provides some professional space
- Recognizing a colleague who would manage well in this challenging situation. Identify how they would be behaving and copy this behaviour, 'in this meeting I will be professional like Nurse Jenkins'
- Disassociating from the emotions of the situation by thinking of something less upsetting. Breathe deeply; do something to take your mind off the upset for a few seconds, re-engage as a resourceful nurse
- Seeing the situation in a scientific way or as a service provider can reduce the emotional labour involved.

Whatever the strategy chosen, it is important to remain outwardly congruent (outward behaviour should be true to the situation) or others may construe that the nurse does not care.

Empathy

Empathy is when a person puts themselves in the other person's position, attempting to understand the world as they see it. Empathy is an emotional response to another person's situation; people often describe feeling a physical sensation when they see someone in a bad emotional or physical state.

It is not uncommon for people to want to laugh if they see or hear others laughing, yawn when they see others yawning and cry when others are upset. We are 'wired' to echo the movements and the expressed emotions of others. By doing this, people feel the same physical feeling, have thoughts that relate to the feeling and behave in ways that relate to the thoughts and feelings. People can influence others with their happy mood or bad temper. Emotions are 'infectious' because people have a tendency to automatically empathize. This is classed as 'emotional contagion' (West & Turner 2009).

For some people, empathizing is not easy. These people are naturally self-orientated. This does not mean they are self-centred; they are more internally focused. People with autism and Asperger syndrome have challenges in empathizing because they have a limited 'theory of mind'. This constrains their ability to attribute thoughts and feelings to other people and to understand that other people's thoughts and feelings are different to their own. This affects their social and communicative competence.

People with autism may feel confused when faced with other people's behaviour, it can seem random and bewildering. Some people with autism will go through life without social connections or needing to be with others, preferring the calm of their own world, routines and structures. Other individuals can be aware that there is a difference in the way they relate to others. This realization of poor psychological connectedness may be challenging and confusing and can result in an increased sense of difference for the individual.

Children with autism show this lack of psychological connectedness with those around them and also in their play; they may find role-play challenging because they cannot attribute behaviours, thought and feelings to others, including toys. The inability to imitate others such as playing 'mum' or 'teacher' stifles the child's development in attributing roles to people, standing in other people's shoes and seeing the world through their eyes, i.e. empathizing (Box 9.15).

? Critical thinking Box 9.15

Sharif

7-year-old Sharif has autism. He is extremely distressed, having hit his head. Sharif needs to attend the Emergency Department, but his mother, who is also very upset, feels that there is no possibility of Sharif cooperating with hospital staff. Sharif is clinging desperately to his red lorry, looking straight ahead and avoiding contact with his mum.

Student activities

- Think of ways in which you could communicate the need to go to hospital to Sharif.
- How would you help his mother to assist in the situation? How would you show empathy to her?

Rapport

Rapport is the connection between two people, where they talk on the same 'wavelength', share the same humour and share each other's pain and sorrow. Couples, family members and lifelong friends often experience deep rapport.

Rapport plays a significant part in developing a therapeutic relationship but this does not mean that without rapport nurses cannot facilitate change in people's health. However, rapport promotes productive relationships and thereby better outcomes for all. There are three different levels of rapport (Table 9.3).

Level three is often associated with being deeply attached to someone. Although most people have the opportunity to feel this depth of closeness during their lives, others are less fortunate. This level of rapport is not appropriate for a nurse to share with a patient/client or carer. Feeling this close to someone negates any possibility of a professional therapeutic

relationship; the nurse would not be a resource for the patient/client/child or carer. Nurses who share this level of rapport with people they work for can experience immense stress, destroy professional trust and can seriously affect the health of the patient/client (see Boundaries are healthy, below).

A working level of rapport gives power to each person in the relationship; it gives the nurse room to provide the correct care within the limitations of their role and responsibilities and encourages them to refer to others when necessary. The professional alliance formed respects the participants for the skills and knowledge they bring to the situation. Importantly, people remain independent of each other; they do not merge into one entity.

Rapport is easier between individuals who share similar life experiences, values, belief systems and language. This is because trust comes easier in these situations. In developing rapport and empathy with patients/clients and carers it is important to realize that people relate to each other on very different levels and to different degrees depending on their circumstances and their ability to comprehend others. Some people have difficulty in understanding how to relate to other people in a healthy way. These difficulties in relating to others may be due to anxiety, anger, confusion or poor relational skills.

Facilitating change

In therapeutic relationships, nurses are trusted to assist change in patients/clients and carers by facilitating the understanding of information. They are also entrusted with the task of helping a person involved in this health process to move from the current state A to the desired state B (Fig. 9.4).

Communication and interpersonal skills underpin facilitation (Box 9.16). A patient/client is unable to move from A to B if they cannot relate to the nurse, i.e. if rapport, trust, the nurse's concern and the nurse's skills in 'being there' for the client are not evident. Nor will they move from A to B if

Table 9.3 Levels of rapport		
Level of rapport	**Description**	**Who**
Level 1	No rapport The beginnings of a connection	Strangers who have just met. They neither need to know each other nor want to People who have spent a little time together and are exploring common ground
Level 2	A connection creating good communication	People are making the effort to understand each other socially, professionally Finding out about each other and using interpersonal skills to express ideas, needs, to investigate and gather evidence either on a social or professional level; this might be from meeting someone for the first time and realizing you both enjoy the same music Sales people may have excellent communication skills and are adept at creating rapport at speed because that is when you are most likely to purchase their product You could be working with a family who are being educated regarding the health of their child who has a long-term illness
	Good connection, good communication, mutual feelings of relating well	The people involved are actively listening to each other, good eye contact, personal space is within 3 metres
Level 3	Excellent connection, relaxed, easy communication, parties sense a physical closeness	People involved feel the other person really knows them, feels they can share everything, almost as if the other person automatically knows what they are thinking They can pre-empt the other person's next move

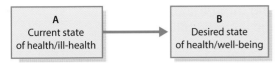

Fig. 9.4 • Facilitating change from the current state to the desired state.

? Critical thinking   Box 9.16

Nurse–patient/client relationship and care delivery

1. Rosa telephoned the GP surgery in a very agitated state. She tells the practice nurse that she has just done a pregnancy test and it's positive. Rosa and her partner wanted a baby, but they didn't think it would happen so soon and Rosa continued drinking a glass of wine most days.

2. Emily is key nurse to 8-year-old Imran who has leukaemia and his parents Rahil and Muntasir Ahmed. Imran's parents are always with him and are fully involved with the care team. Imran will need long-term care, both at home and in hospital.

3. Simon is running the CBT clinic and has just met Mr Desai who has concerns about his lack of sleep, anxiety and inability to concentrate on his work, which is putting his job at risk.

4. Ali is on a community placement that caters for people with moderate to severe learning disabilities. He is working closely with his mentor and Paul who is experiencing a particularly distressing time due to his parents' divorce. Paul resorts to obsessional behaviours as a coping mechanism for his feelings of anxiety; these behaviours only emerge in times of severe stress.

Student activities

In each case consider:

- What opportunities does the nurse have to develop a nurse–patient relationship with the patients/clients/families?
- What level of rapport could be developed between the nurse and the patient/family?
- How will the nurse develop the patient's/client's/family's trust in them?

---

the nurse does not have the communication strategies to be a resourceful facilitator.

The scenarios in Box 9.16 provide different levels of contact between nurse and patient/client/carer, all of which require different levels of relationship building. No one way fits all and nurses have to accept that while they value good interpersonal communication skills and strategies, not all nurse–patient/client/carer relationships need to be in-depth to be resourceful, but it is vital that some are.

Positive regard

Positive regard is the ability to hold and convey feelings for other people that are not based on negative beliefs about the person. Having positive regard for patients/clients, carers, parents and colleagues enables the nurse to approach others with positive intentions towards them as a valued human being. Maintaining positive regard for people can help nurses manage their thoughts, feelings and behaviours even in

situations where the other person may be behaving in a way that is inappropriate.

Boundaries are healthy

Boundaries are useful and positive rules that enhance resourceful relationships to improve health outcomes. Some nurses find the correct level of boundary between themselves and patients/clients easy to judge, whereas others find it more challenging and many nurses can remember where they 'got it wrong'.

Boundaries begin to develop as soon as the nurse meets the patient/client or carer and explains their role and responsibilities. A clear and concise explanation gives information about what the nurse does, thus enabling the patient/client or carer to begin to develop a picture of why each healthcare professional is involved and, crucially, how they, the patient/client or carer will be involved in the process.

On one level, the public needs to know the roles, responsibilities and level of involvement they can expect from healthcare practitioners, as outlined above. At a deeper level, nurses are enhancing the ability to be in a resourceful position for the people they work with. Boundaries enable nurses to maintain a professional commitment to the public; nurses are resources who offer healthcare, expertise and skills to facilitate change in ways that would be difficult if they became 'friends' with the people they work with. Professional and therapeutic boundaries are safety nets for the protection of everyone involved.

Boundaries also provide clarity for professionals. People working in healthcare often find themselves working across professional boundaries; nurses may overlap with occupational therapists (OTs) or social workers in the same way as they may overlap with traditional nursing roles. For example, supporting people in their own homes with developing independence skills could be facilitated by a nurse, an OT or a social worker, particularly when they work in multidisciplinary teams (MDTs).

Boundaries sometimes go wrong by being unclear, breached, ignored, too stringent or, more seriously, abused. Unclear boundaries do not provide the supportive structure needed for clinicians to deliver the service required. Moreover, lack of clarity disempowers the patient/client and carer because they do not have the information required to be fully involved in their care. Unclear boundaries can lead to breaches of professional conduct (see Ch. 7), including over-involvement or abuse by either the care provider or the person receiving care.

Professionals who are unclear about each other's roles create confusion, which can impede communication and service delivery, meaning that patients/clients and carers suffer. Unclear professional boundaries can lead to missing information, which can have extremely serious consequences such as role confusion, misdiagnosis, incomplete assessments or poor care and health outcomes.

Therapeutic relationship stages

Peplau's (1952) model of the therapeutic relationship described in Varcarolis and Halter (2009) comprises:

- Pre-orientation
- Orientation

- Working
- Termination.

Pre-orientation stage

This occurs before communicating with the patient/client. It is crucial at this stage for the nurse to recognize their beliefs and values regarding the person and their family. This requires the nurse to be mindful of the values and beliefs they hold. Understanding how their blueprint of behaviour (p. 194) may differ from the other person's and how this may affect the therapeutic relationship is important. With this knowledge the nurse can monitor their own behaviour, working towards better understanding and acceptance for others.

This stage allows the nurse to discover information from the patient's/client's notes, the MDT and possibly family members. This information can enhance the communication between nurse and patient/client at the initial meetings. It may also enable the nurse to make informed choices regarding the need to provide immediate care and to manage risk.

Orientation stage

This stage of the relationship can take time. It provides the opportunity to establish roles and responsibilities, boundaries and trust. It is at this critical point that the nurse will discuss confidentiality (see below), times and regularity of meetings, and arrangements for informing each other should it be necessary to cancel a meeting. An important feature of this discussion is for the nurse to have the confidence to talk with the patient/client about how the sessions/meetings will end once the patient/client is ready to move on.

Working stage

During the working stage of the relationship, the nurse enables the patient/client to safely:

- Explore current issues impacting on their lives
- Establish well-formed goals
- Develop problem-solving skills to address the issues
- Identify behaviours that are resistant to change and to facilitate shifts in these behaviours
- Provide a safe place for the client to try out new behaviours and beliefs
- Evaluate progress according to the patient's/client's journey
- Redefine patient/client goals as movement occurs.

Termination stage

With a clear understanding of goals identified and resolved in the working stage, termination of the relationship is a necessary and therapeutic point of the relationship. Termination may also need to occur if the patient/client and nurse are 'stuck' and one or other does not have the resources to move the relationship forward.

It is at this stage that the patient/client and the nurse can reflect on the journey they have both taken. Sharing the feelings that termination arouses in the nurse is valuable to the patient/client. Not only does it teach each person how they can cope with a relationship ending, it gives respect to the patient/client.

Working in partnership with families – confidentiality

Confidentiality is a central concept for nurses (see Chs 6, 7). The Nursing and Midwifery Council (NMC 2008, p 3), provides a clear statement:

- 'You must respect people's right to confidentiality
- You must ensure people are informed about how and why information is shared by those who will be providing their care
- You must disclose information if you believe someone may be at risk of harm, in line with the law of the country in which you are practising'.

The principle of confidentiality is to protect individuals from indiscriminate disclosure and divulgence of their personal information. All people have the right to privacy and to personal information to be protected by the professionals working with them.

Nurses build relationships on trust, ensuring patients/clients develop trust and so enhance the ability to work therapeutically. Nurses ask people to give very intimate and detailed information as part of the nursing process (see Ch. 14).

People need to know that the information they give to health professionals is safe from improper disclosure:

'If the patient or client withholds consent, or if consent cannot be obtained for whatever reason, disclosures may be made only where:

- they can be justified in the public interest (usually where disclosure is essential to protect the patient or client or someone else from the risk of significant harm)
- they are required by law or by order of a court.'

Where there is an issue of child protection, you must act at all times in accordance with the NMC, national and local policies.

Nurses who breach confidentiality are liable to disciplinary action from their employer, action by the regulatory body that could result in their removal from the professional register and ultimately legal action from the patient/client or carer (see Ch. 6).

Nurses have a duty to inform patients/clients and carers of their responsibilities regarding maintaining and possibly breaching confidence. Nurses may initially find this a difficult topic to discuss with someone who has come to them for 'help'. However, having the confidence to clearly outline your role as a nurse and the boundaries of that role, shows the client respect and honesty, thus developing the nurse–patient/client relationship.

Nurses do need to judge whether they should explain the full details of when they would be required to breach confidentiality. For example, a community nurse working to support an adult newly diagnosed with diabetes may find it unnecessary to discuss 'abuse' or 'serious offences'. However, it is acceptable to outline roles, responsibilities and boundaries in a clear and informative manner.

Managing significant information

It is a particularly daunting prospect to tell someone 'bad news' or something that they would find worrying. Managing information that has significance for the person may involve information about serious illness or death. However, just as with the experience of pain, 'significant information' is individual to the person receiving it, e.g. a patient/client being told that their partner has phoned to say they missed the bus and cannot visit today may consider this to be significant. Therefore, it is useful to assume that, because people have different blueprints of behaviour and different internal maps of the world, it is not always possible to know how the person will react.

Most patients/clients, carers and parents want to know the truth, even the bad parts. Managing significant information with a child is very dependent on their age, stage of development and the wishes and involvement of the parents. People with cognitive and communication difficulties, people who speak another language and people in distress need nurses to be sensitive to their communication needs.

In managing significant information with a person who has a cognitive disability, the nurse needs to be aware of the person's cognitive level and their concept of illness or death. It is important that the person is told in a timely manner in terms they can understand, i.e. provided with information that is as meaningful as possible in a mode that is accessible.

Registered nurses who communicate significant information will draw upon their interpersonal skills, rapport and empathy. They will be aware of their verbal and non-verbal communication. They will use skills to match the other person's communication by converging, matching vocabulary, pace and loudness, and being congruent to the message (Kurtz et al 2004). Feedback skills are used by the speaker to ensure that the message has been decoded and understood, to ensure their communication has the desired outcome. Again, having a communication model in mind will help the nurse focus on the communication and outcome.

Different strategies for managing significant information have been developed and most follow a set pattern (Box 9.17) which provides assistance to the nurse and the right level of information to the listener. These strategies can be tailored to all clients, carers and children by adapting language and interpersonal skills in accordance with their communication needs.

Professional relationships

The primary purpose of a professional relationship is to work with other professionals in order to fulfil the needs of the core task, i.e. patient/client care. The components of a professional relationship centre around the professional skills the participants bring to the relationship so that the core task can be met. Professional relationships are enhanced through:

- Understanding roles and responsibilities
- Defined boundaries where appropriate
- Clear communication strategies
- Openness and honesty
- Trust
- Responsibility and accountability accepted by each professional for their area of work.

Strategies for managing significant information	Box 9.17

Preparation

- See the person as soon as possible
- Reduce the levels of external 'noise' and possible interruptions
- Use a comfortable/neutral setting
- Organize family or friend support
- Know the background information
- Check your own feelings – another nurse may be the correct person to give the information.

Starting off

- Gather information about what has happened recently and what information is already known
- Assess the emotions, thoughts and feelings of the person to decide where to start the discussion, how to pitch it and how much information to give
- Outline the need for discussion and a possible process and ask permission
- Ascertain how much information the person wants.

Presenting the information

- Present information clearly. Know what is to be said and what outcome is required
- Present the information in understandable 'chunks', remembering the 'noise' created by stress and distress
- If possible, get clarification that the person has understood
- Be gentle, empathic and acknowledge the person's feelings
- Use accessible language and use silence to enable the person to digest the information
- Be aware of the person's responses. Be attentive to their verbal/non-verbal language that provide clues to their inner feelings and adapt communication/relational skills.

Provide support and clarify next steps

- Have a support plan ready for the person, e.g. specialized resources, family members, social workers, counsellors, etc.
- Explain clearly what happens next
- 'Chunk' the next steps information into understandable sections; support with written or pictorial information as appropriate
- Give clear timeframes where appropriate; for some illnesses, this could be difficult
- Allow the person to look for the best outcome from the information and gently encourage them to focus on the information.

Communication and care coordination within the MDT

It is important to recognize that, despite each person's professional independence, they also relate to each other as a team. This enhances the unity, effectiveness and efficiency of the team and meets the individual need for belonging. Most, though not all, people find this relationship positive (Mullins 2008). Members of the team relate along several dimensions including power, status, liking, communication, roles and leadership (see pp. 212-213) (Buchanan & Huczynski 2004). All the dimensions are communicated through non-verbal, verbal and other communication strategies.

Communication within MDTs requires clear management and facilitation on a number of levels, including:

- Environmental
- Skills and capabilities
- Beliefs and values
- Identity
- Vision or mission (Hall 2000).

Communication within MDTs also requires systems and assertive control and the flexibility to respond to changes. The information should go through as few people as possible to avoid the possibility of distortion (Guirdham 2002).

Nurses empower the MDT and their profession by clearly explaining their roles, responsibilities and professional boundaries to facilitate joint working that provides efficient, effective, evidence-based care (see Ch. 5).

Leadership

There is much literature that discusses the need for good quality leaders in all areas of healthcare and particularly in nursing. Indeed, *leadership and team working* form part of NMC Competency Framework Domain 4: Leadership, management and team working (NMC 2010).

Leaders are identified as those who influence the behaviour of others (Mullins 2008). Nurses as team leaders enable the people they lead to care for patients/clients and carers by:

- Being aware of their needs
- Listening to their views
- Hearing their concerns
- Being able to access their knowledge of their health status.

Team leaders also have to focus on the broader information sources and strategies that inform their practice and that of the nursing team they lead. It is of little surprise that nurses in this position can spend over 80% of their time communicating.

Leadership behaviours

For nurses, their approach to leading will depend on the situation, the individuals and teams around them and the tasks that are required. This author proposes that nurses have a responsibility to evaluate and develop their emotional intelligence skills (see below), because these skills enhance relationships and the care environment and are strongly connected to good leadership. Before looking more closely at emotional intelligence, it is appropriate to consider some styles of leadership. All the styles described below are appropriate in healthcare but when they are utilized depends significantly on the situation.

The plethora of leadership approaches can be daunting when nurses begin to explore the subject. Research by Binney et al (2009) shows leadership has three main elements:

- Leadership occurs between people, i.e. it is a social interactive process that facilitates links between people in organizations
- A leader's behaviour is shaped by the context in which they find themselves leading; as the situation/environment changes, so does the leader's behaviour

- Leaders are most effective when they take their skills to a situation, for the benefit of the individuals, groups and task, when they can relate to others as real people with emotional and cognitive intelligence and life experience that they can draw upon for the benefit of those around them.

It is useful to recognize what types of leadership behaviour are suitable in what situation. In accepting that there is a continuum of leadership behaviour that moves from high levels of control by the leader to high levels of freedom for those who are led, it can provide a framework for nurses to identify effective leaders and also assess their own leadership skills. This continuum in often described in terms of three leadership styles identified by Lewin et al (1939) (Fig. 9.5):

- Autocratic
- Democratic
- Laissez faire.

Adair (2009) focuses on a functional leadership approach where (in this case), as the nurse leader mirrors the characteristics of the nursing profession, they focus their concern on the task, the team and the individual. Communication and interpersonal competence of the leader are key abilities needed to lead individuals as a team to achieve the task. Leadership involves clearly communicating the objectives, aims and purpose of tasks in a manner that engages and motivates individuals and in the process gives the team a common purpose. Leaders find themselves communicating a great deal, often having informal 'chats' that may not be high on information giving but essential to positive relationships within the team. Good leadership involves a level of self-sacrifice, to engage people they need to trust, and to gain their trust leaders often have to show that they would not ask anything of someone else that they would not be prepared to do themselves (Adair 2009). Nurses take a lead in care situations, they all need to be trusted and considered genuine by patients, families and colleagues and this is achieved through skilled and congruent interpersonal and communication skills.

Emotional intelligence

Pre-1990, there was an assumption that intellect or 'rational' intelligence was fundamental to good working relationships and leadership. However, it is now thought that the intellect that is centred on understanding emotions, your own and others' and how these affect other people can enhance working relationships and leadership outcomes.

Emotional intelligence is encapsulated by the way people communicate, the language they use and the nonverbal cues used. Emotional intelligence is made up of a number of skills:

- Self-awareness, insight
- Managing own emotions
- Being aware of personal motivators and what motivates others
- Being able to empathize with others, being perceptive to the emotions of others
- Interpersonal skills in developing rapport, to persuade, to influence others.

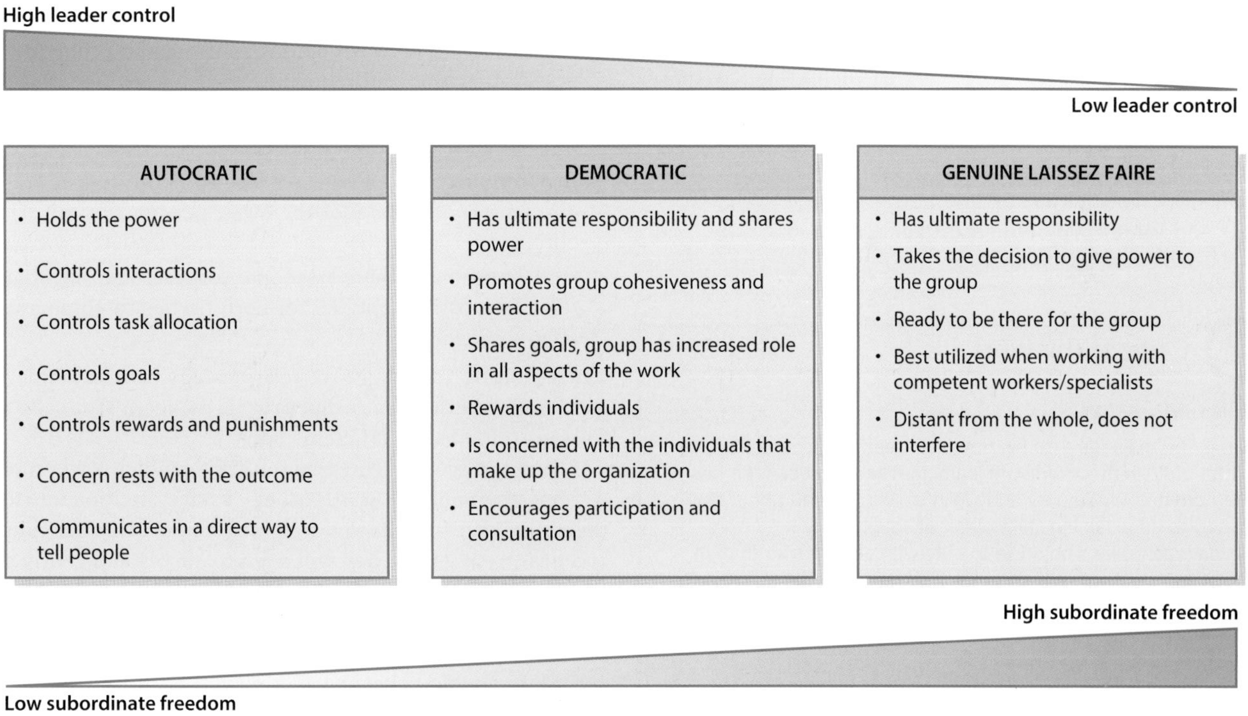

High leader control

Low leader control

AUTOCRATIC	DEMOCRATIC	GENUINE LAISSEZ FAIRE
• Holds the power	• Has ultimate responsibility and shares power	• Has ultimate responsibility
• Controls interactions	• Promotes group cohesiveness and interaction	• Takes the decision to give power to the group
• Controls task allocation	• Shares goals, group has increased role in all aspects of the work	• Ready to be there for the group
• Controls goals	• Rewards individuals	• Best utilized when working with competent workers/specialists
• Controls rewards and punishments	• Is concerned with the individuals that make up the organization	• Distant from the whole, does not interfere
• Concern rests with the outcome	• Encourages participation and consultation	
• Communicates in a direct way to tell people		

High subordinate freedom

Low subordinate freedom

Fig. 9.5 • Leadership styles.

Effective leaders have higher levels of emotional intelligence than leaders who are less effective (Goleman 2006).

Promoting quality and standards

Nurse team leaders develop over time; they evolve skills that shape people and services. But when is a leader a leader? Is a leader always the person in charge? Are those in responsible positions always leaders?

All nurses, including students, need the communication skills to influence the behaviour of others, e.g. educating patients/clients and carers about their health. They also need to influence the behaviour of their colleagues. Nurses use leadership skills to inform, teach and support colleagues and also to challenge each other's practice. The ability to gracefully challenge other people's behaviour in a way that is clear, informative and respectful is an essential aspect of delivering quality interventions and services (Box 9.18).

Relationships with families and main carers

Relationships with main carers and families are as important as the ones with patients/clients. As discussed above, nurses facilitate good relationships with carers by clearly describing their roles, responsibilities and boundaries.

Good relationships with families/carers are vital for the health outcomes of the patient/client. They are also important in ensuring that families/carers are supported in their caring role. Caring for carers has been a low priority for some nurses. However, carers' needs are increasingly being addressed through support and lobbying from carer organizations, government initiatives and patient involvement bodies (see Ch. 3).

? Critical thinking   **Box 9.18**

Promoting quality care – challenging poor practice

- A child has knocked a drink over. The team leader witnesses the accident and sees a colleague ignore the child and walk straight past the mess. The team leader asks politely if they could fetch another drink and clear up the spillage but their colleague says it's not their job and walks off.

- The key nurse has written a care plan with the client, detailing their relaxation exercise programme and how they will request support from staff if needed. The plan has been communicated clearly to the team. When the key nurse returns next day the client is upset because the nurse on duty refused to help with the relaxation exercise despite having time to do so. The client cannot see the point of 'working in partnership' if nothing happens. The key nurse checks the nursing notes where it clearly states that the client had not asked to practise the relaxation exercises.

- A student overhears a resident's daughter asking a colleague why her mother's soiled clothes have not been changed for 4 days. The colleague shrugs and says: 'You'd better write to the home manager.'

Student activities

- Discuss with your mentor what the nurse observing the poor practice/behaviour should do to safeguard the child/client/resident.

- How should the nurse challenge a colleague's practice/behaviour in a way that ensures the problem is not repeated while maintaining their colleague's dignity and showing respect for the individual?

Working with carers enhances the experience of patients/clients. Good support is far reaching and makes a positive difference to people's lives. Any working involvement requires effective interpersonal skills and good communication strategies and systems. For example, the scenario in Box 9.19 requires tact, commitment, courtesy, empathy, rapport, matching language, and understanding how the nurse's and carer's beliefs and values may influence their actions.

 Critical thinking Box 9.19

Colin and Jeanette

Colin is the main carer to his daughter Jeanette who is a young woman of 20 with a moderate learning disability. Jeanette has been admitted for surgery and Colin is very worried about her reaction to hospital. He states that, although he is tired from physical caring, he would like to stay with Jeanette so that he knows she is settled, comfortable and not anxious. He explains that when Jeanette is anxious she can quickly become depressed and introverted, which sometimes results in self-harming behaviour as a coping mechanism.

The nurse admitting Jeanette recognizes that Colin is the expert regarding Jeanette's physical and emotional needs, but realizes that Colin is tired and as main carer, he also has substantial needs.

Student activities

• What communication and interpersonal skills would you utilize in meeting Colin's needs?
• What dilemmas exist for the nurses supporting and caring for Colin and Jeanette?
• Discuss with your mentor how you could agree a plan with Colin, which meets both his and Jeanette's needs.

Barriers to communication

Effective communication skills and strategies are clearly important for nurses. However, it is recognized that such skills are not always evident and nurses do not always communicate well with patients/clients, carers and colleagues. This generalization is reason for concern. The barriers to effective communication outlined below will help nurses to understand the challenges, how these impact on practice and possible strategies to overcome them.

Conflict

Conflict is a common effect of two or more parties not sharing common ground. Conflict management is a skill that nurses need to develop in order to reduce the negative effects of conflict and restore the beneficial effects of harmonious relations. Conflict can be healthy in that it often offers alternative views and values. However, it becomes a barrier to communication when the emotional 'noise' detracts from the task and purpose. We manage conflict in a variety of ways, some are more effective than others (Borkowski 2011):

• Competition – where we enter into a win-or-lose battle
• Avoidance – where we do not confront the problem hoping that this will reduce it
• Compromise – where we negotiate common ground but lose some of our desired outcome
• Accommodation – where we lose some of desired outcome for the sake of the other persons desired outcome
• Collaboration – where we come together and negotiate the best possible options for both parties to come away feeling satisfied.

Nurses aim for collaborative relationships with patients, peers and families. Adopting competitive or avoidant strategies tends to lead to increased problems later.

Often the most frightening result of conflict is when people 'act out' their anger towards others. In this situation, nurses use their therapeutic skills in developing rapport through empathy and positive regard. They will need to clearly and gently direct the situation using active listening skills, summarising, paraphrasing and guiding the angry person into a more managed discussion. Box 9.20 offers specific guidance on dealing with anger and hostile behaviour in a mental health setting.

Dealing with anger and hostile behaviour Box 9.20

• 'Acknowledge the person's anger and the right to their feelings
• Allow the expression of anger in appropriate safe ways – verbalizing anger, discharge of anger in non-destructive acts. Anger is self-limiting unless re-stimulated
• Try and stay calm (use self-coaching and relaxation techniques). Provide psychological containment. Stay in the 'same gear', avoid any tendency to retaliate or appease
• Be aware of your body language. Try not to communicate threatening non-verbal signals
• Don't try to defend the situation or individuals the person is angry about
• Avoid a struggle of wills, someone has to lose. Look for compromise
• Be aware of power issues in the helping relationship and a person's need to rebel, or the need to reclaim power and assert autonomy
• Set limits. Encourage self-restraint. Raise awareness of response cost
• Help the person explore the immediate cause of their anger
• Help the client to engage in problem-solving. Be clear about what you can and cannot do
• Accept that some anger may be projected or displaced onto you
• Don't take unnecessary risks. Be aware of the indicators of high risk. If a person's anger is not subsiding but is in danger of escalating into destructive or violent acts, take whatever action is necessary to protect yourself and others
• Debrief with colleagues after the incident. Decide if you need any additional support'.

(Reproduced from Watkins, P., 2009. Mental Health Practice: a guide to compassionate care, Second ed. Butterworth Heinemann, Edinburgh, p 48, with permission.)

If, in the rare situations that the other person becomes physically aggressive, nurses use 'break-away' techniques and call for assistance. Some nurses are specially trained in physical control techniques such as Control and Responsibility (C&R) and Management of Actual or Potential Aggression (MAPPA). It is the nurse's duty to maintain as safe an environment as possible in such situations.

Task-orientated culture

Nurses work in busy environments; they have to complete a specific amount of work in a day and work with a variety of other professionals, patients/clients and carers. The roles are hard, challenging and tiring. There is a culture to get the work done, to 'do the diary', meet physical needs and ensure that documentation is up-to-date, etc. Some nurses still consider colleagues who spend time talking with patients/clients to be avoiding the 'real' work and lazy.

People like to 'fit in' to the dominant culture and do not want to be outside the group. Nurses and students who might have been confident in spending time with patients/clients in an area where this was valued, when faced with a task-orientated culture have the dilemma of fitting into the group or being outside the group and spending time engaging with clients. However, as evidence shows us, care, engagement and compassion speed up the healing process.

Internal noise, mental/emotional distress

Shannon and Weaver's model (Fig. 9.2, p. 195) refers to internal 'noise'. Fear and anxiety can affect the person's ability to listen to what the nurse is saying. People with feelings of fear and anger can find it difficult to hear. Illness and distress can alter a person's thought processes. For example, if a client is experiencing visual or auditory hallucinations, they can find it very difficult to concentrate on what is being communicated because they are occupied with other stimuli.

Reducing the cause of the anxiety, distress, anger, or visual/auditory hallucination would be the first step to improving communication. This can be achieved in a number of ways and it is for the patient/client and nurse to choose which is likely to be most effective. Ways of reducing internal 'noise' include:

- Choose a quiet environment if possible
- Deal first with the issue that is foremost in the patient's/client's mind before embarking on the nurse's topic
- Ask the patient/client when it would be good for them to talk. Do not assume that you as the nurse are always wanted or the patient/client is always in a position to be with you
- Are you choosing a particularly difficult time to discuss an issue? Consider what is happening for the patient/client at the moment
- Are you the right person to do this? Does someone else have a better nurse–patient/client relationship?
- Is there an optimum time of the day when the patient's/client's treatment is more effective, i.e. when they are less

confused or drowsy, in less pain, experiencing fewer hallucinations, less anxiety, less fear?
- Ensure that the patient's pain has been assessed and pain relief given (see Ch. 23)
- Ensure you have as much privacy as is practically possible
- Let the patient/client know you need to talk to them; give them the subject to be discussed rather than just launching in with no preparation at all
- Ensure you are using the most appropriate level of language
- Check whether the patient/client needs their glasses or a hearing aid.

Difficulty with speech and hearing

People can experience physical difficulties in speech/sign production or understanding speech, such as following a stroke or brain injury; people who are very breathless find it difficult to speak (see Ch. 17). Stroke or trauma may affect brain areas that normally enable the individual to comprehend and produce speech, or the physiology that produces sound. It is the role of the nurse and carers to promote all other communication channels by encouraging the patient/client to draw, write, gesture, point or use a more sophisticated communication tool such as computer-aided speech synthesis. Working in collaboration with the SLT can be very beneficial.

Some patients/clients have problems with hearing, which present barriers to communication. Nurses may need to work with patients/clients who lip-read or use signing. It may be necessary to work with a sign language interpreter or ensure a referral to an audiologist or SLT in order to achieve effective communication (see Ch. 16).

Medication

Medication can have a significant effect on communication; in some cases it can for example cause dry mouth or excess salivation, nausea and indigestion, all of which influence the person's ability and motivation to engage in conversation. If patients/clients are embarrassed or concerned that they will not be able to speak properly or control their mouth, they could be reluctant to speak. In this situation, the nurse needs to reassure the patient/client by offering time, a non-judgemental attitude, fluids and oral care to suit their specific needs, and ensure that all steps are taken to reduce the negative effects of the medication.

Cultural factors acting as barriers

It is important for nurses to think about many of the issues already covered and their own experiences when considering cultural differences in communication and how these can challenge health professionals and service users.

Whenever people discuss difference, there is a tendency to make value judgements regarding those perceived as being different. In this chapter, difference, sameness, foreign, British, multilingual, bilingual, unilingual – all these notions are of difference but in no way is one difference more or less valued than another. This is not to say that 'everyone is the same really' – people are not; everyone holds different thoughts, beliefs and values, and people come from a multitude of cultures and experiences.

When discussing communication difference it must be noted that some examples used to highlight issues are not positive; however, there are other examples that provide ideas for good practice, which nurses are strongly encouraged to employ.

This text can only offer generalizations about language and communication differences; however, nurses need to develop the skills and knowledge to meet individuals' needs. Never assume that because someone is from a certain country or background, they follow a specific faith, support a particular political party or speak a certain language; to assume anything would be to reduce the nurse's flexibility and ability to meet the needs of others.

One of the assumptions that we often make, in a valiant attempt to understand people from other communities, is to ask people about their culture because from our perspective their culture is very different and we expect people to be able to identify their own cultural differences, but can we? (Box 9.21).

 Reflective practice   **Box 9.21**

Differences in culture

How do you define your culture, e.g. what makes your culture different from others – dress code, diet, religion, fasting, specific holy days/holidays?

Student activity

- Reflect on situations when you have asked others about their culture, or when people have asked you.
- Discuss with your mentor how very difficult these seemingly clear enquiries are to answer and how they encourage the development of generalizations about people from other communities and cultures that may not be helpful (Henley & Schott 1999).

Differences in language and communication rules

Despite sharing a great deal, there are differences in the way language is used to communicate. For example, there are differences in prosody, i.e. tempo, speed, rhythm and pitch of speech.

Intonation

Intonation is the way words are said, the degree of emphasis given and the rise and fall of the pitch in a sentence. The singsong of spoken English or a tonal language such as Chinese shows great variety in the application of intonation. However, the raise in the pitch of voice at the end of a sentence indicates the speaker has asked a question and this is true for many languages.

British English speakers and speakers of other languages in the same family tend to use a narrow range of tone in speech; when these speakers hear the intonation of people who use a wider range of tones they can be interpreted as brash or even aggressive.

People who use tonal languages change the meaning of a word by changing the pitch level. The meaning of the word is dependent on the pitch, either rising–falling, or falling–rising. When people with native tonal languages learn 'tune' languages, it may take some time to learn and develop the singsong skills. As a result, they may sound monotone and a little harsh to the ears of a tune language user, resulting in confusion about the emotional content of the statement.

Emphasis

In *British* English emphasizing a word
In British English emphasizing a word
In British English *emphasizing* a word
In British English emphasizing a *word* changes the meaning of the sentence; in language, meaning is changed by the speed of delivery, the loudness or softness of the word. Again there is plenty of room for confusion. This often leads to anxiety, thereby creating 'noise', which affects the message. Emphasizing important information enables the nurse to help the patient/client/child listen to the message in a more useful way, e.g. 'Please tell me if at any time you want me to stop and I will.'

Loudness

A loudly spoken word or sentence suggests urgency or importance in many languages, but it can also suggest submission to authority, as well as authority over the situation. Softly spoken words also have different meanings that include showing respect for the listener and emphasizing the authority of the speaker; in some languages it suggests professionalism and in others it is used to express anger (Crystal 2010). Nurses who meet someone who is culturally Zulu for the first time, may find it odd that they may speak quietly and deferentially to them. This may appear to a British English speaker as if the person is overly polite, shy or may even be hiding something. However, it is the norm to show respect to others in this way using the voice courteously.

Sentence structure

In British English, sentences tend to be structured as subject–verb–object, e.g. 'The nurse answered the telephone'. In other languages there is a topic–comment structure, such as: 'The library is open, I will go in an hour.' The way people structure their conversations also differs from language to language. Some people like to map out the situation before getting to the point to give the listener as much background as possible. Some people would find this difficult to follow and at worst, find the speaker rude and evasive. Other people will get straight to the point and add the context later, which – while time saving – can also be interpreted as brusque. It is important for nurses to know how to present information; if they are unsure whether to get straight to the point with a patient/client, colleague or carer, they should listen to how the person speaks to them. Gently reflecting their style may improve communication.

Taking turns and guggling

British English speakers lower their voices when they are ready for the listener to speak but in Southern Europe, the speaker offers the listener a brief pause in which to speak. British English speakers allow longer pauses in their conversations to give the listener the cue to speak. Clearly people could be confused with the signals and may interpret the long pause or lack of pause as rudeness or poor listening skills.

In some communities, it is acceptable to talk at the same time as the speaker on the same subject as a mark of agreement and listening; this sharing of conversation space is also seen in twin, sibling and close friendship conversations. Again it is a mark of involvement, of closeness. However, some linguistic communities would see this as poor manners and shoddy inter-personal skills. British English speakers tend to like clear turn-taking.

British and other sign language users also take turns in sequence rather than signing at the same time. Signing at the same time as someone else is considered rude, though not as impolite as holding a person's hands when they are signing in order to stop them making their point, no matter how much the listener may disagree.

Guggles are important in some languages (see pp. 204-205); there are even guggles in sign language. However, in some languages, being still, maintaining a passive facial expression, not making a sound and making little eye contact is a sign from the listener that they are listening and attentive.

It is important that nurses do not assume that there is only one way of encouraging people to speak. The Western model of developing rapport in order to work in partnership with others is not the only way. In order to work within the social, interpersonal and linguistic 'rules' most effectively requires an individual who shares the first and preferred language of the person (Henley & Schott 1999). The services of a qualified interpreter may be needed.

Working with interpreters

When the communication barrier is due to the nurse not speaking the patient's/client's language, a third party who speaks both languages will be needed (Henley & Schott 1999).

A person who can speak two or more languages is not the same as an interpreter. Interpreting is a learned skill, and working with an interpreter is also a skill that has to be learned. Furthermore, interpreters are a professional body of people, most of whom work to exacting codes of ethics and professional standards. Interpreters are skilled in enabling each party to understand the culture of the other, particularly where cultural differences would cause misunderstandings.

Without quality interpreting services, people can be misdiagnosed, mistreated, undiagnosed, uninformed, etc. If the interpreter is untrained, these issues are unresolved. Ultimately, this means that people's health suffers, carers are unable to support the process effectively and many service users avoid the health service, believing that they will not receive any sort of service.

SUMMARY

◆ Nurses are encouraged to reflect on their own skills, to develop their awareness and understanding of those with whom they will work.

◆ This chapter introduces the skills that underpin this area of interpersonal communication and relationship.

◆ All nurses can enhance their communication skills and relational skills by using the *Essence of Care 2010 Benchmarking Tools for Communication* (DH 2010) to focus their development.

◆ The benchmarks identify good practice in communicating as expected by clients, colleagues and carers.

◆ Once confident in behaving in ways that produce the outcomes that clients and carers expect, nurses can develop finer communication skills that will truly enhance therapeutic relationships between patients/clients, carers and colleagues and increase the effectiveness of resources.

◆ Good communication skills are the underpinning foundation on which to base all other nursing interventions.

◆ Understanding how language is constructed, learned and what part it plays in the development of 'self' in a social world enables the nurse to monitor, evaluate and adapt their communication to meet the needs of the person.

◆ Recognizing the power of language in developing and sustaining working relationships with others is vital when influencing others ecologically.

◆ Utilizing reflective exercises, wider reading and focused action plans to develop a lifelong learning portfolio of development will help nurses become skilled communicators.

KEY WORDS AND PHRASES FOR LITERATURE SEARCHING

Assertiveness

Body language

Communication barriers

Courtesy

Customer care

Emotional intelligence

Empathy

Interpersonal skills

Listening skills

Positive regard

Proxemics

Self-awareness

Therapeutic relationships

 Useful websites

Empathy and Listening Skills and Psychological Hugs
    www.psychological-hug.com
Language and Culture: An introduction to human communication
    http://anthro.palomar.edu/language/default.htm
The Northern School of NLP and Associated Studies
    www.nlpand.co.uk
All websites accessed September 2012.

References

Adair, J., 2009. Effective leadership, revised edn. Pan Macmillan, London.

Argyle, M., 1994. The psychology of interpersonal behaviour, fifth ed. Penguin Press, London.

Armstrong, D.F., Stokoe, W.C., Wilcox, S.E., 1995. Gesture and the nature of language. Cambridge University Press, Cambridge.

Binney, G., Wilke, G., Williams, C., 2009. Living leadership: a practical guide for ordinary heros, second ed. Pearson Education, Harlow.

Borkowski, N., 2011. Organisational behaviour in health care, second ed. Jones and Bartlett, Sudbury.

Boysson-Bardies, B., 1999. How language comes to children. MIT Press, Cambridge, MA.

Buchanan, D., Huczynski, A., 2004. Organisational behaviour: an introductory text, fifth ed. Financial Times/Prentice Hall, London.

Crystal, D., 2010. The encyclopaedia of language, third ed. Cambridge University Press, Cambridge.

Department of Health, 2010. Essence of care. 2010 benchmarks for communication. Online. Available: www.dh.gov.uk/prod_consum_dh/groups/dh_digitalassets/@dh/@en/@ps/documents/digitalasset/dh_119978.pdf September 2012.

Egan, G., 1998. The skilled helper – a problem management approach to helping, sixth ed. Brooks Cole, Pacific Grove.

Fiske, J., 2010. Introduction to communication studies, 3rd revised edn. Routledge, London.

Fromkin, V.A., Rodman, R., Hyams, N., 2010. Introduction to language, ninth ed. Wadsworth, Boston.

Gibbs, G., 1988. Learning by doing: a guide to teaching and learning methods. Further Education Unit, Oxford Brookes University, Oxford.

Goleman, D., 2006. Emotional intelligence. Bantam Dell, New York.

Guirdham, M., 2002. Interactive behaviour at work, third ed. Financial Times/Prentice Hall, London.

Hall, M., 2000. The source book of magic. Crown House, Carmarthen.

Hargie, O. (Ed.), 2006. The handbook of communication skills, third ed. Routledge, London.

Henley, A., Schott, J., 1999. Culture, religion and patient care in a multi-ethnic society. Age Concern, London.

Holmes, J., 2001. Introduction to sociolinguistics. Longman, London.

Kurtz, S., Silverman, J., Draper, J., 2004. Teaching and learning communication skills in medicine, second ed. Radcliffe Publishing, Oxford.

Lewin, K., Llippit, R., White, R.K., 1939. Patterns of aggressive behaviour in experimentally created social climates. Journal of Social Psychology 10, 271–301.

Mullins, L.J., 2008. Essentials of organisational behaviour, second ed. Pearson Education, Harlow.

Nursing and Midwifery Council, 2008. The code: Standards of conduct, performance and ethics for nurses and midwives. Online. Available: http://www.nmc-uk.org/Publications/Standards/The-code/Introduction/ September 2012.

Nursing and Midwifery Council, 2010. Standards for pre-registration nursing education. NMC, London.

O'Brien, L.M., 2000. Nurse-client relationships: the experience of community psychiatric nurses. Australian and New Zealand Journal of Mental Health Nursing 9, 184–194.

Pinker, S., 2007. The language instinct, third ed. HarperCollins, New York.

Varcarolis, E.M., Halter, M.J., 2009. Essentials of psychiatric mental health nursing. Saunders, St Louis.

West, R., Turner, L.H., 2009. Understanding interpersonal communication, second ed. Wadsworth, Boston.

Wolvin, A.D., Coakley, C.G., 1996. Listening, fifth ed. McGraw-Hill, Boston.

Further reading

Bennett, M., 2001. The empathic healer. Academic Press, San Diego.

Holland, S., Ward, C., 1997. Assertiveness: a practical approach. Speechmark, Oxon.

Sully, P., Dallas, J., 2010. Essential communication skills for nursing & midwifery, second ed. Mosby, Edinburgh.

Tribe, R., Raval, H., 2002. Working with interpreters in mental health. Brunner-Routledge, London.

Sleep, rest and complementary and alternative medicine

10

Ah Nya Plant

LEARNING OUTCOMES

This chapter will help you:

- Understand why rest and sleep are important to maintain health
- Describe the physiological control of sleep
- Describe the stages of the sleep cycle
- Outline factors that affect normal sleep patterns
- Outline sleep patterns in different age groups
- Identify factors that disrupt normal sleep patterns
- Describe some common sleep disorders
- Apply simple measures to promote sleep and rest
- Outline the use of complementary and alternative medicine (CAM) in the promotion of sleep, rest and well-being
- Understand the concept of integrated health
- Describe the range of CAM therapies available
- Understand the need to access these therapies in a safe manner.

Introduction

Thy best of rest is sleep.

(William Shakespeare, *Measure for measure*, Act 3, Scene 1).

Maslow's hierarchy of basic human needs comprises five or seven levels (see Ch. 8). The first level, physical/physiological needs, such as food and water, are necessary for life. These physiological needs, which include sleep and rest, have the greatest priority.

Sleep, relaxation and rest maintain, enhance and restore the person's physiological, psychological and social well-being. Nurses in all care settings are involved in helping and guiding people to attain optimum health and well-being. Nurses promote daily routines and lifestyle that enables the individual to enhance rest by relaxation and sleep. This is important during illness or following injury when the restorative functions of sleep are most needed for reducing stress and promoting healing. Many patients/clients have problems getting sufficient

rest and sleep, especially in hospital or a care home. Inadequate sleep and rest may be caused by anxiety, pain, the environment or specific treatments.

The first part of the chapter provides an overview of sleep, including physiological control, the sleep stages and functions. The factors that cause disturbances of sleep, effects of sleep deprivation and some specific sleep disorders are addressed.

The nursing interventions employed to promote rest and sleep throughout the lifespan are discussed in some depth and include the assessment of sleep, sleep hygiene/pre-sleep routines and the sleep environment, and the role of relaxation, orthodox medications and herbal products in promoting sleep. The outline of relaxation (see Ch. 11) and herbal products used in relation to rest and sleep provides a link to the section about complementary and alternative medicine (CAM).

In the last part of the chapter, the integration of CAM therapies with conventional healthcare is discussed. Information on how some therapies can be accessed, utilized safely to promote rest, relaxation and sleep and examples of the wider uses of CAM are provided.

Sleep, rest and relaxation

Sleep, rest and relaxation, are necessary for well-being and health maintenance. Sleep is an altered state of consciousness, accompanied by a reduction in metabolism and skeletal muscle activity. It occurs naturally in humans and follows a 24-hour biological rhythm (see below).

During sleep, the arterial blood pressure, heart and respiratory rates all decrease and skin blood vessels dilate. Sleep is considered important for restoration and repair of cells and tissues.

Martini and Nath (2009) suggest that the significance of sleep is its impact on the central nervous system. It is already known that proteins are made in neurones during sleep. However, the exact functions of sleep are yet to be explained.

Apart from the brain, all other organs undergo just as effective restoration during relaxed wakefulness (Horne & Reyner

1997). This highlights the importance of relaxation and rest periods during the day, e.g. breaks from work and the need for relaxation and relief from anxiety. Babies and children need a balance between active play and restful relaxed activities such as sitting on a carer's lap to listen to a story and sleep.

Protected time for rest and relaxation is important for patients/clients in hospital and other care settings, thus avoiding exhaustion from long visiting hours and interventions from health professionals (Box 10.1).

⟳ Reflective practice   Box 10.1

Protected rest times

Periods of rest and relaxation are important for everyone but particularly so during illness or following surgery.

Student activities

- Find out what happens in your clinical area or local hospital with regard to having protected rest/quiet times for patients/ clients.
- Reflect on how you would feel if you were unwell and admitted to an area where there is activity throughout the day, visitors, nursing care, treatments and visits to other departments for investigations and therapy. Discuss your feelings with a fellow student.

Sleep can help revitalize mental activities such as learning, memory, reasoning and emotional adjustments. It is especially important for health professionals to have sufficient sleep of good quality. Studies of hospital nurses working extended shifts indicate an elevated risk of patient care errors; a combination of long hours, lack of sleep and fatigue increases this risk (Scott et al 2010). Caruso and Hitchcock (2010) assert that working long hours can lead to sleep problems, declining performance and fatigue-related errors.

Biorhythms

Biorhythms are the cyclical patterns of biological functions unique to each individual, e.g. sleep–wake cycles, fluctuations in body temperature, blood pressure, heart rate, mood and some hormone secretion. Biorhythm cycles may follow a 24-hour day–night (circadian) pattern or a longer period, e.g. the menstrual cycle.

The sleep–wake cycle follows a circadian (Latin: *circa*, about and *dies*, day) or diurnal daily pattern. A 'biological clock' synchronizes the sleep–wake cycle with the 24-hour clock, which determines daily and social activities. It follows a day–night/light–dark rhythm of around 24 hours, thus giving rise to individual sleep patterns and different times for going to bed such as 8pm, midnight or the early hours of the morning.

Physiology of sleep

The physiological control of sleep involves an area in the brain, the reticular formation (RF), sometimes known as the reticular activating system (RAS), other brain structures, various chemicals such as neurotransmitters, neuropeptides and the hormone melatonin (Fig. 10.1). An outline is provided here and readers requiring more detail should consult their anatomy and physiology books.

When a person is asleep, the body is relaxed and they are not conscious of external stimuli such as noise or internal stimuli such as hunger. The stimulating mental activity such as thoughts about events of the day or preparatory work for the next day diminishes as the person begins to feel drowsy and falls asleep. However, if these stimuli are intense, the person wakes up and consciously responds to the stimuli. The sensory nerve pathways receive and convey nerve impulses upwards to

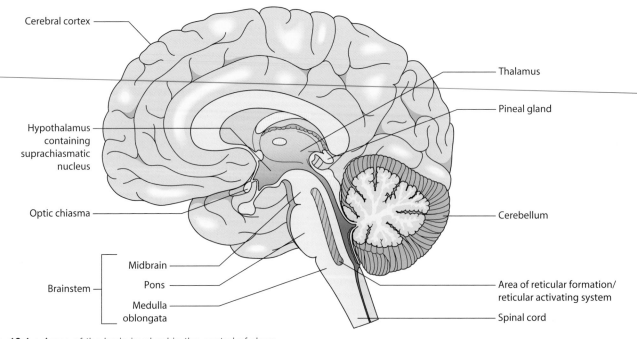

Fig. 10.1 • Areas of the brain involved in the control of sleep.

the cerebral cortex ('conscious brain'). They arise in response to stimuli such as light, noise, pain, temperature and hunger. Likewise, descending messages from the cerebral cortex enable the person to respond accordingly, e.g. getting up to have a snack if hungry or lying awake thinking of a solution to a problem. The balance of impulses to and from the cerebral cortex controls the sleep–wake cycle.

Reticular formation – the reticular activating system

The RF or RAS comprises diffuse neurones found throughout the brain stem (midbrain, pons and medulla oblongata). It has connections with the cerebral cortex, thalamus, hypothalamus, cerebellum and spinal cord. The RAS is important in the control of motor activity, some autonomic functions and the regulation of sensory inputs *en route* to the cerebral cortex.

The RAS controls the sleep–wake cycle, the state of cortical awareness. Ascending sensory impulses, e.g. sound and light, stimulate the RAS and this increases cortical activity and the person wakes. Consciousness is maintained through the activity of feedback mechanisms that involve the RAS, cerebral cortex and skeletal muscles. When the RAS is inhibited, its activity is low and the person becomes relaxed and falls asleep. Thus, a quiet, dark room promotes sleep. Increased RAS stimulation increases its activity and the high level of excitation prevents the person from relaxing and falling asleep. Stimulating factors, e.g. anxiety, being upset, hunger, thirst, physical discomfort and noise can prevent sleep. RAS functioning is inhibited by some drugs, e.g. anaesthetic agents, sedatives, anxiolytic drugs that reduce anxiety, and by alcohol and nervous system problems.

The biological 'body clock'

Normally, adults sleep at night and stay awake during the day. This timing of the sleep–wake cycle that corresponds with darkness and light is a circadian rhythm. The timing is controlled by a group of cells known as the suprachiasmatic nucleus (SCN) found in the hypothalamus in the brain (Fig. 10.1). The SCN, identified as the 'biological clock', is stimulated by visual information from the retina of the eye. Hence light is the primary controlling stimulus for the biological clock's daily rhythm and humans sleep at night.

Melatonin, a hormone secreted from the pineal gland in the brain (Fig. 10.1), is concerned with the regulation of circadian rhythms; melatonin production is controlled by the SCN (Wu & Swaab 2005). The secretion of melatonin exhibits a 24-hour cycle and fluctuates in relation to light. Darkness stimulates its secretion and light inhibits it. Thus, levels of melatonin are high at night but low during the day. Melatonin plays an important role in regulating the sleep–wake cycle. Levels are higher in children than in adults and may explain why children sleep more than adults (see pp. 224-225). Ongoing research into the effects of melatonin include:

- Its effects of lowering body temperature, hence inducing sleep
- Its role in managing/preventing jet lag (see p. 225)

(see pp. 224-225)

- Its relationship to low mood in winter and seasonal affective disorder (SAD) (Box 10.2)
- As a potential treatment with light therapy for circadian disorders related to ageing and in early Alzheimer's disease (Wu & Swaab 2005)
- Its potential as a natural sleeping pill in treating insomnia (sleeplessness) and its possible role in the reproductive function (Widmaier et al 2010).

Neurotransmitters involved with sleep–wake physiology

Several neurotransmitters including monoamines, catecholamines, amino acids and neuropeptides involved in controlling the sleep–wake cycle are produced in the RF and elsewhere in the brain. These substances affect the sleep–wake cycle by influencing the level of activity in the RAS, causing the transition from sleep to arousal to waking and vice versa. Changing levels of neurotransmitters cause the shift from one state to another and give rise to two types of sleep: non-rapid eye movement sleep (NREM) and rapid eye movement sleep (REM) (see below). The neurotransmitters include:

- Acetylcholine (ACh)
- 5-hydroxytryptamine (5-HT) (also known as serotonin)
- Histamine
- Dopamine
- Noradrenaline (norepinephrine)
- Gamma-aminobutyric acid (GABA)
- Hypocretin-1 and -2 (also called orexin-A and -B)

? Critical thinking **Box 10.2**

Seasonal affective disorder (SAD)

The symptoms of SAD include:

- Disturbed sleep, early morning awakening, a desire to oversleep or sleep longer and daytime sleepiness
- Reduced concentration
- Tiredness, lethargy, inability to carry out normal routines
- Low mood and mood swings
- Increased appetite, particularly for carbohydrate and sweet foods
- Reduced libido
- Loss of interest in work, socializing and hobbies. In severe SAD, symptoms may also include:
  - Stress and anxiety and inability to tolerate stress
  - Feeling hopeless, depressed and despairing.

Student activities

A client/patient asks you for some basic facts about SAD:

- Access the NHS Choices website and find out the following:
  - The causes of SAD
  - The types of treatment available for people with SAD
  - The support available for people suffering from SAD.

Resource

NHS Choices – www.nhs.uk September 2012.

Stages of sleep

There are two types of sleep, named according to whether or not the eyeballs can be seen to move behind the closed eyelids, i.e. NREM sleep and REM sleep. For young adults, a normal night's sleep of about 8 hours comprises around 70–80% of NREM sleep, with the remainder spent in REM sleep. Subjects observed during NREM and REM sleep show distinctive features of brain wave patterns, changes in muscle tone, heart rate and breathing.

NREM sleep

NREM (orthodox) sleep, which occurs first, has four stages (Box 10.3). Sleep begins with the person relaxed, feeling drowsy and then proceeds from stage 1 to stage 4. This normally takes 40 minutes. The process then reverses, moving back through NREM stages 3 and 2, followed by an episode of REM sleep. If the sleep is uninterrupted, it continues in this cyclical fashion (Fig. 10.2). In adults, the cycle repeats four to five times in an average night's sleep, each cycle lasting about 90 minutes. However, the time spent in stages 3 and 4 declines as the night progresses and more time is spent in REM sleep. The amount of REM sleep differs between age groups and during the individual's lifespan. In NREM sleep, there is progressive muscle relaxation and reduced muscle tension. Blood pressure, heart and respiratory rates all decrease. The gonadotrophic hormones, which stimulate the ovaries and testes, and growth hormone (GH) are released during NREM sleep. When awakened during NREM sleep, dreaming is rarely reported.

REM sleep

REM sleep is also known as paradoxical sleep, because the brain wave pattern resembles that of the waking state, but paradoxically, the sleeper is difficult to arouse (Box 10.3). During REM sleep, oxygen consumption is high and, when awakened, subjects report that they have been dreaming. In

---

Initiation and characteristics of the different stages of the sleep cycle	Box 10.3

Wakefulness

Alert, awake, eyes open, relaxed, drowsy, feeling tired, eyelids getting 'heavier', eyes may close, head relaxed, droops, lacks concentration and attention, sleepy but not asleep.

NREM (orthodox) sleep

About 50% in neonates, 20% in preschoolers, 70–80% in young adults and variable in older adults:

- Stage 1 – time taken to enter this varies, normally takes about 1–7 min, light sleep, lack of awareness continues, muscles relax, heart and respiratory rates are stable. Easily roused by moderate stimuli
- Stage 2 – lack of sensitivity more marked, muscles more relaxed, becoming more difficult to rouse
- Stage 3 – occurs about 20 min after the person falls asleep, moderate deep sleep occurs and the person is very relaxed and very difficult to waken. Body temperature and blood pressure drop
- Stage 4 – a progression of stage 3. Deep sleep, only strong stimulation such as shaking will rouse. Sleepwalking, talking, nightmares and tooth grinding (bruxism) may occur in some people.

Note: Stages 3 and 4 may also be described together as short wave sleep (SWS) (le May, 2011).

REM (paradoxical) sleep

About 50% in neonates, 20% in young adults and variable in older adults. This stage normally begins at the end of each sleep cycle. Therefore, REM sleep occurs approximately every 90 min, each episode lasting about 10 min. The deepest sleep and greatest relaxation occurs and the person is difficult to rouse. Dreaming occurs, rapid eye movements behind closed eyelids, possibly the person is visualizing and following the events of the dream. There is a marked increase in brain oxygen consumption. Blood pressure, pulse and respiratory rates vary more than during NREM sleep.

Fig. 10.2 • Stages of sleep in adults.

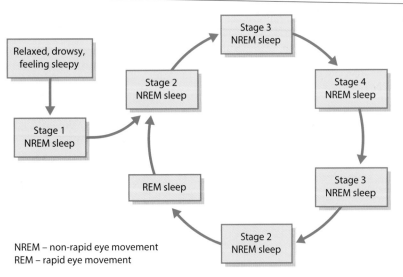

NREM – non-rapid eye movement
REM – rapid eye movement

REM sleep, blood pressure, heart and respiratory rates are increased and irregular. There is rapid eye movement. Although twitches of facial muscles may occur, there is loss of skeletal muscle tone throughout the rest of the body.

Functions of sleep

The functions of sleep are not clearly understood. There are several hypotheses; one suggests that during REM sleep, dreaming enhances the chemical changes that the brain undergoes during learning and memory. Dreams may also provide the expression of concerns in the 'subconscious'.

During sleep, relaxation of skeletal muscles and a reduction in metabolic processes occurs. This helps to conserve energy and, together with the release of GH, growth and cell/tissue repair such as during wound healing are enhanced (see Ch. 25).

The proper functioning of the immune system is linked with sleep. For example, interleukin-1 (a signalling protein produced by some white blood cells), which has an important role in the inflammatory response (see Ch. 25), fluctuates in parallel with normal sleep–wake cycles (Widmaier et al 2010).

Effects of sleep deprivation

Most nurses can relate to the effects of not enough sleep such as lack of concentration, irritability and poor performance of skilled tasks (Box 10.4). An increase in accidents, e.g. driving home after night duty, and domestic and work-related accidents due to impaired judgement and human errors are all related to sleep deprivation.

 Reflective practice   Box 10.4

Sleep deprivation

Think about times when you have not had enough sleep for whatever reason.

Student activities

- Reflect on tasks that you found more difficult, e.g. calculating a drug dose.
- Were you aware of any changes in the way you interacted with other people?
- Discuss with your mentor whether it was likely that your concentration was affected, perhaps during a lecture or a handover report?

Sleep deprivation is associated with reduced function of the immune responses and resistance to infection. It may induce mental health problems and even psychotic behaviour if accompanied by stress.

The effects of sleep deprivation vary in individuals and some examples are outlined in Box 10.5. These effects can become problematic and may cause the individual to seek help. Unresolved poor sleep habits can develop into a chronic problem such as insomnia (see p. 229). The most effective treatment for sleep deprivation is elimination or correction of factors that disrupt sleep patterns. Nurses should be proactive in helping the person to achieve and retrieve lost sleep.

Examples of the cumulative effects of sleep deprivation   Box 10.5

- Loss of appetite
- Headaches
- Feeling cold due to fall in body temperature
- Poor coordination
- Overwhelming desire to sleep
- Tiredness
- Hallucinations
- Irritability
- Mood swings
- Confusion/disorientation
- Increased aggressiveness
- Poor concentration
- Reduced ability to perform skilled tasks
- 'Microsleeps' lasting a few seconds. These may be dangerous, e.g. while driving or operating machinery.

Factors that affect normal sleep patterns

A person's normal sleep pattern is determined by factors that include:

- Genetic make-up – being a 'morning or evening type'
- Individual needs – sleep patterns show huge individual differences
- Culture (Box 10.6) – such as a 'nap' after lunch, or an afternoon siesta in Mediterranean countries and a late evening meal when it is cooler. In many cultures children stay up late and eat with the extended family and this may require adjustments during hospitalization
- Body mass index (see Ch. 19)
- Physical activity
- Age is an important factor and is discussed in more detail below.

 Reflective practice   Box 10.6

Cultural influences on sleep patterns

Consider the cultural influences on the sleep patterns of an adult patient/client.

Student activities

- How does their sleep pattern differ from a typical pattern of being awake all day and sleeping for 8–9 hours at night?
- To what extent have they had to change their sleep pattern since being in hospital/care home or having care at home?
- Reflect with another student on how individual sleep patterns can be maintained in a care setting.

Box 10.7 provides an opportunity to consider your own sleep pattern and the factors that influence it.

Reflective practice **Box 10.7**

Normal sleep patterns

Consider your typical sleep pattern.

Student activities

• How many hours sleep do you normally have?

• How many hours sleep do you need to feel fresh and alert the next day?

• Think about the factors listed in the text. Which ones have been important in determining your sleep pattern?

 Health promotion **Box 10.8**

Helping infants to sleep at night

Many new mums and dads/carers tell their health visitor or practice nurse that they cannot get their baby to sleep at night or that the baby cries excessively. Often this leaves them feeling anxious, unable to cope and worried about doing something wrong; all of which are compounded by the effects of their own lack of sleep.

Student activities

• Using the resources below, prepare a summary of the main advice for parents about getting infants to sleep and dealing with crying.

• Discuss with your mentor the importance of establishing a nighttime sleeping pattern in infants.

Resources

Cry-sis – www.cry-sis.org.uk/sleep.html.

NHS Choices Babies, Crying – www.nhs.uk/conditions/babies-crying/Pages/introduction.aspx.

Family lives (Parentline free 0808 800 2222) and online, available at: http://familylives.org.uk.

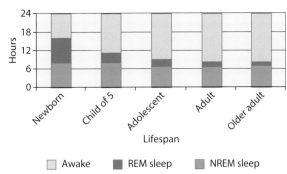

Fig. 10.3 • 'Typical' sleep pattern changes throughout the lifespan.

Sleep patterns during the lifespan

Normal sleep patterns change throughout the lifespan in order to meet the different requirements during growth, development and maturation. The amount of sleep required by a newborn baby is vastly different from that needed by an older adult. The duration, quality and quantity of sleep are all subject to change (Fig. 10.3).

Infancy and childhood

In the first week of life, infants are usually asleep for 16 hours out of the 24 hours, but this is interspersed with waking for frequent feeds. Establishing a sleep pattern is important and a pre-sleep bedtime routine can be introduced as early as 6 weeks. This helps the infant to learn the 'sleep cues' and enhances settling down at bedtime (Box 10.8).

By the age of 3–4 months, a pattern of sleep develops and infants sleep around 8–10 hours during the night and wake up early in the morning. Normally, infants and toddlers have sleeps during the day but the duration reduces and eventually ceases when the toddler reaches the age of 3 years. However, those who are more active will sleep less. Sleep disorders affecting children are outlined later (see p. 229).

Once the child starts school, the amount of daily activity and the overall health of the child will dictate the hours of sleep required. Children aged between 4 and 5 years spend, on average, about 10–11 hours sleeping at night.

Adolescents/young adults

Adolescents and young adults need sufficient sleep to cope with the period of rapid growth that occurs. Most young people are engaged in physical and mental activities at school, college/university or work and socializing in the evenings and at the weekend. Normally by bedtime, they should have no difficulty falling asleep. A small study ($n = 201$) by Owens et al (2010) found that a 30-minute delay in the start to the school day improved sleep duration on school nights and the percentage of students having less than 7 hours sleep decreased by nearly 80% and there was an increase in those achieving at least 8 hours sleep from less than 17% to over 50%. The benefits included a reduction in daytime sleepiness, low mood and fatigue (Owen et al 2010).

However, it is normal for those who extend their activities past midnight to sleep on in the mornings, especially at weekends when they may sleep late only emerging at lunchtime. An average adolescent sleeps 8–9 hours per night but this will vary according to the demands of study, socializing, sport, part-time work, etc.

Adulthood and midlife

During adulthood and midlife, sleep requirements vary between individuals. Most adults have around 8 hours sleep each night. However, some people may need 10 hours, whereas others need as little as 4 hours sleep at night. For some women, hot flushes and night sweats around the menopause can affect their sleep patterns.

Older adults

Sleep patterns and sleep requirements of older adults vary considerably. It is a misconception that older people require less sleep. In fact, the total amount of sleep does not change with ageing. Although the time spent sleeping at night decreases because people wake more often during the night, this loss is offset by an increase in daytime naps and rest time. Also, the quality of sleep deteriorates, as there is a progressive decrease in REM sleep and NREM sleep (stage 4).

The fragmented sleep patterns in older adults may be explained by changes in sleep regulation due to age-related alterations in the circadian rhythm of melatonin secretion. There are changes in both the amount and timing of melatonin rhythm (Skene & Swaab 2003). There may be reduced sensory stimuli and less awareness of time. People with dementia are particularly likely to experience changes in sleep patterns and circadian rhythms (Box 10.9).

 Reflective practice Box 10.9

Sleep patterns in dementia

Frank has dementia and lives with his daughter. She tells you that he does not seem to know whether it is day or night. It is increasingly difficult to get him to go to bed and he wanders about the house at night.

Student activities

- What changes in Frank's sleep pattern, e.g. increased daytime napping etc., might be observed?
- Discuss with your mentor how Frank's daughter might improve his nighttime sleeping pattern?

Chronic illnesses may also interfere with the regulation of sleep and also reduce sleep quality. For example, people who suffer pain due to arthritis may be uncomfortable and woken by pain. Medication may affect sleep patterns, e.g. the person taking diuretic drugs, which increase urine production, may waken several times during the night to pass urine (see Ch. 20).

Factors disrupting normal sleep patterns

Many factors can disrupt normal sleep patterns and affect quality and quantity of sleep. Disruption is usually caused by a combination of lifestyle, psychosocial, physiological, environmental factors, physical and mental health problems and the effects of medication.

Nurses in all care settings can help to eliminate factors which disrupt or prevent sleep and promote those which enhance relaxation, rest and sleep. Disturbing a person's sleep in order to perform observations, give care or medication can be avoided by coordinating care and observations or revising medication timing and where possible, doing observations without waking the person (Box 10.10).

Lifestyle factors

Lifestyle factors and changes in daily routines can disrupt normal sleep patterns. These may include:

- A change in the person's usual pre-sleep routines can prevent sleep. These routines may be disrupted by admission to a care setting
- Anxiety and stressful situations
- A heavy meal late at night can cause discomfort
- Inappropriate diet in infants or colic disrupting sleep for the infant and parents/carers (see Box 10.8)

Ethical issues Box 10.10

Waking a patient/client

Dan, who has severely depressed moods, is an in-patient in an acute mental health unit. He finds it difficult to get to sleep and wakes very early in the morning. Dan went to bed quite early at 10pm and had just fallen asleep when the nurses realize that he has not had his medication.

Student activities

- Consider the choices available to the nurse in charge (see Ch. 7).
- Think about what you would do and discuss this with your mentor.

Jet lag Box 10.11

Travelling through time zones causes the biological body clock and circadian rhythms to be desynchronized with the new environmental timing. Srinivasan et al (2010) describe jet lag as a collection of symptoms. The effects, which are more marked if travelling east, include:

- Symptoms of loss of sleep, e.g. headache (see also Sleep deprivation, p. 223)
- Disrupted sleep pattern, i.e. unable to sleep at night, early waking and daytime sleepiness
- Reduced efficiency
- Reduced appetite
- Reduced alertness
- Reduced cognitive skills
- Fatigue
- Low mood.

Resource

Eastman, C.I., Burgess, H.J., 2009. How to travel the world without jet lag. Sleep Medicine Clinics 4 (2), 241–255.

- Constipation may be a cause of sleepless nights in all age groups (see Ch. 21)
- Waking due to hunger
- Pre-bedtime intake of caffeine contained in coffee, tea, cola-type drinks and chocolate can increase the time taken to fall asleep
- Nicotine from tobacco smoking causes problems falling asleep, staying asleep and may cause daytime sleepiness. Interestingly, nicotine patches may cause a reduction in REM sleep and early morning waking
- Drinking alcohol speeds onset of sleep but disrupts sleep patterns later in the night and affects the quality of sleep
- Longer or different work schedules such as shift changes, working or studying late into the evening. Shift working is discussed further below
- Travel through different time zones leading to 'jet lag' (Box 10.11)
- Overstimulating play, e.g. computer games near to bedtime can prevent children getting to sleep

- Strenuous exercise or energetic play near bedtime. Although fatigue due to moderate programmed exercise/ physical activity can promote relaxation and a good night's sleep, exercise too late in the evening can extend the time it takes to fall asleep (sleep latency)
- Frequent late nights socializing can disrupt sleep patterns.

Shift working

Work routines involving rotational night shifts may cause difficulty adjusting to changes in sleep patterns. The person sleeps against the biological 'body clock', perceives it is time to be awake and active, and may take several weeks to adjust to the new bedtime.

Nurses with changing shift work patterns may report feeling run down, physically exhausted, irritable and have difficulty staying alert when at work. This has consequences for patient safety. Suzuki et al (2004) found significant associations between medical errors, e.g. incorrect patient identification, drug errors, and being mentally in poor health, with night or irregular shift work, and age. A review by Monk (2005) concludes, 'older people have more trouble coping with shift work'. This has important implications for the UK nursing profession, where 63.34% of registered nurses are over 40 years of age and 29% are over 50 (Nursing and Midwifery Council (NMC) 2006).

A systematic review by Wang et al (2011) examined studies investigating a link between shift work and an increased risk of chronic diseases including cancer and cardiovascular disease. Wang et al (2011) concludes that evidence is suggestive for an increase in breast cancer and cardiovascular disease, but epidemiological evidence is inadequate and further research is needed.

Environment

External factors including temperature, ventilation, lighting and the level of noise adversely affect the ability to fall asleep. These factors can be a problem in all care settings, including the person's home. Nurses should be aware that people in care settings need time to adjust to sleeping in a strange environment. People discharged home or being nursed at home can find sleep disrupted, e.g. having their bed downstairs. Examples of external factors that disrupt sleep patterns include:

- Noise caused by other patients, staff, equipment or activity in hospital. Paradoxically, a person may find it difficult to sleep if they move to a quieter environment such as a rural care home when used to city centre noises
- Lighting – some people need complete darkness to sleep, whereas babies and children may need the reassurance of low-intensity lighting
- Temperature – being too hot or too cold. The ward/room temperature may be the problem or the amount of bedding. Infants may sleep better if swaddled in a blanket but overheating has been associated with sudden infant death syndrome, (SIDS) or 'cot death' (increasingly known as sudden unexpected death in infancy, SUDI) (Box 10.12).

Health promotion   Box 10.12

Minimizing the risk of sudden infant death syndrome (SIDS)

SIDS or sudden unexpected death in infancy (SUDI) is also described as a 'cot death', but it is important to remember that unexpected sudden death can occur in a pram, carrycot or elsewhere.

Advice for parents/carers includes:

- Put babies down to sleep on their backs
- Place babies at the foot of the cot to prevent them wriggling under bedclothes (Fig. 10.4)
- For the first 6 months have the baby sleep in a cot in your room
- Do not have your baby in bed with you if you or your partner is very tired, have had prescribed medicines, alcohol or illicit drugs that can make you drowsy, you are a smoker or your baby was born before 37 weeks or weighs less that 2.5kg (5½ lbs)
- Be aware that you could suffocate your baby if you fall asleep and roll on it. The baby could also get trapped between the bed and the wall, or fall out of bed
- Do not sleep with your baby in an armchair or on the sofa
- Do not let your baby get too hot and do not cover the baby's head. Overheating can be caused by having too much clothing or bedding, or having the room too hot
- Babies should never sleep with an electric blanket or hot water bottle. Nor should they be placed to sleep near a heat source or in direct sunlight
- Both parents should not smoke during pregnancy
- Do not let anyone smoke in the home
- Breastfeed if possible as it reduces the risk of SIDS
- The use of a dummy when babies are put down to sleep may reduce SIDS, however some experts do not agree and some babies do not like a dummy. If the baby is breast-fed they should not have a dummy until breast-feeding is well established, after 1 month
- Always obtain advice from a health professional if your baby appears unwell.

(Adapted from: FSID, 2009. Looking after your baby. Online. Available: http:// fsid.org.uk September 2012; NHS Choices last reviewed 2011 Cot death: how to reduce the risk. Online. Available: www.nhs.uk/Livewell/childhealth0-1/ Pages/Cotdeath.aspx September 2012.)

- Poor ventilation – a 'stuffy' ward and odours associated with other people
- Sleeping in a room with strangers
- A strange or uncomfortable bed and bedding
- People who usually share a bed with a partner or a pet animal may find it difficult to sleep alone in a single bed
- A change in normal bedtime routine.

Nurses should be aware that patients/clients might become exhausted when continually disturbed for observations and nursing care. Some health/care units advocate a rest period after lunch when the ward/floor/unit is closed to visitors and only essential observations or procedures are undertaken during this period (see Box 10.1, p. 220). This ensures that patients/ clients are undisturbed and allowed to relax, rest or sleep for a period during the day. In areas such as high dependency or intensive care units, an effort should be made to differentiate

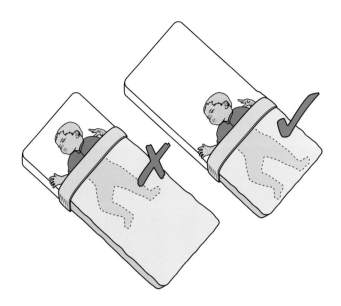

Fig. 10.4 • Feet-to-foot sleeping position. (Reproduced with permission from Fraser, D.M., Cooper, M.A. (Eds.), 2009. Myles textbook for midwives, fifteenth ed. Churchill Livingstone, Edinburgh.)

day from night by, where possible, minimizing noise, light intensity and interventions for a period during the night.

Psychosocial factors

Most people have experienced a sleepless night prior to an interview or an exciting event. A person who is constantly worrying about finances, work or having surgery may find difficulty in falling asleep. Emotional problems and anxiety caused by stress and life events throughout the lifespan, e.g. starting school, a new sibling, moving house, retirement or bereavement, can disrupt sleep (see Chs 8, 11 and 12). Children may worry about being accepted at school or be affected by relationships with siblings and parents. Adolescents and young adults often have anxieties about relationships, their appearance, exams and employment prospects.

Mental health problems

People with mental health problems such as anxiety disorders, bipolar disorder (depressed mood or mania), dementia (see p. 225), eating disorders and disordered thought processes may have disrupted sleep patterns. Sleep disruptions can include hyperactivity, difficulties getting to sleep, early waking and excessive sleeping (hypersomnia).

Physical and physiological changes

Changes such as alterations in body temperature and biological rhythms such as hormonal cycles, can disrupt sleep. Some women experience disrupted sleep patterns in the days before menstruation. The hormonal and physical changes of pregnancy may also disrupt sleep patterns (Box 10.13). These include:

- Nocturia during the early weeks and again towards the end of pregnancy

| ◉ **Reflective practice** | Box 10.13 |

Sleep disturbances during pregnancy

Consider a patient/client, a family member or friend who experienced sleep disturbances during pregnancy.

Student activities

- How has pregnancy affected their sleep?
- Reflect with your mentor on what pregnant women can do to improve sleep quality.

- Difficulties in getting comfortable in bed
- Discomfort such as low back pain and other muscular aches and pains
- Fetal movements
- Dyspnoea
- Nasal congestion
- Restless leg syndrome (RLS)
- Anxiety about labour and coping with a new baby.

Facco et al (2010) found that, compared with baseline early in pregnancy, sleep duration was significantly shorter in the last 3 months of pregnancy, and there was an increase in snoring and RLS.

Sleep disruption can also be associated with the hot flushes and night sweats experienced by some women as oestrogen secretion declines during the climacteric.

Physical health problems

Physical health problems such as pain or discomfort can result in problems with falling asleep or staying asleep. For example, the pain of arthritis, nighttime cramps or RLS and itching/irritation of skin rashes are among the diverse factors that disrupt sleep.

Most nurses can relate to having a cold and the discomfort of nasal congestion, which prevents sleep. People with cardiac or respiratory disorders may be short of breath and may need to sleep sitting up in bed or a chair (see Ch. 17). Those who have episodes of chest pain and irregular heartbeats are often afraid to go to sleep because of the fear of a heart attack at night. People with high blood pressure often feel tired and may wake up very early in the morning.

Pain from a peptic ulcer may prevent sleep or wake the person in the night. Changes in weight for example, severe weight loss and decreased body mass index (BMI) (see Ch. 19) associated with an eating disorder can disrupt sleep. Although people with a higher BMI tend to sleep better, those who are overweight or obese are at risk of sleep apnoea (see p. 229) due to the fat stored around the neck, making breathing more difficult.

Having to get up during the night to pass urine (nocturia) (see Ch. 20) disrupts the sleep cycle and getting back to sleep may be difficult. In older people, nocturia may be caused by heart or kidney disorders, or prostatic enlargement in older men. It is worth noting that this further disrupts sleep in a group who are already sleeping less well at night.

Sleeping in an awkward position due to back injuries, joint deformities or while attached to monitoring equipment in hospital, an intravenous infusion, or having a leg in plaster or in traction can interfere with sleep.

People who cannot change their own position in bed, such as those with severe physical disabilities or following a stroke, can suffer discomfort and disrupted sleep.

Effects of medication

People who take medication, either prescribed or over-the-counter (OTC), herbal products or illicit drugs may experience sleep disruption due to side-effects or interactions with other medication or alcohol, food or beverages. If the medications are required for treatment of chronic illness, e.g. diuretics, it may be necessary to review the dosages and time of administration in order to prevent disruption of sleep. Drug groups that may disrupt sleep include:

- Beta-blockers, e.g. atenolol, may disrupt sleep and cause nightmares
- Diuretics, e.g. furosemide, may lead to nocturia
- Some antihistamines, e.g. chlorphenamine, may cause daytime drowsiness
- Antidepressants, e.g. fluoxetine, may cause sleep disturbances – insomnia or drowsiness.

The effects of caffeine, nicotine and alcohol on sleep patterns are outlined above (see p. 225).

Nurses should educate patients about any medicines that can affect sleep and advise them to read enclosed information and any warning labels (Box 10.14). Patients should be asked to seek advice if sleep disruption occurs.

 Reflective practice Box 10.14

Medicines that disrupt sleep patterns

Think about common medications used for the patient/client group in your placement.

Student activities
- Find out if any of the common medications are likely to disrupt sleep patterns or cause daytime drowsiness.
- Are patients/clients routinely informed about side-effects and interactions with other medicines and alcohol?

Resources

British National Formulary (BNF): www.bnf.org.
BNF for Children: www.bnfc.org.

Both websites accessed September 2012.

Sleep disorders – an outline

Sleep disorders cover a wide range of conditions affecting both adults and children. These include insomnia, snoring, sleep apnoea, narcolepsy, sleepwalking, etc. The commoner sleep disorders are outlined in Box 10.15 but readers requiring more information are directed to Further reading (e.g. World Health Organization 2010). Fuller coverage of the general interventions to promote sleep is provided below and pp. 229-233.

Sleep disorders have physical and psychosocial effects which may include problems with education and study, work and relationships. For example, parents/carers or partners may be prevented from sleeping by snoring, or by anxiety about a loved one who has sleep apnoea or who sleepwalks.

Nurses should be aware of any limitation of skill in this specialist area and advise the person/carer/parent to seek help at a sleep clinic and offer information about support groups, e.g. The British Snoring and Sleep Apnoea Association (see Useful websites, below). Parents/carers should be encouraged to discuss any sleep problems with their health visitor, children's community nurse or learning disability liaison nurse (Box 10.16, p. 230).

Nursing interventions to promote sleep, rest and relaxation

Nurses play a key role in helping patients/clients to obtain sufficient sleep and rest. A holistic nursing assessment that includes normal rest and sleep patterns and pre-sleep routines is central to planning interventions that promote rest and sleep. Patients/clients or parents and carers may be asked to keep sleep diaries where sleep patterns are disrupted. This part of the chapter will consider sleep hygiene/pre-sleep routines/rituals and the sleep environment and the role of relaxation, orthodox medications and herbal medicines in promoting sleep. In all of these measures, it is vital to involve the patient/client/child, parent or carer in the assessment and decision-making about appropriate interventions and in evaluating their effectiveness.

Nursing assessment of sleep

Nurses should know the patient's/client's normal sleep pattern and habits in order to plan appropriate interventions and detect departures from normal. Most people suffer disruptions to sleep patterns at some time. Nurses should note whether there is difficulty in falling asleep, frequent waking during the sleep cycle, early wakening or oversleeping and the degree to which the quantity, quality and consistency of sleep are affected. A holistic assessment should include:

- Culture, beliefs and religious practices which influence sleep pattern
- The person's understanding of the functions and importance of rest and sleep
- Normal pre-sleep routine, e.g. milky drink, warm bath, a child having a bedtime story, reading
- Sleep environment: a light in the child's room, special toys or 'comfort' items, whether the person shares a bed, or sleeps in a chair or have their own room
- Usual bedtime
- Length of time to fall asleep (sleep latency)
- Usual duration of sleep in hours

Sleep disorders
Box 10.15

Insomnia

This includes difficulties in: falling asleep, remaining asleep, going back to sleep after awakening. It may be temporary, last a few nights or may become chronic. The complaint is of insufficient quantity and quality of sleep, but frequently the person sleeps more than they realize. Insomnia can affect any age group and causes tiredness/sleepiness, depression, anxiety, lethargy and irritability during the day. A vicious circle develops where worrying about not sleeping prevents the person from falling asleep.

Management includes interventions to promote sleep, such as good sleep hygiene/pre-sleep routines, reducing anxiety, relaxation and improving the sleep environment (see pp. 231-233). If sleep does not occur it is better to get up, read or have a drink and then go back to bed. Sleeping tablets should only be prescribed in the short term such as during hospitalization for surgery. Specialist help may be needed if the problem is unresolved and becomes chronic.

Buysse et al (2011) found that cognitive behavioural treatment is a simple and effective strategy for chronic insomnia in older people.

Narcolepsy (excessive somnolence)

This results when sleep–wake regulation mechanisms are not functioning properly. It commonly occurs during the young adult years. Excessive daytime sleepiness culminates in a 'sleep attack' where the person exhibits sudden muscle weakness (sleep paralysis), being unable to move and falls to the ground. REM sleep can occur within minutes. The 'sleep attacks', can happen several times a day at inappropriate times, e.g. during meals. The person may experience hallucinations and insomnia.

Narcolepsy requires investigation and treatment by a specialist sleep clinic. Modafinil is used for narcolepsy; for certain types of narcolepsy, clomipramine or sodium oxybate may be prescribed. The person is advised to inform others of the condition. Good sleep hygiene, such as pre-sleep routines and enhancing the sleep environment, is crucial for these patients. Maximum support is needed at home, in the workplace or at school/college.

Sleep apnoea

Sleep apnoea requires investigation and treatment by a specialist sleep clinic. Patients should lose weight and avoid alcohol in the evening. If severe, continuous positive airway pressure (CPAP) may be considered (see Ch. 17). Upper airway surgery may be performed.

Sleepwalking (somnambulance)

This occurs during stage 4 NREM sleep and about 15% of children aged 5–12 years do quiet sleepwalking. After a brief sleep period, they sit up, eyes open, walk purposefully with an unsteady gait and do strange things, e.g. urinating in the wardrobe then proceed directly to bed again. Adults if anxious or stressed, may resume sleepwalking as they once did as children. Sleepwalking may be accompanied by violent behaviour.

Management focuses on ensuring their safety (and that of others) by simply watching while the person is sleepwalking and perhaps guiding them gently back to bed, rather than trying to wake them up.

Sleep/night terrors

These occur in stage 4 NREM sleep. The child sits up and screams, clearly terrified but are unable to vocalize the source of the fear. They may have some recollection but it is usually very brief and quickly forgotten. The arousal is sudden and the body responds physiologically with sweating, increased heart and respiratory rate and the strong feeling of fear (this also occurs in nightmares). The child may appear to be hallucinating and pushing an imaginary object or person away. Sleep terrors may be accompanied by violent behaviour. Parental attempts to console are not recognized and rejected. Eventually, the child falls asleep.

When caring for a patient/client suffering a night terror, it is important to remain calm and reassuring with a quiet, steady voice and be sure that the person is alert and knows who you are prior to touching or comforting.

Nightmares

These occur predominantly during REM sleep. These are dreams that induce a powerful emotional arousal, often causing sudden awakening.

Nurses can provide reassurance by reminding patients/clients where they are and telling them that they are safe, as they may be disorientated on awakening. Sometimes a drink or a chance to talk helps to calm their fears. An increase in the amount of lighting in the room may help.

Bruxism (teeth grinding)

This usually occurs in stages 1 and 2 of NREM sleep. It may occur in children when the first dentition has erupted. In older children, it may be related to anxiety and stress. Bruxism can cause tooth damage and misalignment. Relaxation therapies and talking through anxieties may be helpful (see p. 232 and Ch. 11). Dental and/or orthodontic interventions such as a nighttime mouthguard may be needed to prevent damage to the teeth.

Other sleep disorders

These include jet lag (see p. 225), shift work sleep disturbance (see p. 226), sleep paralysis, nocturnal enuresis (see Ch. 20), those associated with mental health problems (see pp. 225, 227) and neurological conditions such as epilepsy.

Note: Children with Down's syndrome and other learning disabilities may show several sleep disorders, some of which may be due to physical problems, e.g. disordered breathing and sleep apnoea. Sleep deprivation and related daytime behaviour problems are also apparent (Stores 2008).

- Whether they wake in the night
- Waking up time in the morning
- Whether they feel refreshed following a night's sleep
- Does the person feel that their sleep pattern is normal?
- What helps the person to fall asleep or sleep better and what prevents sleep?
- Do they dream or have nightmares?

- Recent changes in sleep patterns – onset and duration of the problem
- Factors affecting their sleep pattern such as being alone in the house or being away from home, menstrual cycle, time of year
- Measures taken to promote sleep if normal patterns are disrupted, e.g. altering bedtimes, complementary

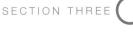

Sleep problems and learning disability

7-year-old Molly has a learning disability. She lives at home, attends school and regularly goes into respite care to give her parents a break. Molly has always been difficult to settle at night but now she becomes distressed at bedtime, pulling her hair and screaming. She only sleeps for 2–3 hour periods and wakes her parents every night. Molly's parents are exhausted and feel that they need help to deal with Molly's sleep problem.

Student activities

- Speak to a learning disability nurse and a health visitor and find out what advice and support they would offer Molly's parents. Ask them if they would consider complementary therapies such as aromatherapy (see pp. 237-238).
- Find out if there is a sleep clinic or special services/schemes, e.g. Sleep Scotland in your area? Sleep Scotland provides help for families with children with special needs whose severe sleep problems can disrupt family life.

Resources

Atherton, H.L., Crickmore, D.J. (Eds.), 2011. Learning disabilities. Towards inclusion, sixth ed. Churchill Livingstone, Edinburgh.
Sleep Scotland – www.sleepscotland.org September 2012.

keep a diary. Initially, this can be for 1 week. The contents can help to identify the main problems and highlight factors that relieve or exacerbate sleeplessness. As a tool, the diary can assess progress and efficacy of interventions used to improve the person's sleep pattern. Initially this can prove tedious to document but once a routine is developed, it becomes easier. In the author's experience, most people who have a severe sleep problem would do nearly anything to resolve it. It is important to accept the person's interpretation of their sleep pattern/sleep disruption, even if it does not agree with your own analysis.

It is important to explain from the outset the aims of the diary and to support and give positive feedback to the person for persisting with the documentation. It is helpful to provide written instructions (prompters of key phrases and questions) for completing the diary (Box 10.17). Children can describe their sleep patterns through age-appropriate documentation, such as colouring books, cartoons depicting children sleeping/ not sleeping, clock faces with movable hands or the use of stickers for hours slept.

therapies, using OTC medicines or herbal medicines or prescribed sleeping tablets
- Do they nap during the day?
- What time is their last large meal?
- Do they have a snack before bed or wake in the night to have a snack?
- Do they smoke or consume caffeine or alcohol in the evening?
- Current lifestyle, work and domestic relationships, social activities including play-rest-sleep patterns for children
- Worries, stress and anxieties, e.g. worries about the health of a loved one, debts, exams
- Ongoing emotional problems such as relationship difficulties
- Usual medication, OTC, herbal medicines, prescribed drugs and use of illegal drugs
- Other therapies, e.g. counselling
- History of conditions, e.g. RLS, migraine or joint pain
- Previous sleep problems, e.g. insomnia
- Recent changes in health status
- Behaviour changes, e.g. a child who is upset at bedtime after the arrival of a sibling, or increasing daytime sleeping in an older adult with dementia
- Change of environment, e.g. moving into a care home
- Changes to routine, e.g. starting school, different work pattern or shift times, travel across time zones or a new baby in the house.

Keeping a sleep diary

When sleep patterns are disrupted or a sleep disorder is suspected, patients/clients, parents or carers are encouraged to

- Use an ordinary diary (day per page) with dates, times and space for writing
- Start the diary on the first day of the week (e.g. Monday) and finish it on the same day, as most people have set routines from the beginning of the week
- Have the diary by your bed
- Note the activity and type of meal, e.g. watched TV, snack, a glass of wine, a pizza, before bedtime, for that day
- Note the time you get into bed that night (with the intention of going to sleep)
- Note separately what time, how quickly or how long you took to fall asleep. If you are too drowsy to write all this down, document the approximate time when you awake or ask your partner (if relevant) to note this down for you
- If you waken during the night, note the time you awoke and what woke you
- If you cannot get back to sleep immediately, note the reason why; note any measures taken to help you to fall asleep again
- Note the time you wake up the next morning and what woke you up
- Note how easy it was and how long it took before you got out of bed
- How did you feel 5–10 min after waking up? For example, did you feel refreshed or very tired? Did you feel like going back to sleep or were you ready to get on with the day's work?
- Note the total number of hours you *think* you have slept and calculate roughly how many hours you really slept
- Note if you had any dreams last night
- Note what your activities are for the day, e.g. important meeting or usual routine day
- Note how you felt for the rest of the day, e.g. fresh, tired, irritable, needed a nap.

Note: Include other relevant information, e.g. upset after a row with partner; period started; really worried about the electricity bill, etc.

Monday 3rd January	
	Busy day at work, got home too late to cook. Had a takeaway curry and 2 large glasses of wine at about 21.00.
22.30	Made a drink of hot chocolate and took it to bed. Tried to look through a magazine but too tired.
23.00	Settled down to sleep.
02.30	Woke up to pass urine.
03.00	Still awake. Not sure when sleep resumed - possibly after 15 min but partner said I 'tossed and turned' for half an hour.
07.00	Woken up by alarm clock, dozed for a few minutes.
07.30	Struggled out of bed, did not feel refreshed. Didn't dream but partner said that I mumbled soon after falling asleep the first time, but he couldn't make out any words. Important meeting at work this morning, very stressful. Felt really tired after lunch. Irritable during the afternoon and snapped at colleagues.

Fig. 10.5 • Sleep diary entry.

Soon, people become familiar with the requirements and 'automatic' documentation occurs. Some people may prefer to use special charts with dates, times and prompters instead of a standard diary. The completion of the diary should coincide with follow-up sessions at the clinic to discuss the results. Figure 10.5 illustrates a typical sleep diary entry.

Improving sleep hygiene and the sleep environment

Simple changes can improve sleep hygiene such as going to bed and getting up at about the same time each day. It is helpful to avoid using the bedroom/bed for other activities such as working or eating. Developing a pre-sleep routine that helps the person to fall asleep and stay asleep is important. This might involve a bedtime story, a milky drink, warm bath, changing into nightclothes, teeth/denture cleaning and passing urine. In care settings, the nurse should try to maintain the person's pre-sleep routine as far as is possible, and offer assistance as required.

People should be given advice about eliminating factors known to disrupt normal sleep patterns (see pp. 225-228). This might include reducing strenuous physical activity in the evening, encouraging quiet play for children, reducing caffeine intake by replacing tea or coffee with fruit teas. Avoiding an excessive fluid intake just before bedtime can minimize nocturia in children and older people. However, they must have sufficient fluids during the day (see Ch. 19). Others may need to eat their main meal earlier in the evening and have a small bedtime snack. A bedtime snack should be available in care settings if necessary. Excessive daytime sleeping or naps may disrupt sleep at night and people may need advice about reducing naps.

Some patients/clients may wish to carry out religious activities such as prayers before sleep, or position their bed to face the correct way, i.e. towards Mecca. Some people will want to see a local religious leader or read from their holy book. These facilities and privacy should be made available.

It is important to promote sleep by ensuring comfort and providing an environment conducive to sleep before medication is considered. The many simple interventions that promote sleep, either at home or care settings, include the following:

- Many adults need a dark environment in order to sleep so having thick curtains drawn is important. Where light is still a problem, such as from streetlights, the person may use an eyemask. Some children can only sleep if there is low intensity light in their room or on the landing/corridor. Some care settings for older adults may also provide minimal lighting to reduce confusion on waking and to reduce the risk of falls if the person gets out of bed
- Reducing noise to a minimum (Box 10.18)
- Check the environmental temperature before bedtime to ensure it is neither too hot nor too cold
- Good ventilation, e.g. opening a window or use of electric fans on summer nights
- Provide a relaxing atmosphere – reduce the lighting in the evening, listen to music, read
- Children can engage in a relaxing/soothing activity before sleep, e.g. colouring, a bedtime story
- Complementary therapies (see pp. 233-238) can be used to enhance relaxation. For example, some herbal products are mildly sedating, e.g. chamomile, lavender and lemon balm (see below and pp. 235-236)
- Where possible, reduce ward/unit activities well before bedtime

 Reflective practice　Box 10.18

Aiming for silence

Sleep can be difficult to achieve if noise levels are too high or if the type of noise changes. Noise will affect sleep in every setting, including the person's home.

Student activities

- Stop and listen to the noise one night in your placement. What types of noise are present?
- Reflect on ways to reduce noise, e.g. talking quietly, reducing the loudness of telephones at night.
- Find out what design/structural features have been used to reduce noise such as double glazing.

- Ensure bedding is adequate and comfortable, and that pillows are arranged for sleep. Some people living in care homes may want to use their own pillows/pillow cases, but always check local policy and safety issues
- Ensure a comfortable sleep position by using, e.g. supportive dressings, splints, extra pillows or a firm mattress if preferred by the patient/client. Older mattresses that no longer support the spinal column should be replaced
- For infants and toddlers ensure that they are clean and dry and change nappies as necessary. Many infants will settle more easily if they have physical contact such as cuddling and touch by gently massaging their head or abdomen or back. Others are comforted by wrapping in a blanket, but beware of overheating (see p. 226). Quiet singing, music or humming may also help to relax the infant/toddler and promote sleep
- Patients/clients who have pain will require analgesics and/ or other pain-relieving measures (see Ch. 23)
- Feeling secure is important in promoting sleep. For example, a child needs to know that parents/carers are downstairs. People receiving care at home need the reassurance of knowing when the care team will visit and how to get help. In hospital/care home, people feel more secure if they know who is caring for them. Therefore the night staff should walk round to see everyone before bedtime.

Relaxation and sleep

Anyone who is suffering from altered sleep or significant sleep disorders often complains of feeling stressed, anxious and tense and unable to relax (Box 10.19). Several research studies have highlighted the efficacy of complementary therapies in inducing relaxation and so offer an important clinical contribution to stress-related sleep disorders. For further coverage of relaxation techniques and their uses in relieving stress and pain, see Chapters 11 and 23.

 Reflective practice   **Box 10.19**

Relaxation and sleep

Think about a patient/client who has difficulties with relaxing and getting to sleep.

Student activities

- What strategies have you seen the registered nurses, family or carers use to help the person relax at bedtime?
- Find out what relaxation therapies, e.g. massage, are available locally.
- Discuss with your mentor how you can promote sleep by helping patients/clients to relax.

In a study by Lichstein et al (1999) participants who received relaxation therapy reported improved sleep efficiency and reduced withdrawal symptoms during a sleep medication withdrawal programme. Harris and Richards (2010) conclude

that both physiological and psychological indicators suggest the effectiveness of two massage techniques in encouraging relaxation in older people.

Other therapies, such as acupuncture, are used for insomnia. However, Cheuk et al (2007) conclude that there is a deficiency of clinical evidence supporting the use of acupuncture for insomnia, and that further high quality research is required. (Herbal medicines are considered below and the wider uses of herbal medicine on pp. 235-236.)

Sleep medications

Orthodox medications may be used to aid rest and sleep for patients/clients who cannot sleep despite the non-pharmacological interventions discussed above. In addition, people may choose to use herbal medicines.

Orthodox medications

The cause of insomnia should be known, e.g. 'sleeping tablets' may be prescribed for a patient who is in hospital following surgery and cannot sleep because of noise. The drugs used to aid sleep include hypnotics (drugs that induce sleep), anxiolytics (tranquillizers that reduce anxiety) and analgesic drugs (painkillers) (see Ch. 23). In addition, the dose of antidepressant drugs can be adjusted and taken at night to improve sleeping in people suffering from depression. However, hypnotic and anxiolytic use has a number of disadvantages, including:

- Changes to the amount of the time spent in different sleep stages
- Daytime sleepiness and a 'hangover effect' with some hypnotics
- Increased risks of falls in older people
- Tolerance develops to hypnotics and for this reason, they should only be prescribed for short periods (preferably 1 week): one or two doses for transient insomnia and no longer than 3 weeks for short-term insomnia (*British National Formulary*, BNF 2012)
- Withdrawal symptoms, rebound insomnia, vivid dreams when discontinued.

Examples of the medications used to aid sleep are provided in Box 10.20 but readers requiring more specific information about indications, side-effects, contraindications, etc. should consult the current BNF.

Herbal medicines

Valerian (*Valeriana officinalis*), hops (*Humulus lupulus*), lemon balm (*Melissa officinalis*), passion flower (*Passiflora incarnata*), chamomile (*Matricaria chamomilla*) and lavender (*Lavandula angustifolia*) have all been traditionally used in herbal medicine for treating restlessness and sleep disturbances.

It is important to advise people to avoid self-medication with OTC products, especially herbal products, which are advertised to promote sleep. These products may interact with the person's prescribed medications. It is safer to consult a

---

Examples of orthodox medication used to aid sleep   **Box 10.20**

- Benzodiazepines, e.g. diazepam, nitrazepam, temazepam; only for severe, disabling and distressing insomnia. Use lowest possible dose for the shortest possible duration (BNF 2012)
- Clomethiazole
- Antihistamines, e.g. promethazine hydrochloride
- Zaleplon, zolpidem and zopiclone
- Antidepressant drugs, e.g. amitriptyline, mirtazapine
- Melatonin may be used for adults aged over 55 years and it may be given to children, including those with learning disabilities, visual impairment and autism, etc., where other treatments have failed (BNF 2012).

Note: Barbiturates are no longer recommended. Hypnotics are not generally used for children.

---

trained herbal practitioner who can advise the person on the appropriate herbal remedy to aid sleep (see pp. 235–236).

Complementary and alternative medicine

Complementary and alternative medicine (CAM) refers to a diverse group of health-related therapies, which are not part of conventional (mainstream) or allopathic medicine. These therapies tend to be health interventions practised by different cultures over thousands of years. Some CAM therapies offered in conjunction with conventional medicine are described as complementary, e.g. aromatherapy (see pp. 237–238), whereas others, such as osteopathy, provide diagnostic information and are offered as an alternative to conventional medicine.

Most CAM therapies differ from conventional medicine management in their philosophies, concepts and principles of care and no one single philosophy is shared by all CAM disciplines. Some CAM philosophies linked to religious practices have evolved over centuries of use and are now incorporated into interpretations of body functions, health and disease. The majority of CAM therapists believe that their view of care embraces all dimensions of the person, so there is less divide between the body, mind and spirit, hence the term 'holistic' is often used.

The emergence, development and regulation of CAM

In the late 1980s and early 1990s, there was an increase in interest and wider use of CAM in the UK by both the general public and health professionals, especially nurses. There were approximately 50 000 CAM practitioners and, of these, 10 000 statutory registered health practitioners offered CAM alongside conventional care (Budd & Mills 2000). People accessed CAM through CAM practitioners, through other health professionals, including doctors, nurses and physiotherapists who offered CAM, or by purchasing OTC products. Surveys conducted in Australia, the United States and Europe suggest that

the public there are equally keen to use CAM. In Europe, however CAM is practised alongside conventional medicine (Department of Health, DH 1996). Surveys on patient/client satisfaction and the popularity of CAM have identified certain themes and characteristics of CAM therapies (Box 10.21).

Perceptions of CAM   **Box 10.21**

- Individualized care
- A combination of treatments tailored to people's specific needs
- CAM therapists were more friendly
- More time spent with each person/client
- Person/client receives more information on their disease and its treatment and in simple language as CAM practitioners are more likely to use everyday language (see Ch. 9)
- Consultations are more thorough and take longer
- Therapists actively listen to the person/client
- Therapists show more interest in other aspects of person's/client's life, not just their physical symptoms, including personality, life experiences and social network and support
- Focus on the person/client, not the disease
- Increased person/client involvement and a wider choice of treatments and management
- Increased touch and less technical equipment
- Increased level of hope and optimism
- Social issues are explored, thus helping the person/client to understand their problem/illness in the context of family and work
- A holistic approach may mean that the person/client can make sense and understand more about the illness because it becomes more personally relevant

(From House of Lords 2000).

This widespread use of CAM raised concerns about having in place rigorous structured regulations to protect public safety and interests. Related issues such as an evidence base for research, adequate training for practitioners, information resources for the public and what prospects there were for NHS provision of these therapies were raised. These concerns prompted a House of Lords Select Committee report (House of Lords 2000) and the then government's response the year after (DH 2001), which noted the wide range of CAM therapies (Box 10.22). Some therapies had complete systems of assessment and treatment whereas others complement conventional treatment with various supportive techniques. While some were well-regulated, others were very fragmented with no consensus about regulation.

Chiropractic and osteopathy are already self-registered and self-regulated which means that their professional activity and education are regulated by Acts of Parliament. Practitioners must be registered with the General Chiropractic Council or General Osteopathic Council, respectively, in order to practise in the UK.

At the time of writing, the introduction of statutory regulation for other CAM disciplines is ongoing following an analysis of responses to a consultation in 2009 (DH 2011).

Categories of CAM therapies	Box 10.22

Group 1 therapies

Acupuncture, chiropractic, herbal medicine, homeopathy and osteopathy. Viewed as the 'big five' in CAM, these offer diagnostic skills, appear to be the most organized and already have an established research base for some aspects of practice. There is increasing NHS provision for some therapies.

Group 2 therapies

Aromatherapy, the Alexander technique, massage, counselling, stress therapy, hypnotherapy, reflexology, shiatsu, meditation and healing. Often used to complement conventional medicine and do not include diagnostic techniques. There is some NHS provision for these therapies, especially in palliative care and with people with a learning disability.

Group 3 therapies (groups 3a and 3b)

3a – Ayurvedic medicine and traditional Chinese medicine (TCM)
3b – Crystal therapy, iridology, radionics and kinesiology

(Adapted from House of Lords 2000).

Integrated medicine

Many practitioners consider the term CAM to be outmoded and that it is more appropriate to use 'integrated medicine' or indeed 'interprofessional healthcare' instead.

Despite the wide diversity of CAM, its popularity and potential role alongside conventional therapies, access to CAM via the NHS remains limited.

CAM therapies

This part of the chapter outlines the scope and main characteristics of the 'big five' CAM therapies: acupuncture, chiropractic, herbal medicine, homeopathy and osteopathy – and others, e.g. aromatherapy, that have been integrated into conventional healthcare.

It does not lay claims for efficacy. Where treatment and conditions are linked, it serves only to highlight that a particular treatment exists rather than the author's or editor's opinion or recommendation.

The language used to describe elements of a particular therapy such as 'vital force', 'holism' and 'energies' are existing terms related to that therapy.

Readers requiring information about other therapies such as humour therapy, shiatsu, massage, therapeutic touch, etc. are directed to Further reading, below (e.g. Mantle & Tiran 2009).

Acupuncture

Acupuncture widely practised in China since the first century BC involves the insertion of small needles into specific points on the surface of the body. Since the 1970s, it is used mainly in the West for pain relief. Currently in the UK, registered medical practitioners and other healthcare professionals practise acupuncture. At present, acupuncture is not statutory regulated, but procedures leading to legislation are in progress (see p. 233).

Acupuncture is part of traditional Chinese medicine (TCM), which includes the use of herbs, diet, massage, acupressure and relaxation through special exercises. The fundamental principles of TCM are based on the belief that a person functions in harmony with the universe. So health, disease and treatment relates to a person's harmony or disharmony with external forces of wind, damp, dryness and cold, and internal anger, excitement, worry, sadness and fear. Elements such as wood, fire, earth, metal and water are used to describe various states of health and illness. Two complementary but opposite forces – yin and yang – if balanced within the body, results in good health. Yin represents cold, damp, darkness, passivity and contraction whereas yang signifies heat, dryness, light, action and expansion. The interaction of yin and yang gives rise to *qi* (pronounced 'chee'). Qi is described as an invisible life energy and is a vital force that flows around the body through meridians or energy channels. There are 12 regular meridians, which run down the body in pairs, six on the left and six on the right.

The meridians are named for the main internal organs through which they pass, e.g. the lungs or kidneys. Disruption of flow on a meridian interrupts circulation of qi and can create illness at any point along it. For example, a disorder in the stomach meridian (passing through the upper gums) could cause toothache. There are about 365 points along the meridians at which qi is concentrated and can enter and leave the body. At these points, acupuncturists insert the acupuncture needles to stimulate or suppress the flow of qi, restoring energetic balance and organ function.

During the first consultation, a thorough interview to establish the presenting problem, past medical history and a physical examination is required. Specific questions and examination would include:

- Inspection of 'trigger points' related to the pain and reflex points on the trunk
- Evaluation of the strengths and weaknesses of the internal organs by examination of the ear, tongue and pulse.

Tiny needles are inserted in the area where the blocked energy to the circulation network is identified (Fig. 10.6) and left in place for 5–20 minutes. To protect the person/client from energy depletion, a much shorter time is used if a person is very tired, frail or old.

Additional stimulation and activation of the acupuncture system is achieved by connecting the needles to a special electrical device, by moxibustion (heating the needles with burning mugwort – an aromatic herb) or by gentle manual manipulation of the needles.

Weekly reviews are scheduled and with good progress, follow-up treatments can be every 4–6 weeks or further apart.

Integration of acupuncture into conventional healthcare

The type of acupuncture adapted and integrated into orthodox healthcare is 'Western medical acupuncture'. It is practised by orthodox medical and other health professionals in the West. In some areas of the UK, it is available from the NHS. The same needling technique as traditional acupuncture is

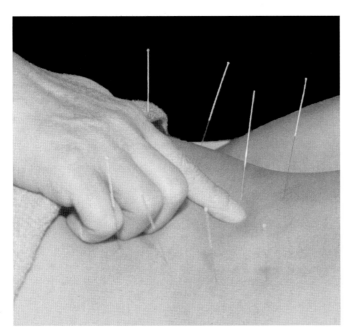

Fig. 10.6 • Acupuncture needles *in situ*. (Reproduced with permission from Zhu, H.Z., 2005. Running a safe and successful acupuncture clinic. Churchill Livingstone, Edinburgh.)

used but works by affecting nerve impulse transmission and the central nervous system. Acupuncture is effective for anaesthetic and analgesic (see Ch. 23) purposes and musculoskeletal complaints (Box 10.23); substance misuse (e.g. smoking cessation), in maternity care, migraine, high blood pressure and digestive disorders. Although traditional acupuncture is a widely accepted therapy, medical opinion is still divided on its efficacy.

 Critical thinking   Box 10.23

Acupuncture in orthodox healthcare

Orthodox practitioners, e.g. physiotherapists and anaesthetists, use acupuncture to relieve pain and induce sleep.

Student activities

- Is acupuncture available in your area of practice?
- Talk to a health professional who uses acupuncture to relieve pain and/or promote sleep.
- What are the contraindications to the use of acupuncture?

(See Further reading, e.g. Mantle & Tiran 2009).

Chiropractic

The term chiropractic comes from the Greek words *cheiro*, meaning 'hands' and *prakticos*, meaning 'doing'. Collectively meaning 'done by hand' or manipulation. Developed in the late nineteenth century by David Palmer, a Canadian osteopath, chiropractic diagnoses and treats disorders of the spine, joints and muscles. Chiropractics use their hands to manipulate joints and adjust muscles by high velocity, short amplitude thrust and gentle soft tissue massage.

These techniques realign nerve supply to affected organs and can be used to treat musculoskeletal complaints by relieving pain, increasing mobility and improving function.

A chiropractic views the body as a mechanical structure with the key being the spine, which links the brain to the rest of the body. Therefore, distortion of the spine affects the body parts and reduced 'nerve flow' leads to disease. Treatment can ease muscle tension caused by stress or those linked to problems in internal organs such as the intestine. When the skeletal structure functions smoothly, the body's natural healing processes keep all body systems working in harmony enabling the body to heal itself from within.

During the initial consultation, a detailed case history of the presenting problem, past medical and surgical history and lifestyle factors are explored. For example, the client is asked about exercise and type of bed used. A full clinical examination entails the person/client adopting different postures, e.g. lying down, sitting and standing.

Diagnostic procedures include X-rays, neurological tests including reflexes, 'motion palpation' to check the spine and use of a rubber-tipped instrument called an activator. The activator delivers a very small thrust to manipulate the vertebrae. The activator can be used for very frail older people and even babies.

Controlled techniques to adjust and 'unlock' any joint problems heard as 'clicks' during the manoeuvres are painless. The first session takes about an hour and subsequent sessions about 20 minutes. Some muscle aches and pains lasting a few days after the treatment are normal. Treatment continues with weekly follow-up visits until the problem is resolved. Chiropractics recommend 'maintenance' visits 6–12 monthly to prevent recurrence. If the problem requires specialist treatment, the person/client will be referred to their GP.

Integration of chiropractice into conventional healthcare

Chiropractice can be used to treat neck, muscle, joint and postural problems, sciatica, migraine, sports injuries and gastrointestinal disorders. However, Walker et al (2010) concluded that currently, there is no evidence that supports or disproves that chiropractic interventions provide a clinically significant difference for pain or disability in people with low back pain when compared to conventional interventions.

In the UK, chiropractics are subject to statutory regulation and must register with the General Chiropractic Council in order to practise. Some orthodox practitioners are trained chiropractics.

Herbal medicine

Over 80% of the world's population use herbs for health maintenance. Herbal medicine, one of the most ancient forms of treatment, is used by every culture to treat disease and promote well-being. This system of medicine uses plants and plant extracts to treat disorders, promote and maintain good health. There are several subcategories practised in the UK, namely Chinese herbal medicine, Tibetan herbal medicine, Ayurvedic herbal medicine and Western herbal medicine (also called phytotherapy or phytomedicine). Chinese herbal medicine is an integral part of and practised with TCM and acupuncture. This chapter focuses on Western herbal medicine.

In 2011, the Secretary of State for Health announced that practitioners of herbal medicine have attained statutory regulation with the Health and Care Professions Council (HCPC) but the commencement date is still to be decided.

Conventional medicine uses laboratory-produced drugs derived from plants, but often refined to isolate a single active ingredient. Herbal remedies differ from synthetic drugs, in that parts of a whole plant are used as the remedy. Western herbal medicine is a holistic treatment system that seeks to restore the body's self-healing mechanism or 'vital force'. Remedies are prescribed, tailored to the holistic needs of the person, not just the symptoms of the illness. Rather than treating symptoms in isolation, the herbal practitioner identifies the cause of illness such as poor diet, an unhealthy lifestyle or excessive stress, which may imbalance the body's delicate homeostatic physiological, psychosocial and spiritual domains. Practitioners attribute disease to a disruption in the body's state of harmony or homeostasis. Herbal remedies promote healing by supporting the body's vital force in its efforts to restore homeostasis.

The herbal practitioner's skills lie in knowing the actions of different plant constituents on specific body systems. For example, a plant, or parts of it, may stimulate the circulation or calm the digestive system.

Herbal synergy is a key factor where parts of whole plants are deemed more effective and gives a better therapeutic effect. For example, meadowsweet (*Filipéndula ulmaria*), used to treat digestive disorders, contains salicylic acid, the basis of the drug aspirin. However, while aspirin can cause gastrointestinal bleeding, meadowsweet contains tannins and mucilage that protect the stomach lining (Mills & Bone 2000).

Herbal remedies are extracted from leaves, flowers, fruits, stems, bark, roots, rhizomes, seeds or exudates (e.g. frankincense resin) and other plant parts which contain a complex mix of active ingredients with medicinal effects. This use of strictly plant products is unlike other herbal traditions (e.g. Chinese herbal medicine) where non-plants materials, such as insects, shells, minerals, animal bone or organs, are also used.

Herbal remedies can be made from combinations of herbs or from a single herb. The remedies can be taken in different ways. These include:

- Infusions of plant parts infused with boiling water (herb teas)
- Tinctures of plant products extracted in alcohol
- Oils
- External applications, e.g. creams.

Every herbal remedy is said to have three effects on the body: to detoxify and eliminate wastes, to strengthen it and help it heal itself and to build up the organs.

The first consultation takes 1½ hours to explore the presenting complaint, past medical history, social history, medications and lifestyle factors. Diet history is an important aspect of the assessment. If necessary, physical examinations related to the presenting complaint, e.g. using a stethoscope to auscultate the lung fields or the heart; or a neurological examination – will be carried out. The management plan is discussed with the person/client. The relevant remedy could be a tincture or a combination of herbs, teas or creams. The first review is normally at 2 weeks and good response to treatment is followed-up at 4–6 week intervals. People's/clients' involvement in their own healing is important and they are advised to actively engage in making lifestyle changes encompassing social context and self-responsibility. Complex cases are referred to the GP or another appropriate health practitioner and the person/client is advised that herbal treatment is not suitable.

Integration into conventional healthcare

In the UK, some hospitals and GP practices have part-time Western herbal practitioners working in the multidisciplinary team. However, people/clients who are using herbal treatment are usually self-funding. In Europe, e.g. Germany and France, Western herbal medicine is practised by conventionally trained physicians and integrated into routine medical care. Herbal medicines can be used to treat a range of conditions including musculoskeletal disorders, menstrual irregularities, anxiety and nervous tension, as well as gastrointestinal upsets. For example, colic in babies may be reduced by the use of dill (*Anethum graveolans*) and fennel (*Foeniculum vulgare*). These may be prescribed as teas for breast-feeding mothers or as tincture drops in juice for older children (Scott & Barlow 2003).

There is a dearth of controlled studies on the efficacy of herbs, especially those used to enhance sleep, and this is an area where nurses can engage in collaborative research with herbal practitioners (Box 10.24).

 Evidence-based practice   Box 10.24

Herbal medicine – safety

Nurses and midwives are required to 'Use the best available evidence' (NMC 2008)

Student activities

- Access *The code: Standards of conduct, performance and ethics for nurses and midwives* (NMC 2008) and access the part relating to the use of complementary or alternative therapies (such as herbal remedies)
- Talk to a herbal practitioner about the evidence, to date, for the safety of herbal medicines used for insomnia.

Homeopathy

Derived from the Greek words *homoios*, meaning 'like' and *pathos*, meaning 'suffering', homeopathy is a system of medicine that uses remedies prepared from plant, mineral and animal substances. These remedies are taken by mouth in tablet, powder or liquid form or applied as creams.

Hippocrates, in the fourth century BC, proposed that a substance which mimics an illness can be used to cure it. This principle of treating 'like with like' was later developed into homeopathy in the eighteenth century by a German doctor, Samuel Hahnemann. This principle of Law of Similars, 'like cures like', means a substance that produces symptoms similar to the disease can be used to cure the disease. Thus, a person's symptom is used as a guide to finding the remedy. For example, being stung by nettles produces a rash, redness and inflammation. The same herb when prepared as a homeopathic remedy can be used to treat allergic reactions producing the same symptoms.

The Law of Potentization in homeopathy states that the more a remedy is diluted, the more potent it is to heal and the 'potential' to cause side-effects is reduced. In a typical dilution, one drop of the 'mother tincture' (preparation of the plant material in alcohol) is diluted in 99 drops of alcohol, and then shaken vigorously in a process known as succussion.

Homeopaths view symptoms of illness as the body using its natural powers of self-healing to fight back. Accordingly, if the body's vital force, which maintains health is under strain, illness can result. Homeopathic treatments stimulate the body's self-healing ability rather than suppress symptoms of the illness.

The first consultation of 1½ hours will cover medical history, lifestyle, diet, physical and emotional factors (e.g. mood, likes and dislikes), sleeping patterns, reactions to weather conditions and personality traits. Exploring the person's/client's problems and needs is essential for prescribing the best matching remedy which may be an animal, plant or mineral preparation, e.g. sepia (cuttlefish ink), aconite (monkshood) and nat mur (sodium chloride) (Phatak 2003). Homeopaths put less emphasis on physical examination and for longstanding problems, several review consultations are necessary where the prescription can be altered according to the changes in the symptoms.

Integration with conventional medicine

Both medically and non-medically qualified practitioners practise homeopathy. Some GP practices can refer people to a homeopathic hospital.

Osteopathy

The term is derived from the Greek *osteon* 'bone' and *pathos* 'disease'. Dr Andrew Taylor Still, a doctor in the nineteenth century, developed this therapy. Osteopaths see the organs of the body as supported and protected by the musculoskeletal system. The bones, joints, muscles, ligaments and other connective tissue provide a framework, which if correctly aligned and working well, results in the tissues and systems of the body being healthy.

The initial consultation of 1½ hours includes looking for reasons behind the fault in the musculoskeletal system. Lifestyle and physical, mental and emotional health are explored. Poor posture or injury can affect the musculoskeletal system, causing pain, strain, impaired nerve function and affect the vital organs. Manipulation of misaligned joints and a focus on soft tissues (muscles, tendons, etc.), treatment to relax muscles and restore joint mobility will be used. Initial weekly sessions until the problem is resolved are followed-up with 4–6 weekly reviews.

Integration into conventional healthcare

Osteopathy was the first complementary therapy to be subject to statutory regulation (Osteopaths Act 1993). The General Osteopathic Council ensures standards of practice. In the UK, osteopaths must be registered with the General Osteopathic Council in order to practise. The therapy is well supported by many GPs who refer people for NHS-funded osteopathy.

Alexander technique

This is a form of education rather than therapy where the person is trained to avoid 'bad habits' of poor posture and learn to readjust body alignment. An Australian actor, Frederick Alexander developed the technique in the late nineteenth century, based on the theory that the way a person uses their body affects their general health.

This technique encourages people to stand, sit and move according to the body's natural design and function. This can be taught on a one-to-one basis to any age group.

During the first consultation, the person goes through a series of movements to assess their posture and body alignment. The first treatment session involves lying down, relaxing the body, and light adjustments are made if necessary. Further sessions entail different movements involved with standing, moving, sitting, lying down, walking and lifting objects. In these sessions, the teacher adjusts posture and re-educates the use of muscles with minimum effort and maximum efficiency. A session lasts 30–45 minutes, usually twice-weekly, and a course may be 15–30 sessions depending on the person's progress.

Integration into conventional healthcare

Although the Alexander technique is not likely to be available on the NHS, most GPs are aware of it and referrals are increasing. It can be used by all age groups and is deemed safe when taught by teachers who have received proper training.

Aromatherapy

Ancient cultures in China, Egypt and India used plant oils combining their medicinal properties with the ancient art of massage. The modern use of plant oils is attributed to a French chemist, Rene Gattefosse, who coined the term 'aromatherapy' in 1937.

Plant material such as flowers, leaves, stems, roots and barks yield oily substances that are refined into 'essential oils'. Distillation (subjecting the plant material to steam until vaporization) is one method of extracting the oils. There are many essential oils, including those extracted from tea-tree (*Melaleuca alternifolia*); common lavender (*Lavendula angustifolia*) and frankincense (*Boswellia carterii*). Other oils – known as 'carrier' or 'base' oils – used with essential oils for making massage blends are: marigold (*Calendula officinalis*) and grapeseed (*Vitis vinifera*) (Mills & Bone 2000).

A few drops of the essential oils diluted in the carrier oil can be absorbed into the body in several ways. These include:

- Through the skin – during massage, a compress or when added to bath water
- Through inhalation – using steam inhalers or a diffuser in a room. Oil molecules enter the nose and reach the brain via the olfactory apparatus and olfactory nerves.

Oils with specific properties can be selected to invigorate or relax the person and induce sleep by influencing mood, emotions and physical well-being (Price & Price 2007). Aromatherapy may be used for simple relaxation but it can be useful in a wide range of conditions that include insomnia, restlessness, stress, anxiety, muscle pain, migraine and other headaches, etc. A small study of aromatherapy using four essential oils (rosemary, lemon, lavender and orange), involving older people with dementia, found that aromatherapy was an effective therapy for dementia (Jimbo et al 2009).

The first session involves a holistic history-taking regarding medical history, lifestyle factors and essential oils likes and dislikes. An essential oil blend is used in a full body massage or selected areas of the body appropriate to the client's needs. Advice about home treatments using oils for baths or diffusers may be recommended as appropriate. An initial consultation and massage session may take up to 2 hours. A course of treatment may entail weekly sessions of 1 hour massage for 4 weeks and fortnightly or monthly thereafter. It is common for clients to have a series of treatment sessions.

Integration into conventional healthcare

Nurses have long promoted the use of aromatherapy as an adjunct to improving patient/client care. NHS settings have protocols for the practice of aromatherapy by registered practitioners. Aromatherapy can be used for people with mental health problems, learning disabilities, in primary care, intensive care, pain clinics, in wound care and palliative care (Box 10.25).

Reflexology

In reflexology therapy, pressure is applied to the feet, and sometimes the hands or ears, to assess the person's health, treat disorders and promote well-being.

Foot massage was practised in China about 5000 years ago and Egyptian tomb paintings depicted men manipulating the feet and hands of others. The basis for reflexology is that there are invisible zones running vertically through the body so that each organ/structure has a corresponding location in the foot and hands, e.g. the urinary tract (Fig. 10.7).

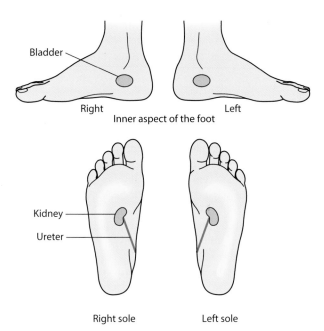

Fig. 10.7 • Reflexology pressure points on the feet.

noting any discomfort, tenderness or pain. This may indicate the source of the person's health problem. If necessary, the person will be referred to their GP.

During a treatment session (45–60 min) a series of movements involving application and release of pressure are used as the practitioner's hands move from one reflex point to another. Several weekly follow-up sessions may be necessary until the health problem is resolved.

Integration into conventional healthcare

Reflexology is used in midwifery practice (Tiran 2010) and many other situations, including pain, cancer care, smoking cessation (Tiran & Mackereth 2011) and can be beneficial in inducing deep relaxation, relieving anxiety and improving sleep.

 Reflective practice   Box 10.25

Aromatherapy in healthcare practice

Think about the patients/clients on your placement.

Student activities

- Find out if aromatherapy is available in this area.
- Reflect with your mentor on situations where aromatherapy might have been helpful in helping a patient/client to rest or sleep.

The theory of reflexology suggests that waste accumulates around reflex points as uric acid and calcium crystals. Treatment of reflex points stimulates natural healing powers by breaking down the waste material and freeing the flow of energy along the zone.

During the first consultation of 1 hour, with the person lying comfortably on a couch, the person's bare feet will be assessed for existing or potential health problems. The practitioner's fingers and thumbs will stimulate reflex points all over the foot,

SUMMARY

- The physiological significance of relaxation, rest and sleep impacts on the emotional, cognitive and physical well-being of the individual.
- Insufficient rest and sleep can contribute to impaired judgement and increased risks of adverse effects on the care of patients/clients.
- The nurse has a crucial role in helping the patient/client to identify, manage and resolve factors contributing to sleep disturbances.
- Simple measures to prevent or alleviate sleep disturbances should be employed and medications such as sedatives should be a last resort.
- Patients/clients with serious sleep disturbances should be referred for specialist advice and management.
- Complementary and alternative medicine used by practitioners with recognized qualifications can be used to promote rest and sleep.
- The nurse should be well informed of up-to-date research findings related to relaxation and sleep and, where appropriate, participate in the research.

KEY WORDS AND PHRASES FOR LITERATURE SEARCHING

Alternative therapies

Biorhythm

Circadian rhythm

Complementary therapies

Diurnal rhythm

Insomnia

Integrated medicine

Relaxation

Sleep

Sleep disorders

Useful websites

BBC – useful information about sleep www.bbc.co.uk/science/ humanbody/sleep

British Snoring and Sleep Apnoea Association www.britishsnoring.co.uk

Complementary Therapies in Clinical Practice (Journal) www.sciencedirect.com/science/journal/17443881

General Chiropractic Council www.gcc-uk.org

General Osteopathic Council www.osteopathy.org.uk

Health and Care Professions Council www.hpc-uk.org

National Sleep Foundation – US website with useful information about sleep and interactive features www.sleepfoundation.org

Narcolepsy Association UK www.narcolepsy.org.uk

Sleep (Journal) www.journalsleep.org

The Royal College of Psychiatrists – Leaflets about Sleep www.rcpsych.ac.uk

The National Center for Complementary and Alternative Medicine (NCCAM) – part of the US National Institutes of Health http://nccam.nih.gov

All websites accessed September 2012.

References

British National Formulary, 2012. Online. Available: www.bnf.org.uk September 2012.

Budd, S., Mills, S., 2000. Professional organisation of complementary and alternative medicine in the United Kingdom. Department of Health, London.

Buysse, D.J., Germain, A., Moul, D.E., et al., 2011. Efficacy of brief behavioral treatment for chronic insomnia in older adults. Archives of Internal Medicine 171 (10), 887–895.

Caruso, C.C., Hitchcock, E.M., 2010. Strategies for nurses to prevent sleep-related injuries and errors. Rehabil Nurs 35 (5), 192–197.

Cheuk, D.K., Yeung, W.F., Chung, K.F., et al., 2007. Acupuncture for insomnia. Cochrane Database of Systematic Reviews 2007, Issue 3. Art. No.: CD005472. DOI:10.1002/14651858.CD005472.pub2 September 2012.

Department of Health, 1996. Complementary medicine and the National Health Service. TSO, London.

Department of Health, 2001. Government response to the House of Lords Select Committee on Science and Technology's report on complementary and alternative medicine. TSO, London.

Department of Health, 2011. Analysis report on the 2009 consultation on the statutory regulation of practitioners of acupuncture, herbal medicine, traditional Chinese medicine and other traditional medicine systems practised in the UK. Online. Available: www.dh.gov.uk/en/Consultations/Responsestoconsultations/DH_124337 September 2012.

Facco, F.L., Kramer, J., Ho, K.H., et al., 2010. Sleep disturbances in pregnancy.

Obstetrics and Gynecology 115 (1), 77–83.

Harris, M., Richards, K.C., 2010. The physiological and psychological effects of slow-stroke back massage and hand massage on relaxation in older people. Journal of Clinical Nursing 19 (7–8), 917–926.

Horne, J.A., Reyner, L.A., 1997. Should we be taking more sleep? Sleep 10, 901–907.

House of Lords, 2000. Complementary and alternative medicine: House of Lords Select Committee on Science and Technology 6th report (session 1999–1900). TSO, London.

Jimbo, D., Kimura, Y., Taniguchi, M., et al., 2009. Effect of aromatherapy on patients with Alzheimer's disease. Psychogeriatrics 9 (4), 173–179.

le May, A., 2011. Promoting sleep. In: Brooker, C., Nicol, M. (Eds.), Alexander's nursing practice, fourth ed. Churchill Livingstone, Edinburgh.

Lichstein, K.L., Peterson, B.A., Riedel, B.W., et al., 1999. Relaxation to assist sleep medication withdrawal. Behavior Modification 23 (3), 379–402.

Martini, F.H., Nath, J.L., 2009. Fundamentals of Anatomy & Physiology, eighth ed. Pearson, San Francisco.

Mills, S., Bone, K., 2000. Principles and practice of phytotherapy. Churchill Livingstone, Edinburgh.

Monk, T.H., 2005. Aging human circadian rhythms: conventional wisdom may not always be right. Journal of Biological Rhythms 20 (4), 366–374.

Nursing and Midwifery Council, 2006. Statistical analysis of the register. 1st April 2005–31st March 2006. Online. Available: www.nmc-uk.org September 2012.

Nursing and Midwifery Council, 2008. The code: Standards of conduct, performance and ethics for nurses and midwives. Online. Available: www.nmc-uk.org September 2012.

Owens, J.A., Belon, K., Moss, P., 2010. Impact of delaying school start time on adolescent sleep, mood, and behavior. Archives of Pediatric and Adolescent Medicine 164 (7), 608–614.

Phatak, S.R., 2003. Concise materia medica of homeopathic medicines. B Jain, New Delhi.

Price, S., Price, L., 2007. Aromatherapy for health professionals, third ed. Churchill Livingstone, Edinburgh.

Scott, J.P., Barlow, T., 2003. Herbs in the treatment of children: leading a child to health. Churchill Livingstone, Edinburgh.

Scott, L.D., Hofmeister, N., Rogness, N., et al., 2010. An interventional approach for patient and nurse safety: a fatigue countermeasures feasibility study. Nursing Research 59 (4), 250–258.

Skene, D.J., Swaab, D.F., 2003. Melatonin rhythmicity: effect of age and Alzheimer's disease. Experimental Gerontology 38 (1–2), 199–206.

Srinivasan, V., Singh, J., Pandi-Perumal, S.R., et al., 2010. Jet lag, circadian rhythm sleep disturbances, and depression: the role of melatonin analogs. Advances in Therapy 27 (11), 796–813.

Stores, R., 2008. (revised) Managing sleep problems in children with Down's syndrome. Down's Syndrome Association Medical Series. Online. Available: http://www.downs-syndrome.org.uk/images/documents/1074/sleep_problems.pdf September 2012.

Suzuki, K., Ohida T Kaneita, Y., et al., 2004. Mental health status, shift work, and occupational accidents among hospital nurses in Japan. Journal of Occupational Health 46 (6), 448–454.

Tiran, D., 2010. Reflexology in pregnancy and childbirth. Churchill Livingstone, Edinburgh.

Tiran, D., Mackereth, P.A., 2011. Clinical reflexology: a guide for integrated practice, second ed. Churchill Livingstone, Edinburgh.

Walker, B.F., French, S.D., Grant, W., et al., 2010. Combined chiropractic interventions for low-back pain. Cochrane Database of Systematic Reviews Issue 4. Art. No.: CD005427. DOI: 10.1002/14651858. CD005427.pub2 September 2012.

Widmaier, E.P., Raff, H., Strang, K.T., 2010. Vander's human physiology: mechanisms of body function, twelfth ed. McGraw-Hill, New York.

Wang, X.-S., Armstrong, M.E., Cairns, B.J., et al., 2011. Shift work and chronic disease: the epidemiological evidence. Occupational Medicine (Lond) 61 (2), 78–89 doi:10.1093/occmed/kqr001 September 2012.

Wu, Y.H., Swaab, D.F., 2005. The human pineal gland and melatonin in aging and Alzheimer's disease. Journal of Pineal Research 38 (3), 145–152.

Further reading

Barnes, J., 2002. Herbal medicine: a guide for health care. Rittenhouse, London.

Ernst, E., Pittler, M.H., Wider, B., 2006. The desktop guide to complementary and alternative medicine. An evidence-based approach, second ed. Mosby, Edinburgh.

Mantle, F., Tiran, D., 2009. A-Z of Complementary and alternative medicine: A guide for health professionals. Churchill Livingstone, Edinburgh.

Mills, S., Bone, K., 2005. The essential guide to herbal safety. Churchill Livingstone, Edinburgh.

National Institute for Health and Clinical Excellence, 2008. Sleep apnoea – continuous positive airway pressure (CPAP). Technology appraisal, TA 139. Online. Available: http://guidance.nice.org.uk/TA139 September 2012.

Payne, R.A., 2005. Relaxation techniques, third ed. Churchill Livingstone, Edinburgh.

World Health Organization, 2010. International classification of disease and related health problems (ICD-10), tenth ed. WHO, Geneva. Online. Available: www.who.int/classifications/en September 2012.

Stress, anxiety and coping

11

Neil Murphy

LEARNING OUTCOMES

This chapter will help you:

- Discuss the functions of stress and anxiety
- Identify the changes in thinking, feelings, behaviour and physiology that may occur in response to stress or anxiety
- Describe ways in which stress and anxiety can impact on health and behaviours
- Identify common work-related stressors associated with nursing
- Identify strategies to manage own work-related stress
- Identify coping strategies patients/clients/carers may use in response to illness
- Discuss how stress may impact on recovery from illness
- Outline strategies used to reduce the negative effects of stress and anxiety on patients/clients.

Introduction

The word 'stress' was originally used by Selye (1956) to describe the 'pressure' experienced by a person in response to life demands. These demands are referred to as 'stressors' and include a range of life events, physical factors (e.g. cold, hunger, haemorrhage, pain), environmental conditions and personal thoughts.

Stress is a reactive state to demands or potential demands made on the adaptive capacities of the mind and body. It is not necessarily unhealthy, as without stress, people would have little motivation to act and could not feel the pleasure of achievement. In many ways, stress should be considered a useful and necessary reaction in that, not only does it motivate action, it also prepares the person to take this action. Selye used the term 'eustress' to describe some of the more useful and adaptive forms of stress which enhanced a person's well-being.

However, if people lack the capacity to deal with the demands made upon them, their coping resources may be overwhelmed. In situations in which a person constantly feels under pressure with little respite, or when people experience severe trauma, the adaptive effects of stress can become harmful and may damage health. To describe these types of stressors, Selye used the term 'distress'.

The first part of this chapter provides a framework for understanding the causes and effects of stress and anxiety and how these can be used to understand the potential effects on health. These ideas are developed to show how nurses, working in different fields of practice, can apply this knowledge and the associated skills to managing their own stress and to reduce the negative effects of stress on their patients/clients/carers.

Nature of stress

People tend to associate both stress and anxiety with negative effects on health. But to understand both where stress comes from and how it will impact upon us, we need to accept that life is stressful and that ambient factors can have an influence. Stress and anxiety do generate unpleasant feelings and can lead to problem behaviours, but people have feelings for a reason, they have a function. Even when the effects of stress and anxiety seem maladaptive, e.g. difficulty with decision-making, they can usually be explained and understood.

A good place to start in understanding stress is to consider ambient stressors and life stressors, including those we experience in our own lives (Boxes 11.1, 11.2).

Examples of ambient and life stress	Box 11.1

Ambient stress

Includes everyday stressors such as housing, nutrition, finances, social life, child care, everyday hassles and disappointments.

Life stress

This is more discrete. The stress has more impact, such as in the relationship break-up, the death of a close friend, job loss, some major trauma.

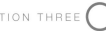

Reflective practice   Box 11.2

A typical day at university

Look back at yesterday and what happened to you throughout the day. Include getting up, the journey to placement or university, study periods and break times.

Student activities

- What ambient stress factors did you experience?
- Did anything really stand out as being particularly exciting or frustrating?
- Can you identify what these factors made you both feel like and think of? Discuss your conclusions with a fellow student.

Identifying why you did these things can be difficult; you need to consider your motivation. For example, if you are successful and become a nurse you will be able to earn a living, in a job, which you (it is hoped) like and which is valued by others. If you do not attend or study, you risk criticism and failure. It is the demands created by the need to succeed and avoid disapproval that motivate people to act, and the anticipation of success can be linked to excitement, pride and pleasure.

It is important to emphasize how central stress is to life; it is perhaps the main reason people do anything. The feelings associated with stress put pressure on people to act. Taking this idea further, it could also be argued that without successful stress management, there would be less pleasure in living.

Understanding emotion

Stress and anxiety are specific emotional states, with four main elements:

- *Cognition:* The way people understand a situation, how they rate their ability to deal with the situation and considerations of different responses relating to 'thinking' or how people process information. Information processing may involve awareness, although some is involuntary and automatic. The term cognition describes all of these processes
- *Affect:* The way people 'feel' in a situation (good or bad) and how intense these feelings are is referred to as 'affect'
- *Behavioural:* What people do and say
- *Physiological:* The internal changes that take place in order to deal with the situation.

All of these elements interact; changes in one will affect other elements within an integrated system. Emotions provide an ideal example of how the mind and body interact.

Common causes of stress and anxiety

The terms referred to earlier of ambient and life stress can lead you to understand the normality of stress in our everyday living and that at times, how impotent you can be in the face of it. The fact that we are commonly a bystander in the face of it, is one way of looking at the causal factors, but we must not lose sight of the fact that we can create a great deal of our own

stress and anxiety by our interpretation of events and in the way that we attempt to cope with them.

In anxiety, a fear-like emotion, it is usually easier to identify specific causes because of the perceived threat. There also seem to be specific types of anxiety responses depending on the nature of the threat (Box 11.3).

Emotional effects of specific threats   Box 11.3

1. Threats to physical safety/personal existence and integrity, fear of death, pain, mutilation and mental health problems. These are often highly specific situations and are frequently associated with feelings of panic, obvious physical symptoms, e.g. breathlessness, and sensations of impending doom; the person is motivated to escape the threat or, in extreme situations, may freeze – the 'fight or flight' response (see pp. 244-246). Feelings of panic are common; however, individuals who experience them so frequently that they interfere with their lives are said to be suffering from panic disorder.
2. Threats to self-image, fear of social appraisal, disapproval and ridicule are felt in many situations and are associated with more generalized anxiety. Symptoms are typically less intense but more pervasive. The person may feel uneasy and lead to an overestimation of negative events, motivating them to avoid situations. Consequently, they may become inappropriately aggressive under pressure to act or comment. Again, these feelings are both common and useful; they help people to learn appropriate social behaviours. When the fears are excessive they inhibit social relationships and lead to generalized anxiety disorder (GAD). This is characterized by 'excessive worry about a number of different events associated with heightened tension' (National Institute for Health and Clinical Excellence, NICE 2011, p 4).
3. Threats associated with the loss of something valued or loved (see Ch. 12) can create changes in behaviour similar to depression. The effect of the loss can become overestimated and the affective responses all-consuming. This may lead to withdrawal from social contact and apathy.

Fear is considered to be the basic reactive emotion leading to the typical 'fight or flight' response and is usually initiated by automatic systems (see pp. 244-246). Anxiety, however, almost inevitably involves conscious judgements or appraisals about situations.

Common themes in understanding what causes stress

Despite the difficulties in identifying individual stressors, there are some common themes that can be identified as causing most people some stress. People need some stimuli to keep them active and motivated. However, the ability to deal with stress differs between individuals and at a certain point, coping resources can fail and performance becomes impaired. There appears to be an optimum level of arousal in which eustress is associated with staying in this optimum range and distress occurs when the stress exceeds the range.

In this model, the arousal (heightened activity including cognitive, affective, physiological and behavioural changes) associated with stress produces the competitive edge; arousal speeds thought processes and quickens reaction. Indeed, when demands are made upon an individual, the increased arousal improves both physical and cognitive abilities in order to meet these demands. However, under- or overarousal is associated with a reduced ability to function effectively.

Change

Change is any event that requires an individual to adapt to an altered situation. Adaptation describes the changes in physiology, cognition and behaviour in response to changes in the environment. Holmes and Rahe (1967) identified a number of life changes (e.g. death of a partner, divorce, separation, serious illness, employment changes) and produced a frequently used scale to measure social readjustment. People who had experienced high-scoring events in the previous year were significantly more likely to become physically ill in the following year than those with low scores. It is important to remember that even events seen as positive still require adaptation and are included as stressors.

Hassles

Earlier, we inferred that ambient stress can be caused by hassles. These hassles were discussed by Lazarus (1981) and identified as events appraised as harmful or threatening. He went on to suggest that opposed to the hassles were uplifts – events appraised as positive.

While people find it easy to identify specific stressful situations, in reality it is the ongoing problems of life that are the really significant causes of stress-related health problems (Box 11.4).

Reflective practice   Box 11.4

Everyday stresses

Think about some of the hassles in your everyday life that cause stress and potentially stress-related health problems. For example, being a long-term carer, reliance on public transport, stressful work, etc.

Student activities

- What hassles cause you stress?
- How does this make you feel and behave?
- Reflect on how everyday stresses impact on patients/clients, parents and carers.
- What uplifts can you identify? Discuss your conclusions with a fellow student.

Stress can be seen as frustration when things do not turn out as planned; a positive slant is for individuals to view these as 'stumbling blocks'.

People

In social situations, people are always aware of others and conscious of the impression they may be making; when there is uncertainty about others' evaluations, they feel self-conscious and anxious. In the same way, the availability of social support is an important protector against the negative effects of stress.

Interpersonal issues are extremely important; the need for acceptance and approval is so powerful it can override even survival needs. People need to feel life has value and meaning. The sense of meaning derives from other people. People appear to devote a great deal of their cognitive resources to dealing with interpersonal issues, which may also be a reflection of, or supported by, some specific inherited elements.

Mediators and the stress response

A number of more general issues also affect the nature and intensity of the stress response. Individual responses to stress and anxiety have both inherited and acquired elements, which interact within the situational context. People clearly differ in a whole range of ways in respect to personality, autonomic reactivity, physical strength, dexterity and intelligence, all of which may affect the stress response. Humans may have certain predispositions that influence stress responses such as learning and remembering. Previous experience is extremely important in moderating a person's reaction to stressors.

Importantly, the way you interpret stress and attribute its effects can affect the way you respond at the time and in the future. Generally, we tend to attribute things that have gone well to internal factors such as ability, but things that have not gone well to external factors such as things outside your control. This can lead to a self-serving bias and should be considered as a defence mechanism for your ego.

The role of the unconscious

Sigmund Freud (1856–1939) suggested that a person's internal mental world was dominated by primitive, often socially and personally unacceptable, drives. In order to protect self-esteem and mental health, these drives were kept out of awareness, in the part of the mind he called the unconscious. However, even though these unacceptable drives were unconscious, they did continue to exert 'pressure' to come into conscious awareness and be acted upon.

In a similar way, the memories of certain emotionally painful early experiences could also be kept out of awareness to defend the conscious mind from the associated pain. To manage the threat of unacceptable memories or impulses coming into consciousness, Freud suggested that people deploy a range of mental strategies he called defence mechanisms (see Ch. 8). Defence mechanisms function by distorting a person's view of reality and have an important role in protecting a person from psychogenic pain. More recent work has emphasized how certain events or experiences, e.g. the experience of illness, activate some of the more primitive unconscious fears that everyone has. Common defence mechanisms include the use of:

- *Humour*: A very common defence used to manage many of the unpleasant realities of nursing
- *Regression*: The reversion under stress to an earlier or more restricted level of psychological development, e.g. a previously continent child who starts bedwetting when admitted to hospital (see Ch. 20)

- *Suppression*: The dismissal of unpleasant thoughts and distraction are conscious defences everyone uses to manage unpleasant thoughts
- *Denial*: A person appears unaware of a stressor that they might reasonably be expected to recognize. For example, a patient/client who professes ignorance about a serious diagnosis, despite clear explanation or who appears totally unconcerned about a serious health problem
- *Displacement*: The transfer of emotion away from the correct person, object or experience to a substitute in order to reduce distress. For example, a man may feel guilty following the death of a neglected parent and finding this emotion too distressing to be recognized, attempts to displace the guilt about his lack of care onto the nurses by accusing them of neglect
- *Projection*: An individual projects their own unacceptable feelings onto another person in order to render their own feelings more acceptable. A nurse who dislikes a patient but who thinks of themselves as very caring might insist that the patient dislikes them, making their own feelings more acceptable
- *Intellectualization*: An attempt to deal with problems by treating them as an academic or theoretical issue and ignoring the feelings that underpin what the person is saying. This distances the nurse from the painful feelings but is often perceived by the patient as uncaring.

A seminal paper by Menzies-Lyth (1959) also identified a number of ways that organizational and social structures can evolve to support an individual's defences. For nurses, these operate as depersonalization (a way of thinking about patients/clients that diminishes their basic humanity and identity). When a nurse relates to a patient/client as an individual, the patient's/client's pain and distress can also be very distressing for the nurse to deal with. It is often suggested that nurses should avoid emotional involvement, which in a similar way diminishes or denies the nurse's basic humanity. There is always some level of involvement for the nurse and finding appropriate ways of managing this can enhance the experiences and rewards of nursing. However, during periods of high work-related stress, there is a tendency to reduce patient-related stress by minimizing the patient's individual distinctiveness, so instead of using names, the patient may be referred to by diagnosis or bed/room number.

There can also be a tendency to make moral judgements, that some patients/clients are more deserving of care than others. Patients/clients who engage in behaviours that are disapproved of may be excluded from good healthcare or treated badly. These groups include people who self-injure, smoke or those who do not cooperate with treatment. Because some types of behaviour would be seen as unethical or even abusive, it is only through using defences such as depersonalization, detachment and denial that nurses can continue to act professionally in ways that do not reflect their personal values.

Identifying stressors

An important function of developing nursing knowledge is that it allows nurses to predict and manage potential problems that may arise. Nurses need to adopt a holistic approach in an assessment to identify stressors, which includes consideration of the following influences:

- Biological
- Psychological
- Interpersonal/social/environmental
- Spiritual.

Stressors in healthcare rarely affect just the patient/client. They affect relatives, friends and of course nurses involved in their care. The way in which a person behaves in response to stress will have a significant effect on their future. People often feel angry and irritable when stressed and if this results in aggressive behaviour, they might alienate the people that they rely upon for care and support, thus increasing future stress.

Box 11.5 outlines some potential stressors that may impact on specific care situations.

(?) Critical thinking   **Box 11.5**

Identifying stressors

- Ted is being discharged home 4 days following a heart attack. He works as a bus driver and his wife works shifts in a factory. He smokes but has previously had good health.
- Rhian, who is 12 years old, is attending the day unit for her next chemotherapy treatment. Following the second treatment, she suffered unpleasant side-effects. On this occasion, her father, who is not known to the staff, accompanies Rhian.
- Pauline has attended the same special school for years. Her parents report that she is increasingly withdrawn and uncooperative. She has been told that now she is 18, her care will be transferred to adult services and she will be moving to a day service.
- The police have brought Joseph, aged 19 years, to the unit following what is described as an attempt to burn down the family home while his parents were asleep. He is very distressed, overactive and excitable and feels everyone is trying to harm him.

Student activities

- Identify the significant stressors that may be present in the scenarios and who is most likely to be affected.
- Discuss this with your mentor.

The effects of clients' and colleagues' behaviours can impact on your stress level. Some of the challenges to the nurse's role caused by stress are outlined in Box 11.6.

The stress response

The term stress response can be described by the adaptive physiological changes that occur to enhance a person's ability to deal with demanding situations. While the adaptive changes are occurring in response to the stress situation, the internal environment, e.g. blood chemistry, must be maintained within a normal range for optimum cell function (see Ch. 19). This ability to maintain the internal environment within the normal range is known as homeostasis. Allostatic load refers to the cumulative cost to the body of maintaining homeostasis while responding to stressors; when these resources are overloaded, then there is a serious risk to health.

When increased mental and physical activity are needed, the necessary physiological responses are regulated by two interdependent control systems:

- The autonomic nervous system (ANS), the part of the nervous system which is generally outside conscious control
- The endocrine system that uses chemical messaging systems (hormones) (Fig. 11.1).

The ANS is divided into the sympathetic and the parasympathetic divisions, but while periods of stress and anxiety lead to a general stimulation of the nervous system, it is the effects of the sympathetic division that predominate.

The sympathetic division is responsible for mobilizing the body's resources in response to stress by releasing the neurotransmitter noradrenaline (norepinephrine) at the effector organs. The adrenal medulla (middle part of the adrenal glands) is also stimulated to release adrenaline (epinephrine) and noradrenaline into the bloodstream. Noradrenaline and

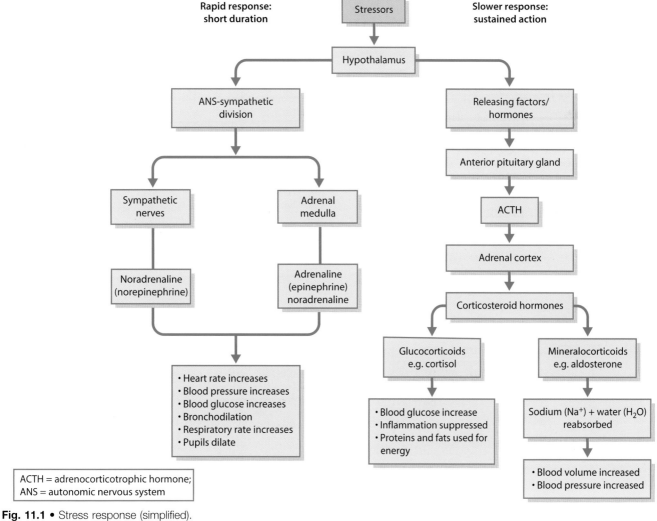

Fig. 11.1 • Stress response (simplified).

ACTH = adrenocorticotrophic hormone;
ANS = autonomic nervous system

adrenaline are related catecholamines, which cause effects that include the 'fight or flight' response of increased heart and respiratory rates, blood pressure, etc.

Releasing factors/hormones from the hypothalamus in the brain stimulate the pituitary gland, which regulates other endocrine structures. Pituitary hormones, e.g. adrenocorticotrophic hormone (ACTH), stimulate the release of corticosteroid hormones from the adrenal cortex (outer part of the adrenal glands). Corticosteroid hormones – known as glucocorticoids, e.g. cortisol – increase the availability of the body's energy resources, alter immune responses and generally prepare the body for action and potential injury. Other corticosteroids, known as mineralocorticoids, e.g. aldosterone, influence sodium and water retention.

Corticosteroids are involved in chronic long-term stress and also influence mood and behaviour. Table 11.1 outlines some effects of the stress response, their adaptive function and the potential impact on health.

To summarize, the sympathetic nervous system and endocrine system coordinate a response that increases available energy, endurance and pain tolerance and enhances the ability to survive injury. However, as this increased state of arousal is often uncomfortable and is costly in terms of resources, there may be negative health effects associated with both acute short-term stress and chronic long-term stress. In acute states, the most significant problems are often due to behavioural changes, whereas the physiological changes occurring in chronic stress appear to increase vulnerability to a range of disorders.

Selye (1956) described the stress response as being triphasic (having three stages): an alarm stage, a resistance stage and an exhaustion stage (Fig. 11.2). Selye's model – the General Adaptation Syndrome (GAS) – was the first real attempt to develop a general theory of stress and clarify the role of stress in health and illness. However, the model focused on the underpinning physiology and failed to adequately address psychological and social factors. Despite these problems, the model has been highly influential in stress research.

Stress-related health problems

A general view of the effects of both stress and anxiety is that they evolved to influence physiology, cognition, affect and behaviour in order to increase the chances of surviving in difficult and dangerous environments. However, life has changed and the evolved mechanisms are less useful in dealing with the complex and enduring stress associated with modern life. Stress depletes physical and mental resources, while reducing behaviour control.

Chronic stress in particular is strongly associated with a wide range of health problems because of physiological and psychological 'wear and tear' and inefficient use of energy. This may be associated with behavioural changes that increase other risks and reduce an individual's ability to deal with new challenges.

In someone with a pre-existing vulnerability, exposure to increased stress may be the stimulus to trigger illness; it may then influence recovery and other health-related behaviours. Those with existing conditions may experience a worsening of symptoms, e.g. anginal pain (see Ch. 17) or increased frequency of migraine attacks.

Sociocultural, psychological and biological variables combine to produce a range of disorders. The interaction between these factors is now widely accepted as the only way to make sense of body functioning. Increasingly, the immune system is becoming the focus for understanding the relationship between stress and illness; an area of study called psychoneuroimmunology.

Managing stress and anxiety

This part of the chapter outlines the general principles and methods that individuals may use in managing stress and anxiety.

The huge variation in the ways that stress presents and the ways it might affect the person mean that a range of techniques need to be considered. The main reason for this variation is attributable to the fact that, after an initial, often automatic reaction to a situation (primary appraisal), people make a series of judgements, which will largely control the responses (secondary appraisal) (Fig. 11.3, p. 249). Box 11.6 (p. 245) asked 'what you should do in a specific situation'; consider now if there may have been another way of coping.

While recognizing the role of physiology, Lazarus and Folkman (1984) suggested that an individual's previous

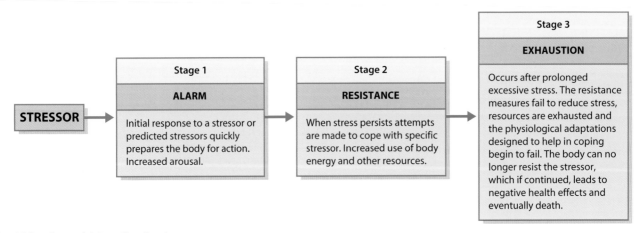

Fig. 11.2 • General Adaptation Syndrome.

Table 11.1 Stress response – effects and potential consequences

Effects	Adaptive function	Acute symptoms	Chronic problems
Physical effects			
Increased heart rate and force	Increase in blood supply to tissues	Palpitations	
Increased blood pressure	As above	Headache	Arterial disease: CHD, stroke (see Ch. 17)
Sodium and water retention	Increased plasma volume and blood pressure in preparation for injury		As above
Redistribution of blood supply	Increased blood supply to body core and large skeletal muscles	Skin pallor Gastrointestinal problems	
Increased respiratory rate and volume. Dilatation of bronchi	Increase in oxygenation	Breathlessness	Changes in blood chemistry Panic
Increased muscle tone	Fast reaction	Trembling	Muscle pain/aches
Immune system stimulation	Migration of leucocytes into tissues Body prepares defences in case of injury	Activation of autoimmune disorders	Slower healing (see Ch. 25) Reduced immune surveillance Increased risks of infection (see Ch. 15) and cancer
Increased platelet adhesiveness	Faster haemostasis in case of injury		
Increase in blood glucose and fatty acids	Increased energy		Weight gain Arterial disease Protein used for energy reduces muscle mass
Increase in basal metabolic rate	Increased energy and endurance	Feeling hot Sweating	Exhaustion Slower healing

Continued

Table 11.1 Stress response – effects and potential consequences—cont'd

Effects	Adaptive function	Acute symptoms	Chronic problems
Cognitive effects			
Increased alertness	Increased vigilance Avoid danger	Jumpy, overreacts	Sleep disturbance (see Ch. 10)
Focus on potential threat	All mental resources available Increased problem-solving	Cannot concentrate on other things Overarousal reduces efficiency (see p. 243)	Memory disturbance
Sensitized to novel, unexpected, unpredictable, intense, uncontrollable events	Reduces risk, avoids danger	Impulsive/automatic 'fight/flight' behaviours	Avoidance behaviours lead to anxiety states Accident risk increases
Context-specific memories	Potential help in problem-solving, recall previous solutions	Intrusive, unpleasant memories Mood links to memories	Negative mood state Past failure affects self-efficacy
Flashbulb memories	Situation labelled as potentially dangerous Reduces exposure to future risk	Memory and mood stay active in consciousness	Non-threatening situations labelled as dangerous Behaviour labelled as unreliable Increases hesitancy and uncertainty
Narrowing of perceptual field	Linked to focusing attention, dealing with threat is the priority	Misses important detail Focuses on irrelevant detail	Memory problems Accident risk increases
Reduced complex problem-solving relates to emotional state	Increased use of rapid automatic responses for danger avoidance	Consequences of behaviour not considered	High levels of arousal significantly impair conscious problem-solving
Rapid associative learning	Rapid identification of potential threats	High potential for association of non-threatening events with danger	Phobias
Emotional effects			
Experienced as a negative affective state	Motivates behaviour to reduce the feelings	Possible aggressive or attack behaviours Inappropriate avoidance/escape behaviours	Feels out of control Relationship or legal problems Use of drugs, alcohol and tobacco
High levels of anxiety; people may freeze	Reduces visibility to potential predators	Unable to function effectively	Reduces self-esteem Other people make judgements of competence
Emotion perceived as evidence for belief	Allows fast responses	People frequently aware that concerns are illogical and feel embarrassed	Maintain self-esteem by using defence mechanisms
Managing stressors is associated with self-esteem	Learn to predict potential for effective actions	Self-esteem linked to beliefs about abilities and value	Low self-esteem associated with many mental health problems

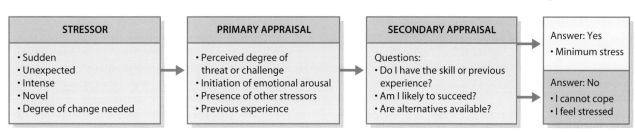

Fig. 11.3 • Primary and secondary appraisal of stressors.

learning and experience significantly affects the way in which they react to life events; others can look at the same event and come up with differing interpretations. In this view of stress and anxiety, it is not the stimulus itself that is problematic, it is the individual's appraisal of the stimulus and their belief about their ability to manage its effect.

This model emphasizes cognition. Judgements are made about the stressor and the person's ability to change their behaviour or thoughts in such a way as to master or reduce the effects of the stressor. These responses are coping strategies, which may be adaptive (managing the event without increasing other problems) or maladaptive (where coping strategies might fail or increase stress). This framework is particularly important in understanding many of the principles of stress management.

Everyone uses ways of minimizing stress and improving rest and relaxation (see Ch. 10), such as socializing, reading, listening to music, holidays, etc. Various coping strategies are discussed below.

Avoidance

Avoidance commonly involves reducing exposure to stimuli that cause stress or anxiety, attempts to ignore the demands/ threats or to suppress the negative feelings. Avoidance is a very common reaction to threat when often the first reaction is to escape, thus avoiding further exposure. To ignore stressors, people might engage in distracting tasks, use defence mechanisms (see pp. 243–244) or simply refuse to recognize the importance of the stimulus. People might try to induce positive feelings, e.g. comfort eating, 'treating' themselves or using stimulant (usually illegal) drugs, sedatives or alcohol.

People frequently resort to sedatives and alcohol to help manage the unpleasant feelings associated with stress and anxiety. They might attempt to 'drown out' overwhelming feelings associated with severe trauma, loss or threat by using a sufficiently high dose to induce insensibility. Sometimes, the use of anxiolytic drugs, e.g. diazepam, can be used in similar ways during short episodes of intense anxiety or distress but, like alcohol, continued use over long periods (can lead to habituation) is associated with a range of health and interpersonal problems. This does not address the causes or problems faced by people and while they might allow a person to cope with an acute and intense trauma, they have no place in long-term management. Continued management in this way can lead to complications and the development of further psychological problems such as depression.

Dealing with the stressor

The most direct approach to dealing with demands is to take action to meet those demands. This approach is often the most adaptive, particularly for low-level stressors when people can use problem-solving and evaluate the potential consequences of their actions. When the stress experienced is associated with very high levels of arousal, problem-solving is impaired and actions may not be well considered.

Among the most effective and easiest interventions nurses can use to reduce anxiety and stress, is to provide useful and understandable information (see Chs 9, 23 and 24). Patients/ clients should know what to expect in relation to illness, recovery and specific interventions. This is important in allowing the person and their family to prepare themselves and recognize the difference between normal and abnormal sensations – without information, every unusual sensation causes anxiety. Nurses may need to adapt information or ways of communicating, and seek help from family and carers when clients find it difficult to understand the situation, e.g. a person with a learning disability or cognitive impairment.

To deal successfully with a range of demands, people learn and use a series of skills. When demands and expectations are predictable, learning useful skills can be structured and planned (Box 11.7).

Reflective practice   Box 11.7

Dealing with stressors

A student nurse may feel anxious about doing something for the first time, e.g. giving an injection. Preparatory information can reduce anxiety and frequent practice with supervision allows the nurse to feel sufficiently confident that eventually little or no anxiety is experienced.

Student activities

• Think about a nursing intervention that caused you anxiety.
• What helped you to feel confident? Discuss this with your mentor.

When people feel confident in their abilities to control and meet demands, little stress is experienced and successful outcomes become more likely. People often experience positive feelings of achievement when they manage challenging situations and their beliefs about their coping abilities are enhanced. Assertion training by increasing skills in negotiation and relating to others may enhance this perception of control.

Explaining that anxiety is a normal response to many situations is also a useful way of giving people 'permission' to talk about anxieties. Again the nurse must be imaginative in finding ways to help people with learning disabilities or dementia to express/communicate their anxieties.

Imposing structure

In situations that involve multiple and complex stressors, the ability to prioritize is important. This could involve making 'to do' lists, prioritizing demands in order of importance and managing the time available to deal with the demands. The principle here is a simple one: for life to be manageable, it needs to be managed (Box 11.8).

 Health promotion   Box 11.8

Time management

Using a diary to note important events, e.g. appointments, submission dates, and keeping track of arrangements is the most effective way of controlling the demands made on time. A diary allows the person to consider the practicalities of accepting extra commitments and to prioritize how much time to devote to each. This allows realistic judgements to be made about how many issues can be addressed in the given time.

The diary is only a tool; the person needs to be able to use the information in negotiating their commitments with others and must be prepared to say no when necessary. These ideas help people to deal with stressors in which direct action is appropriate and likely to be useful.

Controlling the emotion

Strategies are principally about changing appraisals about the situation. This could involve reassessing the importance of an event and reassessing personal ability to cope with the perceived demands. People may deliberately remind themselves of past successes in managing similar events or make positive statements about their coping abilities. Improving self-awareness helps people recognize the stressors that appear particularly important to them and to recognize the effects of stress early, allowing them to address the situation before the feelings become overwhelming.

Most current research supports the view that it is people's beliefs about the situation and their abilities to cope that control emotional reactions. Changing these beliefs can therefore alter the meaning of the situation and the responses to it. Unfortunately, the underpinning beliefs that inform the way in which people appraise threats or demands lead to habitual and automatic responses based on previous experience. Thus, many people are basically unaware of why they feel like they do and as a consequence, do not check the accuracy of their beliefs.

The cognitive therapies provide frameworks to help people understand these principles and techniques for re-evaluating belief systems. This involves helping individuals recognize that it is not the event that causes distress, but their beliefs about the event that lead to the emotional consequences.

Ellis (1994), who developed a cognitive approach called Rational Emotive Therapy, suggests that people evaluate situations by using simple exclamatory statements about the event. Characteristically, they first make an evaluation of the event, which is sensible and rational, followed by an irrational statement about its meaning. It is the irrational statements which have little or no supporting evidence that cause the emotional reaction. Moreover, people tended to have generalized, irrational beliefs that add to stress interpretations (Box 11.9).

Common irrational beliefs   Box 11.9

- Everything we do must be approved of by others
- We must be loved by everyone
- We must be competent and successful in everything
- Certain things are wrong and the perpetrators should be punished
- When things are not as we like, it is a catastrophe
- It is easier to avoid difficulties and responsibilities than to face them
- Past behaviour will determine our present behaviour
- We are victims of our emotions and have no control over them so cannot help how we feel.

Table 11.2 outlines the sequence of events in creating distress and an example of ways in which people can challenge these beliefs and therefore change the feelings.

People need to identify the beliefs that cause problems and then learn to challenge them. A useful strategy is to note the events/situations which cause stress and then try to identify why they are important.

Enhancing coping resources

A wide range of strategies can enhance coping, including:

- Increasing energy reserves by increasing 'wellness' – by taking exercise, good nutrition (see Ch. 19) and adequate rest (see Ch. 10), etc.
- Taking responsibility for self-care of long-term disorders increases control and confidence that enhances coping. Indeed, the person-focused outcome in *Essence of Care 2010 Benchmarks for Self Care* is 'People have control over their care' (Department of Health, DH 2010, p 7)
- Learning new skills that help to deal with demands or feared situations more effectively
- Learning specific skills that induce feelings of calmness and relaxation, these feelings being incompatible with feeling stressed or anxious.

Relaxation techniques

Over the centuries in diverse cultures and under various guises, the ability to relax the body and mind has been seen as an important skill, particularly for those who had to problem-solve and make effective decisions.

Table 11.2 Example of cognitive sequencing

Stage		Example
A	Activating event – actual or inferred, current or predicted	Student has to present course work to peers and lecturers
B	Beliefs – often in the form of rigid and unqualified demands in the form of 'musts', 'shoulds' and 'oughts' Appraisals are often automatic and habitual – people need to learn how to identify them	*Rational appraisal*: • People will be evaluating my performance • I will feel and look anxious *Irrational appraisal*: • My presentation must be perfect or the others will think I am stupid • If they see how nervous I am they will think I'm a useless nurse • If I can't answer questions everyone will know how ignorant I am
C	Consequences – emotional, behavioural and physiological responses to appraisal. Often unpleasant and leads to inappropriate, unhelpful behaviour	Increasing self-focus and anxiety, reducing performance Dry mouth, difficulty speaking, unable to remember points Awareness of each increases anxiety The appraisal becomes a self-fulfilling prophecy and is taken as evidence that the beliefs were right
D	Disputing the disturbance-producing appraisals. Subjecting beliefs to rational evaluation. Questioning the evidence for the belief	Are you the only one who is anxious? Isn't it normal? Would you think badly of someone who is anxious? As a student why do you expect to be perfect?
E	Effective – as in the actions chosen. Those based on rational thinking are more likely to be effective in managing stressors	Seeing anxiety as normal and common and accepting that expectations about their own behaviour are unrealistic help to reduce belief Unpleasant feelings reduced with increased likelihood of appropriate behaviours

If an individual can reduce emotional arousal and focus their thoughts onto problem-solving, then they are better able to more clearly analyse the situations and generate solutions.

The techniques are widely used in healthcare, e.g. pain management (see Ch. 23), insomnia (see Ch. 10), prenatal preparation for labour, even though the underpinning evidence is inconclusive. However, the feelings induced by effective relaxation techniques are usually perceived by clients as pleasant and restful and there is little evidence of side-effects or safety concerns. Using relaxation becomes more effective with regular practice.

Although there are considerable differences between individual relaxation techniques, there does appear to be some common themes. These usually include:

• Control or awareness of the physical body, e.g. position, etc.
• Control of or an awareness of breathing
• A specific mental focus, e.g. words/phrases (a mantra), visual stimuli, candles, prayer mats, mental images/fantasy, physical sensations and a gradual shift from external concerns to internal sensations.

Box 11.10 describes one relaxation technique, but for information about other techniques such as imagery, see Further reading, e.g. Payne & Donaghy 2010. These techniques can be used to help patients/clients or for personal stress management; generally they tend to be most appropriate in situations where direct action or problem solving is unlikely to be helpful.

Complementary and alternative medicine (CAM) therapies

It is important to remember that some CAM therapies (see Chs. 10, 23) are linked to particular faiths and will not be

---

A relaxation technique – the parasympathetic flop   **Box 11.10**

• Sit or stand in a comfortable position, and focus your awareness on how your body currently feels, become aware of muscle tension, areas of discomfort and symptoms of stress

• Become aware of your breathing, consider rate and regularity. Take control of your breathing and begin using slow abdominal or diaphragmatic breathing (breathing deeply, push out the abdomen)

• On each breath out, focus on the feelings you get when all of the chest muscles relax and deliberately think about your other muscles relaxing at the same time. Let your body sag, let your shoulders drop and allow your head to lean forward

• Remain in this state, repeating the breathing exercise until you feel more comfortable and then stretch and start moving quite slowly

• Before finishing, return your attention to your body and breathing; you should find that breathing is slower and your body feels more comfortable

• With practice you should be able to relax more quickly and more deeply.

---

acceptable to all groups. There can also be ethical concerns about using methods that have no evidence-based information for safety and efficacy.

On the other hand, inducing relaxation is perhaps the one area in which many CAM therapies have shown considerable promise. Meditation, massage, reflexology, yoga and tai chi exercises can all be useful in helping a person manage the effects of stress. Massage techniques are particularly useful in children and in individuals with sensory impairment; the fact that they may reduce pain might also lessen the impact of pain as a stressor.

Ability to tolerate stress

Despite the wish for a predictable controllable life, everyone is faced with periods of uncertainty and feelings of helplessness in dealing with the problems of living and indeed dying. There are techniques such as the AWARE technique that improves stress tolerance. The person is encouraged to:

- Accept the feelings, not fight or avoid them. Choose to set aside time to think about the things that worry you. Replace anger, or fear or rejection of the feelings with recognition and acceptance
- Watch it, study the feelings, be a dispassionate observer, learn about them without attempting to change anything. Avoid making judgements of good or bad, watch variations like a bystander
- Act in relation to how you feel; if you want to act anxious then do so, you can also choose to act in different ways. You retain control and choice over behaviour. Slow down if you need to but keep going. The important thing is not to do things simply to avoid the feelings
- Repeat the exercise; the more time spent studying your feelings the better, become an expert in your own experiences. The more the feelings become an object of study the less discomfort you will experience
- Expect good outcomes but be realistic; you cannot eradicate anxiety so do not try. During monitoring you will discover variations; notice the good points and pay attention to increasing control.

The role of the nurse

The nurse's role in stress management and health promotion has extensive coverage in the competency domains (generic and field-specific) and the essential skills clusters (ESCs) of *Standards for pre-registration nursing education* (Nursing and Midwifery Council 2010).

The nurse's role is likely to be influenced by their field of practice. The advice nurses give to individuals in order to enhance coping skills, should be tailored to fit the needs of that person. This will require the use of initiative and development of learning packages for practice, after all, nurses are often ideally placed to educate patients/clients about the nature and effects of stress. The implementation of these skills will promote healthy living that contributes to 'wellness' and increase resistance to the adverse effects of stress.

Global skills in stress management

In all fields of practice, stress management is an essential skill required for nurses in order to be able to function somewhere near their optimum level. Although essential for all fields, mental health nursing has taken something of a lead as an exemplar for self-management and collaborative management of stress and anxiety. Much of the work undertaken by mental health staff is stress related.

Other than the skills highlighted throughout this chapter there are some key approaches that help practitioners to avoid

unhealthy levels of stress and to continue to function in their role. The skill of looking relaxed while you are not is not easy to master. A level of confidence (but not arrogance) is needed and a level of knowledge that addresses most situations.

The awareness that if you look anxious, others around you will pick up on this and start to feel anxious is important. Self-control and an awareness of posture and distance to the stressful event or client is needed. Although potentially anxious inside, it is necessary to actively listen and not to appear defensive. Giving short but pertinent answers is a necessity and in some instances, the use of touch may help someone in distress. Being confident enough to engage the person's attention in order to divert their focus away from the stressor is one of the key skills needed. Once you have their attention, it is important that you have some strategy in mind to offer. This can be helping to establish the level of distress/disruption being experienced, to allowing someone to detail the confusing feelings they have. Someone trying to tell you why they are upset is not always systematic and logical – if they could order it logically, they probably would not have the problem. Being able to listen and maintain appropriate eye contact is one skill, but responding and acting on what is said is equally important (see Ch. 9). Ensuring that you understand what is causing the stress and then being able to reflect this in your own words can help to show that you have listened with empathy and are aware of the process of events and consequences. The final simplistic stage would be the advice and action. Remember that if you cannot act immediately, allocate time to revisit the person. Just a few simple words later on can mean a great deal, especially if it involves something you have said you would do and can demonstrate that you have done so. Ultimately, much of the work needs to be done by the person experiencing the stress with you as facilitator.

Stress and people

This part of the chapter describes the more specific aspects of stress that relate to nurses and nursing. This includes work-related stress, which is extremely important in healthcare settings. Stress affecting patients/clients and their carers is addressed with suggested interventions for reducing its adverse effects. In many instances, the more general information on causes, effects and interventions can be used to inform the nurse's actions, both in self-care and the care of others.

Stress and nursing

Over a period of 12 months from 2009–2010, the estimated prevalence of self-reported work-related stress, anxiety and depression in the UK was 435 000; furthermore, stress was one of the most commonly reported work-related illnesses (the other being musculoskeletal disorders) (Health and Safety Executive 2010).

The nurse's role is inherently stressful due to the unpredictable nature of ill-health. In order to address the chance of the workforce becoming stressed, stress intervention measures should focus on stress prevention for individuals as well as tackling organizational issues (McVicar 2003). The managers of the environment and the nurse require vigilance to identify triggers early and take the necessary steps to remediate the situation. A major contributor to stress is the increased rate of practice and organizational change. Rapid changes to service provision can potentially lead to a stressful working environment (Price 2008).

One important feature is that nursing is fundamentally an interpersonal activity – nurses deal with people. Many of these encounters are with strangers and in situations that are already emotionally charged where patients/clients and their families are frequently anxious, angry or distressed.

In order to understand the potential for stress, it is important to realize that while most nurses would identify angry or aggressive patients/clients as causing stress, there are other less obvious issues to consider. These include:

- People who, despite efforts to help them, fail to recover
- People whose condition affects their verbal and non-verbal communication skills (see Ch. 9)
- People with visible signs of illness, skin lesions or disfigurement
- People who are experts in managing their condition
- People who have been victims of violence or other forms of abuse
- Anxious relatives who complain or become aggressive
- People whose behaviour is bizarre, unpredictable or aggressive
- People whose lifestyle choices may have contributed to their condition, e.g. overeating, smoking, drug or alcohol misuse, high-risk sexual behaviours.

These issues are common to many areas of nursing and often have an emotional impact on the nurses involved in providing care (Box 11.11).

 Reflective practice   Box 11.11

Nurses and stress

Identify a patient/client from a clinical placement who caused you to feel uncomfortable or stressed.

Student activities

- Reflect upon the characteristics of this patient/client that caused your discomfort.
- Think about the people, behaviours or conditions frequently seen in your chosen field of practice which might generate stress and anxiety for you.
- Consider the importance of attitudes and judgements in dealing with patients/clients.
- Talk to your mentor about some potentially damaging consequences of this type of stress and anxiety for nurses and the care they deliver to patients/clients.

There are also significant stressors that arise from the working environment. Those commonly identified by qualified nurses include:

- Increasing demands made upon them
- Lack of resources
- Inadequate staffing
- Shift work conflicts with family commitments
- Poor management.

Whereas student nurses frequently have other concerns, some feel that their role is poorly defined, they change practice areas frequently and need to balance this with assignments. Galbraith and Brown (2011) suggest that stress management programmes for student nurses are important given the high dropout rates.

Burnout

It is no surprise that some individuals working in high-stress environments, particularly if combined with significant external stress and poor levels of support, can feel powerless to contribute effectively at work. This failure of a person's coping resources in the work environment is often referred to as 'burnout'.

Many students start their course with high hopes and expectations; indeed many people still consider nursing to be a vocation in which helping others becomes the person's primary goal in life. While humanity should be thankful that such people exist, they often set themselves unrealistically high goals and expectations, dramatically increasing their risk for burnout.

There is no general definition of burnout but Maslach et al (1996) suggest that it is a syndrome characterized by:

- Emotional exhaustion and excessive tiredness
- Depersonalization (person loses the feeling of their own reality, everything seems dreamlike)
- Reduction in personal accomplishment and the sense of pleasure
- Reduction in morale
- Increased absenteeism
- Changes in interpersonal behaviour and relationship problems
- Increased use of alcohol or drugs
- Reduced concern for, and involvement with, their patients/clients.

Physical symptoms are common and are similar to anxiety:

- Feeling tense all the time
- Muscle pains
- Headaches
- Poor sleep (see Ch. 10)
- Indigestion
- Sweating
- Palpitations.

Patrick and Lavery (2007) identified that in nursing, these factors are prevalent in burnout (Box 11.12) and stated that long hours and unexpected demands have detrimental effects on staff stress levels and consequently levels of burnout. They also suggest that increasing age and fewer working hours were associated with lower levels of emotional exhaustion and depersonalization.

Associated with the potential for burnout is the emotional labour attributed to the caring role. This can affect all levels and as indicated earlier, the toll on not attending to stress levels

Box 11.12

Ethical issues

Dave

You are on placement with Dave, a fellow 1st year student. Over the last month he has become snappy with patients/clients, is often late on duty and looks unkempt. He seems harassed and frequently gets personal phone calls that he either asks others to say that he is not there, or takes them in private.

Student activities

- What do you think might be happening to Dave?
- Identify ways in which you might help Dave. What ethical issues (see Ch. 7) and professional issues should you consider?
- What other actions might you take to reduce the negative effects of this situation?
- Discuss these issues with your mentor.

Resource

Nursing and Midwifery Council, 2008. The code: Standards of conduct, performance and ethics for nurses and midwives. Online. Available: www.nmc-uk.org/Nurses-and-midwives/ Standards-and-guidance1/The-code/ September 2012.

---

can be high. Most nurses only tend to address the stress of caring once it has already had an impact on their functioning. For junior staff, the use of reflection and frequent discussions with mentors, supplemented by pastoral support from university tutors can help to refocus any fears or anxiety. 'A problem shared…' is a good mantra.

Managing work-related stress

However, while nursing is considered to be a stressful job, several important features of the work counter the negative effects of work-related stress. Nursing can be very rewarding work and if there are good supportive relationships, nurses appear to tolerate and cope with potential stressors very well. The ability to discuss work pressures and develop new adaptive skills have been identified as protective so frequently in studies that providing mentorship and clinical supervision

opportunities is considered central to good practice. Another important consideration is that an individual who identifies that they are stressed can use the problem-solving process of care planning to meet their own needs.

Schaufeli and Enzmann (1998) developed a matrix that provides a useful summary of the interventions that can reduce stress-related problems caused through work (Table 11.3).

Traumatic stress

Some events, particularly if they are sudden, intense and life-threatening may so overwhelm a person's coping ability that the capacity to process emotions is impaired. These events include being involved in serious accidents, natural disasters, violent crime or life-threatening illness/injury. In nurses, the sudden unexpected death of a patient, dealing with major incidents/accidents and exposure to threats or violence may generate the same types of response, generally described as an acute stress reaction.

Normal and frequently adaptive responses to extreme stress are shock and denial, both of which 'switch off' the immediate emotional response. Emotional shock is described as feeling stunned, dazed or numb. In health staff dealing with disasters, denial may leave them feeling disconnected from the horror of the situation but more importantly, it allows them to function. However, these initial effects are temporary and because they prevent people making sense of emotions at the time, are typically followed by a number of other effects, which may include the following:

- Feelings are experienced more intensely, often with a sense of threat or danger
- Emotions feel difficult to control
- Vivid memories or 'flashbacks' of the event suddenly and unpredictably come to mind, often associated with intense fear or distress. The 'flashbacks' become a source of anxiety; people might dread them occurring and avoid any potential reminders
- Sleep, eating and interpersonal relationships become disrupted.

Table 11.3 Matrix of organizational stress management interventions

	Primary stress reduction	Secondary stress management	Tertiary stress treatment
Individual perspective	Personal stress Time management Assertiveness Communication	Healthy lifestyles Reflection Clinical supervision Mentorship Relaxation Support	Counselling Intervention from Occupational Health Diet Exercise
Group/team perspective	Team building Team role Clarifying boundaries	Group development Diagnosis and intervention Workload analysis Team supervision	Therapeutic teamwork Renegotiate team role
Organization/systems perspective	Job description Clarify roles Individual performance review	Workload management Risk analysis (see Ch. 13) Employee participation	Employee assistance programmes Cultural change

For the majority, these symptoms will gradually reduce but how they are experienced and their duration, is highly variable.

Managing traumatic stress

Symptoms persisting longer than 6 months are called post-traumatic stress disorder (PTSD), which may require more specialist help. Therapies are based on cognitive behavioural psychotherapy and some people benefit from antidepressants. Even when the symptoms are severe, many people will recover with appropriate help.

The guiding principle in dealing with others who have experienced traumatic stress is to provide a safe, supportive environment with the opportunity to talk if required. The best interventions appear to be in preparing people to deal with potential trauma. Individuals who understand what reactions can be expected, and how feelings of guilt and responsibility are common but usually inaccurate, are less likely to develop long-term problems. For example, training in the management of aggressive clients should not only address the skills involved, they also need to address the psychological effects of aggression on the nurse.

Stress: patients, clients and carers

It is important to remember that many clients are not ill, but may still experience stress, e.g. people having a health 'MOT' or during pregnancy (see pp. 257–258).

Feeling well, being physically fit and well-nourished all contribute to the ability to deal with stressors and contribute to confidence and self-worth. However, when health is compromised, people must deal with the added stress associated with their condition, at a time when their coping resources are also reduced. Illness is a poorly-defined concept: it may describe the presence of a specific disease but the word has much broader connotations. The word can be linked with or used to describe anything that causes evil, harm, pain or trouble, and historically, was used to describe things going badly or getting worse. Even when describing specific conditions, the link is with *disease*, i.e. to have 'no ease'.

Many of the common effects of illness present significant physical and psychological challenges that can reduce or exhaust a person's coping resources. These can include:

- Lack of sleep (Ch. 10)
- Malnutrition and fluid deficits (Ch. 19)
- Toxins such as in infections, treatment side-effects, previous substance misuse or smoking
- Trauma or surgery
- Pain (Ch. 23).

In primary care, the interplay between physical and emotional health is well understood; it is estimated that up to 80% of consultations have a significant psychological component. This provides an example of how anxiety can be adaptive: if people were not concerned about their health they might not seek help.

Yet even when the problem is primarily stress-related the person usually presents with physical symptoms, which can make choosing the best interventions very difficult. Healthcare services also often deal with the consequences of social problems, such as poverty or relationship difficulties, which overwhelm coping resources and adversely affect health.

When admission to hospital is required, it is likely that this will be accompanied by the sense of threat. This may be intensified for people with learning disabilities, children and also for carers of people with complex needs. Again the main mediator of the anxiety experienced will be based on the meaning the person attaches to the condition.

Two related issues, body image and expressing sexuality/sexual identity, can also be highly significant in the person's response to illness.

Body image

Body image is the mental representation people have of their body and physical appearance. The view of physical self is central to a sense of identity, social value and self-esteem. Changes in body image, particularly if they involve loss of function, impaired ability to communicate or visible signs of illness and injury can be particularly traumatic. Where the change is likely to be temporary, individuals may simply detach from the situation, putting their life on 'hold' by adopting the sick role and making no attempt to adapt. This avoidance strategy can be highly adaptive in such situations. However, a change that is likely to be permanent often leads to grief-like reactions, in which initial shock is followed by profound depression and anger. In these cases, adaptation can be difficult and delayed.

Expressing sexuality

Expressing sexuality is linked to gender identity, attractiveness, fertility and sexual functioning and gives a person a sense of value and self-esteem. Changes caused by trauma or illness that impact on these areas appear to have emotional effects much more pronounced than would be expected from just functional loss. The presence of visible lesions, stoma formation or loss of body parts, e.g. female breast, or sudden weight changes are all particularly difficult to cope with. Loss of sexual functioning, factors affecting sexual performance, e.g. erectile dysfunction, and infertility may reduce self-efficacy and increase stress and depression.

Coping with illness

Illness can often highlight major differences in the demands made by the situation and the resources a person has available to deal with them. Coping often involves ongoing appraisals and reappraisals of a situation (making sense of something that does not necessarily make sense) in which individuals may attempt to alter the problem or their emotional responses to the problem.

Attempting to alter the problem is problem-focused coping and depends on the person believing that the problem is controllable or changeable. Ideally, actions should be based on analysis of the situation and planning solutions before the problem is dealt with. However, often actions are based on attempts to confront situations assertively which may involve actions based on anger, thus increasing risk.

Emotion-focused coping strategies that aim to control the emotion are frequently used when the person believes that they cannot change the stressor, either because they believe that they lack the resources/skills or the situation is insoluble, e.g. bereavement (see Ch. 12).

Social support provides emotional support through empathy, understanding, caring, etc., supporting self-esteem and offering practical help or information. People differ in their needs for social support; for those who like to cope alone, social support can be detrimental.

Helping patients/clients and carers to cope – role of the nurse

Although dealing with distressed individuals can be emotionally draining, the nurse needs to maintain an aspect of calm and helpful concern, while showing care and compassion. Nurses can help the person focus on the important issues, provide useful though often limited information, help the person to identify what immediate actions are needed and offer practical help as when acutely stressed, attention and memory may be impaired.

Nurses should anticipate the potential for stress and anxiety in their patients/clients and plan actions to prevent or minimize the more damaging effects. It is important to recognize that many of the anxieties a patient/client may have are realistic and so prevention may be difficult. As there is also the problem that anxiety and stress often affect logical thinking and memory, interventions are best made before feelings become too strong, ideally before the stressful event. Patients/clients and their carers, with appropriate and timely help from the nurse, may cope much more effectively.

Patients/clients/carers may also be reluctant to discuss anxieties, so as to avoid embarrassment; again the nurse can prevent problems by introducing such subjects into conversation. Communicating in this way and with tact, can give the person 'permission' to talk about difficult subjects.

There are important mediators of stress and anxiety that the nurse must consider in planning care. Cognitively, both stress and anxiety reflect feelings of vulnerability. There is a perception that demands/threats will overwhelm a person's ability to cope.

Stress and vulnerable individuals

Children, some people with learning disabilities, those with cognitive impairment and others, who do not understand stressful events and have limited coping resources, will be particularly vulnerable and are more likely to respond differently to life events.

The effects of long-term stress on childhood development have been well documented and have been associated with problems in adulthood. Young children who live in institutions or are maltreated by their family are at danger of developing behavioural or emotional problems (Loman & Gunnar, 2010). This can alter the child's future ability to deal with stress-related events.

In common with adults, stress in childhood may relate to issues other than illness, such as bullying (p. 257). Their behaviour may change, e.g. becoming withdrawn, tearful, depressed, headaches, etc. Children are affected by stress within families such as that caused by abusive relationships and domestic abuse/violence (see Useful websites, below, e.g. Childline; Further reading, e.g. DH 2011; Trevillion et al 2011).

Children have limited experience of dealing with demands and inadequate coping strategies, thus anxiety is a common and frequent experience for children. Young children in particular may also have a very limited ability to communicate their distress to adults. So to understand stress in children, it is important to consider their age, the developmental stage and communication skills.

Children are skilled at judging the emotional state of their parents/carers and can become distressed in response to adult anxiety. This is important for a child who is admitted to hospital, as they already have an increased level of stress caused by the admission and the environment.

Children attempt to make sense of illness and to cope by using much more basic defence mechanisms, such as regression (see p. 243). Nurses assessing stress and anxiety in children often find that behaviour is a better indicator of a child's distress than their verbal reports (Box 11.13).

Age-related stress behaviours   Box 11.13

- *Infant* (birth to 12 months) – sleep problems accompanied by excessive screaming; feeding problems, which may result in weight loss, failure to thrive, etc.
- *Toddler* (1–3 years) – behavioural problems, e.g. difficulties in socializing with other children, may be excessively shy or aggressive (boys are more aggressive than girls)
- *Preschool age* (4–5 years) – social isolation with problems relating to adults and other children
- *Primary school age* – excessive levels of aggression. May exhibit depression. Behavioural problems, e.g. use of violence (learn that violence is a way to resolve conflict)
- *Adolescents* – problems with social interaction and in some cases violent or criminal behaviour.

Children commonly become uncooperative. These behaviours may lead to reduced social support or anger in their carers and so can be seen as maladaptive and damaging. Teenagers in particular can be especially difficult by refusing help and by engaging in high-risk behaviours, which include:

- Smoking, drug or alcohol misuse
- Truancy
- Crime
- High-risk sexual activity
- Self-harm.

Age-appropriate techniques that nurses, parents/carers might use to reduce the child's distress include:

- Distraction – for younger children rattles/toys; in older children involvement in games and music
- Touch

- Massage and imagery
- Relaxation.

Children with long-term problems, e.g. diabetes, when faced with the increased stress associated with the major transition into adolescence, may also start to neglect their condition and increase their health risks.

When caring for people with learning disabilities, there may be problems in both recognizing and helping to manage their stress. Depending on the nature of the disability, the person may have restricted understanding of situations and limited communication skills. In addition, damage to the central nervous system may lead to a reduced tolerance to environmental stimulation, overwhelming their ability to cope. Alternatively, they may become insensitive to stressors, leading to disinhibition and risk taking.

For those with reduced tolerance to environmental stimuli, one approach to reducing distress is the use of Snoezelen. This multisensory stimulation technique utilizes lights, tactile surfaces, music and sometimes essential oils (see Ch. 10) to provide an environment that is soothing and relaxing (Box 11.14). Moreover, the family can be involved in sessions in order to increase their understanding of the patient's/client's feelings, abilities, etc. and enhance family relationships.

 Evidence-based practice   **Box 11.14**

Snoezelen use for people with learning disability or dementia

Advocates for Snoezelen assert that it can reduce challenging behaviour and enhance mood and concentration, although reliable evidence is lacking. The Snoezelen room has also been used to enhance the experiences of women during labour.

Some studies demonstrated a wide range of positive outcomes whereas others reported entirely negative outcomes.

Student activities

- Locate one recent study with positive outcomes and one with entirely negative outcomes and discuss the findings with your mentor.

Many older people with learning disabilities evaluate their sense of value and their abilities by comparison with people of their own age. This can lead to problems with self-concept and an acute sensitivity to perceived criticism. For some clients, the frustrations associated with these social comparisons and their perceived lack of ability may be expressed in low self-esteem, dependency, self-destructive behaviours or difficult behaviours towards their carers. All of these features are associated with reduced ability to deal with potential stressors; the behaviours used in coping often increase stress in both carers and client.

There is still considerable stigma associated with learning disabilities, which can lead to exclusion, rejection and prejudice. Even when prejudice is not present, there can be a general insensitivity to the needs of people with a learning disability, which can add considerably to the stress they experience.

Bullying is a stressor commonly identified in children, people with a learning disability and in other vulnerable adults who are considered different in some way (physically,

culturally, intellectually), especially if they are seen as less able or weak (Box 11.15).

Stress and pregnancy

Pregnancy, albeit a natural event which is usually welcomed, is associated with stress and anxiety (Box 11.16). Importantly, maternal stress levels can affect the unborn infant, as the fetus is exposed to maternal cortisol (for cortisol, see p. 246) which crosses the placenta. Glover (2011) asserts that if a woman suffers stress and anxiety during pregnancy, her infant is more likely to exhibit a range of problems, including attention deficit hyperactivity disorder (ADHD), anxiety, conduct disorder, etc.

'While there remains some debate about what proportion of these effects are due to the prenatal or the postnatal

---

 Reflective practice   **Box 11.15**

Bullying

Bullying takes many forms: young people describe this in a variety of ways, e.g. teasing, being pushed, rumours spread, cyber bullying. In addition, people who behave differently, those with learning disabilities, dementia or mental illness, may be at risk of bullying.

Student activities

- Reflect on types of bullying and solutions
- Which behavioural problems, such as anxiety, may be caused by bullying?
- Discuss with your mentor the agencies/organisations that can help to deal with bullying and its effects.

Resource

Childline – www.childline.org.uk/Explore/Bullying/Pages/Bullyinginfo.aspx September 2012.

 Reflective practice   **Box 11.16**

Stress associated with pregnancy

Scenario 1 – Millie aged 15 years is pregnant, it was not planned and she doesn't know the father's name. She lives with her mother, who doesn't yet know, and four younger siblings. Millie hardly ever does a full week at school.

Scenario 2 – This is Rani's first pregnancy and she is determined to have a natural birth with no pain relief. Her mother and husband urge her to keep an open mind and not dismiss the idea of having pain relief, but she remains adamant that everything will be fine.

Scenario 3 – Caroline aged 41 years and Pete her partner have just had a baby after four miscarriages. Now Pete is back at work, Caroline feels anxious and inadequate. She can't get into a routine, is still in her pyjamas when Pete gets home and can't cope when the baby cries.

Student activities

- Consider the three scenarios and identify the likely stressors in each.
- Discuss with your mentor ways of reducing stress levels in each case.

---

environment, and the role of genetics, there is good evidence that prenatal stress exposure can increase the risk for later psychopathology ...'

(Glover 2011, abstract).

The findings from Glover's paper supports the need to provide appropriate support as part of prenatal care in order to reduce stress during pregnancy. This includes providing factual information and answering questions about pregnancy, labour and infant care, and the teaching of relaxation techniques which can aid the process of childbirth. Such prenatal programmes aim to provide the participants with education relating to the birth and options for pain relief, and importantly to meet other pregnant women and their partners. Certain groups are less likely to attend prenatal programmes, e.g. unsupported mothers, very young mothers, non-English speakers, women who are carers, etc.

Coping with serious illness, chronic problems and disability

There are real differences in the way individuals deal with acute illness and the demands of adapting to chronic illness, disability and life-limiting illness (see Ch. 12). Rather than anticipating recovery, the patient/client and family must learn instead to live with the continued physical, social and emotional effects of their condition.

Having to deal with a serious or life-limiting condition can generate a great deal of anxiety in both the patient and the people to whom they are closest. Following a period of shock or detachment, those involved try to give the situation meaning; they try to make some sense of the value of their life in the face of death.

Preliminary steps could use appraisal of the situation, exploration of the emotions and problems created by the need to adapt to health challenges. Commonly used coping strategies used include an attempt to regain the lifestyle prior to the illness. With people with a cancer diagnosis, a positive life attitude, willingness to fight against the disease and to accept the disease as part of one's life are resources for coping (Kyngäs et al 2008). Ultimately, an attempt to take hold of the things they can control in life is needed. This includes self-management and the control of information given to family and others.

Chronic illness and disability

An acquired disability often means that the client's social roles change and the pressures placed upon the family and carers increase. Throughout, there is a need to adapt to many new situations that affect not only health and functioning but also roles and self-concept. Initially, adaptation is resisted but at some point, the patient/client must learn to accept the changes and work towards the best outcomes. Patients/clients who fail to make these mental changes often become depressed and possibly self-destructive.

Assessment requires a measure/tool that is inclusive, identifies normal functioning and establishes a baseline from which to evaluate the effect of care at a later date. The assessment also needs to address the requirements of the patient's family,

as providing long-term care can have profound effects on family and carers. Long-term interventions include many specialist services and collaborative multiprofessional working (see Ch. 3). However, it is good practice for a specifically named person to act as care coordinator and to engage the patient and family in all aspects of care.

Rehabilitation

Rehabilitation involves learning ways of coping with long-term illnesses or injury. This may involve maximizing physical abilities, learning new skills, problem-solving and changing appraisals about the condition and its consequences. Many conditions may run a prolonged and chronic course, requiring considerable adaptation by the patient/client and those around them. Conditions may be congenital (present from birth), e.g. profound and multiple learning disability requiring life-long help, or acquired (after birth) as in psychosis, multiple sclerosis, spinal injuries, type 2 diabetes, chronic respiratory or heart diseases and arthritis; many of which occur in older adults. Unfortunately, the effects of the increased stress, associated particularly with acquired conditions, may also be instrumental in maintaining or worsening the condition. (A full discussion of rehabilitation is beyond the scope of this book and readers are directed to Further reading, e.g. Ward et al 2009.)

Models in rehabilitation

It is particularly important in long-term care planning that the guiding model is person-centred, holistic and allows for multi-agency collaboration with patients/clients and carers (Box 11.17, and see Ch. 14).

Planning long-term care	Box 11.17

1. Holistic assessment:
   - Learn about the individual and their unique problems
   - Establish their expectations
   - Identify the knowledge they have of the condition
   - Identify current coping strategies
   - Identify social support systems
2. Develop a plan on patient/client goals and those of others involved
3. Identify the strategies for goal attainment and equipment/adaptations needed:
   - Identify potential problems and barriers to achievement
4. Identify a named individual to implement the strategy
5. Work within a timeframe for goal completion
6. Set a flexible review date
7. Provide contact details for the key people involved
8. Ensure that the plan is clear and unambiguous
9. Review outcomes with the patient/client and their carers.

An example of using such an approach is the Wellness Recovery Action Plan (WRAP). The WRAP was developed by Copeland (1997) as a structured system that enables the active monitoring of distressing symptoms in people with long-term mental health problems. However, many of the principles are applicable to most care situations. The development of a WRAP culminates in a plan that aims to modify or eliminate the most distressing symptoms the patient/client identifies. There are five pivotal principles that need consideration when developing a WRAP:

- *Hope:* People must have a reason to make the effort to manage their condition
- *Personal responsibility:* People must recognize that they are not passive recipients of care but actively involved, as a partner
- *Education:* Learning about the illness allows people to make good decisions
- *Self-advocacy:* Aids self-belief, knowing personal rights and seeing that they are respected; setting goals and working to make them happen
- *Support:* Effective support from family, friends and professionals aids in symptom relief.

The development of a WRAP is dependent on framing the wants and needs of the patient/client. Patients/clients, although frequently anxious, do know what they can and cannot do and in developing the plan, the patient/client can begin to recognize the collaborative nature of the nurse–patient relationship. In time, and with help from the nurse, the patient/client becomes the expert in their illness or disability.

SUMMARY

- All nurses require a good understanding of mental health-related problems, including stress and anxiety and stress management.
- Stress and anxiety are complex psychological and physiological reactions an individual has in response to environmental demands or perceived threats.
- While people experience stress and anxiety as unpleasant, it serves a useful and adaptive function in motivating behaviour to reduce the demands or potential risk.
- Although some stress and anxiety are normal and necessary, there are links between stress and health breakdown. Particularly evident in long-term stress.
- High levels of stress almost invariably interfere with a person's ability to function effectively.
- Responses to stress depend very much upon people's beliefs about a situation and their ability to cope. Developing coping strategies and modifying beliefs are the most effective ways to reduce the negative effects of stress.

- Nursing is fundamentally an interpersonal activity in which nurses are frequently in contact with people who are distressed and need help.
- Nurses experiencing high levels of stress are more likely to engage in behaviour which can be damaging to the health of both patients and themselves.
- A range of strategies may be used in the management of stress in both patients/clients and in self-care. Coping styles and strategies will vary from individual to individual and matching the intervention to the individual is an important function of effective nursing assessment.
- All nurses should be able to recognize indicators that might suggest that stress and anxiety are overwhelming a client's resources as more specialized help may be needed.

KEY WORDS AND PHRASES FOR LITERATURE SEARCHING

Adaptation

Coping strategies

Rehabilitation

Stress

Stress at work

Stress in nursing

Stress management

Theories of stress

 Useful websites

BBC www.bbc.co.uk/health/emotional_health/mental_health/mind_stress.shtml

Childline www.childline.org.uk

National Childbirth Trust (NCT) www.nct.org.uk

The American Institute of Stress www.stress.org

The Nursefriendly Stress Resources for Nurses (North American) www.nursefriendly.com/nursing/stress.htm

The Royal College of Psychiatrists www.rcpsych.ac.uk

Stress resources website – www.teachhealth.com

All websites accessed September 2012.

References

Copeland, M.E., 1997. Wellness recovery action plan. Peach Press, Dummerston, VT.

Department of Health, 2010. Essence of care 2010 Benchmarks for self care. Online. Available: www.dh.gov.uk/prod_consum_dh/groups/dh_digitalassets/@dh/@en/@ps/documents/digitalasset/dh_119978.pdf September 2012.

Ellis, A., 1994. Reason and emotion in psychotherapy, second ed. Carol Publishing, New York.

Galbraith, N.D., Brown, K.E., 2011. Assessing intervention effectiveness for reducing stress in student nurses: quantitative systematic review. Journal of Advanced Nursing 67 (4), 709–721.

Glover, V., 2011. Annual Research Review: Prenatal stress and the origins of psychopathology: an evolutionary perspective. Journal of Child Psychology and Psychiatry, and allied disciplines 52 (4), 356–367.

Health and Safety Executive, 2010. Statistics 2009/10 Online. Available: www.hse.gov.uk/statistics/overall/hssh0910.pdf September 2012.

Holmes, T.H., Rahe, R.H., 1967. The social readjustment and rating scale. Journal of Psychosomatic Research 11, 213–218.

Kyngäs, H., Mikkonen, R., Nousiainen, E.M., et al., 2008. Coping with the onset of cancer: coping strategies and resources of young people with cancer. European Journal of Cancer Care 10 (1), 6–11.

Lazarus, A.A., 1981. The practice of multi-modal therapy. McGraw-Hill, New York.

Lazarus, R., Folkman, S., 1984. Stress appraisal and coping. Springer Verlag, New York.

Loman, M.M., Gunnar, M.R., 2010. Early experience and the development of stress reactivity and regulation in children. Neuroscience and Biobehavioral Reviews 34 (6), 867–876.

Maslach, C., Jackson, S., Leiter, M.P., 1996. Maslach burnout inventory manual, third ed. Consulting Psychologists Press, Palo Alto, CA.

McVicar, A., 2003. Workplace stress in nursing: A literature review. Journal of Advanced Nursing 44 (6), 633–642.

Menzies-Lyth, I., 1959. The functions of social systems as a defence against anxiety: a report on a study of the nursing service of a general hospital. Human Relations 13, 95–121.

National Institute for Health and Clinical Excellence, 2011. Quick reference guide generalised anxiety disorder and panic attacks (with or without agoraphobia) in adults. Clinical guideline 113. Online. Available: www.nice.org.uk/nicemedia/live/13314/52601/52601.pdf September 2012.

Nursing and Midwifery Council, 2010. Standards for pre-registration nursing education. Online. Available: www.nmc-uk.org September 2012.

Patrick, K., Lavery, J.F., 2007. Burnout in nursing. Australian Journal of Advanced Nursing 24 (3), 43–48.

Price, B., 2008. Strategies to help nurses cope with change in the healthcare setting. Nursing Standard 22 (48), 50–56.

Schaufeli, W.B., Enzmann, D., 1998. The burnout companion to study and practice: a critical analysis. Taylor and Francis, Philadelphia.

Selye, H., 1956. (revised 1975) The stress of life. McGraw-Hill, New York.

Further reading

Department of Health, 2011. Violence against women and children. Online. Available: www.dh.gov.uk/en/Publichealth/ViolenceagainstWomenandChildren/index.htm September 2012.

National Institute for Health and Clinical Excellence, 2011. Common mental health disorders. Identification and pathways to care. National clinical guideline CG 123. Online. Available: www.nice.org.uk/nicemedia/live/13476/54604/54604.pdf September 2012.

Payne, R.A., Donaghy, M., 2010. Payne's handbook of relaxation techniques, fourth ed. Churchill Livingstone, Edinburgh.

Sharma, A., Sharp, D.M., Walker, L.G., et al., 2008. Stress and burnout among colorectal surgeons and colorectal nurse specialists working in the National Health Service. Colorectal Disease 10 (4), 397–406.

Trevillion, K., Agnew-Davies, R., Howard, L.M., 2011. Domestic violence: responding to the needs of patients. Nursing Standard 25 (26), 48–56.

Ward, A., Barnes, M., Stark, S., et al., 2009. Oxford handbook of clinical rehabilitation, second ed. OUP, Oxford.

12

Loss and bereavement

Karen Strickland   Catriona Kennedy

Introduction

The death of a significant person is the most difficult loss most people will face and nurses have an important role to play in supporting people who are dying and their families. The first part of this chapter explores issues of loss and bereavement, including death, and the impact of different types of loss on people. Consideration is given to bereavement, including understanding grief responses and planning care.

The middle section focuses on the palliative care approach to care, which encompasses care of people with life-limiting conditions such as cancer, chronic heart and respiratory diseases, and some degenerative neurological illnesses. Several members of the multidisciplinary team (MDT) are likely to be involved in the care and support of patients/clients with advanced disease, and their families. However, nurses are generally the health professionals who have most contact. Nurses therefore have a significant role in supporting individuals through illness, at the end stages of life and families who are

bereaved. The skills and knowledge of nurses caring for those with advanced, non-curable illness are crucial to the delivery of high quality care. Strategies for communication and the management of distressing symptoms are discussed. Helping nurses to understand the philosophy of the palliative care approach and the services available is the focus of this section.

The last section is about the care of people facing death; both the person who will die and those closest to them. The Liverpool Care Pathway (LCP) as a framework for providing care around death is presented. Finally, ethical concerns at the end-of-life are identified and the role of the nurse in the last act of care and in the provision of palliative care is identified (see Ch 6).

Loss including death

This section considers factors relating to loss and bereavement. Death of a significant other is recognized as a difficult loss to cope with. Nurses are important in helping people to deal with losses which result from injury, illness and death. Therefore it is important to consider how experiences of loss – expected, planned or unexpected – throughout life prepare individuals to cope.

Types of loss

Loss and change are part of everyday life and everyone will experience both of these during their lifetime. Loss is experienced in the absence of a person, miscarriage/stillbirth, own impending death, an object, body part, a function (e.g. walking), change related to age/milestones, loss of status, loss/change of job/retirement, a move into a care home, or from institutional to community care, or emotion, which was formerly present.

Some losses may be thought of as rather less traumatic than others. However, responses to loss are individual and linked to a range of other personality and lifestyle factors

---

Reflective practice Box 12.1

Reactions to loss

Identify an object you have recently lost, e.g. keys, handbag or breakage of a favourite item, etc.

Student activities

- How did you feel?
- Reflect on a situation when you might have underestimated the impact on a person of what you considered to be a 'trivial' loss.

It is likely that many of the feelings you experienced are similar to those associated with loss through bereavement. Therefore, even apparently trivial loss can result in a range of distressing feelings. It is important that nurses do not assume how people feel about loss, as insignificant loss to one person may be catastrophic to another.

(Box 12.1). For example, non-animal lovers may find it hard to understand why a person is devastated at the loss of a much-loved pet. Loss is an inherent part of any change, even where people have decided to make changes such as getting married or having a child. The losses associated with significant life events are expected and normally occur as the person matures from one stage of life to another and makes decisions about how they want life to develop (see Chs 8, 11). If progress through life's normal milestones is not achieved, then feelings of loss may result. For example, parents whose children do not achieve normal life milestones due to disabilities or illness often find it hard to cope. Similarly, if a couple find they cannot have children, apart from dealing with their own feelings, they may feel pressurized by others who expect them to have children. Therefore, response to loss is shaped by context and culture.

Throughout life, people form attachments and the stronger the attachment, the greater the loss experienced when that attachment is broken. When an attachment is broken, people cope by revising and reconstructing their life, thereby adapting to loss and subsequent change, often with support from family and friends. Professional intervention may be required if an individual cannot cope with significant loss such as a major change in body image or death. For most people, loss associated with life events they have not 'chosen' is the most difficult to cope with.

Bereavement

In most healthcare settings, nurses will encounter patients/clients and/or carers who are experiencing loss or have suffered bereavement (the loss of somebody or something of value, especially through death). It is often the nurse who assumes the role of helping the patient/client or carer. Bereaved individuals need open acknowledgement of the death and opportunities to display expressions of grief and mourning in order to help them come to terms with the loss. To do this effectively, the nurse requires knowledge of what loss is and how people react to and cope with loss. There is also considerable evidence to suggest that professionals working with people who are dying find this enormously stressful (Lockhart-Wood 2001; Skilbeck & Payne 2003). This type of stress has been referred to as the 'emotional labour' of nursing (James 1989). Through understanding the theories relating to the process of dying and grieving, the nurse is better equipped to support patients and carers in their journey.

For the purpose of this chapter, the following definitions (Stroebe et al 2002) will guide understanding:

- Bereavement – describes the situation when a person has died
- Grief – describes the emotional reaction to loss or death
- Mourning – the expression of the emotion which characterizes grief.

Models that describe dying and bereavement demonstrate that these processes usually involve a series of stages and that individuals take varying lengths of time in each stage and may move from one to the other and back again. Thus it is important to remember that each individual's reaction to loss is unique and there is no right or wrong way to grieve.

To date, Elisabeth Kubler-Ross' (1969) 'preparing to die' model of dying has been the most influential. This seminal work was one of the first attempts to explain the process of dying in relation to the emotional and psychological adaptations which accompany the process. This theory made the previously taboo subject of death and dying one that could be openly discussed. For the first time healthcare professionals were able to relate to a theoretical model which made sense of their patients' behaviours and actions. The five stages of this model are:

- Denial
- Anger
- Bargaining
- Depression
- Acceptance.

Anticipatory grief

While Kubler-Ross' model focuses on dying, it has close similarities with the concept of anticipatory grief. Anticipatory grief is grief occurring before death. It differs from post-death grief in its nature and course. Lindemann (1944) was the first to recognize this phenomenon and identified five characteristics of anticipatory grief:

- Guilt – for unresolved issues such as old quarrels
- Somatic (body) distress – physical manifestation of grief, often characterized as feelings of anxiety, sleeplessness, poor appetite, nausea
- Anger (see Kubler-Ross' model)
- Loss of patterns of conduct – inability to carry out daily activities such as getting dressed, work and household chores
- Fixation with the image of the dying person – coping with the changing physical appearance and social standing of the person.

Kubler-Ross noted that common behaviours include denial, reassurance seeking, secrecy about the diagnosis, anger and guilt. There are conflicting views of how helpful anticipatory grief is to the bereavement process, with some authors suggesting that it makes little difference. However, the predominant view is that it helps people to cope and reduces the length of time someone has to adjust to the news of impending death of a loved one. Parkes and Weiss (1983) found that those who have more than 2 weeks to adjust to loss had less difficulty in their adjustment than those who had less than 2 weeks. An alternative argument, however, could be that sudden deaths are more traumatic for the person and invoke a much stronger grief reaction.

One problem, however, is when the dying person appears to live longer than expected; the psychological preparation that goes with anticipatory grief and the state of 'readiness' may be achieved prior to the actual death.

Grief and mourning

Grief and mourning are terms used to describe the emotional reaction to loss or death and the expression of the emotion in relation to this event. Several theories have been proposed to aid understanding of the grieving process, and those of Worden (1991) and Parkes (1998) are two of the most influential. These two theories complement each other (Box 12.2): Parkes' theory describes the feelings and emotions the person affected by the loss is experiencing during different stages; Worden's theory illuminates the process of adjustment that is necessary to regain equilibrium.

 Reflective practice   Box 12.2

Understanding the grief process

Reflect upon the theories of grieving and their relevance to your field of nursing. You may wish to consider a patient/client and their family you have cared for. Although it is difficult to neatly package the actual experience into stages, you may have recognized some of the characteristics that would indicate the stage of grief.

Student activities

- Discuss your reflection with a mentor or colleague.
- How might knowledge of the theories help you support patients/clients and families?

Parkes (1998) describes four components of grief:

- *Numbness*: This relates to the initial reaction to the news of a loss or that a person has died. This component may last for a period of a few hours to a number of days. Following this is the 'pining' component where feelings of grief are evident.
- *Pining*: The person has intense feelings of pining, often described as 'pangs of grief'. The person continues to function with day-to-day essential chores but may seem listless and distant. This component can also have physical manifestations, which include reduced appetite and

weight loss, poor concentration and short-term memory impairment. Insomnia may also be a problem resulting in irritability (see Ch. 10).

- *Disorganization and despair*: This component is characterized by continual ruminations over events leading up to the death. For many, this will lead to a feeling of the need to apportion blame and anger, which is often directed at the healthcare system. If there were any areas for concern, these may become magnified during the grieving process. During this phase, the bereaved person may report hallucinations in the form of hearing or seeing the dead person nearby, especially when they are relaxed or drowsy. Usually these hallucinations dissipate when the person becomes more awake.
- *Reorganization*: Finally, reorganization occurs when the feelings described in the preceding components are resolved and the bereaved person has learned to accept and adapt to life with the loss or without the person who has died. It has been suggested that this component may take a long time to achieve, with some people who have lost someone very close such as a spouse or child not really recovering until well into the second year following the death (Parkes 1998).

Parkes suggests that the components of grief must be worked through to enable the individual to 'let go' of the person they have lost and to be able to move on with their lives. He likens this process to the loss reaction and period of adjustment that people display when they have become disabled through the loss of a body part.

While each of these components is seen to be of equal significance, it is important to remember that people often do not clearly signal when one component is complete and they have moved into the next component. Indeed, the boundaries are often blurred and people may oscillate between components before moving on. Parkes stresses the importance of allowing people to express their emotions and states that repression of grief is harmful and may result in delayed reactions and complicated grieving. Equally, obsessive grieving is harmful and may lead to chronic grief and depression.

Parkes' theory describes the feelings relating to different stages of the grieving process. This is complemented by Worden's theory of 'grief work' which focuses on the tasks that need to be completed to achieve resolution of these feelings. People sometimes talk about someone who has been recently bereaved as being in a 'state of mourning'; however, Worden (1991) suggests that mourning is an active process which has to be 'worked' at. In his seminal work, Worden (1991) asserts that there are four 'tasks' of mourning that must be worked through in order for the person affected by the loss to be able to come to terms with their loss. They are:

- *Task 1 – To accept the reality of the loss*: Even when death is expected, once it has occurred it is often accompanied by a sense of unreality. The first task of mourning is to come to terms with the reality that the person has died. Part of this is also to accept that reunion is not possible and separation is permanent.
- *Task 2 – To work through the pain of grief*: It is necessary to work through the pain of the grief or it will manifest

itself through physical or psychological symptoms or aberrant behaviour such as anxiety or anger outbursts. One of the aims of grief counselling is to help the client work through the pain of the grief and to allow the expression of emotions and feelings to permit resolution so that grief is not carried with them throughout their life.

- *Task 3 – To adjust to an environment in which the person is missing:* Realization that life is different without the dead person occurs from 3 months following the loss. This may involve the gradual coming to terms with living alone and/or raising children alone. It may be that the bereaved individual relied upon the person to do many of the manual tasks around the home or to take care of the finances. Adjustment through learning how to accomplish these tasks alone is an example of what is seen as part achievement of this task of mourning.
- *Task 4 – To emotionally relocate the deceased and move on with life:* This task describes the work of finding an appropriate place for the dead person in the bereaved individual's emotional life, enabling them to move on and live effectively again. Incompletion of this task may for example be characterized by a holding onto the past and making a pact with oneself never to love again.

Factors affecting grief

Many factors influence how people respond to loss and bereavement. Whether the death was expected or sudden has an impact on the bereavement process (see pp. 270–272). However, age, cognitive impairment (e.g. dementia or learning disabilities) and cultural differences are all factors that may influence the process of grieving. Box 12.3 provides an opportunity for you to consider the grief that results from a miscarriage or a stillbirth and the support services available in your area.

? Critical thinking   **Box 12.3**

Miscarriage and stillbirth

The death of an expected infant through miscarriage or stillbirth is a traumatic event for the parents and other family members.

Student activity

- Discuss with your mentor what resources are available locally to support families who experience miscarriage or stillbirth.

Bereavement in children

Bereaved adults caring for a child are often left to support the child. Many are ill-equipped to do so and this often results in a protective instinct to shield the child from the pain of the loss. However, with some support, even very young children are able to grasp the concept of death. Furthermore, studies have demonstrated that children who have suffered bereavement and not been able to express their grief are more susceptible to depression. Thus, helping and supporting the child to grieve is important.

? Critical thinking   **Box 12.4**

Bereavement in children and young people

Domka is dying and she and her husband Andrzej have talked about how they can best prepare their children (Piotr aged 15 and Ruta aged 9) for Domka's death and life without their mother.

Student activities

- Access the Winston's Wish website (see Useful websites, p. 277) and look at the services they offer and the activities and suggestions they have to help children and adolescents who are facing the death of a loved one or who are bereaved.
- Discuss with your mentor how these resources could be used in your field of nursing.

There are a number of interventions that can be carried out in order to help children accept and come to terms with death (Box 12.4). These include:

- Preparing the child for bereavement
- Supporting parents and carers of the child
- Explaining and talking openly about death with the child
- Encouraging the child's participation in mourning, e.g. attending the funeral
- Resumption of normal activities
- Visiting the grave/special place
- Memory boxes/books

(See Useful websites, p. 277, e.g. Childhood Bereavement Network, Winston's Wish).

Bereavement in people with learning disabilities

It is widely accepted that the pattern of bereavement in people with learning disabilities is similar to everyone else, as is the case with people who have dementia. However, Dodd and Guerin (2009) state that people with intellectual disabilities present unique challenges, which include variations in their understanding of death.

In some cases, the grief reaction is delayed and is first manifest by a sudden change in behaviour such as violent outbursts and withdrawal. Due to the delay in response, it is often handled inappropriately using medication or behavioural therapy (Hollins & Esterhuyzen 1997). In her study of the provision of education for carers of people with learning disabilities, Bennett (2003) found that many felt inadequately prepared to provide bereavement support to their clients. This may indicate why people with learning disabilities are sometimes inappropriately managed with medications and behavioural therapies.

People with learning disabilities generally do better if they are adequately prepared for the loss and are supported through the bereavement – with help and support to express feelings of grief with an empathetic confidante.

Complicated grief

While it is acknowledged that each person's course of mourning will be unique, uncomplicated grief is characterized by the patterns and feelings described above. When grief becomes complicated, it can lead to unusual patterns of behaviour. The point where normal grief reactions become complicated is generally considered when the grief reaction becomes prolonged and causes significant disruption to functioning in daily life either by severe depression or the use of maladaptive coping strategies such as alcohol or drug misuse. Complicated grief may become chronic, it may be delayed or exaggerated.

Palliative care

This part of the chapter explores what palliative care is and how palliative care services are organized within the UK. Nurses have an integral role to play in providing patients and families with high quality palliative care. The term palliative care is derived from the Latin word *pallium*, meaning 'to cloak'. Thus palliative care focuses on symptom relief without curing the illness which is causing the symptoms.

Palliative care has been known by many terms over the years. These include terminal care, hospice care, care of the dying, end-of-life care and supportive care (Payne 2008). Problems have arisen with the terminology used previously. For example, Hanks et al (2009) argue that the term 'terminal care' is confusing because it implies there is little that can be done for the patient. This is in stark contrast to the active and sometimes interventionist nature of palliative care, which may include chemotherapy (anti-cancer (cytotoxic) drugs to destroy cancer cells) and radiotherapy (the use of high energy X-rays to destroy cancer cells). Similarly, the term 'hospice care' is misleading as it gives the impression that the approach is limited to those in the care of hospice professionals rather than indicating an approach to care that can be used in any setting and at every stage of the illness journey. This term, however, was first used to denote the hospice movement, which advocated a move away from acute hospital care for patients who were dying of incurable illnesses such as cancer. 'End-of-life' care similarly falls short of what encompasses palliative care as it implies that care is only given when the patient is at a certain stage of their illness. End-of-life care certainly falls within the remit of palliative care but palliative care is much broader, with many authors arguing that it should begin at the time of diagnosis. Palliative care then is essentially care of patients and their families whose illness is no longer curable and should begin when this is known.

What is palliative care?

The World Health Organization (WHO 2004) has provided a useful definition:

Palliative care improves the quality of life of patients and families who face life-threatening illness, by providing pain and symptom relief, spiritual and psychosocial support from diagnosis to the end-of-life and bereavement.

In this definition, the holistic nature of palliative care is evident as it encompasses the multidimensional approach. The WHO outlines the principles that underpin the approach to palliative care, as follows:

Palliative care provides relief from pain and other distressing symptoms. It:

- Affirms life and regards dying as a normal process
- Intends neither to hasten nor postpone death
- Integrates the psychological and spiritual aspects of patient care
- Offers a support system to help patients live as actively as possible until death
- Offers a support system to help the family cope during the patient's illness and in their own bereavement
- Uses a team approach to address the needs of patients and their families, including bereavement counselling, if indicated
- Will enhance quality of life and may also positively influence the course of illness
- Is applicable early in the course of illness, in conjunction with other therapies that are intended to prolong life, such as chemotherapy or radiation therapy, and includes those investigations needed to better understand and manage distressing clinical complications

(WHO 2004).

The WHO definition and the principles of palliative care illustrate the complexity of palliative care. For this reason, it is unlikely that any one healthcare professional will be able to deliver palliative care in isolation, rather it has to be a MDT approach. Members of the MDT may vary in their level of input over the course of the patient's illness but examples of people involved are:

- General nurses
- Hospital-based medical staff
- District nurses
- Learning disability liaison nurses
- General practitioners
- Specialist palliative care nurses and doctors, Macmillan and Marie Curie nurses
- Physiotherapists
- Occupational therapists
- Dieticians
- Psychologists
- Social workers
- Religious figures
- Complementary therapists
- Volunteers.

Furthermore, it is unlikely that palliative care will be delivered in a single place. Thus, health and social care professionals working in hospitals, community, hospices and voluntary sectors must understand the palliative care approach (Box 12.5).

The MDT should have a shared idea of common roles and accepted objectives; in order to achieve these, traditional professional roles may have to be adjusted. There is great value in including family and carers within the team, as many patients express a wish to be cared for in their own homes. Families and carers must be well informed and supported in order for this to happen.

The provision of high quality palliative care is a multidisciplinary endeavour. However, nurses usually work very closely with patients and their families during the course of their illness and in bereavement, and therefore have a central role in providing information, care and support.

Palliative care for children

The WHO (2004) states that palliative care for children is closely related to adult palliative care and provides principles for care of children with chronic non-curable illness. Palliative care for children:

- Is the active care of the child's body, mind and spirit, and also involves giving support to the family
- Begins when illness is diagnosed, and continues regardless of whether or not a child receives treatment directed at the disease
- Requires health providers to evaluate and alleviate a child's physical, psychological and social distress
- Requires a multidisciplinary approach that includes the family and makes use of available community resources
- Can be provided in tertiary care facilities, in community health centres and in children's homes

(WHO 2004).

Overview of palliative care services

Founding of the UK palliative care movement is widely attributed to Dame Cicely Saunders who pioneered the palliative care approach with the opening of St Christopher's Hospice in 1967. However, it took a further two decades for palliative medicine to be recognized as a medical specialty.

The palliative care approach was developed in St Christopher's Hospice with the aim of providing care that was informed by research and was sensitive to the needs of individual patients. Since then, it has proliferated throughout the UK and it is now delivered in a variety of settings:

- Home
- Hospital
- Hospice.

Palliative care has been subdivided into general and specialist palliative care.

General palliative care

This is based on the principles of palliative care and should be a core skill of every clinician. It is widely referred to as 'the palliative care approach'. The aims are to promote both physical and psychosocial well-being and are a vital part of all clinical practice whatever the person's illness or its stage. It includes holistic consideration of the family and domestic carers rather than purely medical/physical aspects.

Specialist palliative care

Specialist palliative care teams are multidisciplinary, available to provide care and advice to general health practitioners in the hospital and community settings. Often, the support they provide transcends both these settings and may provide hospice and community specialist palliative care to complement the general care the patient is receiving.

Palliative care in hospitals

Despite evidence that the majority of terminally ill patients wish to die at home, most people die in an NHS hospital. Reasons for this include:

- The need for continuous nursing care for people requiring considerable physical help
- Increasing numbers of older people who live alone
- Requirement for complex symptom control.

Patients may be under the care of general physicians or surgeons and be nursed in general wards. The palliative care approach should be adopted in such cases and there are established hospital palliative care teams in the majority of UK hospitals.

Hospital palliative care teams are ideally multidisciplinary; however, some specialist nurses still work alone. The role of the MDT is to provide specialist advice and support for patients with complex palliative care needs and support and advice for general staff caring for the patient.

While many palliative care team members will have a background in cancer care, their remit extends to other diseases, e.g. heart failure. They provide advice on issues such as pain and symptom management, emotional support for the patient and family, advice and support to hospital staff and the primary care team, liaison with other palliative care services and bereavement care.

Hospice care

Hospice care developed largely from the work of charitable organizations such as Marie Curie Cancer Care, Sue Ryder and Macmillan Cancer Support. The services provided include:

- Hospice inpatient units
- Hospice beds within hospitals and nursing homes
- Hospice at home
- Day care
- Community palliative care team.

Although hospice in-patient units were initially set up to deal with the needs of patients suffering from terminal cancer, hospice services are increasingly being sought from patients with other terminal illnesses such as motor neurone disease. On the other hand, children's hospices have developed for the needs of a much broader range of diseases, as children most commonly die of degenerative disease (Katz 2008).

Patients are admitted to in-patient hospice care for a variety of reasons, including assessment, rehabilitation, pain and symptom management, short respite stays to help relieve carers and terminal care. The environment is more homely than hospitals, and centres on the individual patient's needs. Families are encouraged to be involved in care where appropriate and visiting tends to be open. Staff normally have access to specialized training and education in palliative care.

The main aim of hospice day care is to enhance the quality of life of the patient, as well as providing respite for relatives caring for the patient at home. The focus of care is on providing support and advice on pain and other distressing symptoms, as well as providing emotional support and rehabilitation, all of which may enable the patient to remain at home. Most day-care units run as multidisciplinary community services where the patient remains under the care of the GP. The role of healthcare professionals in the day-care unit therefore necessitates close liaison with the patient's GP and other members of the primary care team (see Ch. 3).

Hospice at home provides extra care and support to terminally ill patients in their own homes and offers support to relatives and carers. It supplements the services normally provided by district nurses. 'Hands-on' care and support are provided by a team of qualified nurses and auxiliary staff who provide most, if not all, of the nursing care that would be available in an inpatient hospice. This makes it possible for people to spend the last weeks or months of their illness in familiar surroundings, with their family and friends around them.

Marie Curie nurses care for around 50% of all people with cancer who die in their own homes (Marie Curie Cancer Care 2010). They provide free expert nursing care and emotional support to families affected by cancer and other terminal illnesses. They are available for periods during the day and night, which helps to reduce patient stress and anxiety (see Ch. 11) and gives carers the opportunity to rest or sleep.

Community palliative care team

A community palliative care team may consist of specialist palliative care nurses who visit patients and families in their own home, or they may be part of a bigger team such as those in a hospice. Increasingly, hospital and community are becoming more closely integrated and working across the boundaries.

Similar to the other palliative care services described above, the role of the community palliative care team includes providing support and advice on pain and other distressing symptoms, providing emotional support for the patient and their carers and also providing bereavement support. Charities such as Marie Curie Cancer Care and Macmillan Cancer Support have led the way in providing community-based support by providing nursing services.

Communicating with patients and families

Communication is central to high quality palliative care. Communication skills are often regarded as 'something nurses can do' (see Ch. 9). However, in palliative care, effective communication requires considerable knowledge and skill. Kinghorn (2001, p 167) states that 'effective and sensitive communication is the heart of comforting, assessment of need, expression of psychological/social/spiritual distress as planning for what may be perceived to be an undesirable and premature end to life'.

Speaking to dying patients and their families can often be difficult and uncomfortable and conversations focussed on prognosis are usually led by experienced clinicians. However, when involved in routine care of the dying patient it is important to acknowledge that awkwardness when dealing with advanced illness and death is universal, and nurses should not view inabilities as personal failings. However, it is the responsibility of nurses and other healthcare professionals to develop, refine and advance their communication skills. While it is necessary to understand theories of communication, reflecting upon clinical practice to reach new understandings is critical (Box 12.6).

Reflective practice   Box 12.6

Communication skills in palliative care

You may wish to arrange to observe an experienced colleague when they are talking with a dying patient and their relatives or you may already have had this experience.

Student activities

- What was positive and negative about the way the situation was handled?
- What skills and attributes of the clinician were important?

Care and symptom control

There is a variety of symptoms associated with terminal illness, e.g. pain. These are discussed below.

Managing pain in palliative care

Cancer is not synonymous with pain. The WHO suggests that up to 80% of patients with pain may have their pain adequately controlled by following a simple three-step approach to pain management:

- By the mouth – the oral route of administration should be used whenever possible
- By the clock – patients should be prescribed regular analgesia
- By the ladder – a three-step approach has been suggested by the WHO for managing cancer pain (World Health Organization 2005). If a drug fails to relieve pain, then a drug from the next step up the ladder should be used (see Fig. 23.10).

Evidence-based guidelines for the management of cancer-related pain suggest that assessment of pain is crucial to effective management (Scottish Intercollegiate Guidelines Network, SIGN 2008).

The principles of pain management in adults outlined above are equally applicable to children. Assessment of pain is crucial to effective management. Pain assessment self-report scales have been developed specifically for children such as the 'faces scale' (see Ch. 23).

The WHO pain ladder (see Ch. 23) can be used for managing pain in children. However, calculation of drug dosages is complex and should be calculated according to either the weight or the body surface area of the child depending upon the circumstances; in addition, there are average weight-for-age tables that suggest the percentage of the adult dose (Greenstein & Gould 2009).

Breathlessness

Breathlessness (dyspnoea) is an unpleasant and often frightening sensation of being unable to breathe easily (see Ch. 17). It is a very common symptom in patients with all types of terminal illness.

Some causes of breathlessness may be reversible and therefore, accurate assessment of the cause is vital. Reversible causes of breathlessness include:

- Infection
- Anaemia
- Pleural effusion (presence of fluid in the pleural cavity)
- Bronchospasm (spasm of the smooth muscle of the bronchi leading to bronchoconstriction and narrowing)
- Pulmonary embolism (clot in the blood supply to the lungs).

Hypoxia (reduced levels of oxygen in the tissues) may result from any of the above causes. Oxygen therapy is used for hypoxia.

Care of the breathless patient should be individualized and a multidisciplinary approach is essential. Advice from the physiotherapist is often particularly helpful on positioning patients in a bed or chair, control of breathing rate and relaxation methods (see Chs 10, 17). Breathlessness has both physical and psychological elements. Not being able to breathe easily can cause intense fear, which causes the patient and family to become anxious, and the physical symptom worsens. This cyclical pattern requires sensitive support and careful management. Explanation, reassurance and support can help reduce anxiety, along with relaxation techniques (see Chs 10, 11) and anxiolytic drugs, e.g. lorazepam.

Excess respiratory secretions

Excess respiratory secretions often become problematic within the last days or hours of life. The build-up of secretions in the airways is due to the patient's inability to cough up or swallow them. This presents as a noisy gurgle during breathing, often referred to as the 'death rattle', as it is associated with the terminal phase. The patient is usually in a state of altered consciousness at this stage and is not aware of the problem; however, it is particularly distressing for the family.

Careful positioning of the patient on their side may assist in relieving the problem for a short time. The registered nurse may carry out regular oral suctioning. Drugs such as hyoscine butylbromide may also be prescribed to reduce the secretions and hence the distressing sounds. These drugs, which also cause sedation, may be given by subcutaneous injection or via a syringe driver (see Chs 22, 23).

Fatigue

Fatigue is the most common symptom experienced by patients with advanced cancer. It is defined as 'a total body feeling ranging from tiredness to exhaustion, creating an unrelenting overall condition which interferes with an individual's ability to function to their normal capacity' (Ream & Richardson 1996, p 527). Fatigue is a difficult symptom to manage, as it is not merely corrected by rest. There are a number of physical and psychosocial causes of fatigue, some of which can be alleviated. They include:

- Physical factors:
  ○ Anaemia
  ○ Cancer treatments such as radiotherapy, chemotherapy
  ○ Cachexia (emaciation resulting from rapid weight loss, often seen in patients with gastrointestinal or lung cancers as a result of complex metabolic changes)
  ○ Toxic breakdown products from cancer cells
  ○ Coughing
  ○ Breathlessness.
- Psychosocial factors:
  ○ Inactivity
  ○ Insomnia (see Ch. 10)
  ○ Anxiety (see Ch. 11)
  ○ Depression.

Management of cancer-related fatigue is difficult and needs to be tailored to the needs of individual patients. Little research has been done in this area to support management strategies; however, reversible causes such as anaemia should be corrected. Some clinicians report an improvement in fatigue when patients are encouraged to do gentle exercise. It would appear that a balance between periods of rest and activity is the optimum for promoting well-being.

Nausea and vomiting

Patients may feel nauseated and retch for many hours before they vomit or they may not vomit but still suffer the unpleasant sensation of nausea. Nursing care such as ensuring easy access to vomit bowls, tissues and mouthwash, as well as ensuring privacy, can promote the patient's comfort (see Ch. 19). Avoidance of strong odours and food smells can also help to reduce nausea. There are many causes of nausea and vomiting in patients with advanced illness including:

- Drugs, e.g. opioids and chemotherapy
- Toxins
- Radiotherapy
- Constipation (see Ch. 21)
- Pain

- Hypercalcaemia (abnormally high level of calcium in the blood)
- Cough
- Anxiety
- Gastric (stomach) irritation, stasis, 'squashed stomach syndrome' or dilatation.

Some of the causes are reversible and treatment of nausea and vomiting depends very much on the cause. Reversible causes must be identified and treated appropriately through accurate assessment.

Vomiting is initiated and synchronized by two centres in the brain: the vomiting centre, which has overall control, and the chemoreceptor trigger zone (CTZ). Both centres respond to various stimuli (Fig. 12.1). The vomiting centre and CTZ contain receptors able to respond to different stimuli arriving from the cerebral cortex, the vestibular centre (impulses from inner ear and cerebellum) and the gastrointestinal tract depending on the cause of vomiting. The receptors include histamine receptors (H_1), acetylcholine receptors (ACh_m), dopamine receptors (D_2) and those for 5-hydroxytryptamine receptors (5-HT3).

Nurses need to know about the receptors because each type of antiemetic (against vomiting) drug acts in a different way (Table 12.1). Therefore, it is essential to use the appropriate antiemetic drug for the cause of the vomiting and this is usually based on the doctor's assessment. Nausea can be treated with oral drugs; however, alternative routes of administration must be used if the patient is vomiting, e.g. rectal, subcutaneous or intramuscular (see Ch. 22). It is important that the patient with nausea receives regular antiemetic drugs before vomiting occurs. When nausea and vomiting is anticipated, such as with some chemotherapy drugs, antiemetics should always be prescribed and given. (See Useful websites, p. 277, e.g. Palliativedrugs.com.)

Oral problems

Oral hygiene is very important for patients with terminal illness, especially when there is difficulty taking food and fluids or dehydration (see Chs 16, 19). The most common problems encountered are dry or sore mouth, oral thrush (candidiasis) and ulceration.

Constipation

Constipation is a significant problem for patients requiring palliative care and is a particularly distressing symptom. Constipation may also be the cause of other problems such as nausea and vomiting, abdominal pain and cramps, bloating, and faecal soiling and diarrhoea from faecal overflow.

Constipation may have a number of causes, e.g. opioid analgesics. This should be anticipated and a prophylactic laxative prescribed and administered. Immobility, inadequate food and fluid intake, as well as the patient's illness, may all be causes of constipation. As with all symptoms, accurate assessment is crucial to determine the cause of the constipation. The patient's normal bowel habit is recorded in order to assess how this has changed.

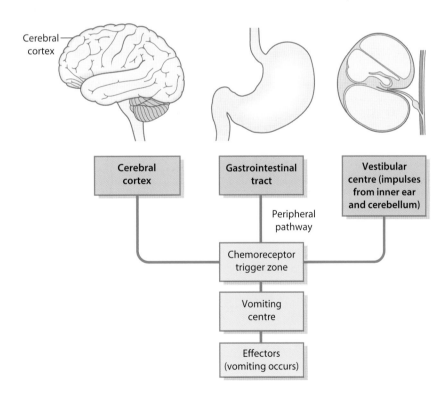

Fig. 12.1 • The vomiting reflex. (Reproduced with permission from Bruce, L., Finlay, T. (Eds.), 1997. Nursing in gastroenterology. Churchill Livingstone, Edinburgh.)

Table 12.1 Commonly used antiemetic drugs

Drug	Site of action	Cause of nausea and/or vomiting
Cyclizine	Acts centrally at the vomiting centre and in the vestibular centre of the inner or middle ear	Useful in managing the vomiting associated with raised intracranial (within the skull) pressure or motion
Haloperidol	Acts centrally at the CTZ	An effective antiemetic for chemical causes such as hypercalcaemia, renal failure or due to opioids
Metoclopramide/Domperidone	Principal site of action is peripherally in the gastrointestinal tract, where it acts by improving gastrointestinal motility	Used to treat motility problems such as gastric stasis or 'squashed stomach syndrome'. Action is blocked by the concurrent use of cyclizine
Levomepromazine	A broad-spectrum antiemetic that has activity at the vomiting centre, vestibular centre and CTZ	Useful in vomiting of uncertain or mixed origin and when other antiemetics have failed. Prescribed in low doses as an antiemetic. Due to its sedative properties is also prescribed in higher doses for terminal agitation at the end-of-life
Ondansetron and Granisetron	Acts centrally at the CTZ	Very effective in the vomiting associated with cancer chemotherapy. Very constipating so not recommended for routine use in palliative care

(Reproduced with permission from Brooker, C., Nicol, M. (Eds.), 2011. Alexander's nursing practice, fourth ed. Mosby, Edinburgh, on the companion website.)

Simple measures may help, such as ensuring privacy and acting promptly to requests for a commode or help to get to the lavatory. Interventions that prevent or alleviate constipation are discussed in Chapter 21. Ensuring adequate fibre and fluid intake where appropriate may help; however, with some patients, this will not be possible if their illness is advanced.

Terminal agitation

Terminal agitation or restlessness is common in patients in the terminal phase of the illness. At this time, the patient may become confused, agitated and may also be hallucinating (a perception of the presence of something which is not there). Care should be taken to identify any treatable causes such as unrelieved pain and constipation. Similarly, if the patient is clear in their thought processes, time should be spent trying to identify if the patient has unresolved issues, as fear and anxiety may exacerbate this symptom.

A quiet, calming environment with familiar surroundings or people known to the patient may help; however, it may be necessary to use sedation to resolve agitation and calm the patient. Opioids can have a sedative effect, although their use in this instance is not appropriate as they may induce further confusion and/or hallucinations. Sedative drugs such as haloperidol and/or midazolam can be administered either as subcutaneous injection or via a syringe driver in order to sedate and calm the patient.

Terminal agitation can be very distressing for relatives to watch; however, a simple and clear explanation as to the reasons for the confusion and the strategies used to try to alleviate it may be helpful in reducing their distress.

Death and dying

It has been identified that the palliative care approach is applicable in the early stages of chronic, non-curable illness. However, at the end-of-life, this is particularly appropriate as it promotes quality of life and comfort regardless of the stage of the illness. In this section, issues relating to death and dying are considered.

Death may result from trauma, or sudden or progressive illness, and nurses have a role in supporting patients and their family and friends during this time. Personal experiences of death vary and the cause, circumstances and support available influence how individuals experience death and dying. The nurse's actions at the time of death can profoundly affect bereavement, grief and adaptation to the loss. The circumstances surrounding death are unique to each individual and family; however, there are likely to be physical, psychosocial and spiritual needs and the requirement for open and honest information.

Sudden death

When a person dies suddenly, this is due to cerebral ischaemia (lack of blood flow to the brain). This can be caused by a stroke, heart attack, cardiac arrest or haemorrhage due to trauma.

Sudden death may result from an acute illness or trauma, accidents or suicide. When death is unexpected, the family and those closest to the deceased are likely to experience profound shock, numbness, disbelief and feelings of chaos and disorder. Sudden death due to accidents, suicide or other trauma is the main cause of death in young adults, particularly males, so meeting the needs of those closest to these patients is challenging (Box 12.7). (See Useful websites, p. 277, for information about sudden unexplained deaths occurring in infancy, e.g. Foundation for the Study of Infant Deaths, FSID).

 Critical thinking   Box 12.7

Sudden death due to suicide

Ben, who was 25 years old, suffered from severe depression. He committed suicide while a voluntary patient in a mental health unit.
    Discuss with your mentor the potential impact of Ben's death on his family and friends and the staff.

Student activities

Visit the Office for National Statistics website (www.ons.gov.uk/ons/rel/subnational-health4/suicides-in-the-united-kingdom/2010/stb-statistical-bulletin.html Released 2012) and find out:

- How many people commit suicide per 100 000 of the UK population.
- How suicide rates vary by age, gender and geographical location.

Crumbie (2007) suggests that grounding sudden death in reality is difficult as there is no preparation for the event. There are three important factors in helping people to cope with their loss: perception of the event, external resources and inner resources.

Perception of the event

People search for information to help attribute cause and seek an explanation for what has happened. Some people may be unable to cope with information immediately following the bereavement, so information giving should be tailored to meet individual needs (see Ch. 9, p. 211). Nurses should also consider where people get support and information once their contact with healthcare professionals has ceased.

External resources

It is important to establish what support is available for the bereaved person. Initially, support is likely to be provided by family and friends. It is therefore important that nurses identify who can be called upon to provide support, e.g. with transport home from the hospital if a close relative has died suddenly. Careful consideration must be given to what information should be given over the phone by the registered nurse who may not know the person and how they are likely to respond, especially if a relative is being asked to come to an emergency department. Dealing with sudden death is demanding and requires sophisticated communication skills (see Ch. 9). Knowing what to say and when is important and nurses need to discern what information to give the bereaved person who may be so shocked they cannot think what to ask.

For hospital-based staff, contact with people who experience the sudden death of a loved one may be limited. For many bereaved people, the full impact of their loss may not be apparent for some time following the death. Untimely, unexpected and traumatic deaths may cause severe and prolonged grieving.

It is therefore important for nurses to be aware of local resources and types of help available and to give this information to bereaved relatives, including information relevant to different faiths. One such source of support is Cruse Bereavement Care, which exists to promote the well-being of bereaved people and help them to understand their grief and cope with their loss (see Useful websites, p. 277).

Inner resources

Individual coping strategies help bereaved people deal with the crisis of sudden death and its aftermath. When a sudden, unexpected death occurs, there is usually no opportunity to be present at the time of death. This is thought to complicate the grieving process and how people cope with the bereavement. One of the most important issues in helping people to accept the reality of the death is knowledge of what happened at the end, and nurses can help (Box 12.8). Relatives may ask if the person suffered or what their last words were and registered nurses should not avoid giving this information or indeed any information they have. Rather than traumatizing relatives, as is often thought to be the case, it is likely that providing information will help them cope with the reality of the situation.

 Critical thinking   Box 12.8

Death of a child

Louisa, the eldest of three children, has recently been killed in a road traffic accident. Her parents are devastated and her mother cannot accept that Louisa is really dead. They have visited the mortuary many times to see Louisa and spend long periods of time there. They are increasingly distressed following each visit.

Student activities

- Consider why Louisa's mother needs to visit the mortuary repeatedly.
- Discuss with your mentor how staff could help Louisa's parents and younger siblings.

Viewing the body is also important in achieving understanding of the loss. Generally, even in traumatic death, relatives who view the dead person, especially if they were not present at the time of death, find this helpful (Wright 1996). Preparation of the bereaved for viewing a loved one is an important nursing role that can help to lessen the impact of seeing significant changes in body colour or trauma.

Expected death and palliative care

Gradual expected death occurs when there is failure of one or more organs and/or systems that maintain the internal environment of the cells (homeostasis). As the internal environment deteriorates, an increasing number of cells and tissues malfunction, leading to system failure. For example, when the respiratory system fails, hypoxia (reduction of oxygen in the tissues) and hypercapnia (increased carbon dioxide in arterial blood) will result in the failure of other organs including the heart and brain (see Ch. 17).

When death is anticipated and expected, patients and families experience profound and individual physical and emotional consequences. Dealing with these experiences is crucial to the process of accepting and responding to the situation. Whatever stage of acceptance and resolution individuals have reached as the end-of-life approaches, appropriate care around the time of death is arguably one of the most challenging and responsible aspects of the nursing role.

One of the issues for nurses involved in caring for patients approaching the end-of-life is that of advance care planning (DH 2008a; DH 2008b; Scottish Government 2008). Advance Care Planning (ACP) is the description for the process of discussing and planning ahead, e.g. in anticipation of some deterioration in a patient's condition (Gold Standards Framework 2011). Advance care planning therefore requires a sensitive attitude and ongoing discussion to explore the uncertain future faced by the patient and their family. Note that the use of advance decisions and advance statements are not the same as advance care planning (see Ch. 6).

Recognizing that death is approaching

Knowing when a patient is likely to die is usually very important for family members, some of whom will normally wish to be present at the time of death. For people of many faiths, it is especially important for the patient to have the next of kin present, as religious rituals must be performed to ensure the dying person passes on to the next life (see Table 12.2, p. 273). Families may ask if they should take a break from sitting at the bedside or when they should contact other family members who live at a distance. An important role of the nurse at the end-of-life is ensuring that family members are alerted to the imminence of death and have privacy to say their goodbyes and grieve. While it is not possible to predict exactly the last stages of life, there are recognized signs that death is imminent (adapted from National Council for Hospice and Specialist Palliative Care Services 1997). They include:

- Profound weakness – usually bed-bound requiring assistance with all care
- Gaunt physical appearance
- Drowsy or reduced cognition – may be disorientated, restless, have difficulty in concentrating and scarcely able to cooperate with carers
- Diminished intake of food and fluids
- Difficulty swallowing medications
- Breathing changes/excess secretions
- Incontinence
- Decreased urine output
- Cold extremities
- Cyanosis.

Causes of death and the need for palliative care

People die in their own home, in a hospital, hospice or a residential/nursing home. Increased life expectancy and the shift from infectious diseases to degenerative diseases such as cancer, heart disease or stroke as causes of death have meant that deaths are concentrated in old age. Many people facing death live alone and lack informal support.

Addington-Hall (1996) surveyed the symptoms experienced in the last year of life in three groups of patients: those with cancer, heart disease and stroke. Symptoms including pain, nausea and vomiting, etc. were prevalent in advanced cancer. People with heart disease had breathlessness and people dying from strokes experienced mental confusion and incontinence. Significantly, this survey revealed that while people with cancer experienced more symptoms, the duration was shorter than for the other two groups. Palliative care is frequently associated with cancer; however, policy directives indicate all patients with advanced, non-curable illness require access to palliative care.

Main causes of death in the UK

The UK population is ageing. The Office for National Statistics (2011a) report that 17% of the population were aged 65 and over in 2010; this was an increase from 15% in 1985. The result was an increase of 1.7 million in that age group. It is projected that 23% of the population will be aged 65 and over in 2035 (Office for National Statistics 2011a). Furthermore, the number of people aged 85 and over has increased to 1.4 million. These population trends correspond with life expectancy (the expectation of number of years of life at birth), which continues to improve. In addition, infant mortality rates continue to fall (Office for National Statistics 2011b).

In the year 2000, around 80% of deaths were of people over 65 years of age compared with 20% in 1901. However, improvement in life expectancy is accompanied by significant rises in the so-called degenerative diseases which can be linked to lifestyle factors such as cancers and cardiovascular diseases. Therefore, the correlation between life expectancy and healthy life expectancy is important, as evidence to date suggests that while life expectancy is increasing, healthy life expectancy is not, and the 'burden of disability' towards the end-of-life is increasing. Cardiovascular diseases and cancer are significant causes of death of adults in the UK, USA and most European countries (Box 12.9). These trends are predicted to continue due to increasingly sedentary lifestyles, obesity, smoking and diets high in saturated fats.

 Critical thinking   **Box 12.9**

Causes of death

Select a cause of death relevant to your chosen field, e.g. suicide/injury undetermined deaths, sudden unexplained deaths occurring in infancy, childhood cancer, maternal deaths or alcohol-related deaths.

Student activities

- Discuss with your mentor where you can access the relevant information, e.g. Office for National Statistics www.statistics.gov.uk
- Find out the number of deaths from your chosen cause in your part of the UK.

Table 12.2 Religious practices around the time of death

Faith	As death approaches	When death is imminent	Immediately after death
Buddhism	Dying person needs opportunities to meditate. A monk or religious teacher should visit the dying person to talk and chant passages of scripture	The ideal is to die in a fully conscious and calm state. A monk or fellow Buddhist may chant to encourage a peaceful state of mind	No special requirements relating to care of the body. Buddhists from different countries will have different traditions
Christianity	Some Christians may want prayers or anointing with oil by a minister or priest	As appropriate, a priest or minister should be notified. Some Christians will wish to receive communion or the last rites.	No special requirements
Hinduism	Hindus may receive comfort from hymns and readings from the Hindu holy books. Some patients may wish to lie on the floor. The family should be present	A Hindu priest may be called to perform holy rites. A dying Hindu should be given Ganges water and the sacred Tulsi leaf placed in the mouth by the relatives. A person should die with the name of God being recited. Hindus often wish to die at home	The family will normally wash the body themselves. If no family member is available, health workers should wear gloves, close the deceased's eyes and straighten the limbs. Jewellery and religious objects should not be removed
Humanism	No special requirements	Needs and preferences of the patient should be agreed and met	No special requirements. Work with patient and family preferences
Islam	Other Muslims, normally family members, join the dying person in prayer and recite verses from the *Quran*. Dying person may wish to face Mecca (south-east in the UK)	The declaration of faith (Shahada) is said	Non-Muslim health workers should ask permission to touch the body and use disposable gloves. The body must be kept covered. Soon after death there is a ritual of washing the body by same sex Muslims. Post-mortems are disliked
Judaism	A rabbi may be called to join the dying Jew in prayer and facilitate confession	The dying person should not be left alone. Jews present will recite psalms and, when death occurs, the Declaration of Faith (Shema)	Health workers should handle the body as little as possible and cover with a white sheet. The Jewish burial society will collect the body and perform a ritual wash before burial. Post-mortems are disliked
Sikhism	A dying Sikh may receive comfort from reciting hymns, a relative or any practising Sikh may do so instead.	A Sikh person should die in the name of God, Waheguru being recited. Some may want to have holy water (Amrit) in the mouth	Health workers should not trim hair or beards and the body should be covered with a plain white cloth. The five symbols of faith should not be removed from the body: • Kesh – uncut hair • Kangha – a comb which keeps the hair bun or jura in place • Kara – steel bangle worn on the left wrist • Kirpan – symbolic dagger worn under clothes • Kaccha – special underpants or shorts

(Adapted from the Open University, 1992. Religious practices wall chart. The Open University, Department of Health and Social Welfare, Milton Keynes.)

Death states

Death may be sudden due to accident or illness, or be 'expected', e.g. when a patient has an advanced non-curable illness such as chronic respiratory disease, cardiovascular disease or cancer.

Death as a process begins with the failure of a body system, which then affects other systems (see above). Medical interventions, which can keep people alive even when vital functions have been lost, have created difficulties in deciding when a person can be declared 'dead'. This is particularly so when brain function is lost and a person's body may continue to function or be supported on a ventilator/respirator. Distinctions are normally made between three states:

- *Permanent vegetative state (PVS)*: The cerebral cortex is irreversibly damaged but the vital centres in the brain stem remain intact so breathing occurs spontaneously, the heart beats and blood circulates. The person's eyes may open and reflexes remain intact, which can make it difficult for relatives to accept that recovery is impossible. Brain cells are extremely sensitive to hypoxia and irreversible damage occurs if the blood supply is interrupted for 2–4 minutes.
- *Brain stem death*: If the brain stem is irreversibly damaged, the patient will be deeply comatosed and breathing will cease unless artificial ventilation is used to maintain life. Brain stem death is confirmed by a series of tests performed on more than one occasion.
- *Certified death*: Once circulatory and respiratory function have permanently ceased, a person can be legally certified as dead (see p. 275).

Care around the time of death

Whether a patient dies suddenly or the death is expected, the actions of those involved in caring for the patient and family are of utmost importance. Care that meets the needs of individuals around the time of death has been shown to impact on how well they cope following bereavement. Providing care when a patient reaches the last stages of life is an important nursing role. Regardless of the clinical area, nurses are likely to care for people who are dying. All nurses therefore require appropriate knowledge to inform care planning.

The Macmillan Gold Standards Framework (GSF) is designed to offer guidance to primary healthcare teams to improve the planning of palliative care so they can meet the needs of patients and carers. While designed for primary care, the seven principles of the GSF provide guidance for nurses involved in caring for dying patients regardless of the clinical setting. Box 12.10 outlines a framework for care.

A framework for palliative care, dying and death	Box 12.10

Communication

- The patient (if able) and carers should participate in decision-making about care
- Time and opportunities should be given for patients and relatives to seek and be given information
- Instructions should be written down and contact numbers given/obtained.

Coordination

- Effective care requires a collaborative approach using palliative care specialists as required, e.g.:
  - Clinical nurse specialists
  - Marie Curie and Macmillan nurses
  - Palliative medicine consultants
  - Hospice/hospital palliative care teams
  - Community physiotherapists and occupational therapists
  - Social workers and counsellors
  - Spiritual advisors
- A primary nurse in a hospice/hospital or a lead district nurse if the patient is at home should coordinate nursing care and collaborate with other team members involved.

Control of symptoms (see pp. 267–270)

- Each patient should have their symptoms, problems and concerns (physical, psychological, social, practical and spiritual) assessed, recorded, discussed and acted upon in accordance with their agenda
- In the last days/hours of life, only medications that control or prevent distressing symptoms should be given. Generally, the only drugs needed in the final stages of life are:
  - Analgesics (usually subcutaneous via a syringe driver)
  - Anticonvulsants
  - Hyoscine for 'rattle'
  - Tranquillizers.

Continuity

- Regardless of where the patient is located, care should be seamless and healthcare professionals should ensure information is transferred, e.g. to out-of-hours service or hospice.

Continued learning

- All healthcare professionals must be committed to continued learning to ensure optimum care for patients and carers and know how to access and appraise evidence on which to base practice.

Carer support

- Emotional support – carers need support, to be listened to and kept informed. They should be encouraged to participate in care as appropriate and in accordance with the wishes of the patient
- Practical support – if the patient is at home, practical support such as night sitters, respite care and equipment, e.g. commodes, should be provided
- Bereavement information about sources of support/counselling should be provided
- Staff support – professional carers need support as caring for dying patients is challenging and emotionally draining. Reflection and clinical supervision are some of the methods by which nurses may receive support (see Ch. 11).

Care of the dying

- Caring for patients in the last days or hours of life requires particular interventions:
  - Stopping non-essential interventions, e.g. wound dressings and drugs, if this would cause considerable discomfort
  - Considering comfort measures
  - Psychological and religious/spiritual support
  - Bereavement planning
  - Communication
  - Care after death.

(Adapted from National Council for Hospice and Specialist Palliative Care Services 1997 and Thomas 2004.)

The Liverpool Care Pathway (LCP) is an integrated care pathway that is used to improve quality of the end-of-life care and the experience of dying in the last hours and days of life. The LCP has been implemented into hospitals, care homes, in the individual's own home/community and into hospices. The LCP is recommended as a best practice model by the Department of Health (DH 2009). (See Useful websites, p. 277, for further information about the LCP.)

Providing support and information around the time of death is important, particularly where a patient may be classified as being either brain stem dead or in a PVS. Tactful handling is required at a time when nurses may be struggling with their own feelings (Box 12.11). Many relatives may not have seen a dead person before so preparation and gentle explanation are necessary.

 Reflective practice   Box 12.11

Personal experience of death

If you have experienced the death of someone close to you, reflect on the things others said or did, both helpful and unhelpful. If you have not experienced the death of someone close, think what might be helpful.

Student activities

- Discuss the helpful things with your mentor or another experienced nurse.

In recent years, several attempts to change the law regarding physician-assisted suicide have been made both within the UK and Scottish parliaments. To date, the law remains unchanged and assisted suicide is a criminal act, however this is an issue which is gaining increasing support from some sections of society (see Ch. 6).

Cultural aspects of dying and death

If nurses are to provide appropriate care at the end-of-life they must understand and meet the spiritual and cultural needs of individuals. Different cultures and societies approach death and grieving differently and nurses need to communicate with patients and families to establish what their needs and wishes are and ensure particular requests are communicated among the MDT. Nurses should establish if patients have any religious beliefs, as some patients may not have a belief or faith. They may, however, have requests for care around the time of death, e.g. humanists who neither believe in a God nor an afterlife but celebrate the life that has been (see Useful websites, p. 277). Table 12.2 provides an overview of religious practices around the time of death.

Caring for people who are dying or bereaved requires knowledge of specific cultural and religious rituals in order to provide culturally aware care. Nurses need to know when and who to contact from the person's own culture or religion to ensure traditional practices are followed and the patient's wishes are met. The best way to ensure appropriate end-of-life care is to take sufficient time to explore and assess the wishes and needs of the patient and family. Integration of cultural issues into care

assessments and care planning is crucial, as is the communication between team members (see Ch. 9). If the patient's needs are carefully assessed, documented and communicated among team members, the experience of dying will significantly improve for those involved (Box 12.12).

 Reflective practice   Box 12.12

Meeting cultural and spiritual needs

In your current/next clinical placement, find out how cultural issues are addressed.

Student activities

Find out if:

- There is access to information about death and dying practices for different groups.
- There are established links with local religious/spiritual leaders.
- Cultural issues and wishes are ascertained, recorded and communicated within the healthcare team.
- Patients/families are able to adhere to cultural/spiritual practices, e.g. fasting times.

Resource

Neuberger, J., 2004. Caring for dying people of different faiths, third ed. Radcliffe Medical Press, Oxon.

 Ethical issues   Box 12.13

Hydration at the end-of-life

The provision of nutrition and hydration is a part of the nursing role and failing to meet these needs may be seen as practice falling short of the standards of the Nursing and Midwifery Council. However, in palliative care, the beneficial effects of hydration are inconclusive and hydration may not be essential for comfort in the last stages and may even cause discomfort by increasing respiratory secretions and urinary output.

The psychological and emotional aspects of hydration must be considered alongside the physiological effects when active hydration is considered as part of care. Deciding whether it is acting in the patient's best interests is complex and requires regular review of the evidence to support clinical decisions, the patient's condition, prognosis and wishes of the patient and the family.

Student activities

- Consider the perspectives of the patient, family and professional staff.
- Discuss with your mentor the issues relating to hydration at the end-of-life.

Resource

Nursing and Midwifery Council, 2008. The code: Standards of conduct, performance and ethics for nurses and midwives. Online. Available: http://www.nmc.uk.org/Publications/Standards/The-code/Introduction/ September 2012.

Royal College of Physicians (RCP) British Society of Gastroenterology, 2010. Oral feeding difficulties and dilemmas. Online. Available: http://bookshop.rcplondon.ac.uk/details.aspx?e=295 October 2012.

Nursing skills Box 12.14

The final act of care/last offices

- Wear appropriate protective clothing for the prevention and control of infection (see Ch. 15). In some circumstances, such as patients with HIV/AIDS, full last offices are not carried out in the ward area. The body is usually labelled, e.g. 'danger of infection', and transported to the mortuary sealed in a protective body bag. The mortuary and undertakers are always informed about the presence of infections. Check local protocols regarding the use of infection labels and body bags
- Insert the person's dentures and use a rolled up towel under the chin to keep the mouth shut prior to the onset of rigor mortis (this should be removed before the family visit)
- Wash the body as necessary and ensure the body is labelled with the patient's details, according to local guidelines
- Remove all intravenous infusions, urinary catheters (drain urine prior to removal), drains, etc. unless the death is associated with a serious accident or suspicious circumstances and is to be reported to the Procurator Fiscal or Coroner. In these instances, all drains etc. are left in place
- Dress the body in a clean gown or pyjamas – consult the family about this. When a child dies they may have chosen a favourite outfit to be worn
- Brush and comb the hair and shave the face if required (if this was their normal preference)

- Ensure removal, recording and safekeeping of jewellery according to local guidelines (checking this is in accordance with the wishes and beliefs of the patient and/or family)
- Cover the body to the shoulders with a clean sheet
- Tidy the area around the bed, removing unnecessary equipment and charts
- Organize chairs around the bed for family members
- Allow the family as much time as they need to say their goodbyes
- Stay with the family to offer support as needed, although you should establish if they want time alone
- Discuss with the family the arrangements for collecting belongings and official documents
- Provide information about local undertakers or other services families may find useful, e.g. Cruse Bereavement Care (see Useful websites, p. 277)
- If a post-mortem is required, this must be explained carefully and sensitively to the family by a registered nurse or a doctor
- Provide information for relatives about registering the death
- Provide the appropriate information, e.g. What to do after a death (Box 12.15)
- Aftercare for family/friends – identify follow-up care and support
- Care of health professionals and other carers. Support systems should be identified and used.

End-of-life ethical issues

Ethical issues at the end-of-life are complex and require careful consideration. Although students are not responsible for making care decisions at the end-of-life, they will be exposed to ethical issues and may contribute to debating issues and plans of care. Decision-making in palliative care is governed by the ethical principles of respect of autonomy, beneficence, nonmaleficence and justice (see Ch. 7).

At the end-of-life, there are numerous issues that present ethical dilemmas for those involved. These include:

- Active nutrition and hydration (Box 12.13; see also Ch. 19)
- Decisions about whether to resuscitate or not (see Ch. 6)
- Extraordinary versus futile treatments
- Withholding and withdrawing treatments (see Ch. 6)
- Hastening death.

Care after death

Certification of death is a legal requirement normally carried out by a doctor. After death, the patient is referred to as 'the body'. The body should receive care – known as 'laying out or last offices or last act of care' – as soon as possible to minimize tissue damage or disfigurement (Box 12.14). If the patient has died at home, the undertaker/funeral director or family is likely to attend to the laying out of the body.

It is important to check with the family as some cultures and faiths have important rituals about how the body is treated

 Critical thinking Box 12.15

What to do after a death

Think about the type and presentation of information needed by family or friends after a death.

Student activities

- Access the relevant information from the websites below.
- Find some information provided by an organization such as Cruse (see Useful websites, below).
- Find out what information is used locally.
- Discuss the different forms of information with your mentor. Think how these may need adaptation if the bereaved person has a learning disability.

Resource

What to do after a death – www.direct.gov.uk/en/ Governmentcitizensandrights/Death/WhatToDoAfterADeath/ index.htm
What to do after a death in Scotland – www.scotland.gov.uk/ Publications/2009/06/24094516/1
Websites accessed September 2012.

after death (see Table 12.2). The family should be asked if they wish to be involved, as many people find it helpful to accept the reality of the death if they are involved in a final act of care.

SUMMARY

- Holistic care at the end-of-life is multidimensional and multiprofessional in focus and embraces the needs of patients and those closest to them.
- Palliative care as an approach is applicable at all stages of the illness journey.
- Nursing care aims to manage physical and psychological needs and difficult symptoms, and involves helping the person and family adapt to, and cope with, the resulting role and lifestyle changes.
- Patients requiring palliative care are cared for in most healthcare settings so all healthcare professionals involved need knowledge of the palliative care approach.
- Caring for individuals who are dying and their families is a challenging, but rewarding, aspect of nursing care.
- Nursing care of the bereaved person is aimed at moving towards accepting the reality and adapting to life.
- Effective communication is central to high quality palliative care.
- Perhaps the most important nursing role is that of 'being alongside' or 'being a companion' to those who are dying and providing comfort for their family.

KEY WORDS AND PHRASES FOR LITERATURE SEARCHING

Bereavement

Death

Dying

Loss

Pain management

Palliative care

Quality of life

Symptom management

Useful websites

British Humanist Association www.humanism.org.uk/site/cms

Cancer Research UK www.cancerresearchuk.org

Childhood Bereavement Network www.childhoodbereavementnetwork.org.uk/index.htm

Cruse Bereavement Care www.crusebereavementcare.org.uk

Foundation for the Study of Infant Deaths (FSID) http://fsid.org.uk

Gold Standards Framework www.goldstandardsframework.nhs.uk

Help the Hospices www.hospiceinformation.info

Liverpool Care Pathway (LCP) www.liv.ac.uk/mcpcil/liverpool-care-pathway

Macmillan Cancer Support www.macmillan.org.uk

Marie Curie Cancer Care www.mariecurie.org.uk

National Council for Palliative Care (NCPC) (many useful publications) www.ncpc.org.uk

Palliativedrugs.com www.palliativedrugs.com/palliative-care-formulary.html

NHS End-of-Life Care Programme (NEoLCP) www.endoflifecareforadults.nhs.uk

Scottish Partnership for Palliative Care www.palliativecarescotland.org.uk

Winston's Wish – For grieving children and their families www.winstonswish.org.uk

All websites accessed September 2012.

References

Addington-Hall, J., 1996. Heart disease and stroke: lessons from cancer care. In: Ford, G., Lewin, I. (Eds.), Managing terminal illness. Royal College of Physicians, London.

Bennett, D., 2003. Death and people with learning disabilities: empowering carers. British Journal of Learning Disabilities 31 (3), 118–122.

Crumbie, A., 2007. Death, grief and loss. In: Walsh, M., Crumbie, A. (Eds.), Watson's clinical nursing and related sciences, seventh ed. Baillière Tindall, Edinburgh.

Department of Health, 2008a. End of life care strategy: promoting high quality care for all adults at the end of life. Online. Available: www.dh.gov.uk/en/Publicationsandstatistics/Publications/PublicationsPolicyAndGuidance/DH_086277 September 2012.

Department of Health, 2008b. Advance care planning: a guide for health and social care staff. Online. Available: www.endoflifecareforadults.nhs.uk/assets/downloads/pubs_Advance_Care_Planning_guide.pdf September 2012.

Department of Health, 2009. End of life care strategy: quality markers and measures for end of life. Online. Available: www.dh.gov.uk/en/Publicationsandstatistics/Publications/PublicationsPolicyAndGuidance/DH_101681 September 2012.

Dodd, P.C., Guerin, S., 2009. Grief and bereavement in people with intellectual disabilities. Current Opinions in Psychiatry 22 (5), 442–446.

Greenstein, B., Gould, D., 2009. Trounce's clinical pharmacology for nurses, eighteenth ed. Churchill Livingstone, Edinburgh.

Gold Standards Framework, 2011. Advance care planning. Online. Available: www.goldstandardsframework.org.uk/AdvanceCarePlanning/ACPandGSF September 2012.

Hanks, G., Cherny, N.I., Christakis, N.A., et al. (Eds.), 2009. Oxford textbook of palliative medicine, fourth ed. Oxford University Press, Oxford.

Hollins, S., Esterhuyzen, A., 1997. Bereavement and grief in adults with learning disabilities. British Journal of Psychiatry 170, 497–501.

James, N., 1989. Emotional labour: skill and work in the social regulation of feelings. The Sociological Review 37 (1), 15–42.

Katz, J.S., 2008. Palliative care in institutions. In: Payne, S., Seymour, J., Ingleton, C. (Eds.), Palliative care nursing: principles and evidence for practice, second ed. Open University Press, Buckingham.

Kinghorn, S., 2001. Communication in advanced illness: challenges and opportunities. In: Kinghorn, S., Gamlin, R. (Eds.), Palliative nursing. Bringing comfort and hope. Baillière Tindall, Edinburgh.

Kubler-Ross, E., 1969. On death and dying. Macmillan, New York.

Lindemann, E., 1944. Symptomatology and management of acute grief. American Journal of Psychiatry 101, 141–148.

Lockhart-Wood, K., 2001. Nurse-doctor collaboration in cancer pain management. International Journal of Palliative Nursing 7 (1), 6–16.

Marie Curie Cancer Care, 2010. Our services. Marie Curie nurses. Online. Available:

www.mariecurie.org.uk/en-gb/who-we-are/services/ September 2012.

National Council for Hospice and Specialist Palliative Care Services (now The National Council for Palliative Care, NCPC), 1997. Changing gear – guidelines for managing the last days of life in cancer. NCPC, London.

Office for National Statistics, 2011a. Ageing. Fastest increase in the 'oldest old'. ONS, Newport.

Office for National Statistics, 2011b. Infant mortality. ONS, Newport.

Open University, 1992. Religious practices wall chart. The Open University, Department of Health and Social Welfare, Milton Keynes.

Parkes, C.M., 1998. Coping; with loss: bereavement in adult life. British Medical Journal 316 (7134), 856–859.

Parkes, C.M., Weiss, R.S., 1983. Recovery from bereavement. Basic Books, New York.

Payne, S., 2008. Overview. In: Payne, S., Seymour, J., Ingleton, C. (Eds.), Palliative care nursing: principles and evidence for practice, second ed. Open University Press, Buckingham.

Ream, E., Richardson, A., 1996. Fatigue: a concept analysis. International Journal of Nursing Studies 33 (5), 519–529.

Scottish Government, 2008. Living and dying well: A national action plan for palliative and end of life care in Scotland. Online. Available: www.scotland.gov.uk/Resource/Doc/239823/0066155.pdf September 2012.

Scottish Intercollegiate Guidelines Network, 2008. Control of pain in adults with cancer. SIGN 106. Online. Available: www.sign.ac.uk/ September 2012.

Skilbeck, J., Payne, S., 2003. Emotional support and the role of clinical nurse specialists in palliative care. Journal of Advance Nursing 43 (5), 521–530.

Stroebe, M.S., Hansson, R.O., Stroebe, W., et al., 2002. Handbook of bereavement research: consequences, coping and care. American Psychological Association, Washington, DC.

Thomas, K., 2004. Caring for the dying at home. Radcliffe Medical Press, Oxon.

Worden, J.W., 1991. Grief counselling and grief therapy. Tavistock/Routledge, London.

World Health Organization, 2004. WHO definition of palliative care. Online. Available: www.who.int/cancer/palliative/definition/en September 2012.

World Health Organization, 2005. WHO's pain ladder. Online. Available: www.who.int/cancer/palliative/painladder/en September 2012.

Wright, B., 1996. Sudden death – a research base for practice. Churchill Livingstone, Edinburgh.

Further reading

Department of Health, 2006. Help is at hand. A resource for people bereaved by suicide and other sudden, traumatic death. Online. Available: www.dh.gov.uk/assetRoot/04/13/90/07/04139007.pdf September 2012.

Department of Health, 2011. National End of Life Care Programme, Improving end of life care. Route to success: the key contribution of nursing to end of life care. Online. Available: www.endoflifecareforadults.nhs.uk/assets/downloads/RTS_Nursing_final_web_version_20110701.pdf September 2012.

Diamond, J., 1998. C: Because cowards get cancer too... Vermillion, London.

Dickenson, D., Johnson, M., Katz, J.S., 2000. Death, dying and bereavement. Open University Press, London.

Ellershaw, J., Wilkinson, S., 2003. Care of the dying. A pathway to excellence. Oxford University Press, Oxford.

Faull, C., Carter, Y., Daniels, L., 2005. Handbook of palliative care, second ed. Blackwell, Oxford.

Gordon, T., 2001. A need for living. Wild Goose, Glasgow.

Holland, K., Hogg, C., 2010. Cultural awareness in nursing and health care, second ed. Arnold, London.

Kennedy, C., 2003. Death and dying. In: Kindlen, S. (Ed.), Physiology for health care and nursing, second ed. Churchill Livingstone, Edinburgh.

Lugton, J., McIntyre, R., 2006. Palliative care: the nursing role, second ed. Churchill Livingstone, Edinburgh.

National Institute for Health and Clinical Excellence, 2011. End of life care for adults quality standard (QS 13). Online. Available: http://publications.nice.org.uk/quality-standard-for-end-of-life-care-for-adults-qs13 August 2012.

Nicol, M., Bavin, C., Cronin, P., et al, 2012. Essential nursing skills, fourth ed. Mosby, Edinburgh.

Picardie, R., 1998. Before I say goodbye. Penguin, London.

Section 4

Developing person-centred nursing skills

Safety in nursing practice

13

Emma Briggs

LEARNING OUTCOMES

This chapter will help you:

- Discuss the importance of health and safety for practitioners and individuals receiving care
- Describe the role of risk assessment in harm reduction and identify common potential or actual risks in a clinical area
- Outline the legislation in place to maintain safety and prevent accidents
- Identify the main nursing considerations in relation to standard infection control precautions (for detail, see Ch. 15), managing aggression, fire safety and principles of moving and handling (for detail, see Ch. 18)
- Describe the principles of first aid and the action required for burns and poisoning.

Introduction

The International Council of Nurses (2010) describes the nursing role as promoting health, preventing illness or caring for ill, disabled or dying people, along with acting as an advocate and promoting a safe environment. An individual's health and their safety are very closely linked, and a fundamental part of nursing care is to identify factors that influence a person's safety. This may include actual factors, e.g. being unable to drink that has led to dehydration and confusion in an older adult, or potential hazards, e.g. if a toddler is given a very small toy, they are at risk of choking.

Healthcare practitioners have a responsibility to look after their own safety and that of the people they work with and care for. Many issues have the potential to affect everyone in a care setting, e.g. poor handling techniques could result in an injury to the patient/client, yourself and/or a colleague. Health and safety is also essential to maintain standards and promote improvements in the quality of patient care as part of clinical governance within the NHS (Ch. 3). Therefore, this chapter emphasizes the health and well-being of everyone concerned through prevention, identifying the risks and eliminating or minimizing them through safe practice. This is achieved by exploring:

- The process of risk assessment
- The legislation in place to maintain safety
- The principles of moving and handling
- Standard infection control precautions
- First aid
- Preventing and managing violence and aggression
- Fire safety.

This chapter explores the fundamental aspects of nursing practice, which are also identified within the Nursing and Midwifery Council's Essential skills clusters (NMC 2010a). These require nursing students to be competent in a range of safety issues, be able to enhance the safety of service users and, identify and actively manage risk and uncertainty in relation to people, the environment, self and others (NMC 2010a, p 19).

Subsequent chapters address harm reduction further, e.g. infection control (Ch. 15), safe administration of medicines (Ch. 22), patient assessment (Ch. 14) and nursing care. These are all elements of safe practice and require further reading to aid your development and understanding. Additionally, a safe practitioner is able to identify and minimize hazards for patients/clients and this requires a number of other qualities and skills. These are highlighted below and their development is encouraged throughout this chapter, while addressing diverse safety topics in order to help you to become a safe practitioner.

A critical or questioning approach

This means that you will ask if something is unclear, or tactfully challenge practice. It is important to develop the confidence to speak up if you do not understand or you think safety may be compromised. It is possible to discuss such concerns with mentors, senior clinical staff or university teaching staff, depending on the situation.

Recognize limitations of knowledge and skills, and seek support

Self-awareness is an essential skill for all nurses and knowing the limitations of your knowledge and clinical skills means that you are less likely to try something beyond your capabilities (which may go wrong). Where you are unsure, always seek support from mentors, read around the topic and speak to teaching staff if necessary.

Evidence-based practice

Nursing practice should be based on interventions that are known to be safe, effective and informed by research findings (see Ch. 5), clinical expertise and the patient's/client's own wishes.

Use of reflection during and after practice situations

Reflection (Ch. 4) is a valuable learning tool which helps to make sense of situations, apply the theory behind a topic, highlight the positive points and identify areas for future action. You should now complete the exercise in Box 13.1 to explore the relationships between nursing, health and safety.

 Reflective practice   **Box 13.1**

Relationships between nursing, health and safety
Student activity

Take a piece of paper and on the left-hand side, write down the main activities nurses do in everyday practice. On the right hand side, write down how this helps the person's health and reduces harm (and is therefore concerned with their safety). The example below should help you to start:

Nursing activity	How this improves health and maintains safety
Helping someone to eat and drink	Provides energy and nutrients for daily life and recovery
	Prevents malnutrition and health deteriorating
	Able to go home more quickly, maintains independence

Risk assessment

Risks are taken in our everyday lives: some result in positive gains such as winning a lottery; others have negative outcomes, e.g. taking part in a contact sport can result in injury. Risks are also managed regularly to reduce the likelihood of negative outcomes occurring, e.g. wearing seatbelts and having airbags decrease the risk of injury in the event of a car accident.

In clinical practice, there are many potential and actual hazards that can cause harm to patients/clients and staff. Nurses need to identify hazards and reduce the likelihood of harm occurring. This may be as simple as mopping up water on the floor to stop people slipping or more complex, such as using an electric hoist to help clients who cannot stand to transfer from the bed to a chair safely. Much of nursing practice focuses on helping people to remain safe and this section explores the way in which risks are identified and reduced to minimize potential harm. The principles of risk assessment are discussed here, illustrating common issues across all fields of nursing practice. However, people receiving care may have unique health issues and require an individual assessment (see p. 283).

Risk assessment principles

A hazard has been defined by the Health and Safety Executive (HSE 2006a, p 2) as 'anything that can cause harm, e.g. chemicals, electricity, working from ladders' and a risk as 'the chance, high or low, that somebody will be harmed by the hazard'. It is important to understand the relationship between hazards and risks. A lightning strike presents a serious hazard that can result in death but the risk, or likelihood, of it happening to an individual in their lifetime is very small. Even when you know what the hazards and risks are, other factors can increase or decrease a risk. Going out into wide, open spaces during a thunderstorm may increase the risk of being struck by lightning. When drawing up or giving injections, needles are never re-sheathed because of the potential hazard of a needlestick injury and transmission of blood-borne viruses, e.g. hepatitis B, human immunodeficiency virus (HIV) (see Ch. 15). The risk of a needlestick injury is greatly reduced if nurses adhere to clinical guidelines, but lack of knowledge or understanding about the importance of this increases the risk of an injury. Before reading the rest of this section, complete the activity in Box 13.2.

? **Critical thinking**   **Box 13.2**

Hazards that can cause accidents
Student activities:

Examine a kitchen or bathroom in your placement.

Identify:

- What accidents could happen in the area.
- Potential causes of accidents (hazards) and who could be harmed.
- Any information displayed warning staff of hazards.
- Measures in place to reduce the likelihood of accidents, e.g. temperature controls on hot water taps of baths, or equipment available if an accident occurs, e.g. fire blankets.

It may not be possible to eliminate risks completely but by identifying the hazard, risk and associated factors, the chances of harm occurring can be minimized. This process is called risk management and the first stage is known as risk assessment. There are several reasons why risk assessments are undertaken, including patient/client welfare and ethical and professional responsibilities, including a duty of care to protect vulnerable

Risk assessment in nursing settings — Box 13.3

Step 1: Look for the hazard

- Ward B2 is a surgical ward with four single cubicle toilets. Recently, two patients have fallen in the toilet area and a risk assessment was requested to identify factors contributing to the falls. It was noted that one toilet cubicle was small, the toilet seat low and there were no grab rails for patients to use. The floor was also slippery when wet. This represents a hazard for both patients and staff.

- Sunshine Hospice cares for a range of children and young adults with life-limiting conditions and their families, providing respite, palliative or terminal care. The risk assessment examined three rooms built for toddlers and their families. The cots are at a fixed height (do not move up and down for taller and shorter carers) and on one, the cot side is broken. This is a hazard to any child and all cots pose a risk for parents and staff who have to lean over them to care for children.

- The Richard Smith Education Centre is a school for children and young adults (4–17 years) with learning disabilities and the pupils have a range of abilities and needs in terms of health and social care. The risk assessment is taking place in the new multisensory relaxation room – a room with fibreoptic lights, music and soft furnishings, a technique also known as Snoezelen (see Ch. 11). Children with severe learning disabilities will be regularly transferred from their wheelchairs to the floor to engage in activities. There is currently no equipment to help carers transfer the children who may therefore be tempted to lift them.

- Rosehill House is a residential facility for older adults experiencing mental health problems, including dementia. The largest bathroom on the first floor is the most frequently used by staff helping clients to bathe because of the space available. The bath is fitted to the back wall and floor on the left-hand side, and clients have to climb into and out of the bath themselves. Staff have expressed concerns about clients getting into and out of the bath safely, particularly if there is an emergency and they need to get the client out quickly. There is currently no equipment available.

Critical thinking — Box 13.4

Risk assessment

Step 2: Decide who may be harmed and how

Student activities

For each setting in Box 13.3 identify:

- Who may be harmed? Think about the physical and emotional effects.
- How may this occur? What has caused the accident?

The example from Sunshine Hospice is given below to start you off.

Who is at risk of being harmed?

- Any child is at risk of physical injury if placed in the broken cot. This would cause severe distress and pain to the child, the parents and staff
- Fixed height cots mean that staff and parents are at risk of injuring themselves.

How may they be harmed?

- A child in the broken cot may fall out, trapping their fingers or limbs or sustain a major injury that could be fatal
- Staff and parents may injure their backs leaning over fixed height cots and may then be unable to care for the child or continue to work.

people (Ch. 7). Risk assessment is an integral part of health and safety legislation (see p. 284).

The process of risk assessment may sound complicated, but it is essentially an examination of the factors that could cause harm to people in a care environment so that precautions can be taken to prevent injuries (HSE 2006a). The activity in Box 13.2 is the start of a risk assessment, which usually has five stages:

- *Step one*: Look for the hazard
- *Step two*: Decide who may be harmed and how
- *Step three*: Evaluate the risks and decide whether existing precautions are adequate or more should be done
- *Step four*: Record the findings
- *Step five*: Review the assessment regularly and revise if necessary.

These stages are explored in a series of boxes using a moving and handling example from each nursing specialty. The scenarios focus on hazards for staff and patients/clients and follow one of the basic principles, i.e. looking after your joints and your back (not stooping, twisting, reaching or lifting people).

Step one: Look for the hazard

This involves walking round a clinical area to identify what sort of things could cause harm to people, talking to the staff to find out what problems they experience and examining accident and sickness records to identify any particular patterns (HSE 2006a). Examples of this are provided in Box 13.3.

Step two: Decide who may be harmed and how

This essentially refers to the staff and patients/clients involved, but must also include visitors and employees who may be in the clinical area temporarily, e.g. cleaners, contractors (HSE 2006a). Now read Box 13.4, which builds on the moving and handling scenarios above.

Step three: Evaluate the risks and decide whether existing precautions are adequate or more should be done

This stage of the risk assessment involves looking at the likelihood of harm occurring (remember the being struck by lightning scenario?) and deciding whether the risk is high, medium or low. Then the risk has to be made as small as possible by taking precautions (HSE 2006a). This could include using equipment and educating staff so that they are aware of the risks and can take precautions themselves. Box 13.5 gives two examples of how this may be done.

Step four: Record the findings

With each scenario above, the results of the risk assessment must be recorded. Healthcare organizations usually have

---

Risk assessment   Box 13.5

Step 3: Reducing the risks

Ward B2

There have already been two accidents with patients using toilets so the risk of further injury is high. Installing non-slip flooring, grab rails and a raised toilet seat can minimize the risk. Each patient must be assessed for using the toilet; they need to be independent as the area is too small for staff to assist safely. Reviewing staff knowledge of how to deal with a fallen patient would also be a useful exercise.

Richard Smith Education Centre

Staff and pupils are at high risk of injury if pupils are moved to and from their wheelchairs without equipment. Installing a hoist to transfer children safely should reduce this risk. Staff will also need education on use of the hoist.

 Reflective practice   Box 13.6

Risk assessments in practice

Generic risk assessments should be available in each placement.

Student activities

1. Locate some of the risk assessments and policies in your placement, e.g.:
   - Moving and handling
   - Infection control
   - Drug policy and safe storage of medications.
2. Find out what hazards have been identified in your placement and how they have been reduced.

---

specific documentation for this process. Written records also demonstrate that employers have abided by the law (HSE 2006a) and can complete the final stage.

Step five: Review the assessment regularly and revise if necessary

Risk assessments need to be reviewed regularly and when there are any significant changes. A date is often set to remind people when to review the assessment.

The risk assessments described here could be applied to a number of patients/clients or staff and the focus is the specific task, e.g. transferring people from a wheelchair to the floor. This is often referred to as a generic assessment and comes under health and safety law. Therefore, it is the responsibility of the employer to carry this out although senior management may delegate the assessment to a specific individual trained in risk assessment and who regularly works in that clinical area (Box 13.6). Nurses have a duty of care (see Ch. 6) to follow the procedures that reduce the risk, such as using equipment provided and to report situations where safety is compromised.

Individual risk assessments

A person's health and social care needs are unique and nursing assessment (Ch. 14) includes identifying actual or potential hazards that can affect their health. A wide range of assessment

tools have been developed to help nurses and other healthcare professionals identify whether people are at risk of specific factors such as malnutrition or pressure ulcers (Box 13.7 provides some examples of these and sources of further information).

Examples of specific risk assessment tools   Box 13.7

Area of risk assessment	Further information
Falls risk assessment	See Box 13.10 (p. 285)
Early Warning Score (EWS)	See Fig. 14.14 (p. 333)
Nutritional assessment	See Ch. 19
Pressure ulcer development	See Fig. 14.2 (p. 309) and Ch. 25

Most assessment tools offer a checklist and a scoring system, with the overall result giving an indication of the degree of risk, e.g. high, medium or low risk of developing pressure ulcers. The assessing nurse can then decide how to minimize those risks.

Assessment tools are designed to help nurses in practice identify particular risks but they do not replace clinical judgement. For example, a nutritional assessment tool might indicate that a patient admitted for surgery is currently at a low risk of malnutrition (see Ch. 19). However, the patient will spend at least 4 hours fasting prior to surgery (Ch. 24) and thereafter, may not be able to eat or drink for several hours, or experience nausea and vomiting. They will therefore be at higher risk of developing malnutrition and this indicates the importance of regular reassessment.

The discussion on generic risk assessments above highlighted a common issue across all nursing specialties, namely moving and handling. For individual assessments, a number of field-specific issues arise. Risks are taken as part of growing up and everyday life as we develop and learn. This may occur on many different levels, e.g. crossing a busy road, drinking alcohol, starting a new relationship or embarking on a career, and these can often be a case of trial and error. Risk taking is a natural part of life and if people who have learning disabilities or mental health conditions are overprotected, this can lead to social exclusion and infringement of their rights and dignity (Alaszewski & Alaszewski 2000).

To promote social inclusion, people need to be allowed to take reasonable risks to aid their development by promoting independent living and social activities. Risks still need to be reduced to a minimum and agreed by the multidisciplinary team and client but the value of risk-taking should also be recognized. Box 13.8 presents a case study and an opportunity for reflection on a number of issues discussed here.

Health and safety legislation

Legislation plays a major role in promoting safety of individuals and public health in general. This section briefly examines the regulations in place in the UK to prevent accidents and ill-health and also the health and safety responsibilities of employers to protect staff and the public.

Critical thinking Box 13.8

Promoting independent living and social activities

You are on a 4-week placement at a busy day centre for young adults with mild to moderate learning disabilities. Tom is 17 years old and you have been working closely with him for the past week. When he first arrives, he confides in you saying he had an argument with his mum before he left home. You find out that he had asked to go to the cinema with his girlfriend Cheryl who also attends the day centre. His mum had said he was not allowed to go alone with Cheryl as the cinema is 4 miles from home and he and his mum usually travel together on the bus. He has never used public transport alone.

Student activities

- Why do you think Tom's mum is concerned about risks and safety?
- Do you think her concerns are realistic?
- How do you think the issue could be resolved, so that social inclusion for Tom and Cheryl is promoted?

Maintaining safety and promoting health

Wide-ranging legislation exists to promote public health and safety including:

- Supply of clean water
- Food standards
- Environmental protection
- Sewage treatment
- Fire precautions
- Safety standards for manufacturers
- The provision of a National Health Service.

Individual UK countries also publish specific public health strategies (Box 13.9), which focus on reducing death rates from cancer, coronary heart disease and strokes, mental health illness and accidents (Ch. 1). Specific national strategies and targets have followed, e.g. for children, older people, mental health, coronary heart disease, diabetes, and cancer (see www.dh.gov.uk for publications). Preventative measures can maximize people's health and reduce accident rates. For example, the National Institute for Health and Clinical Excellence (NICE 2004) provided guidance on assessing older adults in order to prevent falls and minimizing their recurrence. Falls prevention campaigns have also been launched, aimed at educating older adults. Where accidents do occur, the target is for faster diagnosis and effective treatment to improve

Health strategies in the four UK countries Box 13.9

England: Her Majesty's Government (2010) Healthy Lives, Healthy People: Our Strategy for Public Health in England
Scotland: The Scottish Government (2007) Better Health, Better Care
Northern Ireland: Department of Health, Social Services and Public Safety (2002) Investing for Health
Wales: Welsh Assembly Government (2010) Our Healthy Future.

Health promotion Box 13.10

Falls prevention

Even minor falls can result in loss of confidence, loss of mobility leading to social isolation and increased dependency and disability. The *National Service Framework for Older People* (DH 2001) sets specific targets for reduction in the number of serious injuries resulting from falls and appropriate rehabilitation of people who have fallen. Many multidisciplinary teams have been established to assess individuals and run falls prevention programmes.

Student activities

1. Read the NICE (2004) guidelines about preventing falls in older people. Consider the extent to which they are implemented in your placement.
2. Identify how the elements of a falls prevention programme listed below may help prevent falls in older people:
   - Exercise classes and keeping active
   - Emphasizing healthy eating
   - Wearing appropriate, well-fitting footwear
   - Being aware of changes in health and eyesight
   - Preventing illness
   - Adjustments in the home, e.g. lighting and grab rails
   - Dealing with the fear and anxiety.

Resources

Department of Health, 2001. National service framework for older people. DH, London.
NICE, 2004. Falls: the assessment and prevention of falls in older people. Online. Available: www.nice.org.uk/CG021 September 2012.

health outcomes. By undertaking the activities in Box 13.10, you will find out more about assessment and prevention of falls in older adults.

Nurses across all fields of practice may have a number of roles to play in accident prevention as they come into contact with people at various stages of their lives for health promotion and treatment measures in different settings including the community, hospitals, clinics, schools and walk-in centres. This may be as part of local education or screening programmes on accident prevention for patients/clients or their families. Nurses are also heavily involved in people's care after accidents have occurred and this provides opportunities for assessment and education to prevent further accidents.

Health and safety in healthcare settings

The Health and Safety at Work (HSW) Act (1974) is the main piece of UK legislation that places specific responsibilities upon employers to protect the welfare of people at work and the public. Under this Act, many subsequent regulations have been issued which deal with specific topics such as manual handling and the safe use of equipment. Although employers are responsible for providing a safe working environment, employees (including students) have responsibilities for:

- Following the regulations
- Taking reasonable care of their own safety and that of others

Table 13.1 Main health and safety regulations under the Health and Safety at Work Act (1974)

Regulation	Date	Main aim
Management of Health and Safety at Work	1999	Ensures employers carry out risk assessments, implement changes and appoint qualified people to provide information and staff training
Workplace (Health and Safety and Welfare)	1992	Ensures employers cover range of health and safety issues, e.g. ventilation, heating, lighting, seating, welfare facilities
Health and Safety (Display Screen Equipment)	1992	Lays down requirements for people who work with visual display units (computer screens)
Personal Protective Equipment at Work	1992	Ensures that employers provide protective clothing and equipment for employees
Provision and Use of Work Equipment	1998	Ensures that employers provide safe equipment for use at work
Manual Handling Operations	1992, amended 2002	Lays down requirements for the movement of loads by hand or involving bodily force
Reporting of Injuries, Diseases and Dangerous Occurrences	1995	Employers must report work-related accidents, diseases and dangerous occurrences
Control of Substances Hazardous to Health	2002	Ensures that employers identify hazardous substances, assess risks to health and take appropriate action to reduce risks
Noise at Work	1989	Ensures that employers use systems that protect people's hearing in noisy environments
Electricity at Work	1989	Electrical systems are safe and well maintained
Health and Safety (First Aid)	1981	Ensures employers provide adequate first aid equipment and personnel

(Based on HSE 2003.)

- Implementing any training and education given
- Reporting unsafe conditions.

Health and safety is essentially everyone's responsibility. This section presents the main legislation that applies to clinical practice (Table 13.1) and summarizes the key points.

The HSE enforce health and safety law in the UK under criminal law, as opposed to civil law, which focuses on personal claims for compensation (see Ch. 6). This means that employers may be heavily fined, or worse, for failing to comply with health and safety regulations. The HSW Act (1974) laid out general duties for employers to:

- Provide a safe working environment
- Identify hazards and reduce them
- Provide information and training for employees
- Arrange safe transportation and handling of articles and substances (HSE 2003).

The Management of Health and Safety at Work Regulations (1999) were more specific and require employers to carry out:

- Risk assessments
- Risk reduction
- Risk and accident monitoring
- Health surveillance
- Consultation with staff.

These two pieces of legislation provide the background and general principles for health and safety but it is useful to look at some of the more specific regulations highlighted in Table 13.1 and their implications for clinical practice.

Control of Substances Hazardous to Health (COSHH)

Chemicals and other substances used at work can be hazardous to people's health and employers must control exposure to prevent harm occurring (HSE 2009a). Hazardous substances include chemicals, gases, dust and biological agents (blood and blood products, microorganisms) that can cause illnesses ranging from mild allergic reactions to occupational asthma and death. Risk assessments are therefore carried out and precautions put in place, including:

- Educating staff
- Providing personal protective equipment
- Health surveillance
- Formulating policies for dealing with hazardous substances, e.g. disposal, spillages and emergencies.

Manufacturers must also supply information and warning labels on hazardous substances, both domestic and industrial (Fig. 13.1). These highlight whether the chemical is an irritant, corrosive, highly toxic or flammable and it is important to be familiar with these.

Reporting of Incidents, Diseases and Dangerous Occurrences Regulations (RIDDOR)

Accident statistics, covering the period 2009–2010 (HSE 2010) show that:

| Corrosive | (Very) Toxic | Highly or extremely flammable |

NB Always read the hazard statement on the packaging to understand the hazard

Fig. 13.1 • Hazard signs. (Reproduced with permission from HSE Health and Safety Executive, 2009a. Working with substances hazardous to health: what you need to know about COSHH. HSE, Sudbury.)

- 152 people lost their lives at work
- 26 061 experienced major injuries predominantly through slipping or tripping
- 95 368 received injuries that caused a 3 day or more absence from work.

RIDDOR aims to ensure that accidents and near misses are documented and reported to the HSE so that these can be investigated if necessary and harm reduction measures implemented. Reportable incidents include a patient/client, visitor or member of the public or staff experiencing one of the following:

- A dangerous occurrence or near miss that happens in practice, e.g. collapse of equipment or explosion
- An injury that lasts for more than 7 days or a work-related disease, e.g. a severe allergy
- A major injury, e.g. fracture, amputation, or injuries leading to acute illness, unconsciousness or death.

In nursing practice, all accidents and near misses are documented using the local NHS electronic incident forms that record people involved, details of the incident, the consequences including injuries or ill-health and the remedial action taken. Health and safety representatives then review and report to the HSE as necessary (Box 13.11).

 Reflective practice   Box 13.11

Reporting incidents in placements

Student activities

- Locate the safety or adverse incident forms used in your placement.
- Discuss the types of incidents and events that are documented with your mentor.
- Find out what happens to these forms after they are completed.

In addition to the general targets for reducing accidents in the health service, the National Patient Safety Agency (NPSA) monitors reported patient safety incidents and near misses. As well as advising on particular universal issues, e.g. intravenous infusion pumps, the NPSA collect and analyse confidential incident reports from across the country. This information is then used to advise on preventative measures and to build a culture of safety and learning within the NHS (NPSA 2011).

Equipment used at work

Provision and Use of Work Equipment Regulations (PUWER; HSE 2009b) and Lifting Operations and Lifting Equipment Regulations (LOLER; HSE 2005) are designed to cover a range of industries but both ensure that equipment used at work is:

- Suitable for use
- Well maintained
- Regularly inspected
- Only used by trained individuals
- Accompanied with safety measures such as warning labels and protective devices (HSE 2009b).

In addition, LOLER relates to equipment such as electric hoists that should be tested at 6-monthly intervals and have safe working loads (maximum patient/client weight) clearly marked on them (HSE 2005).

Manual Handling Operation Regulations 1992 (amended 2002)

Moving and handling includes lifting, lowering, pushing, pulling, carrying or moving loads such as inanimate objects, and helping people to move. Nursing involves many of these activities on a day-to-day basis and using incorrect techniques or failing to use equipment provided puts practitioners at high risk of injury. Musculoskeletal injuries occur frequently at work in the UK and have considerable personal and economic implications. An estimated 572 000 musculoskeletal injuries occurred in the period 2009/2010 affecting mainly the back (43%) and upper limbs or neck (40%) (HSE 2010). Many of these injuries are preventable and the Manual Handling Operation Regulations lay out the requirements under health and safety law and the responsibilities of employers and staff.

This section introduces the principles of safe practice but moving and handling must not be undertaken without completing a specific course that addresses the theory of safe handling and allows practice of these techniques. Readers should refer to Chapter 18 for further guidance on helping patients and clients to move.

There are five key stages to planning and executing a handling manoeuvre to reduce the risk to the handler and patient/client.

1. *Avoid unnecessary handling*: Is the manoeuvre really necessary? Can the person do it themselves if given enough time, adequate instructions or the right equipment? Is it necessary to move equipment or boxes?
2. *Assess the risk*: If the task cannot be avoided then assess it using 'Task, Individual, Load and Environment' as a framework (TILE, see below).
3. *Plan the move*: Decide on the most appropriate posture or technique.
4. *Prepare for the move*: Gather the right equipment, number of people required and make sure they are all clear about the technique and the instructions.
5. *Perform the manoeuvre*: Ensure that smooth controlled movements are used and your back is in a natural vertical position.

Moving and handling require an approach similar to other health and safety issues and one of the first stages is a risk assessment. This may be:

- Generic, i.e. referring to a group of people and a particular task or
- Specific, i.e. relating to a particular patient/client and their individual handling needs.

The TILE framework

This helps to think through the move using biomechanics (the study of human movement) and ergonomics (the science of design and fitting the work environment to the worker). Both of these disciplines contribute to the understanding of how to prevent injuries. TILE is discussed below, based on the guidance from the HSE (2004).

The task (T)

Assessing the task means identifying the factors that may cause injury and eliminating or reducing them. The HSE (2004) suggest that the following questions be asked:

- Does the task involve holding or manipulating loads at a distance to the trunk?
  Holding an object close to the trunk means that it is easier to control and there is less risk of back injury compared to holding it at a distance or at arms' length.
- Does the task involve twisting, stooping or reaching upwards?
  Stooping, twisting and reaching greatly increase the risk of injury because they place stress on the lower spine. These actions must be avoided in moving and handling tasks by using legs and feet to move rather than twisting at the trunk and by remaining close to the load or patient/client.
- Does the task involve excessive carrying of inanimate objects across a distance or excessive lifting or lowering?
  Carrying objects over long distances or repetitive lifting or lowering can cause fatigue and increase the risk of injury. Equipment, such as a trolley, reduces the risk of injury from carrying. Also, heavier items should be stacked on shelves at waist height so they are not lifted from the floor or high shelves.
- Does the task involve pushing and pulling?
  Pushing and pulling may be a safer technique than lifting but it can still put the handler at risk of injury. For example, pushing a heavy load along an uneven surface or up a slope could be unsafe.
- Can the load suddenly move?
  If the contents of a half full box are not secure, they may shift during movement so the load needs to be secure to be safe. If the task involves people, there is always a risk of unexpected movements so the likelihood of this occurring is reduced by making sure the patient/client knows their role and what to expect so they do not become frightened or uncooperative.
- Are there sufficient rest periods for handlers?
  The greater the physical effort, the greater the risk of injury, and inadequate rest periods mean that muscles and joints do not get a chance to recover.

- Is the correct equipment available?
  As part of the risk assessment, the equipment available for the task needs careful consideration. There is a wide range of aids available, from sliding (glide) sheets that reduce friction and help people move up in bed, to electric beds and hoists that assist people to sit up, transfer or stand (see Ch. 18). During your moving and handling practical training, you will have the opportunity to practise with a range of equipment. Equipment must be well maintained and checked before each use. It is important to be aware that all equipment has a safe working load, i.e. an upper weight limit for use, usually marked on larger pieces of equipment such as hoists. This is why it is important to document patients'/clients' weight as part of nursing assessment (Ch. 14). Infection control precautions also need to be considered, e.g. whether equipment can be disinfected with alcohol wipes or if special laundering arrangements are necessary.

Individual capabilities (I)

This refers to the assessment of handlers' abilities. Nursing activities should not require great physical strength but general fitness and regular exercise are important as these reduce the risk of injury. We must also assess our ability to be involved in moving and handling on a daily basis. Classroom trainers or clinical staff must be alerted to any pre-existing or current injuries that could prevent you from being involved in safe moving and handling. People with existing injuries and those who are, or have recently been pregnant, require an occupational health assessment.

Inappropriate clothing can restrict movement during handling manoeuvres or encourage adoption of awkward postures to protect the handler's dignity, and both situations increase the risk of injury. Uniform policies include trouser suits that allow freedom of movement and footwear that is flat and provides plenty of grip. It is therefore important to follow local uniform policies.

The load (L)

The manual handling guidelines identify a number of factors for consideration regarding the load (if it is an inanimate object) or the patient/client involved. For objects, it is important to have an indication of their weight. This is often printed on boxes or can be judged by gently rocking the item before deciding whether to lift it. The size of the load is considered and whether it is possible to split it to make handling easier. Other areas to consider are the type of grip to use and whether the item could be too hot or sharp to handle.

Patients/clients should not be lifted because of the risk of injury to the person and the handlers. Nurses must assess people's capabilities and then determine the best technique or equipment to help them move. People vary greatly in shape and size and those receiving healthcare have the added complication of ill-health and attachments such as intravenous infusions and urinary catheters. Therefore, specific assessment must be carried out for each patient/client before carrying out manoeuvres. Care settings including NHS Trusts should have their own moving and handling assessment for patient/clients; some of the key areas that require consideration are outlined in Box 13.12.

Box 13.12

Summary of the TILE assessment for moving and handling

Task (T)

Assess and minimize the risks that cause injury, e.g. holding the load or person away from the trunk, twisting, stooping or reaching, considerable lifting, lowering or carrying distances for objects and pushing or pulling. Assess the need for team handling and think about the range of equipment available including its safe working limits, its condition and last recorded service.

Individual (I)

Assess the capabilities of staff, e.g. their age, gender, height, physical fitness, previous injuries, current or recent pregnancy, training, knowledge or experience, and wearing of restrictive clothing or inappropriate footwear.

Load (L)

- *Objects*: Assess the weight, dimensions, contents (loose, heavy at one end), bulky, harmful (hot or sharp) and whether it is difficult to grasp
- *People*: Assess their mobility and ability to bear weight, physical health, history of falls or confusion, understanding and concordance, attachments (intravenous infusions, catheters) and risk of moving unexpectedly, e.g. first time out of bed, prone to muscle spasms or seizures.

Environment (E)

Includes adequate lighting, temperature (especially extremes of heat and cold), flooring (for slippery or uneven surfaces, carpet, gradient), obstacles and weather conditions if outdoors.

The environment (E)

There are many factors in the environment that can increase or decrease the risk of injury to handlers and patients/clients. It is important to assess whether there is adequate lighting; non-slip flooring; a floor gradient or potential obstacles, e.g. doors, furniture, stairs. Extremes of temperature can also alter people's concentration levels and physical abilities. Moving and handling need to be planned to ensure that none of these factors contributes to an injury. There must be sufficient space to avoid awkward postures or techniques and it is important to be alert to hazards that may cause you and the client to slip or trip.

Moving and handling procedures cannot be completely risk-free but the TILE framework allows major hazards to be identified and reduces injuries to staff and patients/clients through using the correct technique and equipment. Figure 13.2 illustrates a good handling technique for lifting an inanimate load and Chapter 18 examines specific techniques for helping people to move.

First aid

First aid is the initial treatment or assistance given to an individual who is injured or unwell and a first aider provides this assistance, while making sure everyone is safe and no further harm is caused (Austin et al 2011). This section discusses first aid at work, the general principles of first aid and how to deal with some specific emergencies, i.e. burns and scalds, and suspected poisonings.

All employers must provide first aid facilities, equipment and personnel under the Health and Safety (First-Aid) Regulations 1981 (HSE 2003), including:

- First aid boxes
- Trained first aiders who have undergone an HSE approved course
- Specialist equipment if there are particular hazards and therefore a higher risk of accidents.

Green posters may also advertise where the nearest first aid box is located and the names of trained first aiders. Some clinical areas may be better equipped to deal with emergencies than others, e.g. comparing a hospital ward and a day centre for older adults. However, all are required to conduct risk assessments and provide appropriate facilities.

Administering first aid outside placements can be very different, as equipment is not readily available. Also, not all nurses are trained first aiders although they do have knowledge that is useful in an emergency situation. First aid and emergency skills are part of pre-registration programmes as required by the NMC. The NMC (2008) also describe the duty of care that nurses have outside work in an emergency situation. Often nurses are concerned about expectations of them but any first aid provided is judged in relation to the particular circumstances and against what can reasonably be expected from someone with their level of knowledge, skills and abilities (NMC 2008). This means that expectations of an experienced nurse working in an Emergency Department would be much higher than a student nurse who has only completed a basic life support course.

Some people may be concerned about the legal aspects of first aid provided outside the healthcare environment and being held to account if events do not go as well as anticipated. Similar to the NMC guidance, so long as first aiders have acted in the person's best interests and acted within their limits of competence and training, they will be in a safe position.

This section introduces the basic principles of first aid, principles for burns and scalds, poisoning and emergency childbirth, and subsequent chapters deal with other specific situations. As well as reading the information in these chapters, there are other considerations that can help to develop knowledge and confidence. First aid skills are included in nursing programmes and attending a recognized training course to become a qualified first aider may help (see 'Useful websites', p. 301). Remember that first aid should 'do no harm' and that recognizing the limitations of one's knowledge and skills is important; however, you may be the only person present who has attended a basic life support or first aid course and simple measures will often help save someone's life or prevent their condition worsening.

Dealing with incidents, emergencies and prioritizing

Emergency situations can be difficult to deal with as people may be distressed, in pain or confused and there may be more

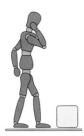

1. Think before handling and lifting
Plan the activity - where is the load going to be placed? Remove obstructions and for long lifts, e.g. from floor to shoulder height, consider resting the load midway

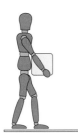

2. Keep the load close to the waist with the heaviest side next to the body

3. Adopt a stable position: feet should be hip width apart with one leg slightly forward to maintain balance

4. Ensure a good hold on the load

5. Moderate flexion (slight bending) of the hips, knees and back at the start of the lift is preferable to stooping or full squatting

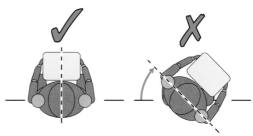

6. Don't flex the back any further while lifting

7. Avoid twisting the back or leaning sideways. Move the feet rather than twisting and keep the shoulders level and facing the same direction as the hips

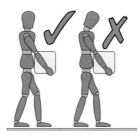

8. Keep the head up when handling, looking ahead

9. Move smoothly. Keep the load under control

10. Do not lift more than can be easily handled. If in doubt seek advice

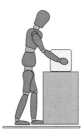

11. Put it down then adjust. Slide the load into its final position if it needs to be precisely placed

Fig. 13.2 • Handling technique for inanimate objects. (Reproduced with permission from HSE Health and Safety Executive, 2004. Manual handling: guidance on regulations. HSE Norwich.)

than one injury or a number of people involved. However, it is important that you remain calm and apply some simple principles (based on Austin et al 2011) that will help to organize your thoughts and decisions on the most appropriate action. The principles of first aid are listed in Box 13.13 and described below.

Assess the situation

Make a brief visual assessment of what has happened, looking for evidence of danger or potential hazards for yourself and the casualty. The most important rule of first aid is that you never put yourself in danger, otherwise you too may become

a casualty. Once you have determined that it is safe, introduce yourself to the casualty or bystanders and ask them to describe what has happened.

Protect yourself and casualties from danger

Can you safely remove potential dangers such as obstructions or switching off electric sockets? Only remove the casualty from the situation as a last resort and only if there is imminent life-threatening danger. Prevent cross-infection through good hand hygiene and using disposable gloves and apron where available.

First aid Box 13.13

Principles of first aid

- Assess the situation
- Protect yourself and casualties from danger – never put yourself at risk
- Prevent cross-infection as far as possible
- Assess the casualty providing comfort and reassurance
- Give early treatment and prioritize injuries:
  - Airway (A)
  - Breathing (B)
  - Circulation (C)
- Arrange for appropriate help.

(Based on Austin et al 2011).

Give early treatment and prioritize injuries

Chapter 16 discusses how to make an initial assessment of a collapsed individual by checking their level of response (see p. 388) and then:

- Airway (A)
- Breathing (B)
- Circulation (C).

If the casualty has more that one problem, e.g. they are unconscious and their arm is bleeding, deal with problems in the ABC order, i.e. make sure their airway is clear, they are breathing and then attend to the source of the bleeding. If there is more than one casualty you will have to prioritize and decide who requires the most immediate attention. Again, use the ABC assessment. Quiet or unconscious casualties often require the quickest attention. You know that those who are crying or shouting at least have a clear airway, are breathing and also have a pulse. However, they will still need reassurance and assessment of their injuries, so encourage bystanders to stay with, and reassure them.

Call for help

In a placement, call for help immediately by shouting and using emergency buzzers where available. You may be asked to put out a 'crash call' – a telephone call to the switchboard that will alert the resuscitation team. Clearly state that there has been a cardiac arrest and give the name and location of the area. The NPSA requested NHS Trusts to standardize their crash call number to '2222' so that the emergency number is always the same. Ensure that you find out the emergency number on the first day of each new placement.

Outside of placements, you will need to telephone 999 (in the UK, 112 in Europe) to summon emergency services, free from public phone boxes and most mobile phones. State the emergency service required (ambulance, police, fire brigade, coastguard) and you will be put through to the appropriate call centre. You will be asked for your name and location and to provide the number of casualties and describe their injuries.

Provide first aid

Provide first aid and stay with the casualty until help arrives. Healthcare professionals will make their own assessment of the situation but your information about the event, your observations and the treatment given are useful.

After the event

Dealing with emergencies can be stressful and you may experience a range of emotions afterwards (Ch. 11). It is also quite natural to reflect on the situation, your role, what went well and what you would do differently if the situation occurred again. You might find it helpful to talk to your mentor or your personal tutor at university, to help make sense of events or for advice about alternative sources of support. Being a first aider in a serious incident can affect people weeks or even months later. Reliving the event in some way, sleeplessness or flashbacks may be a sign that support of a general practitioner (GP) or counsellor may be useful (Austin et al 2011).

Dealing with burns and scalds

Around 100000 people attend Emergency Departments in England annually because of burns and scalds (Health and Social Care Information Centre 2009). Most are caused either by dry heat (e.g. flames) or moist heat (e.g. steam, hot liquids or fat), although industrial and domestic chemicals can also cause burns along with high and low voltage electrical sources, radiation (including sunburn, X-rays and radioactive sources) and extreme cold (e.g. frostbite).

The skin is the largest organ in the body and is discussed in more detail in Chapter 16. The epidermis and dermis make up the two main layers of the skin, and burns can involve both layers; in severe cases, the underlying subcutaneous fat and muscle layers are also affected. Burns are classified according to the depth and percentage of the body surface area involved. Box 13.14 compares the three depths of burn injury: superficial, partial thickness and full thickness.

Types of burn Box 13.14

Superficial

- Only involve the epidermis and heal well
- Redness, swelling and sometimes blistering
- Painful and sensitive.

Partial thickness

- Epidermis and dermis separate, forming fluid-filled blisters
- Redness and swelling
- Painful and sensitive
- Require medical treatment in children and when more than a minor burn in adults.

Full thickness

- Deep burn involving dermal, subcutaneous and muscle layers
- May appear waxy, charred or leathery
- No pain sensation due to damaged nerve endings
- Need urgent medical attention, specialist burns treatment and skin grafts.

The extent of burns may initially be estimated using the 'rule of nines' (Fig. 13.3): the greater the area affected, the

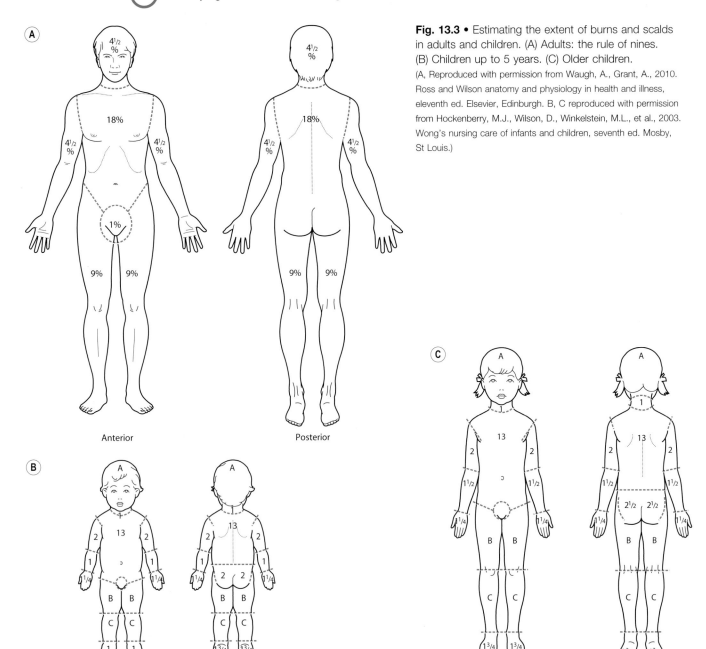

Fig. 13.3 • Estimating the extent of burns and scalds in adults and children. (A) Adults: the rule of nines. (B) Children up to 5 years. (C) Older children. (A, Reproduced with permission from Waugh, A., Grant, A., 2010. Ross and Wilson anatomy and physiology in health and illness, eleventh ed. Elsevier, Edinburgh. B, C reproduced with permission from Hockenberry, M.J., Wilson, D., Winkelstein, M.L., et al., 2003. Wong's nursing care of infants and children, seventh ed. Mosby, St Louis.)

Relative percentages of areas affected by growth

AREA	BIRTH	AGE 1YR	AGE 5YR
A = 1/2 of head	9 1/2	8 1/2	6 1/2
B = 1/2 of one thigh	2 3/4	3 1/4	4
C = 1/2 of one leg	2 1/2	2 1/2	2 3/4

Relative percentages of areas affected by growth

AREA	AGE 10 YR	AGE 15 YR
A = 1/2 of head	5 1/2	4 1/2
B = 1/2 of one thigh	4 1/2	4 1/2
C = 1/2 of one leg	3	3 1/4

greater the risk of shock caused by fluid loss. In adults, medical attention is needed for anything more that a minor superficial burn. A doctor should see children with what appears to be a superficial burn. Medical attention should always be sought for burns affecting the face, groin, hands and feet. When more than 15% burns in adults is present, specialist burns care in hospital is necessary. This figure is 10% burns in children where a modified chart is used to calculate the extent of burns because of the different sizes of children. Box 13.15 describes the first aid management of burns and scalds.

Electrical burns

Extreme caution is required when there are electrical burns to ensure that the casualty is no longer in contact with the source of electricity. It may not be possible to attend to them until it

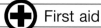

 First aid Box 13.15

Burns and scalds

Recognition

Tissue damage as described in Box 13.14.

Aims of treatment

- Establish and maintain airway, breathing and circulation
- Cool the affected area to remove the heat to limit tissue damage and provide temporary pain relief
- Transfer to hospital if appropriate.

Treatment

- Cool the burn under cool running water (not ice cold as this will damage the skin) for at least 10 minutes
- Remove any rings, jewellery and watches that may cause constriction later on due to swelling
- Do not remove any clothing stuck in the wound
- Cooling gels and sprays are not recommended because of difficulty in controlling the cooling effect
- For large burns, the casualty is at risk of hypothermia because of the cooling effect of the water. Help to keep the casualty warm by covering unaffected areas
- Superficial burns: cover with a non-adhesive dressing
- Partial or full thickness burns: cover the wound with clean, non-fluffy material (to avoid sticking) to reduce the risk of infection and provide protection while being transported to hospital. Kitchen film is ideal (although ensure the skin has been cooled first and discard the outer two layers of the roll of film that may be contaminated).

(Based on Austin et al 2011).

 First aid Box 13.16

Poisoning

Recognition

- Casualty may report history of accidental or deliberate poisoning
- Evidence of empty containers, bottles or syringes (if a drug overdose is suspected, watch out for used syringes in the area or in pockets that could cause a needlestick injury)
- Drowsiness or loss of consciousness
- Nausea and vomiting when poisons have been ingested.

Aims and treatment

- Maintain or establish airway, breathing and circulation
- Identify poison by asking the casualty, if possible, and look for clues in the area
- If unconscious, treat as outlined in Box 16.28, p. 390
- Treat any other injuries found
- Call for help to arrange transfer to hospital without delay, even if there are no symptoms.

Ingested poisons

- The casualty is more likely to vomit and protecting their airway becomes a priority
- Vomiting should not be induced because casualties may inhale the vomit blocking their airway
- If mouth-to-mouth resuscitation becomes necessary, then protect yourself with a specially designed plastic resuscitation face shield (Austin et al 2011).

Inhaled substances

- The danger with inhaled substances, e.g. carbon monoxide gas or smoke, is that the contaminant is still present in the atmosphere
- Work environments where hazardous gases are used have specialist breathing equipment available and trained personnel in case emergencies arise
- If inhalation is suspected, the most appropriate course of action is to summon the emergency services.

has been confirmed that the current has been turned off (Austin et al 2011). Anyone who has experienced an electrical burn must seek medical attention because the current may have interfered with the electrical activity of the heart.

Chemical burns

For burns caused by chemicals splashed onto skin or into the eyes, ensure that the water flushing the area runs away from the body so that it does not come into contact with any other region causing further burns. Unlike burns caused by heat, where clothes should be left untouched, it may be necessary to remove contaminated clothing. First aiders must wear protective clothing including heavy-duty rubber gloves and apron to protect themselves. When arranging for the casualty to be transported to hospital, ensure that paramedics are aware that chemicals are involved.

Burns caused by cold injuries, e.g. frostbite, require different treatment and should not be cooled.

Dealing with poisoning

A poison is any substance that enters the body in sufficient quantities to cause temporary or permanent damage. Poisons may be accidentally or deliberately ingested, inhaled, splashed on to the skin or injected. Signs and symptoms vary according to the amount and type of poison involved and its route of

entry. Box 13.16 shows the principles of dealing with a suspected or known poisoning.

In clinical areas, healthcare practitioners have access to the National Poisons Information Service (www.npis.org) which provides a 24-hour emergency helpline and a toxicology database of known poisons and recommended treatments.

Emergency childbirth

Around 40 weeks of pregnancy, the natural process of childbirth (labour) usually begins and there is time for a woman and their birth partner(s) to make arrangements at home or attend hospital. Occasionally, labour can begin early, progress quickly or a woman may be particularly anxious and need support in obtaining medical assistance, reassurance, privacy and care for her and the baby during and after delivery (Austin et al 2011). The NMC (2010b) requires nurses who work with adults in particular to be able to respond in an emergency to safeguard the well-being of mother and child. Therefore, it is important to understand the normal process and your role in an emergency childbirth. There are three stages of childbirth:

- *First stage*: Contractions begin and put increasing pressure on the cervix until it is fully dilated. This can take several hours in the first pregnancy and is usually shorter in subsequent pregnancies
- *Second stage*: The mother will have a strong urge to push and the baby will pass through the vagina, usually head first. The baby is born at the end of this stage
- *Third stage*: Up to half an hour after delivery, the placenta and attached umbilical cord will be expelled through further contractions.

Now, complete the activity in Box 13.17 and reflect on your role in this situation.

| **Emergency childbirth** | **Box 13.17** |

Student activities

Access the authorized First Aid Manual (Austin et al 2011), read pages 228–229 and answer the following questions:

- What is your role in an emergency childbirth?
- How would you alert the emergency services and what information do you need to tell them?
- How can you reassure and support the mother during the first, second and third stages of labour?

Infection control and standard precautions

Preventing the spread of infection is one of the most important nursing roles and is concerned with safety, preventing ill-health, and promoting health and well-being in individuals or groups of people. This section briefly introduces key concepts of safe infection control practice and Chapter 15 examines them in more detail.

Standard infection control precautions, previously known as universal precautions, were introduced to reduce the risk of transmitting blood-borne viruses such as HIV and hepatitis B to healthcare workers. Both terms describe infection control guidelines that minimize the risk of coming into contact with body fluids (including blood, urine, faeces and other body secretions and excretions), non-intact skin and mucous membranes. The standard infection control precautions outlined in Box 13.18 are used with those receiving care, regardless of their infection status, in order to protect healthcare practitioners and prevent the spread of infection.

There are several routes by which bacteria, viruses, fungi and other infectious agents can be transmitted including inhalation, direct contact, ingestion and inoculation. However, effective handwashing has been repeatedly shown to be the most important factor in reducing the spread of infection. Knowledge of appropriate handwashing techniques (see Ch. 15) and the necessary frequency is therefore essential and shown in Box 13.19.

Many healthcare procedures are invasive, meaning that they use sharp devices that penetrate the skin or body in

---

| **Standard infection control precautions** | **Box 13.18** |

Standard infection control precautions are essential in preventing spread of infection between patients/clients/healthcare professionals and others. These include:

- Hand hygiene, e.g. handwashing and use of alcohol gels; this is the most effective measure
- Personal protective equipment (PPE), e.g. gloves, aprons, masks
- Safe use and disposal of sharps to prevent infection and also needlestick injuries
- Safe management of waste, including spillage, and linen
- Decontamination of patient-care equipment, i.e. cleaning, sterilizing, disinfecting.

Guidelines about each of these topics and further measures, known as additional precautions, are discussed in detail in Chapter 15.

| **When handwashing is carried out** | **Box 13.19** |

Handwashing is undertaken:

- On entering and leaving the clinical area
- Before and after any direct patient contact and between patients, whether or not gloves are worn
- Immediately after gloves are removed
- Before handling an invasive device
- After touching blood, body fluids, secretions, excretions, non-intact skin, and contaminated items, even if gloves are worn
- During patient care, when moving from a contaminated to a clean body site of the patient
- After contact with inanimate objects in the immediate vicinity of the patient
- After coughing, sneezing or using the lavatory.

(Based on World Health Organization, 2007. Standard Precautions in healthcare. Online. Available: www.who.int September 2012.)

---

some way such as needles or surgical instruments. This carries the risk of needlestick injury to practitioners and also transmission of blood-borne viruses after devices have been in contact with patients/clients. Sharps therefore require careful handling and disposal (see Ch. 15). Sharps bins are special containers that conform to British Standard Institute specification, which ensures that they are yellow in colour, puncture resistant, leak-proof, clearly marked with three-quarters lines indicating when they should be closed, suitable for incineration and marked with hazard signs.

In the community, some pharmacies and organizations offer needle exchange programmes for intravenous drug users. These harm-reduction programmes aim to help individuals reduce the risk of contracting hepatitis B or HIV by supplying clean needles and safely disposing of used equipment.

Clinical waste must be carefully managed to ensure that toxic or hazardous materials are handled, transported and disposed of safely. There are regulations surrounding clinical waste that needs to be segregated under the Environmental Protection Act (1990). This includes using appropriate bags for household waste such as paper and flowers, which can be sent to landfill, yellow clinical waste bags for materials contaminated with blood or body fluids, and sharps containers that need to be incinerated. Hospital linen also has a colour coding system which determines how laundry bags are handled (see Ch. 15).

Infection control and standard infection control precautions are an essential part of all healthcare practitioners' everyday practice to ensure the safety of staff, patients/clients and the wider community. Chapter 15 is therefore an important chapter to read. Carrying out the activities in Box 13.20 will help you examine, practice and familiarize yourself with infection control procedures and policies for handling, storage and disposal of clinical waste in your placement.

 Reflective practice　　　　Box 13.20

Standard infection control precautions in practice
Student activities

1. Locate the sharps container(s) in your placement:
   * What information should be documented on the side of the bin, when and by whom?
   * Where are sharps containers placed for collection and disposal?
2. Discuss the measures in place to prevent and deal with needlestick injuries with your mentor.
3. Find out how clinical and non-clinical waste is segregated and disposed of.

Principles of managing violence, anger and aggression

Developing safe practice involves identifying potential risks and minimizing them, and the issue of violence and aggression is no exception. People are at highest risk of this when engaged in work that involves (Royal College of Nursing, RCN 2003; HSE 2006b):

* Dealing with the public
* Providing care and education
* Working with people who are confused, have mental health problems or behavioural challenges
* Working alone
* Handling valuables or medication
* Working with people under stress or those who misuse alcohol or drugs.

Nurses from all fields of practice may be involved in these situations. However, the fear of violence and aggression can be out of proportion to the risks: although verbal aggression or anger is more common and physical harm is comparatively rare (HSE 2006b), both can have detrimental effects on practitioners. This section is about awareness and prevention. Being aware of the factors that can lead to aggression helps to develop the interpersonal communication skills that prevent incidents where aggression may occur and defuse tense situations.

The phrase 'violence and aggression' may hold slightly different meanings for different people but the NHS Security Management Service (NHS SMS 2010, p 1) defines workplace violence as: 'Any incident in which a person is abused, threatened or assaulted in circumstances relating to their work'. A description of non-physical and physical behaviours is provided in Box 13.21.

Types of violence　　　　Box 13.21

Non-physical assault
Definition: The use of inappropriate words or behaviour causing distress and/or constituting harassment (NHS SMS 2009, p 6)

Examples
　Verbal abuse including racial and sexual harassment
　Swearing
　Shouting
　Name calling and bullying
　Insults
　Innuendo
　Threatening gestures or postures
　Harassment, in all its forms
　Threatening use of dogs
　Abusive phone calls

Physical assault
Definition: The intentional application of force against the person of another without lawful justification, resulting in physical injury or personal discomfort (NHS SMS 2009, p 7)

Examples
　Kicking
　Punching
　Head-butting
　Biting
　Spitting
　Scratching
　Use of weapons
　Assault causing physical injury

(Based on Bibby, 1995. NHS Security Management Service, 2009. Tackling violence against staff. Online. Available: www.nhsbsa.nhs.uk/SecurityManagement.aspx September 2012.)

Minimizing violence, anger and aggression

The reasons why violence, anger and aggression occur are complex but for healthcare practitioners, there may be a number of additional factors that contribute to an increased risk of witnessing or being involved in an incident. People receiving healthcare may be anxious, tired, in pain, confused, frustrated by waiting times, under the influence of drugs or alcohol, have mental distress or a history of violence – and all of these predispose to unpredictable behaviour. Nursing often takes place in stressful situations and treatment or facilities may be granted, denied or delayed (RCN 2003).

Over recent years, there has been concern in the nursing media and general press about increases in violent incidents towards healthcare staff. However, this is difficult to illustrate because previously, there was no clear definition, as well as considerable underreporting (Bibby 1995). The national media also focus heavily on serious incidents and often on individuals with mental health problems; however, it is important to be mindful of the stereotypes that can arise from this. Most people with mental health conditions are at greater risk of harming themselves than other people (Jones & Jackson 2004). Mental health symptoms can clearly be a safety issue for an individual that may require support from healthcare professionals (Ch. 9).

The NHS Security Management Services (NHS SMS) has explicit policy and strategies for reducing the number of incidents towards staff. Policies also exist to ensure that incidents are reported and lone workers are protected. Lone working should be avoided where possible but where is it necessary, e.g. in community practice, staff need to be aware of the local lone working policy and adhere to it. Risk assessments are carried out, as in any other clinical area, and specific arrangements made for times when practitioners are out on duty. These include the use of mobile phones to keep in contact, a log of visits and alarm reporting systems where staff can notify a call centre of incidents or threats. A violent patient indicator system can also be used where a violent incident towards NHS staff is documented in the paper or electronic patient records.

Violence, anger and aggression in the workplace have an immediate impact on individuals involved, their colleagues and also potential long-term consequences. NHS Trusts must focus on specific areas including the environment, education provided to staff and methods of communication (DH 2002).

Environment

Examining the environment in which care is delivered can identify factors that may trigger or contribute to aggressive or violent incidents (Box 13.22).

> **Improving the healthcare environment to decrease violence** Box 13.22
>
> - Waiting rooms and reception areas need to be clean and hospitable with clear direction signs and notices
> - Extremes of temperature and overcrowding may contribute to people's discomfort
> - Comfortable seating arrangements should be provided along with measures that relieve boredom, e.g. television or radio (but ensure noise is minimized) and reading materials
> - The environment should be laid out to ensure that areas restricted to patients are locked and that there is a clear line of sight between areas wherever possible
> - Adequate lighting is also needed and closed circuit television (CCTV) can be a useful deterrent against violent behaviour, especially outside, e.g. in car parks
> - Where there is a greater risk of violence, or staff are isolated, a panic button system will alert others to the need for help.
>
> (Based on DH 2002; RCN 2003.)

Although creating a pleasant but safe patient/client environment is important (Box 13.23), this involves a balance between providing a friendly area and adequate security (National Audit Office 2003). In one department, protective glass screens actually increased tension for staff and clients and were therefore removed and replaced with other preventative measures (HSE 2006b).

> ◔ **Reflective practice** Box 13.23
>
> **Providing a safe environment**
> **Student activities**
> 1. Consider your current placement or one you have recently worked in:
>   - Are the waiting and reception rooms clean and spacious, and do they have comfortable seating?
>   - Are direction signs clear?
>   - Are there measures to relieve boredom?
>   - Is CCTV used?
> 2. Discuss your observations with your mentor.

Education

Education ensures practitioners are aware of the safety issues and how to prevent or defuse a situation. Training included in nursing programmes is likely to involve the theory and practice of:

- De-escalation techniques, i.e. methods of preventing and defusing violent behaviour
- Breakaway techniques for some fields of practice, i.e. methods of physically escaping from someone's hold.

In low-risk environments, e.g. operating theatres, staff training may include basic theory and de-escalation techniques. In high-risk areas, e.g. where challenging behaviour is common, or in mental health secure units, training will also usually include breakaway and restraint techniques.

Improving communication and preventing incidents

Safe nursing practice includes promoting effective communication between staff and patients/clients at all times (Ch. 9). Observation and interpersonal skills are often the key to preventing or defusing a situation by first looking for verbal and non-verbal cues that suggest that people may be agitated (Box 13.24).

Awareness of factors that can predispose people to violence, anger and aggression (see above) is useful. Mason and Chandley

---

> **Verbal and non-verbal cues that suggest that people are agitated** Box 13.24
>
> - Awkward or tense posture
> - Facial expressions
> - Hand gestures
> - Increased restlessness
> - Excitability
> - Pacing up and down
> - Speech patterns such as increased speed, loudness, threatening remarks or refusal to communicate or withdrawal.
>
> (Based on Mason & Chandley 1999; RCN 2003.)

(1999) remind readers of the need to be mindful of stereotypes and prejudices that may arise. For example, not everyone with dependence on alcohol or mental distress becomes violent, and external appearances, e.g. tattoos, piercings, do not represent particular attitudes or behaviours.

Interpersonal skills and non-verbal behaviour can help to resolve situations and prevent them from escalating, including maintaining respect and dignity for the people involved and appearing calm and confident. Box 13.25 identifies good practices to help prevent or de-escalate a situation.

 Nursing skills Box 13.25

Preventing and de-escalating potentially violent situations

- Wherever possible, make a good initial contact by introducing yourself, perhaps shaking hands and asking the client their preferred name
- Maintain a relaxed, open posture and ensure that your nonverbal behaviour is not threatening
- Demonstrate that the person has your full attention through your body language, i.e. is directed towards them, and avoid distracting behaviours such as foot tapping, fiddling
- Encourage the conversation by asking open-ended questions and acknowledging their feelings, e.g. 'I can see that you must have been feeling frustrated if you have been waiting' – do not attribute blame
- Try to solve the problem or find someone who can help, but do not make promises you cannot keep. Ask the person what they think could be done to resolve the issue
- Share the problem by using the term 'we', e.g. 'we need to work together on this so that you receive the medication on time in future'
- Avoid behaviours that may escalate the situation, including use of jargon, retaliatory remarks, sarcasm, swearing, ridiculing, trivializing the client's feelings or using phrases such as 'Don't be daft' or 'Calm down'
- If tension continues to escalate, it may be helpful to agree to take a break or change venue. Alternatively, if you feel the patient/client is reacting badly towards you, with their agreement, it may be helpful to refer them to someone else.

(Based on Bibby 1995; Mason & Chandley 1999; DH 2002; RCN 2003.)

If more critical situations arise, these principles still apply and a confident, calm approach is still needed, although it may not be appropriate to intervene. When possible, withdraw from the situation and think about moving other people away from the area too. Being aware of the environment you work in is also important – knowing how to summon help (e.g. other members of staff, security, police) and the general layout of the area along with the exit points. Avoid talking to people in confined spaces or corners if you recognize that a situation may become hostile. It is a good idea to suggest that all concerned move into a more suitable area to discuss the issue. Communication between staff is equally important to ensure everyone's safety. Always inform staff when you are leaving a clinical area, where you will be and when you will return. This is good practice so that if an emergency occurs, e.g. fire or cardiac arrest, colleagues are aware of your location.

Communication between agencies such as emergency departments, police, GPs and social services is also important. The RCN and NHS Executive (1998) describe a case where a district nurse was requested to visit a patient in their home to re-dress a dog bite wound. The gentleman's GP notes revealed reports from the emergency department recording several attendances there following dog bites from his son's bull terrier and also after being involved in fights. Social services documentation revealed that his grandchildren were also on the Child Protection Register. As a result of the communication between agencies, the district nurse arranged wound care at the health centre rather than visiting him at home and advised the gentleman to return to the emergency department for out-of-hours care if necessary, in order to maintain her own safety.

Dealing with and reporting violent incidents

Much of the discussion on violence and aggression has dealt with preventing incidents and defusing or de-escalation. Unfortunately, because of the complex nature of violence it can still occur, despite the use of these techniques. The actions required in these incidents focuses on the immediate responses and then detailed follow-up and evaluation (RCN 2003).

Immediate responses involve dealing with the emotional and physical needs of the practitioner(s) affected. In the case of violent assault, this may mean first aid and people usually experience a range of emotional reactions. This could include a 'crisis' phase where people feel shocked and numb but after the adrenaline has subsided, they feel physically and mentally exhausted (RCN 2003). People need to feel that they are not alone when incidents have happened and healthcare organizations should have support mechanisms in place for staff who have experienced violence. This may include debriefing sessions for staff and patients/clients involved to make sense of events, long-term counselling and follow-up.

An important part of the evaluation is documenting and reporting aggressive and violent incidents using appropriate documentation so that follow-up action can be taken, in order to prevent further incidents. However, staff may not want to document incidents for a number of reasons. These were highlighted by the National Audit Office (2003) who found that some staff thought:

- The incident was accepted as part of the job
- The incident may reflect badly on them
- No action would be taken.

A number of campaigns and education programmes aimed to address these concerns, have highlighted that violence and aggression are not acceptable and do not reflect upon either the individual concerned or their skills. Details of incident documentation include:

- The people involved
- Any known trigger factors and causes
- The location
- Any injuries or absence from work as a result (DH 2002).

It may also be necessary to complete health and safety forms associated with RIDDOR. Given the emotional nature of events, the person completing the form should always receive help from senior staff to recall and document the incident (RCN 2003). It may also be appropriate to inform the police.

The continued care of someone who has become violent is often not considered. They too may be shocked and upset by their behaviour and may wish to discuss the event from their perspective (RCN 2003). Agreements can be drawn up between patients/clients and healthcare organizations regarding antisocial behaviour, discussing terms and conditions under which they will receive healthcare. These written agreements may mean that care is withdrawn if violent behaviour continues; however, it must always be made clear that it is the behaviour that is being rejected, not the person (Taylor 2000).

In extreme circumstances, e.g. a client is seriously endangering their own safety or that of others, other methods may be used to protect them and others. In specialist areas such as forensic mental health nursing, 'time out' and seclusion are used for short periods to help divert aggressive behaviour, reduce sensory stimuli, encourage internal control and disrupt the source of provocation (Mason & Chandley 1999).

However, if more extreme measures are employed, such as observation and restraint, healthcare providers must have clear policies regarding their use and practitioners involved require specialist training. These techniques remain controversial because they prevent a person doing what they want to do, restrict their liberty and, when used inappropriately, can be considered a breach of human rights and abuse (RCN 2008). People have also been injured or have died during physical restraint, which has led to a number of investigations and recommendations for practice.

Where techniques such as observing people at regular intervals (Box 13.26) are used because people have become aggressive or are at risk of suicide, the emphasis is on a therapeutic intervention (rather than a custodial approach) and encouraging positive interactions. A balance needs to be struck between ensuring people's safety and maintaining their privacy, dignity and autonomy (Jones & Jackson 2004).

Restraint

Restraint is a technique that also raises issues of human rights (see Ch. 6) and its use requires careful thought about safety issues. Restraint can include a wide range of explicit and subtle controls such as bedrails (Box 13.27), medication, locked doors, stairgates, arranging furniture to impede movement, controlling language or body language or withdrawal of aids such as walking frames or spectacles (RCN 2008). Most of

---

Risk assessment: bed rails	**Box 13.27**

Bed rails (also known as safety rails or cot sides) are used in hospitals, people's homes and care homes when people, of all ages, are at high risk of falling out of bed. However, they can also be a source of injury and people have climbed over the top and fallen or become trapped between the bars and asphyxiated. Therefore, their use needs careful consideration and the following points are based on guidance from the Medicine and Healthcare Product Regulatory Agency (2011) who provide a poster with practical guidance.

Risk assessment

- *Are bed rails actually necessary and is the person at risk of falling out of bed*?
- *Are the safety rails compatible with the bed and the mattress*? Integral or third party (not designed for a specific bed) are available. The manufacturer's instructions must be followed
- *Is the safety rail fitted correctly*? Is there a risk of entrapment because of the size of the space between the rails and the bed or headboard?
- *Integral bed rails*: Some profile beds have fitted bed rails, usually in two sections, with a gap in the middle. Extra care is needed when adjusting the bed, e.g. moving the head end up to help the person sit up, as there may still be a risk of entrapment
- *Using a safety rail bumper*: Quilted or sponge covers are available to go over the top of safety rails and may reduce the risk of entrapment.

Patient/client factors

- *Is their head or body small enough to fit through the bars or the rail and the mattress*? Children need special types of rail because of their smaller size
- *Are they confused or agitated*? This puts them at greater risk of injury
- *Will they need to get out of bed at night*? Consideration needs to be given to how people will alert staff to the need to get out of bed.

Inspection and maintenance

All bed rails must be inspected before use to ensure that they are working properly and regularly maintained so that they remain in good order.

(Based on Medicine and Healthcare Products Regulatory Agency, 2011. Safe use of bed rails. Online. Available: http://www.mhra.gov.uk/home/groups/dts-pcc/documents/publication/con2025725.pdf September 2012)

Reflective practice   Box 13.26

Close observation

Lucy McFarland is a 22-year-old who has been treated for severe depression for 6 years and has attempted suicide for the second time. She has been admitted to an acute mental health unit and, with Lucy's agreement, staff searched her belongings to remove any articles she may use to harm herself and have been maintaining close observation. This means that staff check her activities every 15 minutes and she is not allowed to leave the unit unaccompanied. This duty is shared by several staff who rotate hourly. The ward is often short staffed and regularly employs agency staff, which means that Lucy often does not know the nurse observing her.

Student activities

- How do you think Lucy is likely to feel about being under close observation?
- How do you think her privacy, dignity and rights may be affected?
- How can staff make the process of close observation better for her?

these practices are unethical and solutions to safety issues must be found that do not affect people's dignity and independence (see Ch. 7). RCN (2008) guidelines contain a range of strategies for nurses to provide patient-centred care.

Specific guidance is available regarding the restraint of children and young people, particularly for painful procedures (RCN 2010). Chapter 7 discusses the ethical issues surrounding restraint in clinical practice in more depth.

Careful consideration needs to be given to the types of situation where restraint (overt or hidden) or seclusion and observation can be used, assessing the risk to the person and their human rights (Box 13.28).

 Reflective practice   **Box 13.28**

Restraint

Terrance Thornton is an 83-year-old man who has developed dementia and has recently moved into a residential home. He is confused in his new surroundings, especially at night when he has been becoming agitated, shouting at staff and prone to wandering. Care home staff installed bed rails to stop him getting out of bed but as a result he is unable to go to the toilet independently. Staff insist on providing continence pads when helping Mr Thornton to get ready for bed.

Student activities

- How are safety rails being used as an indirect method of restraint?
- What are the consequences of using safety rails and what further problems may occur?

Fire safety

Fire represents one of the greatest hazards to people's safety with potentially devastating consequences. There need to be three ingredients for a fire to start:

- A source of fuel
- A source of ignition
- Oxygen (Fig. 13.4).

Removing any one of these ingredients means that a fire cannot start and, by lowering the chances of the three coming together, the risk from fires is reduced.

Similar to many other safety issues, legislation (Regulatory Reform (Fire Safety) Order 2005; this applies to England and Wales although similar regulations apply to Northern Ireland and Scotland) aims to prevent fires by ensuring that employers:

- Carry out a fire risk assessment
- Provide fire detection and warning systems
- Provide an emergency plan and means of escape
- Provide facilities for fighting fire
- Provide fire safety training, normally annual training in healthcare settings.

Fire risk assessment

A fire risk assessment must identify all the fire hazards (e.g. sources of fuel, ignition) and the people at significant risk, especially those who have impaired mobility, sight or hearing. This information is used to identify improvements needed and implement measures to ensure everyone's safety (Department for Communities and Local Government Publications, DCLG 2006).

Fire detection and warning systems

All large buildings must have fire detection systems that trigger an alarm system or alarms that can be activated at fire points, usually by breaking the safety glass. There may be different fire alarm sounds, e.g. continuous for the immediate area (evacuation signal) and intermittent for other sections (alert signal), so it is important to know the local arrangements and when fire alarm testing takes place.

Emergency plans and means of escape

Hospitals are often organized into compartments that provide fire-resistant walls, ceilings and floors for a specified period of

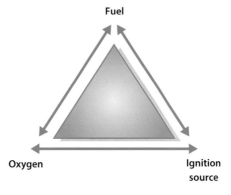

Sources of fuel

- Flammable liquids (paints, varnish, and solvents such as white spirit, petrol, paraffin)
- Flammable chemicals
- Wood, paper or card
- Plastics, rubber or foam
- Flammable gases
- Furniture and textiles

Sources of ignition

- Smokers' materials e.g. cigarettes and matches
- Naked flames
- Electric, gas or oil-fired heaters
- Cooking
- Engines or boilers
- Machinery
- Lighting equipment
- Hot surfaces and obstruction of equipment ventilation
- Static electricity
- Metal impact such as tools striking each other
- Arson

Fuel / Oxygen / Ignition source

Fig. 13.4 • The fire triangle. (Reproduced with permission from Home Office, Scottish Executive, Department of Environment (Northern Ireland) and Health and Safety Executive, 1999. Fire safety: an employer's guide. TSO, London.)

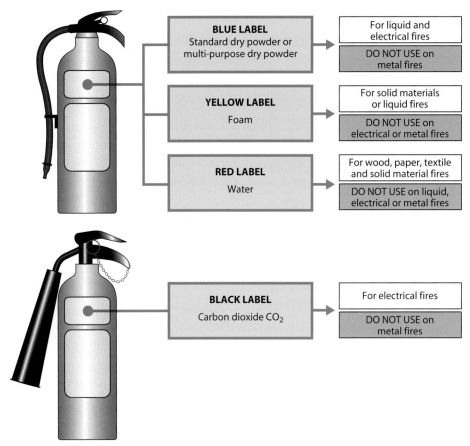

BLUE LABEL
Standard dry powder or
multi-purpose dry powder

For liquid and
electrical fires

DO NOT USE on
metal fires

YELLOW LABEL
Foam

For solid materials
or liquid fires

DO NOT USE on
electrical or metal fires

RED LABEL
Water

For wood, paper, textile
and solid material fires

DO NOT USE on liquid,
electrical or metal fires

BLACK LABEL
Carbon dioxide CO_2

For electrical fires

DO NOT USE on
metal fires

Fig. 13.5 • Types of fire extinguisher (based on Department for Communities and Local Government Publications 2006 Fire and resilience. Online. Available: www.communities.gov.uk/fire September 2012).

time. This reduces damage to buildings and increases survival rates, as initial evacuation is usually horizontal into the next compartment rather than downstairs (DCLG 2006). Emergency plans should discuss evacuation of people of differing mobility and availability of equipment such as evacuation chairs and flat ski sheets for immobile people on mattresses. Local training enables you to understand the arrangements for specific placements.

Facilities for fighting fire

Healthcare premises must provide facilities for fighting fires such as sprinkler systems and hose reels. In addition, fire extinguishers and fire blankets are located in appropriate areas such as kitchens so that people who have been trained to use them can tackle small fires. Figure 13.5 illustrates the different types of fire extinguisher.

Fire safety training

This section has introduced the basic principles of fire safety but within your nursing programme and throughout your career, fire training should be undertaken annually. This ensures that you are aware of local procedures, any new changes and can rehearse emergency situations. Carrying out the activities in Box 13.29 will highlight your fire safety awareness.

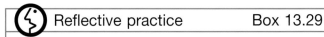

(⚡) Reflective practice	Box 13.29

Fire safety

Student activities

Consider an area of your college or university that you visit regularly and find out:

- Where are the nearest fire exits?
- How are they signposted?
- Where are the nearest points for raising the alarm in case of a fire?
- When are the fire alarms tested?

In each new placement, it is essential to familiarize yourself with the locations of fire points and read the fire action notices that give instructions. You should also:

- Find out how to contact the switchboard or the fire brigade.
- Locate fire extinguishers in the area and correctly identify the types of fire they can be used to tackle.
- Discuss fire evacuation procedures with your mentor.

SUMMARY

◆ Harm reduction in any area of healthcare begins with risk assessment and includes five stages.

◆ Risk assessment can be generic (relating to a group of patients/clients, staff or a particular task, e.g. fire hazards, moving and handling) or specific (examining the needs of individuals).

◆ Health and safety in the workplace is governed by legislation. Nurses must understand this and their responsibilities relating to COSHH, RIDDOR and moving and handling. They must implement training given, follow procedures, use equipment designed to improve safety, take reasonable care of themselves and others, and report any safety concerns.

◆ Standard infection control precautions, especially handwashing, are essential to prevent the spread of infection.

◆ Violence and aggression include verbal and physical abuse towards an individual. Many factors can lead to aggressive behaviour and clinical areas conduct risk assessments to identify contributing factors and implement measures to reduce incidents occurring.

◆ Core safety skills require theoretical knowledge and rehearsal for practice. These include moving and handling, fire safety, resuscitation and de-escalation techniques. They are part of nursing programmes and annual updates are necessary.

◆ First aid requires training and practice that builds the confidence needed to deal with emergency situations. This is included in nursing programmes and other organizations also provide training.

◆ As well as a number of core safety skills, becoming a safe practitioner also means developing a questioning approach, recognizing one's limitations and using evidence-based practice and reflection.

KEY WORDS AND PHRASES FOR LITERATURE SEARCHING

Fire precautions

First aid

Health and safety regulations

Moving and handling/patient handling

Risk assessment

Violence and aggression

 Useful websites

BackCare www.backcare.org.uk

First Aid Training Organizations

British Red Cross www.redcrossfirstaidtraining.co.uk

St Andrew's First Aid www.firstaid.org.uk

St John Ambulance (including Northern Ireland) www.sja.org.uk

St John Cymru www.stjohnwales.co.uk

Health and Safety Executive www.hse.gov.uk

National Patient Safety Agency (future being reviewed) www.npsa.nhs.uk

Royal Society for the Prevention of Accidents www.rospa.com

All websites accessed September 2012.

References

Alaszewski, A., Alaszewski, H., 2000. Risk: empowerment and control. In: Alaszewski, A., Alaszewski, H., Ayer, S. (Eds.), Managing risk in community practice: nursing, risk and decision-making. Baillière Tindall/RCN, Edinburgh.

Austin, M., Crawford, R., Armstrong, V.J. (Eds.), 2011. First aid manual, nineth revised ed. Dorling Kindersley, London.

Bibby, P., 1995. Personal safety for health care workers. Arena, Aldershot.

Department for Communities and Local Government Publications, 2006. Fire and resilience. Online. Available: www.communities.gov.uk/fire September 2012.

Department of Health, 2002. Managers' guide – stopping violence against staff working in the NHS. DH, London.

Health and Safety at Work Act, 1974. HMSO, London.

Health and Safety Executive, 2003. Health and safety regulation: a short guide. HSE, Sudbury.

Health and Safety Executive, 2004. Manual handling: guidance on regulations. HSE, Norwich.

Health and Safety Executive, 2005. Simple guide to the Lifting Operations and Lifting Equipment Regulations 1998. HSE, Sudbury.

Health and Safety Executive, 2006a. Five steps to risk assessment. HSE, Sudbury.

Health and Safety Executive, 2006b. Violence at work: a guide for employers. HSE, Sudbury.

Health and Safety Executive, 2009a. Working with substances hazardous to health: what you need to know about COSHH. HSE, Sudbury.

Health and Safety Executive, 2009b. Simple guide to the Provision and Use of Work Equipment Regulations 1998. HSE, Sudbury.

Health and Safety Executive, 2010. The HSE statistics 2009/10. HSE, Sudbury.

Health and Social Care Information Centre, 2009. Accident and emergency attendances in England (experimental statistics) 2007–2008. Online. Available: www.hesonline.nhs.uk September 2012.

International Council of Nurses, 2010. The ICN definition of nursing. Online. Available: www.icn.ch/about-icn/icn-definition-of-nursing September 2012.

Jones, J., Jackson, A., 2004. Observation. In: Harrison, M., Howard, D., Mitchell, D. (Eds.), Acute mental health nursing: from acute concerns to capable practitioner. Sage, London.

Mason, T., Chandley, M., 1999. Managing violence and aggression: a manual for nurses and health care workers. Churchill Livingstone, Edinburgh.

National Audit Office, 2003. A safer place to work: protecting NHS hospital and ambulance staff from violence and aggression. TSO, London.

National Institute for Health and Clinical Excellence, 2004. Falls: the assessment and prevention of falls in older people. Online. Available: www.nice.org.uk September 2012.

National Patient Safety Agency, 2011. National Reporting and Learning Service. Online. Available: www.nrls.npsa.nhs.uk September 2012.

NHS Security Management Service, 2010. Procedures for placing a risk of violence marker on electronic and paper records. Online. Available: www.nhsbsa.nhs.uk/SecurityManagement.aspx September 2012.

Nursing and Midwifery Council, 2008. Providing care in an emergency situation outside the work environment. Online. Available: www.nmc-uk.org September 2012.

Nursing and Midwifery Council, 2010a. Preregistration nursing education. Annexe 3: Essential skills clusters. Online. Available: http://standards.nmc-uk.org/Documents/Annexe3_%20ESCs_16092010.pdf September 2012.

Nursing and Midwifery Council, 2010b. Standards for preregistration nursing education. Online. http://standards.nmc-uk.org/PreRegNursing/statutory/Standards/Pages/Standards.aspx September 2012.

Royal College of Nursing, 2003. Dealing with violence against nursing staff: an RCN guide for nurses and managers. RCN, London.

Royal College of Nursing, 2008. Let's talk about restraint – rights, risk and responsibility. RCN, London.

Royal College of Nursing, 2010. Restrictive physical intervention and therapeutic holding for children and young people. RCN, London.

Royal College of Nursing and National Health Service Executive, 1998. Safer working in the community: a guide for NHS managers and staff in reducing the risks from violence and aggression. RCN, London.

Taylor, D., 2000. Student preparation in managing violence and aggression. Nursing Standard 12 (14), 39–41.

Further reading

BackCare and Royal College of Nursing, 2011. The guide to the handling of people, sixth ed. BackCare, Teddington.

Glasper, A., Richardson, J., 2010. A textbook of children's and young people's nursing, second ed. Churchill Livingstone, Edinburgh.

Waugh, A., Grant, A., 2010. Ross and Wilson anatomy and physiology in health and illness, eleventh ed. Elsevier, Edinburgh.

The nursing process, holistic assessment and baseline observations

14

Pauline Hamilton   Theresa E. Price

LEARNING OUTCOMES

This chapter will help you:

- Identify the stages of the nursing process and discuss the value of using a problem-solving approach to care
- Discuss how the use of a model of nursing can enhance patient/client care
- Explore the approaches to nursing care used in different settings
- Identify the need for careful documentation as part of nursing practice
- Discuss different nursing assessment strategies
- Explain how body core temperature is assessed using tympanic, oral, axillary and rectal routes, and with different types of thermometer
- Accurately assess and record adults' and children's temperature, pulse, blood pressure, respirations, Early Warning Scores, height, growth and weight, with reference to normal values
- Explain the nursing interventions used to manage pyrexia and hypothermia.

Introduction

This chapter provides an introduction to the nursing process and how it can be applied to different individuals who have varied healthcare needs. It acknowledges the diversity of nursing and provides examples of how the nursing process can be applied in child, mental health, learning disability and adult settings.

The key nursing skills required for holistic assessment are included, with emphasis on the need for effective verbal and written communication skills to promote accurate assessment, followed by effective nursing intervention. Tools that assist in the assessment of individuals are explored, as well as some models of nursing and approaches to care planning.

Assessment of a person's health status includes the measurement of four vital signs: body temperature, blood pressure, pulse and respirations. In addition, a person's weight, height and, in children, the growth rate may be measured. This chapter explains how each of the vital signs is measured and recorded and, for patients who are acutely ill, entered into an Early Warning Score chart (EWS). Assessment of health status usually takes place:

- When a person is admitted to a healthcare system
- If there is a change in health status
- To monitor change as a result of treatment, e.g. administration of medication
- Before, during and after surgery.

The nursing process

Nursing and healthcare delivery systems throughout all fields of nursing are diverse. The philosophies that underpin approaches to nursing vary enormously. In the past, the medical model was prevalent in many areas of nursing. Using this approach, nursing care usually followed the medical diagnosis and was focused on the physical condition of the person. The practice of nursing is based on interpersonal relationships (see Ch. 9), with other technical aspects of nursing following.

In recent years, there has been a move away from the medical model, recognizing the individuality of patients/clients and the need to address issues that go beyond the scope of physical care and medical diagnosis. However, medical diagnosis not only affects the needs that people may have, but also has an impact on other aspects of life. Thus, there is an attempt to provide holistic care to all groups of people requiring support from nurses and other healthcare professionals. There is also an increasing body of nursing knowledge available to support different nursing strategies and approaches to care, i.e. evidence-based practice (see Ch. 5). This too has an impact on care given. The decision to utilize a particular approach to care should therefore be based upon the unique needs of the person and family, as well as the nursing context (Department of Health, DH 2010a).

Yura and Walsh first described the nursing process in 1967 as a means of adopting a problem-solving approach to nursing care. The nursing process provides a systematic way of examining people's problems with a view to providing interventions that would move towards resolving the problems. Their view was that nursing comprises more than intuitive care and that a systematic approach would allow further analysis of the problems that people present with and how they might be resolved. It should be noted that problems identified are problems of the person, not nursing problems. Thus, management of these problems should be person centred (Yura & Walsh 1967).

The nursing process can be applied in all nursing settings although the way in which it is applied depends on the health needs of patients/clients, the skills of the nurses and the care environment. The nursing process is cyclical and has a number of stages:

- Identify with the person what the problems are – *assessment*
- Make plans to address the problems – *planning*
- Take steps to manage the problems – *implementation*
- Reflect on what has happened – *evaluation*.

Sometimes a fifth stage is added to the nursing process – the nursing diagnosis stage – which fits between the stages of assessment and planning (Fig. 14.1). The nursing diagnosis stage has been adopted more in North America than in the UK. The North American Nurses Diagnosis Association (NANDA) has provided standardized nursing diagnoses for many situations (NANDA 2008). Nursing diagnosis explains the effect of the medical diagnosis. For example, the patient may have suffered a heart attack (myocardial infarction) and so one of the nursing diagnoses may be 'central chest pain'. Nursing diagnosis has been used to standardize terminology and assist the process of audit, a mechanism to measure quality of care to determine if standards are being met.

The nursing diagnosis stage relates to the diagnosis of nursing issues, which may be based on an underlying medical condition but differs from the medical diagnosis. Medical diagnosis is the identification of disease from examination of symptoms and presenting features, whereas nursing diagnosis is more about gaining understanding of the person's situation, which may have wider implications for the person and also impact on other healthcare professionals (Barker 2009; NANDA 2008). The approach to planning care influences whether or not the nursing diagnosis stage is included. Patterns of care delivery vary and the UK is moving towards multidisciplinary ways of working, with documentation being designed to incorporate multidisciplinary terminology.

As the nursing process is cyclical in nature, evaluation can lead to reassessment if required. If patient/client goals (see p. 310) have been achieved, care can be stopped relative to the goal, or the plan of care may be modified if the goal has not been fully achieved.

While the nursing process can be applied in different settings, it is helpful to use a tool that will provide further guidance appropriate to the needs of people and the care setting. This can be achieved by the use of a model of nursing (see p. 311). The stages of the nursing process are explored below.

Assessment

The first stage is assessment of the patient's/client's and family's needs. Assessment involves collecting information (data) about the person and using that information to make decisions about what care, support or intervention is required. Decision-making involves organizing and interpreting the information collected. Professional judgement may also contribute towards the decision-making process. Assessment documentation and techniques vary according to the setting, e.g. outpatient, inpatient, short stay, ambulatory care, rehabilitation, day care, primary care based in the home, clinics or surgeries. Risk assessment is discussed fully in Chapter 13; however, it is an integral part of the assessment process.

As assessment is the cornerstone of establishing what a person's needs are, so the quality of assessment is pivotal to the success of the nursing process. Successful nursing intervention hinges on a complete and thorough assessment being undertaken. Even throughout the other stages of the nursing process, the nurse continues to assess the response to care and success of interventions. Thus assessment is an ongoing process. The aims of assessment are to:

- Determine the needs and potential needs of the person and their family
- Gather information on which a plan of care may be based
- Document information that will provide a basis for reassessment and evaluation
- Act as a mechanism for quality care
- Fulfil statutory obligations
- Aid the structure of nursing knowledge.

Best practice in assessing, planning and implementing care can be achieved by incorporating principles from The Department of Health *Essence of Care 2010: Benchmarks for Self Care* into the process of assessment. The document advocates that

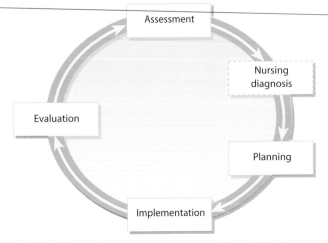

Fig. 14.1 • The nursing process. (Reproduced with permission from Brooker, C., Nicol, M., 2003. Nursing adults: the practice of caring. Mosby, Edinburgh.)

healthcare workers seek the views of the person to inform the care plan (DH 2010b).

Assessment is a complex, time-consuming activity that requires many skills. Assessment of someone's needs should be performed jointly with the person whenever possible. Establishing people's own perspective of their problems helps to create partnership working and assists in providing person-centred care that is holistic in nature. Sometimes, this is not possible due to the nature of the person's problems, e.g. in a high-dependency setting when the patient is unconscious, or in a mental health assessment unit when a client is confused and disorientated.

The information required in any given assessment situation will be determined by the nursing context. Confidentiality must be maintained in all settings (Nursing and Midwifery Council, NMC 2008; see also Ch. 7). Information should be collected systematically to ensure that important issues are not overlooked. A combination of observation, interview and measurement is required to provide a full assessment (NANDA 2008).

Observation is a key nursing skill that informs the overall assessment process. Observing is a form of data collection made by using the senses. Visual observation can relate to all aspects of the person. Someone's general appearance and physical signs such as skin condition can be observed (see Ch. 16). Touch is also used to assess characteristics such as the temperature of a person's skin, presence or absence of pulses or signs of dehydration such as dry, inelastic skin (Barker 2009). Smell can be used to assess dimensions of a person in relation to the environment, such as chemicals in the air. In relation to the person, alcohol may be smelt on their breath or smoke on their clothes.

Interactions with other people can be observed, e.g. verbal and non-verbal communication (see Ch. 9). People's behaviour can also be observed, e.g. their reactions to a particular situation, including emotional signs such as crying. Observations should be systematic to maximize the information gathered.

To complete assessment accurately, practitioners should strive for objectivity. Personal interpretations of observations should be avoided. For instance, when describing a person's physical characteristics, it is desirable to retain objectivity and, where possible, to be specific. For example, blood pressure '180/95' instead of 'blood pressure high', or 'smiles frequently' rather than 'happy'. Essential nursing skills include objective measurement. Equipment is often used, such as a thermometer to measure temperature (p. 323) or a sphygmomanometer to measure blood pressure (p. 328). Height and weight may be measured with the use of a measuring tape and set of scales (p. 334). Quantifiable information is therefore acquired through the use of equipment as well as direct observation.

Information can be collected in a variety of ways, depending on the situation. The initial assessment of people attending an emergency department will differ greatly from the assessment undertaken by a practice nurse who is immunizing a family going abroad on holiday. The practice nurse makes an assessment of what is required for the safety of the travellers in the longer term, whereas the emergency department nurse makes an initial short-term assessment of the person in relation to their priority for treatment.

Holistic assessment

For assessment to be comprehensive, it should be undertaken in a holistic manner. Thus, the following dimensions of need should be assessed (Fawcett 2005):

- Physical
- Sociocultural
- Spiritual
- Psychological
- Emotional.

While people may present to the nurse with similar medical or social problems, it is only by thorough and systematic assessment that includes the physical, psychological, sociocultural, spiritual and emotional dimensions of their lives that a truly individualized plan of care can be developed. It can, however, be difficult to separate the dimensions, as they are all inter-related and can impact on a person's health in different ways (Box 14.1).

 Critical thinking   **Box 14.1**

Holistic assessment

Anna is a young married woman with small children who is undergoing radiotherapy treatment for cancer. She may experience physical side-effects, including fatigue. The fatigue may cause anxiety, as Anna may be less able to look after her children and fulfil family obligations. She may consider not completing the course of radiotherapy to allow the fatigue to diminish. It is only by undertaking a holistic assessment that the impact of the treatment on Anna and her family's lives can be ascertained.

Student activities

- Think about the dimensions of holistic care and try to identify more aspects of Anna's life that may be affected.
- Assuming that Anna's children had left home and the other circumstances were unchanged, identify the potential differences that Anna and her children may face.
- Discuss your ideas with a colleague.

The nurse's role is to identify and react to a person's response to their own situation. Thus, while a medical condition is acknowledged when assessing a patient or client, it only forms part of the assessment. The aim is to acquire the fullest information necessary without gathering irrelevant information.

Priorities of assessment may differ within different fields of nursing. In mental health, assessment may concentrate initially on psychological and social dimensions, since much of the care of people with mental health problems centres on human responses to illness (see p. 316). With children, it is appropriate to use a child and family-centred approach (see p. 317). The benefit of such an approach is that it addresses the needs of the family as well as the child. Learning disability assessment also has unique characteristics, which are discussed later. Nurses working in many settings will meet people with a learning disability as most live in the community and access health services in the usual ways, e.g. though primary care via their GP or practice nurse. What is important is that the principles discussed on page 315 are incorporated into the assessment process.

The nurse will undertake a decision-making process to make sense of the data collected from the assessment and formulate a plan of care. Thus the nurse's assessment of the patient/client will form the nursing history.

Sources of information

Information can be gathered for assessment purposes from:

- The patient/client – the primary source
- Other people or records – secondary sources.

Primary source

The patient or client should be the primary source of information, including children and young people as developmentally appropriate, as it is important to elicit their own perspective of their situation. To successfully interview the patient/client, the nurse needs to be a skilled communicator; questioning, actively listening and eliciting information (see Ch. 9). The nurse's questioning technique will depend on the circumstances. Open questions are often appropriate to encourage the person to respond, however there are times when it is more appropriate to use closed questions, e.g. in the case of an acutely ill breathless patient or a patient in extreme pain.

Questions for the nurse to ask during the assessment interview should be holistic. Factors that encompass an holistic perspective may relate to physical, sociocultural, spiritual, psychological and emotional factors. It is important for the nurse to be aware of factors that may influence the patient or client's situation. Therefore, consideration of these five factors may assist the nurse in formulating appropriate questions to ask the patient or client. Perhaps environmental factors influence the person with asthma and it would be appropriate to ask about the nature of their workplace. An example of how these factors can be incorporated into holistic assessment of breathing can be seen in Box 14.2.

Often assessment is undertaken in difficult circumstances, e.g. emergency admission to hospital is an anxiety-provoking event for patients and their relatives. Crisis intervention within community mental health nursing is another occasion when assessment is required, usually following a series of difficult events leading up to the need for intervention. The initial impression the nurse may have of the patient/client and their family can influence the ease with which the nurse is able to elicit reliable information. If the nurse gives the impression of being disinterested or hurried, it is unlikely that an accurate assessment will be made. Assessment should form the beginning of a trusting relationship between the nurse and patient/client and provides the person with the opportunity of putting their view of their current situation forward. There may be occasions when the patient/client is unable to provide information, through illness, confusion, being too young or having difficulty with communication, e.g. learning disability.

Secondary sources

These are used together with the primary source. Biographical data can be confirmed from previous health records. It is important to confirm the currency of this information in case of changes in circumstances such as someone being widowed or having moved house. Social and medical history can often be confirmed from other health records. Other practitioners can also offer information about patients/clients. For example, key workers of individuals living in residential or nursing homes can provide information if a client is hospitalized. Patient-held records or patient passports are also used, when available. Past medical history is also important to assess along with the current health situation. This can reveal information that may impact on the current situation, such as knowledge of allergic reactions to a drug or relevant information about the person's prior experience. Family members and significant others can also be rich sources of information about the patient/client and how their current situation is affecting their ability to cope with daily living.

Discharge planning

Prevention of early readmission may be avoided if discharge planning is robust enough to support the person on discharge. Inadequate planning and coordination can lead to unnecessary suffering and can also have a major impact on the resources needed to support the person. Preparing a patient/client and their family for discharge from hospital is an integral part of nursing care (DH 2010c). In many cases, discharge is the most important aspect of a hospital admission for the patient/client and their family.

As many hospital admissions are very short, planning for discharge should be incorporated into the initial assessment and pre-assessment stage. During surgical pre-assessment visits (see Ch. 24), people are given information regarding requirements for going home following surgery or other invasive procedures. If a patient lives alone and is unable to have someone stay with them following discharge after day surgery and/or an anaesthetic, an overnight hospital stay may be more appropriate. Thus social, physical, psychological, economic and environmental aspects of assessment are crucial in providing

---

Nursing considerations as part of holistic assessment of breathing	Box 14.2

1. Physical:
   - What is the rate and pattern of breathing?
   - Is breathing affected by activities or environmental factors?
2. Psychological:
   - Is there a need for breathing or relaxation exercises?
   - Is there a chance that emotion may affect breathing?
3. Sociocultural:
   - Are there influences on the person's behaviour, e.g. smoking?
   - What are the person's health beliefs (see Ch. 1) about coughing, expectorating or using inhaled medication?
4. Environmental:
   - Are there factors influencing breathing, e.g. medication, position in bed, home/workplace – dampness, irritants?
5. Politicoeconomic:
   - Are there constraints on resources that affect breathing, e.g. housing issues, financial issues?

relevant information that will inform a safe discharge. With many people being discharged following hospital admission for acute problems, or longstanding chronic problems, complex management plans and packages of care may be required and therefore a coordinated approach to discharge planning is necessary. Early supported discharge teams are in place in some specialties such as orthopaedics and care of older adults. Within these services, there is explicit inclusion of discharge criteria in the care planning documentation. The nurse caring for the patient has a responsibility to ensure that a multidisciplinary approach is taken when required. Therefore, discharge planning is documented as an integral part of care delivery, emphasizing the need for the nurse to work in partnership with other professional groups and agencies (DH 2010c).

The nature of a patient's health needs or presenting problems will inform discharge planning; for hospitalized patients, nurses also need to enquire about the perspectives of carers. Most patients have a network of significant others who can provide information about them; they must also be consulted about certain aspects of care such as the transition from home to hospital, or hospital to home. Without the support of significant others, it is often not possible to achieve a successful discharge. Patient transfer also necessitates careful planning and communication of all involved. DH (2010c) emphasize the importance of involving patients/clients and carers in the process and to help these principles be applied to transfer situations, a best practice template is available (Scottish Government 2009). Box 14.3 summarizes factors that require consideration before transfer or discharge.

Factors that are taken into account before a patient is transferred or discharged　　　　Box 14.3

- Patient and their relatives are aware of transfer/discharge
- Specific care, e.g. wound care is documented
- Appropriate patient education has been undertaken
- Mode of transport appropriate and organized
- Name of person responsible for transfer/discharge
- Social service involvement needed and organized
- Community services needed, e.g. nurse/multidisciplinary team/home care
- GP letter/immediate discharge document/transfer documentation completed
- Medication ready to go with patient
- Follow-up appointment information available
- Aids/dressings/prosthesis are available
- Access to home has been assessed.

The assessment interview

The planned assessment interview that forms the basis of the nursing history can take place in many settings. The health visitor may conduct an assessment of a child's developmental progress at home surrounded by parents and other family members. Alternatively, the assessment might be in a situation of crisis, such as a serious injury following an accident. Whatever the situation, there must be structure to the interview. The focus will be not only on the documentation being used

but also on the person being interviewed. It is important to include both. The use of documentation alone will not allow the whole spectrum of issues to be captured. The first interview allows the nurse to gather baseline information about the person. Comparisons against this will be ongoing. In some settings the interview will be conducted by a doctor and a nurse such as in acute mental health admissions (Barker 2009). The advantage of this is that the client will not have to repeat similar information to different professionals. There is also the benefit of engaging in multiprofessional working, with all health professionals sharing care of the patient to provide a cohesive service (Barker 2009).

Privacy

At all times during the assessment process, privacy must be respected. This may be easier to achieve in some settings than in others, e.g. when an interview room is available. In the patient's/client's home or in a busy department where there are many other people, it may be more difficult to achieve and therefore careful consideration is needed. In the home it may mean asking other family members to leave the room, or in the department it may be necessary to speak quietly behind screens. Other barriers to effective communication need to be identified and remedied, e.g. environmental noise affecting concentration could be avoided by moving to a quieter area. Language barriers may be overcome by the use of interpreters from within the family or the health provider organization. Confidentiality should be maintained if interpreters are being used. It should be recognized that factors affecting the quality of the interaction between the nurse and the person may have an adverse effect on the quality of information provided and the care received (see Ch. 9 and Box 14.4).

 Reflective practice　　　　Box 14.4

Sharing personal information

Before starting your nursing course, you may have had to undergo occupational health screening.

Student activities

- Reflect on the situation where someone you had not previously met has asked you to reveal personal information.
- Consider how you felt about divulging personal information to a stranger.
- How did the approach of the person affect your feelings at the time?

Interpretation of information

The nurse will undertake a decision-making process to make sense of the data collected from the assessment and formulate a plan of care. Nurses need to be aware of their own beliefs, values and attitudes as well as their level of knowledge and competence. Assumptions should not be made about the condition of a patient/client. Unlike BP measurement, not all patient/client observations, can be validated. For example, it is difficult to measure the level of anxiety a patient is experiencing (see Ch. 11). As such, nurses need a degree of self-awareness to ensure that value judgements and assumptions are not made regarding the person's situation.

Staging assessment

The use of a step-wise approach to assessment is sometimes appropriate, with some aspects of the assessment process being undertaken immediately, while others are undertaken later. For example, an older adult being admitted to a care home may have a full assessment undertaken over a period of 1 week to minimize the effects of relocating on their usual routines and ability to adapt. An unconscious child admitted to an emergency department would need immediate assessment to allow priorities of care to be established.

It is sometimes inappropriate to explore every aspect of assessment at the initial interview. In some mental health and learning disability settings, client assessment may be undertaken incrementally as the therapeutic relationship is established. This is also the case in situations when a person is moving into long-term care, e.g. a nursing home. If this is the case, the nurse assessing must take responsibility for ensuring full assessment is completed. This can be useful if the patient/client needs time to adjust to their new situation before discussing sensitive issues with the nurse.

Documentation

Documentation of the nursing process, at each stage, is an important way to communicate to other members of the healthcare team how the patient/client is progressing and responding to interventions. Documentation must be comprehensive and accurately reflect the health status of the patient/client. Accuracy is achieved by recording information precisely, e.g. 'the patient had 150 mL of tea, and toast and scrambled eggs' rather than 'good appetite', as appetite varies from person to person, and also from nurse to nurse, thus making the assessment subjective. It is a professional requirement to record nursing interventions and the information collected to inform the intervention, as nursing documentation is a legal document (NMC 2010a).

Assessment documentation takes different formats according to the setting. Electronic records of care are being implemented gradually throughout the UK as information technology systems are developed to support healthcare delivery (DH 2010c; House of Commons 2007). Patient-held records are also used, especially for people with long-term conditions. Patient-held records can support self-management and self-care, thus increasing patient involvement. For example, in asthma care when a person attends the practice nurse, the GP and an outpatient department, it is useful for them to have one record that can be used by all professionals to improve continuity of care across primary and secondary care settings. Increasingly, multidisciplinary documentation is being developed with the whole team having access to the records. Confidentiality should be maintained at all times regarding documentation, irrespective of the mechanism being used (NMC 2010a).

Single shared assessment is intended to simplify the assessment process, be person-centred and clarify responsibilities between health and social care providers, mainly for older adults in the community. Making this process work, however, requires commitment from all healthcare practitioners to keep the patient/client central to planning of their care. Additionally, this may mean the erosion of traditional professional barriers and boundaries. The underpinning philosophy of shared assessment is that it is 'needs led' rather than 'service led'.

Assessment tools

Assessment tools, as part of risk assessment, form part of the assessment process and those used depend on the specific needs of the patient. Assessment tools, developed by nurses (practitioners and researchers), provide a validated method of eliciting information with a view to minimizing patient/client risk. Tools devised by other professional groups are also used by nurses, e.g. the Glasgow Coma Scale and Paediatric Glasgow Coma Scale (see Ch. 16). An example of a commonly used assessment tool is the Waterlow scale, a pressure ulcer risk assessment tool (Fig. 14.2; see also Ch. 25). This tool is used to predict the level of risk of an individual developing pressure ulcers, taking their overall condition into account (Box 14.5). Early Warning Score (EWS) charts are assessment tools commonly used to monitor patient's vital signs in order to identify deterioration in condition (see Fig. 14.14). Tools should be appropriate to the client group to optimize their effectiveness. Risk assessment (see Ch. 13) should be performed at appropriate times, e.g. when there is a change in the health status of a patient/client. It is important that all staff using an assessment tool are familiar with its use.

⍰ Critical thinking   Box 14.5

Using assessment tools

- 2-year-old Jane has been admitted to a children's ward with suspected meningitis. She has a generalized rash and moving is painful
- Isa Oliver (84) has been admitted to an orthopaedic ward through the emergency department after a fall at home. She has previously been in good health and independent at home. She has a fractured hip and is scheduled for surgery today
- Imad Jumaa (68) lives in a nursing home. He has dementia and poor mobility due to arthritis. He is doubly incontinent and is unable to attend to his own hygiene needs. Imad has difficulty with communication
- Fred Maxwell is 28 years old and has a learning disability. He lives in a house with four other service users who are supported by carers. He also has physical disabilities and mobilizes with a wheelchair. Fred is underweight and his appetite is poor; he needs help with personal hygiene and feeding, and is incontinent of urine.

Student activity

Using the Waterlow scale (see Fig. 14.2), assess the level of risk the people above may have of developing pressure ulcers (see Ch. 25 for further information, including other pressure ulcer risk assessment tools).

Planning

This stage of the nursing process involves identifying the person's problems or needs and what nursing care, intervention or support is required. The care plan should be written down and contain clear statements about how the person's goals will be achieved (see below). The patient/client should also be involved

(A)

WATERLOW PRESSURE ULCER PREVENTION/TREATMENT POLICY
RING SCORES IN TABLE, ADD TOTAL. MORE THAN 1 SCORE/CATEGORY CAN BE USED

BUILD/WEIGHT FOR HEIGHT	◆	SKIN TYPE VISUAL RISK AREAS	◆	SEX AGE		◆	MALNUTRITION SCREENING TOOL (MST) (Nutrition Vol. 15, No. 6 1999 - Australia)		
AVERAGE BMI = 20-24.9	0	HEALTHY	0	MALE	1		A - HAS PATIENT LOST WEIGHT RECENTLY	B - WEIGHT LOSS SCORE	
ABOVE AVERAGE BMI = 25-29.9	1	TISSUE PAPER	1	FEMALE	2		YES - GO TO B	0.5 - 5kg = 1	
OBESE BMI > 30	2	DRY OEDEMATOUS CLAMMY,PYREXIA	1 1 1	14 - 49 50 - 64	1 2		NO - GO TO C UNSURE - GO TO C AND SCORE 2	5 - 10kg = 2 10 - 15kg = 3 > 15kg = 4 unsure = 2	
BELOW AVERAGE BMI < 20 BMI=Wt(Kg)/Ht (m)^2	3	DISCOLOURED GRADE 1 BROKEN/SPOTS GRADE 2-4	2 2 3	65 - 74 75 - 80 81 +	3 4 5		C - PATIENT EATING POORLY OR LACK OF APPETITE 'NO' = 0; 'YES' SCORE = 1	NUTRITION SCORE If > 2 refer for nutrition assessment/Intervention	

CONTINENCE	◆	MOBILITY	◆	SPECIAL RISKS				
COMPLETE/ CATHETERISED	0	FULLY RESTLESS/FIDGETY	0 1	TISSUE MALNUTRITION	◆	NEUROLOGICAL DEFICIT		◆
URINE INCONT,	1	APATHETIC	2	TERMINAL CACHEXIA	8	DIABETES, MS, CVA		4-6
FAECAL INCONT.	2	RESTRICTED	3	MULTIPLE ORGAN FAILURE	8	MOTOR/SENSORY		4-6
URINARY + FAECAL INCONTINENCE	3	BEDBOUND e.g. TRACTION	4	SINGLE ORGAN FAILURE (RESP, RENAL, CARDIAC)	5	PARAPLEGIA (MAX OF 6)		4-6
		CHAIRBOUND e.g. WHEELCHAIR	5	PERIPHERAL VASCULAR DISEASE	5	MAJOR SURGERY or TRAUMA		

SCORE					
10+ AT RISK		ANAEMIA (Hb < 8)	2	ORTHOPAEDIC/SPINAL	5
15+ HIGH RISK		SMOKING	1	ON TABLE > 2HR#	5
20+ VERY HIGH RISK				ON TABLE > 6 HR#	8

MEDICATION - CYTOTOXICS, LONG TERM/HIGH DOSE STEROIDS, ANTI-INFLAMMATORY   MAX OF 4

#Scores can be discounted after 48 hours provided patient is recovered normally

© J Waterlow 1985 Revised 2005*
Obtainable from the Nook, Stoke Road, Henlade TAUNTON TA3 5LX
* The 2005 revision incorporates the research undertaken by Queensland Health.

www.judy-waterlow.co.uk

(B)

REMEMBER TISSUE DAMAGE MAY START PRIOR TO ADMISSION, IN CASUALTY. A SEATED PATIENT IS AT RISK
ASSESSMENT (See Over) IF THE PATIENT FALLS INTO ANY OF THE RISK CATEGORIES, THEN PREVENTATIVE NURSING IS REQUIRED. A COMBINATION OF GOOD NURSING TECHNIQUES AND PREVENTATIVE AIDS WILL BE NECESSARY
ALL ACTIONS MUST BE DOCUMENTED

PREVENTION PRESSURE REDUCING AIDS			Skin Care	General hygeine, NO rubbing, cover with an appropriate dressing

Special Mattress/beds:
10+ Overlays or specialist foam mattresses.
15+ Alternating pressure overlays, mattresses and bed systems
20+ Bed systems: Fluidised bead, low air loss and alternating pressure mattresses
Note: Preventative aids cover a wide spectrum of specialist features. Efficacy should be judged, if possible, on the basis of independent evidence.

Cushions:
No person should sit in a wheelchair without some form of cushioning. If nothing else is available - use the person's own pillow. (Consider infection risk)
10+ 100mm foam cushion
15+ Specialist gel and/or foam cushion
20+ Specialised cushion, adjustable to individual person.

Bed clothing:
Avoid plastic draw sheets, inco pads and tightly tucked in sheet/sheet covers, especially when using specialist bed and mattress overlay systems
Use duvet - plus vapour permeable membrane.

NURSING CARE
General   HAND WASHING, frequent changes of position, lying, sitting. Use of pillows
Pain   Appropriate pain control
Nutrition   High protein, vitamins and minerals
Patient Handling   Correct lifting technique - hoists - monkey poles Transfer devices
Patient Comfort Aids   Real sheepskin - bed cradle
Operating Table
Theatre/A&E Trolley   100mm(4in) cover plus adequate protection

WOUND GUIDELINES
Assessment   Odour, exudate, measure/photograph position

WOUND CLASSIFICATION - EPUAP
GRADE 1   Discolouration of intact skin not affected by light finger pressure (non-blanching erythema)
This may be difficult to identify in darkly pigmented skin
GRADE 2   Partial thickness skin loss or damage involving epidermis and/or dermis
The pressure ulcer is superficial and presents clinically as an abrasion, blister or shallow crater
GRADE 3   Full thickness skin loss involving damage of subcutaneous tissue but not extending to the underlying fascia
The pressure ulcer presents clinically as a deep crater with or without undermining of adjacent tissue
GRADE 4   Full thickness skin loss with extensive destruction and necrosis extending to underlying tissue.

Dressing Guide   Use Local dressings formulary and/or www.worldwidewounds.com

IF TREATMENT IS REQUIRED, FIRST REMOVE PRESSURE

Fig. 14.2 • The Waterlow scale. (Reproduced with permission from Judy Waterlow ©2005.)

in this stage, if possible. The format of the care plan depends on the particular setting. As well as establishing the person's existing problems, any potential problems are also identified. Learning disability nurses may also concentrate on a client's strengths as well as weaknesses.

Prioritizing care

Planning also incorporates prioritizing care according to the needs of the individual and seriousness of the problems. Life-threatening situations such as airway obstruction must be considered and acted upon before wider health needs, such as the desire to stop smoking. Determining priorities is achieved through an understanding of the theory and concepts underpinning nursing. Involvement of the person in this stage of the nursing process also assists in prioritizing care according to their wishes if there are no life-threatening issues. Through communication, mutually agreed goals can be set, based on the person's perception of their situation.

Actual and potential problems

The aims of planning are to:

- Solve actual problems (or meet health needs)
- Minimize the risk of potential problems
- Reduce recurring problems
- Assist in development of coping strategies for problematical health issues
- Build on strengths.

Consequently, nurses need to be able to 'see beyond' the present situation and use their knowledge and expertise to avoid complications and potential problems occurring (Box 14.6). It can be seen from Rashid's situation that the impact of one problem can potentially create many other problems for him that transcend different dimensions of need (p. 311).

Goal setting as part of care planning

Goals are set to enable measurement of the success, or otherwise, of the nursing interventions planned to meet them. Different types of nursing action are often required to meet the goals. For example, different members of the healthcare team may deliver different aspects of the care required. Which member of the team delivers the care to an individual depends on the complexity of their care and on the skills of the members. Competent healthcare assistants may perform some nursing interventions, e.g. they may be able to assist people to maintain personal hygiene. However, for some therapeutic interventions, the registered nurse (RN) would be required to monitor some parameters such as central venous pressure.

Goals can be either short or long term. They should be person centred and achievable. To assist in this, goals should be SMART and incorporate the following characteristics:

- **S**pecific – state clearly what is to be achieved
- **M**easurable – be made quantifiable
- **A**chievable – must be able to be achieved by the patient/client
- **R**ealistic – possible for the patient/client to achieve
- **T**imed – have a time limit by which the goal can be achieved and evaluation undertaken.

A goal could be 'the patient should drink 2.5 L of fluid within the next 24 hours'. Within this goal, it would have been assessed that the patient is capable of taking fluids orally, making it achievable and realistic. It is specific because it states the amount of fluid to be taken, is measurable as fluid intake and is timed as there is a timeframe allocated to its achievement. Box 14.7 provides an example of short- and long-term goals. If goals are unrealistic and unachievable, this can lead to disappointment of both the patient/client and the nurse. As a consequence, the therapeutic relationship may be adversely affected.

Actual and potential problems	Box 14.6

59-year-old Rashid was admitted to hospital with a left-sided weakness and investigations show that he has had a stroke. Rashid is left handed. One of his actual problems is that he is unable to move his left side, which might affect his mobility, skin integrity and independence.

Actual problem

- Unable to move left side.

Potential problems

- Negative impact on self-esteem
- Help required with eating and drinking
- Reduced mobility (see Ch. 18)
- Pressure ulcers (see Ch. 25)
- Deep vein thrombosis (see Ch. 24)
- Muscle weakness
- Limb contractures
- Inability to attend to personal hygiene
- Loss of independence.

Short- and long-term goals	Box 14.7

Eddie has been admitted to the ward with breathlessness. In relation to this, the following goals may be appropriate.

A short-term goal may be:

- To reduce Eddie's respiratory rate to <20 breaths/min within 2 hours

  The goal may be achieved by:
  - Careful positioning in bed; sitting upright, well supported with pillows or leaning on a bed table (see Ch. 17)
  - Administration of prescribed medication (see Ch. 22)
  - Administration of prescribed oxygen therapy (see Ch. 17).

A long-term goal may be:

- To cope with mild breathlessness prior to discharge

  The goal may be achieved by:
  - Education regarding breathing exercises prior to discharge
  - Teaching Eddie to reduce activity that provokes breathlessness
  - Referral to the physiotherapist.

Implementation

Putting the care plan into action forms the implementation stage of the nursing process. Implementation should incorporate current evidence-based practice (Ch. 5). The care plan may encompass physical, psychological, social, emotional and environmental interventions. Implementation may also include activities that are outwith nurses' expertise, e.g. it may be appropriate to refer the patient/client to another healthcare professional such as an occupational therapist for assessment of dressing ability. This referral is the nurse's responsibility and is recorded in the care plan. Such multidisciplinary working and collaboration should assist in providing holistic care.

Evaluation

Evaluation determines if the planned intervention has been effective in achieving the goals set. The goals are reviewed to determine whether or not the patient has met them or is moving towards meeting them. At this stage, the goals can be modified or changed according to the patient's/client's response to the interventions. If a goal has been achieved, this is documented. If a goal has not been achieved, the nurse should question why this is the case, and reassess the patient. Perhaps the goals did not encompass the SMART characteristics or the patient's/client's condition may have changed, making the goals unrealistic. Health needs are dynamic and thus require periodic reassessment. Evaluation is an ongoing action that forms part of the cyclical nursing process. However, evaluation is only possible if clear criteria have been applied to the goals. Evaluation of care can be used as part of nursing audit.

Nursing models

A nursing model, also known as a 'conceptual model', is a tool used to guide nurses as they engage in the nursing process and can be viewed as a practical way of putting the nursing process into action. Central to the use of any nursing model is the need for nurses to have excellent communication skills (see Ch. 9). There are many different nursing models that reflect the diversity of each field of nursing. Therefore nursing models have different philosophical assumptions underpinning them, each with a unique perspective of nursing knowledge and nursing practice and several are explored in the following sections. Most nursing models are based upon four concepts, which are said to form the essential structure of nursing. The relationship that emerges between the nurse and patient/client will depend on these four concepts:

- The person – the nature of the patient/client having a dimension of 'wholeness' or holism
- Nursing – a helping process with interpersonal relationships at its core
- Health – the goal of nursing is to assist people to achieve an optimum state of health, whether or not they are 'ill' (see Ch. 1)
- The environment – the physical constructions of the world and society within it.

Approaches to care planning for adults

Two commonly used nursing models are discussed in this section.

The Roper, Logan and Tierney model for nursing

The Activities of Living model was developed in the UK by Roper, Logan and Tierney who first published the *Elements of Nursing* in 1980. Their work developed some of the central components of Virginia Henderson's earlier definition of nursing (see Ch. 2). There are two parts to this model: the model of living and the model for nursing (Fig. 14.3). Over the years it has been refined, indicating that nursing is a dynamic profession, constantly developing in response to external influences.

According to Roper et al (2000), five interrelated components form the core of the model of living:

- The individual
- Activities of living (ALs)
- Lifespan
- Dependence/independence
- Factors influencing the ALs.

The individual

According to Roper et al (2000), individuality in living acknowledges that each person has a unique way of performing the ALs according to where they are on the lifespan, the degree of dependence/independence they have and the influences of biological, psychological, sociocultural, environmental and politicoeconomic factors. Individuality in living is concerned with how an individual experiences and performs ALs according to their preferences, abilities and attitudes.

Activities of living

Roper et al (2000) suggested that 12 activities are essential for survival:

- Maintaining a safe environment (Ch. 13 + others)
- Communicating (Ch. 9)
- Breathing (Ch. 17)
- Eating and drinking (Ch. 20)
- Eliminating (Chs 20, 21)
- Personal cleansing and dressing (Ch. 16)
- Controlling body temperature (see p. 319)
- Mobilizing (Ch. 18)
- Working and playing (Ch. 8 + others)
- Expressing sexuality (Ch. 8 + others)
- Sleeping (Ch. 10)
- Dying (Ch. 12).

It is evident that the activities cannot be viewed as mutually exclusive as they are dimensions that interlink with each other

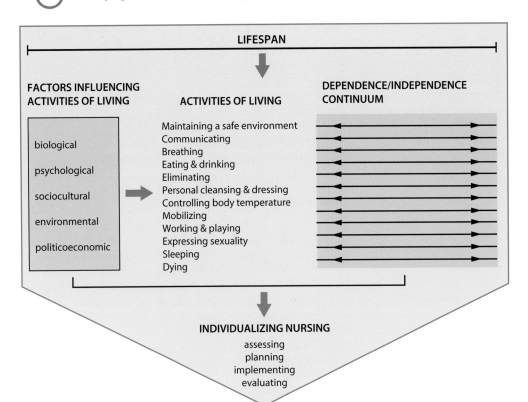

Fig. 14.3 ● The Roper, Logan and Tierney model for nursing. (Reproduced with permission from Holland, K., with Jenkins, J., Solomon, J., Whittam, S. (Eds.), 2008. Applying the Roper Logan Tierney Model in practice, second ed. Churchill Livingstone, Edinburgh.)

? Critical thinking   **Box 14.8**

The relationship between factors influencing activities of living (ALs) and the interdependence of ALs

Jane is 17 years old and lives with her mother and 11-year-old sister. Jane's parents are divorced and her father is not in contact with them. Her mother has chronic arthritis and is physically dependent on Jane to support her with running the house. Jane helps her mother to get into the shower in the evenings and collects her prescriptions. She also does the shopping, cleaning, ironing and supervises her younger sister with homework and getting ready for school. Jane is at college full-time and on Friday evenings, her friends often go the student union then on to a nightclub. Jane is usually too tired to join them.

Student activities

- Think about how Jane may experience social isolation from her peers (working and playing).
- Consider the psychological impact that home circumstances may have on Jane (sleeping).
- Identify ways in which Jane could get additional support to ease her situation (maintaining a safe environment).

(Box 14.8). For example, it is not possible to consider elimination without considering eating and drinking.

Lifespan

The lifespan is considered to be a continuum with changes occurring along it from birth to death. Throughout this time,

every aspect of living is influenced by biological, psychological, sociocultural, environmental and politicoeconomic factors. The five stages of life identified by Roper et al (2000) are:

- Infancy
- Childhood
- Adolescence
- Adulthood
- Old age.

Throughout these periods, levels of dependence and independence vary. An infant is vulnerable and dependent on others for survival and love. Childhood and adolescence are affected by cultural issues, sociocultural norms and subcultures (see Ch. 8) and are dominated by the family. In adulthood, work and family affect lifestyle. In old age, individuals may have an illness that affects their level of independence, e.g. arthritis which can impair mobility.

Factors influencing the ALs

There are five main factors that can influence daily living (Roper et al 2000), as outlined below.

Biological factors

In the context of the model of living, biological factors relate to physical and physiological performance. While there are predetermined genetic influences affecting physical characteristics such as skin colour, hair colour, height or genetically determined diseases such as haemophilia, other factors can also affect physical characteristics and function. In wartime, if a child is deprived of food, growth may be affected, resulting in slower rates of growth and development. Thus, environmental and politicoeconomic issues may also affect physical factors. Biological factors associated with ageing may affect a person's ability to work, thereby impacting on their sociocultural status.

Psychological factors

Mental and intellectual activity begins in childhood and continues through adolescence, adulthood and into older age. The stimuli within these lifespan phases vary. In childhood, development begins through sensory stimuli that can be influenced by family issues such as having siblings who may spend time playing with the toddler. In adolescence, development can be affected by the place of the child in the family and the expectations placed upon them. Thus environmental factors may also influence psychological development. Development across the lifespan is discussed in Chapter 8.

Sociocultural factors

Ideas, values, knowledge and beliefs are embedded within cultural norms of groups within society (see Ch. 8). Thus, many variations exist among the population from which patients and clients will come. Culture is unique to groups of people and can affect the behaviour of individuals. It is important to remember that cultural beliefs may have a profound impact on lifestyle and the responses of people who need to access health services. Dietary practices can have an impact on biological factors; for example, vegetarians may have a low iron intake leading to low blood haemoglobin levels and anaemia. Religion may affect how individuals respond to treatment options, e.g. Jehovah's Witnesses may reject blood transfusion as a treatment option compatible with their beliefs. Therefore sociocultural aspects may impact on biological and psychological factors.

Environmental factors

Environmental factors include housing, the atmosphere, noise and sound. Any of these elements can influence the other factors. Atmospheric pollutants such as carbon monoxide can aggravate respiratory conditions such as asthma, thereby having an impact on biological and psychological factors. Noise pollution can cause anxiety that may impact on psychological and biological functioning, e.g. by causing insomnia and anxiety.

Politicoeconomic factors

The economy, law and the state comprise the politicoeconomic factors that impact on individuals. People are governed by fiscal measures such as the need to pay council tax. Local and national economies also affect people and consequently their behaviour. For example, people on low incomes have limited choices on which to spend their money. Asylum seekers who are given vouchers as part of their financial support may have few choices about where they can exchange them. This may lead to lack of choice and being unable to follow dietary customs, thus impacting on biological and psychological factors.

It can be seen that the main themes of the model are inextricably linked and the activities in Box 14.9 highlight this.

? Critical thinking   Box 14.9

Factors influencing activities of living (ALs)

Groups such as asylum seekers, people with a learning disability and those with chronic illness may have limited control over the five factors that influence ALs.

Student activities

- Think about the impact of the five influencing factors on the three groups of people above. Draw on any experiences you have had in practice, but if you have not encountered such situations, use the information you have read.
- Think of an occasion when one of the five factors that influence ALs has affected your own well-being and how that occasion affected other aspects of your life.

Roy's adaptation model

Sister Callista Roy developed this model in the USA in the 1960s. It has been refined over the years to make it suitable for nursing in the twenty-first century (Roy & Andrews 1999). The basis of Roy's model is that individuals must adapt to a constantly changing environment. The health of the individual is a reflection of that adaptive process. It is a behaviourist model, as it is concerned with the way in which individuals behave in response to changing circumstances. Behaviourism is the study and observation of how individuals behave.

Roy's behaviourist model is based on the following two philosophical assumptions:

- That veritivity (true values and meaning of humankind, the purposefulness of human existence) is the principle of human nature, i.e. individuals exist with a common purpose of humankind
- That humanism is central to the individual, i.e. that human experiences are central to knowing and valuing.

The model is based on the following two scientific assumptions:

- That there are interdependent parts of an individual, working in unity. Control mechanisms are involved in the functioning of the system, and for every stimulus there will be a range of behaviours.
- The capacity and ability of the individual to respond to the stimuli, from both the internal and external environment, relates to the adaptation level.

Within the model, there are three types of stimuli (systems). These are:

- Physiological
- Psychological
- Social.

Roy and Andrews (1999) state that there is an interrelationship between these three systems, with all of them working together to maintain a balance within the individual. For example, if a person is physically unable to drink fluids due to a swallowing problem they may become dehydrated, and thus the internal body environment may be affected. Equally, if someone is

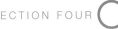

trekking across the desert with no water to drink, their social system is affecting their physiological status as they are unable to access fluid to prevent dehydration. Thus the systems are interrelated and interdependent, interacting with each other at all times.

According to Roy, if an individual adapts to these stimuli, it could be said that they are healthy. Most people cope effectively with constant changes to their internal and external environments. During a heat wave, for example, an individual may drink more fluids, slow down their level of activity and increase the ventilation of their home. An individual who is unable to make these changes, such as a toddler, may be considered to have an ineffective response to the stimulus of heat. If the individual has not adapted to the stimulus, then the role of the nurse is to assist the person to adapt to it. Thus, the focus for the nurse is to identify the stimuli to facilitate adaptation in the individual patient/client. Roy acknowledges the individuality of people and so there will be no complete state of balance applicable to everyone. Therefore, the nurse must recognize the needs of individuals.

Roy discusses the adaptation level of individuals as forming an adaptive range. Behavioural responses to stimuli can be effective, adaptive stimuli or maladaptive. The factors that cause problems of maladaptation are called stimuli and there are three types:

- *Focal stimuli* – the internal or external stimulus immediately affecting the person
- *Contextual stimuli* – any environmental factors contributing to the focal stimuli
- *Residual stimuli* – previous experience or attitudes or beliefs (Roy & Andrews 1999) (Box 14.10).

 Critical thinking   Box 14.10

Thinking about Roy's model

The activities below will help you consider how Roy's approach could affect you as a student nurse.

Student activities

- Imagine you are driving through busy traffic to an appointment with your tutor and you are late. You are approaching traffic lights and they turn red. Think about the effect that focal, contextual and residual stimuli may have on your judgement.
- Your second clinical placement is far from where you live, and the shift patterns there will cause travelling problems. Consider how the focal, contextual and residual stimuli may affect your adaptation to the situation.
- Suggest two behavioural responses to undertaking an assignment. (For example, an adaptive response may be the creation of a mind map to assist your planning, while an ineffective response would be doing nothing.)

Adaptive modes

There are four adaptive modes within Roy's model that serve as a framework for assessment. It is believed that a person's response to stimuli can be observed in these adaptive modes:

- *Physiological adaptive mode* – physiological balance, i.e. homeostasis
- *Self-concept adaptive mode* – psychological integrity, moral, spiritual
- *Role function mode* – social integrity, managing social interaction
- *Interdependency mode* – emotional and affective (moods or emotions) behaviour.

Roy states that these four modes contribute towards the promotion of adaptive goals leading to integration and wholeness. Nursing intervention would be required if there is a need deficit.

Assessment

With Roy's model, assessment is advocated using three stages:

- Stage 1 – examine the adaptive modes; identify if coping is adequate
- Stage 2 – detailed assessment; identify focal, contextual and residual stimuli
- Stage 3 – make a nursing diagnosis based on adaptation status; plan the nursing intervention based on the nursing diagnosis.

Planning

Planning should identify SMART patient-centred goals (see p. 310) that should incorporate the following:

- *Ineffective behaviour to be changed:* For example, if a patient is pyrexial (see p. 321) the goal may be to 'assist patient to regain normal temperature range by providing cool drinks, administering antipyretic medication and monitoring temperature 4-hourly'.
- *Adaptive behaviours to be reinforced:* For example, if a patient has stopped smoking since admission to hospital, the goal may be to 'provide positive reinforcement and assist distraction from smoking through a range of activities such as listening to the radio, reading health education literature and providing access to smoking cessation helpline'.

Evaluation

This involves exploring whether the goals have been met, thus determining if the adaptation response has been achieved effectively or ineffectively. Reassessment occurs at this stage.

Figure 14.4 shows the nursing process as it relates to Roy's adaptation model.

Approaches to planning care for people with learning disability

The focus on the needs of people with learning disability is embedded in national strategies published in the government's White Paper *Valuing People* (DH 2001). The Scottish Executive (2002) published *Promoting Health, Supporting Inclusion,* a strategy document to guide practice and the Welsh Assembly Government (2002) has an equivalent, *Inclusion, Partnership and Innovation.* These strategies, along with societal changes,

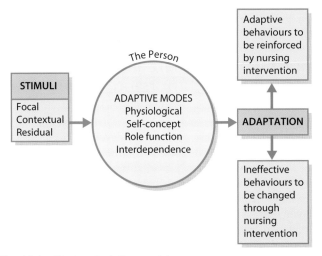

Fig. 14.4 • Roy's adaptation model.

have provided frameworks for the move towards social inclusion for those with learning disability. The underlying key principles of these documents are:

• Rights
• Independence
• Choice
• Inclusion.

Therefore, in order to care for people with learning disability, these key principles need to be included in the planning process. Individuals with learning disability often have complex health needs. While specialist learning disability nurses are in a strong position to begin to assess and meet these needs, generalist nurses may also assess the person's needs if the four key principles above are encompassed in their care.

When planning care for individuals with learning disability, traditional ways of care planning may not always fully encompass these key principles. Many learning disability nurses consider that nursing models are too focused on the medical model. It is important to use an assessment process that fully involves the person.

It is desirable for people with learning disability to achieve citizenship within the communities in which they live. In order to facilitate citizenship, nurses in all settings need to be able to assist people with learning disabilities to make informed decisions about their health and health issues.

As the spectrum of learning disability is very wide, ranging from mild to profound and complex, the only way to plan and provide supportive care is by placing the individual at the centre of the planning process.

Person-centred planning

Person-centred planning is a way of working in partnership with people and their families to achieve personal autonomy, which is pivotal to realizing the policy aims for people with learning disability (Scottish Executive 2004). As people with learning disability often have unmet health needs, another aim in caring for these people is to help the person have more

control over their health (Scarborough & Godsell 2011). For people who have difficulty in articulating their views, an advocate may assist in eliciting their views and thoughts. An advocate may be a paid care-worker or a family member or friend.

Person-centred planning aims to assist people to choose the lifestyle they want. Acknowledgement of the person's disability is made, with acceptance of their need for support on their own terms. The focus is on capacity and capacity building, which means working towards maximizing ability.

Person-centred planning can be achieved by sharing of power between the person, family and professional. Any significant person involved with the client may be involved, e.g. paid support workers or those who act as advocates for the person such as family members. Support workers may be part of the MDT such as learning disability nurses, resource workers, physiotherapists, speech and language therapists, occupational therapists and psychologists. Learning about the person is crucial to developing an understanding of their needs. Careful listening (see Ch. 9) and consultation are essential to fully assess the individual. Person-centred planning is a process that takes time and usually starts with a planning meeting. The key features of person-centred planning are shown in Box 14.11 and some are described in more detail below.

◯ Reflective practice   Box 14.11

Person-centred planning

• The person is at the centre of the planning process
• Family members and friends are partners in planning
• The plan reflects what is important to the person, the capacities of the person and the support that is required
• The plan leads to actions that are about life, reflecting what is possible and not just about services that are available
• The plan results in ongoing listening, learning about the person and further action (see Sanderson 2007).

Student activities

• Reflect on the extent of person-centred planning you have seen used with people with a learning disability
• Discuss this with your mentor.

Resource

Sanderson, H., 2007. Person centred planning. In: Gates, B. (Ed.), Learning disabilities: Toward inclusion, fifth ed. Churchill Livingstone, Edinburgh.

Consulting the person throughout the planning process

If the person with learning disabilities has been involved with planning before, it is sensible to talk to them about how they would like to plan, e.g. whether they want a meeting and, if so, what kind of meeting and how they want to be involved. If they are new to planning, it is important to spend time explaining the purpose of planning and looking at different options. Box 14.12 summarizes how this process may work for an individual.

The person chooses who to involve

Unlike traditional planning, it is for the person with learning disabilities to decide who they want to include in the planning process and how. This is easy to say but, with existing services, this is very different from the way meetings are typically organized. If the people around those with learning disabilities cannot find a way to help them make and communicate that decision for themselves, then they must decide in good faith who they think the person would want to involve. A good starting point is thinking about 'people who know and care about the person', which may well yield a different answer from 'people who provide a service to this person'.

The person chooses the setting and timing of meetings

If a meeting takes place it should be at a time convenient to the person with learning disabilities, with the people they wish to invite and be in a place where they feel 'at home'. The planning should be carried out in a way that is accessible to the person with learning disabilities. Graphics, tapes, videos or photos are often used.

Approaches to planning care in mental health nursing

In common with learning disability nursing, mental health nursing has also been driven by policy development to become user focused. The trend towards community-based care continues with many services provided by mental health nurses. There is emphasis on caring for people who have enduring mental illness such as schizophrenia. The shift away from institutional care has led to examination and scrutiny of approaches to planning and implementation of care. The following key principles underpin care planning in mental health settings:

- Advocacy
- Consent
- Autonomy
- Relationships
- Communication
- User involvement.

In mental health nursing, the approach used is also person-centred (Barker 2009). A person-centred approach builds on the seminal work of Peplau (1952) who espoused the strengths of the therapeutic relationship between the nurse and the person. Building on the work of Peplau is the notion of the professional relationships the nurse has with other professionals as well as the need for a person-centred nurse/person relationship that is not driven by the power of the nurse (Barker 2009).

The Tidal model

The Tidal model (Barker 2009) was initially developed from a study into mental health nursing. It is a multidimensional approach to the provision of mental healthcare. The philosophy is that people can recover from the experience of mental health problems and that nurses can assist clients to return to their daily life. Therefore, the philosophy is about helping people to cope with their problems and find solutions through their own experiences. As it is not about 'fixing them', this model has an empowering approach.

The Tidal model represents the unique contribution that nurses make to the care of people with mental health problems, though it also acknowledges the close relationships with other health and social care practitioners. One of its features is that a care continuum exists. The care continuum straddles the primary and secondary care settings with the premise that the needs of the person should be the focus of care rather than the setting. The assumption is that the need for nursing lies wherever the person is and not within the 'compartments' of primary or secondary care. Other features of the model are:

- Active collaboration with the person and family, if appropriate, to plan and deliver care
- Empowerment of the person through the narrative of illness and health

- Integration of nursing with the services provided by other members of the MDT
- Resolution of problems of living and promotion of mental health through narrative-based interventions in individual and group sessions.

The role of the nurse is two-fold:

- To form a therapeutic relationship with the person and, where appropriate, the family
- To cultivate professional relationships with other workers and professionals who may be involved in the care of the individual.

Barker (1996, p 236) illustrates the core basis of the Tidal model:

> Life is a journey undertaken on an ocean of experience. All human development, including the experience of illness and health, involves discoveries made on the journey across that ocean of experience.
>
> At critical points in the life journey the person experiences storms or even piracy (crisis). At other times the ship may begin to take in water and the person may face the prospect of drowning or shipwreck (breakdown). The person may need to be guided to a safe haven to undertake repairs, or to recover from the trauma (rehabilitation). Once the ship is made intact or the person has regained the necessary sea legs, the ship may set sail again, aiming to put the person back on the life course (recovery).

Barker (1996) asserts that there are three dimensions within the model:

- *World* – the need to be understood, including having the personal meaning of illness and distress validated by others
- *Self* – emotional and physical security
- *Others* – medical, psychological and social interventions, e.g. housing, finance, occupation, leisure.

The aim of assessment and planning within the three dimensions is to allow the person to verbalize their own experience to determine how their needs can be met. The narrative basis of the model suggests that the 'self' of the person-as-the-expert can be explored through careful inquiry by the nurse. Therefore, the therapeutic relationship between the nurse and person is crucial to allow construction of the person's experience through narratives. The care plan should document the needs of the person expressed in their own words rather than in professional language or in the third person. Thus the lived experience of the person can be documented.

The aim of the Tidal model, using a person-centred approach, dovetails with best practice statements regarding engagement with the person to work towards person-centred care (Barker 2009).

Further information about approaches to mental health nursing can be found in Useful websites, p. 335.

Approaches to planning care for children

Partnership in care is advocated as the desired approach to caring for children recommended in the National Service Framework (DH 2003). *Every Child Matters*, the government strategy that followed The Children Act 2004 (HM Government 2004), provides further aspirations and policies about the integrated partnership approach to caring for children across society (see Chs 3, 6). The services that children require change as they develop and encounter illness or vulnerability. The key to providing excellent care is in the relationships that develop between the nurse, the child and the family as well as those that the nurse has with other professional agencies and services. Respecting parents and the family means recognizing that:

- Parents are usually the expert on the child
- Parents may have other children to care for and may need to balance the needs of the other children and the child requiring care
- Parents may have to take time off work to attend outpatient or primary care appointments, or during hospital admission
- Parents may have health issues themselves which may influence their ability to be fully involved with the child
- Healthcare and hospitalization can impose financial hardship on the family (DH 2003).

The Nottingham model (Smith et al 2002) and Casey's partnership model (Casey 2007) are prominent in children's nursing. Both models are based on respect for the wishes of the family and negotiation of care needs. The main differences between them are that the Nottingham model includes the child and the family as 'the client', whereas Casey views the child as 'the client'. However, a partnership approach is central to them both.

The Nottingham model

While the philosophy of this model includes the family members as partners, it is still important to include the child in the decision-making process where possible. By doing this, dignity and respect for the child are maintained. As the model uses a holistic approach, taking account of the wider influences that can affect a child's health, the family's perception of health in relation to the child should be assessed when the history is being taken during admission.

Hospital admission can be very disruptive, not only to the child but also to the wider family. The child may have alteration in normal functioning that spans the physical, psychological, social, emotional and/or environmental dimensions of life (DH 2003). To minimize the trauma associated with hospital admission, a welcoming environment is necessary to enable the process of negotiated care to be established. A routine that allows a child's normal activities to be undertaken in relation to activities of living is encouraged, particularly in respect of education and recreation. Play is an important element of the nursing care provided (see Chs 8, 9) and forms an important aspect of pain management (see Ch. 23). The family or main caregivers should be considered the experts on young children. Their knowledge of the child's behaviour and level of independence can be communicated to the nurse and the plan of care is developed jointly. Assisting the family to retain some control over their lives, while meeting the needs of their child, is desirable. This often means that the family will be involved in direct care giving. To provide this type of family-centred care, the family must have clear guidelines about what to expect from the nurse. Therefore, nurses caring for children need to be excellent communicators. Older children and young people are often the experts about their own conditions and associated care.

If hospital admissions are planned (elective), some of the fear associated with hospital admission can be allayed. Receiving written and verbal information prior to admission may help reduce anxiety for the child and their family. It may also reduce recovery times. Preadmission schemes can also reduce some of the fears and anxiety by providing an opportunity to visit the environment and meet with some of the staff (Smith et al 2002). The Nottingham model follows the steps of the nursing process from assessment, planning, implementing and evaluating care.

Negotiated care

Negotiated care refers to a two-way process between the nurse and the child and their family. The relationship between these people should be based on mutual trust and respect. With each person's contribution being equally valued, an agreed plan of care can be made. The process of negotiation begins at the assessment stage. The level of family involvement should be frequently reassessed as the situation may change, as can the needs of the family. Thus parental participation in direct care delivery may vary over time.

Building an equal partnership

An equal partnership can be developed through the nurse assisting the family to acquire the additional knowledge and skills of caring needed. Equipping the family with knowledge can empower them. Factors that can build the partnership include:

- A positive attitude of the nurse that includes the family in care delivery if desired
- Willingness of the nurse to share information, knowledge and skills
- The ability of the nurse to educate, teach and support others.

Casey's model

This also incorporates negotiated care and partnership building with the child and family. According to Casey (2007), the key elements of paediatric nursing assessment are:

- The nature of the health problem and the child and family's understanding of it
- The developmental effects the health problem has on the child
- The family's situation, its responses to the problem and the nature of the coping
- The wishes of the family and educational needs
- The usual routines of the child
- The child and family's expectations of care and treatment.

Integrated care pathways

As an alternative to nursing care plans, integrated care pathways (ICPs) may be used. ICPs are sometimes called integrated care plans, care protocols or care maps. There has been increasing development of integrated care plans for all groups of people. The focus on providing a high quality service has led to increased use of ICPs as they are based on the current evidence base for best practice. Much of this evidence is informed by the National Institute for Health and Clinical Excellence (NICE) and the Scottish Intercollegiate Guidelines Network (SIGN). The ICP is a single document in which all members of the multidisciplinary team (MDT) record their care. The ICP details expected problems, interventions and outcomes for a specific disorder or group of people. These are devised with explicit agreement by local groups of multidisciplinary and multiagency staff. The aim is to provide a comprehensive service to a group of service users or patients with a specific condition (National Leadership and Innovation Agency for Healthcare 2005).

The MDT agrees on the format of the record that will be used by all professionals, not just one group, e.g. nurses. The pathway anticipates the expected requirements for care and the outcomes for the patient within a specified timeframe. SMART goals (see p. 310) are incorporated into the care pathway. It is still important to have the patient at the centre of the care pathway to ensure that the required standard of care is met. Individual assessment is still undertaken, often based on the assessment process associated with a nursing model. It is important that the philosophy of the assessment meets the needs of the patient/client group. For example, a patient undergoing surgery that may impact on their self-image, such as limb amputation, needs to be assessed psychologically and emotionally to determine their ability to adapt. Thus, the assessment may be based on Roy's adaptation model. So, although the ICP is multidisciplinary, within its development it is vital that the nursing approach is robust enough to incorporate holistic care (Box 14.13).

? **Critical thinking** Box 14.13

Integrated care pathways

Having a single document can help to provide an integrated approach to care, with shared working between professionals encouraging greater understanding of others' roles and responsibilities.

Student activities

Find an ICP used in your placement and then consider the following:

- What benefits are there for the relationships within the MDT when ICPs are used?
- How might the nature of the relationships of MDT members impact on the standard and quality of care given to patients/clients?
- What benefit might there be to patients/clients when ICPs are in use?

The benefits of using ICPs include:

- Enabling monitoring of standards of care
- Transparency of documentation
- Enhanced understanding of other professional roles
- Improved team working
- Explicit goal statements.

Variance

There are often reasons why a patient will not follow the expected path of recovery or response such as the presence of other health issues from any aspect of their life, i.e. physical, psychological, emotional, spiritual, sociocultural or environmental. This does not necessarily mean that the pathway is unsuitable for the patient, but rather it may highlight the unique features of any individual who requires care. If a patient varies from the expected pathway, this is documented on the care pathway, including whether the variance was avoidable or not. For example, other diseases impacting on patient progress is unavoidable whereas a delay in having a test performed is avoidable.

Documentation and record-keeping

Documentation and record-keeping apply to every aspect of nursing intervention. Accurate record-keeping is an essential and integral part of professional practice and personal professional development (NMC 2010a; see also Ch. 7). Records may be required for legal purposes (see Ch. 6) and audit. The quality and accuracy of record-keeping can reflect standards of care.

Timely and accurate records may highlight changes in a patient's/client's condition by providing a graphical record of their health status, demonstrating trends and changes over time, e.g. with charts used for baseline observations (see Fig. 14.14). Clinical observation charts are used to record vital signs and to calculate an Early Warning Score (EWS, see p. 332) which is used to monitor acutely ill patients for signs of deterioration (NICE 2007).

Vital signs

Assessment of a person's health status includes the measurement of vital signs that include temperature, blood pressure, pulse and respiratory rate. These are measures of a person's airway, breathing and circulatory function. In hospital settings, the observations will be recorded on an observations and Early Warning Score chart.

It is of fundamental importance that nurses can competently measure and record the vital signs and respond to change appropriately. The process of measuring, recording and interpreting vital signs demands accuracy. The NMC (2010b) requires student nurses, before the end of progression point 2 (usually at the end of Year 2), to be able to accurately measure and record vital signs and respond to any findings outside the normal range. A further NMC (2010b) requirement is that 'a baseline assessment of height, weight, temperature, pulse, respiration and blood pressure are accurately undertaken using manual and electronic devices'.

This section uses an evidence-based approach to measuring vital signs. A number of factors can influence the information obtained from these measurements, including changes to the environmental temperature or metabolic activity and exercise or eating. Nursing care of people with abnormally high and low body temperature is explained. At the end of this section, measurement of height and weight is described. These measurements indicate general health or underlying illness that may require investigation, monitoring and/or treatment.

Nurses measure, record and interpret vital signs and use the information to plan and implement appropriate nursing interventions as well as to evaluate the effect of care and treatment. Vital signs are usually all measured at the same time.

Body temperature

Core body temperature in health is in the range of 36.4–37.3°±0.2°C. It is measured in degrees (°) Celsius (C), and is relatively constant. Body temperature is an indicator of the balance between the amount of heat being generated by cellular processes and the excess that is lost. Efficient cellular metabolism requires the maintenance of body core temperature and organs that are located within the core, such as the brain, heart and liver, function best around 37°C. This is called the 'set point' and serious problems occur if temperature deviates much from this.

Distribution of body heat

Heat is generated by cellular metabolism; therefore areas of high metabolic activity such as the liver or exercising skeletal muscle have the highest temperatures. The locations that best reflect the body's inner or 'core' temperature are the heart and brain. Peripheral regions, which are nearer to the environment, are cooler as they are more exposed to the lower ambient temperature outside the body. Temperature sensors placed on the skin surface estimate peripheral or 'shell' body temperature. Body core temperature (BCT) can be measured using instruments that may be placed in sites such as the ear canal, oral cavity, axilla or rectum. Figure 14.5 shows body temperature at different sites.

Heat balance

Maintaining body temperature within the normal range requires a balance between heat produced by the body and its loss to the environment. Heat balance is achieved through the interplay of mechanisms that conserve heat and others that promote heat loss.

Heat conservation

When sensors in the hypothalamus detect a fall in temperature they trigger responses that promote heat conservation. These include:

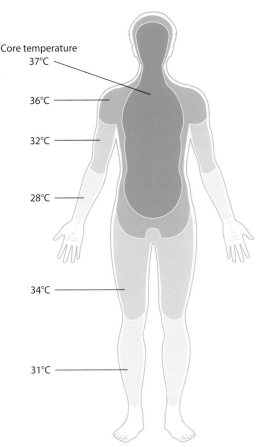

Core temperature
37°C
36°C
32°C
28°C
34°C
31°C

Fig. 14.5 • Body temperature at different sites. (Reproduced with permission from Brooker, C., Nicol, M., 2003. Nursing adults: the practice of caring. Mosby, Edinburgh.)

- *Vasoconstriction* – peripheral blood vessels constrict, diverting blood away from the extremities, thus limiting heat loss from the body to the environment
- *Piloerection* – body hairs are erected, trapping warm air against the body surface (skin)
- *Shivering* – generates heat
- *Reduced sweating* – facilitates heat conservation.

Behavioural responses include putting on more clothes, exercising or moving towards a source of heat.

Heat loss

If core temperature rises above the set point, the body initiates physiological mechanisms that promote heat transfer. These include:

- *Vasodilatation* – dilatation of peripheral blood vessels, which facilitates heat transfer to the cooler environment of the skin
- *Increased sweating* – facilitates heat loss as sweat evaporates from the skin
- *Increased rate and depth of respirations* – promotes heat loss in expired air
- *Decrease in cellular metabolism* – reduces heat production.

Behavioural mechanisms activated by the brain also promote heat loss. These include taking off clothes or wearing lighter clothes, drinking cold fluids or lifting the arms away from the body.

Physiological influences on body core temperature

There are several factors that influence BCT, as outlined below.

Diurnal cycles

BCT varies throughout the day. Variations are normally within a range of 0.5–1.0°C over 24 hours, with the highest point of 37.2°C at around 18:00 hours and lowest (36.7°C) around 06:00 hours. People having their temperature measured daily should therefore have this carried out at the same time each day to avoid normal diurnal variations.

Age

In infants, temperature regulation is labile because their physiological heat-regulating mechanisms are immature, and this can continue until puberty. Babies and small children therefore need to be dressed appropriately for the environmental temperatures around them. Heat production is increased in infants and children due to deposits of brown fat around the neck, back and viscera (the organs within the abdominal cavity). The only role of brown fat is to generate heat, and therefore shivering is not usually observed in this age group. Children also have a higher basal metabolic rate than adults, due to increased tissue growth rates. The consequence of a higher metabolic rate is a higher mean BCT.

Older adults may have a lower mean BCT that is also more influenced by ambient temperature. Therefore, should an older person develop an infection, BCT may not rise significantly. Ageing processes tend to reduce muscle mass, which reduces heat production capability in older adults. Additionally, loss of subcutaneous tissue (insulating fat) and reduced basal metabolic rate influence heat loss and production.

Menstrual cycle

Hormones released throughout the menstrual cycle also influence temperature. Increased cellular metabolism occurs at ovulation and body temperature rises by up to 1°C for the remainder of the cycle.

Other factors

Exercise increases heat production. Stress, pain and illness can also increase body temperature, whereas fatigue and headache can decrease it.

Environmental influences on body temperature

Environmental temperature extremes can raise or lower body temperature. The changes depend on the extent of exposure, air humidity and the presence of convection currents. Smoking cigarettes or cigars can increase oral temperature.

Table 14.1 Pyrexia: phases and nursing interventions

Condition	BCT	Phase	Signs and symptoms	Cause	Nursing interventions
Pyrexia	37.5–39.9°C	1. Chill	Skin is pale and feels cool and dry. Shivering, goose bumps (piloerection). Person complains of feeling cold. BCT rises and rigors may occur during this phase	Constriction of peripheral blood vessels. Immune response triggers heat generation strategies to kill invading bacteria	Keep person covered in light clothing. Add blankets to assist heat conservation
Hyperpyrexia	40.0–42.0°C	2. Plateau	Skin flushed and feels dry. Pulse and respiratory rates elevated. BCT remains high. Dehydration and dry mouth	Set point elevated. Increased cellular metabolism and oxygen consumption	Provide mouthwashes/oral hygiene and fluids or ice chips to suck. Provide an easily digestible diet high in energy to meet increased energy needs. If temperature above 39°C antipyretics and cooling measures may be prescribed
	42–36.4°C	3. Defervescence	BCT initially elevated but returns to normal. Pulse and respiratory rates remain elevated. Skin moist, flushed and hot. Profuse sweating. Dehydration may occur	Vasodilatation of peripheral blood vessels and sweating facilitate heat loss. Dehydration and increased cellular metabolism: contribute to raised pulse and respiratory rates	Provide cool dry clothes and bedding. Sponging with cool water may promote comfort. Continue oral hygiene and fluids as above; a fluid balance chart may be used to monitor hydration status (see Ch. 19). Assess risk of pressure ulcers (see Fig. 14.2 and Ch. 25) as moist skin increases this risk. Continue prescribed antipyretics and cooling measures

Care of people with temperature abnormalities

Body temperature can deviate from the normal range as a result of excess heat production, minimal heat loss or minimal heat production. It may:

- Rise resulting in pyrexia (fever, BCT above 37.5°C) or hyperthermia (BCT above 40°C) due to failure of heat loss mechanisms (see Further reading, Childs 2011)
- Fall, resulting in hypothermia (BCT below 35°C).

Disorders such as heatstroke, hypothermia and frostbite may occur when environmental temperatures are extreme. The first aid for people with heatstroke is outlined in this section.

Caring for patients with pyrexia or hyperpyrexia

Pyrexia is present when elevated temperature readings have been recorded at different times throughout the day, rather than a single raised reading. Pyrexia is often caused by an infection and has three stages. The first stage, during which BCT rises, can induce vigorous shivering or 'rigors'. Shivering generates metabolic heat with a subsequent rise in BCT, which the body uses to mount a response against the invading pathogen. The stages and the nursing care required are outlined in Table 14.1. Elevated BCT increases basal metabolic rate and oxygen consumption and, in hyperpyrexia, there is serious disruption of brain and other organ function. Children under the age of

5 years are prone to febrile seizures and the first aid needed is described Box 16.32 (p. 391).

Two major strategies can be used to manage elevated body temperature:

- Antipyretic medication, e.g. paracetamol, ibuprofen, aspirin (not used for children under the age of 16 years because of the potential risk of Reye syndrome, see Ch. 23) that reduce BCT
- Cooling interventions. The rationales to support cooling strategies are presented in Table 14.2. However, cooling patients remains an area of nursing practice that is ritualistic and lacking in conclusive evidence.

Aggressive forms of cooling such as the use of cooling mattresses or covering the whole body with ice are sometimes required for patients who develop temperatures above 41°C as this may cause serious and sometimes fatal consequences.

Prolonged exposure to hot sunlight or high environmental temperatures can result in the development of a serious condition known as heatstroke where measured BCT can be as high as 45°C. People at risk include:

- Those exercising or engaging in strenuous activity in high environmental temperatures, especially when combined with high humidity
- Children

Table 14.2 Advantages and disadvantages of cooling interventions

Cooling intervention	Advantages	Disadvantages
Fanning – rotary mobile fans blowing over body surface, using a variety of speeds	Perceived patient comfort Convenient Cheap	Shivering and vasoconstriction Spread of airborne microorganisms No evidence to support use in ill patients
Cool water bathing – sponging with cloths soaked in either ice-cool water or tepid water	No shivering Reduction in BCT	Time consuming Discomfort and vasoconstriction with iced cloths
Ice cooling – ice packs applied to areas where major arteries are near the skin surface, e.g. axillae, groins, neck	Surface cooling on area surrounding pack Rapid cooling	Vasoconstriction, which limits heat transfer from core to the skin causing heat conservation
Cooling blankets/mattresses – can be water filled and placed under patient, or air filled and put over patient Temperature controlled thermostat	Rate of fever reduction faster than traditional methods Control over temperature setting	Expensive to buy or rent Uncomfortable, so generally only used on comatose patients No more effective than traditional methods

- Older adults
- Those with co-existing heart disease or metabolic disturbances, e.g. diabetes or hypothyroidism
- Those taking recreational drugs such as Ecstasy, alcohol or medications such as diuretics (see Ch. 22) that may impair heat loss mechanisms.

Recognition of heatstroke and the necessary interventions are shown in Box 14.14.

Caring for patients with hypothermia

Hypothermia is present when BCT is below 35°C. It is described as mild, moderate, severe or profound and can be fatal if untreated. Hypothermia usually occurs accidentally as a result of exposure to low environmental temperatures and people at the extremes of age are the most vulnerable. Awareness of and providing interventions that will minimize the risk factors for hypothermia can often prevent its occurrence. Risk factors in infants, adults and older adults are outlined in Box 14.15.

Hypothermia can also occur in hospital. For example, some anaesthetic drugs lower BCT, as do some interventions, e.g. infusing large volumes of unwarmed fluids or irrigating body cavities with cool fluids in theatre. It is therefore important that temperature is carefully assessed and monitored postoperatively (see Ch. 24).

Restoring low BCT to normal requires careful management. The following parameters should be assessed: blood pressure (see p. 327); heart rate (see p. 325); respirations (see p. 330); oxygen saturation (see Ch. 17); temperature (which should be measured using a tympanic thermometer, see p. 323, or an internal probe) and urine output.

Management involves warming, which can be active or passive depending on the severity of hypothermia; however, it is dangerous to rewarm a patient too quickly. In mild hypothermia, the aim is to increase BCT by 1–2°C per hour and this can be achieved by: closing windows and doors; leaving clothing on if the room is cold, but taking off any wet clothes and wrapping the person in blankets. Other strategies include: wearing a hat to minimize heat loss through the head;

 First aid Box 14.14

Heatstroke

Recognition

Usually there is sudden onset of some or all of the following signs and symptoms:

- Hot dry skin
- Flushed skin
- Headache
- Excessive thirst
- Nausea
- Numbness, tingling, muscle cramps
- Dizziness
- Restlessness
- Mental confusion.

Observations

- Temperature above 40°C
- Tachypnoea (increased respiratory rate)
- Tachycardia (pulse rate >100 b.p.m. in an adult).

Aims of treatment

- To recognize the presence of heatstroke
- To remove the cause
- To reduce body temperature
- To transfer the casualty to hospital.

Treatment

- Remove the source of heat – move casualty into shade or out of the sun
- Lie casualty down and provide reassurance
- Loosen clothing and remove any items of unnecessary clothing if possible
- Sponge with cool water
- Dial 999 (or 112) for an ambulance
- Check and record respiratory rate, pulse rate and level of response.

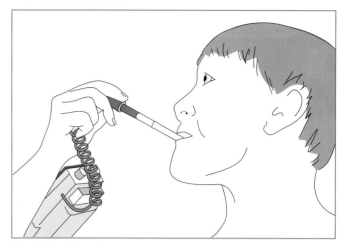

Fig. 14.6 • Oral electronic thermometer. (Reproduced with permission from Nicol, M., Bavin, C., Cronin, P., et al., 2008. Essential nursing skills, third ed. Mosby, Edinburgh.)

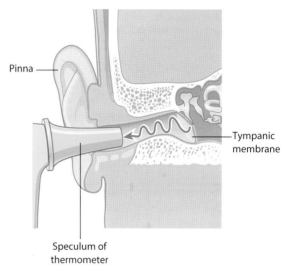

Fig. 14.7 • Using a tympanic thermometer. (Reproduced with permission from Brooker, C., Nicol, M., 2003. Nursing adults: the practice of caring. Mosby, Edinburgh.)

particularly for babies and young children, blowing warm air over the body and warming intravenous fluids in moderate and severe hypothermia.

Body temperature assessment tools

Estimation of body core or peripheral temperature can be made at different sites using a variety of instruments, which include tympanic membrane probes, electronic thermometers and disposable chemical dot thermometers.

Each device has advantages and limitations (see Table 14.3) and therefore individual needs must be assessed. Should intervention to manage abnormal body temperature be required, it is necessary to select a thermometer that can be used to make frequent or continuous measurements. This must be accurate and reliable at the top and bottom of the scale, and be appropriate for the person's age and individual needs.

Electronic thermometers

The electronic thermometer (Fig. 14.6) is a battery-operated device that displays a digital readout of the temperature measured during a preset recording time, usually between 20 and 50 seconds. Attached to the device by a cable is a probe, which is most commonly placed in the mouth, axilla or rectum. Protecting rigid probes with a plastic disposable cover and cleaning them between each use prevents cross-infection.

However, the device requires regular calibration, and the site used to measure temperature influences reliability. For example, the axillary placement is affected by environmental temperature and the oral placement depends on its position within the mouth and the cooperation of the patient.

Tympanic thermometers

Tympanic thermometers measure temperature at the tympanic membrane (eardrum). Because the tympanic membrane is in close proximity to the hypothalamus, measurement here accurately reflects the BCT. The tip of the instrument contains a probe, protected by a disposable sheath, which is placed into the ear. Some manufacturers recommend that the pinna is pulled upward and back for an adult and down and back for a child. This action straightens the external ear canal, creates a seal from external air temperature and facilitates correct insertion of the probe (Fig. 14.7).

The probe detects heat emitted from the tympanic membrane in the form of infrared energy. The resulting signal is processed and displayed as a digital readout. Temperature is measured and displayed within 3 seconds of activation and

Table 14.3 Sites and thermometers – a comparison

Thermometer	Site used	Advantages	Limitations
Electronic thermometer probes	Oral cavity, axilla Rectum	Easy access Good blood supply Well insulated from external environmental influences on temperature	Does not correlate with tympanic or pulmonary artery temperature Not recommended for use with newborns or children
Tympanic membrane thermometer	Auditory canal	Good blood supply Fast measurement (<5 seconds) Easy to use Accurate and reliable	Expensive Ambient temperature may influence temperature within auditory canal Use without specific training may cause unreliability of measurement Poor correlation with oral electronic thermometry Earwax, blood, foreign bodies and other matter in the canal lower the temperature reading so use is precluded in patients who have recently had ear or neurosurgery Hearing aids must be removed before measurement is carried out
Chemical dot thermometers	Oral cavity, axilla, forehead	Ease of access Disposable – reduces cross-infection Low cost	Lacks sensitivity in measuring elevated body temperature Underestimates oral temperature, overestimates axillary temperature Some require 3-minute placement time

the instrument bleeps on completion. The tympanic thermometer measures body temperature accurately between 25° and 43°C.

Tympanic thermometers are widely used in healthcare settings, because they are convenient, easy and quick to use, and reliable. Their limitations are summarized in Table 14.3.

Single-use thermometers

Single-use thermometers, such as chemical dots, are convenient, easy to use, non-invasive and also disposable. The thermometer consists of a plastic strip, with a series of chemically impregnated paper dots, which is placed in the oral cavity or the axilla. The dots change colour with heat. The final reading can usually be taken in up to 3 minutes, depending on the manufacturer's instructions. Their limitations are summarized in Table 14.3.

Glass-and-mercury thermometers

These were used for many years, however risks to health from mercury toxicity and dealing with spillages in healthcare settings means these are now seldom used in healthcare settings.

Thermometer placement sites

Temperature varies widely throughout the body (see Fig. 14.5, p. 320) and it is therefore important to remember that, if a temperature trend is required, the same site is used for each measurement. As a result of site variation of temperature, it is erroneous to believe that one location is more accurate than another. For example, BCT measured at the pulmonary artery is usually higher than the oral or axillary sites because the mouth and skin are exposed to the cooling influences of ambient temperature. In contrast, BCT will be lower than that found in the rectum due to the heat generated from metabolic activity of microorganisms in the rectum. Commonly used sites

for measuring body temperature include the oral cavity, the tympanic membrane, the axilla and the rectum, which are discussed below. Measurement of blood temperature within the pulmonary artery is considered to be the most accurate reflection of BCT – the 'gold standard'. This is because blood returning from major organs to the heart reflects the average temperature of the major internal organs. However, measuring pulmonary artery blood temperature is an invasive technique that is confined to critical care areas as are other sites including the pharynx, oesophagus and bladder.

Oral cavity

The thermometer is placed in the sublingual pocket at the junction with the tongue, which is close to the sublingual artery and therefore equates well with BCT. This site may not be suitable for young children who are at risk from biting the probe, especially if they are afraid and/or uncooperative.

Tympanic membrane

The probe is placed in the auditory canal and can be used for adults or children (Fig. 14.7).

Axilla

An electronic or chemical dot thermometer is placed under the axilla and the arm holds it in place. This site can be used for adults, infants and children. In children, the arm is held gently against the body to keep the thermometer in place.

Rectum

The rectum can be used for adults, although it is not commonly used in children in the UK. It is never used in newborns because of the risk of rectal perforation. If a non-disposable temperature probe is used, a disposable sheath is applied and discarded after use. The thermometer is cleaned according to local policy before and after use.

Skin

A disposable probe attached to the skin surface can be used for adults or children.

Interpreting temperature measurements

The temperature measured should be recorded. In hospitals, this is usually on a clinical observation chart (see Fig. 14.14). Measuring and recording the temperature onto the chart, either every few hours (1–4 hourly) or daily, will reveal a trend for body temperature. If body temperature is elevated above the normal range, then cooling interventions can be initiated (see p. 321). Recording the body temperature every few hours while a patient is being cooled will demonstrate whether the strategy is lowering the temperature effectively. The temperature reading should be entered on the clinical observation chart and also contributes to the Early Warning Score (see Fig. 14.14, p. 333).

Pulse

Nurses frequently perform assessment of the pulse, which is the rhythmic expansion and relaxation of an artery caused by ejection of blood from the left ventricle when it contracts. Knowledge of the rate, volume and rhythm produces information that assists in assessment and evaluation of health status or response to interventions. This section outlines anatomy and physiology of the pulse and explains how it is assessed.

Principal pulse points

The pressure wave, or 'pulse', of blood travelling along some arteries can be felt using the fingers at points of the body, where an artery lies close to a bone (Fig. 14.8). This is the 'peripheral' pulse, and it can be assessed by palpation (gentle compression of an artery using the fingers, against a bone). The most commonly used site is the radial artery at the wrist (Fig. 14.9).

The carotid arteries are located in the neck at each side of the larynx (see Fig. 14.8). They supply blood to the brain and are easily accessible. This is sometimes referred to as a central pulse. However, only light pressure should be applied to one artery at a time, in case the blood supply to the brain is restricted. During cardiopulmonary resuscitation, the carotid artery is palpated by trained healthcare practitioners to detect the return of a pulse (see Ch. 17).

The femoral artery may be used to assess the pulse, especially when the blood pressure is low as peripheral pulses in the arm and lower leg can be difficult to palpate. Peripheral vascular disease restricts blood flow to the lower limbs and it may be necessary to establish the presence of pulses in the legs to confirm blood flow to the extremities. The popliteal, posterior tibial and dorsalis pedis (also known as 'pedal') pulse sites are used to assess whether circulation is present in specific parts of the leg and foot. The popliteal pulse can be difficult to palpate and considerable practice may be required to master this.

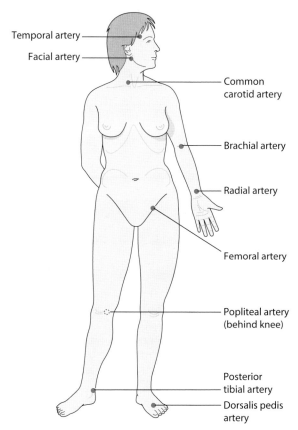

Fig. 14.8 • The main pulse points. (Reproduced with permission from Waugh, A., Grant, A., 2006. Ross and Wilson anatomy and physiology in health and illness, tenth ed. Churchill Livingstone, Edinburgh.)

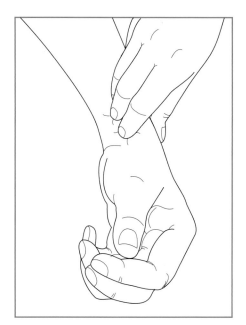

Fig. 14.9 • Taking the radial pulse. (Reproduced with permission from Nicol, M., Bavin, C., Bedford-Turner, S., et al., 2004. Essential nursing skills, second ed. Mosby, Edinburgh.)

Normal pulse rate

The rhythmic pulsation of blood in the arterial system is counted and recorded as the pulse rate (Box 14.16) and normally represents the rate at which the heart beats, i.e. the heart rate. The normal resting rate in adults is between 60 and 100 beats per minute (b.p.m.). In adults, tachycardia is the term given to pulse rates greater than 100 b.p.m.; bradycardia describes a pulse rate below 60 b.p.m.

Nursing skills   Box 14.16

Taking the pulse

Equipment
- Watch with second hand
- Observation chart.

Preparation
- Explain the procedure and seek verbal consent; maintain respect and dignity at all times
- The person should be lying or sitting down. Allow the person to rest for 30 minutes after physical activity, emotional upset or smoking
- Wash hands as per local policy.

Procedure
- Select the pulse site
- Apply pressure gently but firmly with flat fingers until the pulse is palpated
- Count the number of beats for 1 minute using a watch with a second hand. If a regular rhythm is noted, the pulse can be counted for 30 seconds and the number of beats is doubled
- Note further characteristics of the pulse:
  - rhythm (regular or irregular)
  - force or volume
- If the respiratory rate is to be measured, this is usually carried out discreetly while recording the pulse (see Fig. 14.13)
- Wash hands according to local policy
- Record pulse rate on the observation chart (see Fig. 14.14)
- Report and document any changes/abnormalities.

This important skill forms part of Essential Skills Cluster 9 (NMC 2010b).

Factors that affect heart rate

The pulse rate varies depending on the degree of activity within the autonomic nervous system. Stimulation of the sympathetic nervous system and the release of adrenaline increase heart rate, whereas parasympathetic activity decreases it. Due to their higher metabolic rate, children have a faster pulse rate than adults (see Table 14.4).

Stressors such as pain, fear and anger increase the pulse rate as they increase sympathetic activity. The rate also increases with exercise and pyrexia, and may alter due to the effects of medications and some diseases such as those involving the heart, lungs or blood (see Ch. 17). Medication such as digoxin is given to patients with heart failure, to improve myocardial contraction and reduce the heart rate. Salbutamol,

Table 14.4 Pulse rates for children

Age (years)	Pulse rate (b.p.m.)
0–1	110–160
1–2	100–150
2–5	95–140
5–12	80–120
Over 12	60–100

(Reproduced with permission from Mackway-Jones, K., Molyneux, E., Phillips, B., et al. (Eds.), 2005. Paediatric life support: the practical approach, fourth ed. BMJ Books/Blackwell, Oxford.)

used to control the symptoms of asthma, can cause tachycardia.

Assessing the pulse

The radial pulse can be found at the inner aspect of the wrist below the base of the thumb and medial to the radius, or wrist bone. It is palpated by placing two fingers, usually the index and third, and applying gentle pressure on the radial artery (see Fig. 14.9). Measuring the pulse is described in Box 14.16. The regularity and strength are also assessed (see below). Radial, popliteal and pedal pulses may be difficult to locate in adults who are cold or when the environment is cold and those with:

- Peripheral vascular disease, which impairs peripheral circulation
- Low blood pressure (hypotension, see Ch. 17)
- Cardiac arrhythmias (see Ch. 17)
- Peripheral oedema (see Chs 17, 19).

Regularity

When counting the pulse rate, the regularity is also noted, as this reflects the cardiac rhythm. Normally the rhythm is regular as the heart contracts regularly. However, young people may have a rhythm disturbance, known as sinus arrhythmia, which alters with inspiration and expiration. People who have heart disease may have an irregular rhythm due to disordered electrical conduction within the heart, e.g. atrial fibrillation (see Ch. 17). Heart irregularities can be investigated through an electrocardiogram (ECG) (see Ch. 17) and an irregular rhythm should always be reported immediately.

Volume

The force of the pulse is also assessed. The terms used to describe force or volume are:

- *Normal* – the pulse is easy to feel
- *Bounding* – pulse feels 'springy' due to an increase in force of cardiac contraction or circulating blood volume; usually found in the presence of infection
- *Thready* – pulse feels weak, difficult to palpate and difficult to count, which may be due to dehydration or haemorrhage

- *Absent* – indicates a blockage of the palpated artery or, together with other observations such as skin colour, cardiac arrest.

Factors that influence the force of the pulse include the circulating blood volume and the action of hormones on blood vessel walls causing vasoconstriction or vasodilatation.

The pulse reading is recorded on the clinical observation chart and contributes to the Early Warning Score (see Fig. 14.14, p. 333).

Features of the pulse in newborns, infants and children

Pulse rates in children vary with age; normal ranges are shown in Table 14.4. The pulse can be palpated over the radial, brachial or femoral artery. The pulse rate should be assessed while a baby or child is asleep or at rest as crying, eating or sucking increase heart rate.

Apical pulse

The apical pulse is a central measurement, which is the most common method of recording heart rate in infants and young children and also in adults who may have heart disease with rhythm disturbances. The apical (apex) beat is located at the apex of the heart. Measurement of the apex/radial pulse in adults is explained in Chapter 17.

The apical pulse is detected using a stethoscope and listening to heart sounds at the apex of the heart (the pointed end of the ventricle). In children, placement of the stethoscope is dependent on age. The stethoscope is placed:

- At the 4th intercostal space inside the nipple in children under 5 years of age
- At the 5th intercostal space at or inside the nipple for children over 5 years old (Trigg & Mohammed 2010).

Blood pressure

This section outlines what blood pressure (BP) is and the factors that affect it in health; for more detail you should consult your physiology textbook. The equipment needed and how to measure BP are explained. It is important to be familiar with the early material in this section before attempting to practise BP measurement.

BP corresponds to the pressure exerted on arterial walls as blood moves through them. BP measurements provide information about cardiovascular status, which can assist in the diagnosis of disease or evaluation of treatment. Two measurements are made and usually recorded in millimetres of mercury (mmHg):

- *Systolic pressure*, which represents the greatest pressure in the main arteries following contraction of the left ventricle
- *Diastolic pressure*, which is the lowest pressure in the main arteries and occurs at the end of ventricular relaxation while the heart is at rest, before the next cardiac contraction.

The convention for writing blood pressure is to put the systolic pressure first and then the diastolic, e.g. 120/70 mmHg.

Table 14.5 Normal BP values for children

Age (years)	Blood Pressure (mmHg)	
	Systolic	Diastolic
0–2	95	55
3–6	100	65
7–10	105	70
11–15	115	70

(Reproduced with permission from Hull, D., Johnston, D.I., 1999. Essential paediatrics, fourth ed. Churchill Livingstone, Edinburgh.)

Factors that determine blood pressure

BP is determined by several factors including the cardiac output, venous return, blood volume, peripheral vascular resistance (the resistance within arteries and arterioles) and elasticity of large arteries. BP is dynamic, and so varies over the course of the day depending on body demands. For more detail about factors that determine BP and its control, you should consult your physiology textbook.

Blood pressure values

Adult BP is normally in the range of 100–130 mmHg systolic and 60–90 mmHg diastolic. The National Clinical Guideline Centre (NCGC) recommends that optimal BP should be <120/<80 (NCGC 2011). Table 14.5 shows normal BP values for children.

Hypertension (high blood pressure) is defined as systolic blood pressure >140 mmHg or diastolic blood pressure >90 mmHg. The NCGC (2011) recommends that hypertension should be confirmed using 24-hour ambulatory blood pressure monitoring (ABPM) rather than being solely based on measurements taken in the clinic; the use of ABPM is predicted to be more cost-effective for the NHS. Guidance is also provided for home blood pressure monitoring (HBPM) which empowers people to become more involved in the monitoring and management of their hypertension (NCGC 2011).

Hypotension describes BP lower than the normal range of 100 mmHg systolic and/or 60 mmHg diastolic. Hypertension and hypotension are explored further in Chapter 17.

Equipment used for BP measurement

BP is usually measured by non-invasive means, using either the auscultatory or electronic method. The equipment required includes a sphygmomanometer, which may be aneroid or electronic, and an appropriately sized cuff (Table 14.6). BP is sometimes continuously monitored through the invasive method using a catheter inserted into an artery, a technique beyond the scope of this book that is confined to the care of critically ill people.

Table 14.6 Estimated BP cuff sizes

Indication	Width (cm)	Length (cm)	BHS guidelines: bladder width and length (cm)	Arm/leg circumference (cm)
Small adult/child	10–12	18–24	12×18	<23
Standard adult	12–13	23–35	12×26	<33
Large adult	12–16	35–40	12×40	<50
Adult thigh cuff	20	42		<53

(Reproduced with permission from British Hypertension Society, 2011. How to measure blood pressure. Online. Available: www.bhsoc.org September 2011.)

Sphygmomanometers

Mercury sphygmomanometers were used for many years; however, health and safety concerns regarding the use and disposal of mercury in the workplace have emerged and therefore these may no longer be in use in practice. Increasingly common methods of BP measurement are the use of aneroid or electronic sphygmomanometers (Fig. 14.10).

Aneroid sphygmomanometers are less bulky and more portable than other types. They do not use mercury and are a safe alternative that has quickly gained acceptance. However, they have been found to be less reliable as they often underestimate BP. These are not recommended for use in hospitals because they rapidly deteriorate due to high usage and also need frequent calibration to ensure their accuracy (NCGC 2011).

Electronic sphygmomanometers include a pressure sensor within the cuff that registers the systolic and diastolic pressures, which are then displayed digitally. The advantages of these machines are that they require little instruction, eliminate observer bias, and can also display heart rate, mean BP, and the time and date, simultaneously. However, they are often very sensitive to movement and can still be inaccurate in patients with irregular heart rhythms such as atrial fibrillation. No stethoscope is needed and therefore this is not an auscultatory method of BP measurement.

BP measurements may be influenced by a range of factors and all forms of non-invasive BP monitoring have limitations (Box 14.17).

BP cuffs

Some BP cuffs are supplied in two separate parts: the cover (or sheath) and an inner inflatable bladder. Both components should be inspected before use. The cuff should be clean and intact. The tubing attached to both the sphygmomanometer and the inflation bulb should also be intact with no leaks or signs of perishing.

It is important to use the correct size of BP cuff, irrespective of the type of sphygmomanometer used (see Table 14.6). The bladder within the cuff should encircle at least 75–80%, but not more than 100%, of the upper arm. The width of the cuff should be more than 50% of the length of the upper arm. An underestimation of BP will be recorded if the cuff is too

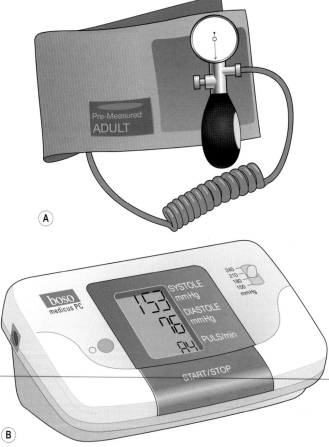

Fig. 14.10 • Sphygmomanometers. (A) Aneroid. (B) Electronic. (Reproduced with permission from Jamieson, E.M., Whyte, L.A., McCall, J.M., 2007. Clinical nursing practices, fifth ed. Churchill Livingstone, Edinburgh.)

large; overestimation of BP will occur if the cuff is too small (NCGC 2011).

Measuring BP

The important points are explained here and BP measurement is outlined in Box 14.18. BP readings are entered on the clinical observation chart and contribute to the calculation of the Early Warning Score (see Fig. 14.14, p. 333).

? Critical thinking

Box 14.17

How reliable is non-invasive BP measurement?

BP is often recorded on a single occasion and one-off readings do not necessarily reveal trends of a person's BP.

- *Variability over the day:* BP varies over the course of a day in order to meet different requirements such as exercise and other activities, e.g. eating, sleeping, smoking.
- *White coat syndrome:* This is an increase in BP ascribed to anxiety or anticipation of BP measurement by healthcare professionals.
- *Postural hypotension:* This is a drop in BP that occurs when standing up from a lying position. It is fairly common in older adults and people receiving antihypertensive medication. In this situation, BP should be measured in both lying and standing positions.
- *Arrhythmias:* Irregular heart rhythms may result in variations in the sounds heard from beat to beat as well as differences in the time between each beat. As a consequence, recordings made using the auscultatory method can be inaccurate.
- *Pregnancy:* BP is monitored closely during pregnancy as hypertension can have serious consequences. In addition, BP can fall when lying supine if the fetus obstructs the inferior vena cava, reducing venous return.
- *Observer error:* The wrong technique or faulty equipment can lead to inaccurate readings.

Student activities

1. Access the National Clinical Guideline Centre and read Clinical Guideline 127 and identify some of the factors that contribute towards a loss of accuracy when measuring BP.
2. BP equipment is frequently used in placements and needs regular checks to ensure that measurements will be accurate. In your placement:
   - Identify the type(s) of sphygmomanometer used.
   - Find out how often they are calibrated and how this is carried out.
   - Identify the different sizes of BP cuffs available and whether they are suitable for use with all the patients/clients there (see Table 14.6).
   - Find out when and how they are cleaned.
   - Examine the cuffs for signs of wear and tear. If they are in need of repair, discuss the further actions required with your mentor.

Resource

National Clinical Guideline Centre, 2011. Hypertension: Clinical management of primary hypertension in adults. Online. Available: www.nice.org.uk/nicemedia/live/13561/56007/56007.pdf September 2012.

 Nursing skills

Box 14.18

Measurement of BP

Equipment

- A sphygmomanometer (see p. 328)
- An appropriately sized cuff (see Table 14.6)
- A stethoscope for auscultatory methods
- An observation chart (Fig. 14.14, p. 333) or medical/nursing notes.

Preparation

- Wash hands as per local policy
- BP measurement should be explained, including the feeling of 'tightness' in the arm, and verbal consent obtained; maintain respect and dignity at all times
- The person should be seated, lying supine for at least 5 minutes, or standing for 1 minute before the procedure begins. They should be relaxed and not moving or speaking
- The arm is supported at the level of the heart (mid sternum) and held straight but relaxed, ensuring that no tight clothing constricts the arm
- The cuff (see below) is applied:
  - with the centre of the bladder marked on the cuff over the brachial artery (see Fig. 14.11)
  - with the lower edge of cuff 2–3 cm above pulsation of the brachial artery
  - in aneroid sphygmomanometers so that the tubing emerges 'up the arm' as movement of the tubing across the antecubital fossa can create artefactual sounds.

Measurement using an aneroid sphygmomanometer

- Estimate the systolic pressure beforehand by:
  - palpating the brachial artery
  - inflating the cuff using the bulb until pulsation disappears
  - deflating cuff until pulsation is felt; the point at which pulsation appears is an estimate of the systolic pressure
- Then inflate the cuff to 30 mmHg above the systolic level, estimated earlier; at this point the brachial pulse will no longer be felt

- Place the diaphragm of the stethoscope over the brachial artery and slowly deflate the cuff at a rate of 2–3 mm/s until you hear regular tapping sounds – this is phase 1, the systolic pressure (see Fig. 14.12)
- Systolic pressure and diastolic pressure are recorded to the nearest 2 mmHg
- Measure diastolic pressure – phase 4 (see Fig. 14.12): abrupt muffling sounds become soft and blowing in quality just before the sounds disappear (phase 5) – this point is recorded as the diastolic pressure
- Completely deflate and remove the cuff to prevent any further compression of the limb
- It may be necessary to repeat the procedure for both lying and standing positions
- Clean the diaphragm of the stethoscope according to local policy
- Wash hands according to local policy
- Record the pressures heard as soon as possible after assessment, noting the position of the patient/client (lying, standing or sitting down) and the arm used. This may be on an observation chart (see Fig. 14.14, p. 333) or in the notes
- Report and document any changes/abnormalities.

Notes: NCGC (2011) recommends that pressures in both arms should be recorded on the first visit and that the arm with the highest BP should be used in subsequent measurements.

This important skill forms part of Essential Skills Cluster 9 (NMC 2010b).

Resources

British Hypertension Society, 2011. How to measure blood pressure. Online. Available: www.bhsoc.org/resources/how-to-measure-blood-pressure/ September 2012.

National Clinical Guideline Centre, 2011. Hypertension. Clinical management of primary hypertension in adults. Clinical Guideline. Online. Available: www.nice.org.uk/nicemedia/live/13561/56007/56007.pdf September 2012.

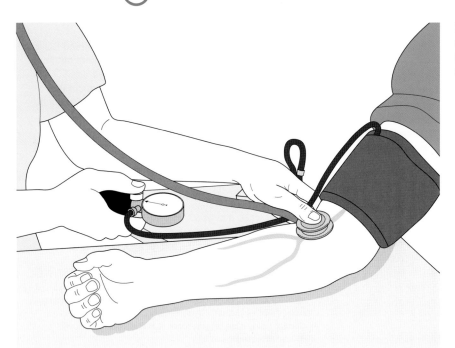

Fig. 14.11 • Stethoscope over the brachial artery. (Reproduced with permission from Nicol, M., Bavin, C., Bedford-Turner, S., et al., 2004. Essential nursing skills, second ed. Mosby, Edinburgh.)

Measuring BP in newborns, infants and children

Although BP may be measured less frequently in children than in adults, consideration must be given to the following:

- It is hard to auscultate the antecubital fossa pulse, so an electronic blood pressure machine should be used in babies and young children
- The lower edge of cuff should be close to the antecubital fossa
- BP should be recorded when a baby is asleep or resting. Crying, sucking and eating increase BP
- Allay any anxiety before measurement. Young children may feel more secure if BP is taken while sitting in a parent's lap.

Further information can be found in Trigg and Mohammed (2010).

Inflating the cuff

Inflation of the cuff compresses the brachial artery (see Fig. 14.11) and the cuff is inflated automatically when using an electronic sphygmomanometer. When an aneroid sphygmomanometer is used, the bladder inside the BP cuff is attached to an inflation bulb with a release valve, which allows the cuff to be inflated manually.

Korotkoff sounds

The auscultatory method relies on the detection of a series of sounds. When using an aneroid sphygmomanometer, a stethoscope with clean, well-fitting earpieces is required. Earpieces are placed in the ears pointing towards the nose. The diaphragm is placed on the brachial artery in the antecubital fossa (Fig. 14.11) to listen to sounds in the brachial artery. These are known as Korotkoff sounds, which are divided into five phases (Fig. 14.12). The first phase can be heard as a clear tapping noise via the stethoscope as the cuff is deflated. This

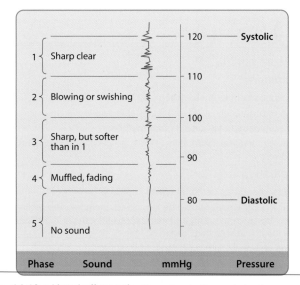

Phase	Sound	mmHg	Pressure
1	Sharp clear	120	Systolic
2	Blowing or swishing	110	
3	Sharp, but softer than in 1	100 / 90	
4	Muffled, fading	80	Diastolic
5	No sound		

Fig. 14.12 • Korotkoff sounds. (Reproduced with permission from Hinchliffe, S.M., Montague, S.E., Watson, R., 1996. Physiology for nursing practice. second ed. Baillière Tindall, London.)

is the systolic blood pressure and represents phase 1. Muffled whooshing noises are usually heard during phases 2 and 3. The sound becomes much more muffled and softer during phase 4 before it disappears at phase 5. The diastolic pressure is normally recorded at the end of phase 4. However, if the sounds continue until 0 mmHg, then the point at which the sounds change at phase 4 is recorded.

Assessing respirations

The accuracy and frequency of recording of respirations is very important. Respiratory rate recording has been shown to be a crucial indicator of serious deteriorations in health status. Decreases in the respiratory rate (<8 breaths/min) and depth have been noted in the hours preceding cardiopulmonary arrest. It has also been suggested that assessment of respiratory rate is not performed as accurately or as frequently as it should be. Additionally, there appears to be an over-reliance on the use of peripheral oxygen saturation monitors to determine respiratory function (Hogan 2006; NICE 2007). However, both respiratory rate and peripheral oxygen saturation are required to calculate the EWS. Analysing and assessing respiratory status requires the observation of several factors, which are outlined below.

At rest, breathing should be regular, effortless and quiet. However, exercise or breathing difficulties may alter the rate, depth, rhythm and/or sound of breathing. Rate and depth of respirations may also change as a result of pain, pyrexia, emotional states and body position, as well as breathing difficulties such as 'shortness of breath' (dyspnoea). They are also influenced by the use of drugs such as nicotine in cigarettes, and opioids, e.g. morphine (see Ch. 23), as well as cocaine and amphetamines. Assessment of respirations is described in Box 14.19.

Respiratory rate

Breathing occurs in cycles. The first phase is inspiration, which is followed by a short pause before expiration (see Ch. 17). The rate and depth of breathing are controlled by the respiratory centre located in the medulla oblongata. Blood levels of carbon dioxide (CO_2) and oxygen (O_2), as well as pH (acidity), are the main influences on respiratory rate. Chemoreceptors located in the brain stem, carotid arteries and the aortic arch monitor and respond to changes in the blood levels of CO_2, O_2

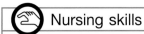

Nursing skills Box 14.19

Assessing respirations

- The patient should be comfortable and relaxed
- Unusually, the patient is not informed that their respirations are going to be counted
- Accuracy and reliability of measurements are increased by counting for a full minute
- Respiratory rate is recorded over 1 minute by observing the rise and fall of the chest wall. If breathing is shallow, it may be easier to count movements using a hand placed lightly on the chest or abdominal wall although the patient may be aware of this
- Each cycle is counted discreetly (Fig. 14.13), usually after taking the pulse
- Other factors also assessed at this time include:
  - Respiratory rhythm (see p. 332)
  - Depth of breathing (see p. 332)
  - Effort of breathing, e.g. use of accessory muscles (see p. 332)
  - Noises associated with breathing (see p. 332)
  - Patient's colour, e.g. presence of cyanosis (see Ch. 17)
  - Presence of cough or production of sputum (see Ch. 17)
- The respiratory rate is recorded on the observation chart (see Fig. 14.14) or patient/client notes
- Any abnormal findings are reported and recorded in the notes.

This important skill forms part of Essential Skills Cluster 9 (NMC 2010b).

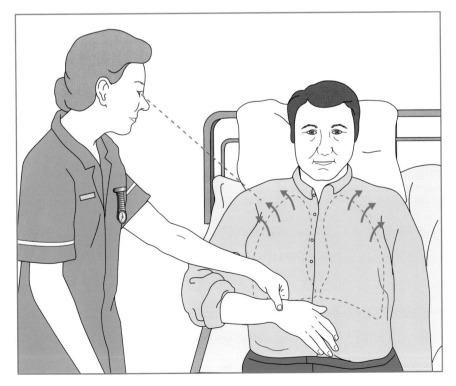

Fig. 14.13 • Monitoring the respiration rate while apparently counting the pulse.
(Reproduced with permission from Nicol, M., Bavin, C., Cronin, P., et al., 2008. Essential nursing skills, third ed. Mosby, Edinburgh.)

Table 14.7 Children's average respiratory rates	
Age (years)	Respirations per minute
Under 1	25–35
1–5	20–30
5–12	20–25
Over 12	15–25

(Reproduced with permission from Hull, D., Johnston, D.I., 1999. Essential paediatrics, fourth ed. Churchill Livingstone, Edinburgh.)

and pH. An increase in blood carbon dioxide levels ($PaCO_2$) and a fall in blood pH (increased acidity) activate the chemo-receptors that respond by increasing the respiratory rate, which increases the elimination of CO_2 and raises blood pH. Breathing can also be influenced by external factors such as pain, emotion or voluntary control. For more information about breathing and its control, you should consult your physiology textbook.

Counting respiratory rate in adults

Respiratory rate is the number of respirations per minute and is recorded as RR. In adults, the normal rate is 12–18 respirations/min. Tachypnoea describes a respiratory rate that exceeds 20/min; absence of breathing is known as apnoea. The respiratory rate is entered on the observation chart (see Fig. 14.14, p. 333) and its calculation into the Early Warning Score (EWS).

Counting respiratory rate in infants and small children

In babies under 12 months old, it is recommended that a stethoscope is used to listen to air movement in the lungs to count the breaths per minute. Average respiratory rates for children are shown in Table 14.7. The child should be relaxed and quiet before measurement is made by lightly placing a hand on their abdomen to count the breaths. If this is not possible, it may be necessary to observe breathing while the child is quietly interacting with a parent or playing.

Respiratory rhythm

Breathing is usually regular in healthy adults. It may be described as regular or irregular and can be influenced, e.g. by emotions such as fear or crying and during breath-holding or panic attacks. Babies often have a less regular rhythm, possibly due to incomplete development of the normal respiratory control systems (see Ch. 17).

Abnormal respiratory rhythms

Alterations in rhythm can also be observed in patients with neurological dysfunction that has impaired the respiratory centre within the brain stem.

Damage or poor blood supply to the brain stem can result in an irregular rhythm and rate called Cheyne–Stokes breathing. In this condition, breathing patterns change between shallow and slow and deep and rapid, with varying periods of apnoea in between. This type of breathing is often present at the end-of-life.

Depth of breathing

The depth of a breath is determined by the volume of air inhaled. In healthy adults, during relaxed breathing, this is about 500 mL and is called the tidal volume. This and other indicators of respiratory status may also be measured by nurses, especially in people with chronic respiratory conditions such as chronic bronchitis and asthma (see Ch. 17).

The depth of breathing is described as normal, shallow or deep and is observed by watching the rise and fall of the chest wall. These are, however, subjective observations and so open to interpretation. Expansion of both sides of the chest should be the same, i.e. 'equal'.

The term hypoventilation is used to describe shallow slow breathing, which implies limited chest movement. Hyperventilation is used to describe fast and deep breathing, and considerable movement of chest wall may be observed.

Deep, regular breaths may be 'Kussmaul' respirations, caused by an increase in blood acidity (low blood pH). This can arise as a result of uncontrolled diabetes.

Effort of breathing

Normally, at rest, breathing is regular, effortless and quiet. During exercise, the breathing pattern becomes more active as body oxygen demand rises and blood carbon dioxide levels increase (hypercapnia). Exercise requires the movement of more air into and out of the lungs, more quickly and forcibly, and also employs the accessory muscles of respiration, i.e. the internal intercostal muscles and the muscles in the neck and shoulders. Forced expiration is facilitated by the abdominal muscles contracting and pushing the diaphragm upwards. Expiration is no longer passive, but becomes forced.

Noises associated with breathing

Although breathing is normally quiet, alterations to breathing patterns can also include changes to the sound of breathing. Whistling noises called wheezing due to constriction of the airways can be heard on expiration in people with chronic lung disease such as bronchitis or asthma. Obstruction of the larynx results in high-pitched noises during inspiration, which are termed stridor.

Children experiencing breathing difficulties can also develop associated vocal noises such as grunting, wheezing and stridor. In addition, they may hold themselves rigidly, have a retracted neck and nasal flaring (Trigg & Mohammed 2010).

Early Warning Score (EWS)

For patients who are acutely ill and at risk of developing a critical illness, vital sign recordings should be entered onto an EWS, Modified Early Warning Score (MEWS) or Track and Trigger chart. Those who are at high risk of deterioration include all patients admitted as an emergency, have a chronic

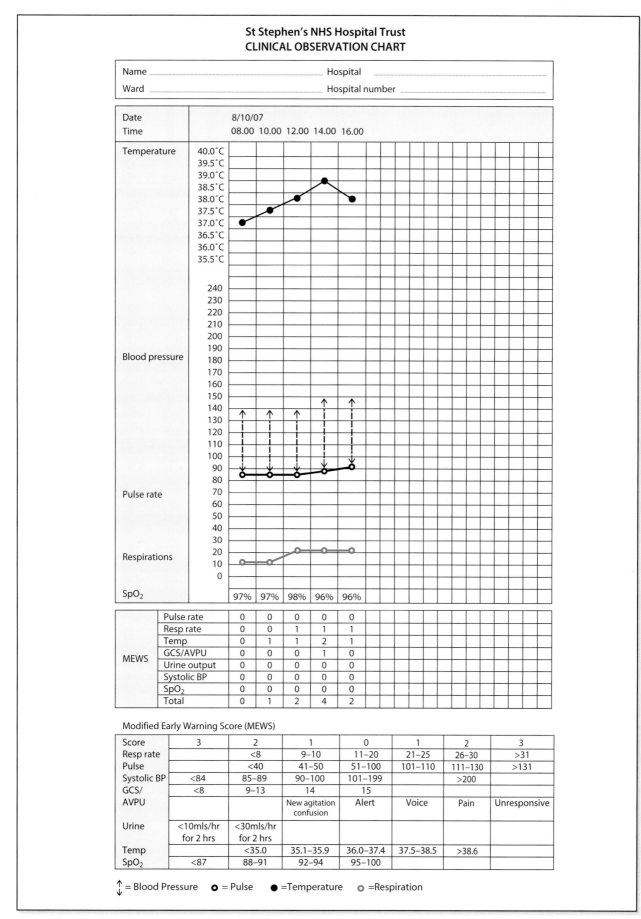

Fig. 14.14 • Clinical observation chart including Early Warning Score (EWS).

health problem, have had surgery and those whose condition may be causing concern or is unstable. However, NICE (2007) recommends that all acute hospital in-patients should have their vital signs recorded and monitored via a track and trigger system. The Royal College of Physicians (2012) has advocated using a standardized NHS National Early Warning Score (NEWS) chart within a year.

The respiratory rate, pulse, systolic blood pressure and body temperature are entered on the EWS chart and awarded a score. Additional information that is scored and required for an EWS includes the patient's hourly urine volumes (see Ch. 20), the Glasgow Coma Score (GCS) or Level of response (AVPU) (see Ch. 16) and the oxygen saturation percentage (SpO_2) (see Ch. 17). The score is calculated by rating each parameter and recording it on the EWS chart (Fig 14.14).

Calling criteria

Once the EWS score is calculated, the assessor is directed towards making a decision about what to do next. This might be to:

- Increase the frequency of patient observations, monitor trends and inform the nurse in charge
- Communicate the results to a senior nurse if the score is 3 in any one category
- Contact the critical care outreach team and the senior nurse to assist in managing the patient's condition if the score is 4 or above *or* increasing by 2 or more *or* the GCS falls by 2 or more *or* if the patient's condition is a cause for concern (NICE 2007).

Height and weight

Measurement of height and weight should be made on admission to hospital or as part of a community assessment. Extremes of weight are associated with health risks. Body mass index (BMI, see Ch. 19) is a useful guide to whether an adult's body weight is appropriate for their height. Knowledge of people's height and weight is needed to calculate drug doses, including anaesthetics, and fluid and nutritional requirements, especially in children.

Children may also be regularly weighed and measured to monitor growth rates and weight gain, which are important in monitoring their health and development. In the UK, children's weight and height should be recorded on the appropriate centile chart produced by the Royal College of Paediatrics and Child Health (2009).

Measuring body weight requires the use of electronic calibrated scales and is recorded in kilograms (kg). A child under the age of 2 should have all clothing removed and placed on scales. Children over 2 years old should have underwear on and asked to sit or lie or stand on the scales.

If serial measurements are made, this should be at the same time each day or week and in similar clothing. Daily weight may be recorded to assess, e.g. fluid loss in response to diuretic drugs. When weight loss is a goal, e.g. in obesity, weight may be monitored weekly.

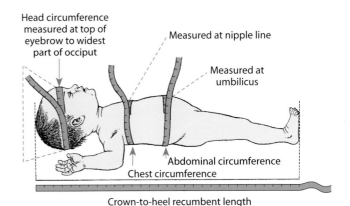

Fig. 14.15 • Measurement of head, chest, abdominal circumference and crown to heel length. (Reproduced with permission from Wong, D.L., Hockenberry-Eaton, M., Wilson, D., et al., 2001. Wong's essentials of pediatric nursing. sixth ed. Mosby, St Louis.)

Children are measured to the nearest centimetre and metres are used for adults; e.g. 65 cm for a child and 1.65 m (165 cm) for an adult.

A fixed measure is used for adults and children over the age of 2 years, standing with the back against a wall or scale. The head should be in the midline and the heels, buttocks and backs of shoulders should touch the wall. A moveable rod is placed on the top of the head, to assist in reading the measurement. For children under 24 months, length is measured instead of height. The child is placed on their back and their head is gently held in the midline. The knees should be held and pushed down until the legs are flat on the table and the child's body is extended (Fig. 14.15). Length, in centimetres (cm), is measured using a measuring tape. In children, the circumference of the head, chest and abdomen may also be measured.

SUMMARY

- The nursing process provides a framework for assessing, planning, implementing and evaluating care.
- Assessment is pivotal to the provision of effective nursing care.
- Assessment is a complex activity that requires various nursing skills including observation, measurement, communicating, documenting, interpreting and decision-making.
- Approaches to care must be tailored to the needs of individuals.
- Assessment of body temperature is required to detect ill health or evaluate patients' progress.
- Methods of thermometry include tympanic, electronic probes and chemical dots. Instruments can be placed in sites such as the ear canal, axilla and mouth, and on skin.
- Assessment of the pulse and BP provides information about general health and cardiovascular status.
- Assessment of respiratory function requires measuring the rate and depth, as well as noting other factors such as effort and noise of breathing.
- Weight and height are not vital signs but are assessed, especially in children, to determine fluid, nutritional or drug requirements.

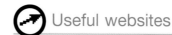

KEY WORDS AND PHRASES FOR LITERATURE SEARCHING

Assessment tool	Nursing process
Early Warning Score	Person-centred care
Blood pressure	Pulse
Body core temperature	Pyrexia
Holistic assessment	Respiratory rate
Hypothermia	Sphygmomanometer
Nursing history	Tachycardia
Nursing model	Thermometry

Useful websites

British Hypertension Society www.bhsoc.org
Tidal model www.tidal-model.com
Waterlow scale www.judy-waterlow.co.uk
National Clinical Guideline Centre www.ncgc.ac.uk
All websites accessed September 2012.

References

Barker, P., 1996. Chaos and the way of Zen: psychiatric nursing and the 'uncertainty principle'. Journal of Psychiatric and Mental Health Nursing 3, 235–243.

Barker, P., 2009. Psychiatric and mental health nursing: the craft of caring, second ed. Hodder Arnold, London.

British Hypertension Society, 2011. How to measure blood pressure. Online. Available: www.bhsoc.org September 2012.

Casey, A., 2007. Partnership model of nursing. In: Glasper, E., McEwing, G., Richardson, J. (Eds.), Oxford handbook of children's and young people's nursing. Oxford University Press, Oxford.

Department of Health, 2001. Valuing people: a new strategy for learning disabilities for the 21st century. TSO, London.

Department of Health, 2003. Getting the right start: National Service Framework for children. TSO, London.

Department of Health, 2010a. Equity and excellence: liberating the NHS. HMSO, London.

Department of Health, 2010b. Essence of care 2010. HMSO, London.

Department of Health, 2010c. Ready to go? Planning the discharge and the transfer of patients from hospital and intermediate care. HMSO, London.

Fawcett, J., 2005. Contemporary nursing knowledge: analysis and evaluation of nursing models and theories, second ed. Davis, Philadelphia.

HM Government, 2004. The Children Act. Online. Available: http://www.legislation.gov.uk/ukpga/2004/31/contents September 2012.

Hogan, J., 2006. Respiratory assessment. Why don't nurses monitor the respiratory rates of patients? British Journal of Nursing 15 (9), 489–492.

House of Commons Health Committee, 2007. The electronic patient record, Vol 1. The Stationary Office, London.

National Leadership and Innovation Agency for Healthcare, 2005. Integrated care pathways: a guide to good practice. NLIAH, Wales.

NANDA, 2008. Nursing diagnosis: definitions and classification 2009–2011. Wiley Blackwell, Indianapolis.

National Clinical Guideline Centre, 2011. Partial update of Clinical Guidelines 18 and 34: Hypertension. The clinical management of primary hypertension in adults. Clinical Guideline 127. Online. Available: www.nice.org.uk/nicemedia/live/13561/56007/56007.pdf September 2012.

National Institute for Health and Clinical Excellence, 2007. Acutely ill patients in hospital: recognition and response to acute illness in adults in hospital. NICE, 2007.

Nursing and Midwifery Council, 2008. The code: Standards for conduct, performance and ethics for nurses and midwives. Online. Available: http://www.nmc-uk.org/Nurses-and-midwives/Standards-and-guidance1/The-code/The-code-in-full/ October 2012..

Nursing and Midwifery Council, 2010a. Record-keeping guidance for nurse and midwives. NMC, London.

Nursing and Midwifery Council, 2010b. Standards for pre-registration for preregistration nursing education. Online. Available: http://standards.nmc-uk.org/PreRegNursing/statutory/Standards/Pages/Standards.aspx October 2012..

Peplau, H.E., 1952. Interpersonal relations in nursing. Putnam, New York.

Roper, N., Logan, W., Tierney, A., 2000. The Roper, Logan and Tierney model of nursing, fifth ed. Churchill Livingstone, Edinburgh.

Roy, C., Andrews, H.A., 1999. The Roy adaptation model, second ed. Appleton and Lange, Stamford, CT.

Royal College of Paediatrics and Child Health, 2009. UK-WHO growth charts: early years.

Online. Available: www.rcpch.ac.uk/growthcharts September 2012.

Royal College of Physicians, 2012. National Early Warning Score (NEWS). Standardising the assessment of acute-illness severity in the NHS. Online. Available. http://www.rcplondon.ac.uk/sites/default/files/documents/national-early-warning-score-standardising-assessment-acute-illness-severity-nhs.pdf August 2012.

Scarborough, K., Godsell, M., 2011. Enabling good health. In: Atherton, H.L., Crickmore, D.J. (Eds.), Learning disabilities: towards inclusion, sixth ed. Churchill Livingstone, Edinburgh.

Scottish Executive, 2002. Promoting health, supporting inclusion. Scottish Executive, Edinburgh.

Scottish Executive, 2004. People with learning disabilities in Scotland: health needs assessment report. Scottish Executive, Edinburgh.

Scottish Government, 2009. Best practice template: admission, transfer and discharge protocol for hospital patients in Scotland. The Scottish Government, Edinburgh.

Smith, L., Coleman, V., Bradshaw, M. (Eds.), 2002. Family centred care. Palgrave, Basingstoke.

Trigg, E., Mohammed, T., (Eds.), 2010. Practices in children's nursing: guidelines for hospital and community, third ed. Churchill Livingstone, Edinburgh.

Welsh Assembly Government, 2002. Inclusion, partnership and innovation: a framework for realising the potential of learning disability nursing in Wales. Briefing paper 3. Welsh Assembly, Cardiff.

Yura, H., Walsh, M., 1967. The nursing process. Appleton Century Crofts, Norwalk, CT.

Further reading

Brooker, C., Nicol, M. (Eds.), 2011. Alexander's nursing practice, fourth ed. Churchill Livingstone, Edinburgh.

Childs, C., 2011. Maintaining body temperature. In: Brooker, C., Nicol, M. (Eds.), Alexander's nursing practice, fourth ed. Churchill Livingstone, Edinburgh.

Cook, K., Montgomery, H., 2010. Assessment. In: Trigg, E., Mohammed, T. (Eds.), Practices in children's nursing: guidelines for hospital and community, third ed. Churchill Livingstone, Edinburgh.

Holland, K., Jenkins, J., Solomon, J., et al. (Eds.), 2008. Applying the Roper, Logan and Tierney model in practice, second ed. Churchill Livingstone, Edinburgh.

Jamieson, E.M., McCall, J.M., Whyte, L.A., 2007. Clinical nursing practices, fifth ed. Churchill Livingstone, Edinburgh.

Nicol, M., Bavin, C., Cronin, P., et al, 2012. Essential nursing skills, fourth ed. Mosby, Edinburgh.

Nicol, M., Brooker, C., 2011. Nursing practice – the essence of caring. In: Brooker, C., Nicol, M. (Eds.), Alexander's nursing practice, fourth ed. Churchill Livingstone, Edinburgh.

Waugh, A., Grant, A., 2010. Ross and Wilson anatomy and physiology in health and illness, eleventh ed. Churchill Livingstone, Edinburgh.

Preventing the spread of infection 15

Gill Loughty McCrossan

LEARNING OUTCOMES

This chapter will help you:

- Explain the relationship between microorganisms and infectious diseases
- Distinguish between nosocomial, community-acquired and iatrogenic infections
- Describe the chain of infection and give examples of factors involved at each stage
- Define common terminology related to infectious diseases
- Identify the key elements of standard infection control precautions and additional precautions
- Explain how and when standard infection control precautions are used in nursing practice
- Describe the purpose of isolation precautions
- Explain the principles of aseptic technique
- Outline the nurse's role in specimen collection.

Introduction

Infections acquired as a result of healthcare have a major impact on patients/clients and healthcare providers. For patients/clients an infection causes anxiety and discomfort, delays recovery and may result in long-term morbidity (ill-health) or even death. Quality healthcare is a basic expectation; the public and government reasonably expect that people will not acquire disease because of their treatment or care. Control of infection is a shared responsibility in all healthcare settings; however, nurses stand in the front line of clinical practice because of their close 'hands on' contact with patients/clients. Therefore in accordance with The Nursing and Midwifery Council's: *The code: Standards of conduct, performance and ethics for nurses and midwives* (NMC 2008), nurses and midwives must ensure that no action they undertake is detrimental to the safety and well-being of those in their care. In addition, one of the five NMC (2010) Essential Skills Clusters, in which nursing students must demonstrate competence is 'Infection prevention and control'. Progression criteria for pre-registration nursing programmes require that students can promote safe care delivery by following local and national guidelines for the prevention of infection. Nurses must therefore understand why infections occur, how they are transmitted, and the precautions necessary to prevent their spread.

This chapter provides an overview of microorganisms and outlines surveillance and reporting mechanisms of some infectious diseases. It considers the sequence of events that spread infectious diseases and the key features of disease development. The body's defence mechanisms are briefly considered. The next section focuses on the practices required to prevent and control the spread of infection, exploring standard infection control precautions and then additional precautions, including isolation precautions and aseptic technique. Finally, it examines the nurse's role in the collection of microbiology specimens for the laboratory.

Overview of microbiology

Microorganisms are tiny living organisms only visible under a microscope, apart from some fungi. Categories of microorganisms include: algae, fungi, protozoa, bacteria, mycoplasma, rickettsia, chlamydia, viruses and prions. Microorganisms are found in:

- Soil
- Water
- Air
- Vegetable matter
- Animals and humans.

For microorganisms to survive in any environment, they must have suitable physical and chemical conditions, nutrients and freedom from hostile competitors. The human body is populated by an extraordinary number of microorganisms, an estimated 1×10^{14} bacteria compared with 1×10^{13} body cells (Tortora et al 2009). These microorganisms (referred to as normal flora or commensals) can benefit the host by providing nutrients, aiding in food digestion and preventing the establishment of more dangerous microorganisms. Normal flora do not populate the entire human body but are located in certain regions, e.g. the skin, mucous membranes and the intestinal tract. Some areas of the body are normally completely devoid of microbial populations, e.g. the urinary tract, blood and the lungs.

Epidemiology of infectious diseases

Infectious diseases are caused by microorganisms and those that cause infectious disease are known as pathogens. An infectious disease that is transmissible from one person to another is called a communicable disease. Communicable diseases range from relatively mild illnesses such as the common cold to debilitating and potentially fatal conditions such as human immunodeficiency virus/acquired immune deficiency syndrome (HIV/AIDS), tuberculosis and malaria which together account for an estimated 274.3 million cases worldwide (World Health Organization, WHO 2011a). Communicable diseases are categorized according to their frequency and distribution:

- *Endemic*: Always present within a population of a particular geographic region. The number of cases may fluctuate over time, but the disease never dies out completely. Globally 331 human deaths have been caused by the highly pathogenic avian influenza A virus (avian flu H5N1) since 2003 (European Centre for Disease Prevention and Control (ECDC) 2011). Other examples include tuberculosis, sexually transmitted infections, chickenpox and mumps.
- *Epidemic*: The sudden outbreak of an infectious disease that spreads rapidly through a population, affecting a large number of people at the same time, e.g. influenza. In hospitals, an epidemic does not necessarily involve large numbers and is recognized when two or more patients in the same ward/unit are infected by the same organism, e.g. Norovirus (winter vomiting virus) and *Clostridium difficile* (Health Protection Agency, HPA 2008).
- *Pandemic*: A worldwide spread of a new disease, e.g. H1N1 (swine flu) rapidly established itself as the dominant influenza strain in most parts of the world in 2009–2010. The most recent pandemics include HIV and H1N1 (WHO 2009a; WHO 2010).

Healthcare-associated infections (HAIs)

Infectious diseases (infections) can be divided into two categories:

- HAIs, also known as nosocomial infections – those acquired within hospitals or other care facilities. In hospitalized patients, iatrogenic infections are frequently caused by invasive procedures and indwelling medical devices which bypass the body's first line of defence (Fig. 15.1).
- Community-acquired infections – those that are present or incubating at the time of hospital admission whereas

an HAI manifests itself 72 hours or more after admission, and includes infections not apparent until after discharge.

A hospitalized patient may have either type.

Prevalence, surveillance and reporting of HAIs

In England, HAIs affect 8.2% of the total inpatient population (Department of Health, DH 2007). Approximately 9% of patients entering acute wards in Scottish hospitals will develop an infection during their hospital stay with the costs of HAI in Scotland estimated at £183 million/year (Health Protection Scotland, HPS 2007).

Clostridium difficile infection (CDI) and meticillin resistant *Staphylococcus aureus* (MRSA) are the most common HAIs with the growing resistance of many organisms to antibiotic drugs exacerbating the situation. Surveillance is adopted to reduce the incidence and consequence of HAI in hospitals and to increase compliance with infection control guidelines. Surveillance includes investigation and survey at a local level and allows ongoing monitoring of the effectiveness of prevention measures (HPA 2011a). All hospitals must maintain compliance and surveillance activities, e.g. audit, care bundles and ward-based education to demonstrate that infection prevention and control are integral to the quality assurance of healthcare provision. Reporting mechanisms also enable demographic details to be obtained, e.g. age, gender and geographical distribution, which allows comparisons to be made between local/national and hospital/community-based infection rates. As a result of surveillance and reporting methods, a 57% reduction in MRSA cases and 48% reduction in CDI between 2008 and 2011 have been identified (HPA 2011a,b). Further data are also shared through the Global Influenza Surveillance and Response System (GISRS) and WHO (2011b) who track and report on all influenza viruses of pandemic potential, e.g. H1N1 and H5N1.

Key infections occurring in the UK are under constant surveillance with robust reporting measures in place. For example, the establishment of voluntary and mandatory reporting measures and a zero tolerance culture for infections has demonstrated a decreased incidence of some bacteria outlined above and a significant increase in others. Unlike CDI and MRSA, *E. coli* bacteraemia has increased by 36% since 2006. Constant surveillance is of particular importance with this organism due to the concern over its resistance to key antimicrobial preparations (HPA 2010a; HPA 2011c).

All patients have a right to expect clean and safe care and every healthcare worker has a responsibility to ensure that a zero tolerance approach to infection is maintained and to comply with all activities that promote the prevention and control of infection.

Chain of infection

The spread of infectious diseases follows a sequence of events that can be compared to a chain with six links, frequently referred to as the 'chain of infection' (Fig. 15.2). If all links remain intact and in the correct sequence, then the infection

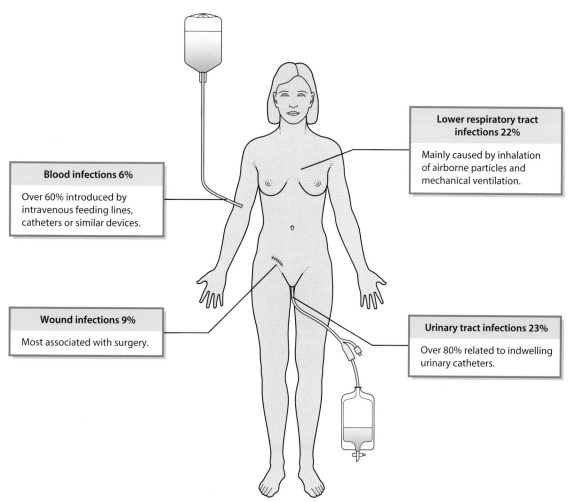

Blood infections 6%

Over 60% introduced by intravenous feeding lines, catheters or similar devices.

Lower respiratory tract infections 22%

Mainly caused by inhalation of airborne particles and mechanical ventilation.

Wound infections 9%

Most associated with surgery.

Urinary tract infections 23%

Over 80% related to indwelling urinary catheters.

Fig. 15.1 • Types and incidence of healthcare-associated infections.

will be transmitted. Therefore understanding the characteristics of each link of the chain provides the fundamental knowledge necessary to break the links and prevent and control infection.

Infectious agent (pathogen)

The relationship between humans and microorganisms is usually one of balanced conflicts between the host's ability to resist infection and the ability of the microorganism to cause disease. Some microbial species are very adept at avoiding or surviving the body's defence mechanisms. For example, some possess surface structures that attach and anchor them to host cells. Others produce toxins (poisons) that target specific body cells and tissues. A few species manufacture enzymes that dissolve the host's tissues, e.g. necrotizing fasciitis – 'flesh-eating bacteria'.

Reservoirs

Pathogens are provided with nutrients and suitable environmental conditions for their survival and multiplication within a 'reservoir', which may be human, animal or non-living (Fig. 15.2), however the principal reservoirs for most infectious

diseases are human carriers. A carrier is someone who is, or has been, colonized with a particular pathogen and can transmit it to others who may then become ill. Various carrier states exist:

- *Temporary*: Those with clinical signs and symptoms of an infectious disease are obvious reservoirs who can transmit the pathogen to others including during the incubation period. Pathogens may continue to be shed during the convalescent period that follows the disappearance of symptoms.
- *Passive*: These carriers shed infectious microorganisms but do not show any signs and symptoms of the disease. For example, one third of women infected with gonorrhoea remain asymptomatic (Gould & Brooker 2008) and, unaware that they have the disease, remain untreated and therefore continue to infect other people.
- *Active*: Following full recovery from the disease, active carriers may shed organisms for long periods of time, e.g. carriers of *Salmonella typhi* (that causes typhoid fever) may shed the bacterium for their entire lives. Carriers of hepatitis B maintain the virus in their bloodstream and can transmit the disease to others by items contaminated with their blood or body fluids.

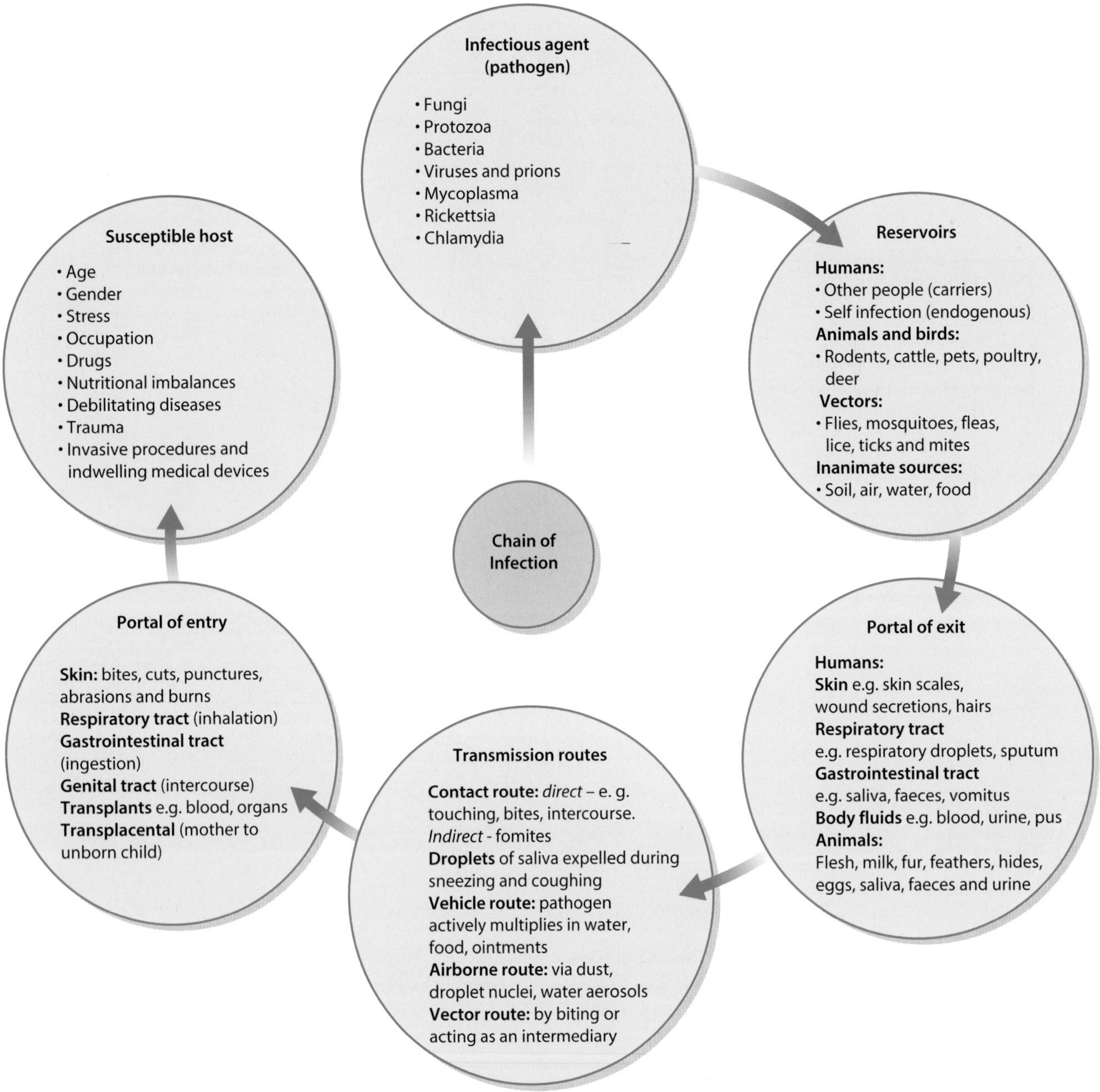

Fig. 15.2 • Chain of infection.

Humans can also become infected with microorganisms that are part of their natural flora. This is referred to as an endogenous infection and occurs when the normal flora that inhabit one site are transferred to another, e.g. when microorganisms from the colon gain access to the normally sterile urinary tract and cause a urinary tract infection.

Portals of exit and entry

The portal of exit is the route by which a pathogen leaves its reservoir. Some pathogens may leave the host using more than one exit route. Portal of entry refers to the path by which an infectious agent invades a new host. The portal of entry is usually the same as the portal of exit (Fig. 15.2).

Transmission of infection

To cause disease, a pathogen must be able to survive transfer from its reservoir to a susceptible host (Fig. 15.2). In HAIs, the following routes are frequently implicated.

Contact transmission

This is direct, when pathogens are transferred by bodily contact between an infected and uninfected person, e.g. to nurses during moving and handling procedures. Indirect contact transmission occurs when fomites (inanimate objects) act as intermediaries in the transfer of pathogens, e.g. contaminated instruments such as electronic thermometers. Contaminated hands of healthcare personnel may also transmit infection indirectly. Correct handwashing technique and changing of gloves between patient contacts are essential to prevent transmission of infection by this route.

Droplet transmission

This occurs when an infected person (the reservoir) releases contaminated respiratory secretions into the air when coughing, sneezing and talking or during procedures such as suctioning and bronchoscopy. Infected respiratory droplets are propelled short distances (usually a metre or less) and can enter the nasal passages, mouth and conjunctiva of another person or they can settle on inanimate objects in close proximity to the infected person.

Airborne transmission

This route involves the dissemination of tiny dried particles (usually 5 μm or less) of evaporated respiratory secretions (called droplet nuclei). In contrast to droplet transmission in which the particles travel only short distances, in airborne transmission the particles may remain suspended in the air for long periods and can be widely dispersed on air currents. When inhaled by susceptible people, their small size allows them to penetrate the lungs from where they can initiate infection.

Susceptible host

The human body has numerous defence mechanisms for resisting the entry and multiplication of pathogens (see Fig. 15.4), which normally prevent infection unless the pathogen is particularly virulent (liable to cause disease). Lack of resistance to infectious diseases is known as susceptibility. A number of factors reduce an individual's resistance to infectious diseases (Box 15.1).

Infectious disease and associated terminology

There are several possible outcomes when an individual encounters pathogenic microorganisms:

- The pathogen may be eliminated by the body's defence mechanisms
- It may reside in the body without causing any symptoms of disease (colonization)
- After successful invasion, it multiplies and causes an infectious disease.

Infectious diseases are often classified according to their severity, duration and the extent by which they spread throughout the body:

- *Local infection*: Occurs when pathogens are limited to a single body site or system. The signs and symptoms vary depending on the system affected (Box 15.2).
- *Systemic infection*: Pathogens spread from the site of entry via the blood or lymphatic vessels to other tissues and organs. In diseases such as measles and chickenpox, the viruses initially invade the upper respiratory tract and then spread to the skin causing a rash and skin vesicles, respectively.
- *Opportunistic infection*: Arises from microorganisms which are not normally pathogenic in healthy people. However,

---

Susceptible hosts	Box 15.1

Age

Congenital infections develop during gestation, while neonatal infections occur in the first 28 days of life. The source of the microorganisms may be the mother's vaginal flora, other infected neonates in a baby unit or the hands of hospital staff. As children grow up, they encounter an increasing variety of social environments and may consequently develop common childhood infections. At the other end of the age spectrum, older adults are prone to infections, mainly due to failing immune responses and chronic diseases.

Gender

Anatomical differences between males and females explain why urinary tract infections are more common in females than males because the shorter female urethra provides microorganisms with easier access to the bladder.

Stress

Prolonged physical or emotional stress alters the body's hormonal balance and reduces resistance to disease. Stress increases the output of cortisol from the adrenal cortex, which suppresses both inflammatory and immune processes.

Occupation

Infectious disease is a persistent hazard of certain occupations, usually when there is increased exposure to pathogens. Healthcare professionals are frequently exposed to patients/clients shedding virulent human pathogens; veterinary surgeons, agricultural workers and those working in meat processing industries are likely to have a higher incidence of diseases spread by animals, and sex industry workers are prone to infections transmitted by sexual intercourse.

Drugs

Both recreational and prescribed drugs can increase susceptibility to infection:

- *Smoking* predisposes to respiratory infections by damaging the epithelium
- *Alcohol*, in excess, increases susceptibility
- *Corticosteroid drugs* suppress inflammatory and immune responses
- *Antibiotic drugs* destroy the normal body flora, encouraging opportunistic infection by extraneous microorganisms
- *Immunosuppressant drugs* lessen the risk of organ rejection following transplantation; however, they suppress the immune response, leaving the person susceptible to opportunistic infections.

Nutritional imbalance

Infections may also be linked to vitamin and protein deficiencies, which partly explains why many infectious diseases are higher in parts of the world where undernutrition is widespread.

Chronic diseases or trauma

Normal defences can be delayed or suppressed by diseases, e.g. leukaemia, diabetes, kidney and liver diseases, and AIDS. The risk of infection may be increased by some therapies, e.g. radiotherapy and chemotherapy, which can severely depress white blood cell counts. Trauma, e.g. burns, damages the body's surface defences, predisposing to invasion by microorganisms.

Characteristics of local infections — Box 15.2

System affected	Signs and symptoms
Skin	Inflammation: redness, pain, swelling and heat
Respiratory tract	Increased respiratory tract secretions Cough Sore throat Difficulty in breathing (dyspnoea)
Urinary tract	Pain on passing urine (dysuria) Frequency Urgency Urine appears cloudy, possibly 'bloody' and may have a 'fishy' smell
Gastrointestinal tract	Abdominal pain Nausea Vomiting Diarrhoea Poor appetite
Central nervous system	Confusion Drowsiness Stiff neck Headache Intolerance of light (photophobia)

The four phases of an acute infectious disease — Box 15.3

1. *Incubation*: The incubation period is the interval between contact with the pathogen and development of the symptoms and signs of disease. In some diseases the incubation period is always the same whereas, in others, it is variable, e.g. the common cold: 1–2 days; influenza: 1–3 days; tetanus: ranges from 2 to 21 days. During this period there are no signs or symptoms.
2. *Prodromal*: During this time, the person feels 'out of sorts' but is not yet experiencing actual symptoms of the disease. Early signs and symptoms are present but are vague, e.g. fatigue or malaise, mild fever, and some may feel that they are 'coming down with something'.
3. *Illness*: The illness period, or acute phase, is when signs and symptoms of the disease are present, e.g. fever, muscle pains, photophobia, sore throat.
4. *Convalescence*: As the patient's immune response and other defence mechanisms overcome the pathogen, the person gradually regains strength and health is usually restored. Sometimes the convalescent period can be lengthy and, although the individual may recover from the illness itself, permanent damage can be caused by destruction of tissues in the affected area, e.g. deafness may follow middle ear infections.

in those with compromised immune systems caused by illness, treatments or invasive procedures, normally harmless microorganisms may become pathogenic. Hospitalized patients are especially susceptible to these infections and may need to be nursed in a protected environment (see Protective isolation, p. 358).

- *Acute infectious disease*: Develops quickly but lasts for a relatively short period of time, e.g. influenza. Usually follows a set pattern comprising four stages: incubation, prodromal, illness and convalescence (Box 15.3).
- *Chronic infectious disease*: Progresses slowly and has a long and often indeterminate duration, e.g. tuberculosis, hepatitis C, syphilis.
- *Latent infectious disease*: Arises from microorganisms that remain dormant in the body for long periods, but then become active (usually when the person is experiencing physical or psychological stress), e.g. the herpes virus which causes cold sores and the chickenpox virus that may re-emerge later in life causing shingles.

Expected signs of infection may not always be obvious therefore nurses need to be alert to subtle changes in behaviour that may indicate presence of an infection (Box 15.4).

Host defence mechanisms

If microorganisms never encountered resistance from the host, then people would be constantly ill and die from infectious diseases. In most cases, however, host defence mechanisms are very effective at keeping microbial invaders out. They can be thought of as an army consisting of three lines of defence. If the enemy (the pathogen) breaks through the first line of

 Reflective practice — Box 15.4

Changes in behaviour indicative of an infectious disease

Student activity

Consider the changes in behaviour that may be exhibited by the following patients/clients during the prodromal stage of an acute infectious disease:

- A 4-year-old boy
- An adult with a moderate learning disability
- An elderly patient with diabetes.

defence, it will encounter and should be stopped by the second line of defence. If the pathogen manages to escape the first two lines of defence, there is a third line ready to attack it.

The first two lines of defence are referred to as nonspecific resistance and comprise external defences and the inflammatory process. The third line of defence is specific to particular microorganisms (called specific resistance) and involves white blood cells (B- and T-lymphocytes) and the production of antibodies that protect the host from one particular foreign substance (Fig. 15.3).

External defences

The integrity of body surfaces forms an effective barrier to the initial lodgement or penetration by microorganisms. This first line of defence to microbial invasion depends on mechanical, chemical and microbial barriers that combat any attack (Fig. 15.4).

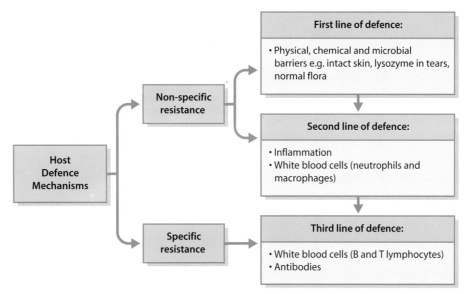

Fig. 15.3 • Overview of the defence mechanisms.

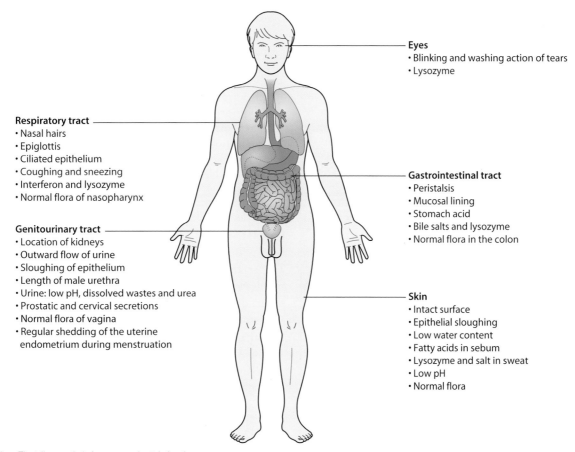

Fig. 15.4 • First lines of defence against infection.

Inflammation

Inflammation is the second line of defence and is triggered when injury or infection damages tissues. The cardinal signs of inflammation are:

- Redness
- Swelling
- Heat
- Pain.

Loss of function can also occur as a consequence of swelling and pain. In apparent contradiction to the signs and symptoms observed, the inflammatory response is beneficial because it attempts to initially destroy the pathogen and then, if possible, remove it and its by-products from the body. Inflammation limits spread in the body by confining the pathogen to one specific area. Finally, the process repairs and replaces damaged tissues.

Specific resistance

The third line of defence is the body's immune response, which is triggered when antigens enter the body. An antigen is any material that the body recognizes as foreign, including pathogenic microorganisms, transplanted tissues and allergens, e.g. pollen, food components and drugs. Two processes work together to combat and destroy a specific antigen: cell-mediated immunity and humoral immunity.

This type of immunity results in the production of antibodies and usually confers lifelong resistance to the antigen. For further discussion of these processes, readers should consult their physiology textbook.

Development of immunity

The formation of antibodies is the basis of immunization against disease and can be either active or passive.

Active immunity

This provides long-term protection against specific microorganisms. It occurs following an infectious disease when antibodies are produced within the body (called *natural active immunity*) or when the person receives a vaccine which stimulates the immune system to produce specific antibodies against a particular agent (called *artificial active immunity*) (Box 15.5).

Critical thinking	Box 15.5

Childhood immunization

Encouraging immunization against common childhood illnesses is an important UK health policy.

After reading adverse publicity about the measles, mumps and rubella (MMR) vaccine, a mother is concerned about having her child vaccinated.

Student activities

- Identify the reasons for encouraging childhood immunization
- At what age is the combined vaccine given?
- Consider how you would deal with this situation.

Resource

Royal College of Nursing (RCN), 2004. Childhood vaccination factfile. Online. Available: www.rcn.org.uk/_data/assets/pdf_file/0005/78629/002467.pdf September 2012

Passive immunity

This provides temporary protection against microorganisms. *Natural passive immunity* is acquired by the developing fetus when it receives maternal antibodies *in utero*, or by baby when it receives maternal antibodies contained in colostrum and breast milk. *Artificial passive immunity* is acquired when a person receives antibodies contained in anti-sera or gamma globulin, e.g. hepatitis B immune globulin is given to protect those who have been exposed to the hepatitis B virus.

Infection control

Infection control refers to the numerous measures that are taken to prevent infections from occurring in healthcare facilities and aims to destroy or remove sources of pathogenic microorganisms by:

- Interrupting the transmission of pathogens
- Protecting people from becoming infected.

These measures break links in the chain of infection. Two tiers of infection control measures are in operation:

- Standard infection control precautions are used for the care of all hospitalized patients at all times, regardless of their diagnosis or presumed infection status (infection is not always detected). They reduce the risk of transmission of pathogens present in blood, body fluids, secretions and excretions, non-intact skin and mucous membranes.
- Additional precautions are necessary during clinically invasive procedures (referred to as aseptic technique), e.g. surgery or insertion of an intravenous cannula or urinary catheter. They are also required to prevent the spread of communicable diseases that are transmitted by airborne, droplet or contact routes. These are referred to as 'isolation precautions' and are always used in conjunction with standard infection control precautions. An overview of the principles of infection control is shown in Figure 15.5.

Standard infection control precautions

This section explores standard infection control precautions, which provide guidelines on:

- Hand hygiene
- Personal protective equipment, e.g. gloves, aprons, masks
- Safe use and disposal of sharps
- Safe management of waste and linen
- Decontamination of patient-care equipment, i.e. cleaning, sterilizing, disinfecting.

Hand hygiene

Many infections are spread by contact and the hands are the major vehicles in transfer of potential pathogens in healthcare settings from:

- One patient/client to another
- A contaminated object to a patient/client
- Healthcare personnel to a patient/client or vice versa.

In the mid-nineteenth century, Ignaz Philipp Semmelweis identified handwashing as the most important feature in preventing transmission of infection in healthcare facilities.

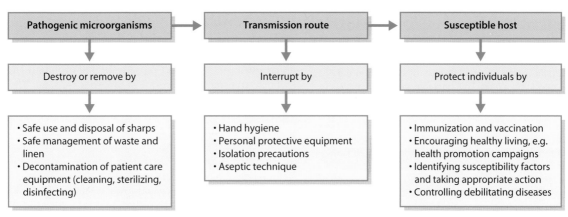

Fig. 15.5 • Principles of infection control.

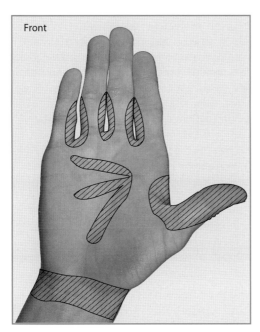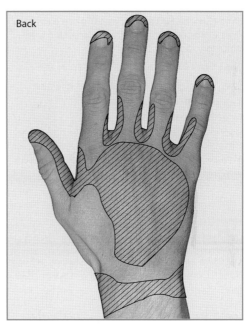

Fig. 15.6 • Areas of hands prone to harbouring microorganisms. (Reproduced with permission from Inglis, T.J.J., 2003. Microbiology and infection, second ed. Churchill Livingstone, Edinburgh.)

Infection control research and guidelines from national and international organizations continue to acknowledge handwashing as the most effective measure in reducing the incidence of HAIs (Pratt et al 2007).

The purpose of handwashing is to remove potentially pathogenic microorganisms from the skin. These may be:

• Resident microorganisms (normal flora) that are difficult to remove as they reside in the deep layers of the skin, hair follicles and sebaceous glands (see Ch. 16)

• Transient microorganisms, which represent recent contamination of the hands. They usually colonize the superficial layers of the skin and are acquired during contact with patients/clients and contaminated objects. Transient microorganisms found on the hands of healthcare personnel are frequently implicated as the source of healthcare-associated infections. Fortunately, they are easily removed by routine handwashing (WHO 2009b).

Indications for handwashing

Hands must be washed whenever there is a chance that they may have become contaminated and any time when there is a risk of transmitting infection to others (Box 13.19, p. 294). Figure 15.6 shows the areas of hands prone to harbouring microorganisms. It is important to be aware that handwashing is one of the most important infection prevention practices and, if not washed at appropriate times, the hands can put patients, residents and clients at risk (Box 15.6). Furthermore, contaminated hands can be a danger not only to the practitioner but also to their colleagues, friends and family members.

Types of handwashing and preparations used

There are three types of hand hygiene used in clinical settings, each of which uses different preparations and is appropriate in different situations.

Handwashing with liquid soap and running water (social handwashing)

Plain soap has detergent properties and effectively removes dirt, most organic substances and transient flora from the skin. Handwashing with soap from a dispenser and water for 10–15 seconds followed by rinsing in running water is used routinely in clinical areas (Box 15.7). If the hands are heavily soiled with dirt, blood or other organic material, e.g. when gloves have been torn, handwashing for several minutes may be necessary (Pratt et al 2007).

Handwashing with antiseptic preparations and running water (aseptic handwashing)

Antiseptic preparations, e.g. chlorhexidine, povidone iodine and triclosan, have the same action as plain soap with the additional benefit of killing or inhibiting the growth of resident microorganisms. Some antiseptics continue to perform these actions for several hours after the hands are washed. Washing the hands with an antiseptic preparation is appropriate in high-risk situations, i.e. before invasive procedures or contact with clients who have compromised immunity and are therefore highly susceptible to infection (Box 15.7).

Alcohol-based hand rubs

These contain 70% alcohol and emollients (moisturizing agents to counteract the drying effect of alcohol) and some contain an antiseptic. They act rapidly and kill or inhibit the growth of both transient and resident microorganisms. Their use can offer a practical and acceptable alternative to handwashing in certain clinical situations, e.g. between surgical cases in high-volume settings (Fig. 15.7, p. 348). However, alcohol gels are ineffective if hands are visibly soiled with dirt, blood or organisms, for example *Clostridium difficile*. In such clinical situations alcohol hand rub must not be used as an alternative to soap, but it can be applied after washing to rid hands of non-clostridial organisms (DH 2009; WHO 2009b).

Personal protective equipment

Personal protective equipment (PPE) includes disposable gloves, gowns, aprons, eye protection and masks. They are worn to protect staff and patients from pathogenic microorganisms in both healthcare and community settings during exposure prone procedures. The decision to use or wear PPE is based on a risk assessment (see Ch. 13) associated with a specific patient care activity or intervention (NICE 2003) (Fig. 15.8, p. 348).

Disposable gloves

The purpose of wearing gloves is to:

- Reduce the risk of healthcare personnel acquiring infections from patients/clients
- Prevent natural flora or transient contamination from the hands of healthcare personnel being transmitted to patients/clients.

Gloves are worn for:

- All activities that carry a risk of exposure to blood, body fluids, secretions or excretions, e.g. when giving injections, emptying catheter bags or disposing of bedpans, performing mouth care (NICE 2003).
- Contact with sterile sites; such as catheterization, broken skin and mucous membranes, e.g. wound care, and invasive procedures, e.g. surgery.

Types of gloves and their uses

Gloves are available in a variety of materials including natural rubber latex (NRL), synthetic latex and vinyl. The appropriate type of glove is determined by the activity to be undertaken:

- Latex gloves are used for procedures requiring a high degree of dexterity such as catheterization
- Vinyl gloves, which are looser fitting, are appropriate to wear when giving injections or cleaning up spillage.

Gloves can be either sterile or non-sterile and selection is based on the type of activity to be undertaken. Sterile gloves must be worn for any contact with sterile sites and invasive procedures (see above); non-sterile gloves are suitable for activities involving contact with body fluids, e.g. handling urine and sputum.

Nursing skills Box 15.7

Handwashing

Prerequisites to handwashing

- Remove wrist and hand jewellery prior to handwashing because it harbours dirt and the skin underneath is more heavily colonized with bacteria
- Keep nails short, as skin below the fingernails harbours high concentrations of bacteria
- Avoid wearing artificial nails, extensions or chipped nail polish, all of which have been shown to increase bacterial counts and

impede visualization of dirt under the nails (NICE 2003; WHO 2009b).

Handwashing with soap and water

Hands are rubbed together vigorously for a minimum of 10–15 seconds, paying particular attention to the tips of the fingers, thumbs and areas between the fingers (see below).

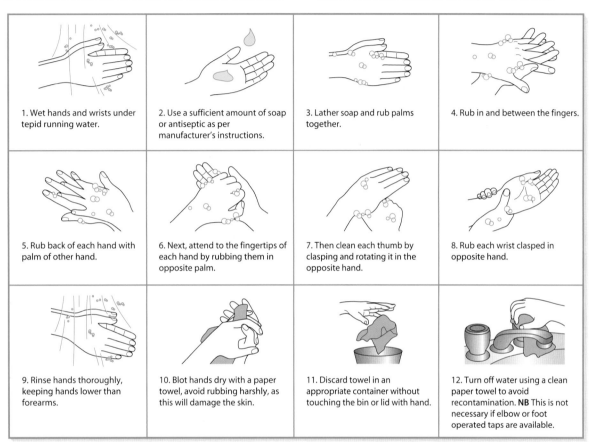

1. Wet hands and wrists under tepid running water.

2. Use a sufficient amount of soap or antiseptic as per manufacturer's instructions.

3. Lather soap and rub palms together.

4. Rub in and between the fingers.

5. Rub back of each hand with palm of other hand.

6. Next, attend to the fingertips of each hand by rubbing them in opposite palm.

7. Then clean each thumb by clasping and rotating it in the opposite hand.

8. Rub each wrist clasped in opposite hand.

9. Rinse hands thoroughly, keeping hands lower than forearms.

10. Blot hands dry with a paper towel, avoid rubbing harshly, as this will damage the skin.

11. Discard towel in an appropriate container without touching the bin or lid with hand.

12. Turn off water using a clean paper towel to avoid recontamination. **NB** This is not necessary if elbow or foot operated taps are available.

Skin care

Regular hand decontamination can cause skin dryness. The regular use of moisturizing hand cream increases skin hydration and replaces depleted skin fats. If a particular soap, antiseptic preparation or alcohol product causes skin irritation, the occupational health team should be consulted (WHO 2009b).

Removal of gloves

Gloves are changed and discarded as follows:

- After contact with each patient
- When performing separate procedures on the same patient if there is a risk of cross-contamination, e.g. mouth care followed by a dressing change
- As soon as they are damaged, e.g. torn or punctured
- On completion of any task not involving patients but requiring the use of gloves
- Before touching any other items, e.g. worktops, pens, telephones.

It is important that gloves are always treated as single-use items and discarded following removal. Wearing gloves does not replace the need for handwashing because gloves may have small defects, may be torn during use or the hands may have become contaminated during removal. Therefore, hand hygiene is essential before their use and after their removal.

Health risks associated with glove use

Pratt et al (2007) advise that gloves should not be worn unnecessarily as their prolonged and indiscriminate use may lead to skin sensitivity and adverse reactions including latex allergy.

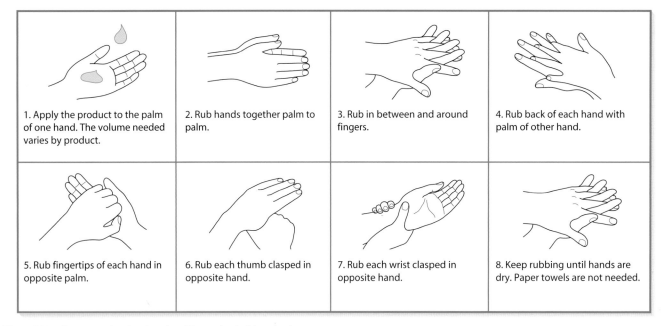

Fig. 15.7 ● Decontaminating hands with an alcohol hand rub. (Reproduced with permission from the Government of Ontario, Canada.)

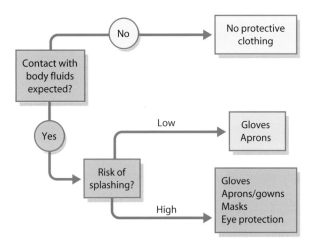

Fig. 15.8 ● Protective clothing risk assessment and selection.
(Reproduced with permission from Wilson, J., 2001. Infection control in clinical practice, second ed. Elsevier, Edinburgh.)

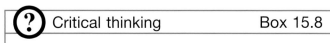

? Critical thinking   **Box 15.8**

Contact with latex in the healthcare environment

You are caring for Mary who states that she is allergic to natural rubber latex.

Student activities

- Identify items in your placement that contain natural rubber latex.
- Consider nursing interventions and treatments where contact with natural rubber latex is likely.
- Find out how a latex allergy is diagnosed.

Gowns and aprons

The purpose of wearing water-repellent protection is to:

- Prevent the user's clothing or skin from becoming contaminated with microorganisms which may subsequently be transferred to others
- Prevent the user's clothing or uniform becoming soiled or stained
- Prevent direct transfer or dissemination of microorganisms from the user to others.

When to wear gowns and aprons

Water-repellent gowns are used for procedures where there is a risk of extensive splashing of blood, body fluids, secretions or excretions onto the skin or clothing, e.g. in the operating theatre, dealing with trauma cases in the Emergency Department and during childbirth.

Disposable plastic aprons are worn to protect the front of the uniform from soiling, wetting or contamination that may occur during procedures involving close or direct contact with patients/clients such as:

Symptoms of latex allergy occurring in sensitized people are variable and usually begin within minutes of exposure but sometimes may develop hours later. Mild reactions include skin redness, itching and urticaria (rashes). Occasionally more severe reactions, e.g. nasal congestion, wheeze and eye irritation may develop. Immediately life-threatening anaphylactic shock is a rare first sign of latex allergy.

Many products containing natural rubber latex are found both in the home (e.g. balloons, erasers and condoms) and healthcare facilities, e.g. elastic bandages, urinary catheters, bath mats and hand grips; therefore patients/clients may also have developed allergies and sensitivity at home which may put them at risk within a healthcare facility (Box 15.8). NICE (2003) advise that any sensitivity to natural rubber latex in patients, carers or healthcare personnel must be documented and alternatives gloves made available.

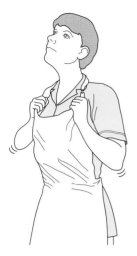
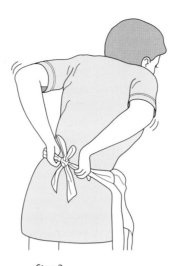
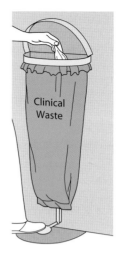

Step 1.
Grasp apron by
neck band and tear

Step 2.
Break waist tie

Step 3.
Carefully dispose into clinical waste
bin and wash hands

Fig. 15.9 • Removing a disposable apron.

- Bed making
- Bathing
- Wound care
- Dealing with spillages
- Preparation and serving of food.

In many healthcare facilities, different coloured aprons are used for different activities. Plastic aprons must be worn as single-use items, i.e. for one procedure or episode of patient care (NICE 2003). Care should be taken when removing aprons (Fig. 15.9).

Masks and eye protection

The purpose of masks and eye protection is to protect the wearer where there is a danger of pathogens in blood or other body substances splashing, splattering and spraying onto the mouth, nose and eyes, e.g. dental and operating theatre procedures, airway suctioning, obstetrical procedures.

Eye protection equipment, such as face shields, goggles and spectacles, must be optically clear (scratch- and mark-free), anti-fog and distortion-free, close-fitting and shielded at the sides. They are identified either as reusable after cleaning or for single-use only.

Masks are worn to protect health care practitioners in situations where microorganisms may be transmitted from patients via the airborne route. It is recommended that if healthcare workers are likely to be exposed to either tuberculosis, H1N1 or severe acute respiratory syndrome (SARS) a particulate filter personal respiratory protection device (close-fitting masks capable of filtering 0.3 μm particles) should be used (WHO 2007). In cases where human to human droplet transmission is possible (e.g. H1N1, H5N1), standard and additional droplet precautions must be taken if working within 1 metre of the patient (WHO 2009c). Masks are also indicated when caring for susceptible clients, e.g. people with compromised immunity (Pratt et al 2007). However, unless the mask fits closely

around the mouth and nose, microorganisms can escape around its edges (Wilson 2006). Furthermore, if worn for long periods, its filtering efficiency is impaired because moisture collects in the fabric and interrupts the passage of air through the mask. Guidance on the correct use of masks is provided in Box 15.9.

 Nursing skills   Box 15.9

Correct use of masks
- The mask should fit snugly over the face, the coloured side facing out and the metal strip at the top
- Position the strings to keep the mask firmly in place over the nose, mouth and chin
- Mould the metallic strip to the bridge of the nose
- Do not touch the mask again until it is removed
- Remove the mask by its ties
- Discard as clinical waste according to local policy
- If the mask is damaged or soiled, replace it immediately.

(Adapted from Health Protection Agency 2009).

Safe use and disposal of sharps

In healthcare settings, injuries from needles or other sharp instruments pose a serious danger in transmitting blood-borne viruses such as HIV and hepatitis B and C to healthcare personnel. These infections can be potentially life threatening but are preventable.

What are sharps?

The term 'sharps' refers to any sharp instrument or object used in the delivery of care including: hypodermic needles, suture

Health promotion | Box 15.10

Safe handling and disposal of sharps

National and international guidelines are consistent in their recommendations for the safe use and disposal of sharp instruments and needles.

Handling sharps

- Minimize handling of sharps
- Do not carry used sharps by hand or pass them to another person.

Sharps containers

- Sharps containers should be located in all areas where sharp objects are used, e.g. treatment rooms, operating theatres, labour and delivery rooms, laboratories
- Containers are located in a safe position – not on floors where they could be kicked over – and out of reach of members of the public, in particular small children. To avoid damage by heat, sharps containers should not be placed near radiators or in direct sunlight (Pratt et al 2007).

Disposing of sharps into sharps containers

- Immediate and safe disposal of sharps into appropriate, puncture-proof sharps bins
- Do not dismantle needles from syringes or other devices, but discard as a single unit
- Place sharps point downwards into yellow sharps container
- Ensure containers are securely closed when three-quarters full
- Ensure containers are disposed of in accordance with local policy
- Needle safety devices must be used where there are clear indications that they will provide safer systems of working for healthcare personnel (NICE 2003).
- Secure and close sharps container prior to removal for incineration.

First aid | Box 15.11

Managing needlestick injuries and exposure to body fluids

Healthcare facilities have protocols to follow if a sharp injury or exposure to body fluids occurs.

First aid

Following any accidental exposure to blood or other body fluids by needlestick, another sharp object or a splash of fluid then:

- Wash the needlestick or cut with soap and water
- Flush splashes to the nose, mouth or skin with water
- Irrigate splashes to the eyes with clean water or saline.

There is no evidence to show that using antiseptics or encouraging the wound to bleed reduces the risk of a blood-borne infection. However, many organizations and healthcare facilities within the UK suggest that this should be carried out as a first aid measure.

Management

- Inform the charge nurse immediately
- Attend the Occupational Health Department, Emergency Department or other designated treatment facility. Prompt reporting is essential as post-exposure treatment is sometimes recommended and should be started as soon as possible.

Whether post-exposure treatment is indicated following exposure to blood or other body fluids depends on a number of factors including:

- The infection status of the person whose blood or body fluids are involved
- The type of exposure, e.g. a splash to the skin versus a deep puncture wound
- Whether or not the casualty has been vaccinated against hepatitis B
- Time elapsed since exposure
- The availability of needed drugs or other therapy.

Documentation

- Complete the relevant documentation for reporting accidents (see Ch. 13).

---

needles, scalpel blades, lancets, stitch cutters, broken glass, razor blades.

Most reported sharps injuries involve nursing staff; however, other healthcare personnel including doctors, laboratory, domestic and portering staff may also be involved (NHS Scotland 2005). First aid for needlestick injuries is described in Box 15.11 (see below).

How injuries occur

Many injuries occur when staff are using and disposing of sharps, e.g.:

- Recapping hypodermic needles after use. This is one of the major causes of sharp object injuries
- Manipulating used sharps which can cause blood inside to splatter or an accidental injury
- Carrying unprotected sharps
- Sharp items are found in areas where they are unexpected, e.g. on surgical drapes, bed linen or clinical waste
- Sudden movement by a client at the time of an injection causes a healthcare practitioner to be accidentally stuck.

Preventing sharps injuries

The assessment and management of risks associated with the use of sharps is paramount in health and safety promotion as well as in infection control. Injuries from sharps can be avoided by handling and disposing of them safely (Box 15.10).

Managing injuries and exposure to body fluids

Exposure to blood from a sharps injury, bite or splashing into the eyes, mouth or broken skin must always be followed up because of the risk of infection from blood-borne viruses (Box 15.11).

Management of waste

Safe management of healthcare waste is a crucial aspect of infection control. It is a statutory requirement for

Table 15.1 Categories, containment, treatment and disposal of waste from clinical areas

Clinical hazardous waste	Container colour and disposal
Items soiled by blood or other body fluids: Include wound dressings, swabs, disposable gloves and aprons, materials used to clean up spillages; contaminated waste from patients with transmissible infectious diseases, e.g. tuberculosis and *Salmonella* including disposable nappies	Yellow or orange bag Incineration or heat disinfection followed by landfill
Sharps	See Box 15.10 p. 350
Pharmaceutical products and chemical wastes: Include expired and unwanted medicines, cartridges from drug infusion devices, cytotoxic drugs	Collected by ward/community pharmacist who makes arrangements for disposal
Body waste products: Include urine, faeces, body secretions and excretions, plus disposables used for their collection, e.g. bedpans, bedpan liners, vomit bowls	Discharged into sewerage system via sluice, lavatory or macerator
Sanpro – sanitary products waste: Includes disposable nappies, incontinence pads, stoma bags, urine containers	Yellow bag with black stripes May be incinerated or sent direct to landfill

Domestic (non-hazardous) waste	Container and destination
General waste: Includes dead flowers, used hand towels, food (small quantities only), paper wrappings from packs, magazines and newspapers	Black bag at source although some facilities may use clear, green, buff or white bags Sent direct to landfill
Glass bottles and jars	When empty, place in a strong box, mark box 'Glass with Care'; put into designated container, recycling unit or landfill
Aerosols, pressurized containers, batteries: May pose a safety and/or environmental risk, i.e. may contain CFCs, prescription medicines, flammable liquids or be explosive in nature	Placed in separately identified containers

(Adapted from DH 2011.)

healthcare facilities to comply with international, national and local legislation and regulations that relate to the segregation, handling, transportation and final disposal of waste.

Classification of waste

Waste generated from healthcare facilities is classified as clinical or non-clinical waste.

Clinical (hazardous) waste

This is generated from many sources including healthcare, veterinary and pharmaceutical establishments. Because of its hazardous, infectious or dangerous content it may be harmful to healthcare personnel, members of the public and the environment. Consequently, special precautions are required to treat and dispose of it safely (DH 2011).

Domestic waste

A considerable proportion of the waste generated in clinical areas is not hazardous to those who come into contact with it and can be safely disposed of as household waste. Therefore it is important that this waste is not sent for incineration in order to minimize both disposal costs and damage to the environment (Table 15.1).

Safe handling of clinical waste in healthcare facilities

Disposing of waste safely and economically depends on correct segregation of different types of waste at the point of generation. Waste is bagged, packaged or containerized and must clearly indicate the contents (Box 15.12, p. 352).

Safe handling of clinical waste in people's homes

The amount of clinical waste generated by patients/clients in their own homes is much smaller and can usually be disposed of as normal household waste. Used needles, e.g. those used by people with insulin-dependent diabetes, must not be discarded as household waste. Instead, arrangements with local hospitals, clinics, pharmacies or local authorities need to be made regarding their disposal. Healthcare personnel, e.g. community nurses and dialysis technicians, who generate clinical waste while treating patients in their homes are obliged by the Health and Safety at Work Act 1974 to transport and dispose of the waste safely (see Box 15.13, p. 352).

Management of linen

Used linen, e.g. clothing, towels, sheets, pillowslips, should be laundered between patient use and when visibly soiled.

In healthcare facilities, linen that is soiled with blood, excreta or other body fluids, or contaminated with microorganisms from infectious patients, needs to be handled carefully in order to prevent:

- Contamination of the skin and clothing of healthcare personnel
- Transfer of microorganisms to other patients/clients and environments.

Laundering should remove evidence of previous use and significantly reduce microbial counts so that the risk of infection to subsequent users is negligible (Table 15.2, p. 352).

Safe handling of linen

To prevent the risk of cross-infection, it is important that linen in healthcare facilities is handled in the same way for all patients/clients. PPE should be used when handling linen, as follows:

Nursing skills · Box 15.12

Safe handling of clinical waste

Dealing with clinical waste bags

- All infectious waste (other than contaminated sharps, glassware or sharp-edged waste) must be disposed of into leak-resistant clinical waste bags
- Gloves and aprons should be worn when handling clinical waste bags and containers
- Clinical waste bags must be suspended in an appropriate container, e.g. a foot-operated lidded bin, and the containers positioned at the point of generation
- Bags must not be filled more than three-quarters full and loose contents should never be transferred from bag to bag or compacted by hand. This will avoid injuries from concealed sharps that may have inadvertently been discarded with clinical waste
- All bags must indicate their origin and be labelled with the name of the facility, e.g. hospital ward or department, and the date
- Bags must be sealed at the point of production with a plastic tie, closure or heat sealer. Staples should not be used as they result in puncture holes
- Waste must not be allowed to accumulate in corridors or other undesignated areas because it could cause harm to others.

Dealing with spillages

- Appropriate PPE, e.g. non-sterile vinyl gloves and plastic apron, must be worn
- Any spilled fluid must be mopped up with absorbent material, e.g. paper towels
- Carefully place contaminated material in a new clinical waste bag, together with all other spilled clinical waste matter
- Seal and label the bag, and dispose of in line with local policy
- Disinfect the spillage area according to local policy, e.g. hypochlorite
- Remove protective clothing and wash hands.

(Adapted from DH 2011).

- Plastic aprons when making or changing beds, to prevent contamination of uniform or clothing by potential pathogens, and discarded afterwards
- Gloves when handling linen or clothing that is soiled with blood, body fluids, secretions and excretions to prevent contamination of the hands. Following their removal, gloves are disposed of and the hands washed.

Safe handling of soiled linen

Linen is handled with minimal agitation and shaking to avoid the dispersal of microorganisms into the air and onto people or objects in the vicinity.

- Heavily soiled linen is rolled or folded to contain the heaviest soil in the centre of the bundle. Large amounts of solid soil, e.g. faeces, are removed with a gloved hand and toilet tissue and discarded into a bedpan or lavatory for flushing.
- Containment is achieved by placing linen immediately into a collection bag at the site of generation. It should not be temporarily placed anywhere else, e.g. on floors, bed tables, lockers or chairs. The collection bag should be of sufficient quality to contain the wet/soiled linen and prevent leakage during handling and transportation. Bags should not be overfilled, as this may prevent closure or increase the likelihood of the bag splitting during transit to the laundry.
- Linen is never rinsed or soaked due to the risk of splashing body fluids onto the skin or mucous membranes.
- Ensuring that sharps and other objects are not inadvertently discarded into linen bags minimizes the risk of injury to portering and laundry staff. A tracking system

---

Reflective practice · Box 15.13

Management of clinical waste

Student activities

- Identify how clinical waste is managed within your community placement from the point of generation to disposal.
- Review practices in relation to clinical waste within your placement.
- Discuss your observations with your mentor.

Table 15.2 Laundering of hospital linen

Category	Description	Bag type and colour	Laundering process
Used	Normal usage or visibly soiled by blood, body fluids, secretions and excretions	White linen or clear plastic	Sorted before disinfection by washing at 65°C for 10 min or 71°C for 3 min
Infected	Linen used by patients with certain infectious diseases or as advised by the infection control team. Also includes reusable nappies	Red outer bag, containing an inner water-soluble bag	Not sorted prior to washing. Water-soluble bag placed unopened in the washing machine and dissolves during the washing process. Disinfected by washing at 65°C for 10 min or 71°C for 3 min

(From NHS Executive 1995).

requires each collection bag to be tagged with the name of the ward/department. This establishes a system whereby extraneous objects found in linen can be returned to the sender.

By careful handling of used linen the nurse can break the chain of infection, thereby protecting patients from HAIs (Box 15.14).

◉ **Health promotion**   **Box 15.14**

Breaking the chain of infection using standard infection control precautions

Staff Nurse Jones was assigned to care for Mr Green, a patient who had an open draining wound on his left lower leg. When a sample of pus was sent to the laboratory for analysis, the microorganism meticillin resistant *Staphylococcus aureus* (MRSA) was isolated. Prior to making Mr Green's bed, Staff Nurse Jones washed his hands. Clean linen and a collection bag for linen were placed at the patient's bed. To remove the soiled linen from the bed, Staff Nurse Jones took the following actions:

- Washed his hands
- Wore non-sterile gloves and a disposable plastic apron
- Handled the sheets by the outermost edges so that the soiled area was folded into the centre of the bundle
- Held soiled linen away from his uniform and placed it directly into the linen collection bag
- Removed the gloves and discarded them directly into a waste receptacle
- Washed his hands.

Staff Nurse Jones applied principles of infection control to contain the infectious microorganisms at many points in the chain of infection as shown below.

Link in the chain	Nursing action to break the chain
Infectious agent: MRSA microorganism *Reservoir*: Mr Green's infected wound	Staff Nurse Jones knew the infected wound contained microorganisms that could easily be transmitted to other patients by indirect contact
Portal of exit: Exudate draining from the open wound	Staff Nurse Jones used proper handwashing techniques, wore protective gloves and handled the linen correctly
Mode of transmission: Healthcare workers' hands frequently transfer MRSA by indirect contact	Proper handwashing, gloving and careful handling of used linen
Portal of entry	Microorganisms isolated using standard infection control principles
Susceptible host	None, due to Staff Nurse Jones' adherence to infection control measures

---

Decontamination of patient-care equipment

Patient-care equipment can act as an intermediary (fomite) in transferring infectious microorganisms from one person to another. It is therefore important that shared or reusable patient-care equipment is decontaminated, i.e. made safe by removing, inhibiting or destroying microorganisms, after use. The term 'decontamination' includes sterilization, disinfection and cleaning. These methods confer different levels of microbial safety on items processed.

Levels of decontamination

The appropriate level of decontamination depends on the risk that equipment may present in transmitting infection. The following factors are critical to that interrelationship:

- The presence of microorganisms, i.e. their numbers and virulence
- The type of procedure to be performed, i.e. invasive or non-invasive
- The body site where the instrument or equipment will be used, e.g. penetrating tissue or used on intact skin.

The risk of transmission can be categorized as high, medium, low or minimal.

Cleaning

This is a physical process that involves decontaminating an item or surface with a detergent solution followed by thorough drying. Cleaning contributes to infection control because it physically removes organic materials, e.g. blood, other body fluids, soil or dust, in which microorganisms can survive. Although cleaning does not necessarily destroy microorganisms, it significantly reduces their numbers and is suitable for low and minimal risk items.

Unless cleaning is carried out competently, infectious microorganisms may be redistributed to other sources and sites (Box 15.15). Cleaning is also essential prior to disinfection and sterilization, otherwise microorganisms trapped in organic material may survive further processing (Centers for Disease Control and Prevention, CDC 2008).

Sterilization

Sterilization is the complete destruction of all living microorganisms including bacterial spores (spores are a resistant casing produced by several species of bacteria that enables them to survive in adverse conditions, e.g. heat, cold, drying, and exposure to most chemicals). When something is sterile, it is devoid of microbial life.

Creutzfeldt–Jakob disease (CJD) and variant CJD present serious cross-infection risks as the microorganisms resist normal decontamination methods. It is important to refer to local policy regarding decontamination.

Sterilization is necessary for all high-risk procedures, e.g. surgical and invasive procedures; using steam, dry heat, ethylene oxide gas, automated chemical systems and irradiation. Sterilized items need to be stored correctly and checked prior to opening (Box 15.16).

Disinfection

Disinfection is the destruction or removal of microorganisms to a level that is unlikely to cause infection. It does not

Maintaining a clean environment | Box 15.15

Good cleaning practices

Although environmental cleaning in most healthcare facilities is the duty of cleaning staff, nursing staff have ultimate responsibility to ensure that the standard of cleaning adheres to national guidelines. As nurses are often required to clean patient-care equipment (e.g. blood pressure equipment, washbowls) and blood and body fluid spillages, it is important that they understand fundamental cleaning principles. PPE, i.e. gloves and aprons, are worn for cleaning and once the task is completed, the hands are washed before carrying out other duties.

Cleaning solutions

When detergent is dissolved in water, it breaks up and dissolves or suspends grease, oil and other foreign matter, thus facilitating its removal. Detergents are available in various forms, e.g. powders, liquids, sprays, gels and wipes. Cleaning solutions:

- Become contaminated almost immediately during cleaning and their continued use transfers increasing numbers of microorganisms to each subsequent surface cleaned (CDC 2008)
- Are used instead of hand soap for patient-care equipment, because fatty acids contained in the soap react with the minerals in water, leaving a residue or scum that is difficult to remove (CDC 2008)
- Are disposed of into a sluice or sink in the dirty utility area. They must not be discarded into washbasins (WHO 2004).

Cleaning cloths

- Cleaning cloths and mop heads can be another source of contamination, especially if left soaking in used solutions. Washing after use and allowing them to dry before re-use minimizes contamination (CDC 2008)
- The same cloth must never be used to clean different areas, e.g. toilets and kitchens
- Disposable, colour-coded cloths are often available for use in different areas (WHO 2004).

Drying after cleaning

This is essential because bacteria thrive in moisture. Weber et al (2010) showed that *C. difficile* cells may remain viable for up to 6 hours on moist surfaces.

Cleaning the hospital environment

This is carried out routinely to ensure a clean, dust-free hospital environment. Visible dirt contains microorganisms and cleaning helps to eliminate them. The main methods of removing organic materials are:

- *Dry cleaning*, e.g. sweeping, dusting is not recommended because it increases airborne bacterial counts
- *Wet cleaning* using detergent and hot water is more effective.

The frequency of wet cleaning required depends on the situation, e.g.

- Areas visibly contaminated with blood or body fluids must be cleaned immediately
- Isolation rooms and other areas that have patients with known transmissible infections should be cleaned with a detergent/disinfectant solution at least daily
- All horizontal surfaces and toilet areas should be cleaned daily (WHO 2004).

Reflective practice | Box 15.16

Storing and checking sterile items
Student activities

Identify a range of sterile items in your placement:

- How are sterile items wrapped?
- Where are sterile items stored?
- What checks must be made before opening a sterile item?
- Why should sterile items be used immediately and, if they are not, discarded?

guarantee complete removal of all microorganisms because bacterial spores can still survive, i.e. some forms of microbial life may still be present after disinfection.

Disinfection is necessary for all medium-risk procedures and for equipment used for those with transmissible infections, e.g. following direct contact with mucous membranes, body fluids or other potentially infectious material. Low risk items within the clinical area (e.g. hoists, blood pressure cuffs and mattresses) also require disinfection following contact with people with known infections. Disinfection can be achieved by thermal and chemical methods.

Thermal disinfection is suitable for items that can withstand heat and moisture but do not need to be sterile. Examples of thermal disinfection equipment used in clinical settings include bedpan washers, dishwashers and laundry machines. Although not frequently used in hospitals, boiling is sometimes used to disinfect medium-risk equipment, e.g. feeding bottles, vaginal specula, ear syringes.

Numerous chemical disinfectants are available to decontaminate equipment and the environment (Table 15.3), although in healthcare facilities, the number available is strictly limited. Furthermore, the use of chemical disinfectants is regulated by the Control of Substances Hazardous to Health (COSHH) Regulations (Health and Safety Executive, HSE 2002) which are designed to protect against risks to health from hazardous substances in the workplace (see Ch. 13). Each healthcare facility has an infection control policy/manual that gives information about procedures for decontamination (Box 15.17).

Additional precautions

These are used in addition to the standard infection control precautions discussed above; aseptic technique and isolation precautions are explained in this section.

Aseptic technique

Patients in healthcare facilities often acquire infections as a result of invasive clinical procedures which breach the body's

Table 15.3 Chemical disinfectants used in healthcare facilities

Group	Characteristics and uses	Precautions

70% Alcohol solutions, e.g.
    Cliniwipes
    Azowipes
    Mediswabs
Hand gel preparations
	Effective, rapid acting disinfectants and antiseptics.
	Poor penetrative powers – should only be used on clean surfaces.
	Active against bacteria and not spores.
	Virucidal activity variable.
	Commonly used for skin disinfection and as agent for rapid disinfection of physically clean hands
		Flammable: use in well-ventilated areas, keep away from heat sources, electrical equipment, flames, hot surfaces.
		Toxic: avoid inhalation

Chlorine-releasing agents Strong sodium hypochlorite solutions Hypochlorite powders, e.g. Domestos®, Chloros®, Milton®, Presept®, Haz-tabs®	Chlorine-releasing agents are rapidly effective against viruses, fungi, bacteria and spores. Recommended for hazards of viral infection, e.g. Hepatitis B, C, HIV	May damage certain materials, e.g. some plastics, rubber, metals and fabrics. Must not be mixed with acids including acidic body fluids such as urine
Phenolic Carbolic acid e.g. Clearsol®, Stericol®, Hycolin®	Active against a wide range of bacteria. Fungicidal, but limited virucidal and sporicidal activity. Poor penetration of organic material e.g. blood, pus, faeces, milk	Absorbed by rubber and plastics. Can cause severe burning of the skin or mucous membranes

---

Reflective practice   Box 15.17

Control of Substances Hazardous to Health (COSHH)

Student activities

In your current placement:

- Locate COSHH guidelines and the infection control policy/manual.
- Select two chemical disinfectants used in practice and, from the COSHH guidelines, identify their uses, associated hazards and first-aid treatment recommended in the case of accidental ingestion or inhalation.
- Reflect on the relevance of COSHH guidelines to your own practice.

(Reproduced with permission from the Government of Ontario, Canada.)

---

normal defence mechanisms, making the tissues vulnerable to invasion by microorganisms. For example:

- Blood infections (septicaemia) after the insertion of an intravenous catheter
- Wound infections following surgery
- Urinary tract infections related to the insertion of an indwelling urinary catheter
- Lower respiratory tract infections, e.g. pneumonia, postoperatively.

Aseptic technique is often referred to as 'sterile technique' or 'no-touch technique'. It includes practices used to render and keep objects and areas sterile, i.e. free of all microorganisms including bacterial spores. Aseptic technique is routinely carried out in a wide range of hospital and community settings.

Indications for aseptic technique

Aseptic technique is carried out during any invasive clinical procedure that enters or penetrates a vulnerable body site such as the vascular system, a sterile body cavity or tissue. Examples of invasive clinical procedures include:

- Wound care
- Insertion of an intravenous cannula or urinary catheter
- Vaginal examinations during labour
- Medical procedures, e.g. lumbar puncture, endoscopy
- Surgical operations and suturing wounds.

Components of aseptic technique

The components of aseptic technique include all the key elements of standard infection control precautions and also focus on:

- Careful preparation of the patient, environment and equipment
- Using an antiseptic solution to decontaminate the hands and the patient's skin (Box 15.18)
- Using only sterile equipment and supplies, e.g. drapes, swabs, instruments, sutures, fluids, catheters
- Creating a sterile working area known as the 'sterile field' where everything within the defined radius is sterile
- Maintaining a sterile working area by safe working practices that prevent contamination of the equipment and supplies.

The principles of aseptic technique are shown in Box 15.19.

Clean technique

Clean technique is a version of aseptic technique. The goal of clean technique is to exclude pathogens from a susceptible site, whereas that of aseptic technique is to exclude all microorganisms (Burton & Engelkirk 2007). When used in conjunction with a 'no-touch' technique (not touching the susceptible body area with non-sterile items), clean technique is used for:

Antiseptic agents   Box 15.18

Antiseptic agents (antiseptics) are chemical solutions that reduce or destroy microorganisms on the skin or mucous membranes without causing damage or irritation. They are used to clean the skin before invasive procedures and also as hand cleansing agents for healthcare workers.

- Antiseptics are used in accordance with the manufacturer's directions, which are designed to ensure that, when used as directed, the antiseptic agent meets its stated efficacy. Like chemical disinfectants, the use of antiseptics is regulated by COSHH Regulations (HSE 2002)
- Liquid soap dispensers should never be 'topped up', as they are a potential source of contamination because bacteria can multiply within many products. They should be completely replaced, including the dispensing nozzle (Wilson 2006)
- As antiseptics do not have the same destructive powers as chemicals used for disinfection of inanimate objects, they should *never* be used to disinfect equipment or environmental surfaces (CDC 2008).

- Injecting medications
- Removal of sutures and drains (see Ch. 24)
- Endotracheal suctioning
- Venepuncture and intravenous cannulation.

Clean technique includes all the key elements of standard infection control precautions including:

- Thorough handwashing before and after the procedure
- Wearing suitable PPE
- Using and disposing of sharps safely
- Appropriate cleaning, disinfection and sterilization practices
- Correct disposal of waste.

Isolation precautions

Microorganisms cause a wide variety of infections and, for most, standard infection control precautions are adequate to prevent their transmission to healthcare personnel and other patients. However, for patients known to have, or are suspected to have, highly transmissible infections or are colonized by dangerous pathogens, additional precautions are needed. In the past, these were referred to as 'barrier nursing', but are now known as isolation precautions. Some healthcare facilities use the term 'source isolation' to indicate that the patient is

---

 Nursing skills   Box 15.19

Principles of aseptic technique

Aseptic technique may vary slightly but the basic principles are always the same.

Preparation

- *Environment*: Preferably use a treatment room for the procedure; if not available, the procedure may be performed at the patient's bedside. Ensure that the door or screens are closed to reduce the likelihood of cross-infection by deterring others from walking in and out of the area and to provide privacy
- *Trolleys*: Those used for aseptic procedures must not be used for any other purpose. They should be cleaned daily with detergent and water and dried with paper towels and wiped with 70% isopropyl alcohol solution before use (CDC 2008)
- *Supplies*: Collect the requisite dressing pack, supplementary packs, lotions and any other items required, checking their expiry dates and for damage and sterility (see Box 15.16). Place all supplies on the bottom of the clean trolley
- *Patient*: Explain the procedure to the patient to obtain their consent and cooperation. Position the patient appropriately and comfortably so that the procedure can be performed easily.

Opening sterile packs and supplies and organizing the work surface

- Wash hands or disinfect clean hands with an alcohol-based hand rub
- Place the pack to be opened on the centre of the trolley top. The outside wrapping is not sterile and therefore it is important that the pack is opened correctly to prevent contamination of its contents. Open the inner wrapping,

handling the corners only: the opened area forms the 'sterile field'. Henceforth only sterile items can come in contact with this area. The open 'sterile field' must lie flat on the trolley top and never be flattened with the fingers

- Gently slide supplementary packs onto the sterile field ensuring that the outside wrappers do not touch the sterile field. If they do, consider the area contaminated
- Sterile lotions are poured slowly and directly into a gallipot. When pouring liquids the bottle must be positioned clear of the sterile field
- Before organizing the work surface, decontaminate hands again and wear sterile gloves (or use sterile forceps) throughout the procedure.

Maintaining a sterile working area during the procedure

- The area around the procedure site should be surrounded with sterile drapes
- Ensure that only sterile items come into contact with the susceptible site
- Do not allow sterile items to touch non-sterile objects; if in doubt about the sterility of an item or area, consider it contaminated.

Discarding supplies

- After completing the procedure, discard any used sharps immediately into a sharps container and then all waste into a clinical waste bag
- Discard protective clothing into the appropriate waste receptacle
- Wash hands to prevent cross-infection to others.

---

the source of the infection and to distinguish them from 'protective isolation', p. 358, the precautions which may be required for patients who are highly vulnerable to infection.

Principles of isolation nursing

The theory and practice of isolation nursing focus on interrupting the transmission route of microorganisms. Consideration is given to the following elements:

Patient accommodation

A key component of isolation is the appropriate placement of the patient. Some healthcare facilities have infectious disease or isolation units where patients are nursed in single rooms with en-suite facilities, controlled airflow systems and cared for by a team of specialist infection control practitioners. In the UK, there are several regional high-security units for treating patients with highly communicable infections, e.g. Lassa fever and Ebola fever.

In other healthcare facilities, patients are isolated in single rooms within a ward. These settings are less appropriate than isolation units due to the close proximity of other patients and the frequent contact that healthcare practitioners have with both infected and non-infected patients. When a single room is unavailable, patients with the same microorganism may share a room, a practice referred to as 'cohorting'.

Patient movement

A practice that impinges on isolation measures is moving isolation patients/clients between wards or other healthcare facilities. This practice interferes with measures to prevent, control and contain infection and should be avoided. If a patient has to be moved, then it is important that the receiving unit/ward is notified of their impending arrival and the infection control measures required (CDC 2011).

Psychological effects of isolation

It is important to safely deliver care to people who require to be nursed in isolation or protective isolation settings and also consider ethical issues relating to confidentiality when caring for people with infectious diseases. Whatever the degree of isolation, it can be a disturbing experience for the patient (Box 15.20). Many patients express feelings of loneliness, anxiety

and boredom when isolated and may also have higher levels depression, lowered self-esteem and sense of control which may be due to less frequent or shorter episodes of direct contact than with patients not in isolation (Abad et al 2010). In order to promote patients' well-being they need to be informed about their condition, its symptoms and treatment at the time of isolation and monitored closely for any adverse effects of isolation. Maintaining patient confidentiality is also an important concern in isolation nursing (Box 15.21).

 Ethical issues   **Box 15.21**

Maintaining confidentiality

Isolation procedures are necessary to reduce the risk of infection to healthcare personnel and other patients. However by their very nature, they may indicate the type of infection, resulting in a breach of patients' confidentiality.

Student activities

Read the NMC (2008) *Code* and Chapter 7. Then think about the questions below.

- Who has the right to know why a patient is in isolation?
- Consider whether the patient's right to confidentiality is more important than the right of others to protect themselves.
- Discuss your ideas with your mentor.

Categories of isolation

The three categories of isolation (transmission-based precautions) are:

- Airborne precautions
- Droplet precautions
- Contact precautions.

These precautions may be combined for diseases that have multiple routes of transmission, e.g. chickenpox which can be transmitted both by the airborne route and by direct contact with vesicle fluid or respiratory secretions.

Whether used alone or in combination, transmission-based precautions are always used in addition to standard infection control precautions. Extra care is also taken when handling equipment, sharp items, linen and waste.

Airborne precautions

Airborne precautions are necessary for infections transmitted by the inhalation of droplet nuclei, e.g. tuberculosis, measles, chickenpox, H1N1. Isolation (transmission-based) precautions are as follows:

- The patient is nursed in a single room that has a negative atmospheric pressure, i.e. the air flowing into the room is extracted to the outside of the building, not into other patient areas. The door must be kept closed for the air extraction system to operate effectively
- If a single room is not available, the patient may share a room with another patient who has the same infection
- People entering the room must wear masks unless they are known to be immune to the pathogen

---

 Reflective practice   **Box 15.20**

The impact of isolation

Susan is 20 years old and has a mild learning disability. She is admitted to hospital for investigations. Three days later she develops a fever and a vesicular skin rash. Suspecting that she may have contracted chickenpox and to prevent the transmission of the virus to others, Susan is isolated in one of the ward's single rooms.

Student activities

- Think about how Susan may feel.
- Consider how you would explain the reason for isolation nursing and the precautions needed to Susan.
- Think about how you could minimize the psychological effects of isolation.

- Movement of the patient from the room is limited to essential purposes only. On leaving the room the patient must wear a mask in order to protect others
- The patient is reminded to cover their mouth and nose when coughing or sneezing
- Gloves and plastic aprons are used when handling respiratory secretions
- Hands are washed before entering and after leaving the room.

Droplet precautions

Some infections are transmitted by contact with respiratory secretions and large droplets expelled during coughing and sneezing, e.g. mumps, diphtheria and whooping cough. These infections are also spread by direct contact with contaminated items in the patient's immediate environment. Isolation (transmission-based) precautions are as follows:

- Special air handling and ventilation are not required to prevent droplet transmission
- Patients are nursed in a single room (or in a room with another similarly infected patient)
- Masks are worn when working within 1–2 metres of the patient and used by patients if transportation is necessary (HPA 2008; HPA 2010b)

- Gloves and plastic aprons are used for contact with infective material
- Hands are washed before entering and after leaving the room.

Contact precautions

Infections are transmitted by direct contact with patients or by indirect contact with surfaces or equipment, e.g. MRSA, C. *difficile*, winter vomiting virus and some skin and respiratory infections. Isolation (transmission-based) precautions are as follows:

- A single room is preferable and essential when the source patient contaminates the environment or cannot assist in maintaining infection control precautions to limit the transmission of the infection, e.g. infants, children and some people with a learning disability or dementia
- Gloves and plastic aprons are worn for contact with infective material from the patient or their immediate environment
- Hands are washed on leaving the room (Box 15.22).

Protective isolation

This type of isolation is also known as 'reverse barrier nursing' or 'neutropenic isolation'. Certain patients are at increased risk

---

 Health promotion Box 15.22

Breaking the chain of infection using transmission-based precautions

Two young children in a paediatric unit start vomiting and have profuse diarrhoea. Suspecting that the condition may be infectious, both children are moved into a double room and contact isolation precautions initiated. The room has its own toilet facilities and supplies of hand soap, disposable gloves, paper towels, plastic aprons, yellow waste bags, a laundry bag and patient-care equipment. One nurse is assigned to care for both children and wears gloves and a disposable plastic apron when in contact with faeces and vomit, e.g. when changing soiled bed linen and assisting the children with personal hygiene. Following each care activity, the nurse removes her gloves and discards them directly into the waste receptacle and thoroughly washes her hands. The nurse applied principles of infection control to contain the infectious organism at many points in the chain of infection as shown below.

Link in the chain	Nursing action to break the chain
Infectious agent: Presently unknown. Could be *Salmonella, Shigella*, Norovirus, etc. Awaiting confirmation from the laboratory	Interrupted the microorganisms' transmission route by implementing contact isolation precautions
	Cohorted the two children with a similar infection in the same room with its own en-suite facilities
	Assignment of one nurse to care for the two children to reduce the risk of transmitting the infection to others in the unit
Reservoir: Gastrointestinal tract	The nurse was aware that the microorganisms could easily spread to other children by direct/indirect contact
Portal of exit: Diarrhoea	Faeces and vomit were discarded directly into the en-suite lavatory
Mode of transmission: Direct contact, especially via the hands of the children and healthcare personnel. Indirect contact with contaminated surfaces/equipment	The nurse wore gloves and disposable apron for all contact with body excretions and used proper handwashing techniques following removal of gloves and apron
	Linen was handled carefully and placed directly into the laundry bag
	Waste was discarded into a yellow waste bag
	Visitors were instructed to wash their hands before leaving the room
	All patient-care equipment was decontaminated before it was removed from the room
Portal of entry: Mouth	The nurse ensured that both children carefully washed and dried their hands following each episode of diarrhoea
	The nurse encouraged the children to refrain from putting fingers and objects into their mouths
Susceptible host	The infection was not transmitted to other children in the unit due to adherence to infection control measures.

of microbial infections from both endogenous and exogenous sources. This is due to compromised defences such as in severe burns, leukaemia, organ transplants, immunosuppressed states and radiation treatment. Premature infants are also highly susceptible to infection. Isolation (transmission-based) precautions are as follows:

- These patients are nursed in a total protected environment (TPE)
- TPE includes a private room (with shower and lavatory) where vented air entering the room is passed through high-efficiency particulate air (HEPA) filters. The room is under positive pressure to prevent corridor air from entering when the door is opened
- The room must be thoroughly cleaned and disinfected before the patient is admitted
- All items coming into contact with the patient are disinfected or sterilized beforehand
- People entering the room must wear appropriate PPE determined by local policies
- Although standard infection control precautions, e.g. hand hygiene and PPE, are necessary before patient contact, masks are rarely required
- No special precautions are required for the disposal of waste and linen.

Specimen collection

Many different specimens are collected from patients and used to diagnose or follow the progress of infectious diseases. The most common clinical specimens that nurses take for sending to the microbiology laboratory are listed in Box 15.23.

Specimens taken by nurses	Box 15.23
These commonly include: • Cervical and vaginal swabs • Conjunctival swabs • Faeces and rectal swabs • Nasal swabs • Pus from a wound or abscess • Sputum (see Ch. 17) • Throat swabs • Urine (see Ch. 20).	

It is important that the specimen is of the highest quality and collected safely:

- Whenever possible, specimens should be obtained before antimicrobial therapy begins. If this is not possible, the laboratory is informed of the antimicrobial agent(s) prescribed
- The most appropriate time to collect specimens is during the acute stage of a disease, i.e. when the patient is experiencing symptoms. Some viruses, however, are more easily isolated during the prodromal stage, or onset, of the disease (see Box 15.3, p. 342)

- Timing of the specimen is very important, e.g. urine specimens should reach the laboratory within 2 hours of collection (Wilson 2006). Sputum specimens need to be obtained before a patient uses an antiseptic mouthwash, which can adversely affect the results
- The specimen obtained must be representative of the infection, e.g. a patient with pneumonia must provide a specimen of sputum and not saliva
- Specimen collection should always be performed with care and tact to avoid harming the patient or causing discomfort or embarrassment
- If patients are to collect specimens themselves, e.g. sputum or urine, they need to be given clear and detailed collection instructions.

Collection of clinical specimens

When collecting clinical specimens for microbiology they must be collected in a manner that maintains the dignity of the patient and prevents their contamination with either the patient's/client's or healthcare professional's microorganisms. It is important therefore, that standard infection control precautions are implemented:

- Handwashing before and after the procedure
- Wearing PPE, i.e. gloves and aprons.

Sterile containers are always used for the collection of specimens (Fig. 15.10). Care needs to be taken to avoid contaminating the inside of the container or its lid when collecting the specimen, and to ensure that the outside of the container is not contaminated by the contents. The container's lid should be closed tightly to prevent leakage during transportation to the laboratory.

A sufficient quantity of material must be obtained to provide enough for all the diagnostic tests required. The specimen container is labelled and accompanied by a request form. As a minimum, labels should contain the patient's name, hospital identification number, ward number/name or the requesting doctor's name, the specimen type and the date and time of collection. The specimen container is placed in a double

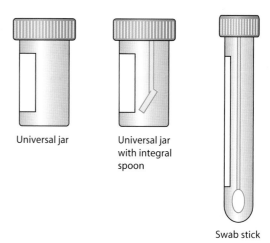

Universal jar

Universal jar with integral spoon

Swab stick

Fig. 15.10 • Examples of specimen containers.

self-sealing bag with one compartment containing the request form and the other the specimen.

When specimens are regarded as infection hazards, the specimen container and request form are labelled with biohazard labels.

Transport of specimens

Specimens should be delivered to the laboratory promptly so that the results accurately represent the number and types of organisms present at the time of collection. If delivery to the laboratory is delayed, the pathogens may die or any indigenous flora (non-pathogens) may overgrow, inhibit or kill the pathogens. If the specimen cannot be transported to the laboratory immediately then it may be refrigerated at 4°C (Prieto & Kilpatrick 2011). However, the refrigerator must be used for specimens only – it must not contain foods or medicines. Blood cultures are never refrigerated but stored at body temperature, in an incubator if necessary.

SUMMARY

- ◆ The range of infectious diseases changes rapidly and in recent years new diseases have emerged.
- ◆ Microorganisms can only survive when their growth conditions are favourable.
- ◆ Inappropriate use of antibacterial drugs increases bacterial mutation and development of resistant strains.
- ◆ A zero tolerance approach for all healthcare-associated infections, along with prevalence surveillance has demonstrated a reduction in the incidence of hospital acquired infections.
- ◆ Healthcare-associated infections are preventable but widespread.
- ◆ Standard infection control precautions are used when caring for patients/clients regardless of whether they have an infection or not.
- ◆ Effective handwashing is the single most important feature of infection control in healthcare settings.
- ◆ Education of all healthcare staff is of paramount importance in preventing the spread of infections and managing those who are affected.
- ◆ Nurses must keep abreast of current evidence and infection control policies and follow them consistently in nursing practice.

KEY WORDS AND PHRASES FOR LITERATURE SEARCHING

Asepsis

Cross-infection

Decontamination

Drug resistance

Handwashing

Infection control

Needlestick injuries

Patient isolation

Respiratory tract infections

Sterilization

Urinary tract infections

Workplace infection risks

 Useful websites

Centers for Disease Control and Prevention www.cdc.gov

Health Protection Agency www.hpa.org.uk/

Health Protection Scotland www.hps.scot.nhs.uk/

Health and Safety Executive www.hse.gov.uk

Infection Prevention Society www.ips.uk.net

National Electronic Library of Infection www.neli.org.uk/ IntegratedCRD.nsf/NeLI_Home1?OpenForm

National Institute for Health and Clinical Excellence (NICE) www.nice.org.uk

National Patient Safety Agency www.npsa.nhs.uk

World Health Organization www.who.int/en

All websites accessed September 2012.

References

Abad, C., Fearday, A., Safdar, N., 2010. Adverse effects of isolation in hospitalised patients: a systematic review. Journal of Hospital Infection 76, 97–102.

Burton, R.W., Engelkirk, P.G., 2007. Burton's microbiology for the health sciences, eighth ed. Lippincott, Williams & Wilkins, Philadelphia.

Centers for Disease Control and Prevention, 2008. Guidelines for disinfection and sterilization in health care facilities. Online. Available: www.cdc.gov/hicpac/pdf/ guidelines/Disinfection_Nov_2008.pdf September 2012.

Centers for Disease Control and Prevention, 2011. Guideline for the prevention and control of Norovirus gastroenteritis outbreaks in health care settings. Online. Available: www.cdc.gov/hicpac/pdf/ norovirus/Norovirus-Guideline-2011.pdf September 2012.

Department of Health, 2007. The third prevalence survey of healthcare associated infections in acute hospitals in England 2006. DH, London.

Department of Health, 2009. *Clostridium difficile* infection: How to deal with the problem. DH, London.

Department of Health, 2011. Safe management of healthcare waste. DH, London.

European Centre for Disease Prevention and Control, 2011. Rapid risk assessment: Potential resurgence of highly pathogenic H5N1 avian influenza. Online. Available: http://ecdc.europa.eu/en/publications/ Publications/1109_TER_risk_assessment_ H5N1_bird_flu_resurgence.pdf September 2012.

General Register Office, 2010. *Clostridium difficile* deaths. Online. Available: www. gro-scotland.gov.uk/statistics/theme/ vital-events/deaths/cdiff/index.html September 2012.

Gould, D., Brooker, C., 2008. Infection prevention and control: applied microbiology for healthcare, second revised ed. Palgrave Macmillan, Basingstoke.

Health and Safety Executive, 2002. The
Control of Substances Hazardous to Health
Regulations (COSHH). Online. Available:
www.legislation.gov.uk/uksi/2002/2677/
made/data.pdf September 2012.

Health Protection Agency, 2008. *Clostridium
difficile* infection: How to deal with the
problem. Online. Available: www.hpa.org.uk/
web/HPAwebFile/HPAweb_C/
1232006607827 September 2012.

Health Protection Agency, 2009. Information on
face masks and respirators. Online. Available:
www.hpa.org.uk/Topics/InfectiousDiseases/
InfectionsAZ/
SevereAcuteRespiratorySyndrome/
Guidelines/sars040Facemasksandrespirators
FAQ/ September 2012.

Health Protection Agency, 2010a. Healthcare-
associated infections and antimicrobial
resistance: 2009/10. HPA, London.

Health Protection Agency, 2010b. Introduction
to preventing infections in a care home
environment (DVD). Online. Available:
www.hpa.org.uk/carehomesdvd September
2012.

Health Protection Agency, 2011a. Summary
points on meticillin resistant *Staphylococcus
aureus* (MRSA) bacteraemia. HPA,
London.

Health Protection Agency, 2011b. Summary
points on *Clostridium difficile* infection
(CDI). HPA, London.

Health Protection Agency, 2011c. *Escherichia
coli* bacteraemia in England, Wales and
Northern Ireland, 2006–2010. HPA,
London.

Health Protection Scotland, 2007. NHS
Scotland National HAI Prevention Survey,
Volume 1. Online. Available: www.
documents.hps.scot.nhs.uk/hai/sshaip/
publications/national-prevalence-study/
report/full-report.pdf September 2012.

National Institute for Health and Clinical
Excellence, 2003. Infection control:
prevention of healthcare-associated
infections in primary and community care.
NICE, London.

NHS Executive, 1995. Health Service
Guidelines: Hospital laundry arrangements
for used and infected linen. NHS Executive,
London.

NHS Scotland, 2005. Needlestick injuries:
sharpen your awareness. Scottish Executive,
Edinburgh.

Nursing and Midwifery Council, 2008. The
code: standards for conduct, performance
and ethics for nurses and midwives. NMC,
London.

Nursing and Midwifery Council, 2010.
Standards for preregistration nursing
education: annexe 3 – essential skills
clusters. Online. Available: http://standards.
nmc-uk.org/Documents/Annexe3_
%20ESCs_16092010.pdf
October 2012.

Office for National Statistics, 2011. Deaths
involving *Clostridium difficile*: England and
Wales, 2006 to 2010. Online. Available:
www.ons.gov.uk/ons/rel/subnational-health2/
deaths-involving-clostridium-
difficile/2006-to-2010/statistical-
bulletin.html September 2012.

Pratt, R.J., Pellowe, C.M., Wilson, J.A., et al.,
2007. Epic 2 National evidence based
guidelines for preventing healthcare-
associated infections in NHS hospitals in
England. Journal of Hospital Infection 65
(Suppl 1), S1–S64.

Prieto, J., Kilpatrick, C., 2011. Infection
prevention and control. In: Brooker, C.,
Nicol, M., (Eds.), Alexander's nursing
practice, fourth ed. Churchill Livingstone,
Edinburgh.

Scottish Government, 2008. Independent
review of *Clostridium difficile* associated
disease at the Vale of Leven Hospital from
December 2007 to June 2008. Online.
Available: http://library.nhsggc.org.uk/
mediaAssets/C%20Diff%20Inquiry/
Independent%20review.pdf September
2012.

Tortora, G.J., Funke, B.R., Case, C.L., 2009.
Microbiology: an introduction, tenth ed.
Benjamin Cummings, San Francisco.

Weber, D.J., Rutala, W.A., Miller, M.B., et al.,
2010. Role of hospital surfaces in
transmission of emerging healthcare-
associated pathogens. In: Rutala, W.A., (Ed.),
Disinfection, sterilization, and antisepsis.
Association for Professionals in Infection
Control and Epidemiology Inc, Washington
DC.

Wilson, J., 2006. Infection control in clinical
practice, third ed. Baillière Tindall,
Edinburgh.

World Health Organization, 2004. Practical
guidelines for infection control in health care
facilities. WHO, Geneva.

World Health Organization, 2007. Infection
prevention and control of epidemic- and
pandemic-prone acute respiratory diseases in
health care. WHO, Geneva.

World Health Organization, 2009a. Strategic
Advisory Group of Experts on Immunization
– Report of the extraordinary meeting on
the influenza A (H1N1) 2009 pandemic.
Weekly Epidemiological Record 8430,
301–304.

World Health Organization, 2009b. WHO
Guidelines on hand hygiene in health care.
First global patient safety challenge clean
care is safer care. Online. Available: http://
whqlibdoc.who.int/publications/2009/
9789241597906_eng.pdf September 2012.

World Health Organization, 2009c. Infection
prevention and control in health care for
confirmed or suspected cases of pandemic
(H1N1) 2009 and influenza-like illnesses:
Interim guidance. Online. Available:
www.who.int/csr/resources/publications/
SwineInfluenza_infectioncontrol.pdf
September 2012.

World Health Organization, 2010. Global alert
and response: What is a pandemic? WHO,
Geneva.

World Health Organization, 2011a. World
Health Statistics. WHO, Geneva. Online.
Available: www.who.int/whosis/whostat/
EN_WHS2011_Full.pdf September 2012.

World Health Organization, 2011b. Global
Influenza Surveillance and Response System
(GISRS). Online. Available: www.who.int/
influenza/gisrs_laboratory/en September
2012.

Further reading

Brooker, C., Nicol, M., 2011. Alexander's
nursing practice, fourth ed. Churchill
Livingstone, Edinburgh.

Burton, R.W., Engelkirk, P.G., 2007. Burton's
microbiology for the health sciences, eighth
ed. Lippincott Williams and Wilkins,
Philadelphia.

NHS Quality Improvement Scotland, 2008.
Healthcare associated infection standards.
NHS QIS, Edinburgh.

Nicol, M., Bavin, C., Cronin, P., et al., 2012.
Essential nursing skills, fourth ed. Mosby,
Edinburgh.

Personal care, sensory impairment and unconsciousness

16

Anne Waugh

LEARNING OUTCOMES

This chapter will help you:

- Discuss the factors that may influence a person's appearance and personal hygiene
- Describe health-promoting activities that relate to aspects of personal care
- Outline the contribution of the *Essence of Care 2010* (Department of Health, DH 2010) in helping people with their personal hygiene
- Explain the nursing interventions that may be needed to assist a person with their personal care in a dignified and respectful manner
- Explain the nursing interventions that will assist communication with people with hearing and/or sight impairment
- State the first aid priorities for assessing a collapsed or unconscious casualty
- Describe the nursing interventions that may be used in caring for an unconscious patient
- Identify relevant sources of information for providing client education on topics included in this chapter.

Introduction

The first section of this chapter explores a range of activities involved in maintaining personal hygiene and appearance, and the factors that may affect them. These activities include many fundamental aspects of care, some of which are highlighted in the *Essence of Care 2010* (DH 2010), emphasizing that a working knowledge of these aspects of care is an important nursing role and also one in which a nurse can 'make a difference'. Sometimes the responsible registered nurse, who remains accountable for the care that clients or patients receive, may delegate these activities to others in the team. In other cases they may form part of a community care package provided to meet social needs or are carried out informally by carers for a relative. Appropriate nursing interventions are discussed to enable holistic assessment and planning when people

need help to maintain their personal hygiene and appearance. In each part of this chapter underpinning anatomy and physiology are briefly reviewed to provide the basis for assessing people's health status and recognizing the presence of abnormalities.

In the middle section, the senses of vision and hearing are outlined and nursing interventions that will help people with sight and hearing impairment in community and hospital settings are explained.

The final section considers unconsciousness and the related first aid interventions. The nursing care required by an unconscious person is then explored with the following aims:

- To introduce the idea that assessment and planning of integrated care for a person with substantial physical needs occurs by combining several fundamental nursing skills explained in this and other chapters of the book
- To show how a holistic, compassionate and person-centred approach to care is largely based on combining fundamental nursing interventions appropriately to meet individual needs.

Personal hygiene and appearance

In this section, factors affecting people's personal hygiene and appearance are considered and health promotion activities involving nurses are explored. When assistance is needed, maintaining dignity is paramount during nursing interventions. These are discussed using the evidence base, where available, and a range of activities to promote inquiry is included.

For most people, maintaining their appearance and personal hygiene is an important aspect of their daily routines that, once learned, is often taken for granted to a greater or lesser extent. Different activities are involved, including:

- Showering, bathing and washing
- Care of the hands, feet and nails
- Care of the eyes, ears and nose

- Hair care
- Facial hair care and shaving
- Dressing
- Maintaining dental health and oral hygiene.

Personal grooming extends to choosing the clothes worn, hair styling and the application of cosmetics and jewellery. The way in which a person chooses to present themselves to others is an integral part of their personal identity and sexuality.

Children and some adults may need temporary or ongoing assistance with some or all of the activities listed above. Personal hygiene is important for both health and social acceptability and, in most cultures, it is expected that people should be clean and odour free.

Attempts to improve fundamental aspects of care in all settings and for all patient groups saw the development and recent revision of the person-centred best practice statements in the *Essence of Care 2010* (DH 2010). Those relevant to nursing interventions discussed in this chapter include:

- Personal hygiene
- Principles of self-care
- Respect and dignity.

The best practice statements, or benchmarks, come with a resource pack to help healthcare professionals rate their practice against them. By identifying and then improving aspects of current practice nurses can work towards meeting these benchmarks. The best practice statements that relate to personal hygiene are shown in Box 16.1.

Best practice statements   Box 16.1

Personal hygiene

- 'People are assessed to identify the advice and/or care required to maintain and promote their personal hygiene
- People's care is planned, implemented, continuously evaluated and revised to meet needs and preferences
- All personal hygiene care and advice is given in an environment that is safe and appropriate to meet People's needs and preferences
- People have toiletries to meet their needs and preferences
- People receive the care and assistance they require to meet personal hygiene needs and preferences
- People and carers are provided with the knowledge and skills to meet personal hygiene needs and preferences'

(From DH 2010, p 8).

Structure and functions of the skin

The skin completely covers the body, providing a waterproof barrier between the external environment and underlying internal structures. It is self-renewing and self-repairing and consists of three layers (Fig. 16.1):

- The *epidermis* is constantly renewed as the deeper cells divide and migrate upwards in about 50–70 days before being shed as flat, keratinized cells from the skin surface.

- The *dermis* lies underneath the epidermis and consists of connective tissue. Structures found in this layer include blood and lymph vessels, nerve endings, sweat and sebaceous glands and hairs.
- The *subcutaneous layer* consists mainly of adipose tissue (fat) and varies in thickness. It provides insulation, cushions the underlying structures and acts as a long-term energy source.

Normal skin flora

Following birth, the skin surface becomes colonized by commensal bacteria which form the normal skin flora (see Ch. 15). They do not normally cause harm unless they gain entry to a part of the body normally protected by the nonspecific defence mechanisms or in someone who is susceptible to infection, e.g. when the immune system is compromised following cancer chemotherapy. In hospital, normal flora (commensal bacteria) are replaced by hospital strains that are more likely to be pathogenic (causing illness) and resistant to many antibiotics. This predisposes people to the development of hospital-acquired infection (HAI, see Ch. 15).

Appendages of the skin

These include hair and hair follicles, different types of glands and the nails. Sebaceous glands are present on most parts of the body and become much more active at puberty. They secrete an oily substance, called sebum, which keeps the hair soft and pliable and the skin supple. Sweat glands are also widely distributed throughout the skin and they secrete sweat that consists mainly of water and sodium chloride (salt). Secretion of sweat is increased when either environmental or body temperature is high and by sympathetic nerve stimulation. Excessive sweating leads to dehydration (see Ch. 19). Specialized sweat glands that become active at puberty are found in the axillae and anogenital region. They secrete sweat together with other substances as an odourless milky fluid. When normal skin flora act on this fluid, the result is a bad smell, sometimes referred to as 'body odour'.

Functions of the skin

Intact skin acts as a nonspecific defence mechanism by providing a waterproof physical barrier plus chemical (acid mantle) and biological barriers that together protect against microorganisms, chemicals and physical trauma.

Control of body temperature (Ch. 14) is an important function of the skin, with heat loss determined by the amount of blood circulating through its vast capillary network.

The skin is also a sensory organ with specialized receptors for touch, pain and temperature. Sensation is mediated by the nervous system (Fig. 16.2, Box 16.2) and provides important information about one's environment. It protects people from potentially dangerous situations, e.g. burns from very hot objects. The automatic response to touching something very hot is immediate withdrawal from the hot item. Children learn a great deal about keeping safe through cutaneous sensation.

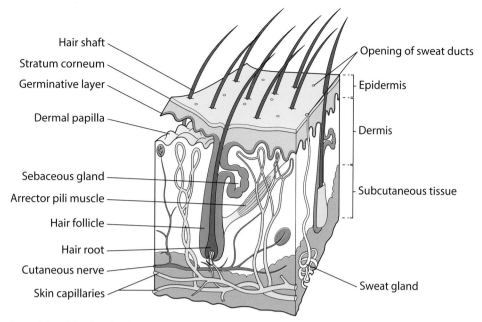

Fig. 16.1 • The structure of the skin showing its appendages. (Reproduced with permission from Waugh, A., Grant, A., 2010. Ross and Wilson anatomy and physiology in health and illness, eleventh ed. Churchill Livingstone, Edinburgh.)

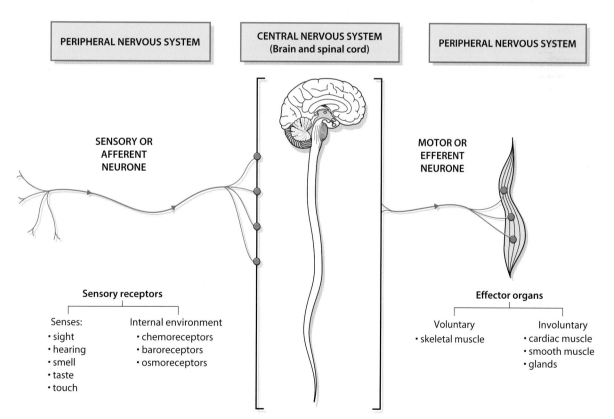

Fig. 16.2 • The functional components of the nervous system. (Based on Waugh, A., Grant, A., 2010. Ross and Wilson anatomy and physiology in health and illness, eleventh ed. Churchill Livingstone, Edinburgh.)

The nervous system — Box 16.2

The nervous system consists of two parts:

- The central nervous system comprising the brain and spinal cord
- The peripheral nervous system that includes all other nerves (see Fig. 16.2).

The nervous system controls and integrates body functions. Put simply, sensory receptors in the peripheral nervous system respond to stimuli either inside the body or in the external environment. This results in generation of nerve impulses that travel to the central nervous system via sensory nerves. After processing in the central nervous system, responses – again in the form of nerve impulses – are conducted through motor nerves to effector organs in the peripheral nervous system, i.e. muscles and glands. Responses may be either voluntary or involuntary.

For a detailed explanation of the nervous system you should refer to your anatomy and physiology textbook.

When something causes pain, they quickly learn not to repeat the behaviour. Impaired sensation puts people at risk from environmental hazards, e.g. stepping into a very hot bath causes scalds.

Limited absorption and excretion of certain substances takes place through the skin. Some drugs are absorbed through the skin, e.g. those contained in transdermal patches (Ch. 22).

Assessment of the skin

A person's skin condition contributes to their body image and the Western media encourages people to see healthy skin as an attractive attribute. A major threat to healthy skin is from overexposure to the sun either through occupational or leisure activities (Box 16.3). People who have skin conditions often consider themselves unattractive to others and suffer from low self-esteem.

Health promotion — Box 16.3

Preventing skin cancer

Skin cancer is usually the result of too much exposure to the sun. In the UK, rates are increasing as many people do not take the required precautions.

Risk factors

- Skin characteristics: burns easily, fair, freckled, many moles
- Previous skin cancer: oneself or a family member
- History of severe sunburn.

Advice

The SunSmart campaign (Cancer Research UK 2009) advises the following actions to reduce the risks:

Stay in the shade between 11.00 and 15.00 hours

Make sure you never burn

Always cover up: wear T-shirt, hat and sunglasses

Remember to take extra care with children

Then use sunscreen – factor 15 or above

Careful observation of a person's skin provides clues about body temperature, hydration and general health. This can be undertaken informally while speaking to them or while recording vital signs when the observant nurse will look at exposed body parts, e.g. the face and extremities. More information can be gained when clothes are removed, e.g. when assistance is needed with activities of living. Formal assessment is needed in some situations, e.g. to assess the risk of pressure ulcers (see Ch. 25) and when a person's primary problem is a skin disorder. The characteristics of normal skin are:

- Colour is normal for racial group
- Warm to touch
- Dry surface
- Intact surface.

Knowing the normal characteristics will alert the nurse to the need to report any abnormalities, e.g. redness, clammy skin, rashes, signs of scratching, that may be present. Conditions affecting the skin may need First Aid treatment e.g. burns and bites or stings (Box 16.4). Signs of scratching may indicate a parasitic infestation.

First aid — Box 16.4

Bites and stings

Animal and human bites

Any bite that breaks the skin poses an infection risk and medical treatment is required. Rabies, in countries where it is present, is a serious health risk.

Treatment

- Reassure the casualty
- Wash the bite wound(s) with soapy water and pat dry with clean gauze swabs
- Cover with a sterile dressing
- Elevate the affected area if possible to minimise swelling
- Arrange for medical review in all cases, and hospitalization if the wound is large or deep.

Insect stings

Bee and wasp stings are usually painful and accompanied by inflammation at the site but are not usually dangerous.

Treatment

- Reassure the casualty
- The sting, if present, can be removed by gently scraping the skin surface with the side of a fingernail. Tweezers should not be used as they may squeeze the sting and cause release of more poison into the site
- Elevate the affected part if possible and apply an ice pack for at least 10 minutes
- Monitor vital signs and observe for signs of allergy; e.g. wheezing, intense itching, pale skin and weak pulse; as anaphylaxis is a rare but very serious complication which requires immediate hospitalization.

Infestation

This is invasion by a parasite that lives on a host, e.g. head lice (pp. 375–376 and Box 16.16) and scabies (Box 16.5). Other infestations include body lice that are rare in developed

Scabies Box 16.5

Scabies is caused by a small parasitic mite *(Sarcoptes scabei)*, which is acquired from another person during close physical contact, e.g. prolonged hand holding or sexual intercourse. The female burrows along the epidermal layer of the skin, laying eggs and leaving faeces behind. Areas where the skin is thin, including the finger webs and ankles, are commonly affected. As adult mites develop, they feed and burrow, eventually through most areas of the skin, and chemicals in their excreta cause intense itching. The burrows can often be seen on the skin.

Treatment

- Application of pesticide lotions after bathing
- Laundering of clothes and bedding in a domestic washing machine

Itching can continue for some weeks until the outer layer of the skin is replaced although the mites will have been eradicated.

countries but sometimes found in rough sleepers who lack facilities for personal hygiene and washing clothes, and pubic lice, also known as 'crabs', which are spread by close contact such as sexual activity and can be recognized by their two large hind claws.

Factors influencing appearance and personal hygiene

Many factors that affect people's preferences and routines are considered below. Knowledge of these helps the nurse assess a person's needs so that holistic interventions can be planned and carried out when independence is not possible.

Physical

Many physical factors influence a person's independence in these activities, leaving them with limited ability to undertake some aspects of self-care through to complete dependence on others to meet their needs. These include frailty, impaired movement or inability to use a limb, unconsciousness, difficulty balancing for any length of time and sight impairment.

Consideration of general mobility will indicate whether assistance to get to the bathroom or the use of a hoist or other equipment is necessary (see Ch. 18). In care settings, equipment such as an intravenous (i.v.) infusion will reduce a person's independence in carrying out activities related to maintaining appearance and personal hygiene.

Breathless and debilitated people may be able to carry out some of the activities required but find trying to complete the whole process themselves exhausting.

If a person is in pain, this will affect both their motivation and ability to undertake or tolerate these interventions. When this is the case, it is important to assess their pain and provide analgesia beforehand.

Psychological factors

Most people feel clean and refreshed after a bath or shower. Someone who is depressed, debilitated or lethargic may not have the interest or energy to engage in maintaining their own appearance and hygiene. This may affect dressing and wearing clean, presentable clothes or extend to complete neglect of personal hygiene. The nurse may need to gently encourage these people to attend to their grooming (Box 16.6). This is also important in people with low self-esteem, low mood or altered body image.

Nursing skills Box 16.6

Strategies for encouraging personal hygiene

- Provide encouragement by ensuring warmth and privacy for showering or bathing
- Encourage participation by providing opportunity and choice in both buying and use of own toiletries, cosmetics and clothes
- Provide motivation by giving praise for improvements in appearance
- Act as a good role model by ensuring your own standards are appropriate
- Remember that if a person refuses to undertake personal hygiene activities, their wishes must be respected (NMC 2008).

Social, cultural and religious factors

Cultural and religious norms often influence individual practice (see NHS Education for Scotland 2006). Religious requirements may include personal hygiene activities, e.g. Hindus and Muslims require their hygiene needs to be met by nurses of the same sex. In Western cultures communal bathing or showering practices vary although in the UK separate facilities for men and women are usually provided, e.g. swimming pools, and nudity is considered offensive in many cultures.

Environmental factors

In Western countries, living accommodation normally includes an indoor lavatory and a fitted bath or shower. Access to and using the bath, shower and lavatory may require the installation of adaptations (see pp. 370–371).

Economic factors

When income is low, people may be unable to afford adequate heating for the bathroom or hot water for showering. Similarly, there may be little money to spend on basic hygiene items including soap, shampoo, toothbrush and toothpaste.

Lifespan factors

At particular stages of the lifespan there are characteristics affecting both independence in personal hygiene activities and the hygiene activities required.

Infancy

In infancy a parent/carer carries out bathing and personal hygiene. Infants do not produce sebum (p. 364) and therefore their skin is susceptible to maceration (softening of the skin caused by continual exposure to moisture) and this predisposes to nappy rash (Box 16.7).

Childhood

During childhood, independence in toileting, washing and dressing is usually established using significant others as role models, as physiological development and maturation of the body systems take place. Through socialization, children learn that personal hygiene is undertaken in privacy or only in the presence of close family members. However, not everyone achieves independence in these activities. For example, children with severe physical or (profound and multiple learning disabilities) may always be dependent, to some extent, on others.

Puberty

Puberty occurs during adolescence and is accompanied by physical and emotional changes that focus attention on personal grooming and hygiene. Increasing under-arm perspiration

develops, necessitating the use of a deodorant. Girls start to menstruate (p. 372) and in boys, there is growth of facial hair.

At this time, there is often experimenting with clothing, hairstyles, cosmetics and jewellery while striving to develop an individual personality and sexual identity. Standards of hygiene may change as development influences the young person's body image and perceptions of self (see Box 16.6, p. 367).

Older adults

In older adults, the physical changes of normal ageing influence appearance and personal hygiene routines. Age-related changes affecting the skin may impact on nursing interventions and include:

- Dryness
- Thinning, making it more easily traumatized
- Wrinkling
- Longer regeneration time.

To a greater or lesser extent, hair turns white as the colour pigment melanin is replaced by air. An older person may find they can no longer reach their toenails and may require help to cut them. Toenails become thicker and often grow abnormally, which may necessitate the services of a podiatrist. Gum disease, which frequently originates in childhood, can result in loss of teeth and the need to wear dentures (p. 379). Physical frailty can make getting into a bath both difficult and unsafe. When this is the case, or there is visual impairment or reduced dexterity, home adaptations and/or aids may be required (pp. 370–371).

Assisting with bathing, washing and showering

Nursing assessment identifies a person's usual routines and preferences in order to understand their habits (see Ch. 14). This includes the frequency, time of day and what the individual can do independently so that holistic and individualized care can be given as required.

When helping people with bathing and washing, it is important to recognize common nursing practices that may not be conducive to maintaining healthy skin, e.g. use of soap.

Assisting a person with their personal hygiene provides a good opportunity for communication. The nurse can identify not only their preferred hygiene practices but also all other aspects of their general well-being and progress. For a dependent person, activities related to personal hygiene can be used to preserve personal choice and individuality when this is not possible in many other aspects of their lives. When a person refuses to undertake any activity, including those concerned with personal hygiene, their wishes must be respected even if this causes the nurse frustration (Nursing and Midwifery Council, NMC 2008).

Maintaining privacy and dignity

It is important to remember the importance of privacy and dignity when considering any aspect of personal hygiene, whether assistance is needed or not. The *Essence of Care 2010*

Evidence-based practice Box 16.9

Skin care

The skin is afforded chemical protection by the acid mantle (p. 364) and has a protective lipid barrier that may be impaired by exposure to hot, cold or windy environments and the use of soap products or other irritants (Benbow 2010). It is often dry, especially in older people, and repeated washing further impairs this barrier.

The effects of conventional soap include:

- An alkaline pH that neutralizes the effects of the protective acid mantle
- Depletion of natural skin oils
- Dehydration (Jamieson et al 2007)
- Irritating constituents that cause allergies in some people. In particular, perfumes and alcohol can irritate the skin and, when these are constituents of wipes and other skincare products, they must be used with caution.

Emollients

These oil-based substances are applied to hydrate and soften dry skin. They act by reducing water loss through the skin surface and include:

- Soap substitutes that clean the skin but do not have the side-effects of conventional soap outlined above
- Ointments, which can be more effective than creams but are more greasy and may stain clothes and bed linen making them less acceptable
- Oils added to the bath that float on the surface or disperse as fine droplets; however, they make the bath surface slippery, constituting a potential hazard for those with mobility problems.

Barrier creams

These include creams, ointments and, more recently, barrier films that protect the skin from exposure to excessive water and irritants e.g. urine, faeces and wound exudate. They include chemicals that may irritate the skin and must also be used with caution.

Student activities

- Reflect on your placements so far and consider the extent to which skin care has been evidence based.
- Discuss your experiences with your mentor or a peer.

best practice statements (DH 2010) are shown in Box 16.8. These extend to client preference, and simple, thoughtful interventions such as ensuring bedside screens are completely closed and gowns meet at the back when mobilizing, will maintain people's privacy and dignity. New NHS modesty gowns are available to replace backless gowns; these are cotton T-shirts with poppers up each side that enable quick and easy access for interventions when needed. When assisting people to carry out activities involved in maintaining personal hygiene it is important to remember that they are likely to feel embarrassed and helpless.

Washing and drying the skin

The skin is usually cleaned by washing with soap, or soap substitute, then rinsed and gently patted dry, with particular attention to skin folds and crevices, e.g. under the breasts and between the buttocks. Gentle patting causes less friction than rubbing and reduces skin flora and skin infection (Jamieson et al 2007). If moisture remains in skinfolds, either through sweating or inadequate drying, irritation and breaks in the skin can develop. This is known as intertrigo. Nursing practices need careful thought to ensure they do not worsen dry skin which is a common problem, especially in older people (Box 16.9).

Skin conditions can be painful and people with skin disorders may use prescribed preparations for washing. These people may also feel particularly self-consciousness if they need help with washing because skin problems can affect self-esteem and body image (see Chs 8, 11, 12 and 21). Children may experience additional problems with peer acceptance.

Bathing and showering

A shower is more compact than a bath. It requires less water and is therefore more economical and environmentally friendly. Skin debris is rinsed away more easily by showering than bathing and, for this reason, Muslims and Hindus use running water for washing whenever possible.

Sometimes, people need the nurse's guidance about how they can have a bath, e.g. waterproof covers are available for plaster casts or a limb can be covered in polythene to keep a wound dry while bathing. Planning is important when assisting patients to ensure:

- All equipment needed is assembled
- Appropriate intervention is provided
- Privacy, dignity and respect are maintained
- Heat loss is minimized
- Safety is maintained (Box 16.10).

Bathing, washing and showering is tailored according to individual needs and preferences. When assistance is needed, timing may require planning to fit in with other scheduled treatment or therapies. The timing of analgesia, when needed, should ensure effective pain relief during these activities. People should have their own toiletries and follow their preferred routines where possible (see Box 16.1, p. 364). Before

Health promotion — Box 16.10

Safety in the bathroom

To prevent scalding

- Water temperature should not exceed 43°C (Jamieson et al 2007) and is checked before a person is assisted into a bath or shower.

To prevent slips or falls on wet surfaces

(involving the physiotherapist and occupational therapist as required):

- Assess the person's ability to get into and out of the bath or shower independently
- Assess the person's ability to bathe or shower independently
- A non-slip mat should be used in the bath or shower
- A clean, absorbent bath mat should be used when stepping out of a bath or shower
- Dry wet floors promptly.

To call for help when required

- Leave a call button nearby when a person is left alone.

Note: People with a history of seizures must not be left alone in the bath.

Nursing skills — Box 16.11

Principles of bathing infants and children

- Ensure the bathroom is warm and draught free
- An infant should be held securely with their head supported on the nurse's arm or hand during bathing (Fig. 16.3) and the free hand used for washing and rinsing
- Infants quickly lose heat and heat loss is minimized by avoiding prolonged exposure during bathing
- Water temperature must be carefully checked, either by dipping your elbow into it or using a lotions thermometer, to prevent scalds
- A non-slip mat is used in the bath or shower to prevent slips and falls
- Infants and young children must never be left unsupervised in the bathroom to prevent accidental drowning
- Bathtime is usually a 'fun time' to be enjoyed by both children and carers
- School-age children may need encouragement to take a bath or shower
- Children often dislike having their hair washed as they hate having shampoo suds in their eyes. This can be avoided by providing them with a folded flannel to cover their eyes during hairwashing.

taking someone to the bathroom, the nurse should check it is vacant, clean and warm and provide the opportunity for the person to use the lavatory. A mechanical hoist or other equipment may be needed to transfer a person to the bathroom or into the bath (see Chs 13, 18). Safety in the bathroom is an essential nursing consideration and measures taken to prevent accidental slips or falls are shown in Box 16.10. Principles of bathing infants and children are outlined in Box 16.11. A towel is wrapped round the person on leaving the bath or shower to keep them warm and maintain their dignity.

After bathing or showering, other aspects of personal care are carried out, including the use of talc, deodorant and moisturizer if desired; oral hygiene; shaving and styling the hair. Many women apply cosmetics to complete their appearance.

The bath or shower is then thoroughly cleaned according to local policy and left tidy for the next person.

Bathing aids

Bathing aids are often used in care settings and home adaptations can also be provided to enable people to remain independent at home (Fig. 16.4). Home assessment is carried out by an occupational therapist and suitable aids identified. Grab rails can be fitted to the walls to assist people getting into and out of the bath; electric bath lifts lower a person into the bath and raise them up again when required. Hoists can be provided at home although assistance from a carer is needed to use this. A shower with a seat can also be installed for people who find standing difficult.

Bedbathing

A bed bath is needed to maintain personal hygiene when a person is unable to use the bath or shower or is confined to bed. These people are usually quite dependent and may also be unconscious or confused.

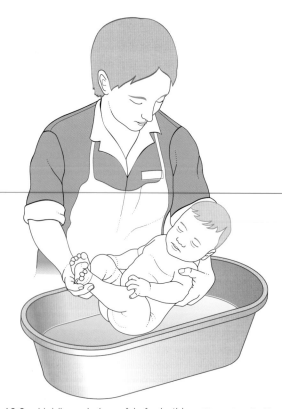

Fig. 16.3 • Holding a baby safely for bathing. (Reproduced with permission from Trigg, E., Mohammed, T.A. (Eds.), 2010. Practices in children's nursing: guidelines for hospital and the community, third ed. Churchill Livingstone, Edinburgh.)

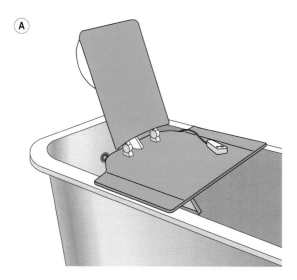

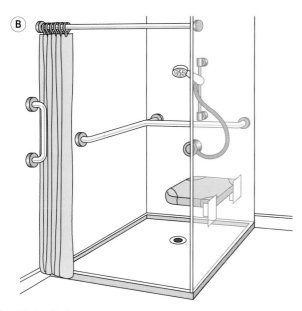

Fig. 16.4 • Bathroom adaptations: (A) Electric bath lift. (B) Accessible shower.

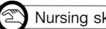

Nursing skills   Box 16.12

Principles of giving a bedbath

- Explain to the person what you are going to do and gain their consent to carry out the bedbath
- Follow local infection control policies for handwashing, disposal of laundry, etc.
- Clear the bed area to make space for equipment needed
- Assemble all equipment so the bedbath can be completed without interruption
- Screen the bed space or close the door to provide privacy and avoid embarrassment
- Offer the opportunity to use a bedpan or commode before starting, to promote comfort
- Use the bedbath as an opportunity for communication, to observe the condition of the skin and to assess general progress and well-being
- Assist the person to remove their nightclothes and cover them with a sheet or blanket to preserve their warmth, modesty and dignity
- If two nurses are present, one washes and rinses the skin and the other dries and applies toiletries according to the person's routine and preference
- The face is usually washed first – ask if soap is used for this. Where appropriate, independence can be encouraged by asking the person if they would prefer to do this themselves
- A second facecloth or disposable cloth is used for the rest of the body (see below for washing perineal area)
- Expose only the part being washed at any time to reduce heat loss and maintain dignity
- The further limb is washed first so that the second nurse can dry the limb nearer to them as the second limb is being washed. This also prevents splashing of the clean, dry limb while the second one is being washed. The extremities can be immersed and then washed in the bowl
- The perineal area is washed using a disposable cloth from the front backwards to prevent cross-infection from the anal area (Fig. 16.5). After the area is dried, the water is changed and used cloths discarded
- The back is usually washed last. It is important to remember to wash between the buttocks and gently wash the perianal area
- When the person is confined to bed, wet or soiled sheets are changed
- Assist the person into clean bedclothes
- A person confined to bed is then given assistance as required to carry out their other hygiene routines including shaving, cleaning their teeth, hair styling, nail care, etc. These are all much easier when the person is able to sit upright
- Ensure the person is comfortable and has their call bell, drinks, etc. within reach before leaving the area
- Ensure that all equipment is cleaned or disposed of according to local policy.

This affords the opportunity for a period of one-to-one communication. The patient should be encouraged to participate as much as their condition allows. Choice of nightclothes and use of a person's own toiletries will enable a person confined to bed to have some involvement in their care. The principles of bedbathing are outlined in Box 16.12. When the bed bath is complete, other aspects of personal care are carried out, including oral hygiene, shaving and hair styling.

Perineal care

When possible, the patient should be offered the opportunity to carry out personal perineal care themselves. This is often referred to as 'washing between the legs' or 'down there'. Many nurses find carrying out perineal care embarrassing, especially when caring for people of the opposite sex. A dignified and professional attitude will help to put both the nurse and patient at ease. The nurse must also consider cultural needs, e.g.

Muslims wash their genitalia in running water after passing urine or faeces. Nurses can provide a jug of water for washing if the person is confined to bed.

Microorganisms normally resident in the bowel are the most common cause of bladder infection (cystitis). This condition is more common in females whose urethra is shorter and therefore more easily reached by ascending microorganisms

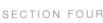
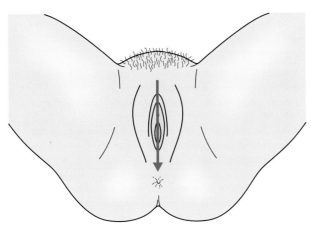

Fig. 16.5 • The perineal area: washing from front to back.

(see Ch. 20) and for this reason, the perineal area is washed from front to back (see Box 16.12 and Fig. 16.5).

Normally, in the male infant the preputial space is incompletely developed, causing the foreskin or prepuce to be adherent to the glans penis. As it is not easily retracted, phimosis (tight foreskin) is normal in early infancy. Through normal development and erections these early adhesions gradually disappear, and the foreskin separates. The foreskin softens and becomes retractable by 2 years of age. Attempts to retract the foreskin for washing, etc. before this age must be avoided. However, in uncircumcised men and older male children, the foreskin is carefully retracted and the glans gently washed and dried before the foreskin is repositioned.

Menstrual hygiene

Menstruation occurs in women between the menarche (first menstruation) during puberty and the menopause (cessation of menstruation). In most women, menstrual periods last around a week and occur about every 28 days. During menstruation, there is vaginal blood loss that can be heavy to begin with and then reduces. A supply of sanitary pads or tampons is required to absorb menstrual loss. This may need to be provided in care settings, together with handwashing facilities for dependent people. In Western society, managing menstruation is a private, personal activity that is generally a taboo subject.

Effective preparation for puberty includes education about the menstrual cycle, explaining that menstrual blood loss is normal, and providing the opportunity to practice using sanitary protection occasionally. Clients with learning disabilities may be unable to manage menstruation independently and some may refuse to wear sanitary protection.

Care of the feet, hands and nails

Assessment of the feet is important because problems can often be treated if detected early; without treatment, mobility can become severely restricted. Older people should always be asked if they are able to cut their own toenails as many have difficulty reaching them. The effects of ageing on the feet include thickening of the nails and development of calluses and hard skin.

Local policies must always be consulted before trimming nails, because some people are always referred to a podiatrist (healthcare professional responsible for managing conditions affecting the feet and/or lower limb) for treatment and cutting of their toenails. 'At-risk' people include those with diabetes mellitus (usually known as diabetes) and poor circulation caused by peripheral vascular disease. It is important that people with diabetes are taught how to look after their feet properly to prevent even minor damage that can progress to serious complications, including gangrene (Box 16.13).

◍ Health promotion   **Box 16.13**

Foot care for people with diabetes mellitus

The following care will protect your feet from damage and ensure you identify any problems that occur promptly:

- Wash and carefully dry your feet every day, paying attention to the areas between the toes.
- Inspect your feet when drying them, looking for:
  - Cuts or sores
  - Changes in colour e.g. blackening, blueness, redness, whiteness of part or all of foot
  - Swelling, warmth, pain, cracks or bleeding
  - Report any ulcers, corns, calluses, blisters, ingrowing toenails or other problems to your foot care specialist (podiatrist)
  - Do not cut your toenails with scissors
  - Visit your podiatrist for regular checks at recommended intervals, usually between 1- and 6-monthly, and when toenails require cutting
  - Never walk around barefoot, to avoid even minor injury
  - Ensure your shoes are spacious and well fitting to reduce the risk of corns and calluses developing.

(Based on National Institute for Health and Clinical Excellence 2004).

Care of the nails is best carried out after a bath or shower; alternatively, the hands or feet can be soaked in a bowl of warm water for 15 minutes to allow the nails to soften. A nailbrush can be used to remove obvious matter. The area under the nails is carefully cleaned using an orange-stick or nail file before the hands or feet are dried thoroughly. After drying, the cuticle is gently pushed backwards to prevent it growing over the nail.

Toenails are cut straight across with scissors or clipped using nail clippers. If difficulty is encountered because they are tough, the person should be referred to a podiatrist. Fingernails are usually trimmed using scissors and then filed to the shape of the finger with an emery board. Hand cream and nail varnish are then applied if wished.

Care of the eyes

Anatomy and physiology of the eye is reviewed on pages 380–382 but the importance of the accessory structures of the eye is considered here in order to understand eye care. This may also include care of spectacles, contact lenses or an artificial eye.

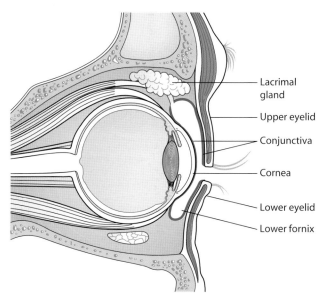

Fig. 16.6 • Accessory structures of the eye. (Reproduced with permission from Waugh, A., Grant, A., 2010. Ross and Wilson anatomy and physiology in health and illness, eleventh ed. Churchill Livingstone, Edinburgh.)

Labels in figure:
- Lacrimal gland
- Upper eyelid
- Conjunctiva
- Cornea
- Lower eyelid
- Lower fornix

Nursing skills   Box 16.14

Principles of eye care

- Prepare the patient by explaining what you are about to do
- Follow local infection control protocols, e.g. handwashing
- Always use a new sterile eye care pack
- The patient should sit or lie down with their head tilted backwards
- Ask the patient to close their eyes
- If there is an infected eye, clean the non-infected eye first
- Gently swab the lower eyelid with a lint-free swab, lightly moistened with sterile sodium chloride 0.9% from the inner canthus outwards
- Take care to ensure the swab does not rise above the lid margin opening the eye as corneal damage may occur
- Use each swab only once
- Repeat swabbing until all the crusting has gone
- Dry away excess solution with a dry swab
- Prescribed medication may then be instilled into the eyes (see Ch. 22)
- Wash your hands.

Accessory structures of the eye

These include the eyebrows, eyelids and eyelashes (Fig. 16.6). Together they protect the delicate structures at the front of the eye, especially the cornea, from sweat, dust and other foreign bodies. For example, when a speck of dust enters the eye, copious amounts of tears are produced and the eye waters profusely in an attempt to wash it away. The conjunctiva is a delicate membrane that protects the cornea and also lines the eyelids.

Tears are continually produced by the lacrimal glands and spread across the cornea during blinking, lubricating it and keeping it moist. They contain an antibacterial enzyme, lysozyme, which protects the eye from infection and drains away through a duct into the nose. The areas where the upper and lower eyelids join are known as the medial (inner) canthus and lateral (outer) canthus.

Eye care

Ensuring the eyes are clean and free from crusting is part of any general hygiene routine and is normally accomplished when washing one's face. Secretion of tears and blinking keep the eyes clean and moist while awake. Unconscious people are at risk from damage to the cornea because the blink reflex is lost and their eyes are therefore kept closed (see p. 392).

Eye care is required is some situations, e.g. presence of discharge. Sometimes it is an aseptic procedure (see Ch. 15) carried out by trained staff for people who have had surgery or trauma to the eye. In other situations, it is a clean procedure (see Ch. 15) (Box 16.14).

Spectacles

Spectacle lenses are made from glass or plastic material and should be kept clean using the cloth provided. They can be washed in soapy water and gently dried using a soft cloth to prevent scratching. They should be stored in their case (labelled with the person's name in care settings) to protect them from scratching and to minimize risk of physical damage when not in use.

Glass lenses are relatively heavy although lighter lenses made from shatterproof material are safer, especially when people are in situations where an object may hit their eyes. Irrespective of the type of lenses, spectacles should be checked for comfort and fit by checking the sides and bridge of the nose and the back of the ears for signs of soreness. A person may have different pairs of glasses for reading and watching TV, and care should be taken to ensure the correct pair is in use.

Contact lenses

Contact lenses are thin transparent discs inserted onto the cornea to correct refractive errors of the eye. They float on a layer of tears and can be hard, soft or gas permeable. The solutions required for the care of the different types of lenses vary and are used according to the manufacturer's instructions. Each lens is kept in a separate labelled container as the two lenses may have different prescriptions. Using disposable contact lenses eliminates the need for cleaning and storage.

Handwashing before insertion or removal is essential to minimize the risk of infection or introduction of foreign bodies that will cause inflammation of the conjunctiva (conjunctivitis) or corneal ulcers. Contact lenses are normally removed at night and should not be used when a person is receiving ophthalmic (eye) medication.

Artificial eyes

An artificial eye, or ocular prosthesis, is required after removal of an eyeball e.g. following trauma or removal of a tumour.

People usually prefer to carry out care needed themselves. If assistance is needed, advice from the nurse specialist or ophthalmology department should be sought.

Care of the ears

In order to carry out safe care of the ears it is necessary to be familiar with two important structures: the external auditory (or acoustic) canal and the eardrum (tympanic membrane) (see Fig. 16.12). (Anatomy and physiology of the ear and hearing is outlined on page 384.)

It is important to wash the skin covering the external ear as part of bathing or showering. Children often forget to wash behind their ears (Trigg & Mohammed 2010). The ears should be cleaned daily by gentle insertion of the corner of a moist flannel and rotating it into the external auditory canal. Nothing else should ever be inserted into the ear (except a tympanic thermometer or an otoscope). Cotton buds and other objects should not be used to try to remove wax because they can push it further into the external auditory canal and also damage the eardrum (Harkin 2011). Hearing impairment may occur when there is build up of wax in the external auditory canal. Excess wax can be removed by irrigation (previously called syringing), a procedure that requires specific training. Any discharge from the ear is abnormal and should be reported immediately.

Young children are prone to putting small items into their ears. A foreign body can cause deafness when the external auditory canal is blocked and may also damage the eardrum. Foreign bodies in the ear are most common in children but they also occur in adults, especially those who unadvisedly use cotton buds or other objects to remove earwax. The first aid interventions required should this occur are:

- Do not attempt to remove the foreign body unless it is a live insect, which can sometimes be removed by gently pouring tepid water into the casualty's ear
- Reassure the casualty and stay calm
- Organize transfer to hospital.

Hearing aids

Action on Hearing Loss (formerly RNID (The Royal National Institute for Deaf People), 2012a) estimates that 1 in 10 adults in the United Kingdom (that is 4 million people) would benefit from using a hearing aid. However, only 1 person in 30 does.

Adapting to using a hearing aid takes time and initially, it is worn for short periods that are gradually increased. Hearing aids are described as analogue or digital, depending on the technology they use. Digital hearing aids process sounds better than analogue hearing aids. The NHS provides, repairs and replaces certain hearing aids free of charge, although some people choose to buy their own.

Hearing aids are battery operated and are worn in or around the ear. They amplify sounds but do not restore natural hearing. There are three main designs: body-worn, behind-the-ear and in-the-ear.

Body-worn aids have a small box that can be clipped to clothing. People with severe hearing impairment often use

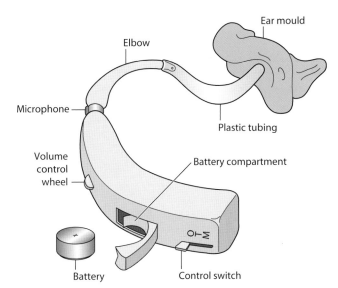

Fig. 16.7 • Behind-the-ear hearing aid. (Reproduced with permission from Gates, B. (Ed.), 2007. Learning disabilities: Towards inclusion, fifth ed. Churchill Livingstone, Edinburgh.)

these as they provide the most powerful amplification. They are also widely used by people who also have poor vision and those who find using the controls of behind-the-ear models difficult. In-the-ear aids are not suitable for people with severe hearing loss. The behind-the-ear aid is the most commonly used (Fig. 16.7). They have a small control switch with letters that mean:

O = aid is turned off

M = microphone is on and will amplify sound

T = induction loop, used to pick up radio signals without interference of background noise when an induction loop system is installed (see p. 387).

The microphone detects sound and must be kept clean and dry. The volume control wheel can be adjusted to suit different environments although this requires reasonable manual dexterity. The battery compartment opens, allowing the small battery to be changed. These should be kept out of children's reach as they can swallow them or poke them into their ears or nose. The plastic tubing transmits sound to the ear mould that is specially made for the wearer and should fit snugly. The plastic tubing and ear mould are wiped with a tissue after use. They are disconnected from the elbow and washed in soapy water and dried at least weekly. The plastic tubing needs to be replaced every few months.

Care of the nose

The nose does not normally require special care. Gentle blowing into a tissue removes excess secretions and debris. The use and prompt disposal of tissues is encouraged in care settings to reduce the risks of cross-infection. Harsh blowing should be avoided as it can cause damage to the eardrum and nasal mucosa. When there is a tube situated in the nose, for example a nasogastric tube, there may be accumulation of secretions that can be gently removed using moist swabs or cotton buds.

Children are prone to inserting small objects into their noses causing pain, trauma, blockage and, some days later, infection. The first aid interventions are:

- Do not try to remove the object as it may be pushed further into the nose, worsening any damage
- Reassure the casualty and stay calm
- Encourage the casualty to breathe normally through the mouth
- Organize transfer to hospital for safe removal of the foreign body.

Hair care

The appearance of a person's hair contributes to their self-esteem, personal identity and sexuality. It also provides an indicator of their well-being and is usually clean and shiny. When tangled, dull or unkempt, this suggests low self-esteem, low mood or that the person is physically unable to carry out hair care independently.

Most people style their hair using a brush or comb, at least daily. Fine-toothed combs are suitable for short hair; broader toothed ones are better for people with long or curly hair. People with impaired movement of the shoulders or poor handgrip find hairbrushes or combs with large handles easier to use. Brushing keeps the hair clean by removing dead epithelial cells and dust from the scalp and hair.

Haircutting is usually carried out at regular intervals and its style contributes to a person's individual and cultural identity. This aspect of personal hygiene is one of the least private and is normally carried out communally at a hairdressing salon. For people unable to get out, arranging for a hairdresser to visit them at home or in a care setting often provides a psychological boost. Hair cutting must never be undertaken without consent of the person involved because some people never cut their hair for religious or cultural reasons, e.g. Sikhs and Rastafarians. Nurses should be aware of the religious and cultural hair care needs of people in their care. Examples of these are outlined in Box 16.15.

Hairwashing

Hairwashing frequency varies considerably between individuals; younger people commonly wash their hair daily although many others wash their hair less often. Without washing, the hair becomes greasy as dried sweat and sebum accumulate.

Hairwashing can be carried out as a separate activity or during showering or bathing. Debilitated people often appreciate help with this at a sink in the bathroom. Helping someone style their hair provides a good opportunity for one-to-one communication and improves their self-esteem. It is important to include the person in decisions about styling when possible to avoid unwanted or inappropriate consequences. Chemotherapy and radiotherapy often cause alopecia (hair loss) and people receiving these treatments are given individual advice about hair care. When hairwashing with shampoo and water is not possible or practical, dry shampoo can be used instead.

Hair care – cultural and religious needs Box 16.15

People of certain faiths keep their hair covered, including:

- Muslim women
- Jewish orthodox women
- Sikh men wear turbans and some Sikh women will also cover their hair.

Moreover, in Sikhism, two of the *Symbols of faith* (the '5 Ks') are to do with the hair:

- *Kesh:* The hair of both sexes is left uncut and worn in a bun (jura)
- *Kangha:* The bun is held in place by a comb known as the kangha. The kangha is of major significance and people will want to wear it or have it with them at all times.

(*Note*: the other *Symbols of faith* for Sikhs are the *kara* (steel bangle), the *kirpan* (symbolic dagger) and the *kaccha* (shorts/underpants).

African-Caribbean people tend to have brittle, crinkly hair and use wide-toothed combs to reduce discomfort and breaking. Pomade is an oil-based product used to enhance shine and smoothness of this type of hair. It is rubbed into the hands and then applied to the hair and scalp. Damp hair may be braided or pleated, but loosely because it tightens as it dries.

Hairwashing can also be carried out in people confined to bed (see Nicol et al 2012).

Head lice

The presence of head lice *(Pediculus capitis)* is also known as pediculosis but, importantly, the presence of nits (the empty cases that remain stuck to the hair after the eggs have hatched) does not indicate current infestation.

Eggs, commonly known as nits, are laid by adult females and firmly cemented to hair shafts near the scalp. The eggs hatch after 7–10 days, mature in 6–14 days and adult insects live for about 1 month. Adult lice are 2–4 mm long (about the size of a sesame seed) and found in the hair with peak prevalence in children between the ages of 4 and 11 years. They are usually found behind the ears and round the hairline. Infestation is often accompanied by intense itching of the scalp and scratching can cause secondary infection.

Fortunately, head lice do not transmit disease to people but their presence causes considerable stigma and social distress. This is compounded by widespread myths and misconceptions about the means of spread and treatment. They affect people from all socioeconomic groups and show no preference between clean or dirty hair. Head lice cannot swim, jump or fly. People who have been in close contact with an infested person should be identified and treated if lice are found. They are spread by direct contact with an infested person and cannot survive for long away from the host. There is no conclusive evidence to support the commonly held belief that spread occurs through sharing of combs, hats and pillows (NHS Clinical Knowledge Summaries 2011). Treatments are summarized in Box 16.16. Continued presence of head lice after any treatment may be the result of non-compliance with or incorrect use of treatment, or reinfestation.

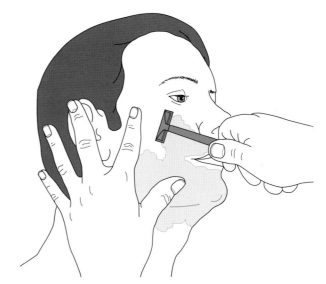

Evidence-based practice   Box 16.16

Treatment of head lice

Treatment can be chemical or mechanical.

1. Chemical treatment involves the use of pesticides or herbal preparations applied to the hair and scalp. There is widespread resistance to some pesticides, whose use is therefore ineffective, and so treatment options require:
   * Consultation of local policies
   * Discussion with a health professional or pharmacist for community settings.

   After chemical treatment, the hair is carefully combed using a fine-toothed comb to remove remaining lice and nits. Two treatments are used 7 days apart.

2. 'Bug busting' is a mechanical treatment using a fine-toothed detection comb to remove head lice from wet hair after conditioner has been liberally applied. This is repeated every 4 days for at least 2 weeks.

Increasing concern about the effects of pesticides, especially on children, is encouraging research into the effectiveness of different treatments. However, all treatments have advantages and disadvantages (NHS Clinical Knowledge Summaries 2011).

Resource

NHS Choices Birth to five. Head lice. Online. Available: www.nhs.uk/planners/birthtofive/pages/headlice.aspx September 2012.

(Adapted from NHS Clinical Knowledge Summaries 2011).

Fig. 16.8 • Shaving. (Reproduced with permission from Nicol, M., Bavin, C., Cronin, P., et al., 2012. Essential nursing skills, fourth ed. Mosby, Edinburgh.)

Care of facial hair

A moustache and beard need daily grooming. Electric trimmers can be used when requested but trimming or removal should never be undertaken without the person's permission as any facial hair may have personal, cultural or religious significance. In frail or debilitated people, gentle wiping or washing after meals easily removes any food debris.

Shaving is best carried out after bathing when the skin is softer. It forms part of many men's daily hygiene routines and being unshaven makes many feel unclean. An unkempt appearance can quickly develop, especially in the eyes of people's relatives.

Many men use an electric shaver, which is a safe, convenient method that is encouraged in those people who are prone to bleeding because they are taking anticoagulant medication or have a clotting disorder. Electric shavers are never shared because of the risk of cross-infection.

Wet shaving is other men's personal preference. When assistance is required, the person's usual routine should be followed. The face is washed and shaving cream applied and worked gently into the skin until lather is formed. Shaving is carried out using small, firm strokes of the razor in the direction of hair growth over taut skin and the razor is rinsed frequently. People often make facial movements that tighten their skin during shaving to provide a closer shave. The face is usually shaved before the neck. Assistance if needed can be provided by the nurse (Fig. 16.8). Any moles or other lesions should be avoided. After shaving, the face is washed thoroughly. Shaving

and the use of aftershave contribute to men's personal identity and sexuality.

Some women have more facial hair than others. Excessive facial hair can result from drugs, some endocrine conditions or reduced oestrogen secretion after the menopause. Facial hair in women can be removed either with appropriate depilatory creams or waxing, or disguised using bleaching agents. On no account should it be plucked or shaved unless this is what the woman usually does. Permanent removal, using electrolysis, is sometimes undertaken.

Dressing

The clothes people wear often reflect their traditions and culture. There are cultural differences in acceptable modesty, especially regarding women who may be expected to wear skirts, cover their legs or cover their faces. Some Muslim women are traditionally clothed from head to foot. Clothes also reflect one's mood and communicate individuality.

Contemporary clothing is normally made from material that can be easily laundered. The type of clothes worn also depends on the context – working clothes often differ from those worn on informal social occasions. Formal social occasions, such as weddings and funerals, often have specific dress codes.

The type and amount of clothes in a person's wardrobe is largely determined by their personal income but also by their hobbies and interest in appearance.

When deciding what to wear, the type of activities to be undertaken and ambient temperature need to be considered. In a cold environment, several thin layers provide more insulation and therefore warmth than one thick layer. This has the additional advantage of allowing the wearer to take off one layer at a time as the temperature increases. In hot environments, thin, pale-coloured clothes made from natural fibres are often preferred because they reflect light and absorb more sweat than synthetic materials. In some situations, special clothing is required to maintain health and safety, e.g.

UK law requires that crash helmets be worn when riding motorcycles.

Everyone should have their own clothes wherever they live. People should be offered choice when selecting clothes to wear, although sometimes assistance is needed in making appropriate choices.

Help may be needed with dressing, e.g. if there is a weak limb or side, the affected limb is put into blouses, shirts or trousers first. The same strategy is used when equipment such as i.v. infusion is in use.

Dressing aids

Adaptive devices or aids are available to make dressing easier, especially for people who have difficulty bending or have poor manual dexterity. They can be used to assist with many different items of clothing including socks, stockings, tights and jackets. Fastening clothes can be made easier by using:

- Velcro® closures
- Button hooks
- Zip pullers
- Reachers/pick-up sticks
- Dressing sticks.

The Disabled Living Foundation (2008) demonstrates many of these items. People with visual impairment sometimes use a tactile code such as sewing differently shaped buttons on the inside of garments or sewing tags in different places to tell what colour their clothes are. Those people who have red–green colour blindness may also have a system to distinguish colour, especially of their socks.

Prostheses

Dentures are discussed later in this chapter (p. 379).

People may use a prosthesis or accessories for cosmetic or clinical reasons. For example, a wig can be used for a change of appearance but in other situations it is worn to hide alopecia, or hair loss, which may occur naturally or following cancer treatment. People who wear wigs for the latter reasons can be self-conscious, both when wearing them and also if they need to be removed for any reason.

An artificial limb may affect a person's ability to carry out bathing and showering independently. External breast prostheses are sometimes used following surgical removal of a breast (mastectomy). Many women find them difficult to adapt to because they feel mutilated and unattractive after surgery (see Chs 12, 24).

When it has been established that a person uses a prosthesis, the nurse should adopt a tactful approach to identify how and when it is used and any impact it may have on their ability to carry out personal hygiene activities. It is important to consider the person's dignity and ask them before removing it for any reason.

Summary – personal hygiene

In summary, assisting someone with personal hygiene and dressing can initially appear simple but tailoring help to meet individual requirements can prove more complex. Box 16.17 provides an opportunity to consider aspects of personal care and the factors that can influence it.

 Reflective practice   Box 16.17

Factors that influence personal hygiene and appearance

Manjit Singh Dhillon is a Sikh client you meet during a home visit with the district nurse. He is 85 years old and recently widowed. He is frail and appears rather unkempt. His clothes are also in need of laundering. During your visit Mr Dhillon tells you about the importance of the symbols of Sikhism (the 5 Ks).

Student activities

- Find out about the items that he referred to as the '5 Ks' (see Box 16.15 and NHS Education for Scotland 2006).
- Think about how help with showering or washing will need to be modified, so that Manjit is able to change his shorts (kaccha) in accordance with the teachings of his faith.
- Reflect on the other factors that may be influencing his ability to carry out appropriate personal hygiene and maintain his appearance.

Resource

NHS Education for Scotland, 2006. A multi-faith resource for healthcare staff. NES, Edinburgh. Online. Available: http://www.nes.scot.nhs.uk/media/3720/march07finalversions.pdf.pdf August 2012.

Dental health and oral hygiene

This section reviews anatomy and physiology needed to understand the importance of a healthy mouth and teeth. The care required to maintain oral health is considered and the nurse's role in maintaining dental health and oral hygiene discussed.

Oral care is a basic hygiene need in both healthy and sick people. The teeth are essential for biting and chewing a normal healthy diet. For many people, having attractive teeth is an important aspect of their personal appearance and self-esteem.

Anatomy and physiology: the mouth

The mouth, or oral cavity, is the first part of the digestive tract (see Chs 19, 21). The tongue consists of voluntary muscles that enable speech, chewing and swallowing and is covered with mucous membrane. Taste buds are present there and the sense of taste relies on the presence of saliva for dissolving chemicals in food to activate the taste receptors. The cheeks and gums are also lined/covered with mucous membrane. The lips are involved in speech and non-verbal communication.

Salivary glands

Three pairs of salivary glands secrete saliva into the mouth. Saliva is essential for a healthy, comfortable mouth and is composed mostly of water. Its effects include lubrication of the mouth and washing away food particles from the teeth. It contains an antibacterial enzyme, lysozyme, that minimizes

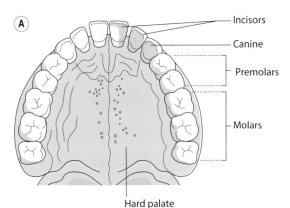

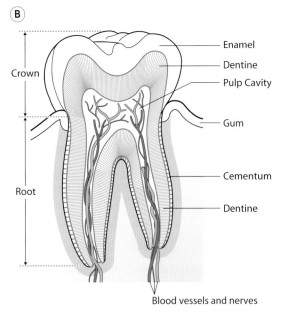

Fig. 16.9 • (A) Types of teeth (second dentition). (B) Structure of a tooth. (Reproduced with permission from Waugh, A., Grant, A., 2010. Ross and Wilson anatomy and physiology in health and illness, eleventh ed. Churchill Livingstone, Edinburgh.)

oral infection and another that begins digestion of dietary carbohydrate.

Teeth

Teeth enable people to eat solid food. At birth there are 10 temporary teeth in each jaw, which normally erupt between the ages of 6 months and 2½ years. These teeth form the primary dentition. From around 6 years they are shed and, in time, are replaced by 32 permanent teeth, known as the secondary dentition. There are four different types of teeth (Fig. 16.9A), their shapes being suited to their functions. The incisors and canine teeth are used to bite and tear food; the posterior premolars and molars, with their broader, flat surfaces, are used for chewing and grinding food. The four posterior molars are commonly known as the 'wisdom teeth'.

All teeth have the same basic structure (Fig. 16.9B). The crown protrudes through the gum, or gingiva, and the root lies embedded in the jawbone. A hard layer of dentine surrounds the central pulp cavity that contains blood vessels and nerves. The crown has an outer coating of enamel, while the root is held firmly in its socket by a layer of cementum and the periodontal ligament.

Maintaining oral health

Dental health promotion aims to reduce tooth and gum disorders and preserve people's natural teeth. Establishing good oral care and dietary habits therefore begins in childhood (Box 16.18).

Health promotion   Box 16.18

Maintaining healthy teeth and gums

- Visit your dentist at least yearly for dental examinations – free NHS treatment is provided for susceptible groups including children, women during and after pregnancy, older adults and unemployed people
- Use fluoride toothpaste; children's toothpaste contains lower levels of fluoride because they are renowned for eating it
- Brush your teeth at least twice daily and preferably after meals and sugary snacks
- Mouthwashes freshen the breath and can dislodge food debris
- Limit food and drinks containing sugar to mealtimes; using a straw for fizzy drinks delivers fluid to the back of the mouth, avoiding the teeth
- Renew your toothbrush every 2–3 months.

(From British Dental Health Foundation 2010a).

Teething can be a troublesome time for both infants and their parents. It only occurs during eruption of the primary dentition that begins from around 6 months. Some infants experience drooling and may bite on hard objects while teething, although others can be very irritable.

Regular visits to the dentist from an early age enable discovery of the characteristic smells and sounds of the dental surgery through non-threatening situations. Toothbrushing by parents should begin when the teeth erupt and continuing assistance and then supervision is needed until 7 years of age.

Eating habits should include sugary foods only at mealtimes and non-sugary foods such as cheese or fresh vegetables for snacks between meals. Sugary drinks should never be put in babies' feeding bottles to avoid the risk of dental caries (decay), especially at night. Sugar-free medicines are widely available and encouraged for the same reasons.

During childhood and adolescence, falls and trauma can damage the teeth and mouth. Measures to minimize potential hazards and resultant injuries should be considered, including:

- Non-slip mats in the bath or shower
- Supervising children when using play equipment
- Mouthguards for contact sports.

The mouth has an extensive blood supply and trauma that causes damage to teeth is likely to be accompanied by profuse bleeding from damaged oral tissues.

Oral care

Effective oral care moistens and cleans the mouth, removes unpleasant tastes and freshens the breath.

Toothbrushing and flossing

Dental health and oral hygiene are maintained by brushing the teeth with toothpaste at least twice daily and ideally also after meals and sugary snacks. This is the most effective way of removing plaque (a sticky film of bacteria that forms on the teeth) and food debris from the teeth and maintaining healthy gums. A small or medium size brush with soft or medium bristles will make it easier to clean the back teeth that can be hard to reach. The toothbrush is held at 45° to brush all surfaces of every tooth. The amount of toothpaste needed is the size of a pea and brushing should be undertaken for 2 minutes.

Toothbrushing is followed by daily interdental cleaning with special brushes or by flossing from around 8 years of age. To do this, dental floss is inserted between each tooth in turn and a seesaw action used to pull the floss backwards and forwards between the surfaces. This removes food debris and plaque from the gums and spaces between the teeth that a toothbrush cannot reach. Flossing reduces gingivitis (inflammation of the gums) but should be undertaken with care by people receiving radiotherapy or chemotherapy because their gums are prone to inflammation, bleeding and infection.

People with poor manual dexterity can hold large-handled toothbrushes more easily. Electric toothbrushes tend to have larger handles and also reduce the manual effort needed to brush the teeth.

Care of dentures

Dentures should fit well and provide a good cosmetic appearance. Ill-fitting dentures cause discomfort, difficulty with eating and inflammation, candidiasis (thrush) or ulceration of the gums and oral mucosa.

They can be cleaned using a toothbrush and non-abrasive denture toothpaste, although the British Dental Health Foundation (2010b) suggest that a soft nailbrush and ordinary soap are also suitable. Brushing should be carried out over a sink containing water or a soft towel to prevent damage if they are dropped. All surfaces should be carefully cleaned. The person's gums and palate are also brushed and the mouth well rinsed. After brushing, the dentures may be soaked in an effervescent denture cleaner to remove staining and bacteria, however dentures should not be soaked in these solutions overnight (British Dental Health Foundation 2010b). Dentures are more easily inserted when they are wet and therefore do not need to be dried.

Removal of dentures can be embarrassing, as people usually feel self-conscious without them and may have difficulty in speaking clearly. Some people sleep with their dentures *in situ* while others prefer to keep them in a denture pot at the bedside. They should be soaked in water to prevent warping or cracking. Denture pots should be labelled in care settings to avoid mix-ups.

People who wear dentures should still visit the dentist for examinations to ensure they continue to fit well and to detect any oral problems, e.g. oral cancer, at an early stage.

Tooth and gum disorders

Disorders include dental caries, periodontal disease and malocclusion.

Dental caries

Discoloration and then cavities, or caries, develop in the teeth when bacteria present in plaque convert sugars into acids that slowly dissolve tooth enamel. The most susceptible periods are between 4 and 8 years (primary dentition) and between 12 and 18 years (secondary dentition).

If plaque is not removed by brushing, it hardens forming tartar (dental calculus). This cannot be removed by toothbrushing and accumulation results in gingivitis. The gums become reddened, ulcerated and prone to bleeding when the teeth are brushed. Dental calculus can only be removed by a dentist or dental hygienist.

Periodontal disease

This results from long-standing gingivitis and becomes increasingly common from the third decade, although it often originates in childhood. There is destruction of the periodontal structures that support the teeth and this causes considerable tooth loss in later life. Prevention is by encouraging good dental health from childhood (see Box 16.18).

Malocclusion

Malocclusion occurs when the upper and lower teeth do not meet normally; because they are uneven, overcrowded or overlapping or when the jaw does not develop normally. Biting and chewing are difficult, there is abnormal wear on the teeth, trauma to oral mucosa and the teeth may also have a poor cosmetic appearance. Orthodontic treatment involving the use of dental 'braces' is usually required in the teenage years to correct this.

Oral assessment and oral hygiene

The mouth has a role in eating and drinking, taste and breathing, and verbal and non-verbal communication, including intimate self-expression. If the mouth is causing discomfort, this can have a detrimental psychosocial impact in addition to other consequences including loss of taste, loss of appetite and resultant constipation.

Assessment provides a baseline that enables planning and implementation of individualized care and from which oral status can subsequently be evaluated. The oral cavity is carefully inspected using a pen torch and spatula. Signs of a healthy mouth include:

- Oral mucosa, tongue and gums are moist, pink and clean
- Clean, white teeth
- Absence of halitosis ('bad breath')
- Absence of ulcers
- Dentures that, if worn, are well fitting.

Abnormalities such as redness, dryness, ulceration and a dirty or coated tongue are recorded together with the presence of loose, capped or crowned teeth, fixed braces or dentures. A wide range of factors may cause oral problems (Box 16.19) and

Factors predisposing to oral problems	Box 16.19

- Dehydration (see Ch. 19)
- Inability to eat or drink
- Malnutrition
- Mouth breathing
- Oxygen therapy (see Ch. 17)
- Ill-fitting dentures
- Poor cognitive function and self-neglect
- Antibiotics – alter the normal flora of the mouth and predispose to opportunistic invasion of *Candida albicans* causing oral thrush
- Other medication, e.g. phenytoin (used to control epilepsy)
- Cancer treatment – radiotherapy and chemotherapy damage the rapidly dividing cells of the oral mucosa and also predispose to oral thrush
- Underlying medical conditions, e.g. diabetes mellitus.

if a person in your care has one or more of these, oral assessment requires careful consideration.

Oral assessment tools

Several of these tools have been developed, taking the condition of the oral cavity and a variety of risk factors (see above) into account; however, they have not been sufficiently tested for validity and reliability to recommend them for general use.

Oral hygiene: nursing interventions

When assistance is required with oral hygiene, thoughtful nursing intervention can make a difference and it is important to take patient preference into account. The aims of nursing interventions are to maintain or restore oral comfort and promote oral health.

When possible, people should be encouraged to carry out their own oral hygiene. For many people, only assistance to get to a sink, where they can stand or sit and brush their own teeth, may be required. A person in bed or sitting in a chair can often also brush their own teeth when provided with a glass of water and a receiver for collecting waste water.

A Cochrane Systematic review by Brady et al (2006) highlighted the lack of evidence on which to base oral hygiene practice. When nursing intervention is required, an appropriate technique and solution should be selected (Table 16.1). A technique no longer recommended is the use of a swab wrapped round a pair of forceps because this can damage the oral mucosa. Some solutions are also no longer recommended: lemon and glycerine should not be used because the osmotic action of glycerine dehydrates the oral mucosa and acidic lemon juice may damage tooth enamel; hydrogen peroxide damages granulating tissue and should also be avoided. Pieces of fresh pineapple or tinned pineapple chunks contain a protein-digesting enzyme that is believed to clean the tongue. Chewing or sucking them is also refreshing and stimulates salivation.

There is little evidence to support an optimal frequency for oral hygiene although this is suggested to be between 2 and 6 hourly in ill people. It is often appropriate to moisten the mouth with water, a mouthwash or ice chips more frequently.

Medication can be prescribed for oral hygiene, e.g. in people undergoing treatment for cancer who have specialized needs, however sugar-free syrups should be used in people of all ages who require oral hygiene interventions to minimize the risk of dental caries. Chewing gum stimulates salivation and, when sugar-free, does not harm the teeth. A person's fluid status (see Ch. 19) should be reviewed when a dry mouth persists as dehydration is not reversed by providing oral hygiene.

Lip salve or soft paraffin may be used to moisturize and prevent cracked lips. It forms an oily film that reduces water loss by evaporation.

Sensory considerations

When planning care, nurses need to consider the effects of sensory impairments on a person's ability to self-care and the implications for effective communication. This section of the chapter introduces issues related to poor vision and hearing and appropriate nursing interventions.

The eye and vision

The eye is the organ that enables vision and provides people with important information about their environment and those things in it. It is estimated that around 80% of the sensory information perceived is visual.

Anatomy and physiology of the eye (see p. 373 for accessory structures)

The eyeball consists of three layers (Fig. 16.10):

- The outer layer includes the transparent cornea at the front of the eye and the sclera, or white of the eye. The posterior part of the sclera provides attachment for the extraocular muscles that move the eyeball in its socket.
- The middle layer comprises the iris, ciliary body and the choroid. The iris is the coloured part of the eyeball and the pupil its central dark space. The pupil constricts in bright light and dilates in dim light. The lens is a transparent body that lies behind the iris.
- The retina forms the delicate inner layer and contains specialized light-sensitive receptors called rods and cones.

The anterior segment of the eye contains aqueous fluid. As its production and drainage is fairly constant the pressure there also remains relatively constant.

Light rays entering the eyeball are refracted (bent) as they pass through the transparent structures at the front of the eye. The lens focuses the light rays towards the retina where a visual image is formed. This stimulates the light-sensitive receptors of the retina, generating nerve impulses that are conducted to the cerebral cortex. Each eye forms an image and both generate impulses that are transmitted to the brain for processing. Binocular vision provides accurate information about the environment, including the speed and distance of objects. If there is

Table 16.1 Techniques and solutions used for oral hygiene

Technique	Advantages and disadvantages
Toothbrush	Gentle use of a soft, small toothbrush followed by rinsing the mouth can be used when there is no inflammation of the oral cavity. This removes plaque and debris from the teeth and gums, and reduces coating of the tongue. This technique requires the person to be able to swallow, rinse their mouth and void waste water safely
Mouthwash	Providing a mouthwash will refresh the mouth when dehydration or nausea is present and after vomiting. The effect is short lasting and mouthwashes need to be offered frequently. A mouthwash requires the person to be able to swallow; rinse their mouth and void waste water safely (see Solutions, below)
Moistened foamsticks	These are widely used to clean and moisten the oral mucosa but they are not effective in removing plaque from the teeth (see Solutions, below). Although there is a belief within the profession that patients may be at risk from biting off and swallowing or inhaling the foam, there is no evidence to support this. Foamsticks are suitable for use in people who cannot swallow or rinse their mouths out safely
A swabbed finger	A moist swab round a gloved finger is also effective for cleaning and moistening the oral mucosa; however, it may cause compression of food debris and plaque into the interdental spaces. Plaque is not removed. This can be used when a patient is unable to use a mouthwash or swallow safely. This technique is not recommended for children or others who may bite the swabbed finger!
Solutions	
Water and sodium chloride 0.9%	Both are readily available, convenient and economical solutions to use. There is insufficient evidence to recommend sodium chloride 0.9% mouthwashes
Thymol tablets	These are widely used and prepared according to the manufacturer's instructions – normally, one tablet to one glass of water. There is no evidence supporting the benefits of their use and some people find the taste unpleasant
Chlorhexidine gluconate	Used as a mouthwash, this solution reduces bacteria and is effective against plaque. Long-term use can cause reversible staining of the teeth and tongue
Sodium bicarbonate	Careful dilution (1 level teaspoon in 500 mL; Nicol et al 2012) is required when using sodium bicarbonate because it is strongly alkaline and can damage the oral mucosa. It also has an unpleasant taste. There is a paucity of evidence to support its use although it removes mucus and other debris present in the oral cavity. It should only be used with care and when other solutions have proved ineffective
Saliva substitutes	For a persistent dry mouth, these sprays are effective for 1–2 hours

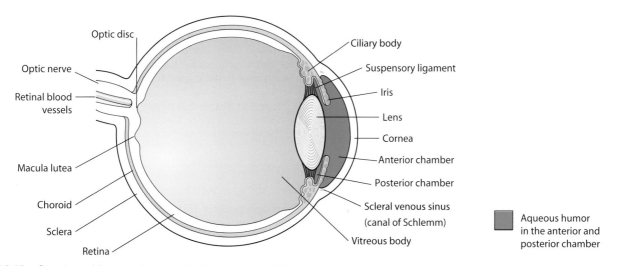

Fig. 16.10 • Structure of the eye. (Reproduced with permission from Waugh, A., Grant, A., 2010. Ross and Wilson anatomy and physiology in health and illness, eleventh ed. Churchill Livingstone, Edinburgh.)

only one eye with vision, less detailed information is perceived. This means that even simple visual judgements, such as putting a cup down safely, are more difficult. Visual perception is complex and interpretation of visual stimuli seldom occurs alone but takes place alongside that of others, e.g. hearing, taste and smell.

Accommodation of the eye describes the changes that take place to allow focusing on near objects, i.e. those closer than 6 m:

- The lens becomes thicker, and must refract more light rays from near objects in order to focus them on the retina. As this requires more effort than distant vision, tiring of the eyes may occur after prolonged close-up activities, e.g. reading
- The pupils constrict
- Both eyes move towards the object being viewed (convergence).

Visual acuity

Eye testing measures visual acuity (VA) to measure visual clarity. The most common method is the 'Snellen type test chart'. The test chart (Fig. 16.11A) is situated in a well-lit area and measurement is carried out 6 m from the chart. This represents 'distant vision', where no accommodation is required. Normal vision is 6/6, meaning that the person can read line 6 at 6 m from the chart. When only the top line can be read, the VA is 6/60. If the top line on the chart cannot be read at this distance, the individual is moved nearer to the chart; if the top line of the chart can be read at 3 m, this is recorded as 3/60. The eyes are tested separately with and without spectacles, if appropriate. For people with learning disabilities or those who cannot speak or read English, alternative charts can

be used such as the Snellen 'tumbling E' chart (Fig. 16.11B). A chart depicting objects of decreasing size (Fig. 16.11C) can be used in prelingual children.

Sight impairment

Box 16.20 outlines some common types of sight impairment and there are many causes. Some causes are reversible, e.g. with spectacles, however others are irreversible. Sight impairment is often found in older adults who have fallen and many people with learning disabilities are found to have refractive errors, or to be blind or partially sighted when their vision is assessed.

Types of sight impairment	Box 16.20

- *Refractive errors:* In the normal eye, light from distant objects is focused on the retina but when this is not the case, corrective lenses can be prescribed to restore normal vision:
  - in *myopia* (shortsightedness) correction requires a biconcave lens
  - in *hypermetropia* (longsightedness) a biconvex lens is used to focus the light rays on the retina
  - in *astigmatism* there is abnormal curvature of part of the lens or cornea and correction is achieved by the use of cylindrical lenses
- *Diplopia:* Meaning double vision, this indicates an underlying problem affecting vision, such as after a stroke
- *Strabismus (squint):* In this condition, a person cannot align both eyes – one or both of the eyes may turn in, out, up or down, and cannot focus simultaneously on a single point. Children with strabismus may initially have double vision. The cause is unknown and it is present at or shortly after birth
- *Presbyopia:* Becomes widespread after the fourth decade as the elasticity of the lens decreases with age and the ability of the eye to accommodate on near objects deteriorates. It is corrected by use of magnifying spectacles for reading
- *Cataract:* This is opacity of the normally transparent lens. It can be congenital or acquired, especially in later life, and is a common cause of blindness worldwide
- *Glaucoma:* Intraocular pressure rises as an abnormality of the production, flow or drainage of aqueous fluid develops. This may be congenital or acquired, and acute or insidious in onset. It may result in blindness if untreated
- *Tunnel vision:* Loss of peripheral vision
- *Diabetic retinopathy:* Disease of the retina in people with diabetes mellitus; a leading cause of blindness
- *Age-related macular degeneration (AMD):* This is a common cause of blindness in people aged over 50 and takes two forms: wet and dry. It affects the macula lutea, an area of the retina needed for seeing fine features and reading.

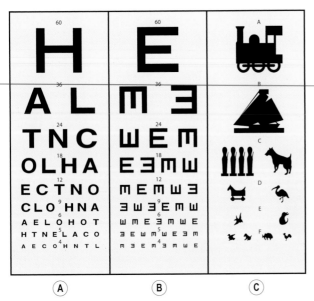

Fig. 16.11 • Snellen test type charts: (A) Snellen letter. (B) Snellen 'tumbling E'. (C) Recognition of objects. (Reproduced with permission from Peattie, P.I., Walker, S. (Eds.), 1995. Understanding nursing care, fourth ed. Churchill Livingstone, Edinburgh.)

Describing sight impairment

For the purposes of registration in the UK, a person can register as 'blind', or 'severely sight impaired', when they can only read the top line of the test chart at 3 m (VA = 3/60) or 'partially sighted', or 'sight impaired', when their VA is 6/60. People who can see further than this in either situation above, may also be eligible for registration when their visual field is very limited. The presence of severe sight impairment does not mean that a person lives in total darkness; many blind and most partially sighted people can recognize a friend at arms length. Less than 10% of blind or partially sighted people are born with impaired vision although sight loss is a common cause of disability in the UK and becomes increasingly common with age. The RNIB, 2010 (formerly The Royal National Institute for the Blind), estimates that 20% of people over 75 years live with registered sight loss, which includes reversible causes such as refractive errors and cataracts, and that the incidence rises to 50% by 90 years of age.

Some people do not like any of the terms 'severely sight impaired' or 'blind', or 'sight impaired' or 'partially sighted' because they feel they are negative and misleading. They may prefer to be described as 'visually impaired' or as having 'impaired vision' or 'visual disability' if they cannot see or are unable to see clearly. It is therefore important to discuss use of terminology with the individual concerned.

Helping people with sight impairment

Nurses should be aware of the common incidence of visual problems, especially in older people who may not have recognized this themselves. They may observe behaviours that suggest sight impairment that warrant further investigation. These include:

- Holding written material very close to the eyes
- Tendency to explore items by touch
- Appearing startled when someone approaches quietly
- Difficulty in establishing eye contact during speech
- Reluctance to move around, especially in a strange environment
- Avoidance of visual tasks or not noticing things that are nearby
- Rubbing the eyes
- Obvious signs of eye problems, e.g. swelling.

It is recommended that people over 60 have their eyes tested annually because eye problems usually develop insidiously and painlessly but can have serious consequences including blindness.

The primary aims when caring for people with visual impairment are maximizing independence and maintaining safety. During childhood, specialized help is needed to support the family in achieving this (Box 16.21). Communicating and maintaining a safe environment are therefore the most important activities that the nurse needs to consider.

Communication

Good verbal communication skills are essential and it is important to use normal speech and maintain eye contact when talking to visually impaired people, as the tone and inflexion convey much more than the actual words used (see Ch. 9). People with visual impairment often compensate by increased perception from their other senses. When approaching a visually impaired person this should be from the side of vision, if there is one. Calling their name will alert them to your approach and identifying yourself and others is essential. When leaving, tell them you are going. A call bell should be left at hand in

Health promotion Box 16.21

Promoting development in children with sight impairment

Aims

1. *To provide support for the child and family:* Information should be provided to enable the family to identify appropriate sources of support and education to meet their needs and to facilitate child development.

2. *To maximize attachment:* From an early stage, bonding between an infant and its parents is reinforced by mutual eye contact which may be absent. Other cues need to be identified to encourage attachment and to facilitate reinforcement. These can be provided in other ways such as speech, touch or cuddling the child.

3. *To achieve optimum development:*
   - Normal motor development leads to independence and relies heavily on visual stimuli. Non-visual cues and stimuli must be provided instead. Later on the child will need to learn to get around independently outside and a cane or guide dog may be introduced to achieve this
   - Development of play and socialization skills also relies heavily on visual stimuli – imitation being a prime example. More time is required to explain what should and can be done and guidance about other stimuli that encourage development of the other senses, e.g. touch and hearing, provided
   - Education needs to take into account the reliance on non-visual cues. Specialist support will be required to facilitate learning and will usually include learning to read Braille.

care settings, as the visually impaired person cannot call to a passer-by for help unless they can hear them. The sense of touch is important for people with visual impairment, especially when this occurs together with hearing problems. Sighted people quickly scan their environment for cues about what is happening around them and the nurse must allow more time for visually impaired people to do this. When describing something being 'over there', a gesture that indicates location often accompanies the words. People with visual impairment may not see these gestures and therefore verbal cues about the location of items can cause confusion. Using more specific language, e.g. the television is beside the window, is helpful.

Written communication can pose challenges for people with sight impairment and simple interventions such as the use of a reading lamp directed towards the material will enhance residual vision, thus assisting reading. Spectacles should always be clean and well-fitting (see p. 373). Many people with visual impairment can read ordinary print but find it is slow and very tiring while others find large print is essential. Books in large print are widely available. Hand-held magnifying glasses can be a useful reading aid. Large writing using a broad, black felt-tipped pen on white paper provides good contrast and is a useful strategy for providing written guidance to people with poor vision.

Many people with sight impairment enjoy audio material. The RNIB provides a Talking Book Service, and recorded audiotapes, cassettes and CDs are also widely available.

Headphones may be required to use audio equipment if others nearby are being distracted by the sound.

Some people with sight impairment use tactile forms of communication. Braille is a system of raised dots that can be learned by touch and produced using a Braillewriter. Moon is another, simpler form of tactile communication used mainly by older people. Both of these methods are effective but only between those people who can understand them.

An increasing range of technology is available to facilitate inclusivity and access to written material through use of computers and the Internet.

Maintaining a safe environment

Many interventions will assist in maintaining a safe environment for everyone, especially for those with sight impairment. Corridors and stairs should always be well lit, well signed and free from moveable and unnecessary items to minimize the occurrence of accidents. This is important at home, in care settings and in public places because many people, especially older people, have some degree of sight impairment although they may not be aware of it.

At home, a sight-impaired person can decide where items are kept and so find them again easily. Orientation to a new environment takes time. Most people will need to be accompanied around a new environment several times before becoming accustomed to new surroundings. Pot-pourri with different fragrances can be used to distinguish areas such as the sleeping area and sitting room. Sight-impaired people should be encouraged to explore parts of their new surroundings by touch. Moving personal belongings should only be carried out after discussion with the person.

Several issues may arise relating to safe use of medication (see Ch. 22). These include difficulty reading small print on labels of the containers, counting tablets and opening blister packs.

People often find bright light and glare uncomfortable, both outdoors and inside on bright sunny days. Wearing ordinary sunglasses may not help because light also reaches the eyes from above and round the sides although wearing a brimmed hat or baseball cap may help. Clip-on tinted spectacles with side shields that can be worn over normal spectacles are useful because they can be quickly removed when going into a dark area.

Services and support

Local authorities maintain registers of blind and partially sighted people to enable planning of services to meet their needs. They provide home adaptations to meet individual needs. After assessment, mobility aids may be provided to provide navigational independence. These include a white guide cane or, for some people, a guide dog supplied in the UK by the charity Guide Dogs.

The ear and hearing

The ear is the sensory organ that enables hearing and provides important information about the environment. The ear also

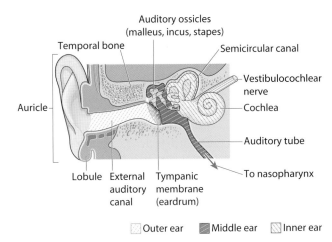

Fig. 16.12 • Structure of the ear. (Reproduced with permission from Waugh, A., Grant, A., 2010. Ross and Wilson anatomy and physiology in health and illness, eleventh ed. Churchill Livingstone, Edinburgh.)

functions in maintaining balance. The anatomy and physiology of hearing is outlined and the nursing interventions that will help a person with hearing impairment are explored here.

Action on Hearing Loss (2012b) estimates there are more than 10 million people in the UK with some type of hearing loss, with numbers increasing as the population becomes older. The numbers are low in children in the UK (45 000) rising to over 70% in those over 70 years.

Anatomy and physiology

The ear consists of three parts (Fig. 16.12):

- The outer ear extends from the auricle (pinna) through the external auditory canal to the eardrum. It is lined with hairs and ceruminous glands that secrete wax.
- The middle ear is an air-filled cavity that transmits sound waves inwards. It contains the auditory ossicles, three tiny bones, which extend across the middle ear to the oval window. Air reaches the middle ear from the nasopharynx via the auditory tube, maintaining equal pressure on both sides of the eardrum. The auditory tube is normally closed but opens during swallowing or yawning.
- The inner ear lies in the temporal bone and contains the specialized receptors involved in hearing and balance.

Sound waves entering the outer ear are funnelled along the external auditory canal to the eardrum which then vibrates. The vibrations are amplified and transmitted across the middle ear to the inner ear where they generate nerve impulses that are conducted to the temporal lobe of the cerebral cortex where hearing is perceived.

Assessment and prevention of hearing loss

Nurses play diverse roles is preventing hearing loss and assessment of people's hearing.

Newborn babies have their hearing assessed through the use of computer-linked equipment – often using otoacoustic emission testing (OAE) in the first few days or weeks after birth. Whenever a hearing problem is suspected, infants and children have specialized investigations (see below) and careful follow-up. Hearing impairment in children is often accompanied by developmental delay and difficulty with speech. Compliance with childhood immunization programmes is recommended as some infectious childhood diseases can cause deafness, e.g. mumps.

Occupational health nurses are involved in preventing noise-induced hearing loss and hearing tests for those who work in a noisy environment. Health and Safety legislation (see Chs 6, 13) requires employers to provide their workers with advice about minimizing the risks of noise-induced hearing loss and provide personal protective equipment, e.g. earmuffs or earplugs, when appropriate. Exposure to regular noise above 100 decibels can lead to noise-induced hearing impairment; this can occur at work or during leisure activities, e.g. shooting. Table 16.2 shows a range of sounds representing various intensities.

Hearing impairment

Interpersonal communication relies heavily on speech and characteristic signs that accompany hearing impairment include:

- Turning one ear towards someone speaking
- Apparent lack of attention or poor concentration
- Inappropriate responses
- Often seeming withdrawn or alone
- No response to sounds in the environment
- Asking for information to be repeated
- Speech which is unusually loud or soft
- Appearing easily startled when someone initiates conversation.

In adults and older children, hearing loss and deafness are usually measured by audiometry. This investigation identifies the thresholds, or quietest sounds, that can be heard across a range of frequencies, or pitches. Hearing thresholds are measured in decibels (dB). The person being tested is asked to respond by pressing a button when they can hear a tone. The level of the tone is then adjusted until it can just be heard and this level is called the threshold. The greater the threshold level found, the greater the hearing loss.

Hearing impairment varies in severity from mild to profound and can be congenital (present from birth) or acquired (onset after birth). Any hearing impairment is likely to impact on people's ability to communicate (see Table 16.2 and Ch. 9). Previously unidentified hearing impairment is most commonly encountered when caring for children and older people. The nurse should be aware that many severely or profoundly deaf people also have other disabilities, including learning disabilities.

There are two types of hearing loss: *conductive*, when sound waves cannot be transmitted to the inner ear, and *sensorineural*, when there is abnormality of the inner ear or vestibulocochlear

---

Table 16.2 Hearing impairment – impact on communication

Decibels (dB)	Typical noise	Severity of deafness (Action on Hearing Loss 2012b)	Impact on communication
140	Jet aeroplane during take-off		
130			
120	Thunder, indoor rock concert		
110			
100	Hearing impairment after prolonged exposure	Profound (quietest sounds heard >95 dB)	BSL is likely to be the first or preferred language. Use lipreading
90	Trains	Severe (quietest sounds heard between 70–94 dB)	BSL may be first or preferred language.
80	Heavy traffic, workshop		
70	Loud radio/television Street noises		Use lipreading and hearing aid
60	Noise in a restaurant		
50		Moderate (quietest sounds heard between 40–69 dB)	Difficulty in following speech without a hearing aid
40	Normal conversation at 1 m		
30		Mild (quietest sounds heard between 25–39 dB)	Difficulty in following speech when there is background noise. Often unaware there is a problem
20	Whisper		
10	Leaves rustling	Normal hearing	None
0	Faintest sounds heard		

(auditory) nerve that transmits auditory impulses to the brain. Some people have both types of hearing loss.

There are many causes of hearing impairment (Box 16.22). Sometimes people develop reversible hearing loss but for most others it is permanent. Accumulation of excess wax in the external auditory canal can cause conductive hearing loss and is common in older people. This can be improved, and sometimes cured, by ear irrigation (p. 374). Hearing loss occurs as part of the ageing process. Known as presbycusis, this is very common in older people who are often unaware of its presence as the onset is insidious and slowly progressive. Ringing in the ears, or tinnitus, is a distressing condition that can also be an early sign of hearing impairment.

Common causes of hearing impairment   Box 16.22

- Pre-term birth
- Infections, e.g. mumps, meningitis, maternal rubella (German measles) during pregnancy
- Accumulation of ear wax
- Older age – known as presbycusis
- Conditions affecting the ear, e.g. repeated middle ear infections (otitis media), Ménière's disease, otosclerosis
- Medication, including aspirin, aminoglycoside antibiotics, e.g. gentamicin
- Ongoing exposure to loud noise, e.g. at work, night clubs.

Describing deafness

It is important to realize that being deaf or hard of hearing can mean different things to different people. People are often comfortable with particular words to describe their own deafness and may feel quite strongly about terms they do not like being used. Action on Hearing Loss (2012b) provides the following guidance:

- Deaf people: generally used term for any degree of deafness
- Hard of hearing people: those with mild to severe hearing loss and also people who have lost their hearing gradually
- Deafened people: those who could hear normally at birth and became severely or profoundly deaf after learning to speak
- Deafblind people: those with very limited hearing and vision (Box 16.23)
- The Deaf Community: used by many people whose preferred language is British Sign Language (BSL) (see Box 16.24) and who consider themselves part of the Deaf Community (where a capital D, emphasizes their Deaf identity).

Communicating with hearing-impaired people

Deaf and hard of hearing people may communicate in different ways depending on the severity of their hearing impairment.

Deafblindness   Box 16.23

Around 95% of what people perceive about themselves and their environment comes through the senses of sight and hearing. Action on Hearing Loss (2012b) estimated there were about 23 000 deafblind people in the UK, some of whom are completely deaf and completely blind, while others have some residual hearing and/or vision.

Facts

- This is also known as dual sensory impairment
- It is sometimes congenital but usually acquired
- Older people are most commonly affected and without appropriate support they can become withdrawn, depressed and isolated. They may lose independence in many areas, including mobility, communication, access to information and enjoying leisure activities
- With appropriate support, deafblind people of all ages can live fulfilling lives at home and in their community. Local authorities may provide guidehelps or communicator guides who help these people take an active part in everyday life
- The organization Sense provides information for people with dual sensory impairment and their carers (see Useful websites, p. 396).

Hearing impairment can be overcome, at least partly, by the use of hearing aids (see p. 374), lipreading, using a computer or sign language. Other strategies used by people with hearing impairment include increased sensitivity to facial expression and other non-verbal behaviours. Some people with mild hearing loss use a hearing aid or lipread. People with moderate hearing loss have difficulty hearing what is said without a hearing aid, especially when there is background noise. People who are more severely deaf may have difficulty following what is being said, even with a hearing aid. Many of these people lipread and some use sign language. Some, but not all, people who are profoundly deaf find that hearing aids are of little benefit and therefore rely on lipreading or sign language (Box 16.24). Nurses will usually need the services of an interpreter when communication is through sign language, especially when detailed or complex information is involved.

It is important to be aware that deaf people often find difficulty communicating in group situations, especially when there are rapid changes in speakers and topics. Box 16.25 provides some tips that enhance verbal communication with people who have impaired hearing.

The unconscious patient

In this section consciousness, assessing levels of consciousness and management of the unconscious casualty are explained. Common conditions affecting the nervous system are outlined and neurological investigations and terminology are highlighted. The final part explores the care of the unconscious person as an example of someone who is completely dependent on others for all aspects of nursing care.

The outcome of unconsciousness can be complete recovery, partial recovery or death, depending on the cause. The

Help for hearing-impaired people   Box 16.24

1. Hearing aids – see p. 374.
2. Lipreading – only about 40% of the spoken word is understood and less when the speaker has a beard, moustache, a strong accent or exaggerated pronunciation. Comprehension is enhanced by the development of increased sensitivity to non-verbal cues including body language, facial expression and gestures.
3. Sign language and finger spelling (see: www.actiononhearingloss.org.uk):
   - British Sign Language (BSL) is a visual–gestural language that uses hand signals, facial expressions and shoulder movements to represent words and ideas, which is widely used by hearing-impaired children and their families
   - Signed English was initially designed to encourage hearing-impaired children with reading, writing and speech, but is also used by people with learning disabilities
   - Finger spelling.
4. Makaton – this is a communication system based on signs, symbols and speech, widely used by both adults and children with communication difficulties including those with learning disabilities. It uses a core vocabulary that focuses on essential daily activities. In the UK, the signs are derived from BSL (Bunning 2011). (See: www.makaton.org for further information.)
5. Other aids for hearing-impaired people:
   - Alerting devices such as lights can be attached to doorbells, alarm clocks and smoke alarms to facilitate communication, enhance independence and promote safety
   - The Action on Hearing Loss website and telecommunication companies provide information about equipment for deaf and hard of hearing people
   - The installation of induction loops helps people with a hearing aid or loop listener to hear sounds more clearly by reducing or cutting out background noise. These systems are widely found in public places including theatres, cinemas, banks, shopping centres and train stations (Fig. 16.13). Smaller systems can be installed at home and are useful for listening to the television
   - Increasingly, specially trained 'hearing' dogs are being used to improve the lives of people with hearing impairments by alerting the person to specific sounds, e.g. smoke alarm, door bell, etc.

Fig. 16.13 • Induction loop symbol.

Nursing skills   Box 16.25

Communication tips for people with hearing impairment

- Gently alert the person to your arrival
- Check the hearing aid, if used, is switched on
- Minimize background noise if appropriate, e.g. television
- Sit or stand at the same level at an appropriate distance from the person – about 1 m if wearing a hearing aid or 1–2 m for lipreading
- Face the person, making sure your face and lips are visible
- If the person lipreads, ensure they are wearing their spectacles, if used
- Speak slowly and clearly using your normal tone and inflection
- Use non-verbal communication skills to reinforce your verbal skills, e.g. hands, facial gestures
- Check that the person is following the conversation by asking them to contribute actively at times
- If you are not understood:
  - try using other words to explain yourself
  - raise your voice slightly but use lower tones, never shout
  - use gestures or writing to enhance understanding.

timescale is variable, lasting from a few minutes or hours to weeks or longer. There are many causes, including:

- Trauma
- Poisons, e.g. alcohol, carbon monoxide, drug overdose
- Seizures
- Stroke
- Cardiovascular conditions, e.g. severe haemorrhage, severe shock, heart attack, cardiac arrest
- Metabolic causes, e.g. kidney or liver failure, severe infection, poorly controlled diabetes
- End-of-life care (terminally ill).

Levels of consciousness

The conscious person is awake, aware of their surroundings and interacts with it, both consciously and subconsciously. This requires normal brain functioning, including the cerebral cortex as well as the brain stem that conducts nerve impulses there for processing. Loss of consciousness is a sign of a serious underlying disorder and nurses must be able to assess an unconscious person and provide appropriate first aid and nursing interventions.

Altered consciousness exists on a spectrum from loss of alertness and drowsiness to coma. These and many other terms used are subjective and therefore unreliable for describing a person's level of consciousness. In order to assess a person's level of response the AVPU scale (see Ch. 14) is used and for level of consciousness the Glasgow Coma Scale (GCS) is used (see Fig. 14.14, clinical observation chart including Early Warning Score (EWS)).

The Glasgow Coma Scale

This scale (Fig. 16.14) relies on scores achieved for three independent measurements:

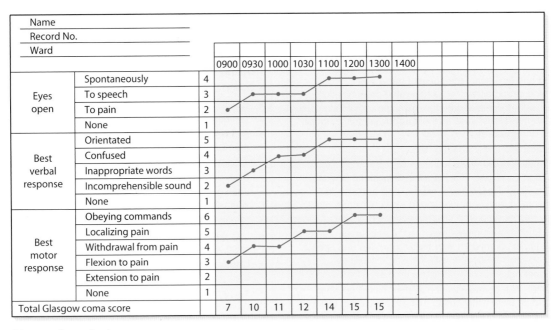

Name															
Record No.															
Ward															
			0900	0930	1000	1030	1100	1200	1300	1400				
Eyes open	Spontaneously	4												
	To speech	3												
	To pain	2												
	None	1												
Best verbal response	Orientated	5												
	Confused	4												
	Inappropriate words	3												
	Incomprehensible sound	2												
	None	1												
Best motor response	Obeying commands	6												
	Localizing pain	5												
	Withdrawal from pain	4												
	Flexion to pain	3												
	Extension to pain	2												
	None	1												
Total Glasgow coma score			7	10	11	12	14	15	15					

Fig. 16.14 • Glasgow Coma Scale.

- Best eye response
- Best motor response
- Best verbal response.

Responses to each of these measurements are added together providing a total score at regular intervals. The best score is the maximum of 15 and the lowest is 3/15. Coma is defined as a score of 8/15 or less but any value under 15 is significant (National Institute for Health and Clinical Excellence, NICE 2007). Changes in the GCS score are important indicators of altering neurological status. A dot for each response is entered in the appropriate box on the chart.

Assessing the level of consciousness using the GCS is shown in Box 16.26. Sometimes it is not possible to assess best eye opening accurately because neither eye can be opened, e.g. when there is severe swelling, and 'C', meaning 'closed', is entered in the bottom box on the chart. The best verbal response involves the person's ability to speak and understand. When a patient has an endotracheal tube in situ or a tracheostomy that prevents them from speaking, a 'T' is entered in the bottom box on the chart.

Assessment of level of consciousness using the GCS is not reliable for children and modifications are required to take expected developmental milestones into account until their language skills have developed (Box 16.27). GCS findings also need careful evaluation to include the presence of a learning disability because developmental milestones may not match those expected for the physical size or age, and verbal communication problems, e.g. the person cannot speak or English is not their first language.

Neurological observations in hospital

This involves GCS measurement, which assesses level of consciousness, together with several other observations including pulse, blood pressure and respiratory rate; the response of the pupils to light; and limb movements. These are recorded on a single chart, known as a neurological observation chart. A full discussion is beyond the scope of this book (see Further reading, below, e.g. Waterhouse 2011).

The unconscious casualty

A collapsed casualty is dependent on the actions of others to maintain life, and providing timely and effective first aid interventions is vital (Box 16.28, p. 390). The principles are always the same although basic life support (BLS) varies depending on age (see Ch. 17).

First aiders should monitor the casualty's level of response, pulse and respiratory rates (see Ch. 14) every 10 minutes, taking a note of them if possible. The condition of a collapsed casualty can change quickly and careful assessment and recording provide important information that will assist in evaluating the casualty's condition, both at the time and later in hospital.

Unconscious or partly conscious people must never be given anything orally because they are at risk from choking or inhaling fluid into their lungs and either of these events will have serious consequences.

People with diabetes may lose consciousness when their condition is poorly controlled. This is usually when blood sugar levels fall below normal, which is often called a 'hypo' – meaning hypoglycaemia. Many people recognize the onset of a 'hypo' and take a sugary drink or snack to reverse it before they become unconscious. If unconsciousness occurs, the person is treated in the same way as any other unconscious casualty. People with diabetes who have been unwell may also lose consciousness, but usually over a longer time, through abnormally high blood sugar levels (hyperglycaemia).

Nursing skills   Box 16.26

Glasgow Coma Scale (GCS) measurements

Best eye opening (maximum score 4)

- Spontaneous opening (4) – eyes open spontaneously as the observer approaches
- Opening to speech (3) – eyes open when addressed by the observer. It may be necessary to raise the voice slightly or gently shake the shoulder in case the casualty is hard of hearing
- Opening to pain (2) – when there is no response to either of the stimuli above, a painful stimulus is applied. The stimulus must be consistent to detect changes accurately
- No eye opening (1) – even to a painful stimulus.

Best verbal response (maximum score 5)

- Orientated (5) – the person is able state their name and where they are and can also answer simple questions about the year, month and date
- Confused (4) – the person can speak but is not fully orientated to time, place and person
- Inappropriate sounds (3) – the person is unable to engage in meaningful conversation
- Incomprehensible sounds (2) – no recognizable words but may consist of sounds, e.g. moaning and groaning
- No response (1) – no sounds are made in response to either speech or painful stimuli.

Best motor response (maximum score 6)

- Obeys commands (6) – the person can do something that involves movement of muscles above the neck, e.g. to stick their tongue out or tightly close their eyes. This means that even if the person has a spinal injury, they can still be assessed accurately and avoids squeezing of the observer's fingers, which can be a reflex action.
- Localizes pain (5) – when the person cannot respond to commands, applying a painful stimulus may elicit a response. The person attempts to locate or remove the painful stimulus (when this has already been demonstrated for their best verbal response, there is no need to reapply another painful stimulus to assess the motor response)
- Withdrawal from pain (4) – the person responds purposefully by withdrawing a limb from the stimulus but does not attempt to locate or remove it.
- Flexion to pain (3) – there is no purposeful response to the painful stimulus and the limbs flex abnormally in a purposeless way
- Extension to pain (2) – the limbs extend, or straighten in an abnormal way, rather than withdraw or flex in response to a painful stimulus.
- None (1) – there is no limb response to painful stimuli.

 Nursing skills   Box 16.27

Adaptation of Glasgow Coma Scale measurements for children

- Best eye opening – carried out as per Box 16.26
- Best verbal response – the adaptations required are:

Best verbal response		Best grimace response – used for pre-verbal infants
Alert, normal babbling, cooing or words used	5	Spontaneous normal mouth and facial movements
Less than usual babbling, cooing, etc. or spontaneous irritable cry	4	Less than normal spontaneous mouth and facial movements or response to touch
Inappropriate crying	3	Vigorous grimace in response to pain
Occasional whimpering or moaning	2	Mild grimace to pain
No vocal response	1	No response

- Best motor response – carried out as per Box 16.26.

(Adapted from NICE 2007).

Common conditions affecting the nervous system

In addition to unconsciousness, there are many conditions that affect the normal functioning of the nervous system (Table 16.3). Related associations/groups providing useful information are listed in Useful websites, below. The following investigations may be used to diagnose or evaluate treatment for disorders of the nervous system:

- X-rays of skull and spine
- Brain scans – computed tomography (CT), magnetic resonance imaging (MRI), positron emission tomography (PET)
- Electroencephalogram (EEG)
- Lumbar puncture (LP) – cerebrospinal fluid (CSF) sampling.

An explanation of some of these investigations along with the nursing care is provided in Woodward (2011). Box 16.29 provides the opportunity to find out what a neurological investigation can involve.

Some of these conditions are very common and you are likely to meet people with them when on placement. Signs and symptoms that can accompany neurological conditions are defined in Box 16.30 (p. 391).

Seizures

These are also known as 'fits' or 'convulsions'. They affect all ages and can be frightening to those around when they occur. This can be at home, in a care setting or outdoors and they are relatively common in some people with learning

There may be evidence of ingestion of drugs or alcohol, e.g. empty bottles or packaging, around an unconscious casualty that will alert the first aider to the possibility of overdose. In either case vomiting can occur and the unconscious casualty is at risk of inhaling vomit unless placed in the recovery position (see Fig. 16.15A, p. 394), when vomit will drain from the mouth, keeping the airway open.

First aid   Box 16.28

The unconscious casualty

Priorities are established using the primary survey:

- **D**anger – Assess the situation for traffic, chemicals, etc; ensure the area is safe for both you and the casualty before proceeding
- **R**esponse – if the casualty appears unconscious, ask them loudly, 'Can you hear me?'

If there is a response:

- Leave the casualty in the position found (if safe to do this) and summon help – dial 999/112
- Treat any serious conditions and monitor level of response, pulse and breathing (Ch. 14)
- Continue monitoring the casualty until help arrives

If there is no response:

- Shout for help
- If possible, leave the casualty in the position found and open the airway
- If this is not possible, turn the casualty onto their back and open the airway
- **A**irway – open the airway (see Ch. 17)
- **B**reathing – assess by looking for the chest rising, listening for signs of breathing and feeling for air movement into or out of the mouth for no more than 10 seconds
- **C**irculation – assess by observing the casualty's colour and feeling for a pulse for up to 10 seconds. Severe bleeding, if untreated, will lead to shock that can be fatal.
  - If the casualty is *breathing normally*, place them in the recovery position (Fig 16.15, p. 394); assess for other life-threatening conditions e.g. severe bleeding and treat as necessary
  - If the casualty is *NOT breathing normally* or there is any doubt whether breathing is normal, begin CPR (see Ch. 17)

See also 'Basic life support – airway maintenance and cardiopulmonary resuscitation', Ch. 17.

(Adapted from St John Ambulance website. Online. Available: www.sja.org.uk/sja/first-aid-advice/life-saving-procedures.aspx September 2012).

 Reflective practice   Box 16.29

Undergoing an MRI scan

Jane is to have an outpatient MRI scan. She has poor short-term memory and becomes confused in new surroundings. Jane keeps asking the staff at the nursing home about what will happen during the test and seems anxious to get more information. She has a moderate hearing impairment and wears a hearing aid.

Student activities

- Find out about MRI scanning.
- Consider how you might feel during this investigation.
- Identify the key information needed by Jane so that she is well prepared for her scan.
- Consider how to provide Jane with information that meets her needs.

Resource

NHS Choices – www.nhs.uk/Pages/HomePage.aspx.

Table 16.3 Common neurological conditions	
Cerebrovascular accident (stroke)	Caused by haemorrhage from cerebral blood vessels or a thrombosis (clot) lodged in a cerebral artery affecting consciousness level, sensation, movement, swallowing, speech and/or vision. One-sided paralysis (hemiplegia) is often present
Confusion (delirium)	Disorientation to time, place or person. This is not an illness but indicates an underlying problem and is common in older people. It is usually reversed when the cause is treated
Dementia	Slow, progressive and irreversible memory loss, disorientation and impairment of reasoning that usually affects older people. The most common form is Alzheimer's disease. Independence declines in the later stages when there is increasing difficulty with speech and performing routine activities
Epilepsy	Recurrent seizures; affects children and adults (see text)
Meningitis	Inflammation of the meninges, usually caused by bacteria or viruses
Multiple sclerosis (MS)	A common cause of disability in people aged under 50 years, characterized by an unpredictable series of relapses and remissions. Onset may be acute or insidious, and blurring of vision or double vision can be early signs. Later, problems with elimination of urine and faeces, speech, vision, fatigue, depression and weakness or paralysis of the limbs are common
Parkinson's disease	Gradual and progressive decline in motor function that results in tremor, rigidity, slowness of movement and difficulty in initiating movement

disabilities. Once started, a seizure is usually short-lived and self-limiting. It cannot be stopped and therefore first aid intervention is based on maintaining a safe environment (Box 16.31, p. 391). A seizure may be accompanied by incontinence of urine and/or faeces.

In children under 5 years, seizures are usually associated with a fever (high body temperature) and are known as febrile seizures (previously 'convulsions'). First aid interventions (Box 16.32, p. 391) therefore aim to reduce the raised body temperature in addition to maintaining safety.

In older children and adults, a warning, or 'aura', often occurs before a seizure, meaning that the person is aware that one is about to take place. After a seizure, there is often a period of drowsiness and disorientation. When recovery occurs

Neurological signs and symptoms   Box 16.30

- Amnesia – loss of memory
- Aphasia – loss of speech
- Ataxia – impaired muscle coordination
- Bradykinesia – slow movement
- Diplopia – double vision
- Dysarthria – difficulty speaking
- Dyskinesia – difficulty with voluntary movement
- Dysphagia – difficulty swallowing
- Dysphasia – difficulty speaking
- Hemiparesis – weakness of muscles on one side of the body
- Hemiplegia – paralysis of muscles on one side of the body
- Paraplegia – paralysis of the lower limbs
- Paraesthesia – abnormal sensation, e.g. tingling
- Photophobia – intolerance of light
- Photophonia – intolerance of sound
- Quadriplegia, tetraplegia – paralysis of all four limbs
- Tremor – involuntary muscle movement usually affecting a limb or limbs.

First aid   Box 16.31

Seizures in adults

Recognition

Sudden collapse, violent muscle twitching, then muscle relaxation followed by a period of unconsciousness and recovery. There are many causes of seizures and several presentations (Woodward 2011).

Aims of treatment

- To maintain a safe environment around the casualty
- To provide care when consciousness returns
- To organize hospital transfer if necessary.

Treatment

- Clear the area of potential hazards
- Ask any onlookers to move away
- Record the time of onset
- Slacken tight clothing, especially around the neck and waist, to assist breathing and place a cushion under the head if possible
- When the seizure is over, observe closely.

After convulsive movements stop

- Roll into the recovery position (see Fig. 16.15A, p. 394), check and record breathing, pulse and level of response (Ch. 14)
- Stay with the casualty until fully recovered
- Record the duration of the seizure.

Do not

- Restrain or move the casualty during the seizure
- Attempt to put anything into the mouth.

Transfer to hospital when

- This is the first seizure
- The seizure lasts for more than 5 minutes
- Unconsciousness lasts longer than 10 minutes.

First aid   Box 16.32

Seizures in children

Recognition

Loss or alteration of consciousness, involuntary muscular twitching, evidence of high fever, not breathing.

Aims of treatment

- To maintain a safe environment around the child
- To organize transfer to hospital
- To minimize carers' anxiety
- To cool the child if feverish.

Treatment

- Place pillows around the child to protect from injury
- Record the time of onset
- If feverish:
  - remove clothing down to underwear
  - tepid sponge the child starting at the forehead working downwards.
- When seizure is over, observe closely.

When seizure has stopped

- Roll the child into the recovery position (Fig. 16.15A or B, p. 394)
- Dial 999 (or 112) for an ambulance
- Check and record breathing, pulse and level of response (Ch. 14)
- Record the duration of the seizure
- Remain calm and provide the child and carer with reassurance until ambulance arrives.

Do not

- Restrain or move the child
- Attempt to put anything into the mouth.

it may be necessary to reorientate the person and explain what has happened.

Nursing the unconscious person

Depending on the cause, nursing care can take place in a variety of settings. These range from a terminally ill person at home to trauma casualties in an intensive care unit. In the latter case, there will also be many technical interventions; however, the principles of nursing care are the same for any unconscious person. These interventions are explained in different chapters of this book and the art of nursing an unconscious person lies in providing coordinated care tailored to meet their individual needs. Assessing, planning and prioritizing the nursing care for an unconscious person is a complex nursing skill that is carried out by an experienced nurse although providing their care often involves other members of the multidisciplinary team (MDT) including student nurses under the supervision of their mentors. There is no 'standard care plan' for nursing an unconscious person although there are many common nursing problems. Table 16.4 (pp. 392-393) uses a problem-solving approach to care planning, to identify common nursing interventions that

Table 16.4 Using a problem-solving approach to plan care for an unconscious patient

Actual/potential problem	Aim	Nursing intervention	Rationale
Maintaining a safe environment			
Emergency situation occurs	To provide rapid and effective intervention	Ensure oral airway, oxygen and other emergency equipment is at the bedside	Equipment needed is readily available if required
Deteriorating condition	To detect and report changes promptly	Carry out EWS (Ch. 14) or GCS and neurological observations (p. 388) as directed	Changes reflect alteration of general or neurological condition
Breathing			
Respiratory or circulatory difficulties	To prevent or detect and report any of the following: • Airway obstruction • Inadequate breathing • Inadequate tissue oxygenation • Circulatory problems To maintain adequate tissue oxygenation	Nurse in the recovery or lateral position (see Fig. 16.15, p. 394) Observe rate, depth and effort of breathing (see Chs 14, 17) Observe skin for pallor or cyanosis Record pulse and blood pressure as advised (see Ch. 14) Administer oxygen therapy as prescribed and maintain safety measures (see Ch. 17)	Maintains patency of the airway and prevents tongue occluding it Identify changes in respiratory function Indicators of decreasing oxygenation Changes indicate changing condition Increases oxygen available for tissues Prevents fire in the area
Communicating			
Unable to communicate verbally Anxiety, fear or disorientation	To provide a safe environment where patient and their relatives understand what is happening	Explain all procedures in simple language before providing interventions Encourage visitors to speak to the patient	Puts patient at ease and provides a calm, therapeutic environment A familiar voice is reassuring
Eating and drinking			
Unable to eat or take oral fluids	To maintain hydration To maintain nutritional status	Administer i.v. fluids as prescribed (see Ch. 19) Administer nasogastric feeding or parenteral nutrition as prescribed (see Ch. 19) Record fluids given on fluid balance chart (see Ch. 19) Observe for signs of dehydration and fluid overload (see Ch. 19)	Provides optimum fluid requirement Meets nutritional requirements which are increased in illness and fever Enables accurate evaluation of fluid balance Enables early detection and adjustment of fluid therapy
Maintaining body temperature			
Infection	To allow early detection of nosocomial infection (see Ch. 15)	Record temperature as directed (see Ch. 14) Send specimens for culture and sensitivity as directed (see Ch. 15)	Increased temperature is an early indicator of infection Allows early identification of pathogenic microorganisms
	To minimize effects of fever	Provide care for a pyrexial patient (see Ch. 14)	Lowers body temperature and promotes comfort
Personal cleansing and dressing			
Cannot undertake these activities independently	To maintain a high standard of personal hygiene	Give a daily bedbath (pp. 370–371) Provide oral hygiene (pp. 379–381 and Table 16.1) Provide hair care (pp. 375–376) Provide eye care (p. 373) and keep eyes closed with hypoallogenic tape or hydrogel pads	Keeps patient comfortable with fresh and clean skin Maintains oral health Keeps hair clean and shiny Keeps eyes moist, clean and closed to prevent corneal damage when corneal reflex is absent

Table 16.4 Using a problem-solving approach to plan care for an unconscious patient—cont'd

Actual/potential problem	Aim	Nursing intervention	Rationale
Expressing sexuality			
Unable to express sexuality or maintain own dignity	To promote individuality	Close screens when carrying out personal care Use preferred routines and own toiletries Dress in own clothing when possible	Maintain privacy, dignity and individuality
Mobilizing			
Problems associated with immobility	To prevent development of pressure ulcers	Assess risk using a validated assessment tool (see Ch. 25) Change position frequently according to risk identified Use of pressure-relieving aids (see Ch. 25) as directed	Identify risk of development of pressure ulcers Prevents prolonged pressure on the skin between firm surface and bony prominences Reduces pressure on skin between bony prominences and a firm surface
	Prevention of deep vein thrombosis (DVT)	Carry out passive exercises as directed (see Ch. 18) Use of other preventive DVT measures (see Ch. 18) Observe for swelling, tenderness or redness of the calves	Reduces venous stasis and promotes circulation in the limbs These are signs of DVT
	To prevent muscle wastage, joint stiffness or contractures	Carry out passive exercises as directed (see Ch. 18)	Exercise of skeletal muscles maintains their tone and reduces muscle wastage Prevents joint stiffness or contractures
Eliminating			
No control over micturition	To maintain intact skin	Keep skin clean and dry – a penile sheath or catheterization and catheter care may be required (see Ch. 20) Record urine output on fluid balance chart	Urinary incontinence predisposes to skin excoriation and breakdown Enables accurate evaluation of fluid balance
No control over defecation	To maintain intact skin To prevent constipation	Wash skin after defecation Record when bowels open in nursing record Increase fibre if possible Administer prescribed laxatives Observe faecal characteristics (see Ch. 21)	Faecal incontinence predisposes to skin breakdown Low fibre diet, insufficient fluid intake and immobility predispose to constipation Signs of constipation, diarrhoea or other abnormalities may be evident
Sleeping			
Frequent nursing interventions disrupt circadian rhythm	To promote circadian rhythm (see Ch. 10)	Plan and implement nursing care in an organized manner	Encourages periods of rest and sleep between nursing interventions
Dying			
Terminal illness	To facilitate a peaceful and dignified death	Support the patient and their relatives (see Ch. 12) Encourage relatives to participate in care if they wish Understand that some patients will not recover	Provides compassion and understanding in the face of a poor prognosis

may be included in the care of an unconscious person. It is based on the Roper, Logan and Tierney model (see Ch. 14) to enable systematic and holistic assessment of a person's actual and potential nursing problems. The many references in Table 16.4 make it easy to find the full explanation of the relevant intervention. Some aspects of nursing care are discussed in more detail below.

The care needed is prioritized and always starts with A, B, C:

- Maintain a clear **A**irway
- Monitor **B**reathing
- Monitor **C**irculation.

Several items of equipment are kept at the bedside of unconscious patients. Some items may not be needed if the patient is having end-of-life care (terminally ill). They are checked each time a new nurse takes over the care to ensure they are still present and in working order in case they are needed in

an emergency. They include: suction equipment, equipment for administering oxygen and an oral airway.

Positioning the unconscious patient

In order to maintain a patent airway the recovery position or lateral position is used (Fig. 16.15). These prevent the tongue moving backwards and obstructing the airway and promote drainage of any secretions from the mouth and respiratory tract.

Recovery position

The recovery position for adults is mainly used in first aid situations when there are no pillows available to support the casualty (Fig. 16.15A). To place someone in this position:

- In a first aid situation, kneel on the ground beside the casualty and remove any large items from their pockets
- Lie them flat on their back with both legs straight

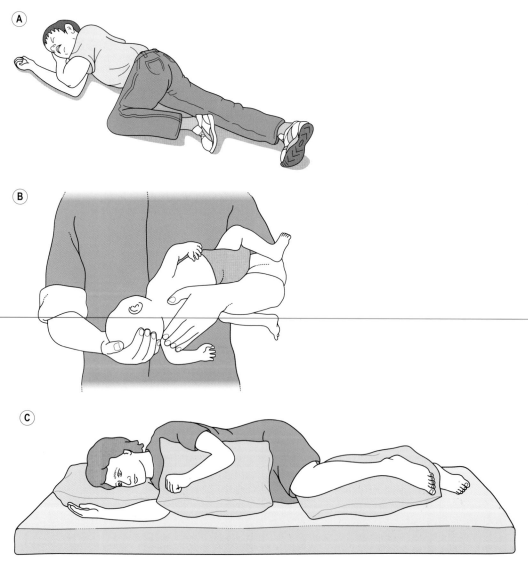

Fig. 16.15 • Positioning the unconscious patient: (A) Recovery position – adults. (B) Recovery position – infants under 1 year. (C) Lateral position.

- Position the arm nearest you at right angles to the body then bend the elbow and place the palm facing upwards
- Bend the upper leg and then roll them towards you until the bent leg is across their body. Keeping the upper leg bent will stop them from rolling onto their front
- Place the back of the upper hand under their cheek in a position that keeps their airway clear.

In infants under 1 year, the recovery position is achieved by the first aider holding the infant on its side with the head inclined downwards (Fig. 16.15B, p. 394).

Lateral position

Nursing care is more easily carried out in the lateral position (Fig. 16.15C, p. 394), which is normally used in care settings. The patient is positioned as follows:

- Head – supported on one pillow
- Torso – the spine is kept straight and a pillow placed behind the back to provide support
- Arms – the lower arm is brought in front of the patient and placed with the palm upwards. The upper arm is bent slightly at the elbow and supported on a pillow
- Legs – the lower leg is kept straight and in line with the spine while the upper leg is bent forwards at the knee and supported on pillows.

Communicating with an unconscious person, their relatives and friends

It is important to provide explanations of interventions before they are carried out just as for any other patient. Normal speech is used when communicating with an unconscious patient. As the person is unable to verbalize any fears, concerns or discomfort, the nurse must be especially alert for and report cues such as restlessness or alterations in vital signs that may indicate pain or changes in their condition. Hearing is the last sense to go and the first to return when consciousness is regained and therefore it is seldom clear to what extent the patient is aware of events around them. In end-of-life care, good communication with relatives plays a large part in helping them come to terms with not only the current situation but also later when the patient dies (see Ch. 12).

Visiting someone who is unconscious is stressful and can be a cause of great anxiety, especially when the prognosis (outcome) is unknown or likely to be poor. Anxiety is reduced when visitors are given clear explanations that enable them to understand and participate in decisions about treatment and care. At least initially, visitors may be limited to close family and significant others to minimize intrusion.

Involvement in the care of their loved one can reduce relatives' feelings of helplessness. Initially relatives can provide information about the person's preferences, lifestyle and hobbies that enables nurses to carry out personal care using preferred routines where possible. They are encouraged to speak to the patient and touch them to provide familiar stimuli and may also be asked to provide some favourite tapes or CDs. They may be asked if they want to participate in aspects of personal care and their wishes must be respected whatever decision is reached.

Planning nursing interventions

Before attending to the patient, consideration is given as to what interventions are required at one time. When the person needs to be turned, this can be followed by oral hygiene, eye care and passive exercises. This will minimize disruption and allow periods of rest, especially important during the night and when seriously ill (Box 16.33).

Reflective practice   Box 16.33

Care of an unconscious patient

Think about an unconscious patient with whose care you have been involved.

Student activities

- Using Table 16.4, identify which nursing interventions were carried out for your patient.
- Discuss the reasons why these were appropriate for that situation, with your mentor or a peer.

SUMMARY

- This chapter provides a discussion of fundamental aspects of nursing interventions relating to personal hygiene activities.
- *Essence of Care 2010* (DH 2010) benchmarks were designed to improve standards of person-centred care and some have been used here to stimulate learning and reflection on nursing practices you have seen on placement.
- The high prevalence of sight and hearing impairment, especially in older people, has been highlighted together with some of their effects on people's lives. Assessment and nursing interventions for people with these conditions has been explored.
- Care of the unconscious patient has been outlined to show that the nursing interventions for a person with complex physical needs are largely based on combining a range of fundamental interventions discussed in this and other chapters.

KEY WORDS AND PHRASES FOR LITERATURE SEARCHING

Blindness

Deafness

Eye care

Hearing aids

Mouth care

Oral hygiene

Personal hygiene

Visual impairment

Useful websites

Action on Hearing Loss (formerly RNID (Royal National Institute for Deaf People)) www.actiononhearingloss.org.uk

Age UK (formerly Age Concern and Help the Aged) www.ageuk.org.uk

Alzheimer's Society www.alzheimers.org.uk

Department of Health www.dh.gov.uk

Disabled Living Foundation www.dlf.org.uk

Epilepsy Action www.epilepsy.org.uk

Makaton Vocabulary Development Project www.makaton.org

Meningitis Research Foundation www.meningitis.org

Multiple Sclerosis Society www.mssociety.org.uk

National Institute for Health and Clinical Excellence www.nice.org.uk

NHS Choices www.nhs.uk/Pages/HomePage.aspx

NHS Clinical Knowledge Summaries (CKS): evidence-based information and practical 'know how' about the common conditions managed in primary care www.cks.nhs.uk/home

NHS Evidence www.evidence.nhs.uk/topic

Parkinson's Disease Society www.parkinsons.org.uk

RNIB (formally Royal National Institute of the Blind) www.rnib.org.uk

Sense – for deafblind people www.sense.org.uk

Stroke Association www.stroke.org.uk

All websites accessed September 2012.

References

Action on Hearing Loss, 2012a. Statistics. Online. Available: www.actiononhearingloss.org.uk/your-hearing/about-deafness-and-hearing-loss/statistics.aspx September 2012

Action on Hearing Loss, 2012b. Describing deafness. Online. Available: www.actiononhearingloss.org.uk/your-hearing/about-deafness-and-hearing-loss/deafness/describing-deafness.aspx September 2012

Benbow, M., 2010. Emollients and ageing skin. Journal of Community Nursing 24 (2), 34–38.

Brady, M.C., Furlanetto, D., Hunter, R., Lewis, S.C., Milne, V., 2006. Staff-led interventions for improving oral hygiene in patients following stroke. Cochrane Database of Systematic Reviews Issue 4. Art. No.: CD003864. DOI: 10.1002/14651858. CD003864.pub2.

British Dental Health Foundation, 2010a. Caring for my teeth. Online. Available: www.dentalhealth.org/tellmeabout/topic/64/2 September 2012.

British Dental Health Foundation, 2010b. Denture cleaning. Online. Available: www.dentalhealth.org/tellmeabout September 2012.

Bunning, K., 2011. Let me speak – facilitating communication. In: Atherton, H.L., Crickmore, D.J. (Eds.), Learning disabilities towards inclusion, sixth ed. Churchill Livingstone, Edinburgh.

Cancer Research UK, 2009. Preventing skin cancer. Online. Available:
www.cancerhelp.org.uk/type/skin-cancer/about/preventing-skin-cancer#smart September 2012.

Department of Health, 2010. Essence of care 2010. Online. Available: www.dh.gov.uk/prod_consum_dh/groups/dh_digitalassets/@dh/@en/@ps/documents/digitalasset/dh_119978.pdf September 2012.

Disabled Living Foundation, 2008. Full list of factsheets. Disabled Living Foundation, London. Online. Available: www.dlf.org.uk/content/full-list-factsheets September 2012.

Harkin, H., 2011. Nursing patients with disorders of the ear, nose and throat. In: Brooker, C., Nicol, M. (Eds.), Alexander's nursing practice, fourth ed. Churchill Livingstone, Edinburgh.

Jamieson, E.M., McCall, J.M., Whyte, L.A., 2007. Clinical nursing practices, fifth ed. Churchill Livingstone, Edinburgh.

National Institute for Health and Clinical Excellence, 2004. Prevention and management of foot problems in people with type 2 diabetes: information for people with type 2 diabetes, their families and carers, and the public Online. Available: www.nice.org.uk/nicemedia/live/10934/29246/29246.pdf September 2012.

National Institute for Health and Clinical Excellence, 2007. Head injury. Triage, assessment, investigation and early management of head injuries in infants, children and adults. Clinical Guideline 56. Online. Available: www.nice.org.uk/
nicemedia/live/11836/36259/36259.pdf September 2012.

NHS Education for Scotland, 2006. A multi-faith resource for healthcare staff. NES, Edinburgh. Online. Available: http://www.nes.scot.nhs.uk/media/3720/march07finalversions.pdf.pdf August 2012.

Nicol, M., Bavin, C., Cronin, P., et al., 2012. Essential nursing skills, fourth ed. Mosby, Edinburgh.

Nursing and Midwifery Council, 2008. The code: standards for conduct, performance and ethics for nurses and midwives. NMC, London.

NHS Clinical Knowledge Summaries, 2011. (minor update) Headlice. Online. Available: www.cks.nhs.uk/head_lice# September 2012.

RNIB, 2010. Key information and statistics. Online. Available: www.rnib.org.uk/aboutus/Research/statistics/Pages/statistics.aspx September 2012.

Trigg, E., Mohammed, T.A. (Eds.), 2010. Practices in children's nursing: guidelines for hospital and the community, third ed. Churchill Livingstone, Edinburgh.

Woodward, S., 2011. Nursing patients with disorders of the nervous system. In: Brooker, C., Nicol, M. (Eds.), Alexander's nursing practice, fourth ed. Churchill Livingstone, Edinburgh.

Further reading

Brooker, C., Nicol, M. (Eds.), 2011. Alexander's nursing practice, fourth ed. Churchill Livingstone, Edinburgh.

Glasper, A., Richardson, J., 2010. A textbook of children's and young people's nursing, second ed. Churchill Livingstone, Edinburgh.

Redfern, S.J., Ross, F.M., 2006. Nursing older people, fourth ed. Churchill Livingstone, Edinburgh.

St John Ambulance Association and Brigade, St Andrew's Ambulance Association, British Red Cross, 2009. First aid manual: the authorised manual of St John Ambulance, St Andrew's Ambulance Association, and the British Red Cross, ninth ed. Dorling Kindersley, London.

Waterhouse, C., 2011. Nursing the unconscious patient. In: Brooker, C., Nicol, M. (Eds.),
Alexander's nursing practice, fourth ed. Churchill Livingstone, Edinburgh.

Waugh, A., Grant, A., 2010. Ross and Wilson's anatomy and physiology in health and illness, eleventh ed. Churchill Livingstone, Edinburgh.

Breathing and circulation

17

Jillian Riley

LEARNING OUTCOMES

This chapter will help you:

- Outline the anatomy and physiology of the heart, circulation and blood, and the respiratory tract and breathing
- Describe some common disorders affecting circulation and breathing
- Describe the first aid treatment for common problems with breathing and circulation
- Describe basic life support procedures in adults, children and infants
- Describe the nurse's role in the assessment of circulation and breathing
- Outline some common diagnostic procedures
- Outline the role of health promotion in the reduction of conditions affecting breathing and circulation, and in minimizing the effects of existing conditions
- Describe the nursing interventions for someone with disorders of breathing and circulation
- Understand the principles of rehabilitation for people with disorders of breathing and circulation.

Introduction

The care of people with problems affecting their breathing and/or circulation takes place in diverse settings, from the home to the acute hospital, and includes people of all ages, from the neonate to older adults. Immense change has occurred over the past decade, through technological advances, the development of new drugs and, possibly more importantly, through the shift in focus from the health professional as expert to the patient as expert involved in self-management and decision-making. These have consequently led to change in the care delivered by nurses, some of which is discussed in this chapter.

Assessment of the patient is an important first step in their nursing management and treatment and so, following a brief review of the structure and function of the heart, circulation, blood and respiratory system, the chapter outlines some of the important nursing observations that may be undertaken as part of a holistic assessment. The chapter also outlines some of the more common disorders and investigations used in their diagnosis.

This chapter describes the ways in which the nurse can contribute towards the health of the person with disorders of breathing or circulation, reduce the effects of illness and maximize quality of life for both the patient and their family. Because disorders of breathing and circulation may at times require emergency treatment, some first aid measures are included. The health promoting activities that help to prevent problems with breathing and/or circulation are also explored.

An overview of breathing and circulation

This section provides a brief outline of breathing and the circulation. Readers should consult their own anatomy and physiology book for more detail. In addition, an outline of common conditions, basic life support, holistic assessment of breathing and circulation and investigations are provided.

Life depends on an adequate and continuous supply of oxygen (O_2) and nutrients to the cells and the removal of the waste products of metabolism. Without this, cells will become starved of oxygen and die. The accumulation of waste products such as carbon dioxide (CO_2) also disrupts cell function and eventually contributes to cell death.

Breathing and circulation are therefore fundamental to life and the cardiovascular system (CVS), blood and respiratory system must work together to supply O_2 to the cells and remove waste CO_2. This requires an adequate intake of air and a good blood supply to the lungs in order for gaseous exchange to take place. Oxygenated blood carries O_2 to the cells and deoxygenated blood, containing CO_2, leaves the cells and is transported to the lungs. The CVS circulates the blood around the body, and to and from the lungs.

Cardiovascular system – outline of anatomy and physiology

The CVS comprises the heart which pumps blood around the body and to the lungs and the circulatory system of arteries, capillaries and veins through which the blood travels.

The heart

The heart is situated in the thorax, within the mediastinum (the space between the two lungs) with its base inclined to the left (Fig. 17.1). It is protected from injury by the bones forming the thoracic cage, the sternum (breastbone) in front, the ribs and the vertebral column behind.

The heart has four chambers and the wall comprises three layers; from outer layer pericardium, myocardium (cardiac muscle) and endocardium (Fig. 17.2). The two upper chambers or atria are the receiving chambers that pump blood into the ventricles. The two lower chambers are thick-walled ventricles that pump blood to the lungs (pulmonary circulation) and to the tissues and cells (systemic circulation). The right and left sides of the heart are divided by the septum.

Valves situated at the entrance or exit of the chambers ensure that the blood flows in one direction. The two semilunar valves are the pulmonary valve at the junction of the right ventricle and pulmonary artery and the aortic valve at the junction of the left ventricle and the aorta. The atrioventricular (AV) valves between the atria and ventricles prevent any backflow of blood from the ventricles to the atria as the ventricles contract. The right AV valve (tricuspid valve) lies between the right atrium and ventricle and the left AV valve (bicuspid or mitral valve) lies between the left atrium and ventricle.

Coronary circulation

Three major arteries supply the myocardium with oxygen: the right coronary, the left anterior descending and the circumflex. They branch to form a dense network of arterioles and capillaries that extend throughout the myocardium and ensure that it is supplied with oxygen, and metabolic waste products are

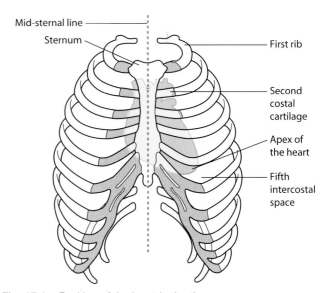

Fig. 17.1 • Position of the heart in the thorax. (Reproduced with permission from Brooker, C., Nicol, M. (Eds.), 2003. Nursing adults. The practice of caring. Mosby, Edinburgh.)

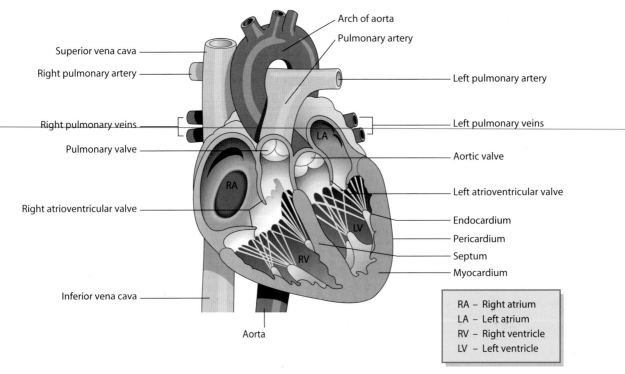

Fig. 17.2 • Heart showing the chambers, valves and blood vessels. (Reproduced with permission from Waugh, A., Grant, A., 2010. Ross and Wilson anatomy and physiology, eleventh ed. Churchill Livingstone, Edinburgh.)

removed. Once the myocardium has been supplied with oxygen, blood returns to the right atrium via the coronary veins and is transported to the lungs for carbon dioxide removal and reoxygenation.

Conduction

The electrical conduction system of the heart has four main structures (Fig. 17.3):

- The sinus node, also known as the 'pacemaker' of the heart, initiates each heartbeat. It normally fires at a rate between 60 and 100 beats per minute (b.p.m.)
- The impulse passes to the atrioventricular (AV) node causing the atria to contract (atrial systole)
- Next the impulse passes down the AV bundle (bundle of His) in the septum and to the right and left bundle branches
- Finally, the impulse passes to the Purkinje fibres. This causes the ventricles to contract (ventricular systole) and eject blood into the aorta and pulmonary artery.

Cardiac cycle

The cardiac cycle is the rhythmic contraction (systole) and relaxation (diastole) of the heart as it fills with blood and pumps it around the body and to the lungs. It comprises a series of stages that occur during a single heartbeat. Normally, the whole cycle is completed in less than 1 second. Once one cycle is completed, the next cycle commences to maintain a continuous flow of blood.

The function of the cardiac cycle is to provide an adequate output of blood from the heart. The amount of blood that is ejected with each heartbeat is referred to as the stroke volume (SV), whereas the term cardiac output (CO) refers to the amount of blood ejected from the heart in 1 minute. Hence the equation:

Cardiac output (CO) = Heart rate (HR) × Stroke volume (SV).

Sinus rhythm

Sinus rhythm is the normal rhythm of the heart. It produces a typical waveform comprising five deflections known universally as P-QRS-T (Fig. 17.4). The deflections depicted on an electrocardiogram (ECG) represent the electrical activity in the heart and correspond to the events of conduction and the stages of the cardiac cycle.

At rest, the adult heart normally beats in response to the sinus node activity at approximately 70 b.p.m. Sinus rhythm describes any heart rhythm with normal complexes that occurs at a rate between 60 and 100 b.p.m. In adults, an HR of <60 b.p.m. is referred to as sinus bradycardia, while an HR >100 b.p.m. is sinus tachycardia.

Systemic and pulmonary circulation

The systemic circulation is the circulation of oxygenated blood from the left ventricle into the aorta then to cells/tissues, and deoxygenated blood back to the right atrium of the heart. The pulmonary circulation is the circulation of deoxygenated blood from the right ventricle to the pulmonary artery then to the lungs, and oxygenated blood back to the left atrium of the heart.

Thus oxygenated blood returning from the lungs enters the left atrium and passes through the left AV valve into the left ventricle (Fig. 17.2). The left ventricle pumps blood into the systemic circulation through the aorta (large artery) and from there to numerous smaller arteries, arterioles and capillaries, which take blood to the rest of the body (Fig. 17.5, p. 400). The coronary arteries supplying the myocardium are the first to branch from the aorta. The arterial blood supplies cells with oxygen and nutrients and returns, carrying carbon dioxide and other waste, to the right side of the heart via small veins (venules) and increasingly larger veins. Deoxygenated venous blood returns to the right atrium in two large veins – the

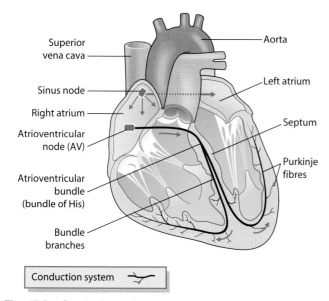

Fig. 17.3 • Conduction pathways. (Reproduced with permission from Brooker, C., Nicol, M. (Eds.), 2003. Nursing adults. The practice of caring. Mosby, Edinburgh.)

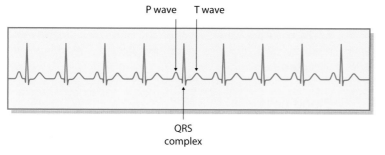

Fig. 17.4 • Sinus rhythm. (Reproduced with permission from Brooker, C., Nicol, M. (Eds.), 2003. Nursing adults. The practice of caring. Mosby, Edinburgh.)

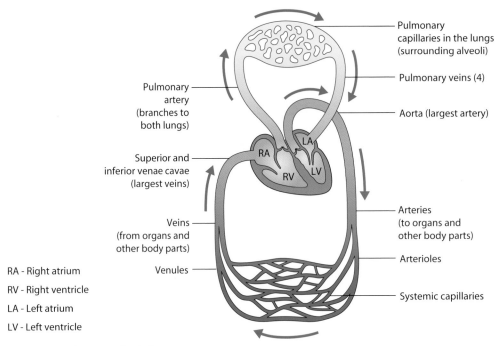

Fig. 17.5 • The systemic and pulmonary circulation.

RA - Right atrium
RV - Right ventricle
LA - Left atrium
LV - Left ventricle

superior and inferior venae cavae – and passes through the right AV valve into the right ventricle.

The right ventricle pumps blood into the pulmonary circulation through the pulmonary artery (Fig. 17.5). The pulmonary artery divides to send a branch to each lung where blood moves through smaller and smaller arteries and arterioles until they reach the pulmonary capillaries. Gas exchange occurs between the blood in the capillaries and the air in the alveoli of the lungs (see p. 403); carbon dioxide moves from blood to the alveoli and oxygen from the alveoli to the blood.

The oxygenated blood is returned to the left atrium of the heart through venules and larger and larger veins that form four pulmonary veins (two from each lung).

An efficient pulmonary and systemic circulation ensures that the body tissues and organs are perfused with oxygenated blood and waste products are removed.

Blood: outline of anatomy and physiology

Blood is a viscous fluid circulating in the blood vessels. It is a connective tissue and forms the main transport system of the body. The colour depends upon the amount of oxygen it is carrying; well-oxygenated arterial blood is bright red, whereas oxygen-poor (deoxygenated) venous blood is darker in colour.

Blood comprises a fluid part called plasma which forms approximately 55%, and the blood cells which form the remaining 45%. Blood is slightly alkaline with a normal pH range of 7.35–7.45.

Blood volume varies according to body size and age. Adult blood volume forms approximately 7–8% of body weight. Females have a smaller proportion than males; however, during pregnancy, the volume increases by between 20% and 40% in order to maintain blood flow through the enlarged uterus and placenta to supply oxygen and nutrients to the fetus and to remove fetal waste products. Infants and children have a greater proportion, which gradually decreases until adult proportions are reached. At birth, the circulating blood volume varies, but is usually around 85 mL/kg. Thus, a newborn weighing 4 kg has approximately 340 mL of blood. The functions of the blood include the following:

- Transports oxygen and nutrients to the cells
- Transports carbon dioxide to the lungs and waste such as urea to the kidneys for excretion
- Helps to maintain fluid, electrolyte and pH balance (see Ch. 19)
- Transports hormones, enzymes and drugs to areas of action
- Distributes heat around the body
- Prevents serious haemorrhage by haemostasis
- Protects against infection with white blood cells and antibodies.

Plasma

Plasma is the straw-coloured fluid found when blood separates. In the vascular system, plasma provides a medium to carry blood cells. Plasma is between 90% and 92% water and dissolved nutrients, gases, electrolytes, hormones, drugs, waste products and proteins such as albumin, globulins and fibrinogen.

Blood cells

There are three types of blood cell: erythrocytes (red cells), leucocytes (white cells) and thrombocytes (platelets).

Erythrocytes (red blood cells)

Erythrocytes are the most numerous of the blood cells and their main function is to carry oxygen. Erythrocytes contain haemoglobin (an iron-containing pigment/protein molecule), which is responsible for carrying most of the oxygen transported in the blood. Iron and some B vitamins (e.g. folic acid and vitamin B_{12}) are essential for the formation of haemoglobin (Box 17.1).

 Health promotion Box 17.1

Iron-rich foods

A balanced diet that supplies sufficient iron is needed for the body to produce haemoglobin. Foods rich in iron include:

- Red meat
- Liver
- Dried fruit
- Nuts
- Beans
- Whole grains
- Fortified cereals
- Leafy green vegetables.

Student activities

Access NHS choices website:

- Which vitamin increases iron absorption from food?
- Which beverages can inhibit iron absorption?
- How can a teenage girl who is strictly vegetarian obtain enough iron from her diet?

Resource

NHS Choices – www.nhs.uk/livewell/goodfood/Pages/ Goodfoodhome.aspx and www.nhs.uk/Livewell/Vegetarianhealth/ Pages/Essentialnutrients.aspx September 2012.

Leucocytes (white blood cells)

Leucocytes are divided into different groups. These include:

- Granulocytes (polymorphonuclear cells) – neutrophils, basophils and eosinophils
- Lymphocytes
- Monocytes.

All leucocytes have a role in defending the body against microorganisms and other foreign particles. Some leucocytes remove foreign particles such as a bacterium or an abnormal cell by phagocytosis, which involves engulfing and digesting the particle; other leucocytes are part of the immune response through the production of antibodies or destruction of abnormal body cells.

Thrombocytes (platelets)

Platelets are fragments of larger cells found in the bone marrow. They are necessary for blood clotting and haemostasis (control of bleeding from small vessels).

Haemostasis

Normally blood flows freely within the vascular system but when there is significant bleeding from a damaged blood vessel, the process of haemostasis normally prevents major blood loss.

Haemostasis involves four overlapping stages:

- *Vasoconstriction:* The diameter of the blood vessels becomes smaller and blood loss is reduced
- *Platelet plug formation:* Platelets clump together at a site of injury and form a 'platelet plug', which can temporarily stop bleeding until blood coagulation processes are initiated
- *Coagulation/blood clotting* (fibrin clot formation): A complex process with many stages requiring 12 clotting factors, whereby inactive prothrombin (a plasma protein) is converted to active thrombin. In the next stage thrombin converts soluble fibrinogen (plasma protein) to insoluble fibrin and forms a fibrous mesh over the cut vessel. This mesh traps blood cells, a fibrin clot is formed and the damaged vessel is sealed
- *Fibrinolysis:* The final stage where the clot is removed by enzymes once healing is complete.

Blood groups

There are two major blood group classifications: the ABO system and the rhesus system.

The ABO system has four main blood groups – A, B, AB and O – which are defined by the presence of antigens (specific proteins) on the surface of the erythrocyte. People with antigen A are blood group A, those with antigen B are group B. People who have both A and B antigens are blood group AB and those without either antigen are group O.

Someone with blood group A will have anti-B antibodies in their plasma, someone with blood group B will have anti-A antibodies, people with blood group O will have both anti-A and B antibodies while someone with blood group AB will have no antibodies. These antibodies will bind to a foreign antigen and initiate the clumping together (agglutinate) of the transfused cells such as occurs if incompatible blood is transfused (see pp. 427–428).

It is important to be aware of the different blood groups in order to ensure that when blood is transfused, blood from the correct group is given to the correct person. Table 17.1 outlines the ABO blood group compatibility.

The rhesus group is determined by a further set of antigens on the erythrocyte. People who have the antigens are rhesus positive (Rh[D]-positive) and those without are rhesus

Table 17.1 ABO blood group compatibility				
Recipient	**Donor**			
	A	B	AB	O
A	Yes	No	No	Yes
B	No	Yes	No	Yes
AB	Yes	Yes	Yes	Yes
O	No	No	No	Yes

(Reproduced with permission from Brooker, C., Nicol, M., 2003. Nursing adults. The practice of caring. Mosby, Edinburgh.)

negative (Rh[D]-negative). Unlike the ABO system there are no preformed anti-rhesus (anti-D) antibodies. However, if a rhesus negative person receives rhesus positive blood they develop anti-D. Although this will not cause a transfusion reaction at the time, any future transfusion will initiate a reaction and the donor erythrocytes will be attacked.

During pregnancy, a rhesus negative woman who has a rhesus positive fetus may become sensitized and develop anti-D antibodies. During a subsequent pregnancy with a rhesus positive fetus the anti-D antibodies can cross the placenta and cause haemolysis (breakdown) of the fetal erythrocytes. This is a serious condition and can lead to fetal death or the baby may suffer brain damage or die after birth. Women are tested for rhesus group during antenatal care. Anti-D is given to rhesus negative women to prevent the sensitization of the immune system. It is given by injection following events that may lead to sensitization such as bleeding during pregnancy, miscarriage and labour.

Respiratory system: outline of anatomy and physiology

The respiratory tract provides oxygen for cellular function and excretes waste carbon dioxide. This is achieved by breathing, where air moves in (inspiration) and out (expiration) of the lungs and by gas exchange in the lungs and at the cells.

Respiratory structures

The respiratory structures (Fig. 17.6) include:

- The nose, pharynx, larynx, trachea and bronchi, which warm, filter and humidify (moisten) air before it reaches the lungs
- The lungs, containing smaller bronchi, bronchioles, alveolar ducts and alveoli where gas exchange occurs.

Nose

The first part of the nasal cavity is lined with skin containing hairs that trap large particles from inspired air. The internal part of the nasal cavity is lined with respiratory mucosa (ciliated columnar epithelium) containing many mucus-secreting goblet cells. The inspired air is humidified by the moist mucosa and warmed by plentiful blood vessels supplying the respiratory mucosa. The sticky mucus traps dust, bacteria and other foreign particles in the inspired air and the cilia then waft these particles towards the pharynx where they are swallowed and so do not enter the lungs.

Pharynx

The pharynx is a funnel-shaped passage with three parts: nasopharynx, oropharynx and laryngopharynx. The process of warming, humidifying and filtering inspired air normally continues in the nasopharynx, which is lined with respiratory mucosa (Box 17.2). The nasopharynx is exclusively respiratory, but the oropharynx and laryngopharynx provide a passage for food and fluids in addition to air.

Mouth breathing	Box 17.2

Mouth breathing, as may occur in patients with nasal obstruction or dyspnoea (difficult breathing), bypasses the normal processes in the nose and nasopharynx that warm, humidify and filter air and leads to an exacerbation of the breathing problems. The respiratory mucosa will be damaged, the cilia cease to function effectively and mucus secretions become dry, crusty and difficult to expectorate (cough up).

The pharynx also contains lymphoid tissue – the nasopharyngeal tonsils in the nasopharynx and the palatine tonsils in

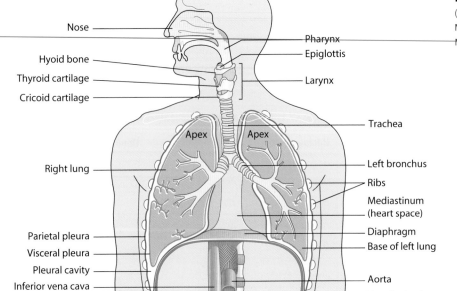

Fig. 17.6 • The respiratory structures.
(Reproduced with permission from Brooker, C., Nicol, M. (Eds.), 2003. Nursing adults. The practice of caring. Mosby, Edinburgh.)

Nose — Pharynx — Epiglottis
Hyoid bone —
Thyroid cartilage — Larynx
Cricoid cartilage —
Apex Apex — Trachea
Right lung — Left bronchus
— Ribs
— Mediastinum (heart space)
Parietal pleura — Diaphragm
Visceral pleura — Base of left lung
Pleural cavity —
Inferior vena cava — Aorta
— Vertebral column

the oropharynx – which form part of the body's defences against invading microorganisms.

Larynx

The larynx (voice box) is formed from cartilage, ligaments and membranes. Inspired air moving through the larynx is warmed, humidified and filtered as it passes from the pharynx to the trachea. The vocal cords, which extend from the front to the back of the larynx, are concerned with sound production. Inspired air must pass through the opening between the vocal cords – the glottis – to enter the trachea.

During swallowing, various reflex mechanisms prevent food or fluids from entering the lower respiratory tract. These include:

- Upward movement of the larynx causes the epiglottis (a small flap-like structure attached to the top of the larynx) to close over the opening into the larynx
- Breathing does not normally occur during swallowing
- The soft palate closes off the nasopharynx.

In addition, if food or fluid does enter the larynx, the cough reflex is normally stimulated (see below and p. 415).

Trachea

The trachea (windpipe) is a continuation of the adult larynx is between 12 and 15 cm in length and formed of C-shaped rings of cartilage that ensure the airway remains open. It divides (bifurcates) to become the right and left main bronchi, with one bronchus going to each lung. The trachea is also lined with respiratory mucosa and continues to warm, humidify and filter air, although warming and humidification is practically complete when air enters the trachea. The mucus continues to trap foreign particles and, in a synchronized process called the mucociliary escalator, the cilia move the mucus with particles upward to the larynx from where it is either expectorated by coughing or swallowed.

Irritation such as that caused by excess mucus or foreign material (food, fluid, etc.) in the larynx, trachea or bronchi stimulates the cough reflex in which a forced expiration expels the mucus and/or foreign material.

Bronchi, bronchioles and alveoli

The processes of humidification and warming in the upper respiratory tract are complete, air is saturated with water and warmed to 37°C and most foreign particles have been removed before it enters the bronchi.

Once the right and left main bronchi enter the lungs they divide into smaller and smaller bronchi, bronchioles and finally the tiny alveolar ducts that lead into the alveoli. The walls of alveolar ducts and alveoli comprise a single layer of simple epithelium, which facilitates gaseous exchange.

The alveoli are very small air sacs clustered together and surrounded by a network of pulmonary capillaries. Special cells in the alveolar walls secrete surfactant (phospholipids) which ensures a moist membrane needed for gaseous exchange and prevents alveolar collapse between breaths. The development of surfactant-producing cells start around 20 weeks' gestation and the amount of surfactant increases until lung maturity at 30–34 weeks (Serci 2009). In the pre-term infant, surfactant

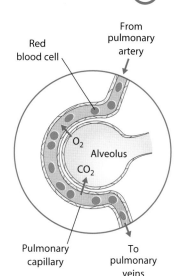

Fig. 17.7 • Gas exchange between alveolus and pulmonary capillary. (Reproduced with permission from Brooker, C., Nicol, M. (Eds.), 2003. Nursing adults. The practice of caring. Mosby, Edinburgh.)

production may be insufficient to maintain patency of the alveoli and lead to respiratory distress (see p. 414).

Oxygen diffuses from the alveolar air, across the very thin layer of cells, the respiratory and capillary membranes into capillary blood (Fig. 17.7). Carbon dioxide leaves the blood and diffuses across the two membranes into the alveoli. The carbon dioxide is excreted during expiration.

For efficient gaseous exchange there must be both adequate ventilation of the lungs and good perfusion with blood.

Lungs

The two lungs are situated within the thoracic cavity, either side of the heart and are protected from injury by the ribs. The right lung is divided into three lobes whereas the left lung is smaller and has only two lobes. Its smaller size is due to the position of the heart in the mediastinum.

A double serous membrane called the pleura lines the thoracic cavity (parietal layer) and covers the outside of each lung (visceral layer). The pleura secretes serous fluid that lubricates the lungs, thus enabling them to move easily as they inflate and deflate. The intact pleura also keeps the lungs inflated.

Breathing (ventilation)

Breathing is the mechanical process by which air moves in and out of the lungs. There are two processes: active inspiration and passive expiration. Expiration is followed by a short pause before the next inspiration. In a normal respiratory cycle (at rest), the amount of air inhaled and exhaled is normally around 500 mL in an adult. This is known as the tidal volume (TV).

During inspiration, the capacity of the thoracic cavity is increased as the diaphragm (muscle dividing the thorax and abdomen) and intercostal muscles (between the ribs) contract. The lungs are stretched, the pressure within the lungs falls and air moves into the lungs.

During expiration, the relaxation of the diaphragm and intercostal muscles leads to an inward and downward movement of the thoracic cage and elastic recoil of the lungs. The pressure in the lungs is greater than atmospheric air and air moves out.

Normal, unlaboured breathing depends on several factors, including compliance, elasticity and airflow resistance.

Common conditions affecting breathing and circulation

Disorders of the CVS, blood and respiratory tract can lead to difficulties with breathing and to circulatory problems. Unfortunately, these are common, e.g. coronary heart disease, a disease that affects both breathing and circulation, accounted for around 88 000 deaths in 2008 in the UK (British Heart Foundation, BHF 2010). Although mortality is decreasing, it remains a major cause of premature death and morbidity. Disorders of the lungs are also common and appear to be on the increase. In 2004 lung diseases led to 117 456 deaths in the UK (British Thoracic Society, BTS 2006).

Diseases that affect breathing and circulation may be acute or chronic and affect all age groups. Some of the more common conditions are outlined below (see Further reading, below, e.g. Brooker & Nicol 2011, Chs 2, 3 and 11).

Common cardiovascular conditions

Cardiac arrhythmias

An abnormal heart rhythm. Some common arrhythmias include:

- Atrial fibrillation (AF) (see p. 411)
- Supraventricular tachycardia (SVT)
- Premature ventricular contraction (PVC)
- Ventricular tachycardia (VT) (see p. 407)
- Ventricular fibrillation (VF) (see p. 407).

Congenital heart disease (CHD)

These are disorders that develop as the heart is formed and present at birth. Common congenital abnormalities include septal defects (hole in the heart) and patent ductus arteriosus (a fetal blood vessel between the left pulmonary artery and the aorta to bypass the lungs). Some defects may be caused by genetic or chromosomal abnormalities such as septal defects in infants with Down's syndrome. Usually congenital defects are treated surgically.

Cardiovascular disease (CVD)

A common condition caused by narrowing of the coronary arteries by atherosclerosis (fatty plaques on the lining layer) with damage to the lining, hardening and eventually a partial obstruction to blood flow through the vessel. Atherosclerosis may be caused by a diet high in saturated fats, hypertension and smoking and exacerbated by obesity and lack of physical exercise (see Boxes 17.5 and 17.7).

CVD can manifest as angina or myocardial infarction (death of tissue) and may eventually lead to chronic heart failure (see below).

- *Angina pectoris*: narrowing leads to a reduction in the blood supply to the myocardium and transient chest pain,

which may radiate to the arms (especially the left), abdomen, jaw, neck and throat. Pain is often induced by exertion, cold weather and wind, emotional stress and sometimes following a large meal. Rest promptly relieves the pain (Box 17.3)

 First aid   Box 17.3

Angina

Recognition
- Chest pain and pain or tingling in the jaw, throat, arms, back or upper central abdomen
- Pain eases with rest and lasts no more than 15 minutes
- Breathlessness.

Aims of treatment
- Encourage a resting position to reduce the workload of the heart
- Pain relief
- Reduce risk of worsening angina.

Treatment
- Encourage the casualty to sit down in a position that eases the pain and breathlessness
- Most people with known angina will have been prescribed sublingual (under the tongue) glyceryl nitrate (GTN), either as a tablet or an aerosol spray to use when they have anginal pain. The casualty should take this as soon as the angina attack starts
- Call for emergency help (dial 999/112) if the pain is not relieved after 15 minutes of using the GTN.

- *Myocardial infarction* (MI) ('heart attack'): usually caused by clot (thrombus) formation where an atheromatous plaque has ruptured – a coronary thrombosis. The coronary artery is occluded and unless the artery is reopened, using thrombolytic drugs that dissolve clots or an invasive procedure such as angioplasty, the myocardium supplied by that vessel will be damaged (infarcted). MI is a common cause of death in Western countries. Approximately 50% of MIs are fatal and, in the majority of these cases death occurs in the first hour after the attack, usually as a result of a cardiac arrhythmia (Webster & Thompson 2011, p 20) (Box 17.4).

Heart failure

The heart fails to pump effectively and is unable to deliver adequate oxygen and nutrients to the cells and tissues. It may occur in one side or both right and left. Heart failure is usually a chronic condition but it can occur acutely. Chronic heart failure is commonly caused by CVD, cardiomyopathy (disease of the myocardium), valvular disease, arrhythmias, hypertension, chronic respiratory disease, etc. (Box 17.5).

Hypertension

This is blood pressure that is persistently 140/90 mmHg or above in adults. Where ambulatory or home blood pressure monitoring (ABPM, HBPM) is used, readings of 135/85 mmHg or above constitute hypertension (National Institute of Health and Clinical Excellence, NICE 2011; see p. 413). In children

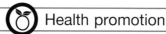

 First aid Box 17.4

Myocardial infarction

Recognition

- Sudden crushing chest pain that is not relieved by rest and lasts longer than 30 minutes. Frequently, the pain comes on when the casualty is resting and this may distinguish it from stable angina. Severe chest pain may wake them from sleep. The pain is usually central, but may radiate to the lower jaw and the left arm. Pain may also be felt in the right arm, throat, back or upper central abdomen
- Sudden light-headedness, dizziness, giddiness
- Nausea and vomiting
- Grey, ashen skin; cyanosis (blue tinge) of lips and extremities
- Sweating
- Cool extremities
- Anxiety, feeling of impending doom
- Breathlessness – copious frothy oral secretions that may be white or pink stained if pulmonary oedema occurs (see p. 416)
- Pulse may be rapid, irregular or weak
- Confusion – as insufficient oxygen is supplied to their brain
- Signs of shock, e.g. pallor, light-headed, extremities cool and moist.

May progress to unconsciousness, or the casualty may stop breathing and the heart stop beating (see Basic life support, pp. 407-410).

Aims of treatment

- Reduce the workload of the heart
- Obtain medical help as soon as possible.

Treatment

- If the casualty is conscious, put in a half-sitting position with knees bent and with head and shoulders supported. Try to allay anxiety
- If the casualty has a history of heart disease and has medication let them take it
- Summon an emergency ambulance by dialling 999/112
- An aspirin tablet (300 mg) should be chewed but only after checking for allergies or history of bleeding
- Continue to monitor condition. If the casualty becomes unconscious, open their airway and check breathing and place in the recovery position. Be prepared to give basic life support if breathing stops or the heart stops.

Note: Patients should be encouraged to seek help at the earliest possible opportunity. It is important that the public are aware of the symptoms of a myocardial infarction and understand that seeking medical help is vital.

Health promotion Box 17.5

Salt intake

A diet containing high levels of salt (sodium chloride) is associated with an increase in blood pressure. High blood pressure (hypertension) is a risk factor for coronary artery disease and for strokes.

The salt content of unprocessed foods is comparatively low, but added salt is present in many prepared or processed foods, e.g. home cooked meals, bacon, cheese, snack foods, ready meals, breakfast cereals, etc. Food products with >1.5 g salt/100 g (0.6 g sodium/100 g) are considered high in salt (NHS Choices 2011).

Adults should be encouraged to keep salt intake within the recommended daily intake. Parents and carers should be aware that the recommended intake for infants and children is much lower than in adults and depends on age. An even lower salt intake may be advised for people who are hypertensive and for those with chronic heart failure. This is because excess salt intake leads to water retention, which increases the blood pressure and leads to the formation of oedema (swelling due to fluid collecting in the tissues, see p. 411).

Student activities

Use the NHS Choices website to answer the following questions:

- What is the recommended salt intake per day for infants, children and adults?
- Find out how to calculate the salt content of a food from the amount of sodium.
- What are the advantages of reducing salt intake?

Reference

NHS Choices, 2011. Salt: the facts – www.nhs.uk/Livewell/Goodfood/Pages/salt.aspx September 2012.

Valvular heart disease

This usually affects the mitral or aortic valves but the tricuspid and pulmonary valves can be affected. The valve may be either stenosed or regurgitant.

Common blood (haematological) conditions

Anaemia

Anaemia occurs when there is a reduced oxygen carrying capacity of the blood, due to reduced numbers of erythrocytes or the amount of haemoglobin, or both. There are several causes including:

- Lack of iron and/or vitamin B_{12} or folate (see Box 17.1)
- Excessive blood loss – acute or chronic
- Abnormal haemoglobin – (see Haemoglobinopathies, below)
- Excessive destruction of erythrocytes – haemolytic anaemia
- Bone marrow suppression – aplastic anaemia

Deep vein thrombosis (DVT)

A DVT is a clot that forms in a vein, usually a large vein of the leg or pelvis, but it can occur in the arm. The predisposing factors are venous stasis (slow blood flow), increased blood stickiness and vein damage. The risk factors for DVT include prolonged immobility (see Ch. 18); increasing age

there is no precise definition for hypertension; however, it is generally agreed to be a blood pressure >130/85 mmHg on three consecutive readings. In the vast majority of cases, no cause is found (Box 17.5). Secondary hypertension may result from a variety of conditions, including kidney disease; endocrine diseases; drugs, e.g. corticosteroids; pre-eclampsia associated with pregnancy (see p. 413).

Rheumatic heart disease

There is chronic inflammation and scarring of the myocardium and heart valve cusps. It usually leads to valvular heart disease.

(>40 years); poor peripheral blood flow; dehydration (see Ch. 19) or clotting disorders. The identification of those at risk and prevention is vital (see Ch. 24). (See Pulmonary embolus, below).

Haemoglobinopathies

The haemoglobinopathies include:

* *Sickle cell disease:* an inherited condition which is due to abnormal haemoglobin, known as HbS. It is seen in individuals from areas where falciparum malaria is common (equatorial Africa, parts of India and parts of the Eastern Mediterranean) and their descendants in Europe, West Indies and the USA. The erythrocytes become sickle-shaped under certain conditions, e.g. hypoxia (reduced oxygen level in the tissues) or dehydration, which leads to reduced oxygen carriage, vessel blockage with pain and infarction and chronic haemolytic anaemia as the abnormal erythrocytes are destroyed in the spleen. At-risk populations should be screened for the abnormal HbS

* *Thalassaemia:* a group of inherited haemoglobinopathies. Thalassaemia can occur in people of all racial groups but is commonly found in people with Mediterranean ancestry.

   The synthesis of globin chains, essential for haemoglobin production, is reduced because of a faulty gene, leading to fragile erythrocytes with impaired oxygen-carrying capacities, which are more rapidly destroyed by the spleen. In thalassaemia major (two faulty genes inherited), there is severe anaemia, jaundice and enlarged liver and spleen; those with the thalassaemia trait (one faulty gene inherited) may have mild anaemia or be asymptomatic.

Leukaemia

A group of malignant diseases affecting the tissues that produce blood cells. Leukaemia leads to anaemia, risk of bleeding and infection. There are several types of leukaemia affecting different leucocytes, e.g. lymphocytic or myelocytic. Leukaemia may be either acute, e.g. acute lymphoblastic leukaemia (ALL) in children or chronic, e.g. chronic myeloid leukaemia (CML) in adults.

 Health promotion   Box 17.6

Self-management in asthma

All people with asthma should have a written self-management plan outlining the daily actions they should take to monitor their condition and identify any deterioration. It should suggest alterations to daily management when their condition deteriorates and indicate when professional help is needed.

A personal asthma action plan is available from Asthma UK, which, if used, should be completed by the patient and their doctor or practice nurse. Any management plan should include the following:

* Record peak expiratory flow rate (PEFR) every morning before medication (see pp. 416–418). If the reading has decreased by 70% of normal then recordings should be taken twice daily. By careful and regular monitoring, it should be possible to recognize when the condition is deteriorating or failing to improve and medical assistance should be sought
* Monitor PEFR recordings twice daily if it deteriorates or there are increased symptoms such as increased wheeze, breathlessness, cough, chest tightness or difficulty sleeping at night
* Use inhalers and other medication as prescribed and use the correct inhaler technique (see pp. 421–423) – the practice nurse should check this on each visit
* Avoid known allergies that trigger an asthma attack, e.g. pets, dust, pollen, etc.
* Smoking cessation
* Avoid contact with people with viral chest infections, as these may trigger an asthma attack.

Student activities

* Access a personal asthma action plan (child under 5 or adult) and consider how it helps patients/parents to manage their condition.
* Discuss with your mentor how some degree of self-management of chronic conditions by patients can influence their feelings of control and improve outcomes and hence, quality of life. However, total self-management will not be an option for all patients, e.g. those with a learning disability or dementia.

Resource

Asthma UK Personal asthma action plan – www.asthma.org.uk September 2012.

Common respiratory conditions

Asthma

Asthma is a chronic condition where inflammation causes spasm of the smooth muscle of the bronchi (bronchospasm), leading to bronchoconstriction and narrowing. There is paroxysmal dyspnoea (difficult breathing) with wheezing and difficulty breathing out, a dry cough and tightness in the chest. The emphasis is on self-management by patients or carers (Box 17.6). An attack of acute, severe asthma is a life-threatening medical emergency.

Bronchiectasis

The bronchi and bronchioles are abnormally dilated and contain copious amounts of foul-smelling purulent (containing pus) sputum. It may be localized or more generalized, when it may be associated with cystic fibrosis (see below).

Bronchiolitis

Inflammation of the bronchioles, usually caused by a viral infection. It occurs mainly during winter months and usually affects infants under 12 months of age.

Chronic obstructive pulmonary disease (COPD)

A group of progressive obstructive lung diseases where airway resistance is increased with reduced airflow, e.g. emphysema, chronic bronchitis or severe asthma (Box 17.7).

* *Chronic bronchitis:* inflammation of the bronchi, defined as a cough with sputum for at least 3 consecutive months in 2 consecutive years. It is frequently caused by tobacco smoke and air pollution.
* *Emphysema (pulmonary):* overdistension of the alveoli leading to rupture and a reduction in gas exchange in the

lungs. It is associated with tobacco smoking, but not in all cases.

Croup

An acute viral infection that causes swelling and/or spasm leading to narrowing of the larynx in children. The child will have harsh-sounding (stridulous) 'croupy' breathing – narrowing of the airway gives rise to the typical crowing inspiration.

Cystic fibrosis (CF)

A genetic disorder affecting the exocrine glands, including those in the respiratory tract and the pancreas. A screening blood test is available for all neonates. Diagnosis may be confirmed by high levels of sodium in sweat. The affected glands produce viscous mucus, which leads to blocked bronchi or ducts, stasis of secretions, infection and fibrosis. The lungs and pancreas are primarily affected, giving rise to repeated chest infections, respiratory problems, digestive problems and eventually heart failure.

Lung cancer

A primary malignant tumour in the lung or bronchi. Smoking is the most important factor in its development but exposure to tobacco smoke, asbestos and environmental pollution are also implicated (Box 17.7). Other cancers, e.g. breast and colorectal, often metastasize (spread) to the lung to form secondary cancers.

Pneumonia

An acute infection of the lung. It may be hospital- or community-acquired or associated with impaired immune responses.

Pulmonary embolism (PE)

A clot that forms in a vein breaks away and travels in the circulation and through the heart to lodge in a pulmonary blood vessel in the lungs (see Deep vein thrombosis, above). It may be fatal or lead to infarction of lung tissue in areas deprived of blood.

Tuberculosis (TB)

A notifiable infectious disease caused by the bacterium *Mycobacterium tuberculosis*. Pulmonary TB is a chronic condition of the lungs, but it also infects other structures such as the lymph nodes, bone, gastrointestinal tract, kidney and causes TB meningitis.

The BCG (bacillus Calmette-Guérin) vaccine is used to protect those at high risk of contracting TB, e.g. infants born in high-risk areas with 40 cases of TB per 100 000 population or higher.

Basic life support – airway maintenance and cardiopulmonary resuscitation

Basic life support (BLS) comprises the first aid measures for maintenance of a clear airway, artificial respiration (e.g. rescue breaths) and chest compressions (external heart massage) in people who have suffered a cardiac arrest (also known as cardiopulmonary arrest), or artificial respiration alone if only breathing has stopped. Cardiac arrest is defined as the sudden cessation of effective output of blood from the heart. There are several forms of cardiac arrest, including:

- *Asystole:* There are no P-QRS-T complexes (see p. 399), the heart is not beating
- *Pulseless electrical activity (PEA):* An electrical rhythm compatible with a cardiac output, but has the clinical signs of a cardiac arrest and therefore no heart rate/pulse
- *Pulseless ventricular tachycardia (VT):* An arrhythmia with rapid ventricular heart rate but insufficient output to produce a pulse
- *Ventricular fibrillation (VF):* An arrhythmia with uncoordinated ventricular activity that produces no output of blood.

The causes of cardiac arrest include myocardial infarction, other heart diseases, hypovolaemia, e.g. severe haemorrhage, electric shock, electrolyte imbalances (see Ch. 19) and severe respiratory problems.

The BLS procedures for cardiopulmonary resuscitation (CPR) outlined below are initiated until the emergency services or hospital cardiac arrest team can start advanced life support (see Ch. 16). The BLS techniques are different for adults, children and newborns. BLS is described using adult procedures and the differences in technique for children and infants (not newborns) are provided later (p. 410).

Adult basic life support

An adult is defined as a person who has reached puberty for the purpose of providing BLS. If the casualty is outside hospital, an emergency ambulance must be summoned by dialling 999/112 (see below). If the cardiopulmonary arrest has occurred in hospital the nurse should know the internal 'crash call' telephone number for summoning the cardiac arrest team. The National Patient Safety Agency (NPSA 2004) advised all NHS Trusts in England and Wales to standardize the internal crash call telephone number to 2222. The 2222 number is also used in Scotland. The vast majority of acute Trusts now use 2222 but until all have converted, individual hospitals may have a different number and all staff should be aware of it.

When initially faced with an adult whom you suspect has experienced a cardiopulmonary arrest, the following procedure should be started immediately:

- Assess for danger.
- If they are unresponsive (no response to gentle shaking or loud speaking – 'can you hear me', etc.). Shout for help and start BLS.
- Open the airway using the head tilt/chin lift method (Fig. 17.8A). Place a hand on the forehead and gently tilt the head backwards. Place the fingertips under the casualty's chin and lift the chin. This is used in the adult to bring the tongue forward to prevent it from obstructing the airway. Using this method in an adult requires the neck to be hyperextended and so should *not* be used when a head or neck injury is suspected. If head or neck injury is suspected in an adult, the jaw thrust method is used. For this manoeuvre, the index and middle fingers are placed under the angle of the lower jaw and steady gentle pressure used to move the jaw upwards and forwards (Fig. 17.8B). The mouth should then open slightly.
- The patient should only be moved if it is not possible to open the airway using this action. In this case turn them gently onto their back.
- Remove any visible obstruction or foreign body from the airway if clearly visible and easy to remove. Do not remove well-fitting dentures.
- Check for normal breathing using the 'look, listen and feel' steps. Spend no more than 10 seconds on these steps.
  - Look at the chest wall and observe any movement
  - Place your ear close to the person's mouth and listen for breath sounds
  - Place your cheek close to the person's mouth to feel any movement of air.
- If there is any indication that the person is breathing, turn them into the recovery position (see Fig. 16.15A) and monitor until help arrives.
- If there is no sign of breathing and you are alone, dial 999/112 *immediately*.
- If not breathing start chest compressions immediately. The heel of your hand should be placed in the centre of the chest. The other hand should be placed on top of the first and the fingers interlocked. Firm pressure is then applied with the heels of the hands (Fig. 17.9A). The

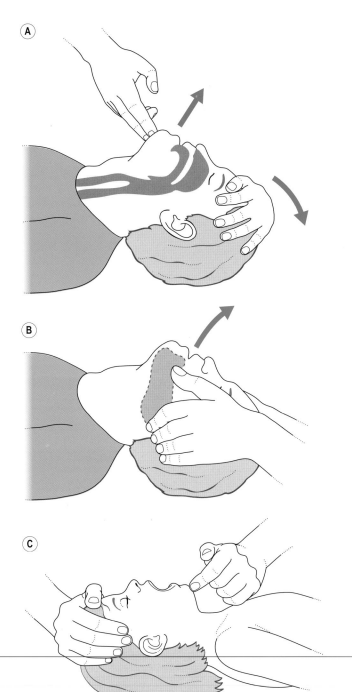

Fig. 17.8 • Opening the airway: (A) Head tilt/chin lift – adult. (B) Jaw thrust – adult. (C) Head tilt/chin lift – child. (A, B reproduced with permission from Mallik, M., Hall, C., Howard, D., 2009. Nursing knowledge and practice. Foundations for decision making, third ed. Baillière Tindall; C, reproduced with permission from Trigg, E., Mohammed, T.A. (Eds.), 2010. Practices in children's nursing. Guidelines for Hospital and Community, third ed. Churchill Livingstone, Edinburgh.)

elbows should be kept straight so that the pressure is exerted downwards. The pressure should be sufficient to depress the sternum by 5–6 cm in an adult. Pressure any greater than this may fracture ribs.

- Thirty chest compressions are performed at a rate of between 100–120/minute followed by two rescue breaths.

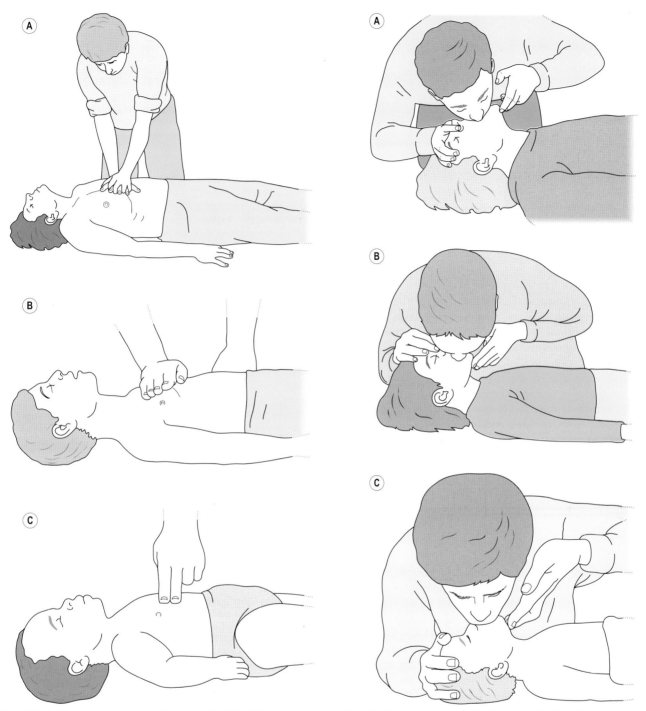

Fig. 17.9 • Chest compression: (A) Adult. (B) Child. (C) Infant.

Fig. 17.10 • Rescue breaths: (A) Adult. (B) Child. (C) Infant.

• Give the casualty two effective rescue breaths. With the airway open, pinch the soft tissue of the nose with the index finger and thumb and open the casualty's mouth a little. Take a deep breath and place your lips around the casualty's mouth and blow steadily into the mouth over 1 second (Fig. 17.10A). While doing this, you should watch to see whether the chest wall rises. Then take your mouth away from the casualty's mouth and watch the chest wall fall as the air comes out. If you don't see the chest wall rise, check the airway is open and give another breath. Do not attempt more

than two breaths before going back to chest compressions.

Note: In hospital, this may be achieved by inserting a plastic airway and using an Ambu bag connected to an oxygen supply to deliver these breaths while waiting for the cardiac arrest team to arrive.

• A lone first aider does 30 chest compressions before two rescue breaths but if two first aiders are present, the 30:2 ratio is used, with one person undertaking chest compression, while the other does rescue breaths and maintains the airway. If more than one rescuer is present,

- another should take over CPR every 2 minutes to avoid fatigue.
- Continue CPR until help arrives or the person starts breathing normally

(Resuscitation Council, UK 2010).

Basic life support for infants and children

A child is defined as a person aged 1 year and up to the age of puberty and an infant as being less than 12 months old for the provision of BLS. The differences between BLS for children and infants and that for adults (see above) are outlined in Box 17.8 (see also chapter 13).

Assessment and observation – circulation and breathing

Assessment and observation form the basis for nursing management and treatment and are therefore key skills to learn. However, observations do not have to be complex, nor require sophisticated equipment. Some of the best skills for assessment and observation are those that involve looking, listening, touching and smelling.

This section covers important areas for the assessment of breathing and circulation and includes assessment of the skin, the heart rate, blood pressure and respiration.

Although assessment is useful, it only becomes a valuable tool if nurses know what to do with the findings. All data should be recorded in the patient's notes and/or on observation charts (see Ch. 14). Where nurses suspect that the data are abnormal, then the person in charge should be notified as soon as possible.

Skin – general assessment

Assessment of the skin provides useful information about both breathing and circulation. Nurses should take every opportunity to assess a person's skin, e.g. while helping them with personal hygiene. More information about skin condition and assessment is provided in Chapters 16 and 25.

In health, the skin should be warm, dry, intact and normal colour for racial group. In people with either very pale or dark skin it may be difficult to notice abnormalities such as pallor or a bluish hue (cyanosis). This explains why it is important to also look at the mucosae, e.g. inside the mouth or the conjunctiva inside the lower eyelid, which in health should be pink and moist.

Changes in skin colour

The colour of the skin, including the nail beds and lips and mucosae can provide valuable information:

- Cyanosis is a bluish hue to skin and mucosae. It is due to hypoxia (reduced oxygen level in the tissues). It may be central cyanosis where the bluish hue affects the lips, the oral mucosa, tongue and conjunctivae, whereas cyanosis affecting the extremities – fingertips, toes, ear lobes or nose – is peripheral cyanosis.

BLS – differences in techniques for children and infants	Box 17.8

- *Assessment of consciousness:* Gently shake the baby or child, speak loudly or call their name if known. They may respond by moving, swallowing, coughing, crying or a verbal response in older children, or breathing (regular breaths more than occasional) may be obvious. If they respond, do not move unless in danger. Check for injuries and get help if necessary. Continue to check condition
- *Opening the airway:* In children and infants the head tilt/chin lift is used but without over-extension because this can cause the airway to close (Fig. 17.8C). Jaw thrust is used if head/neck injury is suspected but this time only the index finger on the lower jaw is used
- *Look in the mouth* and remove any obvious obstruction
- *Check the breathing* as above. If they are breathing, turn them on their side and obtain help. If the child is not breathing, give five rescue breaths. Pinch the nose and place your lips around the child's mouth and blow gently into the lungs (Fig. 17.10B). Only take shallow breaths and do not use all the air in your lungs. While doing this, you should watch to see whether the chest wall rises. As it does so, cease blowing and let the chest fall.

In infants, place your mouth over the infant's mouth and nose and blow gently to give the initial rescue breaths (Fig. 17.10C, p. 409). The amount of air used is that amount that fills your cheeks.

- *Check the circulation* by looking for movement, swallowing, etc. If you have been trained, feel for the carotid pulse in children or the brachial pulse (on the inner aspect of the elbow) in infants.

If the circulation is present, continue rescue breaths for 1 minute before dialling 999/112 for an emergency ambulance

- *If circulation is absent* or the pulse is <60 b.p.m., chest compressions (external cardiac massage) should be started immediately.

For children, the heel of one hand is placed one fingerbreadth above the junction of the rib margin and sternum (Fig. 17.9B). Pressure is then applied with the heel of the hand with the elbows kept straight. The pressure should be sufficient to depress the chest by about one-third of its depth. Fifteen chest compressions are performed at a rate of approximately 100/minute followed by two rescue breaths.

For infants, two fingers are used (Fig. 17.9C) or alternatively, the first aider may put their hands around the infant's chest and place one thumb above the other, one fingerbreadth below the internipple line in the centre of the sternum. Again the chest is compressed to around one-third of its depth.

- *When CPR is necessary* the 15:2 ratio is continued. CPR continues until help arrives.

Resources

Resuscitation Council (UK), 2010. Paediatric basic life support (healthcare professionals with a duty to respond): www.resus.org.uk/pages/pblsalgo.pdf

Note: Separate guidelines are available for Newborn Life Support: www.resus.org.uk/pages/nlsalgo.pdf

All websites accessed September 2012.

- Extremities that are red in colour are also likely to be warmer to touch. This is more commonly found after exercise or when the patient has a high temperature (pyrexia) and the blood vessels in the skin are dilated (vasodilatation) (see Ch. 14).

- Skin may be very white (blanched) when the blood supply has become so severely reduced that the tissues do not have an oxygen supply. If left untreated the skin will become blackened in colour and gangrene is likely to ensue (see Ch. 25).
- Very pale skin may be associated with anaemia. The lips, oral mucosa and conjunctivae will also be pale in anaemia (see p. 405).

Skin turgor and oedema

Assessment of the skin should include turgor and the presence of oedema. Turgor indicates the elasticity of the skin and although this decreases with age, skin turgor may be useful in a holistic assessment of hydration status. Reduced turgor may be an early sign of dehydration (see Ch. 19).

To assess skin turgor, a fold of skin, usually on the back of the hand, is lifted. Once released, it should quickly return to its original position. However, because skin loses its elasticity with age it will not return to its original position so quickly in older people.

Oedema is an abnormal accumulation of tissue fluid between the cells (see Ch. 19). It usually collects in dependent regions such as the legs, ankles/feet or sacral area. For example, if someone spends much of the day sitting in a chair, fluid will collect in the sacral area and ankles. This is partly due to immobility and lack of normal contraction of the calf muscles that squeezes the veins and helps venous blood return to the heart (see Ch. 25). However, dependent oedema is also compounded by gravity, which allows fluid to collect in these areas. Oedema may be seen in people with the following conditions:

- Heart failure
- Venous insufficiency (see Ch. 25)
- Protein deficiency
- Kidney disease
- Liver failure.

However, swollen ankles with some oedema may be found when standing still in hot weather or during pregnancy and are not necessarily a sign of ill-health.

The term 'pitting' is used to describe oedema that remains indented or pitted when lightly pressed. This is frequently a sign of more severe oedema.

Oedema is not usually visible until the body has retained at least 4 L of fluid, which is equivalent to approximately 4 kg of weight gain. In some cases daily weighing is used to monitor fluid retention.

Capillary refill time

Capillary refill time is useful for assessing skin perfusion (blood volume passing through the skin) and cardiac output. Although peripheral areas such as the nail bed may be used, central areas such as the sternum are more useful in people with a poor cardiac output and poor peripheral circulation. To test capillary refill time, two fingers are lightly pressed into the area for a period of 5 seconds. On release, skin colour should return to normal within 2 seconds. If it takes longer for the skin colour to return, capillary refill time is prolonged and it is likely that the person has a low cardiac output.

Heart/pulse rate

When blood is pumped from the heart there is rhythmic expansion and recoil of the arteries in the vascular system. Wherever an artery is near the skin surface this ejection of blood will cause a pulse, which can be felt when the artery is gently pressed against a bony prominence. In adults and older children this is commonly felt at the wrist where the radial artery crosses the forearm bone, the radius (see Ch. 14). In infants and children less than 2 years of age, it is more accurate to assess HR by counting the apex beat of the heart (Kelsey & McEwing 2008) (see also Ch. 14).

The pulse rate should be easily palpated and is a useful measure of the function of the cardiovascular system. The pulse should reflect the HR and varies with age. It is normally between 60 and 80 b.p.m. in adolescents and adults at rest, although up to 100 b.p.m. is considered normal. In the neonate, the HR is faster and is usually between 110 and 160 b.p.m. depending on whether the baby is active, crying, resting or asleep. The HR slows during infancy and childhood to reach adult levels during adolescence (see Ch. 14).

A tachycardia is a heart rate greater than 100 b.p.m. in an adolescent or adult. It occurs in the following situations:

- During and immediately after exercise
- Anxiety, fear
- Pain (see Ch. 23)
- Infection (see Ch 15)
- Pyrexia (see Ch 14)
- Anaemia
- Hypovolaemia (low blood volume)

Bradycardia is a heart rate less than 60 b.p.m. It occurs in the following situations:

- In a fit athletic person
- During sleep
- Hypothermia
- Disorders of the sinus node (the 'pacemaker' of the heart)
- Heart disease, e.g. after myocardial infarction.
- Some drugs used to treat heart disease, e.g. digoxin or atenolol (a beta-blocker).

The volume (force) of the pulse is also assessed, such as thready or bounding (see Ch. 14).

When a pulse is noted to be irregular, it should be reported and documented in the nursing notes and on the appropriate charts. Many heart diseases, such as atrial fibrillation (AF), cause an irregular pulse rate and commonly occur in older people. Further investigations should be undertaken, an apex-radial pulse should be recorded and an ECG performed (Box 17.9).

Nursing skills   Box 17.9

Recording apex-radial pulse (adult)

Note: To record an apex-radial pulse, two members of staff are needed.

Equipment

- Stethoscope
- Watch with second hand
- Observation chart.

Preparation

- Explain the observation and seek verbal consent; maintain respect and dignity at all times
- Ensure that the patient is either sitting or lying and allow time for rest following exertion or a situation that could affect heart rate, such as bad news.

Procedure

- Draw the curtains around the bed space to ensure the patient's privacy and dignity
- One nurse places the diaphragm of a stethoscope over the apex of the heart, at the 5th intercostal space and approximately 12 cm to the left of the midline (see Fig. 17.1); the other nurse locates the radial pulse
- Using the same watch and commencing at the same time, the nurses count the heartbeat for 1 minute
- Help the patient with clothing and replace bedding before opening the curtains
- Clean stethoscope earpieces according to local policy
- Wash hands
- The apex beat and radial pulse recordings are charted in different colours (see local policy)
- Any abnormalities are reported and documented.

If there is a large difference between the two values, it can be concluded that the radial pulse rate does not accurately reflect the heart rate, i.e. there is a pulse deficit. A heart arrhythmia should be suspected and an ECG performed if this is a new sign.

Peripheral pulses

Pulses are found wherever a blood vessel lies close to the skin surface. The radial pulse has been described above. Other peripheral pulses, e.g. femoral artery (see Ch. 14), are assessed in a variety of specific situations.

The electrocardiogram

The ECG waveform depicts the electrical activity of the heart (see p. 399 and Fig. 17.4). It is used to detect arrhythmias and heart diseases such as myocardial infarction. (Readers requiring more information about ECG should consult Further reading, below.)

Blood pressure

Blood pressure (BP) is the pressure exerted upon the wall of the arteries by the circulating blood. It is a useful, non-invasive measurement, widely used in patient assessment (see Ch. 14). BP is usually measured indirectly using a sphygmomanometer (usually aneroid) or an electronic device. BP has two measurements and is measured in millimetres of mercury pressure (mmHg): the upper reading, the systolic pressure and the lower reading, the diastolic pressure (see Ch. 14).

BP is a routine aspect of health assessment in adults and at prescribed intervals for monitoring condition, e.g. during blood transfusion or for hypertension. BP is less frequently recorded as part of assessment in children.

The normal BP range varies with age: in adults the optimum BP is <120 systolic and <80 diastolic, and a normal BP is described as <130/<85 mmHg (Williams et al 2004). In the neonate, BP is normally between 60 and 85 systolic/20 and 60 diastolic mmHg (see Ch. 14).

In addition, there are many factors that normally influence BP throughout a 24-hour period (see Ch. 14). These include:

- Posture
- Activity and exercise
- Emotional state such as fear, anxiety
- Presence of pain (see Ch. 23).

A sustained increase in BP is termed hypertension and in adults this is defined as a BP of 140/90 mmHg or over measured in the clinic (see pp. 404–405). BP tends to increase with age in developed countries. Several lifestyle factors contribute to hypertension (Williams et al 2004). These include:

- Increase in body weight leading to obesity (see Ch. 19)
- Sedentary lifestyle
- Excessive alcohol intake
- Increased salt (sodium chloride) intake (see Box 17.5, p. 405)
- Environmental stress (see Ch. 11).

Hypertension is a serious condition and leads to myocardial infarction, heart failure, strokes, kidney damage and retinal changes, etc. It is important to accurately measure and record the BP (Box 17.10).

A low blood pressure that is insufficient to maintain tissue blood flow and oxygenation is termed hypotension. It may be caused by:

- Dehydration
- Hot weather when the arteries dilate (vasodilatation) and dehydration may also be present
- Heart failure
- Drugs such as beta-blockers
- Serious haemorrhage (Box 17.11)

Hypotension may lead to feelings of dizziness or even fainting (syncope) because insufficient blood and hence oxygen reaches the brain (Box 17.12). Fainting can also be caused by other factors. These include:

- Hot weather or a sudden change in environmental temperature
- Sudden change in body position such as standing or getting out of bed too quickly
- Standing still for a prolonged period, causing the blood to pool in the legs
- Emotional upset such as the sight of blood.

Reflective practice   Box 17.10

Maximizing the accuracy of blood pressure measurement

Measures that help to ensure accuracy include the following:

- Ensure the BP device/sphygmomanometer is 'properly validated, maintained and regularly recalibrated according to manufacturer's instructions' (NICE 2011, p 10)
- Give an explanation about measuring BP to the patient/parent/carer
- Provide a relaxed environment
- Do not record BP if the person has been active – allow them to rest first
- Remove tight clothes that might constrict the blood flow in the brachial artery in the arm
- Position the patient either sitting or lying down, with their arm straight and supported so that the muscles are relaxed
- Use a cuff of the correct size (see Ch. 14)
- Position the device at the correct level
- Record BP in both arms and use the arm with the higher reading on future occasions
- Make a note of the systolic and diastolic readings and record them on the chart and in the notes
- Inform the nurse in charge if the blood pressure has altered by more than 10 mmHg from a previous recording or from the normal BP range for age
- The registered nurse will tell the patient/parent the BP reading, explain any implications and answer their questions.

Student activities

- Think about a recent placement where blood pressure was routinely measured. Which of the measures listed above did you see being used?
- Discuss with your mentor how you might increase the accuracy of blood pressure measurement.

Reference

National Institute for Health and Clinical Excellence (NICE), 2011. Hypertension clinical management of primary hypertension in adults. Clinical guideline CG 127. Online. Available: www.nice.org.uk/nicemedia/live/13561/56008/56008.pdf August 2011.

 First aid   Box 17.11

Minor bleeding, serious haemorrhage and shock

Bleeding ranges from very slight such as after a minor cut up to life-threatening haemorrhage resulting in shock.

Student activities

Using the resource find out about the following:

- First aid for a minor cut/graze and that for severe external bleeding
- Dealing with a nose bleed (epistaxis)
- List some possible signs of internal bleeding
- The signs and symptoms of shock.

Resource

Austin, M., Crawford, R., Armstrong, V.J. (Eds.), 2009. First aid manual. Authorized manual of St John Ambulance, St Andrew's Ambulance Association and The British Red Cross, ninth ed. Dorling Kindersley, London.

 First aid   Box 17.12

Fainting

Recognition

- Pallor
- Weak pulse
- Light headedness
- Stumble or fall suddenly to the ground.

Aims of treatment

- Restore blood flow to the brain by positioning the person so that gravity assists blood flow
- Deal with the cause.

Treatment

- Check and maintain an open airway (see pp. 408, 410) if the person has already fainted
- A person who feels faint should be sat on a chair, leaning forward with their head between their knees, or lying down, with their legs elevated
- Loosen tight clothing at the neck and chest
- Try to ensure fresh air
- Reassure as consciousness returns
- Gradually allow the person to sit up
- Check for injuries if the person fell
- Do not give anything orally until the person is fully recovered, then offer cold non-alcoholic fluids.

Note: If the person does not start to regain consciousness quickly, open their airway and check breathing and circulation (see pp. 408, 410). Put the person into the recovery position (see Ch. 16) and call for medical assistance. If necessary, commence BLS (see pp. 407–410).

Blood pressure during pregnancy

There is a decrease in BP during the first 6 months of pregnancy and then a gradual increase to pre-pregnant levels as full-term approaches (Murray & Hassall 2009). Pregnant women should be followed-up regularly and their blood pressure monitored. Urine should also be examined for proteinuria; an early sign of pre-eclampsia (National Institute for Health and Clinical Excellence, NICE 2010a). High blood pressure in pregnancy is potentially life-threatening for both mother and unborn child.

Later in pregnancy there may be postural hypotension as the enlarging uterus can compress the inferior vena cava when the woman lies supine, thereby reducing the venous return to the heart (Murray & Hassall 2009).

Central venous pressure

Central venous pressure (CVP) records the pressure in the central venous system or the right atrium of the heart and is a useful measurement to assess fluid status. Central venous pressure is measured in the acutely ill and as such is frequently seen in intensive care or high dependency units. However, central venous pressures may also be measured in the patient on the general ward and so it is useful to have some idea of the importance of this measurement (see Further reading, below, e.g. Nicol et al 2012).

Breathing – general assessment

Assessment of breathing includes respiratory rate, depth and rhythm and assessment of the function of the lungs. In infants and children changes in breathing (plus other vital signs) are important indicators of deterioration in their condition (see below and Kelsey & McEwing 2008, Ch. 8).

Normal breathing at rest is silent, even and regular and is the unconscious active inspiration of air followed by passive expiration. However, both inspiration and expiration may become active with the person forcing air in or out of the lungs. Active breathing usually uses accessory muscles of breathing, the abdominal muscles and the muscles of the neck and shoulders. The use of the accessory muscles occurs in normal deep breathing and in a person with breathing difficulties.

Respiratory rate

The respiratory rate should be recorded as one of the first observations in all general assessments (see Chapter 14). In addition, the respiratory rate should be recorded as part of ongoing monitoring of vital signs, as 'respiratory rate is a significant predictor of critical illness' (Butler-Williams et al 2005, p 35). When counting the respiratory rate, breathing should be observed for a 60-second period, with the person at rest. It is also a useful idea to count the respiratory rate without the person being aware and inadvertently altering their breathing rate.

The normal respiratory rate varies with age. The normal adult respiratory rate at rest is usually between 12 and 15 breaths/minute, while it is normal for a neonate to breathe at 30–60 breaths/minute (see Ch. 14).

A respiratory rate that is faster than that expected for age (tachypnoea) is normal when caused by:

- Exercise
- Fear
- Anxiety
- Pain
- Fever.

Disorders of breathing and circulation that cause tachypnoea may include:

- Anaemia
- Heart diseases
- Severe haemorrhage
- Most respiratory illnesses – COPD, chest infection, asthma.

A respiratory rate that is slower then expected for age (bradypnoea) is normal when the person is sleeping; however, it is abnormal when caused by:

- Sedation and opioid analgesics (see Ch. 23)
- Excessive alcohol intake.

Breathing patterns – depth and rhythm

The breathing pattern should be assessed while counting the respiratory rate. When assessing breathing patterns, the nurse should observe features that include:

- *Depth of breathing* (deep, normal or shallow): Very deep, sighing breathing (Kussmaul breathing) is a feature of uncontrolled diabetes with associated acidosis. Sighing breathing occurs with severe haemorrhage. Shallow breathing occurs if it is painful to breathe deeply such as with rib fractures or following abdominal or thoracic surgery (see Ch. 24).
- *Difficulty in breathing* (dyspnoea): Difficult or laboured breathing occurs in a variety of conditions such as: a foreign body in the airway, asthma, COPD, pneumonia, pulmonary embolism, heart failure, severe anaemia and some neurological conditions such as motor neurone disease. Orthopnoea describes difficulty breathing when lying flat. A person with dyspnoea may use the accessory muscles of respiration in an effort to move more air in and out of the lungs. In the adult, these include the abdominal muscles, the muscles of the neck and shoulders and in extreme situations, the person may straighten or arch the back in order to expand the thoracic cage. Pursed-lip breathing is associated with chronic respiratory diseases.

  Accessory muscles of respiration in children include the contraction of anterior chest wall muscles and the nurse should observe for nasal flaring and head bobbing on breathing in.
- *Chest wall movement:* In normal breathing, there is symmetrical chest expansion with both sides moving together. Failure of both sides of the chest to expand simultaneously may be a sign of pneumothorax or serious rib fractures (paradoxical breathing).

  In children asymmetric chest expansion may be a sign of heart failure. Sometimes the chest is sucked inward with each breath (chest retraction/recession). The degree of recession gives some indication of the severity of respiratory distress.
- *Regularity of breathing pattern:* Apnoea is the absence of breathing for a period of 20 seconds or more. This may occur for short periods and be followed by a period of normal breathing. Apnoea occurring during sleep is more common in people who are obese, those with heart failure or chronic respiratory disease (see Ch. 10).

  In full-term infants an irregular breathing pattern can be normal. There is rapid breathing followed by a short period of apnoea. If the baby's colour and HR do not change then this is normal. However, more prolonged abnormal apnoea occurs in very low birthweight infants, especially in those infants born at or before 32 weeks' gestation (MacGregor 2008).

  Cheyne–Stokes breathing is an abnormal breathing cycle characterized by repeated cycles that begin with slow, shallow breathing, gradually becoming abnormally rapid and deep followed by decreasing depth and rate and a period of apnoea. It is usually associated with a poor prognosis and may occur prior to death (see Ch. 12).

Abnormal breath sounds

Normal breathing is silent. Any noise that occurs during breathing is therefore abnormal. The noise may occur either during inspiration or expiration. Abnormal sounds include:

- *Stridor:* A high-pitched noise that occurs on inspiration or expiration and indicates a disturbance to the airflow in the upper respiratory tract. Inspiratory stridor is a feature of epiglottitis (inflammation of the epiglottis), which primarily affects children
- *Stertor:* Snoring sound heard during breathing occurs during sleep and in altered consciousness
- *Wheeze:* A whistling sound heard on expiration and indicates a resistance to airflow in the lower respiratory tract such as occurs in bronchospasm (constriction of the bronchi). Wheezing frequently occurs during an asthma attack (see also p. 406). As it occurs when breathing out it is referred to as an expiratory wheeze. Box 17.13 outlines the first aid for asthma

---

 First aid   **Box 17.13**

Asthma attack

Recognition

- Great difficulty in breathing
- Wheeze on breathing out
- Anxious, restless and distressed
- Difficulty in speaking
- Cyanosis
- Exhaustion.

Note: Cough is a feature in some people.

Aims of treatment

- Relieve breathlessness where possible
- Alleviate anxiety
- Seek emergency assistance if required.

Treatment

- If the person is known to have asthma and has their medication with them, assist them to use their relieving inhaler. Help the casualty to stay calm and relaxed
- Assist the person to sit up (sitting forwards may help) and suggest they take slow breaths
- If this is the first attack the casualty should be seen by a doctor
- If the attack is severe or prolonged, or is not eased by the medication, summon help by dialling 999/112. Check their condition – breathing, airway, pulse and response
- Be ready to open the airway and start BLS
- Stay with the person, reassure and keep them calm until help arrives.

- *Grunting:* A breath sound heard mainly in neonates. It is a serious sign of worsening respiratory function and professional help should be sought immediately
- *Rattle:* A rattle is heard both on inspiration and expiration and is associated with secretions in the lower respiratory tract (see pp. 420–421). Sometimes this is associated with end-of-life (see Ch. 12).

Cough and sputum

In health, regular deep breathing and ciliary action remove normal secretions and inhaled foreign particles. Secretions are generally swallowed but may be coughed up (expectorated). However, when these mechanisms are ineffective or there is an increase in mucus secretion or foreign particles, the cough becomes essential (Jones & Moffat 2002). The cough reflex is part of the protective mechanisms that protect the airway from foreign bodies that either irritate or may obstruct the airway (see p. 403). The cough reflex occurs, e.g. when food or fluid goes the 'wrong way'.

Choking occurs when there is a partial blockage to the upper airway. The person will be anxious, have difficulty breathing and may cough. This may dislodge the foreign body but, if not, urgent treatment may be necessary to prevent asphyxia. This is characterized by severe hypoxia leading to hypoxaemia (reduced oxygen content in arterial blood) and hypercapnia (increased carbon dioxide in arterial blood). Unconsciousness occurs and without effective treatment, eventually death.

Choking has a number of causes but usually occurs when a foreign body, e.g. food such as peanuts, small toys or pieces of toys, loose tooth, pen top, etc., is inhaled. Box 17.14 outlines the first aid for an adult who is choking.

The first aid procedures for choking in infants and children differ from those in adults but obviously it is preferable to prevent choking in the first place by identifying the risks and excluding them whenever possible, such as by choosing toys suitable for a child's age. Box 17.15 provides an opportunity to consider both the prevention of choking in children and the first aid.

A cough may be described as dry or productive. Coughing may be associated with pain in some chest conditions and following chest or abdominal surgery (see Ch. 24). Prolonged coughing can cause muscle pain and may deter patients from coughing. The nurse should assess levels of pain and ensure that effective pain relief is provided (see Ch. 23).

A dry cough is one that develops without the presence of excess secretions. The cough could result from an irritant in the upper airway such as smoke or cold air and sometimes develops into a 'tickly' cough. Some forms of medication cause a dry cough, e.g. some heart medication such as angiotensin-converting enzyme (ACE) inhibitors. A constant dry cough is a nuisance and may result in the person stopping their medication if they think this is the likely cause. Therefore, it is important to listen to the patient's complaints and inform the prescriber so that medication can be reviewed.

A productive cough is one where excess mucus or sputum ('phlegm') is present in the respiratory tract. When the airways are inflamed, as occurs during an infection, there is an excessive secretion of mucus, which then accumulates in the airways. The mucus is usually expectorated by coughing. A productive cough may also be found where ciliary action is ineffective. Smoking is known to damage the cilia, and is responsible for the so-called 'smokers cough'.

The nurse should observe the characteristics of sputum, which include:

First aid Box 17.14

Choking in adults

Recognition

- Struggling for breath
- Difficulty talking
- Pointing to/clutching the throat
- Anxious
- Blueness of the lips and mouth.

Aims of treatment

- Dislodge the foreign body.

Treatment

- Remove debris, dentures and loose teeth from the mouth
- Stand to the side and slightly behind the person, supporting the chest with one hand and lean them well forward
- Use the heel of the hand to give up to five sharp slaps on the back between the shoulder blades (scapulae)
- Check to see if the obstruction is relieved after each back blow
- If the slaps do not relieve the obstruction, attempt abdominal thrusts:
  - Stand behind the person, with both arms around the upper part of their abdomen
  - Ensure the person is leaning forward
  - Place your clenched fist between the umbilicus and bottom of the breast bone (sternum) and grasp it with your other hand
  - Pull sharply inwards and upwards to dislodge the foreign body
- Repeat alternating back slaps and abdominal thrusts if the obstruction remains
- If the foreign body is not dislodged and/or the person is unconscious, summon emergency assistance by telephoning 999/112.
- If the casualty becomes unconscious commence BLS (see pp. 407–410)

Resource

Resuscitation Council (UK), 2010. Choking: www.resus.org.uk/pages/bls.pdf September 2012.

Health promotion and first aid Box 17.15

A. Preventing choking in infants and small children

A friend who has a new baby and a toddler aged 18 months tells you that she and her partner are worried about the risk of choking, as they have heard how easily this can happen in infants and small children. She asks you about how they might reduce the risk as much as possible.

Student activity

- Use the resources below and find out how your friend and her partner can minimize the risk of choking in their children.

B. First aid for choking in infants and children
Student activity

- Access the Resuscitation Council Paediatric Choking Treatment Algorithm and discuss with your mentor the different techniques used for an infant and a child over 1 year.

Resources

Child Accident Prevention Trust – www.capt.org.uk
Resuscitation Council (UK), 2010. Choking – www.resus.org.uk/pages/pbls.pdf
Royal Society for the Prevention of Accidents (RoSPA) – www.rospa.com/homesafety/adviceandinformation/childsafety/accidents-to-children.aspx
All websites accessed September 2012.

---

1. Colour
   - White mucoid such as with a severe 'cold'
   - Yellow or green sputum containing pus (purulent) in bacterial infections affecting the respiratory tract. Common in COPD and CF
   - Red if containing fresh blood or having a 'rusty' appearance if blood is old. Coughing up blood or bloodstained secretions is known as haemoptysis. The amount of bloodstaining can vary from blood streaks to a massive haemorrhage. If bloodstained secretions are new, or develop into a frank haemorrhage, the nurse in charge or the medical team must be notified.
2. Consistency
   - Viscous or sticky secretions, which are difficult to expectorate, may occur in dehydration (see Ch. 19)
   - Copious watery, frothy secretions are characteristic of pulmonary oedema (fluid in the alveoli), which may be due to heart failure. The secretions are generally white but may have a pink tinge.
3. Quantity
   - Increasing or decreasing amounts of sputum should be documented and reported.
4. Odour
   - Foul-smelling sputum may be a feature of bronchiectasis (see p. 406) or lung abscess.

The characteristics of sputum produced during coughing are recorded in the nursing notes and charts and any changes reported to the person in charge.

A specimen of sputum will be sent to the laboratory for microscopy, culture and sensitivity if infection is suspected (see Ch. 15). Box 17.16 outlines the safe and effective collection of a sputum specimen. If the patient is unable to expectorate, a specimen may be obtained during nasopharyngeal/tracheal suctioning (see p. 421) by using a sputum trap.

Peak expiratory flow rate

The peak expiratory flow rate (PEFR) is the greatest rate of airflow out of the lungs and is measured in litres per minute (L/min) during a forced expiration. The normal range for PEFR depends on age, height and gender. It is an important measure of lung function and is frequently used as a guide to monitor the progress of a condition such as asthma or the person's response to their medication. A Wright or mini-Wright peak flow meter is used to measure PEFR (Box 17.17, Fig. 17.11).

Nursing skills Box 17.16

Collection of a sputum specimen

Equipment

- Disposable gloves and apron
- Sterile specimen container and specimen bag
- Request form for microbiology laboratory
- Fresh disposable sputum carton with lid if appropriate
- Tissues
- Mouthwash/teeth cleaning facilities
- Waste bag.

Preparation

- Explain the procedure to the patient to ensure informed consent
- Ensure that the specimen is obtained before the patient uses an antiseptic mouthwash, as this can affect the results (see Ch. 15).

Procedure

- Collect the specimen container, request form and transport bag
- Wash hands and put on plastic apron and non-sterile gloves (Ch. 15) and follow local policy for other protective clothing for specific infections, e.g. tuberculosis
- Ensure privacy to produce a sample
- The physiotherapist may be asked to assist by helping the patient to expectorate
- Ask the patient to cough and expectorate sputum into the sterile container
- Replace the lid on the sterile container and make sure that it is securely closed
- Check that the sample is sputum and not saliva. Observe the sputum and note the characteristics (see above)
- Offer the patient a mouthwash or teeth cleaning facilities, especially if expectorating foul-smelling sputum
- Change disposable sputum carton and observe as required and place in waste bag
- Dispose of used sputum carton/waste bag in the clinical waste bag
- Remove gloves and apron and wash hands
- Label the specimen container with the correct patient information and enclose in a specimen bag with the correctly completed request for investigation form
- Arrange for transfer to the laboratory
- Offer the patient a drink if appropriate
- Record date and time the specimen was collected in the patient's nursing and medical notes.

Nursing skills Box 17.17

Measuring peak expiratory flow rate (see Fig. 17.11)

Equipment

- Peak flow meter and disposable mouthpiece
- Observation chart
- Disposable apron.

Preparation

- Explain the procedure to the patient to ensure informed consent
- Ensure that the reading is taken at the correct time, i.e. before and/or after inhaled medication (see pp. 421–423).

Procedure

- Wash your hands and put on apron
- Attach the disposable mouthpiece and ensure that the meter is set at zero
- Ask or assist the patient to stand or sit upright
- Ask the patient to breathe in as deeply as possible, seal their lips around the mouthpiece and then exhale as forcibly and as quickly as possible
- Make a note of the result and if possible take two more consecutive readings (after resetting the meter to zero) and record the highest. Note: It may only be possible to obtain one reading if the patient is distressed by breathlessness, coughing, etc.
- Ensure that any post PEFR medication is given and recorded (see Ch. 22)
- Check that the patient is comfortable
- If the patient retains the disposable mouthpiece for further use, it is stored dry and covered. Otherwise it is disposed of in the clinical waste according to local procedures
- Chart the results and report any changes or difficulties in obtaining three results.

Further reading

Higgins, D., 2005. Measuring PEFR. Nursing Times 101 (10), 32–33.

Pulse oximetry

Non-invasive pulse oximetry is used to measure the percentage of saturated haemoglobin in the arterial blood and gives a useful indication of the amount of oxygen in the peripheral blood. Oxygen saturation monitoring is frequently undertaken, either continuously or as a periodic measurement. The normal oxygen saturation range is 95–98% (see Ch. 14).

The pulse oximetry device comprises a probe connected to a monitor (Fig. 17.12). The probe should be placed where it is in close contact with the blood such as the nail bed or ear lobe. Arterial oxygen saturation (SpO_2) along with pulse rate can be monitored (Ball 2011). Pulse oximetry has limitations and results must be interpreted carefully.

Recent research recommends that pulse oximetry be used to screen newborn babies to identify congenital heart defects that were undetected with antenatal ultrasound scans (Ewer et al. 2011).

Arterial blood gas analysis, an invasive procedure, may be used in critically ill people to directly measure the amount of oxygen and carbon dioxide in the blood and other parameters that include blood pH (see Ch. 19).

Pain associated with breathing or circulation problems

Pain is abnormal and, if present, may indicate circulatory or breathing problems. It can be caused by a variety of conditions and may be either cardiac or non-cardiac in origin. As with any pain, it is important for the care team to identify the cause so that appropriate pain relief and management can be planned (see Ch. 23).

1. Fit disposable mouthpiece to peak flow meter

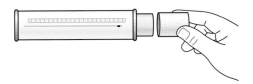

2. Ensure patient stands up or sits upright and holds peak flow meter horizontally without restricting movement of the marker. Ensure the marker is at the bottom of the scale

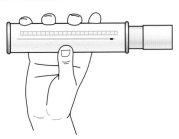

3. Ask patient to breathe in deeply, seal lips around mouthpiece and breathe out as quickly as possible

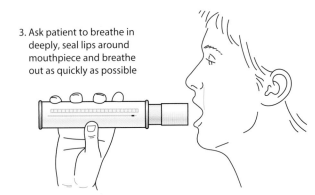

4. Repeat steps 2 and 3 twice more. Choose and record the highest of the three readings

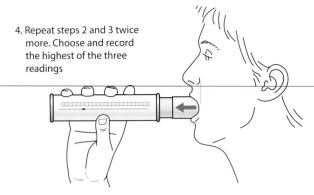

Fig. 17.11 • Recording peak expiratory flow rate. (Reproduced with permission from Brooker, C., Nicol, M. (Eds.), 2003. Nursing adults. The practice of caring. Mosby, Edinburgh.)

The following points should be considered when assessing the person with pain associated with breathing or circulation problems:

• *Precipitating factors:* For example, does the pain become worse with exercise, in cold weather, with deep breathing or movement?

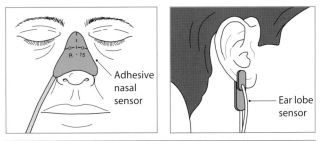

Adhesive nasal sensor

Ear lobe sensor

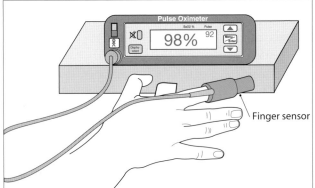

Finger sensor

Fig. 17.12 • Pulse oximeter and probe. (Reproduced with permission from Nicol, M., Bavin, C., Cronin, P., et al., 2008. Essential nursing skills, third ed. Mosby, Edinburgh.)

• *Location of pain:* Cardiac (heart) pain is frequently central and may radiate to the back, arms and jaw. Pain caused by circulatory disorders, such as peripheral vascular disease, will occur in the limbs

• *Description of pain:* Cardiac chest pain may be described as a heavy sensation, aching or crushing. If chest pain is described as a sharp pain on inspiration it is likely to be caused by pleurisy (inflammation of the pleura) rather than angina or a myocardial infarction

• *Intensity of pain:* It is useful to use a pain assessment tool and ask the patient to grade their pain. In children, facial expressions can be very useful for the assessment of pain and pain assessment tools used with children often include faces (see Ch. 23)

• *Factors that relieve the pain:* For example, cardiac chest pain may subside on resting or stopping the activity that caused it, or by a change of position, e.g. a person with pericarditis (inflammation of the pericardium) may obtain relief by leaning forward. Chest pain that is muscular in origin may be relieved by a warm or cold compress.

It is important, however, to remember that it is not always easy to ascertain answers to questions about levels and sites of pain. People with a learning difficulty or speech problems can find it difficult to describe pain or its location, while a child's response to pain is linked to their developmental stage (see Ch. 23).

Common investigations – breathing and circulation

There are many different investigations used to identify disorders affecting breathing and circulation and some of these are outlined in Box 17.18. Box 17.19 provides an opportunity to find out what a cardiac investigation can involve.

Common investigations – breathing and circulation   **Box 17.18**

The following investigations may be used to diagnose or evaluate treatment for disorders affecting breathing and circulation.

- Blood tests – full blood count (FBC), erythrocyte sedimentation rate (ESR), urea and electrolytes, arterial blood gases, blood clotting tests, cardiac enzymes, lipid screening, e.g. cholesterol comprising high-density lipoprotein (HDL) and low-density lipoprotein (LDL)
- Chest X-ray
- Scans – computed tomography (CT), magnetic resonance imaging (MRI), ultrasound/echocardiogram
- Coronary angiogram and cardiac catheterization
- Electrocardiogram (ECG)
- Respiratory function tests – including spirometry, e.g. forced vital capacity (FVC), forced expiratory volume in 1 second (FEV_1), peak expiratory flow rate (PEFR) (see pp. 416–417, 418)
- Sputum specimen for microbiological or cytological examination
- Bronchoscopy.

A simple explanation of some of these investigations accessed on the NHS choices website (www.nhs.uk/Pages/HomePage.aspx) will help you provide patients with information; for a more detailed nursing explanation, see Further reading, below, e.g. Brooker & Nicol 2011).

 Critical thinking   **Box 17.19**

Having an echocardiogram

14-year-old Leroy is booked to have an echocardiogram. He is anxious about the investigation and that it will show something that will stop him playing football.

Student activities

- Find out what happens during an echocardiogram.
- Discuss with your mentor how you would provide Leroy with all the information he needs.

Care of the person with breathing and/or circulation problems

Breathing and circulation problems may affect people of all ages and causes range from respiratory problems such as poor oxygenation, cardiac causes when the heart fails to pump oxygenated blood around the body, or blood disorders when there is insufficient oxygen delivered to the body tissues and organs due to a low haemoglobin level (see pp. 404–407). Problems associated with breathing and circulation such as dyspnoea (see p. 414) or profound fatigue may impact upon all aspects of life: physical functioning and daily activities, and psychological and social aspects.

This section of the chapter outlines the basic, but essential, aspects of care needed by patients who have breathing and circulation problems, helping with expectoration, inhaled medication, oxygen therapy, respiratory support, blood transfusion and rehabilitation.

Communication and relief of anxiety

Breathlessness is extremely frightening and may increase anxiety, which in turn makes the patient more breathless (Prigmore 2005). Communication is both important yet difficult. Communication is a two-way process and this is difficult for the person who is struggling for breath, has a breathing tube, e.g. tracheostomy (opening in the trachea), requires continuous oxygen therapy or who is too breathless to form words (Box 17.20). The nurse must maintain a calm appearance, use gentle touch and appropriate eye contact to provide reassurance. Additionally, alternative communication strategies should be employed such as a pen and pad or a word or picture board. Giving the patient time to express their feelings is clearly important and the nurse should use both verbal and non-verbal cues to ensure that they do not feel rushed. When talking is very difficult, the use of closed questions that do not require long answers may also be useful (see Ch. 9).

 Reflective practice   **Box 17.20**

Breathlessness

Ron, who has COPD, is very breathless and finds talking increasingly difficult. He feels helpless, anxious and exhausted.

Student activities

- Reflect on the difficulties that Ron may experience with communicating his physical and emotional needs.
- Consider the impact of severe breathlessness on Ron's ability to interact with his family and friends.

Positioning to relieve breathlessness

Patients feeling breathless should be supported by pillows in an upright position, either in bed or in a chair. This will increase their lung expansion, which assists gaseous exchange in the alveoli. Breathing may also be easier if they lean forward slightly on pillows placed on a bedside table (Fig. 17.13).

The breathless person is likely to feel anxious if laid flat. However, if they are comfortable lying down, they should lie with their back straight, again to assist with chest expansion. Opening a window may also help someone who is struggling to breathe.

Personal hygiene and skin care

Patients may need help with personal cleansing and dressing depending on how breathless they are and the degree of fatigue caused by poor oxygenation and the constant struggle to breathe (see Ch. 16). They may need extra time to wash

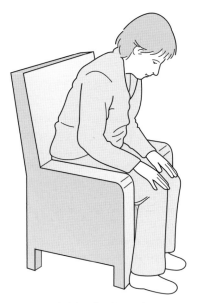

Sitting in chair leaning forward

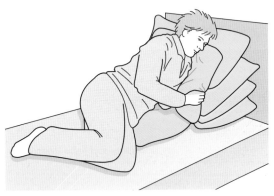

High side lying

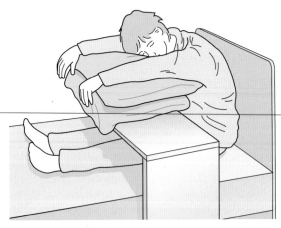

Upright positioning in bed leaning forward
onto pillows or bedside table with pillows

Fig. 17.13 • Positions for relieving breathlessness. (Reproduced with permission from Brooker, C., Nicol, M. (Eds.), 2003. Nursing adults. The practice of caring. Mosby, Edinburgh.)

and also the opportunity to rest during personal hygiene. Additionally, if mouth breathing (see Box 17.2), they will have a dry mouth and require oral hygiene, mouth washes and ice to suck.

Patients with breathing difficulties are likely to have poor oxygenation and consequently some degree of tissue hypoxia. This, combined with factors such as underlying disease, reduced mobility, sliding down from the upright position and poor nutrition, will make them susceptible to pressure ulcers. It should therefore be assumed that any person with a breathing problem is at risk of developing a pressure ulcer and scoring using a pressure ulcer risk tool should be used so that appropriate measures to prevent their occurrence can be implemented. Regular repositioning, mobilization and the use of pressure-relieving devices should be considered (see Ch. 25).

Nutrition and hydration

The breathless patient frequently finds it difficult to eat because of a dry mouth and may also feel nauseated, particularly if they are swallowing secretions. The provision of small, frequent meals helps the breathless person maintain an adequate dietary intake (see Ch. 19). Adequate nutrition to cope with the increased work of breathing is essential in the person with a chronic breathing problem who may also require a high protein diet. The dietitian should be consulted.

Mouth breathing makes their mouth dry and uncomfortable. Additionally, the patient may have an increased respiratory rate or pyrexia (see Ch. 14) that will increase fluid loss from the body. Attention to adequate hydration in the breathless patient is essential, not only for their overall fluid balance, but also for their comfort. A dry mouth rapidly leads to cracked lips and discomfort (see Ch. 16) and dehydration (see Ch. 19) and will lead to viscous secretions. Plugging of the airways may result.

Helping the person with expectoration

Increased and/or viscous secretions make breathing more difficult and the nurse should work with the physiotherapist to assist expectoration and maximize breathing effort.

Breathing exercises and coughing

Secretions can be moved and expectorated by deep breathing exercises and coughing. The patient should be encouraged to increase their fluid intake so that they can more easily expectorate the secretions. It is important to provide the patient with clean sputum cartons with lids as required and mouth washes/teeth cleaning facilities after expectoration. A specimen of sputum may be requested (see p. 417). The nurse should advise the patient to avoid swallowing secretions, as this can lead to nausea.

Patients with chest infections or those who are susceptible to an infection, e.g. postoperatively or with rib fractures, should be encouraged to breathe deeply at intervals. The nurse must ensure that effective analgesics are administered to allow this without pain. Deep breathing with expansion of both lung bases is easiest with the spine straight. This is either in the upright sitting position or with the back straight when lying flat. This will expand the lung bases and facilitate gaseous exchange and clearance of basal secretions.

Breathlessness is extremely frightening and breathing exercises may control and help the person restore their normal breathing pattern during an attack of breathlessness or following a bout of coughing. Usually, the patient will find these exercises easier if they are in a half side-lying position. They should be encouraged to breathe out gently while relaxing their shoulders and upper chest. When breathing in, this should also be gentle, and they should feel their lower ribs and upper abdomen expand. They should be encouraged to breathe gently, with minimal effort. Patients prone to panic attacks and attacks of breathlessness should be encouraged to practise this technique. Learning to sing may also be beneficial. Singing requires control of breathing and posture and a small study has reported improvements in health-related quality of life and a reduction in anxiety (Lord et al 2010).

'Huffing' and coughing are useful techniques to help expectorate secretions. Huffing is thought to be less tiring than coughing and so it is useful to teach this to someone with chronic respiratory disease.

To teach the patient to huff you should ask them to take in a medium breath. They then open their mouth and force the air out (as if breathing on a mirror to clean it). They should then take a few gentle breaths before repeating the sequence two or three times. The secretions should then be in the upper airway and cleared by coughing.

Postural drainage

Sometimes postural drainage is needed to remove secretions, particularly in patients with chronic respiratory disease. In these circumstances, the person lies in bed with the foot of the bed elevated. Gravity then assists the movement of secretions from areas of the lungs. Alternatively, the patient can lie on their side with pillows placed under their waist to gently tip their head down. The physiotherapist will modify the patient's position to drain secretions from particular lobes or lung segments.

In small children with bronchiectasis or cystic fibrosis, a parent or carer may perform postural drainage.

Suctioning

In some circumstances, it may be necessary to use suction to remove secretions from the airway. This is more likely when there is an artificial airway such as an endotracheal tube (a plastic tube introduced through the mouth or nose into the trachea to secure/maintain the airway) or tracheostomy tube (Fig. 17.14, Box 17.21), the person is sedated or unconscious, when there is a poor cough reflex as may occur following a stroke or head injury, or when the patient is too weak to expectorate.

Tracheostomy   Box 17.21

A tracheostomy is a surgical opening into the trachea through the front of the neck. The tracheostomy is kept open with a tracheostomy tube (Fig. 17.14). It facilitates breathing, oxygen therapy or clearance of secretions and may be short or long term. Common reasons for a tracheostomy include:

- Long-term mechanical ventilation (see p. 426)
- Improving respiratory efficiency
- Absent laryngeal reflexes, e.g. following a stroke or head injury
- Sputum retention
- Head or neck injury or surgery
- Upper airway obstruction.

Further reading

Harkin, H., 2011. Nursing patients with disorders of the ear, nose and throat. In: Brooker, C., Nicol, M. (Eds.), Alexander's nursing practice, fourth ed. Churchill Livingstone, Edinburgh.

Suctioning should only be undertaken by someone who is competent to do so. The nurse should therefore have been taught how to undertake the procedure and observed in order to confirm competence. Patients and parents can also be taught how to perform suctioning when long-term assistance with clearing of secretions is required, e.g. a child or adult discharged home on home ventilation (see p. 426). (See Further reading, below, about suctioning, e.g. Nicol et al 2012; Higgins 2005.)

Inhaled medication

Inhaled medication is frequently used in the management of respiratory diseases such as asthma or COPD because the drug acts more quickly when it is administered directly to the site of action. Drugs administered in this way include

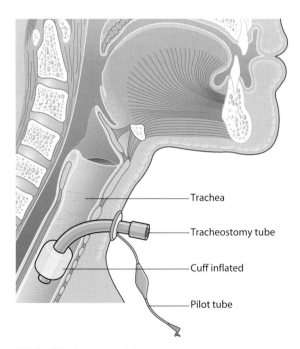

Fig. 17.14 • Tracheostomy tube. (Reproduced with permission from Brooker, C., Nicol, M. (Eds.), 2003. Nursing adults. The practice of caring. Mosby, Edinburgh.)

Labels: Trachea / Tracheostomy tube / Cuff inflated / Pilot tube

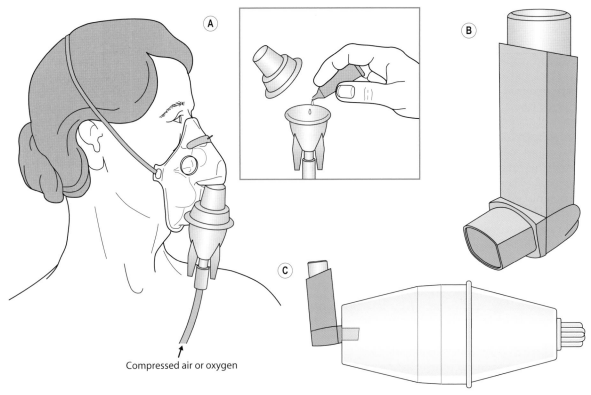

Fig. 17.15 • (A) Nebulizer. (B) Metered-dose inhaler. (C) Inhaler with spacer attached. (A, reproduced with permission from Nicol, M., Bavin, C., Bedford-Turner, S., et al., 2004. Essential nursing skills, second ed. Mosby, Edinburgh.)

bronchodilators (e.g. formoterol fumarate), antibiotics or corticosteroids (see Ch. 22).

There are various ways to administer inhaled medication, including:

- Nebulizers
- Dry powder inhalers
- Metered-dose inhalers.

Nebulizers

A nebulizer (Fig. 17.15A) can be used to administer medication or to liquefy secretions with 0.9% sodium chloride solution. The drug is inhaled and is rapidly absorbed through the alveolar blood supply. It therefore acts quickly and side-effects associated with oral intake are avoided. Most nebulizers require a flow of gas and will be administered either with compressed air or oxygen. The nebulizer breaks up the solution so that it is inhaled as small droplets suspended in a gas. The use of a nebulizer is outlined in Box 17.22.

Dry powder inhalers

A dry powder inhaler releases medication as the person breathes in. The patient places their mouth around the device and breathes in. The flow generated by their breath releases the medication into particles that can be inhaled. These inhalers are easy to carry around and are therefore convenient to use at work, at home, out and about or at school.

The nurse should ensure that patients are able to use their inhaler effectively. Inhaler technique should always be checked by the practice nurse or GP or before hospital discharge and on a regular basis in clinic.

Metered-dose inhalers

Metered-dose inhalers (Fig. 17.15B) are also available for inhaled medication and are frequently used by people with asthma. The inhaler is designed to deliver a dry powder and the medication, which is forced into the lungs.

Before use, the inhaler is shaken to distribute the powder evenly within the gas. The cap is removed and the inhaler is held upright. To be effective, the patient should breathe out gently and then place their mouth around the mouthpiece of the inhaler. As they start to breathe in, the canister top should be pressed to release the medication. The breath should be slow and deep, and held for approximately 10 seconds. Usually, the prescribed dose is for more than one 'puff', in which case the subsequent doses should be taken after approximately 30 seconds.

Using the inhaler requires a degree of coordination and may therefore not be suitable for children, some people with learning disabilities, some older people or those with poor dexterity (Box 17.23). Spacer devices are available which are easier to use (Fig. 17.15C). They comprise a large and, usually, cone-shaped device, onto which the inhaler is fitted and are thought to be effective when used with regular breathing.

Nursing skills Box 17.22

Use of a nebulizer

Equipment

- Nebulizer – mouthpiece or facemask (Fig. 17.15A)
- Air cylinder if piped supply not available
- Nebulizer/drug solution and prescription sheet.

Preparation

- Explain the procedure to the patient to ensure informed consent
- Ascertain whether PEFR measurements are required before and after drug administration
- Wash your hands and follow local infection control procedures
- Ensure that the patient is in the upright position or on their side with their back straight.

Procedure

- Check the medication and the patient's identity against the prescription sheet
- Place the medication, which is normally diluted with 2–3 mL of 0.9% sodium chloride solution, or the sodium chloride solution alone in the nebulizer base and then reassemble
- Ensure that the mouthpiece or facemask is securely connected to the nebulizer. It is preferable to use a mouthpiece to deliver the solution as there is less wastage
- The gas is adjusted to a flow rate of between 4 and 5 L/minute to ensure the medication is vaporized and a fine spray is seen coming out and a hissing sound heard
- The patient is helped to use the mouthpiece/facemask and encouraged to breathe deeply to ensure the solution reaches both lung bases
- Following use, the nebulizer and mouthpiece/facemask should be washed under running water and left to air dry. The equipment is stored dry in a polythene bag at the patient's bedside. It should be changed every 24 hours to prevent infection
- Ensure that all the solution has been vaporized and assist the patient as necessary, e.g. with expectoration or repositioning
- Record the nebulized drug administration and report any changes in condition.

Note: When more than one medication is prescribed for the nebulizer, they should not be mixed and should be administered one after the other, with the bronchodilator (if prescribed) given first. This will open the airways and facilitate more effective treatment with the second drug. Each nebulizer should be labelled according to the medication use.

Resource

Kelly, C., Lynes, D., 2011. Best practice in the provision of nebuliser therapy. Nursing Standard 25 (31), 50–56.

 Critical thinking Box 17.23

Rosie

4-year-old Rosie needs to have inhaled medication to control her asthma symptoms.

Student activities

- Think about how you would explain the use of the inhaler and spacer to Rosie and her parents.
- How will Rosie's level of understanding and motor skills influence the way you explain how to use the inhaler?

Resource

Kelsey, J., McEwing, G., 2008. Clinical skills in child health practice. Churchill Livingstone, Edinburgh, Ch. 16, pp. 170–174.

Oxygen is a potentially hazardous gas. It supports combustion and therefore requires certain precautions:

- Electrical devices should be used with caution when oxygen therapy is in use; this includes electrical shavers and children's toys
- Smoking should not be allowed in the vicinity of oxygen
- Oil, grease, alcohol-based solutions and other flammable solvents should be kept away from the vicinity.

Additionally, the administration of high levels of oxygen can be dangerous and may lead to:

- Eye damage in preterm infants – retinopathy of prematurity (previously known as retrolental fibroplasia)
- Lung damage with fibrosis in preterm infants
- The retention of carbon dioxide in people with COPD whose stimulus to breathe is decreased oxygen in their blood (normally the stimulus to breathe is a rising carbon dioxide level in the blood).

Problems associated with oxygen therapy

There are various physical, psychological and social problems associated with oxygen therapy, many of which are similar to those experienced by patients who are breathless (see pp. 419–421) (Box 17.24). The problems include:

- Noise of gas flow
- Drying of airway mucosa – prevented by humidification (see pp. 425–426)
- Dry eyes – ensure that facemask fits well over the nose to minimize leaks
- Dry mouth – provide adequate fluid intake (see Ch. 19) and oral hygiene (see Ch. 16)
- Difficulties with eating and drinking – consider the use of nasal cannulae
- Nausea – give antiemetics drugs as prescribed
- Plastic smell from oxygen mask
- Soreness caused by facemask or nasal cannulae – the nurse must check regularly for soreness over the nose, the ears or around the nostrils and take steps to prevent skin damage such as adjusting straps to avoid pressure

Oxygen therapy

Oxygen is a drug and should always be prescribed, except in an emergency situation such as cardiopulmonary arrest. The prescription should indicate the oxygen concentration, e.g. 24%, and flow rate in L/min. This includes oxygen delivered by any method, e.g. by mask (face or tracheostomy), nasal cannulae or an incubator, etc. Oxygen is given, usually in the short term, to relieve hypoxia while the underlying cause of the problem is urgently sought.

> **?** Critical thinking   Box 17.24

Piotr

15-year-old Piotr has required continuous oxygen therapy for the past 2 days. The bridge of his nose is sore and he does not want to wear the facemask any longer. His mouth is dry, he has no appetite and is reluctant to drink. Piotr is very quiet and does not want to see visitors.

Student activities

- Why do you think he feels like this and what can the nursing staff do to help?
- Consider the physical, psychological and social problems associated with Piotr's oxygen therapy and write a care plan that will address the specific problems.
- Consider with your mentor how these problems could have been foreseen and prevented.

- Feeling isolated – provide appropriate contact
- Fear – a facemask is frightening and may lead to feelings of claustrophobia – minimize by providing information and explanation
- Communication problems (see p. 419)
- Patients removing the facemask – provide information about reasons for oxygen therapy. Consider changing to nasal cannulae
- System disconnection, especially in a confused patient or young child – the nurse should regularly check system integrity.

Oxygen administration systems

Oxygen is supplied via a piped system or in standard colour-coded cylinders (black with a white top) (Fig. 17.16).

Oxygen can be administered in a variety of ways (Fig. 17.17), including:

- Face and tracheostomy masks
- Nasal cannulae/prongs
- Headboxes and incubators.

The administration method chosen will depend upon age, the reason for administration, whether it is short or long term and where possible the patient's preferences. For example, an infant may not tolerate an oxygen mask and so a headbox or incubator may be used.

Oxygen may be given as a short-term treatment, e.g. post-operatively. However, long-term oxygen therapy (LTOT) may be needed for a patient with COPD or heart failure, and arrangements must be made for oxygen therapy to be supplied at home (Box 17.25).

Fixed performance Venturi systems (high-flow)

Fixed performance facemasks deliver a high flow of gas achieved by directing atmospheric air to mix with the oxygen (Fig.17.17A). Masks are available that provide oxygen at various concentrations, e.g. 24%, 28%, 35%, and the oxygen flow rate is set between 4 and 8 L/min according to the manufacturer's instructions. Specific high-flow masks are available

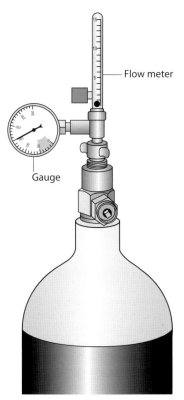

Fig. 17.16 ● Oxygen cylinder. (Reproduced with permission from Nicol, M., Bavin, C., Cronin, P., et al., 2008. Essential nursing skills, third ed. Mosby, Edinburgh.)

for use with tracheostomy tubes. Humidification should be used with high-flow masks.

Variable performance systems

These systems use a low-flow mask, e.g. a Hudson mask, and are frequently used either in the emergency situation or for a person recovering from an anaesthetic (Fig. 17.17B). With an oxygen flow rate of between 6 and 10 L/min, a concentration of up to 60–70% can be given.

Nasal cannulae/nasal prongs

Nasal cannulae/prongs are small plastic tubes, which are inserted into each nostril to administer oxygen (Fig. 17.17C). Oxygen flow rates of approximately 2 L/min are used. Higher flow rates may cause drying of the nasal mucosa, which will damage the delicate mucosal lining.

The system enables the patient to also breathe room air and so does not require an elaborate humidification system. Their use also enables the patient requiring oxygen to eat, drink or talk and is therefore useful alongside a standard oxygen face-mask for short-term use. Nasal cannulae are available in small sizes for infants and young children.

Headbox, body/trunk box

A headbox is suitable for infants up to 8 months of age requiring oxygen therapy (Kelsey & McEwing 2008).

The clear plastic headbox is placed around the infant's head and neck. Humidified oxygen is delivered into the box and the infant breathes air with a higher oxygen concentration (Fig.

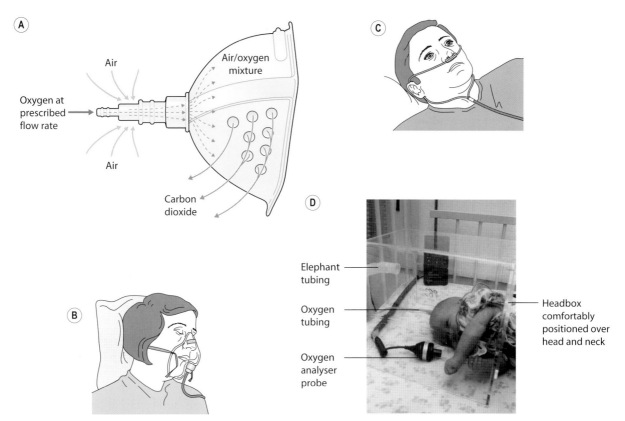

Fig. 17.17 • Oxygen delivery systems: (A) Fixed performance, high-flow Venturi system mask. (B) Variable flow – Hudson-type mask. (C) Nasal cannulae/prongs. (D) Delivery of humidified oxygen via a head box. (A, reproduced with permission from Brooker, C., Nicol, M. (Eds.), 2003. Nursing adults. The practice of caring. Mosby, Edinburgh; B, C, reproduced with permission from Nicol, M., Bavin, C., Bedford-Turner, S., et al., 2004. Essential nursing skills, second ed. Mosby, Edinburgh; D, reproduced with permission from Trigg, E., Mohammed, T.A. (Eds.), 2010. Practices in children's nursing. Guidelines for Hospital and Community, third ed. Churchill Livingstone, Edinburgh.)

Long-term oxygen therapy	Box 17.25

Long-term oxygen therapy (LTOT) is supplied at home for patients who meet certain criteria, e.g. 'People receiving LTOT should breathe supplemental oxygen for at least 15 hours/day' (NICE 2010b, p 11). Such patients could have heart or lung disease.

Oxygen concentrators should be used to provide the fixed supply at home for LTOT (NICE 2010b). Oxygen concentrators remove nitrogen from room air to provide a high concentration of oxygen for the patient.

In addition, ambulatory oxygen is supplied to patients having LTOT who want to continue with treatment outside their home.

17.17D). The clear nature of the headbox means that the infant can see out while also being observed for signs of deterioration such as increased respiratory rate.

Incubator

An incubator is useful for the pre-term or sick baby where the percentage of oxygen in inspired air can be easily controlled while also providing a stable temperature. These are frequently used for the very ill or preterm neonate.

Continuous positive airway pressure (CPAP)

CPAP is increasingly used to correct hypoxaemia and improve oxygen saturation. A tight-fitting mask is placed around the mouth and nose and positive pressure is applied throughout both inspiration and expiration in a spontaneously breathing patient. Not all patients are able to tolerate CPAP and air swallowing can lead to gastric distension with vomiting and aspiration. Careful monitoring of the patient is important with checks made on respiratory rate and effort, oxygen saturations, blood pressure and heart rate.

Because the mask needs to fit securely, the skin condition should also be checked. The bridge of the nose is liable to pressure from the tight-fitting mask. A small piece of DuoDERM® or protective material placed over this area may increase patient comfort. Additionally, it is important to ensure that there is no air leak around the eyes, as the high-flow oxygen can dry and irritate the eyes and cause conjunctivitis.

Humidification

Water vapour is present in atmospheric air so when breathing atmospheric air humidification is dependent upon the environmental humidity. Normal air humidity is between 40% and 60%. Further water vapour is normally added to inspired air as it passes through the upper airways (pp. 402–403). However,

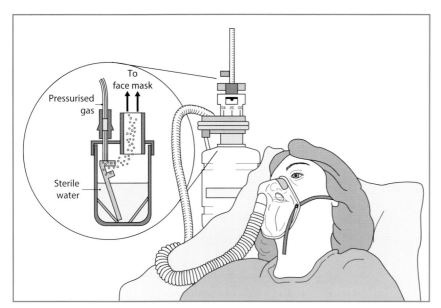

Fig. 17.18 • Humidification of oxygen.
(Reproduced with permission from Nicol, M., Bavin, C., Cronin, P., et al., 2008. Essential nursing skills, third ed. Mosby, Edinburgh.)

humidification of inspired air is impaired in situations that include:

- Breathing in cold dry air, as with piped oxygen, particularly so with high-flow oxygen therapy
- Mouth breathing (see Box 17.2)
- Upper respiratory tract infection
- Dehydration (see Ch. 19)
- When the upper airways are bypassed as occurs with tracheostomy or endotracheal tube.

Various hot-and cold-water devices are available for the humidification of inspired air and an example is shown in Figure 17.18.

Respiratory support – artificial ventilation

This term refers to the process whereby a mechanical device (a ventilator) ventilates the lungs with gases. It can be delivered through an endotracheal or tracheostomy tube, which is attached to a ventilator that pushes oxygen into the lungs.

Non-invasive intermittent positive pressure ventilation (NIPPV) is given through a tight fitting mask that covers the mouth and/or nose and is attached to a mechanical ventilator that pushes oxygen into the lungs. It is useful in nocturnal hypoventilation, a syndrome related to sleep apnoea (see Ch. 10). It is also used in severe muscle fatigue, neuromuscular weakness, COPD and in severe heart failure. NIPPV may be used almost continuously or on a sporadic basis for someone who only requires support at night. It is therefore increasingly used at home for both adults and children who require longer-term assistance with breathing. However, if this is to be effective it is essential that not only do the family receive accurate information beforehand, but they also receive adequate support. People on home ventilation understandably worry that they may suffer equipment failure and back-up systems and emergency plans should be decided upon in advance.

Care of patients requiring a blood transfusion

Blood transfusions can be life saving but they are expensive and can be hazardous. The risks associated with a blood transfusion using donor blood include transfusion reactions, fluid overload and also the risk of acquiring variant Creutzfeldt-Jakob disease (vCJD).

A blood transfusion may be required for a variety of reasons, including:

- Anaemia
- Preoperative preparation
- Postoperatively if blood loss is excessive, despite efforts made during surgery to prevent/minimize blood loss
- Haemorrhage causing hypovolaemia, such as after a road traffic accident
- Blood diseases requiring transfusion of clotting factors or platelets.

For the person with anaemia, or awaiting major surgery where blood loss is expected, every attempt should be made to improve haemoglobin levels through measures including oral iron supplements and a diet rich in available iron (see Box 17.1, p. 401).

In the UK, transfused blood is usually obtained from a healthy volunteer donor. Donors are asked a series of health questions and have a check on their haemoglobin level to ensure that the donation will be safe for both donor and patient. All donated blood is screened for hepatitis B and C, human immunodeficiency virus (HIV) and syphilis. In addition, other tests may be performed, e.g. if the donor has recently returned from certain countries. The blood is stored in a blood bank at around 4°C and labelled with the blood group and type.

Whole blood is transfused but various blood components, e.g. platelets, may be used in specific situations (Box 17.26).

Blood and blood products   Box 17.26

- *Whole blood* transfusions are given to people who have acute serious haemorrhage, e.g. resulting from trauma, gastrointestinal haemorrhage, surgery, etc.
- *Packed cell or plasma-reduced blood* transfusions are used when the transfusion is given to raise the haemoglobin level. This ensures that erythrocytes are given without the risk of fluid overload
- *Red cell concentrate* given to people with a low level of haemoglobin
- *Platelet concentrate* is given to people with bleeding problems where they lack platelets, e.g. leukaemia
- *Fresh frozen plasma (FFP)* is used when clotting factors are needed and may be given to the person who is bleeding following surgery. A concentrate of clotting factors known as cryoprecipitate is obtained from FFP
- *Other coagulation factors*, e.g. factor VIII or IX for patients with haemophilia (inherited bleeding disease where either factor VIII or factor IX is deficient).

Prior to transfusing blood, the recipient's blood should be cross-matched in the laboratory to ensure ABO blood group and rhesus factor compatibility with that of the donor (see Table 17.1, p. 401). This is done to prevent a transfusion reaction where the donor erythrocytes clump together (agglutinate) and block small blood vessels.

Monitoring during blood transfusion

Prior to commencing a blood transfusion it is important to obtain baseline recordings of temperature, pulse rate, blood pressure and respiration rate. These should then be repeated according to local policy during the transfusion, e.g. recorded every 15 minutes for the first hour and thereafter recorded hourly if the person is well and shows no adverse effects until the unit of blood is transfused. The observations should be recommenced at 15-minute intervals with each new unit of blood. The early signs of a transfusion reaction, including fever and rigors, should be observed. If a severe reaction occurs, BLS (see pp. 407–410) may be required. At the first sign of a reaction the blood transfusion should be stopped and the nurse in charge informed. Fluid balance is monitored and recorded and this includes recording the volume of blood transfused. It is generally assumed that a unit of whole blood is 500 mL and a unit of packed red cells is 300 mL. For more accurate recording of fluid volume, the unit of blood should be weighed.

When monitoring fluid balance (see Ch. 19) it is also important to record urine output. If a transfusion reaction occurs, the donor erythrocytes agglutinate and can cause kidney damage. If the patient complains of loin or back pain, a sample of urine should be observed and tested for haematuria (blood in the urine).

Fluid balance is of particular importance in older people, the very young or those with cardiac or respiratory failure, when circulatory overload may lead to hypertension and pulmonary oedema. This is characterized by increasing respiratory rate, dyspnoea and agitation.

Documentation is vital. All observations should be clearly recorded. In addition, the start and finish times of each unit of blood should be documented.

Ensuring transfusion safety

Due to the danger associated with the transfusion of incorrect or incompatible blood and other complications, hospitals and community settings have their own strict blood transfusion policy that must be observed. Although blood should be administered at room temperature it should be removed from the blood bank fridge no more than 30 minutes before transfusion, and, preferably, only 15 minutes prior. The local policy regarding the checking procedure on removal from the blood bank and prior to commencing the transfusion, including patient identification, must be undertaken and a qualified nurse should always take responsibility for this procedure.

The safe disposal of equipment is essential. Gloves should be worn when handling blood or intravenous administration sets to protect staff from blood-borne diseases (see Ch. 15).

When completed, the transfused blood packs should be returned to the laboratory if a transfusion reaction is suspected. Otherwise, the disposal of blood bags should be in accordance with the local policy. Due to concerns over vCJD, any blood products or blood waste must be incinerated.

Transfusion complications

Complications associated with blood transfusion include:

- Blood incompatibility (Box 17.27)
- Febrile reactions

Blood incompatibility   Box 17.27

Transfusion of the wrong or incompatible blood is extremely serious and can lead to life-threatening complications, e.g. kidney failure. It may occur because a mistake has been made with blood samples or the vital bedside checks have not been followed.

Signs and symptoms

- Flushing
- Pain at the cannulation site, abdomen, loin or chest
- Agitation
- Fever
- Shivering
- Hypotension
- Tachycardia
- Nausea and vomiting
- Wheeze
- Headache
- Chest tightness
- Oliguria (reduced urinary output)
- Haematuria.

When a transfusion reaction is suspected, the registered nurse should immediately stop the transfusion and obtain urgent medical assistance. The intravenous access should be kept patent with 0.9% sodium chloride solution. The haematologist should be contacted and any remaining blood returned to the laboratory for investigation.

- Allergic reactions
- Circulatory overload
- Acute bacterial reactions due to contaminated blood
- Delayed complications such as delayed haemolysis (breakdown of erythrocytes), viral infections and iron overload (particularly with regular blood transfusion such as in patients with thalassaemia).

(See Useful websites and Further reading, below, for more information, e.g. British Committee for Standards in Haematology, Nicol et al 2012.)

Alternatives to donated blood transfusion

Blood transfusion is not without risk and it is best to avoid the need wherever possible. Some people for personal or religious reasons, e.g. Jehovah Witness, refuse blood transfusions. Apart from blood conservation through minimizing loss, the alternatives to the transfusion of donor blood include:

- Autologous transfusion – a patient having planned major surgery may donate their blood about 4 weeks prior to surgery.
- Plasma and volume expanders – albumin, gelatin solutions or modified starch solutions may be used as volume expanders.
- Every effort should be taken during the pre, intra and post-operative period to reduce blood loss and the need for blood transfusion.
- Erythropoietin (growth factor for erythrocyte production) can be given intravenously as recombinant human erythropoietin and may be a useful adjunct to good nutrition and iron supplements (Margereson & Riley 2003).

Home-monitoring in patients with conditions affecting breathing or circulation

Patients with a long-term condition such as chronic heart failure or chronic respiratory disease are encouraged to self-care: self-monitor their condition and to self-manage. Where patients wish to, they can also be taught how and when to make changes to their management. For example a patient with heart failure can be taught to increase their diuretic for a period of 3 days if they notice signs and symptoms of increased fluid volume (such as weight increase or swollen ankles). Patients with COPD may be taught to take a course of antibiotics when they notice a change in the colour of their sputum.

Telemonitoring is increasingly being used to support patients develop such self-care skills. It also provides professional monitoring to the patient in their home. Such systems include the installation of simple home monitoring equipment in the home. This could include a weighing scale, blood pressure cuff, oxygen saturation probe or peak flow meter. The patient is asked to use this equipment regularly and the monitored data are automatically transmitted (by the telephone line or internet/wi-fi) for review. These systems are most effective when the review is undertaken by a healthcare professional with sufficient knowledge to know how to respond to the data (Riley & Cowie 2009). Telemonitoring has been shown to reduce hospital admission, can be used to support hospital-at-home strategies and provides close patient follow-up and monitoring. It is increasingly being used for patients with long-term conditions affecting their breathing or circulation and its use is likely to increase enormously over the next few years.

Rehabilitation for conditions affecting breathing or circulation

Rehabilitation for people with conditions affecting breathing and/or circulation aims to restore someone to as normal a situation as possible, e.g. for the breathless person, the ability to function in normal activities of daily living such as washing, dressing, cooking and shopping and return to work if possible. This will include issues such as managing their symptoms, advice to prevent worsening of their condition, increasing exercise tolerance and improving psychosocial coping.

Rehabilitation programmes are provided for people after a heart attack (myocardial infarction), for those with stable heart failure and COPD. Programmes should use a holistic approach to focus on the needs of each individual but are likely to involve education, exercise, and counselling and support. For example, a programme for a breathless person will include:

- *Education:* For the breathless person, this should include information regarding the cause of their breathlessness, strategies to reduce it and lifestyle advice that may prevent the condition worsening, e.g. smoking cessation.

  Singing may be a useful strategy to reduce anxiety and improve breathing for some patients (Lord et al 2010). This should be taught by a trained singing teacher to ensure correct breathing techniques are taught.
- *Exercise:* Includes teaching breathing exercises and exercises for muscle strength. Respiratory muscle training will reduce the effort required for breathing and hence the fatigue associated with breathlessness. Breathing exercises to reduce anxiety and distress also play an important part as does exercise training to assist with the activities of daily living. The specialist nurse, physiotherapist and occupational therapist should all work together to ensure that the exercises are appropriate for recovery.
- *Counselling and psychosocial support:* For most people with a chronic illness, social support is an important factor in helping them to cope (see Ch. 11). Positive support can provide emotional, informational and functional support and so help improve self-esteem.

SUMMARY

- Problems with breathing and circulation are common. They reduce quality of life and account for many thousands of premature deaths in the UK.

- Health-promoting activities that include smoking cessation, a balanced diet, weight control and exercise reduce the risk of developing problems with breathing and circulation and minimize the effects of existing conditions.

- All healthcare staff should be familiar with basic life support procedures for infants, children and adults.

- Nurses should be able to respond to an acute situation and provide first aid for disorders affecting breathing and circulation.

- Holistic assessment of breathing and circulation is central to the planning of appropriate nursing interventions.

- Many nursing interventions can alleviate distressing symptoms, such as breathlessness.

- Promoting self-management is key to improving the health of people with breathing and circulation disorders.

- Nurses play a key role in providing regular monitoring and follow-up to the patient in their home in order to reduce the risk of hospitalisation and to managing chronic disorders of breathing and circulation.

- Rehabilitation programmes for people with conditions affecting breathing and/or circulation aim to restore someone to as normal a situation as possible.

KEY WORDS AND PHRASES FOR LITERATURE SEARCHING

Basic life support

Blood transfusion

Breathlessness

Cardiopulmonary resuscitation

Chronic respiratory diseases

Coronary heart disease

Oxygen therapy

Rehabilitation

Self-care

Smoking cessation

 Useful websites

BBC www.bbc.co.uk/health

British Committee for Standards in Haematology – Guidelines www.bcshguidelines.com

British Heart Foundation www.bhf.org.uk

British Thoracic Society www.brit-thoracic.org.uk

NHS choices www.nhs.uk/

NHS Evidence www.evidence.nhs.uk/topics

All websites accessed September 2012.

References

Ball, C., 2011. Recognising and managing shock. In: Brooker, C., Nicol, M. (Eds.), Alexander's nursing practice, fourth ed. Churchill Livingstone, Edinburgh.

British Heart Foundation, 2010. Coronary heart disease statistics. Online. Available: www.bhf.org.uk/publications/view-publication.aspx?ps=1001546 September 2012.

British Thoracic Society, 2006. The burden of lung disease, second ed. Online. Available: www.brit-thoracic.org.uk/Portals/0/Library/BTS%20Publications/burdeon_of_lung_disease2007.pdf September 2012.

Butler-Williams, C., Cantrill, N., Maton, S., 2005. Increasing staff awareness of respiratory rate significance. Nursing Times 101 (27), 35–37.

Ewer, A.K., Middleton, L.J., Furmston, A.T., et al., 2011. Pulse oximetry screening for congenital heart defects in newborn infants (PulseOx): a test accuracy study. Lancet 378 (9793), 785–794.

Jones, M., Moffat, F., 2002. Cardiopulmonary physiotherapy. BIOS Scientific, Guildford.

Kelsey, J., McEwing, G., 2008. Clinical skills in child health practice. Churchill Livingstone, Edinburgh.

Lord, V., Cave, P., Hume, V., et al., 2010. Singing teaching as a therapy for chronic respiratory disease–a randomised controlled trial and qualitative evaluation. BMC Pulmonary Medicine 10, 41.

MacGregor, J., 2008. Introduction to the anatomy and physiology of children, second ed. Routledge, London.

Margereson, C., Riley, J., 2003. Cardiothoracic surgical nursing: current trends in adult care. Blackwell, Oxford.

Murray, I., Hassall J., 2009. Change and adaptation in pregnancy. In: Fraser, D.M., Cooper, M.A. (Eds.), Myles textbook for midwives, fifteenth ed. Churchill Livingstone, Edinburgh.

National Institute for Health and Clinical Excellence, 2010a. Hypertension in pregnancy. The management of hypertensive disorders in pregnancy. Online. Available: www.nice.org.uk/nicemedia/live/13098/50416/50416.pdf September 2012.

National Institute for Health and Clinical Excellence, 2010b. Chronic obstructive pulmonary disease. Quick reference guide. Online. Available: www.nice.org.uk/nicemedia/live/13029/49399/49399.pdf September 2012.

National Institute for Health and Clinical Excellence, 2011. Hypertension: Clinical management of primary hypertension in adults. Clinical guideline CG 127. Online. Available: http://www.nice.org.uk/nicemedia/live/13561/56008/56008.pdf September 2012.

National Patient Safety Agency, 2004. Patient safety alert 02. Establishing a standard crash call telephone number in hospitals. Online.

Available: www.npsa.nhs.uk September 2012.

Prigmore, S., 2005. Assessment and nursing care of the patient with dyspnoea. Nursing Times 101 (14), 50–53.

Resuscitation Council (UK), 2010. Adult basic life support. Online. Available: www.resus.org.uk/pages/blsalgo.pdf September 2012.

Riley, J.P., Cowie, M.R., 2009. Telemonitoring in heart failure. Heart 95, 1904–1908.

Serci, I.G.J., 2009. The fetus. In: Fraser, D.M., Cooper, M.A. (Eds.), Myles textbook for midwives, fifteenth ed. Churchill Livingstone, Edinburgh.

Webster, R.A., Thompson, D.R., 2011. Nursing patients with cardiovascular disorders. In: Brooker, C., Nicol, M. (Eds.), Alexander's nursing practice, fourth ed. Churchill Livingstone, Edinburgh.

Williams, B., Poulter, N.R., Brown, M.J., et al., 2004. British Hypertension Society Guidelines. Guidelines for the management of hypertension: report of the fourth working party of British Hypertension Society, 2004 – BHS IV. Journal of Human Hypertension 18, 139–185.

Further reading

Brooker, C., Nicol, M. (Eds.), 2011. Alexander's nursing practice, fourth ed. Churchill Livingstone, Edinburgh (Chaptres 2, 3, 11).

Higgins, D., 2005. Tracheal suction. Nursing Times 101 (8), 36–37.

Moore, T., 2003. Suctioning techniques for the removal of respiratory secretions. Nursing Standard 18 (9), 47–53, Quiz 54–55.

[Erratum 2003, Nursing Standard 18(13):31].

Moore, T., Woodrow, P., 2009. High dependency nursing care, second ed. Routledge, London.

Nicol, M., Bavin, C., Cronin, P., et al., 2012. Essential nursing skills, fourth ed. Mosby, Edinburgh.

Sheppard, M., Wright, M., 2006. Principles and practice of high dependency nursing, second ed. Baillière Tindall, Edinburgh.

Waugh, A., Grant, A., 2010. Ross and Wilson anatomy and physiology, eleventh ed. Churchill Livingstone, Edinburgh.

Mobility and immobility

18

Christine Donnelly

LEARNING OUTCOMES

This chapter will help you:
- Appreciate the roles that the musculoskeletal system plays in producing movement
- Describe the first aid interventions for fractures, dislocations, strains and sprains
- Understand the principles of safe handling and moving as applied to people
- Discuss the benefits of mobility across the lifespan
- Explain the principles of nursing care that will reduce the hazards of immobility
- Describe the roles of nurses, physiotherapists and occupational therapists in assisting people regain mobility.

Introduction

This chapter focuses on human movement and its importance to health. An overview of the musculoskeletal system and its role in movement is provided in the first section along with first aid for musculoskeletal injuries and the principles of nursing care for people with casts. The second section explores factors that influence balance, posture and movement. Development of the spinal curves and the importance of maintaining them are described. In the next section, the principles of safe handling and moving that were introduced in Chapter 13 are extended to moving patients/clients, including the use of equipment such as hoists, glide sheets and transfer boards. Helping people to mobilize, including the use of walking aids and wheelchairs, is explored. In the final section the benefits of mobility and the hazards of immobility are introduced and the problems that people of all ages may experience due to immobility are explained. Active and passive exercises are described. This chapter refers to others that provide more detail about potential hazards of immobility such as pressure ulcers (Ch. 25), deep vein thrombosis (Ch. 24) and constipation (Ch. 21). A multidisciplinary approach is normally taken to provide care for people with mobility problems and usually involves at least a physiotherapist and occupational therapist (OT) as well as the nursing team, and their role in promoting mobility is described.

The musculoskeletal system

This section outlines the anatomy and physiology of the bones, muscles and joints, and the role of the musculoskeletal system in mobility. You should refer to your physiology text for more detail of the related anatomy and physiology and to Chapter 16 for a fuller explanation of disorders affecting the nervous system. First aid for fractures, dislocations, sprains and strains is described and the principles of nursing care for people with casts are explained. An overview of common disorders of muscles, bones and joints is included.

Muscles

There are three different types of muscle tissue: voluntary (skeletal), involuntary (smooth) and cardiac. Although their structure differs they all have the following characteristics:
- *Contractility*, the ability to shorten
- *Extensibility*, the ability to lengthen
- *Excitability*, the ability to respond to nerve stimulation
- *Elasticity*, the ability to stretch and return to its original length.

The structure and function of voluntary (skeletal) muscles

Voluntary muscles

Unlike other types, voluntary (skeletal) muscles can be moved voluntarily to allow movement and are those in the body that are attached to two bones with a movable joint between them. One of the bones is usually more stationary at a given moment

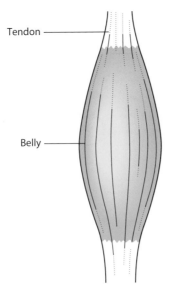

Fig. 18.1 • A typical skeletal muscle. (Reproduced with permission from Greig, J., Rhind, J., 2002. Riddles's anatomy and physiology. Churchill Livingstone, Edinburgh.)

than the other to allow movement to take place between them. Before a skeletal muscle can contract to bring about movement it must be stimulated by a nerve impulse.

Muscles come in different shapes and sizes depending on their function, and they usually have a thicker belly and a tendon at each end for attachment to bone (Fig. 18.1). Postural muscles help to keep the upright posture or maintain positions for sustained periods of time and do not tire quickly; examples include the muscles of the abdominal wall, buttocks and thighs. Active muscles are involved in movements such as typing, running and blinking. These muscles respond appropriately to the tasks they perform but tend to tire quickly (Box 18.1). First aid interventions for strains and sprains, and their subsequent neurovascular checks, are provided in Boxes 18.2 and 18.3, respectively. Common muscle disorders are outlined in Table 18.1. (p. 434)

Fascia

Fascia is formed from connective tissue, one of the four basic tissues in the body (the others being muscular, nervous and epithelial). Superficial fascia refers to the fatty tissue under the skin and deep fascia refers to the tissue that surrounds muscles, tendons and other organs. The superficial and deep fascias are connected to each other, and the deep fascia that surrounds muscle bellies and tendons is continuous throughout the body. It is incredible to think that the connective tissue surrounding the brain (the meninges) is connected to the fascia in the feet (Myers 2009). This is the reason why people with painful knees can be diagnosed with back problems. If the fascia has been damaged in one area, the effects can often be found elsewhere in the body. Fascia is the body's natural shock absorber; without it the body could not absorb and disseminate forces to reduce the risk of injury.

Your jumper (see Box 18.1) is a good analogy for the reactions that occur in the fascia when it is shortened or 'knotted' through

---

 Reflective practice Box 18.1

Understanding the musculoskeletal system
Student activities

1. Using skeletal muscles:
   • Try clenching your fist and see how quickly you begin to feel discomfort.
   • Now think how long you can hold a poor sitting position without moving. These differences between muscles are important when exploring patient/client immobility of all ages.
2. Fascia:
   • Try this if you are wearing a jumper or T-shirt. Grasp the hem at one side, gathering a couple of inches of the hem together, and pull down on the jumper. Observe how the stress lines from the pulled section spread upwards to the shoulder on the same side and also across to the opposite shoulder as well as along the hem towards to other hip.
3. Effects of postural habits on fascia:
   • Stand in front of a mirror and look at your posture, both front and side views. What do you notice about your posture? You may see that you have one shoulder higher than the other or that your head tends to lie towards one side or that your shoulders and hips are not aligned. This may be due to apparent leg lengthening or the way you carry your rucksack or bag. Do you have a habit of putting your bag on the same shoulder? Does your bag stay more easily on one shoulder than the other? Take a mental note of your own postural habits.
4. Consider the effects on your health of particular postural habits by using what you have learned from activities 1 and 2.

 First aid Box 18.2

Strains and sprains
Recognition
• Pain
• Reduced function, especially if a joint is affected
• Swelling and bruising.

Treatment (acronym RICE)
• **R**est and support the injured limb in the most comfortable position
• **I**ce is applied to reduce pain and swelling. A pack of frozen vegetables wrapped in a clean tea towel, laid on the affected area for short periods, is very effective
• **C**ompression is applied to reduce swelling. Apply a bandage or compress to the affected limb. The compress can be soaked in arnica solution, which reduces bruising, made by mixing 10 drops of mother tincture with 250 mL cold water
• **E**levate the affected limb on pillows to reduce swelling
• Check for adequate circulation (see Box 18.3)
• If the casualty is in severe pain or cannot use the affected limb, send to hospital
• Take the casualty to hospital if the pain and swelling do not subside within 24 hours.

Nursing skills   Box 18.3

Neurovascular checks

These are also sometimes referred to as circulation, sensation and movement (CSM) checks, which are carried out to confirm that a cast, bandage or other intervention does not restrict the local circulation. They are carried out as a first aid measure, following discharge with a new cast and in hospital settings.

The frequency is determined by the type of intervention, the extent of damage, any local policy and reduced over time if observations are within expected levels for the particular patient. Any abnormalities (trends or sudden changes) are reported immediately to the charge nurse. The area, often an extremity, distal to the cast is checked for:

- *Temperature:* The area should be warm. Cool or cold fingers are abnormal and may be the result of restricted blood supply to the area.
- *Colour:* The area should be pink. Mottling and white or bluish colour is abnormal and results from impaired blood supply to the affected area.
- *Sensation:* There should be normal feeling in the area. Any tingling, alteration or loss of sensation is abnormal and may be due to compression of nerves due to local swelling.
- *Movement:* The amount of movement of the area. Although this may be restricted, any decrease in previous movement is abnormal.

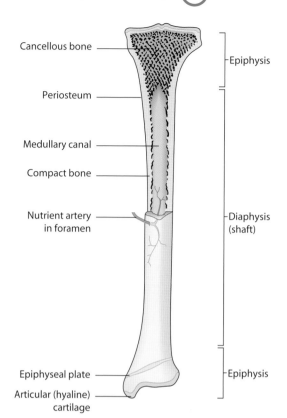

Fig. 18.2 • A typical long bone. (Reproduced with permission from Waugh, A., Grant, A., 2006. Ross and Wilson anatomy and physiology in health and illness, tenth ed. Churchill Livingstone, Edinburgh.)

injury. Have you ever felt knots in your shoulder muscles? Did this affect the arm on that side? The effects of postural change may be distant from the original injury. Knowing that fascia is continuous throughout the body helps to understand some of the problems faced by patients/clients who are immobile or trying to regain mobility following illness or injury. The postural characteristics identified earlier have arisen because the muscles and their surrounding fascia have adapted to your habits and protect the shoulder joint from further injury.

These changes are seldom seen in children because their muscles are more elastic and the fascia returns to a near normal position. They also recover more easily from injuries and awkward movements without obvious lasting effect. Fascia stiffens with age. The longer-standing a postural habit, the more the fascia adapts to the preferred, habitual and adaptive position. Understanding that everyone has habits that affect the underlying muscles and tissues, also helps to appreciate mobility difficulties that people may have. This knowledge not only helps nurses to move patients/clients more appropriately but also helps them to understand why someone may complain of hip pain when the problem may originate in their shoulder. Likewise, the fascia in the feet and ankles receive constant pounding through walking, standing, running and wearing ill-fitting shoes that leads to the development of adaptive postures throughout the leg, hips, spine, neck and head, even to the extent of affecting the joints of the jaw that leads to clenching of the teeth.

Bones

Bones are dynamic, living structures with nerve and blood supplies. The main functions of bones are to:

- Support soft tissue and provide attachment for muscles
- Protect internal organs from injury
- Allow movement at joints as the muscles attached to them contract.

A typical long bone, such as those of the limbs, has a shaft and two epiphyses (Fig. 18.2). Bone growth takes place at each end of the shaft at the epiphyseal plate. This region consists of cartilage until bone growth is complete, when it ossifies. Muscle tendons attach to the outer covering of bone, the periosteum. Hyaline cartilage replaces periosteum at the ends of long bones that form synovial (movable) joints.

Prenatally and during early childhood, the long bones consist mainly of cartilage which is then gradually replaced by bone tissue. This process is called ossification and takes place initially in the bone shaft and at the epiphyses after birth. Several hormones, including growth hormone and thyroid hormones (thyroxine, tri-iodothyronine), are important in growth and development of bones, especially in infancy and childhood, and excessive or impaired secretion results in abnormal bone development. In time, ossification is sufficient to allow walking to be achieved. Although cartilage offers some protection to the vital organs, it behaves like stiff plastic, having a degree of flexibility, rather than the rigid hardness of bone. As a result, children's vital organs are more prone to injury if they fall or are shaken than those of adults, and their bones tend to bend, rather than break, causing greenstick fractures (see Fig. 18.3).

At puberty, there is a growth spurt due to increased production of the sex hormones testosterone and oestrogen. By the

Table 18.1 Disorders of the musculoskeletal system

Disorder	Causes and effects
Muscles	
Cerebral palsy	This condition is primarily neurological but is characterized by neuromuscular abnormalities It can be caused by brain damage due to hypoxia either before or during birth and results in impaired coordination and muscle control Intellect can be unaffected but because clients cannot articulate words easily, care must be taken not to assume this is the case although learning disability is sometimes present
Muscular dystrophies	This is a general term used to describe genetically inherited conditions that lead to skeletal muscle wasting without any nerve damage Congenital muscular dystrophy can be present at birth or manifest within the first 6 months of life Signs include generalized muscle weakness and poor head control Duchenne muscular dystrophy is a rapidly progressive condition that only affects boys and is often fatal during adolescence; it is present from birth but may not become evident until around 4 years of age Many muscular dystrophies are congenital (present from birth)
Strains	Strains occur during overexertion of all or part of a muscle, e.g. the calf muscles during jogging and other keep-fit exercises. If a muscle is not warmed up adequately and too much work is demanded of the fibres, it becomes exhausted, and tightens and shortens The signs of muscle strains and the interventions required are shown in Box 18.2
Apraxia; bradykinesia; dyspraxia	Other terms used to describe problems with movements experienced by patients/clients include: *Apraxia:* The inability to produce coordinated movements *Bradykinesia:* This refers to unusually slow movement, especially the starting and stopping of movements *Dyspraxia:* Partial loss of the ability to produce coordinated movements
Bones	
Fractures	A fracture is a break in the continuity of a bone, usually caused by excessive force being applied to it In simple fractures, the skin remains intact; however, in compound fractures the broken bone protrudes through the skin Figure 18.3 shows different types of fracture: Spiral fractures are common in footballers and skiers because they tend to have the foot fixed in one position, and if the leg and body rotates sharply around it, this causes the bone to fracture (Fig. 18.3B). In comminuted fractures (Fig. 18.3C) there are many bone fragments due to severe damage at the fracture site Fractures are diagnosed by X-ray investigation: they can be difficult to diagnose in children because their bones are softer and are more likely to bend than to break. Fractures of this type are called greenstick fractures (Fig. 18.3D) because the characteristics are similar to bending a green twig. The outer layers of the twig split, while the soft wood underneath only bends Some fractures occur around the epiphyseal plate (see Fig. 18.2). When there is still active bone growth, it is important that these fractures are carefully managed to ensure even growth of bone. Uneven bone growth along the epiphyseal plate will lead to problems with joint alignment, which in turn may cause mobility problems Box 18.4 shows the signs of fractures and the first aid treatment required
Osteoporosis	This condition is characterized by bone fragility, porosity and an increased risk of fractures, especially of the wrist, vertebrae and hip, particularly in women In the UK, one in two women and one in five men over the age of 50 will suffer a fracture due to osteoporosis (see the National Osteoporosis Society website: www.nos.org.uk) Box 18.5 outlines some of the measures that can be taken to maintain bone density, which will reduce the effects of osteoporosis
Rickets and osteomalacia	These conditions are often referred to as 'sick bones' and result from vitamin D deficiency; both terms refer to the same condition, known as rickets in children and osteomalacia in adults In the UK, people most at risk of vitamin D deficiency are those who get little exposure to sunlight; vulnerable groups include people who cover their limbs for cultural/religious reasons, e.g. Muslims, especially women and children, and older adults who are housebound or resident in nursing homes Lack of vitamin D can lead to generalized bone pain and muscle weakness In children there may be enlarged bone ends, particularly in the wrists, that cause lasting deformity

Continued

Table 18.1　Disorders of the musculoskeletal system—cont'd

Disorder	Causes and effects
Joints	
Arthritis	Inflammation of joints associated with pain, swelling and restricted movement
Osteoarthritis	A degenerative disorder usually of weight-bearing synovial joints that commonly accompanies the ageing process, usually due to 'wear and tear' or less often following a previous injury
Rheumatoid arthritis	This condition also affects most body systems. Initially the affected synovial joints are often the fingers and wrists; later the larger joints, e.g. the hip, also become affected
Dislocations	These occur when bones are displaced and the joint can no longer function They may be caused when excessive force is placed on a bone, pulling it out of alignment, or excessive pulling on a joint that causes the ligaments to tear A partial dislocation (subluxation) requires the same treatment as a full dislocation (see Box 18.4)
Sprains	Sprains arise when damage to the ligaments that surround a joint occurs (see Fig. 18.4) Damaged ligaments weaken a joint and may leave it prone to further injury or dislocation Damage around the joint may also cause bleeding within it A common cause of sprains to the neck is a whiplash injury commonly sustained in car accidents. This results from a sudden jerking back of the head and neck causing damage to the ligaments, vertebrae and nerves in the neck region Signs of sprains and the first aid treatment are shown in Box 18.2
Movement and gait	
Parkinson's disease	Named after Dr James Parkinson (1755–1824) who first identified this progressive neurological disorder; this affects movements such as walking, talking and writing It is typified by tremor, muscle rigidity or stiffness and bradykinesia that typically cause hesitancy in walking, characterized by a shuffling gait and the absence of arm swinging, accelerated walking which can result in falls and difficulty in carrying out fine motor movements such as buttoning a shirt
Parkinsonism	This describes the symptoms of Parkinson's disease that occur, e.g. following a stroke, or as a side effect of medication, e.g. chlorpromazine for severe mental distress

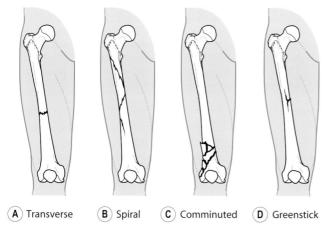

(A) Transverse　(B) Spiral　(C) Comminuted　(D) Greenstick

Fig. 18.3 • Types of simple fracture. (Amended with permission from Dandy, D.J., Edwards, D.J., 2003. Essential orthopaedics and trauma, fourth ed. Elsevier, Edinburgh.)

late teenage years, ossification is largely complete. Bones are not fully hardened until their growth stops at about 18 years in females and 25 years in males. Once bone growth is complete, bones continue to replace old tissue with new, a process known as remodelling. For example, the lower third of the femur (thigh bone) replaces itself every 4 months in young adults. Following a fracture, new bone tissue is laid down to

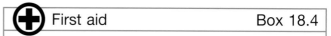

First aid　　　Box 18.4

Fractures and dislocations

Recognition

The cardinal signs of a fracture or dislocation are:

- Pain
- Swelling
- Possible deformity
- Loss of function.

Treatment

This follows the RICE principles outlined in Box 18.2:

- Immobilize the affected limb
- If a bone is protruding through the skin, cover with a clean, wet cloth and place a strand-free dressing round the protruding bone until it is higher than the bone before applying a bandage
- Do not give the casualty anything to eat or drink in case an anaesthetic is required
- Casualties with suspected fractures or dislocations must be sent to hospital.

repair the break. Box 18.4 describes the treatment required for fractures.

Bone mass reaches its peak around 30 years of age and begins to decline after 35–40 years. It is important to maintain a lifestyle that maximizes bone density in order to reduce the effects of reduction in later life, which is excessive in some people, leading to osteoporosis (Box 18.5). The hardness of adult bone protects vital organs such as the brain, spinal cord, heart and lungs from injury. Bone disorders are outlined in Table 18.1.

 Health promotion   Box 18.5

Promoting bone health

To promote bone mass:

- Eat a calcium-rich diet with foods such as milk, cheese and yoghurt (low fat varieties are high in calcium)
- Take regular weight-bearing exercise such as walking, jogging or aerobics for 20 minutes at least three times per week. It is important to be aware that excessive exercise in those with a low body weight and/or eating disorders may result in low oestrogen levels, which means that optimal bone mass is not achieved, predisposing to osteoporosis
- Give up smoking
- Limit alcohol intake to 21 units/week for men and 14 units/week for women
- Avoid consuming excessive amounts of retinol (vitamin A) that is found in fish and dairy products as it is thought to increase the risk of fractures in later life. Vitamin A found in vegetables as carotene is safe.

Student activities

Visit the National Osteoporosis Society website and find out:

- How hormone replacement therapy affects bone density.
- Why older adults are advised to increase their intake of calcium and vitamin D.
- The current treatment strategies for people with osteoporosis.

Resource

The National Osteoporosis Society website – www.nos.org.uk September 2012.

Care of people wearing casts

This section introduces the roles of casts in immobilizing joints and fractured bones and the principles of nursing care are outlined.

People should be as fully participant in their care as possible, particularly as they will need support and encouragement to adapt to their altered body image, whether it is temporary or permanent and regardless of age. This can be particularly challenging during puberty, which brings about body changes that can be difficult enough for adolescents to deal with, without the added complication of being 'different' from their peers because they have to wear a bulky plaster.

Patients who have sustained simple fractures (see Table 18.1 and Fig. 18.3) usually have the fracture immobilized using a lightweight Plaster of Paris (PoP) cast. Plaster of Paris may be used initially as it is cheap and easily removed; particularly if the cast is replaced after a few days when swelling has reduced. It is usually replaced with a harder-wearing, lightweight, waterproof plaster such as thermoplast or fibreglass impregnated

with polyurethane. The principles of care are the same, whichever type of plaster is used (Box 18.6).

 Nursing skills   Box 18.6

Care of people wearing casts

- Once a plaster has been applied, the affected limb is supported on a waterproof pillow, covered by a towel to absorb moisture. The pillow also provides gentle elevation to reduce swelling.
- Fingers or toes are cleaned to remove any debris so that CSM checks (see Box 18.3) can be carried out at regular intervals and any changes or abnormalities reported.
- The person should be encouraged to change their position hourly so that the plaster dries evenly, on all sides.
- When assisting the person to move their affected limb, only the palms of the hands should be used. This avoids causing indentations from thumbs or fingers on the inside of the plaster that could cause pressure on the skin underneath, leading to a pressure ulcer.
- Nothing should ever be inserted inside a plaster to relieve itching, e.g. knitting needles or rulers. These can damage the skin or become lodged in the plaster, causing ulceration, infection or pressure damage.
- The plaster should be kept dry during personal hygiene activities by covering it with a plastic bag. This is also important for waterproof plasters, because the lining material is not waterproof.
- Physiotherapists or experienced nurses supply people with appropriate walking aids if a lower limb is in plaster and teach patients how to use them correctly.
- People wearing casts can usually be discharged early with an out-patient appointment so that progress can be monitored.
- Education plays a vital role in compliance with treatment as the person must be able to care for their own limb and plaster, and identify early warning signs of complications. It is important to involve people in their care and to provide the necessary information both verbally and in writing. Nurses should confirm that the person understands what is required of them and that emergency contact numbers are prominently displayed on the information sheets.

Care of patients requiring treatment with external fixators or traction is beyond the scope of this book but is explained in titles in Further reading, below, e.g. Lucas (2011).

Joints

Joints, or articulations, occur between bones. They hold the bones securely together but may also allow movement. Some joints hold bones together very tightly and do not permit movement, e.g. the sutures of the skull, whereas others, e.g. the hip and shoulder joints, allow a range of movement. The focus here is on synovial joints because they are most involved in body movement. It is these movable (synovial) joints that cause most discomfort and pain, and that most often affect mobility if they become diseased or out of alignment.

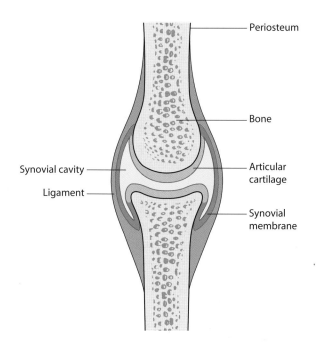

Movements possible at synovial joints   Box 18.7

Movement	Definition
Flexion	Bending, usually forward but occasionally backward, e.g. the knee joint
Extension	Straightening or bending backward
Abduction	Movement away from the midline of the body
Adduction	Movement towards the midline of the body
Circumduction	Movement of a limb or digit so it describes the shape of a cone
Rotation	Movement round the long axis of a bone
Pronation	Turning the palm of the hand down
Supination	Turning the palm of the hand up
Inversion	Turning the sole of the foot inwards
Eversion	Turning the sole of the foot outwards

(From Waugh, A., Grant, A., 2010. Ross and Wilson anatomy and physiology in health and illness, eleventh ed. Churchill Livingstone, Edinburgh.)

Fig. 18.4 • Typical synovial joint. (Reproduced with permission from Waugh, A., Grant, A., 2006. Ross and Wilson anatomy and physiology in health and illness, tenth ed. Churchill Livingstone, Edinburgh.)

At synovial joints (Fig. 18.4), the bone ends are covered in hyaline cartilage, which aids movement between the bones. The joint cavity is lined with synovial membrane and inside is a small amount of synovial fluid, which lubricates the joint. Ligaments consist of white, fibrous tissue and hold the bones together. They are not very elastic and so restrict the amount of movement available and stabilize the joint. Joints are further supported and protected by surrounding muscles, which prevent dislocation (see p. 435) and help to maintain upright posture. Ligaments attach to the periosteum of bones and cross the joint cavity. Twisting a joint, e.g. the ankle, may stretch and tear the ligaments and is known as a sprain.

Muscles work together in antagonistic pairs to allow movements at a joint. Contraction of one of a pair of antagonistic muscles brings about one specific movement and the opposite movement is caused by contraction of the opposing muscle, e.g. the biceps and triceps in the upper arm.

Box 18.7 lists the types of movement available at some joints and Figure 18.5 illustrates some of them. Knowing these movements is important for carrying out passive exercises (movements of joints initiated by an external force, e.g. physiotherapist or nurse, to exercise muscles and joints, see p. 452) or encouraging patients/clients to practise active exercises (movements initiated by an individual that exercise muscles and joints, see p. 452). When caring for people with mobility problems it is important to know the range of movements available at different joints so that they are not moved into positions that could be harmful. This is particularly important when caring for unconscious patients, or following joint replacement surgery. Common joint disorders are outlined in Table 18.1.

Posture, balance and movement

For purposeful movement the body must move in a synchronized manner with the nervous system (see Ch. 16) and musculoskeletal system working together to ensure that movements are smooth and coordinated, and of the appropriate force for the intended task. To understand why problems with movement occur, it is necessary to understand how normal upright and adaptive postures develop, and the principles of human movement and balance. This section explores these areas.

Development of the spinal curves

Babies are born with one 'C' shaped spinal curve, which is convex posteriorly. They are unable to control movement of the head, arms or legs and depend on natural reflexes to bring about movement. For example, the rooting reflex where, in response to lightly touching the side of the cheek, a baby turns its head to that side and begins to suck until the reflex disappears, usually around 3–4 months of age. The head and spine must be well supported when young babies are moved. At about 6 weeks, babies' eyes begin to follow colours and movements. This is accompanied by reflex movements in the back of the neck that strengthen the muscles there. Gradually, the neck muscles become bulkier and stronger, and begin to pull the cervical vertebrae and associated muscles into a secondary concave curve, the cervical curve (see Fig. 18.6). This enables the head to move from side to side. As babies learn to turn their heads, the muscles around the neck strengthen further and they begin to hold their heads steady on their shoulders for short periods. This is the first stage in developing head control. Gradually thereafter, the shoulder muscles strengthen, enabling the muscles of the upper arm to become stronger, leading to more purposeful movements of the upper limbs.

At about 3–6 months, the baby learns to sit up, but the back is still very rounded. At this age, the baby begins to roll from side to side, increasing the risk of childhood accidents (Box 18.8). This rotational movement around the spine develops the muscles of the lower back, leading to the development of the

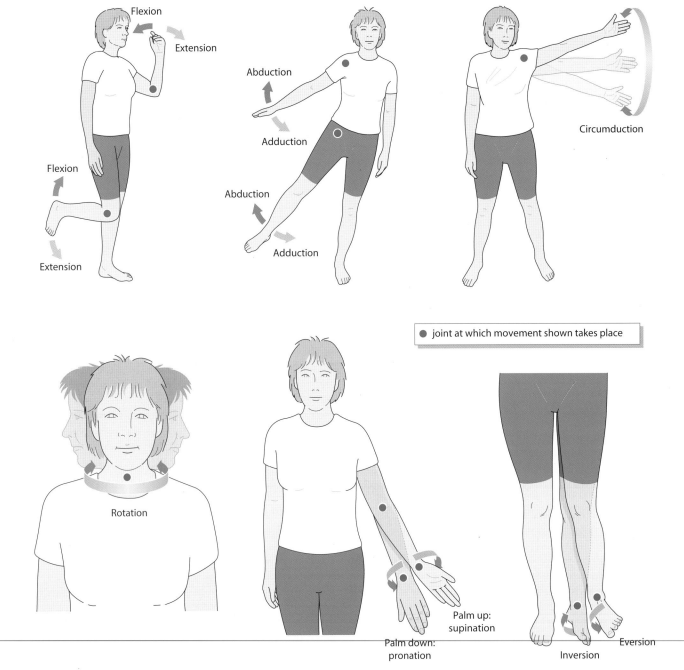

Fig. 18.5 • Main movements possible at synovial joints. (Reproduced with permission from Waugh, A., Grant, A., 2006. Ross and Wilson anatomy and physiology in health and illness, tenth ed. Churchill Livingstone, Edinburgh.)

secondary concave lumbar spine (see Fig. 18.6), which in turn allows the pelvic girdle to be suspended in its correct position at the bottom of the spine.

Only when the spine has achieved the lumbar curve can the child begin to walk and graduate to the toddler stage. Eventually, the muscles of the upper and lower legs and feet begin to strengthen and the child develops the upright posture. The spinal curves bring the centre of gravity into a straight line (see Fig. 18.6), which allows the body weight to be evenly distributed and helps to maintain balance in all movements.

The thoracic and sacral curves are known as primary curves because they retain the initial convex 'C' shape. The cervical

and lumbar curves are known as secondary curves because they develop a concave curvature. A child with severe cerebral palsy, who has poor head control, is unable to learn how to make meaningful movements with the rest of their body.

Adaptive postures

Adaptive postures occur over time because the fascia either shortens or lengthens in response to repeated, sustained tension in the underlying muscles, leading to discomfort and pain. This may be as a result of an underlying mechanical problem, such

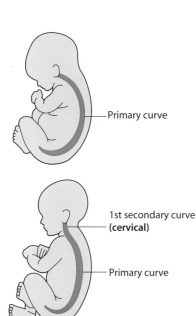

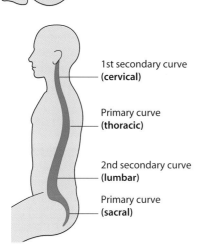

Fig. 18.6 • The spinal curves. (Reproduced with permission from Waugh, A., Grant, A., 2006. Ross and Wilson anatomy and physiology in health and illness, tenth ed. Churchill Livingstone, Edinburgh.)

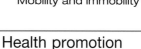 **Health promotion**   Box 18.8

Preventing childhood accidents

From the time that babies can roll over, at 3–6 months of age, they are at risk of rolling off a surface if left unattended. A child's environment needs to be organized to minimize the risk of accidents.

- Children under the age of 5 and people over 65 (particularly those over 75) are most likely to have an accident at home
- 0–4 year olds have the most accidents at home; boys are more likely to have accidents than girls
- Falls are the most common accidents in the home
- Childhood injuries are closely linked with social deprivation and are most common in children from poorer backgrounds (RoSPA).

Student activities

Visit the RoSPA website (www.rospa.com September 2012) and find out:

- The reasons why children of different ages are at risk from accidents.
- The precautions that will minimize accidents to children of different ages at home.

- Weak abdominal and back muscles that allow the pelvis to tilt forward and exaggerate the lumbar curve
- Standing bearing most of the weight through one leg and foot, rather than spreading it equally between both legs and feet causes the spinal curves to move out of alignment leading to an adaptive response in the neck in order to keep the head and eyes in alignment
- Sitting at a computer for long periods also affects the curves of the lower back and neck. If health and safety guidance is not followed (Box 18.9), people will find their spine moves out of alignment, affecting their posture. The trend for computer games and careers in IT encourages many people to spend long hours at the computer, often without much thought of how this will impinge on their long-term health
- Tall children tend to droop their shoulders and keep their heads down, to avoid standing 'head and shoulders' above their classmates and develop 'round shoulders'
- Carrying heavy school bags on one shoulder can also lead to adaptive shortening of fascia and muscle tissue around that shoulder.

The incidence of low back, neck and shoulder problems arising in schoolchildren has increased so much that some European countries demand that children use bags with straps for both shoulders and that they are fitted with wheels so that the bag can be pulled rather than carried if it is heavy. Lockers should also be provided in schools, so that pupils only have to carry the books required for one class at any time.

Peer pressure (see Ch. 8) and the need to conform to fit in with a group can have lasting effects on people's posture and mobility. Teenagers tend to slouch, when both standing and sitting, and girls may also slouch because they are embarrassed by the development of breasts, and comments made by others. It can therefore be difficult to maintain a good posture if it

---

as having one leg shorter than the other (true shortening), or a postural habit such as sitting poorly while using a computer or persistently carrying bags over one shoulder. Gilbert (2010) provides an excellent insight into these problems based on 40 years' experience as a physiotherapist. He has identified that of all the patients he has treated for musculoskeletal problems, 95% of these have resulted from apparent leg lengthening, which is easily treated by a series of physiotherapy stretching protocols called 'kinetic chain release' (KCR). Factors that influence the development of adaptive postures include:

- Apparent leg lengthening (as opposed to true shortening of leg bones), which affects most of the population. This occurs when the fascia in the feet, ankles, knees, hips and spine shorten as a result of postural habits, pulling the leg and heel up from the ground. The pelvis tilts to one side to enable the heel to strike the ground again and this has the effect of apparently lengthening one leg. It is treatable and correctable

 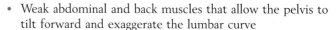

Health promotion Box 18.9

Recommended position for sitting at a computer

These nine steps should be followed when you sit at a computer or workstation:

1. Sit well back in the seat, and adjust the angle and height of the backrest so that your back is well supported.
2. Make sure that the small of your back is well supported.
3. Adjust the height of your chair so that your forearms are approximately horizontal when you use the keyboard.
4. Check that your wrists are in a neutral position.
5. Check that your feet are flat on the floor or use a footrest to take the pressure off the back of your thighs.
6. Make sure the area under your desk is free of clutter so that your feet can move freely.
7. Check that the height and angle of the screen allow you to hold your head in a comfortable position with the top of the screen at eye level.
8. Use a document holder if you do a lot of copy typing.
9. Make sure that your work area is large enough to accommodate your books and other study materials so that you have enough space to support your arms when you are not using your keyboard.

Student activities

Visit the Working-Well website (below) and work through the exercises there to ensure your workstation is correctly organized.

(From: Working-Well – www.working-well.org)

makes an individual stand out from the crowd. However, posture is more than just the ability to stand or sit in a good upright position; it is a balanced action of muscles to maintain all parts of the body in positions that do not involve undue strain, and from which immediate coordinated action of any part of the body is possible.

Normally, babies and toddlers do not have problems with posture unless they are born with an abnormality that predisposes to problems with mobility and/or true leg shortening, such as cerebral palsy, developmental dysplasia of the hip (previously called congenital dislocation of the hip), a shortened leg bone or a missing limb. However, as children grow older, they become more aware of adult habits and often copy them. This is when problems with adaptive posture can begin.

Effects of gravity on height

As two-legged upright beings, humans are constantly at the mercy of gravity trying to pull them nearer to the ground. During the course of a day, people lose height as the spine continually counteracts the effects of gravity on their bodies. Water loss from the intervertebral discs (the pads of cartilage between the vertebrae) is another contributing factor. However, after a night's sleep, the discs swell again and by the morning, height is regained. Therefore, when measuring a patient's/client's height and weight (see Ch. 14), it is advisable to do this at the same time of day, so that the same conditions prevail. This is particularly important when children are being assessed and/or treated for problems with growth and development.

Effects of ageing on the spinal curves

As part of the normal ageing process, the effects of gravity begin to take their toll on the musculoskeletal system. The 'elderly people crossing' road sign depicts older adults walking with stooped posture and using walking sticks. Although not appropriate for the majority of older adults, this sign clearly demonstrates the combined effects of adaptive posture and gravity on the musculoskeletal system. There is, however, nothing wrong with stooped posture, as long as the position is not sustained for lengthy periods, as this will encourage development of an adaptive posture. Anatomically, the stooped posture is exactly the opposite of the upright posture. In the upright posture, the muscles classified as extensors (that act to straighten joints) are active, whereas in a stooped posture the flexor muscles (that act to bend joints) are active. Movement between both of these postures is recommended in order to ensure good blood flow to each group of muscles. Regular changes in posture increases blood flow to, through and from the muscles and improves oxygen exchange (see Ch. 17) between the blood and the muscles; at the same time, waste products are removed from the muscles. This maintains optimum health of the muscles and their surrounding fascia. Try to move regularly between the upright and slouched postures while reading the rest of this chapter.

Movement

Movement is brought about by the actions of muscles on joints. Some muscles act on more than one joint and these are the most active in producing movements. Single joint muscles are the deeper, postural muscles (e.g. soleus) and two-joint muscles are the more superficial, active muscles (e.g. gastrocnemius) (Fig. 18.7). This arrangement of muscles helps to produce coordinated movement. (For a more detailed explanation of the mechanics and physiology of human movement, see Further reading: Myers 2009).

Gait

Gait is the term used to describe the manner in which people walk or run. A person's gait can be analysed in a laboratory, which can assist in the diagnosis and treatment of mobility problems such as arthritis and apparent or true leg lengthening. Gait varies depending on:

- People's movement habits
- The ways in which individuals' muscles and fascia have adapted to their habits over time
- Age
- The presence of disease or abnormalities that affect nerves, bones, muscles and/or joints.

Balance is the key to walking. The balance reflexes do not begin to develop until about 6 months of age and as toddlers begin to walk, at around 12–13 months, their gait is quite different from that of adults. Children under the age of about 2 years walk with flat feet and their legs more widely apart. About the age of 4 years, children begin to develop the arm swing. As the

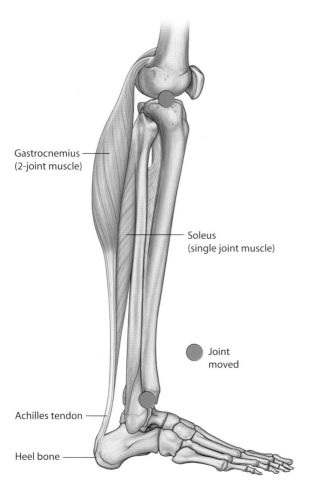

Gastrocnemius
(2-joint muscle)

Soleus
(single joint muscle)

Joint
moved

Achilles tendon

Heel bone

Fig. 18.7 • One- and two-joint muscles of the lower leg. (Reproduced with permission from Drake, R.L., Vogt, W., Mitchell, A.W.M., 2005. Gray's anatomy for medical students. Churchill Livingstone, Edinburgh.)

more balanced adult gait of striking the ground with the heel first and swinging the arms develops, the pace of step and step length increase. This is often lost in Parkinson's disease (see Table 18.1, p. 434). If someone has a particular way of putting one foot down on the ground, the other foot has to alter its pattern of movement to accommodate for this, leading to the development of an adaptive posture.

As posture is about maintaining dynamic balance, whatever happens in one part of the body affects the movement in another. A Trendelenburg gait is characterized by leaning to the affected side every time the opposite leg swings through to take a step, which is caused by unilateral weakness of hip abductor muscles (gluteals). In older adults, the pace of walking and the step length generally decrease. Older adults often suffer from gait disorders that have many causes, one of which may be a fear of falling (Caby et al 2011).

Age and disability are the two major factors contributing to changes in gait because both affect posture and balance. Degenerative changes around the hip also tend to reduce stride length. People gradually lose the ability to maintain their balance as they age; therefore, in order to provide a larger base for support to maintain balance, the width of the step also increases slightly.

The joints tend to stiffen with age, which reduces the range of movement. If this happens around the ankle it becomes more difficult to lift the foot free from the ground, leading to dragging of the toes that can predispose to falls. Finally, joint stiffness also affects the spine, leading to loss of rotation and arm swing. Reduction in both of these elements slows the walking speed.

Joint problems that affect gait may be reversible with surgical intervention and include arthritic joints, flat foot (pes planus) and bunions (hallux valgus). Foot drop is another cause that arises from compression damage to the peroneal nerve caused by, e.g. a prolapsed ('slipped') intervertebral disc. Joint and muscle pain will affect gait. Pain in the hip(s) or knee(s) causes people to spend less time weight-bearing on the affected joint. Fibromyalgia (muscle, tendon and joint pain) and myasthenia gravis (an autoimmune condition) are disorders that both result in weakened and easily fatigued muscles that can impair mobility. Parkinson's disease (see Table 18.1, p. 434) is a common condition that affects both movement and gait.

Many problems with gait can be attributed to problems with the feet, which is why it is important to refer people with foot conditions, especially older adults, to a podiatrist. These include many easily treatable and reversible conditions such as corns and calluses, nail deformities, verrucae, athlete's foot and other fungal infections.

Efficient handling and moving (EHM)

Many people can be encouraged to move themselves with help, such as verbal encouragement or a hand placed over the muscle groups to be moved, and further intervention is not needed. Good handling and moving skills are paramount to the health and safety of nurses and their patients/clients, and are essential to assist people to move safely when they cannot move unaided. Nurses who understand the principles of human movement can apply them not only to care safely for people with mobility problems, but also to protect themselves from injury. Understanding the stages of human development, including ageing, also enables nurses to predict, to some extent, the needs of people of all ages (see Ch. 8).

Details of the current legislation and the principles of safe handling and moving are explained in Chapter 13. This section extends this to include the safe handling and moving of people including:

* Moving people in bed
* Using equipment to assist moving
* Helping people to use walking aids.

Another important text to read is *The Guide to the Handling of People* (Backcare and Royal College of Nursing 2011), which details all the moves that can be executed safely (too numerous to mention in this chapter); those that are condemned because they pose a very high risk to nurses and patients/clients, and how equipment can be used to minimize handling and moving injuries. Suggestions are given about the best way of applying the principles of safer moving but it is beyond the scope of this chapter to cover every potential situation that nurses might come across.

It is important to understand the difference between *efficient* handling and moving, and *effective* handling and moving:

- An efficient movement is one that achieves its goal using the appropriate amount of muscle effort for the demands of the task
- An effective movement usually involves more force than is required to produce the desired action.

Efficient movement is therefore preferable, as it is less likely to result in injury to either nurses or patients/clients. Two safe approaches to EHM are:

- *Ergonomic* – which involves taking a risk assessment approach (see Ch. 13) to reduce the risks of the procedure to the minimum by redesigning the environment or equipment to enable safer working conditions, e.g. using profiling beds to reduce the amount of patient handling
- *Biomechanical* – this practises bending of the knees and keeping the back straight to maintain the spine in its strongest position.

Principles of safe handling and moving

In order to minimize the risk of injury to either practitioners or patients/clients, it is important always to:

- Apply the approach taught in your university, according to local policy
- Carry out a risk assessment before handling and moving either people or inanimate loads by using the acronym TILE:
  - *Task:* whether it requires unusual skills or knowledge, can it be mechanized, is it necessary or can it be achieved by other means
  - *Individual:* in terms of practitioner experience, knowledge, height and weight
  - *Load:* in terms of patient/client height, weight, physical and mental capabilities
  - *Environment:* assess the space, height of working surfaces and the presence of uneven floor surfaces or carpets; remove unnecessary equipment.

The principles of efficient movement are covered in Chapter 13.

Equipment

There are many devices available to assist in moving people. Commonly used equipment and its potential uses are described below. Use of mobility aids such as walking frames, walking sticks and wheelchairs is explained on page 448.

Glide sheets

Glide sheets, also known as slide sheets (Fig. 18.8A) are often used to help people move in bed or in a chair. There are many different styles, but they all work on the same principle of reducing friction between the skin and the bed or chair surface when they are placed under a surface contact area, e.g. the sacrum, heels, shoulders, head. Some glide sheets enable movement to occur in several directions, i.e. up, down, side-to-side and in a circular movement. These are commonly referred to as multiglide sheets, which are made of thin, low-friction material. Others allow movement in one direction only and are referred to as one-way glide sheets. Typically, a glide sheet looks like a sleeping bag, but is open at both ends and has a slippery inner surface. Once in position, it is possible to move a person using minimal force. Some glide sheets have handles to enable handlers to take hold of the sheet rather than placing their hands on the person.

Transfer boards

These are generally fairly solid, although some are more flexible than others, and are used to assist in transfers between different pieces of equipment or furniture such as chairs, beds, baths, wheelchairs, trolleys and car seats. They are often referred to as lateral transfer boards since the person being moved usually moves in a sideways direction. Depending on the nature of the transfer, a smaller or larger board may be used. Glide sheets are often used together with transfer boards as they reduce the handler effort required. Some transfer boards are manufactured with glide sheets attached. These can be useful for bathing. Figure 18.8B shows a small transfer board used for sitting transfers, while larger transfer boards are available for use in bed transfers.

Hoists

Mechanical and electrical hoists are widely used to assist people into and out of bed and chairs. Mechanical hoists usually require more handler effort to operate than electrical hoists. Another benefit of electrical hoists is that patients/clients can be given the control box and, following instruction and supervised practice, they can operate it themselves. Many people with paraplegia (who have paralysis and functional loss of their trunk and lower limbs) are able to move themselves independently using electrical hoists. There are many different styles and sizes of hoists and it is important to learn how a particular hoist works before using it to move people.

Some hoists are used only to assist people into a standing position for a short period of time, e.g. to assist with toileting, or while their personal hygiene is being attended to and/or their clothing is being adjusted.

Standing and raising hoist

Figure 18.8C shows a standing and raising appliance (commonly called a SARA hoist), which is used only for standing transfers. These standing hoists should only be used when the person being moved can take some of their body weight through their feet. If there is any doubt about this, standing hoists must be avoided and a passive lifting hoist that will take the whole body weight used instead. Each hoist clearly displays a safe weight that must not be exceeded.

Passive lifting hoists

Passive lifting hoists are suitable for use in situations where there is any doubt about a person's ability either to move

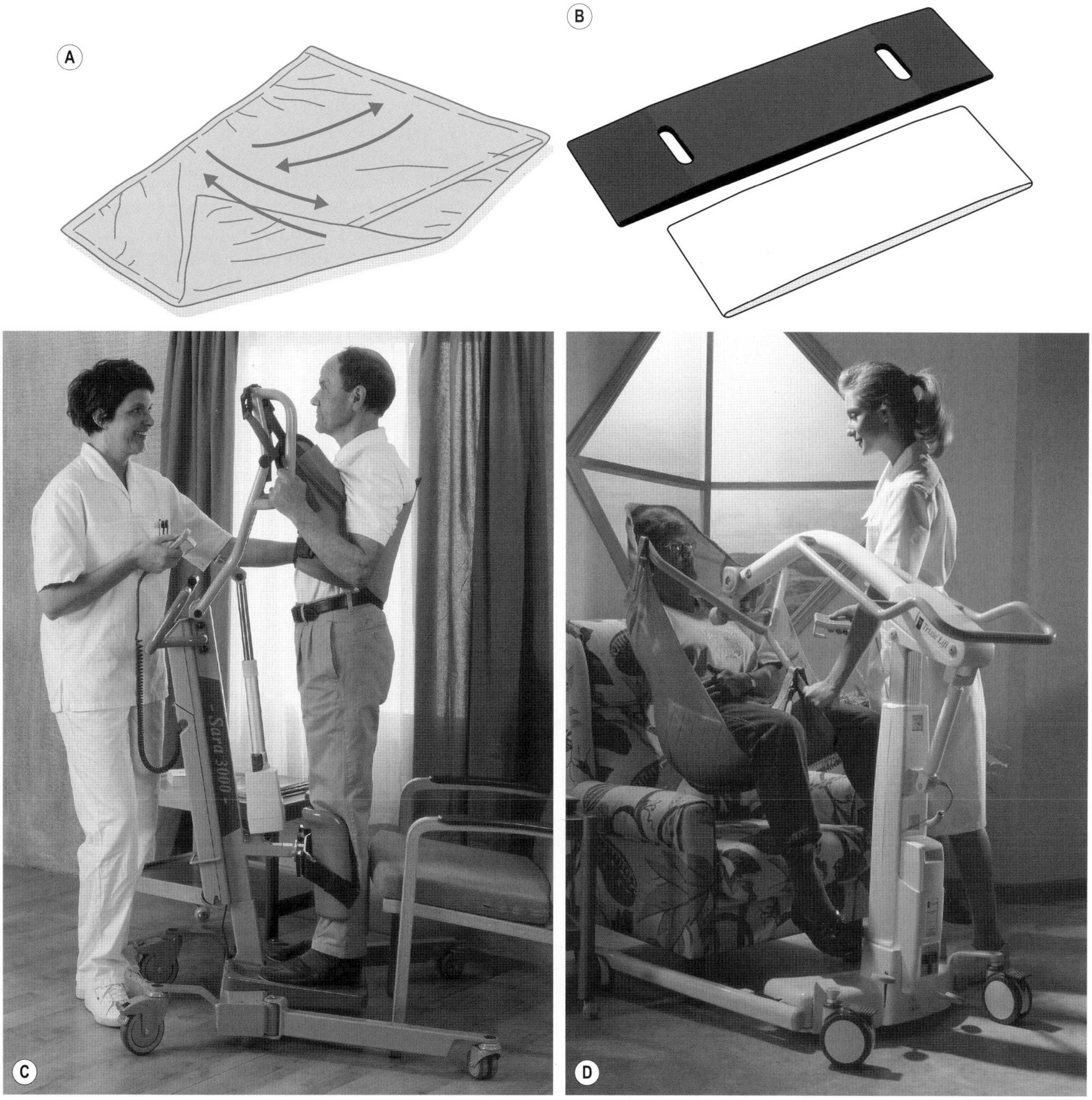

Fig. 18.8 • A range of handling and moving equipment: (A) Glide sheet. (B) Small transfer boards. (C) Standing and raising (SARA) hoist. (D) Trixie hoist. (Hoists reproduced with permission from ARJO.)

independently or to comply with instructions. Passive lifting hoists use slings, made of soft but strong material, that are applied to the patient/client before being attached to the hoist. Disposable slings are sometimes used to minimize cross-infection (see Ch. 15); otherwise the slings are laundered according to the manufacturer's instructions and local policy. Some slings are also suitable for bathing and toileting. Figure 18.8D shows a Trixie hoist with its slings. Slings are not interchangeable and the correct ones for a specific hoist must be used following the manufacturer's guidelines. Slings are available in a range of sizes and the most appropriate size should

be used. A correctly fitted sling adds to the security of a patient/client during the transfer.

There are also hoists that enable people to be raised off the bed in a lying position. These are used for people with spinal injuries who are not allowed any flexion of the spine and in operating theatres.

Hoists can appear very frightening to people who have never been moved in this way before. Nurses should take time to discuss with patients/clients why they are being moved using a hoist, describing how it will benefit the individual and nursing staff involved. Chapter 13 (pp. 285–286) identifies the Health and Safety regulations that must be followed when using equipment such as hoists.

Accessories

Sometimes it is not necessary to use hoists and slides when moving people, and equipment described in this section can be used to assist mobility.

Rope ladders

Rope ladders attached to the end of the bed can be useful for assisting people to move themselves into a more comfortable position independently. Patients/clients need to have good upper limb and head control to be able to pull themselves up into a sitting position.

Turning discs

These consist of two discs that rotate against one another and are designed either for people to sit on or to place under their feet. They are used to assist with turning and can be used independently or with assistance. Generally, it is better to use turning discs with lighter people as the weight of heavier patients/clients can interfere with the turning mechanism.

Using equipment to move people

Nurses must familiarize themselves with any equipment used in people's homes, nursing homes and wards before using it. It is also useful to have experienced being moved using the equipment so that clear explanations can be given. Practical classes at university provide the opportunity to experience being moved in a hoist under close supervision and it is a good idea to use these opportunities. These sessions can also be used to discuss with the trainer if a particular piece of equipment is appropriate for a specific care setting. Observing demonstrations using healthy volunteers who cannot represent your specific patient's/client's needs may not necessarily identify problems with equipment that may be encountered in practice.

Checking equipment

Always check that the equipment is in good working order before using it to move people. Chapter 13 outlines the Lifting Operations and Lifting Equipment Regulations (LOLER) for checking equipment safety on a regular basis. Common faults include:

- Deflated tyres on wheelchairs
- Missing or incorrectly fitting footplates on wheelchairs
- Brakes that are difficult to operate
- Low power or flat batteries on electric hoists
- Tears in slides
- Loose nuts and bolts
- Worn-out slings
- Damaged surfaces on transfer boards.

Risk assessment

Initial assessment of a patient's/client's mobility needs must be carried out by an experienced practitioner and appropriately documented in the nursing notes. Physiotherapists and OTs may be involved in this process, which provides a broad indication of the equipment that may be required to move the patient/client. This part of the patient/client records must be read carefully before any handling and moving activities are carried out. If you are unsure about what is expected, it is essential to seek advice from your mentor to prevent injury to either patients/clients or nurses by carrying out procedures incorrectly (Box 18.10).

⚖ Ethical issues   Box 18.10

Condoning unsafe practice

Jootun and MacInnes (2005) examined the extent to which undergraduate students correctly apply taught principles when handling and moving people during placements. They identified many factors that influence practice and which can promote the continuance of unsafe practice. In today's society where litigation is increasing and patients/clients are more informed about their care and codes of practice, it is important to carefully consider the ethical dilemmas that may arise each time a patient/client is moved.

Student activities

- Identify factors found by Jootun and MacInnes (2005) to predispose to unsafe handling and moving practice
- Have you ever been asked to carry out a manoeuvre that is condemned because it carries a high risk of injury?
- Would you make the manoeuvre because it can be easier than refusing, or would you defend your position and refuse to assist?
- Think about the implications for the nurse and a patient/client if harm occurred during a condemned manoeuvre
- Discuss your findings and thoughts with your mentor.

Resource

Jootun, D., MacInnes, A., 2005. Examining how well students use correct handling procedures. Nursing Times 101 (4), 38–40.

As there is a possibility of litigation when things go wrong, it is always advisable to err on the side of safety. A person in bed is unlikely to suffer harm by waiting a few minutes longer while the appropriate preparations for moving them are made.

Although an initial assessment will have been undertaken, a patient's/client's condition can change at any time. It is therefore important that each time the person is being moved, further assessment of both their needs and the handler's capabilities is carried out.

Effective communication

Handling and moving people requires effective communication skills (see Ch. 9). Pacing of explanations is important, so that too much information is not given at once or causes anxiety or confusion. Children, like anyone else, should not be patronized when equipment is being used; they should also be told what is happening and what to expect. People who are frightened do not cooperate easily and inappropriate explanations may lead to breakdown in the nurse–patient/client relationship. Some people are unable to understand explanations about handling and moving equipment, e.g. those with dementia or severe learning disability. In such cases, an empathetic approach and careful handling and moving must be used.

It is good practice to explain what moving a person will involve and to describe any equipment and what it does before bringing it to the bedside. Patients/clients should direct the speed of moving activities. People with poor vision should be encouraged to touch and handle equipment before it is used so they can get a sense of what will be happening to them.

Finding the most suitable equipment

Sometimes it can be difficult to find the ideal piece of equipment to move a patient/client safely, e.g. where there is apraxia or dyspraxia (see Table 18.1, p. 434). In these situations, physiotherapists must be resourceful in finding and using the right equipment to meet very specific individual needs. Foam wedges, mats and padding are often used to reduce the risk of injury from the equipment itself. These clients can become very agitated and, since they have little or no control over the movements of their limbs, can also be at high risk of injury as can those assisting in the manoeuvre. It is particularly important that only the palms of the hands are used when supporting limbs. Gripping must be avoided as this causes strong contraction of the underlying muscles, making control of the limb even more difficult.

Handling and moving people

This section addresses key issues of moving people with or without equipment. Details about how to carry out specific manoeuvres can be found in the *Guide to the Handling of People* (BackCare and Royal College of Nursing 2011). Nursing patients/clients in bed usually involves handling and moving them to carry out their care, e.g.:

• Moving patients onto and off the bed in a supine position
• Moving patients up the bed
• Sitting patients up in bed
• Turning patients
• Inserting and removing bedpans
• Changing clothing, bedding or dressings
• Transferring a patient to the commode or wheelchair
• Preparing patients to stand up
• Putting patients to bed.

Helping people to move in bed has been identified as carrying a higher risk of injury than other handling and moving activities. For this reason, it is important that all necessary steps are taken to reduce the risk of injury and to follow handling and moving guidance documented in the nursing care plan.

When moving people in beds or chairs, it is important to be aware that the spine is the central axis around which all movement occurs. If a patient/client who has lost power of their arms is required to move one of their hands, the nurse should work from the shoulder girdle. This is because the muscles of the shoulder girdle are postural muscles; built for power, rather than the smaller muscles of the hand, which are built for fine movements. If the hand is moved first, the handlers must bear the load of the whole arm, whereas moving the shoulder first allows the arm and hand to be moved with less effort. Likewise to move a person's foot, the move is started from the hip.

It is often necessary to support patients'/clients' limbs on pillows while they are being moved in bed. This must be carried out in a manner that both supports and protects the limb, and does not cause pain. Limbs should be supported underneath, either in the palm of the hand or across the forearm, while pillows are being positioned. The limbs should be supported in natural positions (Fig. 18.9) that do not put joints into positions that could result in pain or loss of function. Feet should not be left hanging off the ends of pillows and wrists should be supported in neutral positions.

Turning a person in bed

This technique is used to move patients/clients in bed to minimize the risk of twisting their spines while changing bed linen, placing hoist slings in position or turning them (to minimize the risk of pressure damage, see Ch. 25).

Regaining balance

When a person has been immobile for a period of time, none of the body systems work to their full potential and a programme of gradual mobilization is required to enable independence again. After a couple of days in bed with a viral illness, even young people may feel quite unsteady on their legs, dizzy and not up to their usual energy levels, and find carrying out even simple tasks tiring. The dizziness experienced after a lengthy period of lying down can be due to postural hypotension. For this reason, people who have been nursed in a supine position (lying flat) are sat up gradually, so that the cardiovascular system can adjust to the new position.

For patients/clients nursed on a profiling bed, the head of the bed is gently raised a little at a time. Giving the control box to the patient allows them to raise the head of their bed to a position with which they feel comfortable. They may raise the head of the bed further at a rate they can tolerate, until they are able to sit upright. At this stage they will still need to be supported with pillows and backrests. Thereafter they will need to relearn how to sit up unsupported and regain their sitting balance.

Once sitting balance has been regained, the patient/client can progress to standing and walking. The key points to be aware of are whether or not the patient/client can move from sitting to standing unaided and, once standing, whether or not they will have standing balance. Mobility aids and hoists can be used to assist people to stand and walk.

Helping a person to sit up in bed

The most efficient equipment to assist a patient to move from the lying to the sitting position is an electric powered, height

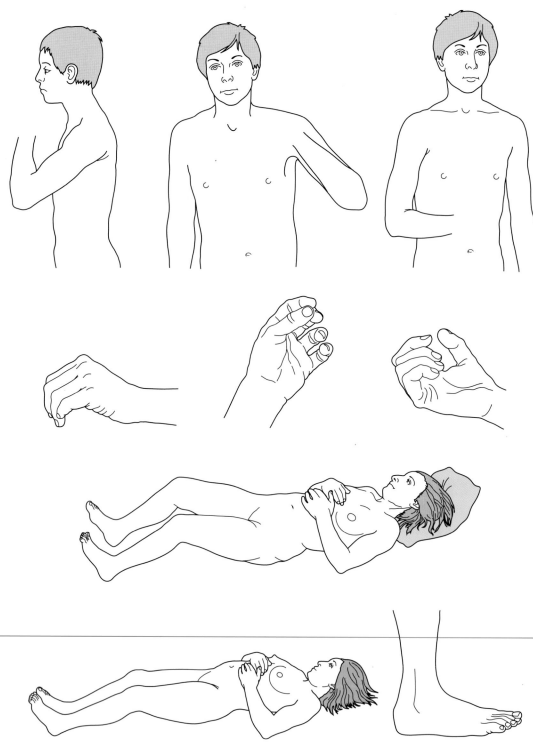

Fig. 18.9 • Resting positions of the limbs. (Reproduced with permission from Peattie, P.I., Walker, S., 1996. Understanding nursing care, fourth ed. Churchill Livingstone, Edinburgh.)

adjustable, profiling bed. If profiling beds are not available, other equipment can be used on non-profiling beds such as:

• Pillow lifters
• Mattress elevators
• A knee break, which supports the patient's knees in a flexed position in bed
• Passive lifting hoists with slings (see pp. 442–443).

Patients/clients can be encouraged to move themselves in bed using equipment designed for the purpose, e.g. rope ladders or slides, or a combination of these.

As patients recover and become more mobile, the nursing care plan is altered to reflect their improving mobility. People should be encouraged to help themselves to sit up by rolling onto their sides, taking their weight through their elbows and pushing themselves up into a sitting position. During any of the aforementioned procedures, the nurse should initially stay beside the patient to offer support if needed and to give advice and encouragement. Once patients have gained confidence in carrying out the move, and the nurse is satisfied that they are capable of moving themselves safely, observation can be carried out from a distance.

Helping a person to get out of bed

Ensure that there is enough space to work safely, taking into account the size of the chair and the amount of space required for turning the patient/client. Box 18.11 explains how to select a suitable chair; however, in reality, choice may be limited. Initially the bed should be level with the upper thigh while the patient/client is being dressed. Once the person is ready to be moved into a sitting position, the bed is lowered to allow their feet to touch the floor. Always check that the brakes are securely applied before helping a person to move. Do not lean against the bed when moving someone as the wheels may slip on the floor.

 Nursing skills Box 18.11

Choosing a suitable chair

Smith (2011) considers that the following factors should be taken into account:

The seat

- *Height:* Should correspond with the leg length of the seated person, should allow the feet to be flat on the floor with the thighs level and should be firm to help the seated person push up.
- *Depth:* Should correspond to the length from the back of the hips to the front of the knee (a lumbar support will increase this measurement).
- *Angle:* The seated person's hips should be level with their knees. If the hips are higher, a footstool should be used to raise the feet and to reduce pressure on the back of the thighs.

The back

- *Height:* Depends on whether a head support is required. Chair wings impede conversation and encourage slouching to the side, but may reduce draughts.
- *Headrest:* Should be tilted slightly backwards to provide comfortable support. A vertical headrest tends to push the head forward, causing neck pain.
- *Armrests:* If present, these should come well forward so that the person can grasp or push down on them to assist moving to the front of the chair before standing. They should provide support for the elbows without distorting the shoulder position.
- *Chair legs:* Front legs should be vertical and the rear legs angled slightly backwards. There should be a minimum of 13 cm clearance under a chair to accommodate hoists.
- *Style:* Reclining armchairs, supportive chairs, riser and adjustable chairs all promote comfort and independence. Riser chairs have features that assist people to move from a sitting to a standing position with minimal assistance.

Well-fitting, lightweight slippers should be put on to prevent the person slipping when their feet reach the floor. Shoes should always be worn with socks, to maintain dignity and to prevent chafing of the feet; however, they can add considerably to the weight of the legs, making them more difficult to move.

The nursing care plan will indicate what equipment to use and how much assistance a patient/client needs to get out of bed and sit in a chair. All equipment requires the assistance of at least one nurse. This includes:

- Passive lifting hoists (see Fig. 18.8D) with slings for people who cannot weight-bear
- Partial weight-bearing hoists and walking harnesses
- SARA hoists (see Fig. 18.8C) for people who have some ability to weight-bear
- Turning discs with frames for people who have good upper body strength and are able to weight-bear. People using these must be able to hold the frame to pull themselves up into a standing position.

Some patients/clients require only minimal assistance to stand up from the side of the bed. These people must have good sitting balance and be able to support themselves while sitting at the edge of the bed with their feet flat on the floor. Always allow patients/clients to dictate the speed of the move; it is important that people feel in control and that their needs are respected. People who have had strong analgesics may not be as quick-thinking as usual and should be given short, concise instructions that are easily understood. It is also important to be aware that some drugs may cause postural hypotension, a drop in blood pressure that may cause dizziness or fainting when standing upright.

Physiotherapists can provide specific advice to nurses about positioning themselves to help particular patients/clients.

Helping a person to stand up from a chair

Standing a patient up from a chair is different from standing a patient up from a bed. The main differences are that nurses must accommodate the arms of the chair and the height of the chair is usually fixed. Equipment that may be used includes:

- Riser seats
- Blocks to raise chairs (the chair legs are slotted into raised blocks that increase the height of the chair)
- SARA hoists (see Fig. 18.8C).

Key points to follow when assisting people to stand from chairs are shown in Box 18.12.

Helping people to mobilize

The differences in gait in children, adults and older people (see p. 440) must be taken into account when assisting people to walk. It can be difficult to walk alongside someone who has an altered gait. Helping people with walking carries an increased risk of injuries (Brooks & Orchard 2011). Allow people with visual impairment to use familiar arm holds for walking, e.g. taking hold of the sighted person's left arm around the elbow and walking slightly behind. Equipment used to assist people with walking includes walking sticks, walking frames and crutches. These are all measured and fitted to the person's

---

 Nursing skills   Box 18.12

Principles for assisting people to stand from chairs

1. Risk assessment using TILE (see p. 442).
2. The nurse stands to the side of the person, with the outer foot pointing in the direction of intended movement, ready to take a step as the person moves.
3. The person's hips are brought close to the edge of the seat.
4. Positioning the person's feet with one foot slightly in front of the other enables a pushing action to assist standing, without the person losing their balance.
5. The person is asked to keep their head in a relaxed upright position, looking forwards.
6. The nurse should be ready to assist, if required, by placing their nearest arm across the person's back, either between the shoulder blades or lower down the back if required, allowing the palm of the hand to make contact to prompt standing. The nurse's other arm should be moved into a position that allows the palm of the hand to cradle the person's nearest shoulder or take a palm to palm hold.
7. Simple instructions are used to direct the movement.
8. The person is encouraged to raise their head to initiate the standing movement and use the armrests to push themselves into a standing position.
9. Simultaneously, the nurse raises their own head and takes a step forward with the leading foot so that on completion of the movement both the nurse and the person are balanced.
10. Before releasing their hold on the person, the nurse checks that the person's weight is equally distributed between both feet and that they have control of their balance.
11. If the person is unable to stand, the nurse's hands will slide off the shoulder and back, leaving the person in a sitting position. The situation should be reassessed and equipment used to move the person from the chair.

---

height by the physiotherapist or registered nurse. Wheeled walkers may be used for children. If a person needs manual assistance with walking, an assessment is carried out and documented in the care plan. This takes account of whether the individual:

- Can control their arms and upper body
- Can maintain balance while standing
- Has an upright or stooped posture
- Can comply with instructions
- Has ever used, or currently uses, walking aids
- Has breathing or respiratory problems that affect their stamina
- Is suffering pain and how this affects their mobility
- Has suitable footwear, e.g. slippers, boots, shoes. Well-fitting, supportive shoes are preferable and reduce the potential for falls (see Ch. 13).

The following factors should also be considered and assessed prior to mobilizing a person:

- Is the individual expected to walk a long distance?
- At what speed will someone desire to walk? For example, is there an urgent need to use the lavatory? If this is the case, it is safer to take the person on a wheelchair and allow them to walk back.

- What are the prevailing floor conditions, e.g. linoleum or carpet?
- Does the individual have attachments such as an intravenous infusion or a urinary catheter?

Walking frames

Walking frames are widely used and come in many shapes and sizes according to the function for which they are required. Some walking aids have wheels and are known as 'rollators'. They may have a shopping basket attached so that they can be used to carry light bags. In hospitals, walking frames often have rubber stoppers on the ends of the legs so that the frames do not slip on the floor. Sometimes walking frames are used temporarily as people regain full fitness. For others, they are always used to maintain peoples' safety and independence, especially those who:

- Have the ability to weight-bear but may tire easily
- Have a history of falling
- Have painful joints
- Lack confidence.

Walking sticks

Walking sticks or tripods (that have one handle and three feet) provide a similar function to walking frames, but are less bulky. They are often used as a first measure when people become aware that their balance is deteriorating. Many people purchase walking sticks without any advice from a physiotherapist or OT. Most are height adjustable and should be set at a comfortable height that allows the elbow to be held in a slightly flexed position. The correct height for the stick is identified by measuring the distance from the person's wrist to the ground while they are wearing their normal outdoor shoes. Normally, the stick is used on the side to which the person is most likely to fall, but this is not a hard and fast rule, and physiotherapists or OTs can assess people to advise on individual requirements. Physiotherapists also measure clients for crutches and tripods so that they are given the correct height of appliance.

Wheelchairs

Wheelchairs offer a degree of independence to some users, but many others are dependent on being pushed around. It is important to understand what a person's expectations are when discussing the use of a wheelchair. The following general principles are useful:

- If people are completely dependent on others pushing the wheelchair, then it is best to use one with smaller wheels (Fig. 18.10A). This makes it easier for the handler to push the wheelchair outside, because the tyres are not inflatable.
- If people wish to move the wheelchair independently, it is better to have larger, inflatable tyres so that the wheels can be turned more easily, causing less damage to the hands (Fig. 18.10B).

Choosing the correct width of wheelchair is important to ensure that the patient/client will not slip out of it. It is also necessary to consider the width of doorways if the wheelchair is for home use. Sometimes it is necessary to remove doors to enable access to rooms. All new buildings must comply with

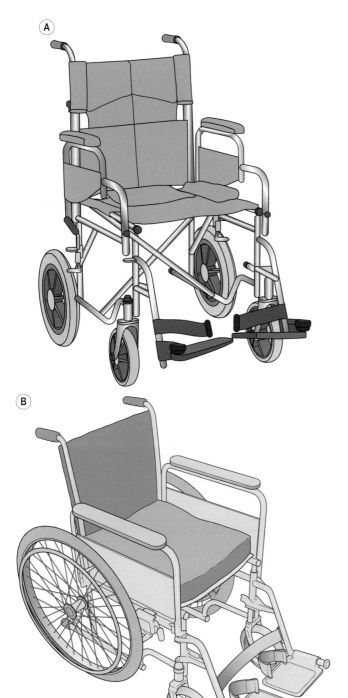

Fig. 18.10 • Wheelchairs: (A) Small wheeled. (B) Large wheeled.

extensions, leg extensions and foot plates can all be adapted to meet individual patient's/client's needs. Many younger people have lightweight frames and wheels on their wheelchairs, particularly if they are likely to be involved in sporting and keep-fit activities. Different types of padded seat are available to reduce the effects of pressure (see Ch. 25). Box 18.13 provides information about checking and storage of wheelchairs.

Wheelchairs	Box 18.13

Safety checks

Ensure that:

- All tyres are inflated
- Both footplates are attached and in good condition
- Heel straps are correctly fitted to footplates
- Both brakes are working
- The chair is clean
- Any additional attachments such as padding, head support or leg extensions are securely in place and in good condition.

Storage

- Chairs can be folded for storage.
- Empty chairs are easier to move if they are left unfolded and a wheelbarrow action is used. Take hold of the handles from underneath and raise the back wheels slightly from the floor so that only the front wheels are in contact with the floor.

Falls

Cryer and Patel (2001) identified that in the community, one-third of people over the age of 65 and 50% of people over the age of 80 will fall at some time. Some of these falls will result in fractures. Dealing with a falling patient is challenging. There are many factors that predispose to falls, including:

- Postural hypotension
- Dizziness
- Alterations in gait
- Stroke
- Fear of falling
- History of previous falls
- Sight and hearing problems
- Poor footwear
- Hazards in the environment
- Poor lighting
- Polypharmacy (Ch. 22)
- Steps and stairs
- Use of alcohol and recreational drugs.

As falls are common, it is very important to be aware of the main predisposing factors in order to prevent or minimize their occurrence. Prevention of falls is explored in Box 13.10 (p. 253). Older adults who are admitted to hospital following a fall are referred to a gerontologist (a physician who specializes in the care of older adults) for further investigation of their physical health and home circumstances. Falling is often the first indication of an underlying problem. It may be the sign of

national building regulations, e.g. the Scottish Building Standards Agency (2011), to ensure that they have wheelchair access through at least one door and, thereafter, into at least one toilet and one public room on the ground floor.

Wheelchairs can be designed to suit the specific needs of individual patients/clients. Sometimes the whole seat is moulded around the person's body to accommodate their body shape which offers support in the correct places such as the head, thorax, hips, knees and feet. Back extensions, head something simple, e.g. a person requires spectacles, or it may be the result of something more serious such as postural hypotension. Gerontologists carry out physical and psychological investigations to identify the cause of falling and the measures required to remedy the situation.

As part of the multidisciplinary team (MDT), gerontologists work in conjunction with nurses, OTs, physiotherapists and social workers to provide the support needed to enable people to return home. By reducing polypharmacy (see Ch. 22), treating previously undiagnosed conditions and putting appropriate mobility aids into the home, many older adults can be enabled to continue to live at home. The benefits of living at home in familiar surroundings far outweigh those of living in supported accommodation, e.g. nursing homes. Moving people from their familiar environment can cause confusion and increase the risk of falls. It is also more cost-effective to provide support in people's homes than in long-term supported care.

Care of people who have fallen

Normally, nurses walk to the side and slightly behind patients/clients when they are escorting them (see p. 447). This means that if a patient/client loses their balance, the nurse can move behind them and begin to control their descent to the ground. However, this should only be undertaken if the following criteria are present:

- There is enough space to enable the nurse and patient to move
- There is no significant height difference between the nurse and the patient
- The patient is not much heavier than the nurse
- The patient is not resisting being handled
- The patient is falling backwards towards the nurse.

Alternatively, the nurse must clear any furniture if possible and allow the patient/client to fall to the ground, particularly if the person is falling away from the nurse.

Once on the ground the patient/client is safe and the situation must then be assessed to find the best means of assisting them to stand up again. It may be necessary to make a patient comfortable on the ground until the requisite help arrives. People should always be assessed for injuries incurred before being moved.

The patient/client may be able to stand up unaided or to follow instructions that will help to do this. Some people will have previously been taught how to do this by the physiotherapist. Small children may be lifted manually, but otherwise inflatable cushions or hoists (see pp. 442–444) should be used if patients cannot assist themselves to stand. An incident form is completed according to local policy (see Ch. 13).

The benefits of mobility and hazards of immobility

In order to maintain good health, it is important to exercise regularly as there are many benefits of mobility that are often taken for granted (see below). Both weight-bearing exercise (e.g. walking, running, cycling) and non-weight-bearing

exercise (e.g. swimming) should be encouraged. Weight-bearing exercises involve overcoming the effects of gravity and are good for maintaining and developing bone mass (see p. 451). Non-weight-bearing exercises, such as swimming, can also be carried out in a hydrotherapy pool (Box 18.14) where the body weight is supported, the effects of gravity are greatly reduced and the joints can be moved more easily.

Health promotion   Box 18.14

Hydrotherapy

Hydrotherapy is the use of water to promote health and well-being. The water can be iced, cold, tepid, hot or steam and can also be used as compresses, inhalations or baths. Hydrotherapy has been used since the days of the ancient Greek philosopher Hippocrates, who promoted the health benefits of taking a bath.

Cold-based hydrotherapies such as ice packs and cold compresses decrease normal activity, constricting blood vessels and numbing nerve sensation, whereas heat has the opposite effect. Sometimes, treatment involves both cold and heat being applied alternately to a painful area to rapidly promote local circulation.

Exercising painful muscles in a warm hydrotherapy pool is beneficial because water overcomes the effects of gravity, making it easier to move. People do not have to be able to swim to take hydrotherapy. Movements are carried out gently and slowly. The acts of getting into the water and floating, moving the arms or walking through the water help to increase the range of movements and build up muscle strength. A complication of hydrotherapy may be the desire to work too hard. Being in a warm, pain-free environment can lull people into a false sense of security and they may move themselves into a range of movement with which their fascia and muscles are not familiar, causing discomfort. Frequent, short sessions are better than occasional longer sessions.

People with arthritis and chronic back pain benefit from hydrotherapy. Hydrotherapy can also have a calming effect and it is often used for people with learning disabilities and associated dyspraxia.

Student activities

Find out about:

- Hydrotherapy facilities available for patients/clients in your placement.
- Activities for particular groups of people at your local swimming pool.

Sometimes complete immobility is enforced, such as during bedrest or coma, while application of a plaster cast confers immobility of the affected limb. Immobility can be short or long lasting. In these situations, it is important to be alert for signs of the many potential hazards of immobility, discussed later in this section. Short-term immobility is less likely to be associated with potential hazards. This section explores the benefits of mobility and the potential hazards of immobility across the lifespan.

Benefits of mobility

Keeping mobile is one of the best ways to keep fit. A 20-minute, brisk walk every day will improve the fitness of all body systems, especially the cardiovascular and musculoskeletal systems. Specific health benefits include:

- Maintaining/increasing bone density, muscle bulk, the thickness of articular cartilage and joint movement
- Maintaining/improving the circulation and prevention of deep vein thrombosis
- Maintaining/improving respiratory function; deep breathing keeps the lungs free from infection
- Preventing constipation by increasing the transit rate in the intestines
- Assisting in achieving all the activities of living
- Improving mental well-being
- Maintaining independence and social interaction.

The Paralympics clearly show that exercise and fitness can be accessible to everyone and that many people are able to overcome severe disabilities to keep fit although they need to remain vigilant about the hazards of immobility, especially the development of pressure ulcers.

Children

Play normally provides the exercise that children's body systems need to grow and develop in a coordinated manner. Further intervention is unnecessary in children who are able to play actively by participating in, for example, cycling, running, ball games and other weight-bearing activities. However, children who have sedentary hobbies such as playing computer games and watching television will begin to feel the effects of lack of exercise. In addition to becoming overweight, normal muscle bulk does not build up and there may be changes to the normal curvature of the spine. These may have lasting effects on children's health, especially the musculoskeletal system, in later life.

Teenagers

Teenagers also need to exercise and should be encouraged to participate in formal exercise in order to develop their bones and muscles. Weight-bearing activities such as walking, running, dancing, skiing, football and rugby help to increase bone mass during adolescence and delay the loss of bone mass thereafter (see below). During exercise, bones accommodate to the stresses that are applied to them, so that those who exercise regularly have denser bones containing more minerals. Bones alter in shape as extra material is laid down at the points of maximum stress. Swimming is an excellent sport for health in general but, as it is not a weight-bearing activity, it does not affect bone mass. It is, however, very good for developing muscle tissue and the cardiovascular system.

Aerobic, anaerobic and resistance exercises are all good for promoting general health and well-being. Aerobic exercises involve using large muscle groups, rhythmically, over a period of at least 15–20 minutes, and the muscles have sufficient oxygen to fully utilize fuel molecules and release the energy required for contraction. These exercises are generally low in intensity and long in duration and include walking, cycling, jogging or swimming. Anaerobic exercises require muscles to work very hard in the absence of oxygen and are usually high in intensity and short in duration, e.g. sprinting, squash. The limited duration of this type of exercise is due to the accumulation of lactic acid because fuel molecules cannot be fully utilized without oxygen. Resistance exercise – also called strength training or weight training – increases muscle strength, mass and tone.

Cross-training, i.e. training for different events at the same time, such as cycling, swimming and running, develops all the body muscles at the same rate and people report fewer injuries during exercise. In addition, greater body flexibility is present because one group of muscles is not being built up at the expense of others. Cross-training for any sport prevents people from becoming muscle-bound, which can lead to injury (Hoeger & Hoeger 2011). For example, runners who only exercise to build up their stamina for running often find their hard-worked muscles become prone to sprains and tendons prone to inflammation. Their other muscles become weaker in comparison and therefore more prone to injury. This is seen when Olympic athletes, who have spent years training for a particular event, pull up with a calf or hamstring (the posterior thigh muscles) injury in the most important race of their lives.

Adults and older adults

As people age, the benefits of exercise continue to increase (Box 18.15). The more the muscles and fascia have adapted to postural habits, the less flexible people become (see p. 432).

Health promotion   **Box 18.15**

Exercise and older adults

Hoeger and Hoeger (2011) recognize the importance of exercising in people of all ages, including older adults, and there are many ways in which communities meet this need:

- Afternoon dances for people who prefer not to go out after dark
- Guided walking/exercises in shopping centres
- Fitness and swimming sessions for older adults.

Student activities

- Visit the websites below and identify the benefits of exercise in older adults.
- Visit the Age Scotland website and find out what activities help to prevent health issues in older adults.
- In your placement, identify people who encourage patients/clients to participate in exercising, e.g. an activity coordinator.
- Find out about activities specifically for older adults in your town.

Resources

Department of Health, 2011. UK-wide advice on activity and fitness levels. Online. Available: www.dh.gov.uk/en/MediaCentre/Pressreleases/DH_128211.
Age Scotland – www.ageuk.org.uk/scotland/.

Both websites accessed September 2012.

Hazards of immobility

There are many and diverse potential hazards of immobility (Box 18.16). The effects of immobility are the same across the

Hazards of immobility   Box 18.16

- Poor circulation that may predispose to deep vein thrombosis
- Poor respiratory function that may predispose to chest infections
- Development of pressure ulcers (see Ch. 25)
- Loss of bone density (osteoporosis)
- Joint stiffness
- Muscle wasting
- Constipation
- Potential loss of mental well-being, e.g. depression
- Boredom, isolation
- Impaired social interaction
- Loss of independence that may affect all the activities of living.

lifespan although children tend to recover more quickly from a period of immobility.

It is very important for nurses to recognize that people with limited mobility, or who are immobile, may be at risk of developing physical or mental health problems (such as depression) as a direct result of the change to their physical capabilities. The risk of these problems developing increases if the period of reduced mobility is prolonged. Early detection of hazards of immobility (Box 18.16) allows appropriate interventions to be implemented to reduce or minimise their effects. In general, the risk of developing problems associated with immobility increases with a person's age, the presence of other health problems and the period of immobility. Bedrest, which confines patients to bed, is sometimes prescribed for therapeutic reasons, for example:

- Some medical interventions, e.g. traction, require this
- To prevent the increase in oxygen demand needed during exercise
- To provide rest for seriously ill or debilitated patients.

Following a period of bedrest or restricted mobility, a programme of planned return to full activity may be required (see pp. 453–454). This often involves several members of the MDT, especially the physiotherapist and OT whose roles are described on p. 454. Falls pose a potential risk in many situations and helping people who have fallen is explained on p. 450.

Maintaining healthy joints and muscles

When not used, the joints stiffen and the skeletal muscles waste, and both will limit movement when mobility can be restarted. It is therefore important to maintain the range of movements available at joints and the condition of skeletal muscles when mobilization is not possible. Active and passive exercises can be carried out in bed in these situations. Active exercises are those initiated by people themselves without aid, e.g. flexing and extending the fingers. Passive exercises are those initiated by carers who move a person's joints through the normal range of movements. It is important to know the normal movements at joints so that they are not moved into

abnormal and potentially harmful positions. Active and passive exercises help to:

- Increase blood flow to, through and from the muscles and fascia
- Encourage blood flow in general, reducing the risk of deep vein thrombosis
- Promote healing and maintain or improve muscle function
- Stimulate the lymphatic system to drain excess tissue fluid and remove potentially harmful microorganisms.

Active exercises

Whenever possible, people are encouraged to actively exercise all their joints themselves. Encouraging patients/clients to meet their own hygiene needs, dress themselves and walk around are all good ways of encouraging active exercises. Safety is always important and it may therefore be appropriate to stay nearby so that patients/clients are not overreaching, e.g. to pick things up, which may affect their balance and result in a fall. When caring for older adults, it is important to give them enough time to carry out such activities. When nurses intervene too quickly or provide too much assistance, this not only reduces people's capacity for self-care but also increases dependence on others. Sometimes physiotherapists organize classes that promote movement and provide regular exercise.

Patients/clients who are confined to bed are often able to carry out active exercises but may need encouragement to move each joint through its full range of movement on a regular basis during waking hours. In addition to keeping the joints and their associated muscles functioning, carrying out active exercises also helps to pass time and gives people some active control over their recovery. Some patients may wish to use weights in order to provide resistance and make the muscles work harder, or they may be taught specific exercises by the physiotherapist. Patients who have undergone mastectomy (removal of breast tissue) or surgery to the elbow should be encouraged to brush their hair using the affected arm to keep the associated shoulder in good condition. Some patients prefer to have the screens drawn round their bed while they are exercising; always check with people first.

Passive exercises

Passive exercises are usually carried out by the physiotherapist or nurse, but sometimes by the patient themselves. When carrying out passive exercises, the joint is supported in the palms of the hands and is moved gently within a given range proximally (towards the centre of the body) and distally (away from the centre of the body). Over time, the range of movement (ROM) is increased. Often patients can resume active exercises, but sometimes active movement may never return, e.g. in people with paraplegia. It is essential that all passive movements are carried out gently and assessing ('sensing'), through touch, the range of movement available at the joint. As soon as resistance to a movement is felt, or the patient expresses discomfort, the joint is returned to its normal resting position (see Fig. 18.9). It is important that the elbow joint is not passively stretched, as it is easily damaged. You must observe a skilled practitioner performing passive movements before attempting them yourself.

Prevention of deep vein thrombosis

Deep vein thrombosis (DVT) occurs when the flow of blood through the deep veins of the legs and pelvis is slowed and blood clots form within those veins. Damage to blood vessel walls and coagulation problems are also implicated in DVT formation, which sometimes occurs in healthy people on long haul flights, causing 'economy class syndrome'. DVT is dangerous because fragments of the clot may become detached and travel in the veins, through the right side of the heart and lodge in a pulmonary artery in lungs causing pulmonary embolism, which can be fatal. The risk of DVT is reduced by carrying out active or passive exercises (see above) and preventing dehydration (see Ch. 19) during periods of immobility.

Preventing chest infection

When mobility is restricted, the benefits of deep breathing that occur during exercise are lost and deep breathing must be actively encouraged. The aim of deep breathing exercises is to improve the flow of air to the bases of the lungs so that they are well ventilated. This helps to prevent the build-up of fluid or respiratory tract secretions within the lungs and the development of a chest infection. Deep breathing (see Ch. 17) also encourages coughing, the reflex which helps to clear the air passages of sputum and potential pathogens. Deep breathing exercises are encouraged in patients/clients who are confined to bed or a chair and those who can walk only short distances.

Pressure ulcers

This complication of immobility, which is almost always preventable, is discussed in depth in Chapter 25. Nursing intervention is key to the prevention of pressure ulcers.

Constipation

Constipation can be prevented by anticipating the dietary and fluid needs of immobile patients/clients and providing an appropriate intake. Peristalsis (the contraction of smooth muscle that moves contents along the digestive tract) is reduced when mobility is limited, predisposing to constipation. The diet should be high in fibre to stimulate peristalsis. In adults, 1.5–2 litres of fluid are required daily to maintain hydration and achieving this can be a nursing challenge (see Ch. 19). Prevention and management of constipation is discussed in Chapter 21.

Maintaining well-being

Limited mobility will often restrict the social interactions that patients/clients are used to and it is necessary to find out the type of activity that will help people to pass the time to prevent boredom or isolation and maintain social interaction. In children, this will include therapeutic play, which is essential to achieving developmental milestones when long-term treatment or intervention is necessary.

People adapt to restricted mobility in different ways and patients/clients should be assessed for changes in their usual:

- Emotional reactions to situations
- Behaviour
- Sleep patterns (see Ch. 10).

Coping mechanisms (see Ch. 11) adapt according to circumstances and changes in these and the features above may indicate difficulty in adjusting to a new situation. People should be encouraged to express their experience of limited mobility and interventions can be provided to minimize its impact. Answering the call bell promptly provides social interaction and will reduce feelings of isolation.

Caring for people confined to bed

Comfort is very important to people who are confined to bed for long periods of time and even apparently small things like a wrinkle or crease in the sheet can become a major issue. As people confined to bed move around, the sheets become wrinkled and lying on these folds can cause pressure damage (see Ch. 25). Children tend to wriggle around a lot and therefore their sheets need to be checked at regular intervals to ensure they are dry, flat and wrinkle free. After eating, sheets should be discreetly checked in people of all ages to ensure they are free from crumbs. Bottom sheets should be changed daily, but this may be more difficult in the home environment than in hospitals with laundry facilities. A district nurse, social worker or orthopaedic liaison nurse can advise about community laundry facilities.

Making sure that drinks and food are easily accessible is also important. Tables and trays must be positioned at the appropriate height and angle to allow the person to be as independent as possible with eating and drinking. It may take slightly longer to arrange the furniture but the effects are three-fold because, as well as promoting independence, it encourages active exercises and improves mood by providing some diversional therapy. Reading, drawing, sewing, jigsaws, crossword puzzles or watching television also provide distraction from the boredom of lying in bed. Support pillows and foam wedges can be used to help people confined to bed to maintain a good position and feel supported in order to engage with any of these diversional activities.

Help will be required with toileting and personal hygiene and taking a basin of warm water to the bed to allow someone to wash their hands in after using a urinal or bedpan is far more satisfying for the patient than being handed a damp facecloth to wipe their hands.

Many local authorities provide a 'care at home' service which can be accessed through the local social work department. They can also provide special beds, toilet aids, walking aids, hoists and glide sheets to help care for the person confined to bed.

Regaining mobility

A person's independence should always be maximized and therefore nursing care aims to enable people to return to their full capacity as soon as possible. However, some people may have less mobility and independence than they previously enjoyed. For others, chronic conditions such as low back pain may result in ongoing mobility problems. The principles of rehabilitation are explained in Chapter 11. The MDT brings together professionals with different skills to help people regain mobility and independence following illness or injury. This section outlines the roles of the different professionals that work together to promote mobility, health and well-being.

Physiotherapy

Physiotherapists are the key healthcare professionals involved in assessing which aids should be used to improve mobility and which exercises patients/clients should be practising. Many people attend physiotherapy departments (either as inpatients or outpatients) where a greater range of equipment is available to facilitate active exercising. This may include hydrotherapy (see Box 18.14). Much of the equipment within hospital physiotherapy departments is not available in the community although physiotherapists may recommend going to a local gym that offers suitable activities.

Physiotherapists are also involved in teaching people with mobility problems or a history of falls how to prevent them in future (see Ch. 13) and how to get themselves up from the floor if they do fall (see p. 450).

Following a stroke, patients are often taught to carry out passive exercises (see p. 452) themselves on their affected limb, e.g. a hand and arm, using their unaffected hand. This helps them to regain their awareness of their affected side, which is often lost as a result of the stroke. Enabling patients to carry out passive exercises means that when they are not working directly with the physiotherapist they can continue to exercise the affected limb. This also helps to promote independence and gives people a feeling of involvement in their recovery. Passive exercising improves the blood supply to the affected area, helping to keep the muscle tissue and fascia supple. The repeated movements also provide feedback to the nervous system, thereby improving neuromuscular well-being.

Hot wax can be used for exercising the hands, e.g. to increase movement in rheumatoid arthritis. The heat from the wax helps to relieve pain, and as the wax cools and hardens it provides resistance for the muscles, making them work harder to achieve the same movements of extension and flexion. The hands can also be exercised using soft squeezy objects or a bowl of sand.

Occupational therapy

The OT is a healthcare professional who provides activities and exercises to encourage movement and increase independence. OTs help people to regain independence with activities of living such as personal hygiene and dressing as well as carrying out activities in the home, e.g. making tea, washing up and cooking. OTs also provide advice about communication systems that enable people who are at risk of falls to raise the alarm if they fall at home.

Home assessment

Physiotherapists and OTs often carry out home assessment visits together. Patients are taken home and observed moving and carrying out normal daily activities in their familiar environment. The OT and/or physiotherapist may recommend home modifications including handrails, raised toilet seats, over-bed tables, trolleys on wheels and other gadgets that enable people to continue to live at home safely and independently.

SUMMARY

- Understanding how the musculoskeletal system develops and its involvement in movement and posture underpins the nursing care of people with mobility problems.
- Many conditions can affect the development and maintenance of an upright posture and normal gait.
- It is essential to be familiar with the principles of safe EHM before being involved in moving either inanimate loads or people.
- Handling and moving equipment such as hoists, wheelchairs and walking aids should be used appropriately in promoting independence for clients with mobility problems.
- Exercise has many benefits and should be encouraged throughout the lifespan to optimize health.
- Immobility has many associated hazards that can often be prevented by providing appropriate nursing interventions.
- Active and passive exercises should be used to maintain and improve neuromuscular well-being and to promote mobility.
- Nursing care needs to be individualized to enable people to maximize or regain independence in mobility and other aspects of their lives.
- Mobility problems in older adults account for a high proportion of falls; however the consequences of falls, e.g. fractures, account for a large proportion of mobility problems in the over 65s.
- Members of the MDT bring specific expertise to promoting independence with immobile patients/clients.

KEY WORDS AND PHRASES FOR LITERATURE SEARCHING

Ageing/aging
Cast/Plaster of Paris
Falls
Fractures
Immobility
Orthopaedics
Osteoporosis
Traction

 Useful websites

Age UK www.ageuk.org.uk
Disabled Living Foundation www.dlf.org.uk
National Osteoporosis Society www.nos.org.uk
Royal Society for the Prevention of Accidents (RoSPA) www.rospa.com
Working-Well www.working-well.org
All websites accessed September 2012.

References

BackCare and Royal College of Nursing, 2011. The guide to the handling of people, sixth ed. BackCare, Teddington.

Brooks, A., Orchard, S., 2011. Core person handling skills. In: Smith, J., (Ed.), The guide to the handling of people, sixth ed. BackCare, Teddington.

Caby, B., Kieffer, S., Hubert, M.D.E.S., et al., 2011. Feature extraction and selection for objective gait analysis and fall risk assessment by accelerometry. BioMedical Engineering 10 (1). Online. Available: www.mendeley.com/research/feature-extraction-selection-objective-gait-analysis-fall-risk-assessment-accelerometry/ September 2012.

Cryer, C., Patel, S., 2001. Falls, fragility and fractures. The Alliance for Better Bone Health, London.

Gilbert, H., 2010. Kinetic chain release. Online. Available: www.youtube.com/watch?v=55QYy4s2XDc September 2012.

Hoeger, W.W.K., Hoeger, S.A., 2011. Lifetime physical fitness and wellness, ninth ed. Thomson Wadsworth, Belmont CA.

Myers, T., 2009. Anatomy trains, second ed. Churchill Livingstone, Edinburgh.

Scottish Building Standards Agency, 2011. Online. Available: www.scotland.gov.uk/Topics/Built-Environment/Building/Building-standards September 2012.

Further reading

Jester, R., Santy, J., Rogers, J., 2011. Oxford handbook of orthopaedic and trauma nursing. OUP, Oxford.

Lucas, B., 2011. Nursing patients with musculoskeletal discorders. In: Brooker, C., Nicol, M., (Eds.), Alexander's nursing practice, fourth ed. Churchill Livingstone, Edinburgh.

Petty, N.J., 2004. Neuromusculoskeletal treatment and management: a guide for therapists. Churchill Livingstone, Edinburgh.

Waugh, A., Grant, A., 2010. Ross and Wilson anatomy and physiology in health and illness, eleventh ed. Churchill Livingstone, Edinburgh.

Promoting hydration and nutrition

19

Chris Brooker

Introduction

Ensuring that people have sufficient fluids and nutrition that meets their needs is a basic, but vital role of the nurse. Healthy body function, recovery from illness and eventually life itself, depend on being able to access fluids and nutrients. Nurses not only help people to eat and drink during illness but they also have an important role in educating people about eating and drinking for optimum health. Although families, healthcare assistants (HCAs) and students undertake considerable 'hands on' care, the registered nurse (RN) remains accountable for all nursing interventions (see Ch. 7). The nurse works within a multidisciplinary team (MDT) that includes, among others, dietitians, specialist nutrition and intravenous therapy nurses and catering staff, to promote hydration and nutrition.

Inadequate or inappropriate fluid and nutrient intake impedes recovery from illness and surgery, lengthens hospital stay and can lead to complications that include delayed wound healing, pressure ulcers, weight loss, low mood, infection, dehydration and poor oral hygiene. Moreover, malnutrition increases mortality and healthcare costs (Jefferies et al 2011).

The importance of providing people of all ages with food and drink is emphasized by the Royal College of Nursing (RCN, 2007), Age UK (2010) and the Department of Health (DH 2010).

Education about and help to access healthy balanced diets is imperative given the increasingly high prevalence of overweight and obese children and adults (see p. 477).

This chapter is in two parts: maintaining fluid, electrolyte and acid–base balance, and nutrition. However, it is important to understand that all of these are closely linked and that none can ensure well-being without the others.

Skilled promotion of hydration and nutrition is a fundamental nursing role that really can 'make a difference' to the well-being of people in your care.

Maintaining fluid, electrolyte and acid–base balance

This part of the chapter outlines the maintenance of fluid, electrolyte and acid–base balance, some common disorders and investigations. Nursing interventions such as assessment of hydration, helping with drinking and the principles of intravenous infusions are covered in some depth.

The amount of water and electrolytes, e.g. sodium, potassium, in the body compartments and acid–base balance are controlled by interdependent mechanisms that keep levels fairly constant within narrow limits. Normal body function depends on homeostasis, i.e. maintaining water, electrolyte levels and acid–base balance in the internal environment within the normal range. Therefore, dynamic homeostatic mechanisms are required to respond to continually changing conditions within the body.

Body fluids and fluid compartments

The amount of water as a percentage of body weight decreases with age (Fig. 19.1). For example, a newborn has around 75% water, whereas an average adult male has around 60% and an older adult between 45% and 50%. The amount of body fat and gender also influence water content. Fat (adipose tissue) contains less water than muscle tissue. Body water is lower in older adults because muscle tissue is replaced by fat; obese people and women, who generally have more fat than men, also have less body water.

Body water is distributed between two fluid compartments:

- Extracellular fluid (ECF), which comprises the fluid between the cells, is also known as interstitial or tissue fluid, plasma (i.e. the fluid part of blood) and lymph
- Intracellular fluid (ICF) is present within all body cells.

In adults, the split is approximately two-thirds ICF to one-third ECF (Fig. 19.2). The fluid distribution in infants and very young children is characterized by more body water in the ECF. This fluid distribution and the increased rate at which ECF is exchanged means that there is an increased risk of dehydration if fluid is lost.

The body surface area also differs in infants and children who have proportionally greater surface areas than adults. Therefore, they lose more water through the skin, which has important implications for fluid balance and intravenous (i.v.) fluid therapy (see p. 469). The immature kidneys of infants/small children cannot excrete or conserve sodium, acidify urine or produce concentrated or dilute urine (Wilson 2011). In addition, they have a higher metabolic rate that produces more waste products for excretion in the urine. Conditions that increase metabolic rate also increase heat production and hence the amount of water loss through the skin.

Electrolytes

Electrolytes are substances such as sodium chloride (described in chemical notation as NaCl), which, when dissolved in water, dissociate into electrically charged particles called ions that conduct electricity. Some ions have a positive charge (cations), e.g. sodium (Na^+), and others are negatively charged (anions), e.g. chloride (Cl^-). In body fluids the main electrolytes are sodium, potassium, calcium and magnesium with a positive charge, and bicarbonate, chloride and phosphate that are negatively charged. The ECF and ICF have different electrolyte compositions; sodium is mainly in the ECF whereas most potassium is in the ICF. The proportions of electrolytes, e.g. sodium and chloride, in the ECF and ICF of infants and young children differ from those in adults. Table 19.1 shows the normal range for serum electrolyte levels in adults. Electrolytes in body fluids and are necessary for:

- Maintaining osmotic pressure, e.g. sodium
- Transmission of nerve impulses and muscle contraction, e.g. sodium, potassium, calcium
- Blood coagulation, strong bones and teeth, e.g. calcium
- Release of neurotransmitters, e.g. calcium
- Enzyme function, e.g. magnesium
- Acid–base balance, pH homeostasis, e.g. bicarbonate.

Fig. 19.1 • Water as a percentage of body weight. (Reproduced with permission from Brooker, C., 1998. Human structure and function, second ed. Mosby, London.)

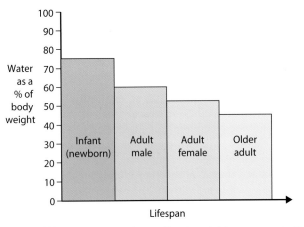

Fig. 19.2 • Distribution of body water in a 70 kg adult male. (Reproduced with permission from Waugh, A., Grant, A., 2010. Ross and Wilson Anatomy and Physiology in health and illness, eleventh ed. Churchill Livingstone, Edinburgh.)

Table 19.1 Serum electrolytes – normal reference values (adults)	
Electrolyte (chemical notation)	**Reference range (serum)**
Sodium (Na^+)	135–143 mmol/L
Potassium (K^+)	3.6–5.0 mmol/L
Calcium (Ca^{2+})	2.1–2.6 mmol/L
Magnesium (Mg^{2+})	0.75–1.0 mmol/L
Chloride (Cl^-)	97–106 mmol/L
Phosphate (PO_4^{2-})	0.8–1.4 mmol/L
Bicarbonate (HCO_3^-)	22–28 mmol/L

Notes: Urea (normal range 2.5–6.4 mmol/L) is usually measured along with electrolytes. Normal ranges may vary slightly on a local basis.

Movement of water and electrolytes

Water and electrolytes and other substances continually move between the ECF and ICF in order to:

- Maintain homeostasis of the internal environment
- Allow oxygen (O_2), nutrients and other metabolic substances to enter cells
- Allow waste products to leave cells for excretion by the lungs (see Ch. 17) and kidneys (see Ch. 20).

This movement occurs through a number of processes, including osmosis, diffusion, filtration and active transport.

Osmosis

Osmosis is the movement of water through a semipermeable membrane. Pores in the membrane allow the movement of water molecules in either direction. Water moves when there is a difference in its concentration on either side of the membrane. The direction of movement is from high water to low water concentration. This means that water will move from a weak solution to a stronger, more concentrated solution until equilibrium is reached, i.e. the water concentrations are the same on either side of the membrane. Osmosis occurs when equilibrium cannot be achieved by the movement of electrolytes or sugars (solutes) across the semipermeable membrane.

The force that opposes the movement of water by osmosis is known as the osmotic pressure; this increases with the concentration difference on either side of the membrane. The concentration of particles that contribute to the osmotic pressure in a litre of fluid is termed the osmolality of a solution. The movement of water stops when the opposing pressures (i.e. concentrations) on either side of the membrane are identical. The solutions are then described as being isotonic. In the body, an isotonic solution has the same osmolality as plasma. A solution with a higher osmolality than plasma is termed hypertonic; one with a lower osmolality to plasma is hypotonic. Osmosis is vital in maintaining water distribution within the fluid compartments.

Diffusion

Diffusion involves the movement of gases and solutes from an area of high concentration to an area of lower concentration, i.e. down a concentration gradient. In the body, diffusion down a concentration gradient takes place within cells or body fluids and also across semipermeable membranes. The latter allow small particles to pass through but hold back larger particles, e.g. proteins.

Diffusion is described as passive because it does not use chemical energy (adenosine triphosphate (ATP)). The end result of diffusion is equal concentrations on both sides of the membrane, i.e. equilibrium. Diffusion is important for the movement of O_2, carbon dioxide (CO_2), electrolytes, nutrients, hormones and waste products such as urea.

Filtration

The passive process of filtration provides another means by which the fluid compartments and the concentration of substances within body fluids are maintained; again there is a gradient difference either side of the membrane, but this time it is pressure rather than concentration. The pressure that forces water and small molecules through membrane pores is known as the hydrostatic (fluid) pressure. Filtration is important in the formation of tissue fluid and urine (see Ch. 20).

Active transport

Active transport is a process requiring chemical energy (ATP) to move substances:

- Against a concentration gradient
- Where no concentration gradient exists
- That are unable to diffuse through membranes.

Substances transported in this way include nutrients and electrolytes, e.g. the sodium-potassium exchange pump in cell membranes where sodium ions (mainly in the ECF) are pumped out of the cell and potassium ions (mainly in the ICF) are pumped into the cell against their concentration gradients.

Acid–base balance

The pH (hydrogen ion concentration or the acidity) of blood and other body fluids must remain within a narrow range for normal cell function. For example, the normal pH range of ECF is 7.35–7.45. Small deviations outside this range are associated with serious physiological disruption because pH is a logarithmic scale and a change of 1 represents a 10-fold change in hydrogen ion concentration.

Acids are ingested on a daily basis and metabolic processes continuously produce acidic substances including CO_2 (which, when dissolved, increases the acidity of a solution), lactic acid and ketoacids. Various interdependent homeostatic mechanisms function to maintain acid–base balance. These are:

- Chemical buffers (substances that limit pH change) that act immediately to counteract changes in pH (see Waugh & Grant 2010)
- Excretion of CO_2 by the lungs (respiratory regulation through rate and depth of breathing operates within minutes)
- The kidneys, which provide long-term regulation by excreting hydrogen ions (H^+) and by conserving or excreting bicarbonate ions (HCO_3^-) in processes occurring over many hours.

If these homeostatic mechanisms fail, acid–base balance is disrupted. When the pH of arterial blood rises above 7.45, i.e. becomes more alkaline, this is known as alkalaemia. The process leading to low levels of acid (excess of alkali) is termed alkalosis. When the pH of arterial blood falls below 7.35 this is known as acidaemia. *Note*: the blood is still alkaline but the pH is closer to the acid range. The process that results in the excess acid is termed acidosis.

Homeostatic mechanisms attempt to restore normal blood pH by either excreting more or less CO_2 from the lungs or by changing the amount of H^+ or HCO_3^- excreted in the urine.

Acid–base imbalances, which are often associated with fluid or electrolyte imbalances (see below), can be life-threatening.

Disorders of acid–base balance

The acid–base disorders alkalosis and acidosis can have either a respiratory or a metabolic cause. Seriously ill patients may develop a mixed disorder.

Alkalosis

- Respiratory alkalosis is due to overbreathing (hyperventilation) that results in a net loss of CO_2. Hyperventilation can be a feature of panic attacks
- Metabolic alkalosis is caused by excessive loss of acids from the GI tract, e.g. vomiting of gastric (stomach) acid, or by excessive ingestion of alkaline indigestion medicines.

Acidosis

- Respiratory acidosis is due to inadequate breathing (hypoventilation) and the build-up of CO_2
- Metabolic acidosis is caused by failure to excrete H^+ in kidney failure, the production of excess acids, e.g. in type 1 diabetes or the loss of alkali, e.g. diarrhoea (see Further reading, below, e.g. Cowen & Ugboma 2011).

Normal fluid and electrolyte balance

The kidneys regulate fluid and electrolyte balance in response to hormone levels. Healthy people take in most fluid by drinking but there is water in food, e.g. soup, fruit and ice-cream, and chemical processes in the body also produce water. Electrolytes are obtained from food and fluids, e.g. sodium from salt added to processed foods. Fluids and electrolytes are excreted from the body in urine, faeces, sweat, through insensible perspiration and during respiration (Table 19.2).

Factors that regulate normal fluid and electrolyte balance

Hormones such as aldosterone and antidiuretic hormone (ADH) maintain fluid and electrolyte homeostasis by their actions on the kidneys (see Ch. 20). Also very important in the regulation of fluid balance is the sensation of thirst. If fluid is lost or intake inadequate a person feels thirsty and usually responds by drinking fluids. However, certain groups of people are unable to respond to thirst: infants, small children, people with mobility problems and other physical disabilities, unconscious patients, people with profound and multiple learning disabilities or dementia and older adults (who may not experience thirst) are all at risk of fluid depletion (Box 19.1).

Reflective practice   Box 19.1

Responding to thirst

Think about people you have nursed.

Student activities

- Identify those who had potential or actual problems in responding to thirst. Your list may include some obvious examples such as small children, people with poor mobility living at home, or someone with other physical disabilities; however, other examples might be someone with dementia who spends the day wandering in the care home, or a person with severe mental distress.
- Did the person you identified receive adequate fluids? (see Tables 19.2, 19.3).
- What nursing measures were used to improve their fluid intake?
- Reflect with a peer or your mentor about how effective the nursing measures were.

Common disorders of fluid and electrolyte balance

Disorders of fluid and electrolyte balance can cause serious and sometimes life-threatening effects.

Common disorders of fluid balance

Disorders of fluid balance can be divided into two main types:

- *Isotonic imbalances* involving a proportional increase or decrease of both water and electrolytes and hence the osmolality of the ECF may be unchanged
- *Osmolar imbalances* where water only is increased or decreased without a proportional change in electrolyte concentration (mainly sodium) and hence the osmolality of ECF is affected.

An outline of fluid balance disorders is provided in Box 19.2.

Electrolyte imbalances

Electrolyte imbalances involve either increases or decreases outside the normal range. Many factors can affect electrolyte levels.

Frequently more that one electrolyte is affected and is accompanied by a fluid imbalance; sometimes there is also loss of acid–base balance. Box 19.3 outlines some important electrolyte imbalances.

Factors that can lead to fluid and/or electrolyte imbalance

Many physical, psychological and social factors lead to imbalances in body fluids and electrolytes. Nurses must be able to identify and minimize the impact of factors that increase the

---

Table 19.2 Average water balance over 24 hours in adults	
Input (mL)	**Output (mL)**
Drinks 1700	Urine 1500
Fluid from food 1000	Faeces 100
Metabolic water 300	During respiration 500 Skin (insensible loss and sweat) 900 in health
Total 3000	Total 3000

Common disorders of fluid balance Box 19.2

Isotonic imbalances

- *Fluid volume deficit* occurs when both water and electrolytes are lost. It can arise through vomiting, diarrhoea, sweating, drainage from the GI tract and the use of diuretic drugs (increase urine production). Fluid may also move into the 'third space', where it is lost from the ECF but remains in the body, e.g. the abdominal cavity. Fluid volume deficit is not dehydration, which correctly describes an osmolar disorder (see below).
- *Fluid volume excess* occurs when there is an increase in both water and electrolytes (usually sodium with water retention) in the ECF. Fluid moves into the interstitial spaces causing generalized tissue water-logging (oedema) or pulmonary oedema (fluid in the alveoli of the lungs, see Ch. 17). This can occur when i.v. fluids containing sodium are overinfused and in people with heart failure and liver disease. The mechanisms that give rise to oedema are:

  - Decreased plasma proteins leading to a reduction in plasma osmotic pressure which is needed to 'pull' interstitial fluid back into the venous side of the capillary network. This can be a feature of some kidney diseases and occurs when dietary protein is deficient (see p. 482)
  - Increased venous hydrostatic pressure caused by venous congestion, e.g. with chronic heart failure, which prevents interstitial fluid returning to the circulation at the venous side of the capillary network
  - 'Leaky' capillaries that allow protein to leak out into the interstitial spaces, e.g. in inflammation. This increases the osmotic pressure in the tissues and because less fluid returns to the bloodstream it collects in the interstitial spaces as oedema
  - Impaired lymphatic drainage – some interstitial fluid normally returns to the circulation through the lymphatic system. Obstruction to lymphatic drainage, e.g. cancer involving the lymph nodes, means that the excess fluid remains in the interstitial spaces.

Osmolar imbalances

- *Hyperosmolar imbalance (dehydration or water depletion)* occurs when water intake is inadequate or fluid loss is excessive. Without a proportional loss of electrolytes it is accompanied by a disturbance in electrolyte balance, especially sodium levels which rise. Loss of water from the extracellular compartment increases the osmolality of the ECF, which becomes hypertonic and fluid moves out of the cells in order to restore the osmotic equilibrium of the ICF and ECF. The overall result is cellular dehydration, which seriously disrupts cell function.
- *Hypo-osmolar imbalance (fluid excess or 'water intoxication')* occurs when ECF water increases without an increase in electrolytes. This can be caused by excessive water intake such as occurs in some severe mental health problems or from inappropriate secretion of ADH. This time the ECF is diluted, its osmolality decreases and, because it is hypotonic compared with the ICF, the movement of fluid is into the cells adversely affecting their function.

Common abnormalities of blood electrolyte levels Box 19.3

Hypernatraemia

Increased blood sodium concentration, caused by excessive loss of water without electrolytes owing to polyuria (increased urinary volume), high salt intake, excessive sweating or inadequate water intake.

Hyponatraemia

Decreased blood sodium concentration, caused by vomiting, diarrhoea, sweating and burns; diuretics, heart failure, kidney disease and diabetes mellitus, or a failure to excrete water or excess intake.

Hyperkalaemia

Increased blood potassium concentration, caused by reduced urine output, e.g. in kidney failure, or excessive prescribed potassium supplements.

Hypokalaemia

Decreased blood potassium concentration, caused by excessive urine output, misuse of laxatives, diarrhoea and vomiting over a prolonged period, starvation.

Age

People at the extremes of age are at increased risk of fluid and electrolyte imbalance. In infants and small children this is because of the distribution of fluid in the ECF and ICF, their immature kidneys, greater body surface area and higher metabolic rate (see p. 456). In older adults the risk of imbalances is increased by the reduced percentage of body water, declining kidney function and inability to access fluids or respond to thirst (see p. 460).

Fasting

People who are having investigations or procedures that require a general anaesthetic can develop fluid depletion if they are fasted for unnecessarily lengthy periods (see Ch. 24). Some groups, including those aged 80 or over admitted for surgery, may well be dehydrated on admission. Indeed, evidence of preoperative dehydration was found in one-third of patients (National Confidential Enquiry into Patient Outcome and Death, NCEPOD 2010).

During the religious festival of Ramadan, all healthy Muslims over the age of 12 years are required to fast between dawn and sunset (Box 19.4).

Fluid and electrolyte loss

Vomiting and diarrhoea and excessive sweating, such as during heavy work or exercise, leads to problems with fluid and electrolyte balance. In addition, hot weather leads to an increased fluid requirement, especially for those exercising strenuously.

Alcohol and excessive caffeine drinks

Alcohol, tea, coffee, cocoa and 'cola' drinks increase urinary output (diuresis) and may contribute to fluid depletion.

risk of people developing problems. These factors include those that prevent a person responding to thirst (see p. 460) as well as the following:

High level of dependency

Those with some physical disabilities and/or profound and multiple learning disabilities may be completely dependent on others for their fluid intake, as they may not be able to ask for or access fluids (Nursing and Midwifery Council 2010 – specifically 'Julie's story'). Some also have problems with chewing, swallowing (see below), muscle tone and posture and the reflexes that protect the airway.

Mental health problems

People experiencing severe mental distress may be unable to maintain an adequate fluid intake because their mood is so profoundly depressed, or they may be experiencing serious manifestations, such as hallucinations, which pervade all aspects of life to the exclusion of self-maintenance activities. Drugs used for some forms of mental distress can lead to fluid and electrolyte imbalances, e.g. lithium carbonate.

People with dementia or confusion may not remember to drink or will have forgotten how to prepare drinks. Insufficient fluid intake worsens confusion and a vicious circle of increasingly severe fluid depletion and worsening confusion ensues.

Immobility and lack of manual dexterity

Older people and those with conditions such as severe arthritis, or following a stroke, may be unable to prepare drinks safely or to carry them from the kitchen. Dealing with hot drinks can be hazardous, particularly when people find it difficult to hold a cup or mug due to tremor or deformity of the hands.

Swallowing problems (dysphagia)

Swallowing problems are very common after a stroke and the risk of choking or inhalation of fluids or food into the respiratory tract is present. It is essential that oral fluid and food be withheld until a speech and language therapist (SLT) or specially trained nurse carries out a full assessment. (For an outline of swallowing, see p. 468 and the Royal College of Speech and Language Therapists website: www.rcslt.org.)

Fear of incontinence

People may restrict their fluids in an effort to prevent nocturia (passing urine at night) or incontinence (see Ch. 20). Nurses should encourage people to compensate by increasing fluid intake earlier in the day.

Drugs

Drugs – including diuretics, e.g. furosemide, can lead to fluid depletion and loss of electrolytes, especially potassium.

Breathlessness (dyspnoea)

Breathlessness can lead to fluid depletion because insensible water loss increases during mouth breathing. The administration of oxygen without humidification also worsens oral drying. A person with severe breathlessness will have little energy for drinking and will be unable to access fluids.

Serious organ disorders

Heart, liver and kidney failure all lead to severe fluid and electrolyte retention, e.g. sodium and potassium. It may be necessary to restrict fluid intake (p. 468) and foods containing particular electrolytes, e.g. sodium (see Table 19.5, p. 478).

Lack of access to clean water

Many people in developing countries and those affected by natural disasters or wars do not have clean water piped to individual homes. Often, people spend many hours a day collecting water, or have no alternative to drinking from dirty sources such as rivers contaminated by untreated sewage.

Nursing interventions: promoting and maintaining hydration

Although the *Essence of Care 2010* benchmark of best practice: 'People receive the care and assistance they require with eating and drinking' (DH 2010, p 8) appears to state the obvious, this does not always happen. This part of the chapter covers nursing assessment and some investigations used to evaluate fluid and electrolyte status. It describes how nurses can help people to drink sufficient fluids. Other interventions covered include caring for people with fluid imbalances and those with nausea and vomiting.

Most people maintain fluid balance with oral fluids. This is ideal, as it maintains normality, is non-invasive and has fewer complications. Where this is not possible, e.g. severe vomiting, unconsciousness or dysphagia, other ways of providing fluid are needed. Box 19.5 outlines other routes and some are discussed below (p. 469).

Assessing hydration

Assessing hydration is a vital component of a holistic nursing assessment, which includes careful observation. It is important to consider all aspects of the person's life such as their normal fluid and food intake and the drinks they normally prefer. The nurse needs to be aware of physical, social or psychological factors that may disrupt fluid and electrolyte balance to identify those people who are at risk of potential or actual

Routes for the administration of fluid

Enteral fluids

People unable to drink sufficient fluids or have swallowing problems but who have a functioning GI tract, can have fluid needs met by the enteral route. This may be through a:

- Nasogastric tube – passed though the nose and oesophagus into the stomach
- Nasoenteric tube – passed into the small intestine via the nose and oesophagus
- Gastrostomy tube – inserted through the abdominal wall into the stomach (see Fig. 19.16).

The enteral route is usually used to provide both nutrients and fluids (see p. 485).

Subcutaneous fluids (hypodermoclysis)

Fluid infused subcutaneously (see p. 468) is increasingly used to manage mild to moderate dehydration and in the short-term to relieve thirst in end-of-life care (Royal College of Physicians 2010).

Rectal fluids (proctoclysis)

Fluid infused into the rectum. Fluid, e.g. tap water or sodium chloride 0.9%, is infused and slowly absorbed into the circulation. Proctoclysis is useful for maintaining hydration in end-of-life care (Royal College of Physicians 2010).

Intravenous fluids

Sterile intravenous fluids (see p. 469) are infused into a vein to maintain fluid, electrolyte and acid–base balance or to correct imbalances, administer drugs and provide nutrients (see also Parenteral nutrition, p. 487).

Intraosseous fluids

This involves the introduction of fluids and drugs into the marrow (medullary) cavity of a long bone, e.g. the tibia. It is used for children in some emergency situations (see Trigg & Mohammed 2010).

problems. The nurse documents the findings from this assessment in the nursing records and ensures that any abnormal findings are reported immediately to the RN. In addition to the nursing assessment, blood and urine tests are used to assess hydration, they include:

- Blood tests:
  - Measurement of serum urea and electrolytes (see Table 19.1)
  - Serum albumin (normal range 36–47 g/L)
  - Packed cell volume (PCV) or haematocrit measures the percentage of red blood cells and from this the amount of fluid in the blood.
- Urine tests:
  - Routine urinalysis (see Ch. 20)
  - Measurement of urine osmolality
  - 24-hour urine collection for electrolyte estimation.

Skin

Normally, when skin is pinched and released it returns immediately to its normal position, as the elastic tissue recoils. This feature is termed turgor. People who have a fluid volume deficit may have reduced skin turgor and the pinched up portion remains raised for longer. Skin turgor is not always reliable in the assessment of older people who have less elastic tissue or in people who have recently lost weight. The skin may appear dry.

The presence of oedema (see p. 468) can indicate fluid volume excess with accumulation of fluid in the interstitial spaces. Generalized oedema affects dependent parts of the body, the feet and ankles (standing or sitting) and the sacral area when confined to bed. On waking, some people may have puffiness around the eyes (periorbital oedema) after lying flat. When oedematous tissue is compressed with a finger and stays indented, this is termed 'pitting oedema'.

Fontanelles

Assessment of the anterior fontanelle (often called the 'soft spot' by parents) in the skull is a guide to hydration in infants. The fontanelles are membranous spaces present between the skull bones in newborns. The diamond-shaped anterior fontanelle is located between the frontal and two parietal bones and closes up during the 2nd year of life. A triangular posterior fontanelle is situated at the junction of the occipital and two parietal bones. This closes within weeks of birth.

The anterior fontanelle can be observed and gently felt with the flat part of a finger. In healthy, well-hydrated infants, the fontanelle is level with the skull bones. A sunken fontanelle can indicate fluid volume deficit while a bulging fontanelle may suggest fluid volume excess, or it can be due to increased pressure inside the skull (raised intracranial pressure).

Weight

Accurate daily weight assessment (see Ch. 14) can give a good indication of the amount of fluid lost or gained, especially oedema.

Sunken eyes

Sunken eyes can indicate a moderate to severe fluid volume deficit. It occurs because interstitial fluid is lost from the periorbital tissue.

Mouth

The condition of the oral mucosa, which is usually pink and moist, is a good indicator of hydration status (see Ch. 16). Fluid depletion leads to a dry mouth, coated tongue and viscous (thick) saliva. Thirst is an important regulator of fluid balance (see p. 460) and people with fluid depletion will usually say that they are thirsty. It is important to remember that a dry mouth may have other causes, e.g. oxygen therapy, mouth breathing and some drugs.

Behaviour

Behaviour can give valuable clues about hydration. Lethargy, anxiety or confusion may occur in fluid depletion and acid–base imbalance. Infants and small children may exhibit irritability. Some infants are quiet and show little interest in their surroundings or a favourite toy or game.

Bowel function (see Ch. 21)

Fluid volume deficit or dehydration can cause constipation. Serious fluid, electrolyte and acid-base imbalance can result from severe or prolonged diarrhoea.

Urine output and specific gravity (see Ch. 20)

The volume and colour of urine are important indicators of hydration. Small volumes (oliguria) and dark concentrated urine with a high specific gravity (SG >1.030) are features of fluid volume deficit. Infants and toddlers have fewer wet nappies than normal. Concentrated urine may have a stronger odour than usual.

Blood pressure

A fall in blood pressure (BP) accompanies fluid volume deficit. In severe situations the person will have a low BP (hypotension) while lying down. However, in milder cases, the fluid volume deficit may only be apparent because of a marked decrease in BP upon standing up from the sitting position (postural hypotension). An increasing BP may be a feature of fluid overload such as during i.v. fluid therapy (see Box 19.12, p. 473).

Pulse

An increase in pulse occurs in fluid volume deficit because there is less fluid in the vascular system (hypovolaemia). Fluid volume excess normally also causes a raised pulse.

Respiration

The respiratory rate, effort and depth can change in response to fluid, electrolyte and acid–base imbalance. For example, a person with fluid volume excess can develop pulmonary oedema (see Box 19.2, p. 461), which causes dyspnoea and a cough with frothy sputum.

Skin temperature

Cool extremities may indicate a decrease in intravascular volume but there are also many other factors that influence skin temperature (see Ch. 14).

Central venous pressure

Central venous pressure (CVP) estimates the pressure of blood in the right atrium of the heart. Used in seriously ill patients to assess hydration status and inform fluid replacement therapy, it is always interpreted in conjunction with other observations such as pulse, BP, respirations and urine output (see Further reading, below, e.g. Cowen & Ugboma 2011).

Fluid balance charts

Fluid balance charts (fluid intake and output charts, or just fluid charts) are used to record all fluid intakes and outputs over a 24-hour period (Box 19.6). The amounts for intake and output are totalled daily and the fluid balance calculated at the same time each day, often at midnight, or at 06:00 or 08:00 hours. A positive balance exists where the intake exceeds output. This situation occurs when fluid intake is increased to rectify fluid volume deficit and dehydration (see p. 469), whereas a negative balance exists when output exceeds intake. This occurs, e.g. when treatment with diuretics is used to

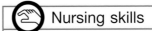

Nursing skills   Box 19.6

Maintaining fluid balance charts

Placing a sign above the bed or on the door ensures that the patient, family and all staff are aware that the person is having fluid intake and output measured and recorded.

- All oral intake is measured and in some circumstances, this also includes milk on cereals, soup and ice-cream
- Nasogastric, gastrostomy, intravenous, subcutaneous and rectal intake are recorded on the intake side of the chart (Fig. 19.3)
- Fluid output from urine (measured hourly in serious illness), vomit, aspirate from a nasogastric tube, diarrhoea, stomal fluid, e.g. ileostomy, ileal conduit (see Chs 20, 21), or wound drain are all recorded on the output side of the chart (Fig. 19.3). The 'Other' column is used to record output other than urine or vomit and the nature of the fluid is specified. For accuracy, it is sometimes necessary to weigh articles, e.g. nappies, wound dressings. The difference between dry and wet weight in grams approximately corresponds to millilitres of urine or drainage
- All measurements of intake and output are charted immediately to ensure that charts are accurate and up-to-date
- Inappropriate or imprecise terms such as 'up to toilet' should be avoided
- Many people who are independent in oral fluid intake and elimination take responsibility for noting what they have drunk and measuring their urine. Disposable jugs for measuring urine are made available
- Nurses monitor fluid charts at regular intervals, the frequency depending on the person's condition.

Note: Nurses should know the volumes of jugs and drinking vessels such as cups, glasses and drinks cans used in community settings or ward (Fig. 19.4 p. 466).

Note: See Further reading, below, e.g. Cowen & Ugbama 2011, p 587, for possible sources of error in fluid balance charting.

rectify fluid volume excess. A record is also kept of the daily fluid balance over several days so that trends can be assessed.

Oral fluids

The average healthy adult needs a fluid intake of 1.5–2.0 L per day. Most of this fluid should be water, as excessive caffeine-containing drinks such as tea, coffee and colas cause diuresis. There are, however, many situations when more than this is needed such as when a person has a urinary catheter *in situ* (see Ch. 20), strenuous exercise, sweating and diarrhoea and vomiting.

Older people may need a higher intake because their kidneys become less efficient in producing concentrated urine. Moreover, older people may be less sensitive to and/or responsive to thirst. Fluid intake may need to increase further when body temperature is raised and in hot weather to prevent dehydration.

Daily fluid requirements for children are determined by weight. Infants have a greater fluid requirement per kg of body weight than do older children (Table 19.3, p. 466). Infants and

Fluid balance chart

Hospital/Ward: **ST. SWITHINS**						Date: **01.01.08**	
Hospital number: **1234567**							
Surname: **SMITH**			Forenames:		**FRANK**		
Date of birth: **01.01.1949**			Sex:		**MALE**		

	Fluid intake			Fluid output			
Time (hrs)	Oral	IV	Other (specify route)	Urine	Vomit	Other (specify)	
01.00	NBM	B/F 500				WOUND DRAIN	
02.00		N/SALINE 0.9%					
03.00							
04.00							
05.00		↓					
06.00		5% Dex		400	90		
07.00		1000					
08.00							
09.00	↓						
10.00	30 water						
11.00	30 water						
12.00	30 water			500			
13.00	30 water						
14.00	30 water						
15.00	30 water						
16.00	30 water						
17.00	30 water						
18.00	60 water	5% Dex		450			
19.00	60 water	500					
20.00	60 water						
21.00	60 water						
22.00	100 TEA						
23.00							
24.00		↓		350	50		
TOTAL	580ml	2000		1700	140		

KEY:
NBM = NIL BY MOUTH
B/F = BROUGHT FORWARD

ALL MEASURMENTS IN MILLILITRES (ML.)
TOTAL INPUT   =   580 + 2000 = 2580 ML.
TOTAL OUTPUT = 1700 + 140 = 1840 ML.
BALANCE = +740 ML.

Fig. 19.3 • A fluid balance chart. (Reproduced with permission from Nicol, M., Bavin, C., Cronin, P., et al., 2008. Essential nursing skills, third ed. Mosby, Edinburgh.)

small children have very little fluid reserve and are at increased risk of fluid and electrolyte depletion (see p. 458). For example, infants and children with diarrhoea lose water and the electrolytes sodium and potassium (Box 19.7).

Helping people to drink

Whether a person receives adequate oral fluid or not can depend on simple interventions, advice and encouragement provided by nurses and other members of the MDT. For example, just having a glass of fresh water within reach at all times will influence fluid intake.

Success in achieving the goals set for fluid intake depends on providing individualized care that meets the person's needs. Most people maintain their fluid intake independently and nurses must be sensitive to the feelings of those who need help with drinking. When helping people to drink, the nurse should consider points that include the following:

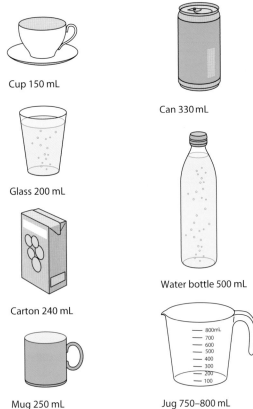

Cup 150 mL

Can 330 mL

Glass 200 mL

Water bottle 500 mL

Carton 240 mL

Mug 250 mL

Jug 750–800 mL

Note - always check the labels and the volume of drinking vessels, as volumes vary

Fig. 19.4 • Typical volume of a cup, glass, juice carton, mug, drinks can, water bottle and jug.

Table 19.3 Daily fluid requirements for children[a]		
Body weight (kg)	**Fluid needed per day**	**Worked example**
1–10	100 mL/kg	An infant weighing 7.5 kg needs $100 \times 7.5 = 750$ mL of fluid/day
11–20	1000 mL plus 50 mL/kg for each kg >10 kg	A girl aged 2½ years weighing 13.0 kg needs $1000 + (50 \times 3) = 1150$ mL of fluid/day
>20	1500 mL plus 20 mL/kg for each kg >20 kg	A boy aged 10 years weighing 30 kg needs $1500 + (20 \times 10) = 1700$ mL of fluid/day
		A girl aged 14 years weighing 50 kg needs $1500 + (20 \times 30) = 2100$ mL of fluid/day

[a]Not suitable for neonates. (Developed from Wilson, D., 2011. Balance and imbalance of body fluids. In: Hockenberry, M.J., Wilson, D., (Eds.), Wong's nursing care of infants and children, ninth ed. Mosby, St Louis).

- *Safety in the home, community settings and in hospital:* The occupational therapist (OT) can assess the person to ascertain their ability to safely heat water and prepare hot drinks. Safety and independence can be enhanced by the provision of aids that include tippers for kettles and teapots for pouring, or a small volume kettle that is easier to lift (Fig. 19.5). The physiotherapist will be involved where people have mobility and balance problems.
- *Swallowing ability:* The SLT or specially trained nurse undertakes a swallowing assessment if there is any doubt

about the safety of giving oral fluids, such as following a stroke.

Swallowing involves three stages: *oral*, which is under voluntary control followed by *pharyngeal*, which commences when the food bolus enters the pharynx. At this point, swallowing becomes involuntary as pharyngeal receptors stimulate the swallowing centre in the brain, which in turn initiates the swallowing reflex. Protective mechanisms normally guard the airway during swallowing. Should these mechanisms fail, the cough reflex functions, in a conscious person, clearing the airways if food does enter. During the *oesophageal*

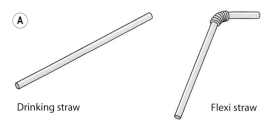

Drinking straw   Flexi straw

Some drinking straws have a non-return valve.

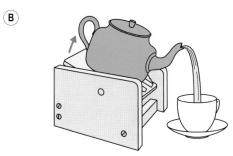

Teapot/kettle tipper.

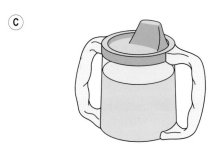

Drinking mug – two handles and wide base for stability.
The handles are shaped for ease of use.

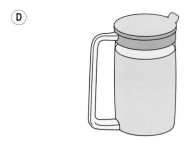

Drinking mug – one handle and conventional spout.

Fig. 19.5 • Aids to independence in drinking: (A) Drinking straws.
(B) Teapot/kettle tipper. (C) Drinking mug – two handles.
(D) Drinking mug – one handle. (Reproduced with permission from Roper,
N., Logan, W.W., Tierney, A.J., 1985. The elements of nursing, second ed.
Churchill Livingstone, Edinburgh.)

stage, the bolus is moved downwards towards the stomach by waves of smooth muscle contraction and relaxation, known as peristalsis.

- *Assessment of the mouth and teeth* (see Ch. 16): A sore mouth, e.g. presence of mouth ulcers, can prevent a person from drinking. Make sure that dentures are clean and in place before offering drinks.

- *Position:* Where possible, the person should sit upright, as this makes swallowing easier.
- *Preferences:* Ask about favourite drinks and the usual timing of these, as preferred fluids are usually more acceptable. Always ascertain whether the person takes sugar or milk in their tea or coffee and never put sugar in drinks without asking. Infants and small children should always be offered sugar-free drinks. However, if sugary drinks are consumed, children should be helped or encouraged to clean their teeth afterwards (see Ch. 16).
- *Temperature:* Ensure that drinks are served at the correct temperature – that hot drinks are hot and cold drinks are cold. At home, providing hot drinks in a vacuum flask will keep them hot for several hours. This is especially useful if the person has mobility problems and family or carers visit during the day. Adding ice or cooling drinks in the refrigerator often increases palatability.
- *Variety:* Tap water can be monotonous; offer variety with carbonated water or water flavoured with fruit juices. People with electrolyte imbalances may need to avoid some fluids, e.g. yeast extract drinks containing high levels of sodium, or someone who needs potassium may be encouraged to drink fruit juices; instant coffee also has high levels of potassium but contains caffeine.
- *Changing water jugs:* This should be done every few hours, as water is not very palatable at room temperature. Try to keep water jugs away from radiators and out of direct sunlight. When jugs are changed, always check that the fluid consumed has been recorded on the fluid chart.
- *Accessibility:* Fluids must always be within reach.
- *Providing encouragement and reminders to drink:* This can increase people's fluid intake (Box 19.8).
- *Drinking aids:* These are sometimes needed (Fig. 19.5) and include:

 Health promotion   Box 19.8

Encouraging people to drink sufficient fluids

Nurses set a goal for the daily intake and, together with the patient/client, parent or carer, plan the timing of drinks to achieve this. People need to know how many cups/glasses will provide the required daily volume, as trying to visualize a specific volume, e.g. 1.5 L, can be difficult (see Fig. 19.6). Encouragement can be as simple as asking, 'would you like another drink?' or pouring and offering a drink. Planning an activity that involves a child can encourage them to drink. For example, adding stickers to a card for each drink or by colouring in a chart with the required number of cups/glasses.

Student activities

- Identify a group of patients/clients, e.g. adults with a learning disability, children in the school reception class (see Table 19.3), people with dementia living in a nursing home, and devise a plan that ensures that they obtain sufficient fluids.
- Discuss the plan with your mentor.

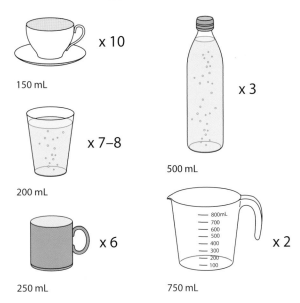

150 mL × 10

500 mL × 3

200 mL × 7–8

250 mL × 6

800mL
700
600
500
400
300
200
100

750 mL × 2

Note – always check the volume of drinking vessels/jugs, as these may vary

Fig. 19.6 • Checking volume. How much is 1.5 L?

- ○ drinking straws (straight, flexible and those with a non-return valve)
- ○ mugs with large handles and wide bases
- ○ mugs that can be used while lying down
- ○ feeding bottles with teats for small children who still use bottles. Although older children usually use cups, during illness they may want to use a bottle again.
- *Providing acceptable volumes:* It is often easier for people to have several small drinks from their favourite glass or china cup (Fig. 19.6). Standard vessels full of fluid put off many people.
- *Providing physical help* if needed and ensuring that the appropriate aids are available and sitting level with the patient/client when assisting.
- *Involving specialist nurses,* e.g. nutrition specialists, stroke specialists when appropriate.

Fluid restriction

Sometimes fluid intake is restricted, e.g. in kidney failure. The person needs to know the exact volume prescribed and the reason for the restriction. The points above about helping a person to drink, including timing and spacing of drinks, small vessels, favourite drinks, are especially important in this situation.

A person having restricted fluids is likely to have a dry mouth and complain of being thirsty. The nurse can minimize discomfort by offering crushed ice or an ice cube to suck to moisten their mouth while still adhering to the restriction.

Caring for the person with fluid imbalance

Fluid depletion

Fluid volume deficit or dehydration requires specific nursing care. The skin will be dry with reduced skin turgor (see

p. 463), which increases the risk of pressure ulcers. Lethargy, caused by fluid depletion, reduces mobility and so increases the risk of skin breakdown. The risk should be assessed using a validated rating scale and appropriate preventive measures put in place (see Ch. 25). Because oral condition is often affected and the mouth is dry, mouth care (see Ch. 16) and mouthwashes are needed until hydration improves. Fluid depletion predisposes to constipation and, when possible, oral fluids, a fibre-rich diet and physical activity are the preferred interventions (see Ch. 21). Lack of fluid can lead to confusion and nurses must be alert to the risks associated with increasing confusion and disorientation, e.g. falls.

Oedema

Oedematous, swollen tissue is easily damaged and this increases the risk of infection and pressure ulcers (see Chs 15, 25). It is important that the risk is minimized by ensuring that neither nurses' nor clients' fingernails, rings or watches damage the skin, and scratching is avoided. After washing, swollen tissue should be gently patted dry rather than rubbed. People with ankle and leg oedema are advised to elevate the leg(s) in order to encourage drainage of the excess fluid, or move about or exercise the ankles and feet to use the skeletal muscle 'pump' in the calves to increase venous return to the heart. Other measures include use of support stockings, if prescribed, and avoiding clothing with tight elasticated parts, e.g. socks, trouser legs, and anything else that will impair venous return.

Caring for the person who is vomiting

Prolonged or excessive vomiting can be distressing and may lead to fluid, electrolyte and acid–base imbalance (see p. 460). People often experience nausea before vomiting; there may be pallor, sweating and excess watery saliva. The causes of vomiting include:

- Gastrointestinal tract distension or irritation, e.g. bacterial toxins, excess alcohol
- Motion sickness
- Pain (see Ch. 23)
- Drugs, e.g. chemotherapy
- Unpleasant sights or odours
- Fear
- Anxiety.

The care needed by a person who is vomiting is outlined in Box 19.9.

Subcutaneous fluids (hypodermoclysis)

Subcutaneous infusion of isotonic fluids is increasingly used for fluid replacement and the maintenance of hydration in older adults, end-of-life care and long-term care. It is used to:

- Maintain hydration when people have an inadequate oral intake
- Rehydrate people with mild to moderate short-term fluid and electrolyte deficits.

Suitable infusion sites include the thighs, abdomen, and over the scapula and the chest wall. The site is only chosen after

Nausea and vomiting

- Ensure privacy, e.g. drawing screens
- Provide a vomit bowl and tissues. At home, an old washing-up bowl can be used to protect bedding, especially with small children
- Remove dentures and place in a labelled denture container
- Provide physical comfort and maintain dignity; hold the vomit bowl or wipe the person's mouth
- Encourage the person to sit upright and breathe deeply. Those lying down or who have altered consciousness should be placed in a lateral position to protect their airway (see Fig. 16.15C). Suction equipment should be close to hand
- Provide a clean vomit bowl before removing a used one
- Provide a mouthwash and help with teeth cleaning
- Help the person to wash their hands and face, particularly if they have been sweating
- Change clothing and bedding as necessary
- Remove the covered vomit bowl to the sluice, measure the vomit and chart on the fluid balance chart. Observe the vomit: colour, odour, undigested food and presence of blood (haematemesis). The type of vomiting, e.g. projectile, accompanied by nausea, related to drugs or food intake or pain, is reported and documented.

Ensure that an appropriate antiemetic drug, e.g. metoclopramide, is administered as prescribed. Antiemetics should always be given in anticipation of expected vomiting such as with some anticancer drugs.

Note: Always wear gloves and a plastic apron if time allows. Vomit is acidic and can damage the skin. Damage can occur, if for instance, an infant or unconscious person's face is resting on vomit-stained bedding. Infants who regurgitate may have vomit in the neck creases and nurses must ensure that the skin is washed and gently patted dry.

discussion with the patient and consideration of comfort, ease of access, mobility and skin condition.

Fluid replacement using hypodermoclysis at home or in long-term care establishments can avoid the need to admit frail older people to hospital for rehydration with intravenous fluids.

The infusion is administered via a butterfly cannula or peripheral plastic cannula, inserted by a RN into the subcutaneous tissues. The cannula is secured with a transparent occlusive dressing for easy observation. The site is changed after 2 L of fluid or according to local policy. Intravenous administration ('giving') sets are used and a RN checks the infusion fluid, e.g. sodium chloride 0.9% or glucose 5%, before commencing a new bag. The giving set is changed according to local policy.

The infusion rate depends on individual needs but the recommended maximum is 2 L in 24 hours or 125 mL/hour into a single site. The prescribed flow rate of subcutaneous fluids can be controlled with a volumetric infusion pump or regulated by gravity and the flow control clamp (flow controller) on the administration set tubing (see Fig. 19.8, p. 470). The enzyme hyaluronidase may be administered to facilitate subcutaneous fluid absorption (Lybarger 2009), either injected via the cannula or added to the infusate.

Fluid overload is unusual but local side-effects include swelling, discomfort or inflammation. Nurses or carers should inspect the infusion site for these, as it might be necessary to change the site. The advantages of subcutaneous infusion include:

- Suitability for most settings, including people's homes
- Convenience, as infusion can be fitted round people's routines, e.g. overnight without disruption to daytime activity
- Cost-effectiveness, because nurses, family or the patient themselves can set up and manage the infusion.

Intravenous fluids

Intravenous (i.v.) infusion of sterile fluid into the circulation is very common in hospitals and is increasingly used in the community. Most nurses will, at some time, care for patients having i.v. fluids (colloquially referred to as a 'drip'). The principles of i.v. fluid therapy and some of the nursing interventions are outlined in this section. Detailed information about the care of i.v. infusions, including those aspects that only a RN may undertake, is provided in Further reading, below, e.g. Dougherty & Lister 2011; Nicol et al 2012.

Intravenous fluid therapy is used when the oral or enteral routes are inappropriate, e.g. following major surgery, serious burns, severe vomiting. Blood transfusion is discussed in Chapter 17. Intravenous therapy is used to:

- Maintain fluid, electrolyte and acid–base balance
- Replace fluids and correct imbalances
- Administer drugs, e.g. pain relief, antibiotics, anticancer drugs
- Provide parenteral nutrition (p. 487).

Most i.v. fluid therapy is short term and can be infused into a peripheral vein in the dorsum (back) of the hand or the forearm, or a scalp vein in infants. Peripheral veins are not suitable for long-term therapy because inflammation can block the vein (see p. 473). For long-term therapy and when irritant or hypertonic solutions are used, fluid is infused into the superior vena cava (a large central vein) where blood flow is sufficient to dilute the fluid and prevent damage to the vein (see Parenteral nutrition, p. 487).

Equipment

Bags or bottles of intravenous fluid are administered through sterile, single-use items of equipment, namely an administration ('giving') set attached to a cannula inserted into the vein (Fig. 19.7).

The type of administration set used depends on the fluid being infused and the safety needs of certain groups. A standard administration set (Fig. 19.8A) is generally used for clear fluids. Blood and blood products are always administered through a set with an integral filter above the drip chamber (Fig. 19.8B; see also Ch. 17). An administration set with a burette (Fig. 19.8C) can be used when drugs or small volumes of fluid are infused. A burette set must always be used with infants, children and others at risk of fluid overload, e.g. frail older people, to prevent accidental infusion of excess fluid (see p. 473). Volumetric infusion pumps (see p. 472) or syringe

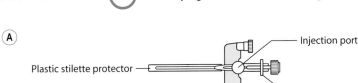

Fig. 19.7 • Intravenous cannulae: (A) Cannula used when i.v. drugs are administered with the infusion or post-infusion. (B) Cannula used for short-term i.v. infusion (also the type of cannula used for hypodermoclysis). (Reproduced with permission from Jamieson, E.M., Whyte, L.A., McCall, J.M. (Eds.), 2007. Clinical nursing practices, fifth ed. Churchill Livingstone, Edinburgh.)

Plastic stilette protector

Injection port

Guard

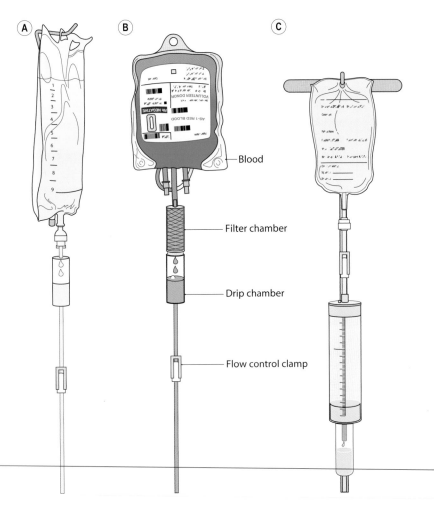

Fig. 19.8 • Types of intravenous administration set: (A) Standard administration set. (B) Blood administration set. (C) Burette (paediatric set). (C: Reproduced with permission from Nicol, M., Bavin, C., Cronin, P., et al., 2008. Essential nursing skills, third ed. Mosby, Edinburgh.)

Blood

Filter chamber

Drip chamber

Flow control clamp

drivers (Ch. 23) are frequently used and always when precise accuracy is required.

Crystalloids and colloids

Fluids for i.v. infusion are divided into crystalloids and colloids. A crystalloid is a clear solution that moves between the bloodstream and the tissue fluid. They are used intravenously to maintain hydration and electrolyte balance and some are supplied with potassium chloride (KCl) added. Examples of crystalloid solutions include:

- Sodium chloride 0.9%
- Glucose 5%
- Sodium chloride 0.18% and glucose 4%.

Colloid solutions contain particles (solutes) that stay in the blood because they are too large to pass through capillary membranes and are used to increase blood volume. Examples include:

- Synthetic solutions containing dextrans or gelatin, e.g. Gelofusine®, or starch, e.g. hetastarch
- Human albumin solution
- Blood and blood products (see Ch. 17).

Principles of care for infusions

The overriding principle is the safety and comfort of the person having i.v. fluids.

The non-dominant arm should be used to site the i.v. infusion whenever possible, thus maximizing independence and minimizing inconvenience. The person may be more comfortable if a pillow with a waterproof cover is used to support the arm or a lightly bandaged single-use splint is applied. The arm may also need to be immobilized using a 'splint designed specifically for use with i.v. therapy' (RCN 2010, p 19). Splints are used according to local policy, if there is a risk of the cannula becoming dislodged such as with small children or adults who are restless or confused.

It is also important to note that Muslims use the left hand for personal cleansing and the right hand for feeding. This has important implications for the siting of i.v. infusions and the wishes of the patient must be taken into account.

Once the i.v. cannula has been sited, it is secured in place with a sterile cannula dressing (Fig. 19.9). The fluid container is connected to an appropriate administration set and fluid is 'run through' to expel air from the tube before connection to the cannula. The tubing is anchored to the arm. The date of cannula insertion and type of administration set is recorded in the nursing notes. A peripheral cannula is removed (or re-sited) after 72–96 hours or before if there are problems; and within 24 hours if the cannula was sited in an emergency where aseptic technique was breached (RCN 2010).

An i.v. infusion is an invasive procedure so aseptic technique and standard precautions must be in place to prevent the entry of contaminants such as microorganisms, and to protect the staff from potentially infected body fluids (see Ch. 15). The closed system only protects if it is kept closed and when it is necessary to open the system, e.g. to change the fluid bag, it is vital that the nurse adheres to the precautions outlined above. Figure 19.10 illustrates the potential routes for contamination.

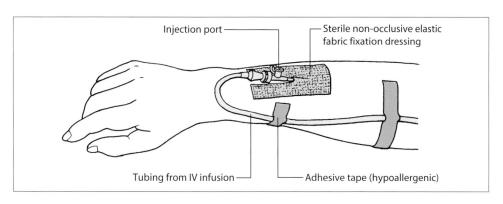

Injection port

Sterile non-occlusive elastic fabric fixation dressing

Tubing from IV infusion

Adhesive tape (hypoallergenic)

Fig. 19.9 • Cannula dressing and securing the tubing. (Reproduced with permission from Jamieson, E.M., Whyte, L.A., McCall, J.M., (Eds.), 2007. Clinical nursing practices, fifth ed. Churchill Livingstone, Edinburgh.)

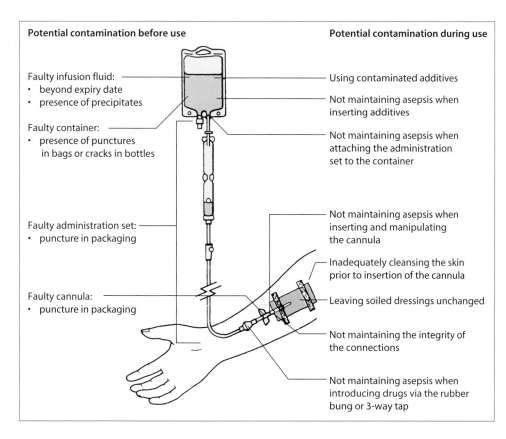

Potential contamination before use

Potential contamination during use

Faulty infusion fluid:
• beyond expiry date
• presence of precipitates

Faulty container:
• presence of punctures in bags or cracks in bottles

Faulty administration set:
• puncture in packaging

Faulty cannula:
• puncture in packaging

Using contaminated additives

Not maintaining asepsis when inserting additives

Not maintaining asepsis when attaching the administration set to the container

Not maintaining asepsis when inserting and manipulating the cannula

Inadequately cleansing the skin prior to insertion of the cannula

Leaving soiled dressings unchanged

Not maintaining the integrity of the connections

Not maintaining asepsis when introducing drugs via the rubber bung or 3-way tap

Fig. 19.10 • Potential routes for contamination during intravenous infusion. (Reproduced with permission from Jamieson, E.M., Whyte, L.A., McCall, J.M., (Eds.), 2007. Clinical nursing practices, fifth ed. Churchill Livingstone, Edinburgh.)

Intravenous fluid bags are changed using aseptic technique every 24 hours. Usually, administration sets are changed every 72 hours for peripheral i.v. fluids and this is recorded in the nursing notes. The cannula site is inspected regularly for signs of inflammation such as redness, swelling and pain that may indicate the development of phlebitis (inflammation of a vein), infection or other complications (see Box 19.12, p. 473). The dressing around the cannula is changed aseptically if it has become loose, wet or bloodstained. Otherwise, the dressing is usually left undisturbed until the cannula is re-sited or removed (according to local policies).

All fluids for i.v. infusion are prescribed and a RN must check that the correct fluid is administered to the correct person. Some areas require that two nurses (one registered) check i.v. fluids. The outer wrapping is removed from the bag and it and the fluid are checked for:

- Expiry date
- Damage or leakage
- Discoloration of the fluid
- Clarity
- Absence of particles.

The type and volume of fluid, e.g. 500 mL of sodium chloride 0.9%, is checked against the prescription sheet and the person's identity band is checked. When a bag of i.v. fluid is commenced, the details including the batch number are recorded in the nursing records. In addition, i.v. fluid volumes are recorded on the fluid intake and output chart. The principles of changing infusion bags are outlined in Box 19.10.

Flow rate calculation and regulation

Nurses are responsible for calculating and regulating the flow rate of i.v. fluids. The flow rate can be regulated by gravity and the flow control clamp (flow controller) on the administration set tubing, or by an infusion pump.

The flow rate is checked at least hourly. Factors that may reduce or stop the flow rate include:

- Kinking of the administration set tubing
- Fluid container too low; overcome by raising the container
- Cannula position in the vein; often overcome by gently changing the position of the hand or forearm.

Intravenous infusion pumps are increasingly used to regulate the flow rate. They should be used:

- For accuracy when i.v. drugs or small volumes of fluid are prescribed
- When a risk of rapid overinfusion exists or people are at risk of fluid overload, e.g. infants, children, frail older people and those with heart failure.

Most models have audible alarms that alert the nurse to situations that include 'infusion complete', 'air in line' and 'flow obstructed'. It is imperative that alarms are never turned off. RNs are responsible for using pumps safely in accordance with the manufacturer's instructions. RNs receive training for each type of pump used in their area and are competent in their use. Nurses who are unsure about a particular pump must seek help and advice from an experienced colleague. Student nurses

Nursing skills   Box 19.10

Infusion bag change

Safety is paramount when undertaking a bag change. The key principles are:

- Changing the infusion bag means that the closed system is breached, thereby increasing the risk of infection
- Wash and dry hands
- Bags are changed before the fluid level falls below the spike of the administration bag; thus preventing the formation of air bubbles in the tubing leading to the cannula
- The new bag of fluid is in date and in good condition (see text)
- Fluid type and the person's identity must be checked by a RN.

The bag change is explained and a visual check of the cannula site made, observing for the presence of complications (see Box 19.12).

- Close the flow control clamp (flow controller) on the administration set
- Take the empty bag from the i.v. stand and remove the administration set from the bag, taking care to avoid contamination of the spike
- Take the protective plastic from the inlet port of the new bag of fluid and insert the spike of the administration set. This is twisted until completely inserted (Fig. 19.11)
- Hang the new bag on the i.v. fluid stand and regulate the flow control clamp to administer the prescribed flow rate (see Box 19.11)
- Check the flow rate at least hourly by using a watch with a second hand, if regulated by gravity and the flow control clamp
- Check that the patient has no discomfort at the cannula site and observe for signs of overinfusion causing fluid overload, i.e. rising pulse, BP and respiratory rate (see Box 19.12)
- The used infusion bag and packaging are disposed of in the clinical waste
- Wash hands before completing the documentation (see local policy) and the fluid balance chart
- Report and record any problems.

(Based on Nicol et al 2012).

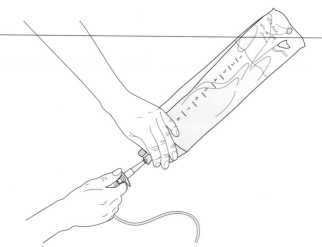

Fig. 19.11 • Changing the infusion bag – inserting the administration set spike into a new bag. (Reproduced with permission from Nicol, M., Bavin, C., Cronin, P., et al., 2008. Essential nursing skills, third ed. Mosby, Edinburgh).

may only deal with pumps under direct RN supervision. The formulae used to calculate flow rates in drops/minute and millilitres per hour are outlined in Box 19.11.

 Critical thinking Box 19.11

Calculating i.v. flow rates

Infusion flow rates are calculated in one of two ways: drops per minute or millilitres per hour.

Drops per minute

Used for infusions regulated by gravity and roller clamp on the administration set and for regulatory devices that use drops per minute and it is vital that the flow rate remains constant. Each type of administration set (see Fig. 19.8) has a specific 'drop factor' (drops/mL):

- Standard administration set; 20 drops/mL for crystalloids
- Standard administration set; 15 drops/mL for colloids
- Blood administration set; 15 drops/mL
- Burette (paediatric set); 60 drops/mL.

The calculation is:

$$\text{Flow rate (drops/min)} = \frac{\text{volume of fluid (mL)} \times \text{drop factor (number of drops/mL)}}{\text{time (min)}}$$

Worked example

Tom has been prescribed 1000 mL of sodium chloride 0.9% in 8 hours. A standard administration set is used.

$$\frac{1000 \times 20}{480} = \frac{20\,000}{480} = 41.6 \text{ drops per minute (rounded up to 42)}$$

Millilitres per hour

Millilitres per hour are used when the i.v. flow rate is regulated by a volumetric infusion pump or syringe driver. The calculation is:

$$\text{Flow rate (mL/hr)} = \frac{\text{volume of fluid (mL)}}{\text{time (hr)}}$$

Worked example

Jyoti has been prescribed 500 mL of glucose 5% in 6 hours via a volumetric infusion pump.

$$\text{Flow rate} = \frac{500}{6} = 83.3 \text{ mL (rounded down to 83)}$$

Student activities

- When you are helping to care for a person having i.v. fluids, ask if you can be involved in the calculation and regulation of flow rates. Try to do this for flow rates being regulated by both a gravity/roller clamp and an infusion pump.

Resource

Gatford, J.D., Phillips, N., 2011. Nursing calculations, eighth ed. Churchill Livingstone, Edinburgh.

Complications associated with i.v. therapy Box 19.12

Local complications

- Phlebitis, which is inflammation of the lining of the vein, e.g. chemical irritation from drugs injected/infused. When associated with clot formation it is known as thrombophlebitis
- Infection due to contamination at several sites (see Fig. 19.10). Infection and phlebitis both cause redness, swelling and pain
- Infiltration occurring when fluid infuses into the tissues ('tissuing') instead of the vein. There is swelling around the cannula site, which may be painful. Sometimes, but not always, the infusion stops
- Extravasation is infiltration causing local tissue damage. Necrosis (tissue death) may occur when a vesicant (highly irritant) substance leaks out of the vein, e.g. cytotoxic drugs, diazepam, glucose 50%, etc. Dougherty (2010, p 48) warns that 'Nurses are not always aware of the vesicant nature of the everyday medications they administer, often falsely believing that it is only cytotoxic drugs that are of concern…'.

Systemic complications

- Circulatory overload occurs when fluid, especially sodium chloride 0.9%, is infused too rapidly. The increase in blood volume can lead to heart failure and acute pulmonary oedema (see Box 19.2, p. 461 and Ch. 17). The patient's BP, pulse and respiratory rate increase. They have dyspnoea and a cough with frothy sputum. This risk is reduced by regular checks on the flow rate (as overinfusion often happens when arm position affects the flow rate) and through the use of infusion pumps (see above)
- Fluid volume deficit due to inadequate fluid prescription or excessively slow infusion rate
- Septicaemia (multiplication of bacteria in the bloodstream) due to spread from a local infection at the cannula site
- Rare but life-threatening events that include an air embolism when an air bubble enters the vein and reaches the heart or a pulmonary embolism (a blood clot, known as an 'embolus', travels through the heart to block a pulmonary artery).

Reference

Dougherty, L., 2010. Extravasation: prevention, recognition and management. Nursing Standard 24 (52), 48–55.

Nutrition

This part of the chapter explores health-promoting activities and nursing interventions such as feeding, that help people to obtain the correct nutrients in sufficient quantities to meet individual needs. The importance and scope of these are illustrated in the benchmarks of good practice in *Essence of Care 2010* (DH 2010) (Box 19.13). In addition, an overview of the gastrointestinal (GI) tract, the principles of nutrition and healthy eating throughout the lifespan are important in ensuring that nurses can meet the nutritional needs of people in their care.

The gastrointestinal tract

An overview of structure and function is provided. Readers are encouraged to consult their anatomy and physiology book for

---

Complications of i.v. therapy

Complications associated with an i.v. infusion may be local or systemic and range from minor to serious and life-threatening. Box 19.12 provides an overview of common complications; those specific to blood transfusion are discussed in Chapter 17.

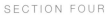 Reflective practice   Box 19.13

Using benchmarks of best practice

Student activities

- Reflect on the following benchmark statements in relation to what you observe at mealtimes in your placement.
- Discuss your observations with your mentor.

Benchmarks of best practice – food and drink (DH 2010, p 8)

1. *People* are encouraged to eat and drink in a way that promotes health
2. *People* and carers have sufficient information to enable them to obtain their food and drink
3. *People* can access food and drink at any time according to their needs and preferences
4. *People* are provided with food and drink that meets their individual needs and preferences
5. *People's* food and drink is presented in a way that is appealing to them
6. *People* feel the environment is conducive to eating and drinking
7. *People* who are screened on initial contact and identified at risk receive a full nutritional assessment
8. *People's* care is planned, implemented, continuously evaluated and revised to meet individual needs and preferences for food and drink
9. *People* receive the care and assistance they require with eating and drinking
10. *People's* food and drink intake is monitored and recorded.

more details (see also Chs 16, 21). The GI tract has a basic, four-layer structure that is modified at various points according to the function of that part. For example, the presence of villi (microscopic projections) in the mucosa of the small intestine increases the surface area available for the absorption of nutrients.

Parts of the gastrointestinal tract

The GI tract is essentially a tube starting at the mouth and ending at the anus (Fig. 19.12). The individual parts and their specific functions are:

- Mouth (see Ch. 16) – ingestion, the teeth enable chewing (mastication), saliva secreted by the salivary glands allows taste (see below) and some chemical digestion of food, and the first stage of swallowing take place here
- Pharynx (nasopharynx, oropharynx and laryngopharynx) – only the oropharynx and laryngopharynx are common routes for food, fluid and air. Swallowing, which is a multi-stage process (see p. 466) involves the mouth, pharynx and oesophagus
- Oesophagus – a tube that conveys food/fluid from the pharynx to the stomach, but has no role in digestion or absorption
- Stomach – in adults, can comfortably hold 1.5 L of food/fluids. However, in infants and children capacity is much smaller. For example, a newborn has a capacity

of 15–30 mL, which has implications for volumes of feed and frequency of feeding. In addition, the gastro-oesophageal sphincter is underdeveloped, predisposing to regurgitation. The stomach churns and mixes food with gastric juices and some digestion and limited absorption takes place
- Small intestine (duodenum, jejunum and ileum) – the duodenum is continuous with the stomach and the ileum leads into the large intestine. Secretions from the pancreas and bile from the gallbladder both enter into the duodenum. Chemical digestion is completed in the small intestine by enzymes from the pancreas and those secreted in the intestinal juice, and nutrients are absorbed
- Large intestine, rectum and anal canal (see Ch. 21).

Overview – general functions of the gastrointestinal tract

The GI tract, plus the secretions from various accessory organs – salivary glands, the liver (gallbladder and bile ducts), and the pancreas (Fig. 19.12) – are concerned with five main activities:

- Ingestion of food
- Movement of contents through the tract by peristalsis
- Digestion of food by mechanical means (chewing) and chemically through the action of enzymes secreted by glands and accessory organs. Enzymes break down the nutrients (protein, carbohydrate and fat) into small molecules
- Absorption of the end products of digestion, minerals, vitamins and water, mainly through the walls of the small intestine into the blood or lymph vessels
- Defecation (see Ch. 21).

Smell and taste

The senses of smell (olfaction) and taste (gustation) are intricately linked and both are important for appetite and nutritional intake. You should consult your own anatomy and physiology book for more detail. Being able to smell and taste food:

- Increases appetite and enjoyment of food
- Increases the variety of foods eaten and helps to ensure a balanced intake of nutrients
- Stimulates digestive secretions
- Affords some protection against eating food that is 'rotten'. Additionally, reflex gagging or vomiting can occur if foul-tasting food is eaten.

Conversely, unpleasant odours can decrease appetite (Box 19.14).

Alterations to smell and taste

Alterations include a reduction in the sense of smell (hyposmia) or complete loss of smell (anosmia). Problems can be

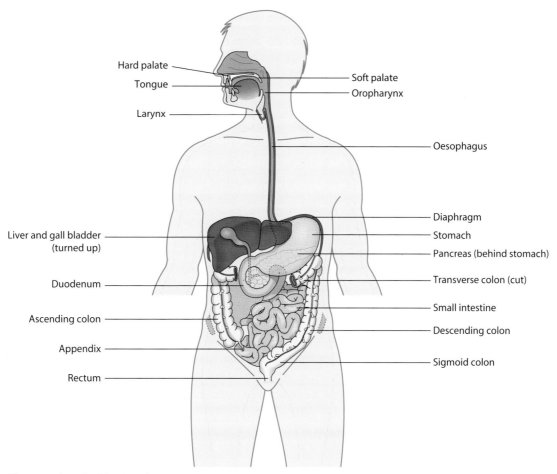

Fig. 19.12 • The gastrointestinal tract and some accessory organs. (Adapted from Waugh, A., Grant, A., 2006. Ross and Wilson anatomy and physiology in health and illness, tenth ed. Churchill Livingstone, Edinburgh).

 Reflective practice   Box 19.14

Smell, taste and appetite

Think about situations when your appetite was affected by smell, e.g. a favourite meal being cooked.

Student activities

- Identify situations where an odour or problem with the sense of smell decreased a patient's appetite
- Reflect on ways of minimizing the impact of unpleasant odours.

Disturbances in smell and taste   Box 19.15

- Some people with epilepsy experience an aura, when they perceive a strange smell or taste immediately before a seizure
- Taste may be changed with cancer
- Hallucinations (false perceptions) may affect any sense including smell (olfactory) or taste (gustatory), e.g. a person may 'smell' burning or taste 'poison' in their food
- Drugs that may affect taste include the anti-arrhythmic amiodarone, lithium, ACE inhibitors such as captopril, and the antibiotics clarithromycin and metronidazole.

---

temporary, such as with a common cold, or may be permanent, e.g. after head injury.

Taste, and hence appetite, can be impaired if a cold affects the olfactory receptors in the nose. Taste can be affected by a dry mouth, e.g. fluid deficits (p. 461), and when oral hygiene and/or dental health is poor (see Ch. 16).

The senses of taste and smell diminish with normal ageing as there is gradual loss of taste and olfactory receptors. Older people may complain that 'modern food' has no taste and this can contribute to a poor appetite. Suggesting stronger flavours and aromas, seasoning and different textures may improve the taste of meals.

Smell or taste can be affected by disease or as a side-effect of some drugs (Box 19.15).

Nutritional and upper gastrointestinal tract disorders

Some disorders, e.g. obesity, eating disorders, upper GI tract disorders and other conditions that impact on nutrition, are outlined in Table 19.4, Boxes 19.16, 19.17 and the Useful websites, p. 489, provide information including related organizations and groups.

Table 19.4 Common nutritional disorders and other conditions affecting nutrition

Obesity (see Box 19.16)	The World Health Organization (WHO 2006) defines overweight and the classes of obesity according to body mass index (BMI) *Note*: BMI is further discussed in Box 19.23. Obesity is very common in developed countries and in England almost 25% of adults were obese in 2008 (NHS Information Centre 2009). It represents a major public health problem leading to type 2 diabetes, hypertension increasing the risk of heart attack or stroke, joint problems and psychosocial problems. *Note*: Obesity is a feature of Prader–Willi syndrome, a rare chromosomal disorder characterized by overeating (hyperphagia).
Eating disorders (see Box 19.17)	Conditions in which a person's eating behaviour and nutrient intake is inappropriate for their needs: • *Anorexia nervosa* characterized by distorted body image and a deliberate restriction of food intake resulting in severe weight loss, malnutrition, endocrine disorders and electrolyte disturbances (see p. 460), etc. • *Bulimia nervosa* where weight is controlled by periods of restricted eating, vomiting, purging and binge eating. Weight usually remains stable and within normal range. • *Binge eating* characterized by periods of binge eating but without periods of food restriction or purging which result in the development of obesity.
Nutritional deficiencies	Deficiencies may involve a single nutrient such as poor iron intake leading to anaemia, lack of vitamin D, or protein-energy malnutrition (PEM) in which the person is deficient in both protein and energy.
Failure to thrive (FTT)	An infant or child fails to develop and grow at the expected rate. This may result from disorders such as heart defects, cystic fibrosis or have causes that include mother-child attachment difficulties, poor knowledge of nutrition, nutrient deficiency (e.g. iron), family stress, psychosocial problems.
Food intolerance	Abnormal reaction, e.g. colic, diarrhoea, to a food which is non-immunological. Examples include lactose (milk sugar) intolerance caused by a deficiency in the enzyme lactase.
Food allergy	An abnormal immunological response to food, e.g. peanuts, which can be severe and life threatening. Signs and symptoms include swelling of the mouth and throat, breathing difficulties, skin rashes and GI tract upsets.
Malabsorption	Deficient absorption of nutrients from the GI tract caused by diseases of, or surgery to, the small intestine, or lack of digestive enzymes or bile salts. There is FTT in children and in adults there is weight loss and fatty stools (steatorrhoea).
Diabetes mellitus (see Chs 1, 16, 20 and 25)	Diabetes mellitus is characterized by hyperglycaemia (elevated blood glucose) and can be due to an absolute or relative deficiency of insulin or a decreased sensitivity to insulin. There are two main types: type 1 usually affects people under 40 years of age and is always managed with insulin injections and diet; type 2 (see Obesity above) mainly affects people over 40 years of age and may be managed by diet, oral hypoglycaemic drugs or insulin, or a combination of these.
Mouth problems	These include: • Cleft lip and cleft palate • Gum hyperplasia (overgrowth), a side-effect of the drug phenytoin used to control seizures • Abnormal eruption of teeth • Infections, e.g. candidiasis (thrush) • Mucositis (inflammation of the oral mucosa) caused by cancer treatment
Diaphragmatic hernia (hiatus hernia)	Protrusion of part of the stomach through the diaphragm into the chest. May be asymptomatic or cause reflux of stomach contents and oesophagitis (inflammation of the oesophagus). May be congenital or acquired.
Gastro-oesophageal reflux disease (GORD)	An incompetent/malfunctioning gastro-oesophageal sphincter allows the stomach contents to enter the oesophagus on inspiration, resulting in vomiting, oesophagitis, scarring, stricture (narrowing) and possibly aspiration pneumonia. GORD can occur with enteral feeding (see p. 485).
Peptic ulceration	A non-malignant ulcer in those parts of the GI tract exposed to gastric juice; usually the duodenum or stomach.
Cancer	Cancer can affect the mouth, oesophagus and stomach but rarely occurs in the small intestine (see Ch. 21 for colorectal cancer).

Health promotion Box 19.16

Obesity

Obesity is a major public health issue in the UK; the morbidity and mortality from obesity-related diseases (see Table 19.4) consume a large proportion of health budgets and cause considerable social and personal problems.

In England, almost 25% of adults were obese in 2008 and 42% of men and 32% of women were overweight (NHS Information Centre 2009). In the same year, the prevalence of obesity in children aged 2–15 years was 16.8% in boys and 15.2% in girls, and 14.6% of boys and 14% of girls were classed as overweight (NHS Information Centre 2009).

The Scottish Government describes obesity as having 'reached epidemic proportions and its prevalence is increasing' (Scottish Intercollegiate Guideline Network, SIGN 2010, p 1).

Student activities

- Reflect with your mentor on the obesity-related problems in your own field of practice.
- What health promoting measures prevent obesity in children and adults, assist overweight or obese individuals to lose weight and achieve/maintain normal weight?

Reference

Scottish Intercollegiate Guideline Network (SIGN), 2010. Management of obesity. Guideline 115. Online. Available: www.sign.ac.uk.

Resources

Milligan, F., 2008. Child obesity 1: analysing its prevalence and causes. Nursing Times 104 (32), 26–27.

Milligan, F., 2008. Child obesity 2: recommended strategies and interventions. Nursing Times 104 (33), 24–25.

Milligan, F., 2010. Primary care screening and brief counselling for overweight or mildly obese children does not improve BMI, nutrition or physical activity. Evidence Based Nursing 13 (1), 8–9.

NICE, 2006 (modified 2010). Obesity: the prevention, identification, assessment and management of overweight and obesity in adults and children. Online. Available: www.nice.org.uk.

Yilmaz, J., Povey, L., Dalglish, J., 2011. Adopting a psychological approach to obesity. Nursing Standard 25 (21), 42–46.

 Critical thinking Box 19.17

Eating disorders

A friend asks you about eating disorders. She wants to know some basic facts and where to get information and help.

Student activities

- Access the websites below and prepare a summary for your friend and find out what help is available in your area.

Resources

Eating Disorders Association (beating eating disorders) – www.b-eat.co.uk.

BBC – http://www.bbc.co.uk/health/emotional_health/ mental_health/mind_eatingdisorders.shtml.

National Centre for Eating Disorders (NCFED) – www.eating-disorders.org.uk.

National Institute for Health and Clinical Excellence (NICE), 2004. Quick reference guide: eating disorders, CG9. Online. Available: www.nice.org.uk/nicemedia/ live/10932/29217/29217.pdf.

All websites accessed September 2012.

Principles of nutrition and the healthy diet

A healthy diet comprises the correct nutrients in appropriate amounts. This varies during the lifespan and following injury or disease. For instance, a healthy diet for a toddler differs from that needed by an older adult or someone with diabetes.

Nutrients provide energy and molecules for functions such as muscle contraction, growth, tissue repair and replacement, and for health maintenance. The nutrients are divided into:

- The energy-yielding *macronutrients* needed in relatively large quantities – carbohydrates, fat and proteins
- The *micronutrients* needed in relatively small amounts – minerals (including trace elements) and vitamins.

Individual foods usually contain several nutrients, e.g. potato provides carbohydrate, protein, minerals and vitamins and also indigestible fibre.

As water is essential for ingestion, digestion, absorption and nutrient utilization, an adequate fluid intake is vital (see p. 464 (adults) and Table 19.3, p. 466 (children)). In addition, a healthy diet should also contain fibre or non-starch polysaccharide (NSP) (see below).

The energy value of food is measured in the SI unit kilojoule (kJ) but in food labelling the kilocalorie (kcal) content is often shown too. Energy requirements vary greatly between people and depend on:

- Gender – adult men need approximately 170 kJ (40 kcal) per square metre of body surface area every hour, i.e. 170 kJ/m^2 per hour, whereas women need 155 kJ (37 kcal).
- Size
- Physical activity
- Health status, e.g. major surgery or serious injury increases energy requirements.

Although alcohol is not a nutrient its consumption can substantially increase the total energy intake, as 1 g of alcohol yields 29 kJ (7 kcal). Alcohol misuse may cause health and social problems that include:

- Obesity
- Deficiency of B vitamins
- Liver damage
- Hypertension (high blood pressure)
- Damage to other organs, e.g. heart, brain
- Fetal alcohol syndrome (FAS)
- Relationship problems
- Job loss
- Financial difficulties.

Box 19.18 provides an opportunity to investigate the recommended 'safe limits' for alcohol.

An outline of the main nutrients and their functions in the body, and food sources is provided below.

Macronutrients

Carbohydrates

Carbohydrates may be sugars – monosaccharides (glucose, fructose and galactose), disaccharides (maltose, lactose and sucrose) or polysaccharides such as starch or glycogen. During digestion, carbohydrates are mainly broken down into glucose, the body's major energy source. Each gram of carbohydrate yields 16 kJ (3.75 kcal). Some is used immediately, some stored as glycogen in the liver and skeletal muscles, but any excess is converted to fat.

Carbohydrates are obtained from sugar, pulses, yam, potato and other vegetables, fruit, cereals such as wheat, oats, rice and maize, plus flour-based products, e.g. bread, pasta and chapattis.

NSP is indigestible plant material, e.g. cellulose and other polysaccharides, that ensures steady absorption of glucose from the intestine, gives a feeling of fullness, adds bulk to the faeces and decreases the time waste remains in the large intestine (see Ch. 21). Good sources of NSP include: wholegrain cereals, pulses, vegetables and fruit. An average intake of 18 g/day is suggested for adults. Children should have proportionally lower NSP intakes, and children under 2 years of age should not have NSP-containing foods at the expense of energy-rich foods that are needed for normal growth (DH 1991).

Fats

Fatty acids are classified as saturated, monounsaturated or polyunsaturated according to their chemical structure. Fats are emulsified by bile salts in the small intestine and broken down

by enzymes into glycerol and fatty acids. The fatty acids are used as a stored energy source, to form lipid substances such as prostaglandins and phospholipids, and as a source of the fat-soluble vitamins A, D and E, and cholesterol. When 1 g of fat is oxidized, it yields 37 kJ (9 kcal), i.e. twice as much energy as that produced by 1 g of protein or carbohydrate and although this makes it valuable when energy requirements are high, excessive intake in sedentary children and adults leads to obesity. However, children under 2 years of age should be given full-fat dairy products.

Fat is obtained from full-fat dairy products, margarine, ghee, cooking oils, fried foods, cakes, biscuits, crisps, pastry, chocolate, meat, oily fish, nuts, pulses and seeds.

Proteins

Proteins are formed from various amino acids. These are released during digestion to provide the amino acids required for protein synthesis, tissue growth and repair and, under certain conditions, for energy. Each gram of protein yields 17 kJ or 4 kcal.

The reference nutrient intake (RNI) for protein in adults is between 45 g and 55.5 g/day depending upon gender and age (DH 1991). However, this increases during growth, pregnancy, lactation and illness.

Protein is obtained from both animal and vegetable sources, e.g. meat, milk, cheese, fish, eggs, nuts, pulses, tofu and cereals. It is, however, vital that vegetarians and vegans obtain a balanced intake, as some cereals are deficient in the amino acid lysine and some pulses are deficient in methionine.

Micronutrients

The micronutrients are the minerals and vitamins required by the body in relatively small amounts. They are necessary for

Table 19.5 Minerals and dietary sources

Mineral	Dietary sources
Calcium	Hard water, milk/milk products, sardines, bread, soya beans, lentils, sesame seeds
Iodine	Seafood, milk, dairy products, eggs, meat, iodized salt
Iron	Offal, red meat, egg yolk, cereal products, pulses, vegetables, cocoa, dried fruit, potatoes
Magnesium	Nuts, seeds, cereals, cereal products, potatoes, green vegetables
Phosphorus (phosphates)	Many animal and vegetable proteins
Potassium	Vegetables, potatoes, fruit juices, bananas, dried fruit, instant coffee granules, Marmite®, meat, fish
Sodium	Common salt, cereal products, meat products, vegetables, cheese, sauces, pickles, snack foods, ready meals
Zinc	Meat and meat products, milk, eggs, cereals, bread, pulses, nuts

many vital body functions, e.g. iron for haemoglobin synthesis, vitamin K for blood clotting. An outline of minerals is provided in Table 19.5 and vitamins in Table 19.6. (See Further reading, below, e.g. Geissler & Powers 2009.)

Recommendations for a healthy balanced diet

A healthy, balanced diet is one that provides all the nutrients outlined above in the correct proportions (Box 19.19). Eating a variety of different foods is likely to provide a balanced diet.

It is convenient to classify foods of similar composition and nutrient content into five food groups (Fig. 19.13):

- Fats, oils and sugars including confectionery – use sparingly
- Proteins – meat, fish (oily fish containing omega-3 fats), eggs and vegetarian alternatives (serving: 1 egg; 80 g lean meat)
- Milk and dairy products (serving: 50 g hard cheese; 250 mL milk)

Health promotion · Box 19.19

Healthy packed lunches

The promotion of healthy eating in schools, together with other measures, is important in reducing the number of children who are overweight or obese.

Student activities

- Plan 5 days of packed lunches for primary school children that provides a balanced healthy intake
- What other measures in schools can help to promote healthy eating and prevent obesity?

Resources

British Nutrition Foundation. Healthier packed lunches. Online. Available: www.nutrition.org.uk/attachments/107_BNF%20 Healthier%20packed%20lunches%20leaflet.pdf.
NHS Choices – www.nhs.uk/Livewell/childhealth6–15/Pages/ Lighterlunchboxes.aspx.

All websites accessed September 2012.

Table 19.6 Vitamins and sources

Vitamins	Sources
Fat-soluble	
Vitamin A	Liver, kidney, oily fish, egg yolk, full fat dairy produce Green, yellow, orange and red fruit and vegetables, e.g. broccoli, carrots, apricots, sweet potatoes, tomatoes
Vitamin D	Oily fish, egg yolk, butter, fortified margarine Action of sunlight on the skin
Vitamin E	Widespread. Best sources are nuts, seeds, vegetable oil, egg yolk, some cereals
Vitamin K	Many vegetables and cereals Also synthesized by intestinal bacteria *Note:* Requires bile in the intestine for absorption
Water-soluble	
Vitamin B_1 – Thiamin	Milk, liver, eggs, pork, fortified breakfast cereals, vegetables, fruit, wholegrain cereals
Vitamin B_2 – Riboflavin	Milk, milk products, offal, fortified breakfast cereals Destroyed by sunlight
Vitamin B_3 – Niacin	Meat, fish, pulses, wholegrains, fortified breakfast cereals Can be synthesized from an amino acid in the body
Vitamin B_5 – Pantothenic acid	Liver, eggs, cereals, yeast, vegetables
Vitamin B_6 – Pyridoxine	Meat, fish, whole cereals, eggs, some vegetables
Biotin (B group)	Widely distributed in many foods, e.g. offal, egg yolk, legumes Can be synthesized by intestinal bacteria
Vitamin B_{12} – Cobalamins	Animal products, meat, eggs, fish, dairy products, yeast extract, fortified breakfast cereals Strict vegetarians and vegans may require dietary supplements *Note:* Requires intrinsic factor secreted by the stomach for absorption
Folates/folic acid (B group)	Green vegetables, fortified breakfast cereals, yeast extract, liver, oranges Supplement recommended prior to conception and during first 12 weeks of pregnancy (see p. 480)
Vitamin C – Ascorbic acid	Citrus fruits, blackcurrants, green leafy vegetables, potatoes, strawberries, tomatoes Content decreases with storage Destroyed by cooking in the presence of air and by cutting and grating raw food

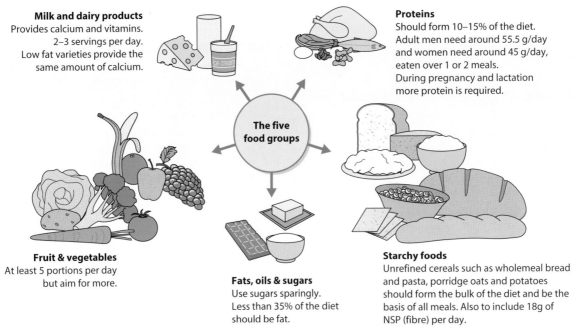

Milk and dairy products
Provides calcium and vitamins.
2–3 servings per day.
Low fat varieties provide the
same amount of calcium.

Proteins
Should form 10–15% of the diet.
Adult men need around 55.5 g/day
and women need around 45 g/day,
eaten over 1 or 2 meals.
During pregnancy and lactation
more protein is required.

**The five
food groups**

Fruit & vegetables
At least 5 portions per day
but aim for more.

Fats, oils & sugars
Use sugars sparingly.
Less than 35% of the diet
should be fat.

Starchy foods
Unrefined cereals such as wholemeal bread
and pasta, porridge oats and potatoes
should form the bulk of the diet and be the
basis of all meals. Also to include 18g of
NSP (fibre) per day.

Fig. 19.13 • Food groups and proportions in a balanced diet for most adults.

- Fruit and vegetables (serving: medium apple; 125 mL orange juice; 1 tablespoon of raisins; 3 heaped tablespoons of peas)
- Starchy foods – cereals, bread and potatoes (serving: 1 slice of bread; 30 g cereal).

The list above starts with foods that should be eaten in small amounts or, in the case of confectionery, only very occasionally and ends with the starchy foods, which should provide around one-third of the daily energy requirement. NHS choices (2011) recommends that most adults should:

1. 'Base your meals on starchy foods
2. Eat lots of fruit and veg
3. Eat more fish
4. Cut down on saturated fat
5. Cut down on sugar
6. Eat less salt
7. Drink enough water
8. Don't skip breakfast'.

Specific lifespan requirements: supplements and advice

People may also require nutritional supplements at particular times during the lifespan or because of their lifestyle choices. These include:

- *Preconception, pregnancy and breast-feeding*: women planning to become pregnant should be normal weight, eat a balanced diet and continue this during pregnancy. Those who are obese are encouraged to lose weight before becoming pregnant as dieting during pregnancy may harm their baby (National Institute for Health and Clinical Excellence, NICE 2010).
  - Women are advised to take folic acid supplements before conception and for the first 12 weeks of pregnancy to reduce the risk of neural tube defects, such as spina bifida
  - Women who are planning to be, or are pregnant, should always ask the pharmacist about the safety of over-the-counter medicines, and check its safety with the healthcare professional who prescribes a drug
  - They should limit their intake of vitamin A supplements which has been linked to congenital defects. Pregnant women are advised to avoid herbal products
  - Vitamin D supplements should be taken during pregnancy and breast-feeding, and extra protein while breast-feeding. (See Further reading, p. 490, e.g. NICE 2008).
- *Infants and children*: from 6 months to 5 years, children should have a supplement containing vitamins A, C and D.
- *Other groups needing vitamin D*: people with darker skin and those who are seldom exposed to sunlight, e.g. cultures where people are always covered, people aged 65 years or over, the housebound and residents in care/nursing homes.
- *Women of child-bearing age*: may have iron deficiency and need to take supplements.
- *Vegans and vegetarians*: need to ensure that they obtain sufficient vitamins B_{12} and D, iron, selenium and omega-3 fats from their diet or consider supplements.

Infant feeding

Breast milk is the perfect food for healthy infants. It contains all the essential nutrients in proportions that meet growth and development needs of infants during the first 6 months. The milk produced during the first 3 days after birth is known as colostrum. It contains antibodies, and because it is less rich than mature breast milk, it meets the needs of newborns. Mature breast milk is usually produced by the 4th day. The maternal antibodies in breast milk protect infants while their own immune systems develop. The results from a large observational study suggests that breast-feeding is also associated with improved cognitive development (Quigley et al. 2009). In addition, there are advantages to the mother that include better bonding with her infant and ready availability of feeds (Box 19.20).

Health promotion   Box 19.20

Infant feeding

You have been asked to assist your mentor with a parent education session about infant feeding.

Student activities

- Make a list of important areas to include about breast-feeding, including when it is not safe, and bottle-feeding.
- Discuss ways in which the information could be presented with your mentor.

Resources

BBC. Baby feeding. Online. Available: www.bbc.co.uk/health/physical_health/child_development/baby_index.shtml.

Department of Health, 2011. A step-by-step guide to preparing a powdered formula feed. Online. Available: www.dh.gov.uk/prod_consum_dh/groups/dh_digitalassets/documents/digitalasset/dh_129346.pdf.

NHS Choices. Feeding your baby. Online. Available: www.nhs.uk/planners/birthtofive/pages/feedingyourbabyhub.aspx.

All websites accessed September 2012.

Notwithstanding the known benefits of breast-feeding, the rates in the UK and Ireland are among the lowest in Western Europe (Spencer et al 2010). Mothers in disadvantaged groups, e.g. teenagers, have the lowest breast-feeding rates.

Bottle-feeding with infant formula milks may be used by choice or where a contraindication for breast-feeding exists, e.g. infants who need special formula milk or mothers who are severely undernourished. Bottle-feeding has several disadvantages that include increased episodes of diarrhoea and the potential for over- or underfeeding. Maintaining high standards when cleaning and sterilizing bottles and other equipment, and preparing and storing feeds is vital (Box 19.20).

Weaning is the gradual introduction of solid food to the milk-only diet of infants. The current UK advice is that weaning should start when the infant is 6 months old. However, Fewtrell et al (2011) raise the question as to whether the previous WHO advice that infants are exclusively breast-fed for 6 months should be changed and infants be weaned earlier, perhaps introducing solid food between 4–6 months of age.

Breast-feeding or formula is continued during weaning. First weaning foods are:

- Puréed fruits and vegetables with no added salt or sugar, e.g. banana and cooked apple, yam, carrot and potato
- Non-wheat gluten-free cereals, e.g. maize, rice and sago, mixed with breast or formula milk.

During the next 6 months, the variety, frequency and amount of solid food is increased so that by the age of 1 year the infant is having three family meals a day and around 600 mL of milk.

(See Further reading, p. 490, e.g. NHS Choices 2011; Townsend & Pitchford 2012.) Infants under 12 months of age must not be given cow's, sheep's or goat's milk because it contains too much protein and salt, is not easily digested and does not contain sufficient iron and other nutrients.

Factors that affect food intake and appetite

Several physical, psychological, cultural and social factors affect food intake. Nurses must be able to identify the factors that increase the risk of people developing nutritional problems including malnutrition caused by excessive or inadequate food intake (see p. 483). Many of these factors are outlined below and some are explored further in the section about helping people to eat. These include:

- Limited access to food shops – without a car, it is difficult to visit out-of-town supermarkets and take advantage of a range of foods, special offers and bulk-buying
- Inadequate cooking facilities, e.g. bed and breakfast accommodation
- Poor knowledge about a 'balanced' diet, menu planning, food shopping and meal preparation and cooking (Box 19.21)

Health promotion   Box 19.21

Understanding healthy eating

Think about a group of vulnerable clients you have met while on placement. You might choose:

- Adults with a learning disability in supported living within the community
- Young people leaving the care of the local authority to live independently
- Families with children living in bed and breakfast accommodation
- Homeless people using night shelters.

Student activities

- Discuss with your mentor how you would help clients to understand the components of a healthy diet?
- What activities, such as menu planning, shopping and meal preparation, are needed to achieve a balanced intake?

- Poverty reduces the opportunity to eat a balanced diet, as people on limited incomes may select fatty cheaper food that satisfies hunger in preference to healthier options such as fruit and vegetables
- The environment is important. Indeed, one of the benchmarks of best practice is that 'People feel the environment is conducive to eating and drinking' (DH 2010, p 8; see also Box 19.13). In care settings, there should be a dining area, adapted utensils and the area should be quiet during mealtimes; inappropriate activities, e.g. ward rounds, treatments, should be stopped. Protected mealtimes (see p. 484) are good practice
- Preferences – if people are offered foods they dislike it is unlikely that their intake will be adequate (Nursing and Midwifery Council 2010 – specifically 'Joseph's story')

- People with specific religious/cultural needs will not eat properly unless they are confident that the food offered has been prepared in accordance with their faith and that the ingredients are acceptable. For example, Hindus neither eat beef nor other food that has been in contact with beef, and vegetarians may refuse foods containing gelatin (Box 19.22)

? Critical thinking   **Box 19.22**

Meeting religious and cultural dietary needs

Vijay Lal Sharma has told the staff in the care home that he does not eat beef. On Sunday, the residents are served roast beef for lunch and the care assistant is surprised when Vijay declines to eat the alternative main course provided for him. Vijay explains that he is worried that his meal may have been in contact with the beef in the kitchen or during serving.

Student activities

- When people first come to your placement, what questions are asked regarding their dietary needs?
- What facilities exist in your placement for preparing meals that are acceptable to people such as Vijay who have special dietary needs?
- Look at the menus for a week – is there always a strict vegetarian choice?

Note: Animal products such as gelatin can be present in foods, e.g. desserts, which might be assumed to be vegetarian.

- Mental health problems, e.g. low mood, eating disorders (see Table 19.4, p. 476) and dementia, can affect appetite, intake or the motivation to prepare and eat food. Low mood may lead to overeating or reduced appetite and weight loss. Moreover, 'people with mental health problems may be particularly vulnerable to some effects of poor diet, such as obesity, due to the side-effects of medication' (O'Carroll & Park 2007, p 191)
- Food/drug interactions, e.g. grapefruit juice with lacidipine (a calcium-channel blocking drug); amine-containing foods such as mature cheese, yeast extract, etc. with monoamine oxidase inhibitor (MAOI) antidepressants.
- Physical problems such as altered consciousness, sore mouth, ill-fitting dentures or dysphagia (see p. 462). Immobility, lack of manual dexterity and dependency that lead to difficulties with shopping, preparing and cooking food, sitting up to eat, cutting up food and feeding
- Conditions affecting nutrition (see Table 19.4), including nausea and vomiting
- Changes in taste and smell sensation (see pp. 474–475).

Malnutrition in vulnerable people

It is a shocking fact that vulnerable people can become malnourished while living in the community or in hospital. Over 3 million people in the UK are either malnourished or at risk of becoming so, with over 90% of cases in the community (Elia & Russell 2009). People whose diets are deficient in protein and energy and/or have increased nutritional needs, e.g. following major surgery, are at risk of protein-energy malnutrition (PEM). It is vital that those at risk of malnutrition are identified on admission to healthcare and this is discussed below.

O'Regan (2009) suggests the use of brightly coloured food trays to highlight those who need help with feeding. The 'Red Tray' system ensures that nurses arrange for vulnerable people to be assisted, perhaps by a volunteer, monitor what is eaten and plan regular assessments.

Independence in eating

For most infants, achieving independence in feeding starts around 9–10 months when they handle food to explore textures and put food in their mouths. During the next 12 months or so, children learn to hold a spoon and use it to transfer food into their mouth. Early attempts at feeding are often accompanied by frustration and mess, as food is dropped. It is important to encourage self-feeding while laying the foundation for good habits such as washing children's hands prior to eating.

Some people cannot achieve full independence in feeding, e.g. people with dementia or profound learning disability and/or physical disability. Nurses must explore ways of maintaining clients' dignity by ensuring that they have as much independence as is possible. For example, offering these people choice, providing 'finger food', e.g. sandwiches or pieces of fruit or raw vegetable, which can be held without requiring cutlery or manual dexterity will maintain their dignity and independence (for help with eating, see p. 484).

Nursing interventions – maintaining nutritional status

Nursing interventions are often vital in helping people maintain or improve their nutritional status. This section outlines:

- Nutritional screening and assessment
- Helping people to eat
- Nutritional support.

Nutritional screening and assessment

The assessment of nutritional status requires a holistic approach that embraces physical, social, emotional, spiritual and psychological aspects. It is essential that people are screened on their first contact, e.g. first home visit, out-patient appointment or on admission to a care home or hospital, to identify those with existing malnutrition and those at risk of malnutrition (see below). Thereafter 'People who are screened on initial contact and identified at risk receive a full nutritional assessment' (DH 2010, p 8).

People at risk must be referred to a dietitian or specially trained RN for a full nutritional assessment, 'using a validated evidence-based tool and appropriate referral is undertaken for people who are identified initially as at risk of malnutrition or as morbidly obese' (DH 2010, p 17). Nutritional assessment includes:

- Anthropometric measurements, e.g. weight, height/length, body mass index (BMI), skinfold thickness, mid-upper arm circumference (MUAC), waist measurement, waist circumference : hip ratio, or waist circumference : height ratio assesses whether fat distribution is intra-abdominal or subcutaneous.

- Use of nutritional screening audit tools
- Biochemical indicators, e.g. serum albumin.

Nutritional screening audit tool

The Malnutrition Universal Screening Tool (MUST) (BAPEN 2003) is one such screening tool. MUST uses a five-step approach for adults in all settings:

1. Calculation of BMI (Box 19.23)
2. Ascertain the percentage of unplanned weight loss
3. Estimate the effects of acute illness
4. Add up the scores for steps 1, 2, 3 for malnutrition risk score
5. Implementation of management guidelines and/or local policies to plan care for those at nutritional risk such as screening frequency or referral.

Stratton et al (2004) found a high prevalence of malnutrition in hospital in-patients and out-patients (using MUST) and agreement beyond chance between MUST and most other tools studied. MUST was quick and easy to use in these groups.

Nutritional screening and assessment in infants and children

This is specialized and includes:

- Regular recording of weight, length/height and head circumference on a standard growth centile chart. BMI becomes relevant once the child is 2 years old and is recorded on a BMI-for-age centile chart
- Developmental milestones (see Ch. 8)
- Food history
- Biochemical indicators.

Common investigations

The following may be used to identify upper GI tract disorders affecting nutrition:

- Blood tests – full blood count, iron and folic acid levels
- X-rays – plain abdominal and chest X-ray, barium meal (swallow) and follow-through
- Endoscopy – pharyngoscopy, oesophagoscopy, gastroscopy, duodenoscopy
- Scans – ultrasound scan (USS), computed tomography (CT), magnetic resonance imaging (MRI)
- Urea breath test for the diagnosis of *Helicobacter pylori* (a bacterium linked with peptic ulceration and gastric cancer)
- Gastric acid studies
- Faecal occult blood (see Ch. 21).

Nurses must provide information about investigations that takes account of a person's ability to understand and retain facts, e.g. modification may be required for a child, or someone who does not read or understand English, or has a learning disability or cognitive impairment. (For more information

---

Body mass index Box 19.23

Body mass index (BMI) is a measurement calculated using body weight and height. It is used to ascertain whether an adult is within a healthy weight range for their height. A limitation of BMI is that it does not differentiate between a muscular physique and obesity.
BMI is weight (in kg) divided by the height squared (m²):

$$BMI = \frac{Weight\ (kg)}{Height\ (m^2)}$$

Worked example
Jane weighs 53 kg and is 1.57 m tall:

$$\frac{53}{1.57 \times 1.57} = \frac{53}{2.46} \quad BMI = 21.5$$

Interpretation of BMI:
- Underweight <18.50
- Normal range 18.50–24.99
- Overweight ≥25.00
- Obesity ≥30.00 (WHO 2006).

Notes: BMI <20.00 is significant in the MUST screening tool (for BMI for classes of obesity, see WHO 2006).
- When it is impossible to measure a person's height other measurements can be used to estimate height, e.g. forearm (ulna) length (BAPEN 2003)
- In situations where neither height nor weight is known, BMI can be estimated from MUAC, e.g. where MUAC <23.5 cm the BMI is likely to be <20.00 (BAPEN 2003).

---

about specific investigations, see Useful websites, p. 489, e.g. NHS Choices; NHS Evidence.)

Helping people to eat

Helping people to meet their nutritional needs may involve the patient/client, family, volunteers and appropriate members of the MDT, including dietitians, specialist nurses, doctors, OTs, SLTs, physiotherapists, ward hostesses, porters and laboratory staff.

Making appropriate healthy choices

Nurses should assist people who need help to choose from a menu. Some people may be unable to read or understand the menus. Moreover, a person with a learning disability or dementia may not remember what they had ordered when the meal is served and will need reminders.

Others may need explanations about the most suitable items if they have cultural or religious needs or are prescribed special diets, e.g. reducing.

Environment and mealtimes

Nurses must ensure that the environment is conducive to eating. Basic activities that encourage eating include:

- Encouraging people to eat in a separate dining area away from bed areas
- Encouraging people at home to use mealtimes to socialize by inviting friends to a meal or attending a day centre

- Ensuring that breast-feeding mothers have support and facilities for washing and privacy as appropriate
- Ensuring that bedpans, commodes and vomit bowels, etc. are removed
- Protected mealtimes – ensuring that the ward/unit is quiet and treatments or visitors do not disrupt mealtimes (National Patient Safety Agency 2007, modified 2009)
- Helping people to wash their hands beforehand
- Helping people to rinse their mouth or clean dentures if necessary
- Helping people to sit up, ensuring that bed tables are at the correct height and the food is within easy reach. Those unable to sit up to eat need individual solutions to allow them to eat
- Providing appropriate crockery and cutlery such as non-slip mats for plates or plate guards and large handle cutlery for people who only have the use of one arm. The OT can provide appropriate utensils (Fig. 19.14)
- Ensuring that food is served at the correct temperature
- Ensuring that the plate/tray of food looks attractive, for instance by placing food carefully and wiping away gravy stains
- Helping people with poor sight by describing the contents of the plate. Using a clockface, e.g. the meat is at 6 o'clock, can be useful
- Providing help and encouragement, when required, during mealtimes (see Red Tray system, p. 482)
- Making sure that meals are available if a person misses a mealtime.

Food fortification

This involves modifying the nutrient quality of the diet and may be advised for people who have small appetites and cannot consume large volumes of food at a single meal. Fortification can be useful for older people. Measures for people who are malnourished or those at risk of malnutrition may include:

- More frequent but smaller meals
- Using full-fat dairy products
- Using milk powder to fortify full-fat milk, cereals and puddings
- Fortifying soup with milk, milk powder or cream

Nursing skills — Box 19.24

Feeding dependent people

Ensure that you have sufficient time to feed the person and that this time is protected.

- Ask if they need to use the lavatory or commode
- Attend to oral hygiene as required (Ch. 16). If worn, ensure dentures are clean and in place
- Prepare the immediate environment and prepare and position the person
- Offer handwashing facilities and wash your own hands
- Protect the client's clothing with a table napkin or paper towel. Plastic, material or towelling bibs compromise people's dignity and should never be used
- Ensure the food is what the person likes and that, where possible, they have chosen it from the menu themselves
- Ensure that food is at the correct temperature and consistency, e.g. pureed for people with dysphagia. If it is necessary to purée the meal, each component should be served separately (never mixed together).
- Only have one course on the tray at a time – people can feel overwhelmed by the sight of several plates of food. Reducing portion sizes or using smaller plates can be less off-putting for those with small appetites
- If the person's mouth is dry, offer sips of water before feeding
- Choose appropriate cutlery and try to use the correct utensil for the food. Using a spoon for the entire meal is not conducive to maintaining dignity
- Remember cultural/religious needs, e.g. Muslims use the right hand for eating and to pass anything in the left hand could cause offence
- Seat yourself level with the person and at an angle that facilitates two-way communication and also allows help with eating
- Where communication is difficult, set up a system whereby people can give you information such as 'ready for more'
- Always describe the food before feeding for people with visual impairment
- Never use pepper and salt or sauces without asking first and checking any special dietary requirements, such as restricted salt
- Feed small amounts and allow time for chewing and swallowing; offer drinks as appropriate
- Do not hurry the person but do not offer food that has become cold
- Inform the RN about the amount of food and fluid taken and record it in the nursing notes and appropriate charts.

Notes: Where possible, encourage/help people to feed themselves. When feeding children, nurses may need to involve play as an activity or therapy; older children might like to listen to music or watch television.

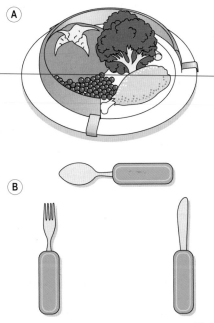

Fig. 19.14 ● Adaptations for eating: (A) Plate guard. (B) Cutlery with large handles.

- Increasing energy by adding sugar, jam or dried fruit to cereals and desserts
- Providing high-energy protein snacks between meals, e.g. cheese/biscuits, peanut butter.

Feeding

Feeding older children or adults should only occur when all other options have been tried and proved ineffective. Sometimes, it is enough to be with people at mealtimes to encourage them to feed themselves, thereby maintaining their independence and dignity.

Independence can be increased for people who cannot use cutlery or have dementia, by providing 'finger foods' (see p. 482). However, there are people who need to be fed and although feeding is a basic nursing skill, it requires time and competence to do well (Box 19.24). Often, family members want to help and many wards/care homes have volunteers who help. The RN monitors the amounts eaten and, using a nutritional screening audit tool (see p. 483), decides whether nutritional requirements can be maintained by oral feeding alone or whether nutritional support is required (see Box 19.26).

Clients requiring special diets

Some people are prescribed a special diet as part of managing particular conditions such as reducing for obesity, or they may have chosen a particular diet for religious/cultural or ethical reasons (Box 19.25).

 Critical thinking   Box 19.25

Individual diets

Reduced phenylalanine

Gluten-free

Diabetic

Reducing

High-protein

Low-protein

High-fibre

Low sodium

Vegan

Vegetarian

Kosher

Halal

Student activities

- Choose three diets from the list that you have encountered during placements and find out why they were used and what they involved.
- How do you think having a special diet affects people's lifestyles, e.g. a child who has a special diet going to a birthday party?

(See Further reading, below, e.g. Geissler & Powers 2009; NHS Education for Scotland 2006.)

Nutritional support

Nutritional support is required to prevent or rectify malnutrition when people cannot eat enough food or absorb or utilize enough nutrients to meet their needs. Box 19.26 outlines different types of nutritional support. However, it is important to maintain normal diet and eating activity as much as possible. The type of nutritional support used depends on:

- GI tract function
- The underlying reason for malnutrition
- Other factors, e.g. altered consciousness.

Types of nutritional support   Box 19.26

Texture modification

People who find chewing and/or swallowing difficult may benefit from food that is mashed, liquidized or puréed (see Box 19.24) and thickening fluids may also be helpful. These changes are initiated in collaboration with the SLT and only after a full swallowing assessment (see p. 466).

Sip feeding

This is provision of nutritious drinks at regular intervals, in place of food, or to supplement the diet in order to meet nutritional needs. Nutritionally complete feeds are produced commercially, e.g. Ensure®, Fortisip®, and may contain extra minerals and vitamins. Many proprietary feeds are specially prepared for specific conditions such as kidney failure. When using proprietary feeds it is vital to follow the manufacturer's guidelines for storage and to check the expiry date.

Enteral feeding

Tube feeding is used for people who have some GI tract function, but are unable to swallow or obtain sufficient nutrition by the oral route. A nutritionally complete liquid feed is used to meet nutritional requirements.

Parenteral feeding

Parental feeding (outside the GI tract) involves the i.v. infusion of sterile nutrient solutions, which require no digestion, directly into the circulation (see p. 487).

The provision of optimal nutritional support requires collaboration between members of the MDT, especially the specialist nutrition nurse.

Enteral feeding

It is usual to use a nasogastric (NG) tube for short-term feeding. For long-term feeding, a percutaneous endoscopic gastrostomy (PEG) tube is inserted through the abdominal wall into the stomach and held in place by a balloon or flange. PEG tubes are frequently used for home enteral tube feeding. PEG feeding is used in situations that include:

- Dysphagia, e.g. following a stroke
- Palliative care
- Unconsciousness (see Ch. 16)
- Adults and children with profound and multiple learning disabilities
- Children with chronic conditions, e.g. cystic fibrosis, cerebral palsy.

Other feeding routes include nasoduodenal or nasojejunal tubes, or jejunostomy tubes (inserted into the jejunum through the abdominal wall).

Nursing skills   Box 19.27

Nasogastric feeding (adult)

- Explain the procedure and obtain consent
- Wash hands, put on a plastic apron
- Check the person's identity
- Make sure that the person is comfortable and if possible sitting upright
- Check the nose and face for signs of pressure or soreness
- Check the feeding tube position according to local protocols before every feed. This should involve aspirating a small volume of gastric contents and checking the pH using a reliable pH testing strip (0–6 with half point gradations) (National Patient Safety Agency, NPSA 2005). The sample of aspirate should not be obtained within an hour of medication or feeding as this can produce inaccurate results. Some anti-ulcer drugs and previous gastric surgery can also affect results. A 20 mL syringe is used to aspirate a fine-bore NG tube, whereas a 50 mL catheter-tip syringe is used to aspirate a wide-bore NG tube (Ryle's type). Avoid creating excess suction when aspirating the tube, otherwise the gastric mucosa could be damaged. A pH of 5.5 or below indicates that the tube is in the stomach (NPSA 2005). When a fine-bore tube is first passed an X-ray is used to confirm the correct position before the guide wire is removed
- The tube is flushed with at least 30 mL of sterile water (Nicol et al 2012)
- Prepare the prescribed feed and enteral administration set according to the manufacturer's guidelines. If a separate container is being used, pour the feed into the bag or reservoir and attach the administration set. Sometimes sterile water is given using this method
- Run the feed through the tubing in order to expel the air and then clamp the tubing using the roller clamp
- Connect the administration set to the NG tube securely
- Commence the feed. In gravity delivery adjust the roller clamp to deliver the prescribed flow rate. If a pump is to be used, insert the administration set according to the manufacturer's instructions and open the roller clamp (Fig. 19.15). The pump is switched on and set at the prescribed rate
- Make the person comfortable and attend to hygiene needs, e.g. mouth and nostril care
- Observe for signs of GORD, nausea or dyspnoea, and diarrhoea
- On completion of the feed, flush the NG tube with at least 30 mL of sterile water to clear feed from the tube
- Record volume of feed given on the fluid chart and document in the nursing records
- The administration set must be changed every 24 hours to minimize the risk of bacterial contamination and growth. Label the new administration set with the date and time and record this in the nursing records
- When a second container of feed is due to start, ensure that the first does not empty completely, allowing air to enter the administration set. Should this occur it would be necessary to disconnect the administration set and run the new feed through as described above.

(Adapted from Nicol et al 2012).

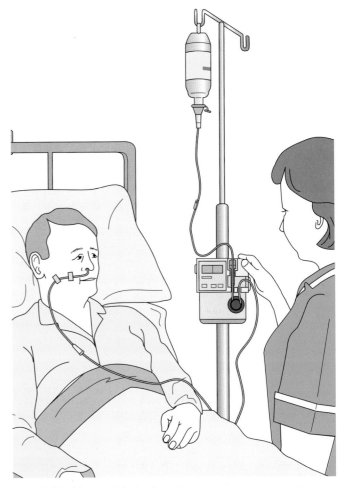

Fig. 19.15 • Nasogastric feeding via a pump. (Reproduced with permission from Nicol, M., Bavin, C., Cronin, P., et al., 2008. Essential nursing skills, third ed. Mosby, Edinburgh).

used to empty the stomach, e.g. after gastric surgery or when the bowel is obstructed. (Information about inserting an NG tube is covered in Further reading, p. 490, e.g. Nicol et al 2012).

Enteral feeding in infants and small children is complex and readers are directed to Further reading, below. In addition, prolonged lack of oral feeding can lead to developmental delay, e.g. problems learning appropriate social behaviour at mealtimes (Trigg & Mohammed 2010).

Enteral feeding must employ clean procedures to avoid bacterial contamination of the feed and/or administration systems, which can lead to diarrhoea. Nurses must ensure that manufacturers' guidelines are followed in respect of storage, the temperature for administration and the expiry date. Enteral feeds can be delivered by:

- Bolus feeds given by syringe through a feeding tube at spaced intervals during the day. Disadvantages include discomfort caused by the volumes needed at each feed to meet nutritional needs (200–400 mL in adults). Moreover, absorption of large volumes takes longer and increases the possibility of high residual volumes remaining in the stomach when the next feed is due, which can lead to nausea and vomiting.

Small-bore NG feeding tubes should be used in preference to wider-bore NG tubes. People find small-bore tubes more comfortable and easier to tolerate. Wider-bore NG tubes are

- Gravity feeding is delivered by an intermittent or continuous drip method. Very careful monitoring is needed to ensure that the person receives the prescribed feed volume and that rapid delivery of a large volume does not occur. This can cause gastric distension, gastro-oesophageal reflux disease (GORD) and aspiration of stomach contents into the respiratory tract.

- Continuous pump-controlled feeding with a 4-hour rest period during the night is the preferred method as it is associated with fewer complications, e.g. diarrhoea and GORD.

Boxes 19.27 and 19.28 provide an outline of Nasogastric feeding, and Caring for a gastrostomy site and PEG tube feeding.

 Nursing skills Box 19.28

Caring for the gastrostomy site and PEG feeding
Caring for the gastrostomy site

- After insertion of a PEG tube the site is treated as a wound (see Chs 15, 25). Local policies vary, but most recommend cleaning with sterile sodium chloride 0.9%, or sterile water, and applying lint-free gauze and a dry dressing.

- Dressings are usually changed twice weekly; however, if the site is discharging it is redressed daily. Once the site has healed, there is no need for a dressing

- Temperature and pulse rate should be monitored for 1 week after tube insertion to detect infection (see Ch. 14)

- The site around the tube is observed daily for signs of inflammation, e.g. redness and swelling, excoriation (soreness), leakage of gastric contents or excessive movement of the tube

- Once the site is healed it is important that the skin disc/guard surrounding the tube (Fig. 19.16) is lifted daily and slid round the tube so that the area can be washed with warm soapy water, rinsed and then dried thoroughly. The tube should then be rotated to prevent necrosis caused by pressure from the retention balloon in the stomach. The skin disc/guard is then replaced

- Following healing, people are able to bathe or shower providing the gastrostomy tube is closed. The site is dried thoroughly afterwards.

Note: There are several types of gastrostomy tube, two of which are illustrated in Figure 19.16.

Principles of giving a PEG feed

Many general aspects of care are the same as those needed when giving a nasogastric feed (see Box 19.27).

- Intermittent feeds can be given when others are having a meal in order to create as 'normal' a situation as possible. However, continuous feeding has been shown to reduce the incidence of diarrhoea

- It is advisable for the person to be sitting up (unless the feed is given very slowly) to prevent GORD

- Remove the cap from the feed container and, maintaining asepsis (see Box 19.10, p. 472), open the administration set, attach it to the feed container according to the manufacturer's instructions, and close the roller clamp

- Hang the feed container on the infusion stand

- Run the feed through the tubing to expel the air. Leave the cap on the end of the tubing to maintain sterility

- Flush the PEG tube with sterile water according to local policy

- Insert the tubing into the pump, take the plastic cap from the distal end of the tubing and attach it to the PEG tube. Open the roller clamp and switch on the pump

- Set the prescribed flow rate and turn on the pump

- Check that no feed is leaking at the connection of the PEG tube and that the feed is running

- Check at regular intervals that the feed is running as prescribed

- Observe for nausea, vomiting, discomfort or diarrhoea

- When the feed is complete the administration set is disconnected and the PEG tube flushed with sterile water according to local policy

- Document details of the feed in the nursing records and record feed volume given and water used for flushing on the fluid chart

- The administration set must be changed every 24 hours to minimize the risk of bacterial contamination and growth. Label the new administration set with the date and time and record this in the nursing records.

Note: When flushing the PEG tube, care should be taken when connecting the syringe, to avoid damaging the connection. A 20 mL (or larger) syringe should be used for flushing the tube, as the pressure exerted by a smaller syringe is too great. When a PEG tube is not being used for feeding regularly, it should be flushed twice a day, to keep it patent (open).

(Adapted from Nicol et al 2008).

Parenteral nutrition

Parenteral feeding into a vein should only be used when enteral feeding is unsuitable, e.g. when the GI tract is non-functional or cannot fully meet nutritional needs. It may be supplemental to oral/enteral feeding, or total (TPN). Sterile nutrient solutions are delivered via a volumetric pump into a central vein; however, a peripheral vein may be used short term, i.e. up to 1 month, for both supplementary parenteral nutrition and TPN. A large central vein is used when hypertonic solutions, e.g. glucose 10–50%, are infused to avoid damaging peripheral veins (see Box 19.12, p. 473). Parenteral nutrition is used for people of all ages and enables children with a variety of conditions to survive. TPN is used in situations that include:

- Severe impairment of GI tract function, e.g. major resection of small intestine, severe inflammatory bowel disease (IBD), children with short bowel syndrome (SBS)

- People with cancer treated by drugs and radiotherapy

- Increased metabolic requirements e.g. serious illness, severe burns.

Parenteral nutrition requires collaboration between the patient/parents or carer and members of the MDT, in particular the specialist nutrition nurse, specialist i.v. therapy nurse, dietitian, pharmacist, doctor and laboratory staff. Management is complex and readers are directed to Further reading, below, for further information, e.g. Kelsey & McEwing 2008; Nicol et al 2012; Trigg & Mohammed 2010).

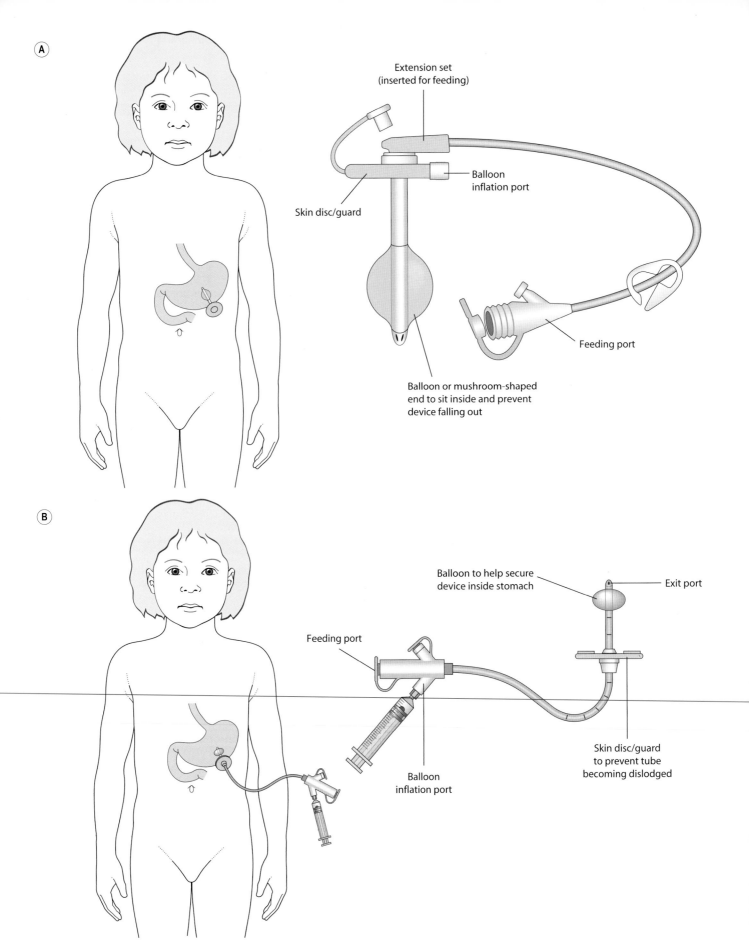

Fig. 19.16 • Types of gastrostomy tube: (A) Skin level 'button' or 'key' device. (B) Percutaneous endoscopic tube. (Adapted from Trigg, E., Mohammed, T.A., (Eds.), 2010. Practices in children's nursing, third ed. Churchill Livingstone, Edinburgh).

SUMMARY

◆ Nursing interventions are fundamental to promoting hydration and nutrition.

◆ *Essence of Care 2010* (DH 2010) best practice benchmarks concerned with eating and drinking are used to underpin nursing practice.

◆ Nurses have important roles in preventing fluid and electrolyte imbalance and malnutrition, especially in assessment of fluid and nutritional status.

◆ Nursing interventions for people with problems associated with drinking and eating range from simple interventions to more complex skills.

◆ The partnership between the person/parents/carers and the MDT is important.

◆ The importance of promoting hydration and nutrition is paramount; the nurse's role is central in ensuring that people in their care receive sufficient fluids and nutrients.

KEY WORDS AND PHRASES FOR LITERATURE SEARCHING

Acid–base balance
Dehydration
Electrolytes
Enteral feeding
Fluid balance
Hydration
Malnutrition
Nutrition
Nutritional assessment/support
Parenteral feeding/nutrition

 Useful websites

BBC www.bbc.co.uk/health/healthy_living/nutrition
British Association for Parenteral and Enteral Nutrition www.bapen.org.uk
British Nutrition Foundation www.nutrition.org.uk
National Obesity Forum www.nationalobesityforum.org.uk
NHS Choices www.nhs.uk/livewell/Pages/Livewellhub.aspx
NHS Clinical Knowledge Summaries (formerly Prodigy) (clinical topics, e.g. obesity, eating disorders) www.cks.nhs.uk

NHS Evidence Topics – A–Z. Online www.evidence.nhs.uk/topics
NHS Quality Improvement Scotland (NHS QIS) www.nhshealthquality.org
National Institute for Health and Clinical Excellence www.nice.org.uk
Royal College of Speech and Language Therapists www.rcslt.org
All websites accessed September 2012.

References

Age UK, 2010. Still hungry to be heard. Online. Available: www.ageuk.org.uk/Documents/EN-GB/ID9489%20HTBH%20Report%2028ppA4.pdf?dtrk=true September 2012.

BAPEN, 2003. Malnutrition Advisory Group. The malnutrition universal screening tool (MUST). Online. Available: www.bapen.org.uk September 2012.

Department of Health, 1991. Dietary reference values for food energy and nutrients for the United Kingdom. HMSO, London.

Department of Health, 2010. Essence of care 2010. Benchmarks for food and drink. Online. Available: www.dh.gov.uk September 2012.

Elia, M., Russell, C.A., 2009. Combating malnutrition: Recommendations for action. BAPEN. Online. Available: www.bapen.org.uk/pdfs/reports/advisory_group_report.pdf September 2012.

Fewtrell, M., Wilson, D.C., Booth, I., et al., 2011. Six months of exclusive breast feeding: how good is the evidence? British Medical Journal 342, c5955.

Jefferies, D., Johnson, M., Ravens, J., 2011. Nurturing and nourishing: the nurses' role in nutritional care. Journal of Clinical Nursing 20 (3–4), 317–330.

Lybarger. E.H., 2009. Hypodermoclysis in the home and long-term settings. Journal of Infusion Nursing 32 (1), 40–44.

National Confidential Enquiry into Patient Outcome and Death, 2010. An age old problem: A review of the care received by elderly patients undergoing surgery. Online. Available: www.ncepod.org.uk September 2012.

NHS choices, 2011. Eight tips for healthy eating. Online. Available: www.nhs.uk/Livewell/Goodfood/Pages/eight-tips-healthy-eating.aspx September 2012.

NHS Information Centre, 2009. Statistics on obesity, physical activity and diet: England, 2009. Online. Available: www.ic.nhs.uk September 2012.

NHS Information Centre, 2010. Statistics on alcohol: England, 2010. Online. Available: www.ic.nhs.uk/webfiles/publications/alcohol10/Statistics_on_Alcohol_England_2010.pdf September 2012.

National Institute for Health and Clinical Excellence, 2010. Weight management before, during and after pregnancy. Public Health 27 Online. Available: www.nice.org.uk September 2012.

National Patient Safety Agency, 2005. Patient safety alert. Reducing the harm caused by misplaced nasogastric feeding tubes. Online. Available: www.npsa.nhs.uk September 2012.

National Patient Safety Agency, 2007 (modified 2009). Protected Mealtimes review – findings report. Online. Available: www.nrls.npsa.nhs.uk/resources/patient-safety-topics/patient-treatment-procedure/?entryid45=59806 September 2012.

Nicol, M., Bavin, C., Cronin, P., et al., 2008. Essential nursing skills, third ed. Mosby, Edinburgh.

Nursing & Midwifery Council, 2010. Safeguarding adults 'Doing our Best' (a series of short films). Online. Available: http://www.nmc-uk.org/Nurses-and-midwives/safeguarding-film-one-an-introduction/ September 2012.

O'Carroll, M., Park, A., 2007. Essential mental health nursing skills. Mosby, Edinburgh.

Office for National Statistics, 2012. Alcohol-related deaths in the United Kingdom, 2010 Online. Available:

www.ons.gov.uk/ons/rel/subnational-health4/alcohol-related-deaths-in-the-united-kingdom/2010/stb-alcohol-related-deaths.html September 2012.

O'Regan, P., 2009. Nutrition for patients in hospital. Nursing Standard 23 (23), 35–41.

Quigley, M.A., Hockley, C., Carson, C., et al., 2009. Maternal health: Breastfeeding is associated with improved child cognitive development: evidence from the UK Millennium Cohort Study. Journal of Epidemiology and Community Health 63, 8.

Royal College of Nursing, 2007. Nutrition Now Campaign RCN principles for nutrition and hydration. Online. Available: www.rcn.org.uk/nutritionnow September 2012.

Royal College of Nursing, 2010. IV therapy forum: standards for infusion therapy, third ed. RCN, London.

Royal College of Physicians/British Society of Gastroenterology, 2010. Oral feeding difficulties and dilemmas. Online. Available: http://bookshop.rcplondon.ac.uk/contents/pub295-ca2ff0c8-85f7-48ee-b857-8fed6ccb2ad7.pdf September 2012.

Spencer, R.L., Greatrex-White, S., Fraser, D.M., 2010. Practice improvement, breastfeeding duration and health visitors. Community Practice 83 (9), 19–22.

Stratton, R.J., Hackston, A., Longmore, D., et al., 2004. Malnutrition in hospital out-patients and in-patients: prevalence, concurrent validity and ease of use of the 'malnutrition universal screening tool'

('MUST') for adults. British Journal of Nutrition 92 (5), 799–808.

Trigg, E., Mohammed, T.A., (Eds.), 2010. Practices in children's nursing, third ed. Churchill Livingstone, Edinburgh.

Waugh, A., Grant, A., 2010. Ross and Wilson Anatomy and Physiology in health and illness, eleventh ed. Churchill Livingstone, Edinburgh.

Wilson, D., 2011. Balance and imbalance of body fluids. In: Hockenberry, M.J., Wilson, D., (Eds.), Wong's nursing care of infants and children, ninth ed. Mosby, St Louis.

World Health Organization, 2006 (updated 2011). BMI classification. Online. Available: http://apps.who.int/bmi/index.jsp?introPage=intro_3.html September 2012.

Further reading

Cowen, M., Ugboma, D., 2011. Maintaining fluid, electrolyte and acid-base balance. In: Brooker, C., Nicol, M., (Eds.), Alexander's nursing practice, fourth ed. Churchill Livingstone, Edinburgh, pp. 575–593.

Department of Health, 2007. Improving nutritional care. Online. Available: www.dh.gov.uk/en/AdvanceSearchResult/index.htm?searchTerms=improving+nutritional+care September 2012.

Dougherty, L., Lister, S., 2011. The Royal Marsden Hospital manual of clinical nursing procedures, eighth ed. Wiley-Blackwell, Oxford.

Geissler, C., Powers, H., 2009. Fundamentals of human nutrition. Churchill Livingstone, Edinburgh.

Green, S., 2011. Nutrition and health. In: Brooker, C., Nicol, M., (Eds.), Alexander's Nursing Practice, fourth ed. Churchill Livingstone, Edinburgh, pp. 595–615.

Kelsey, J., McEwing, G., 2008. Clinical Skills in Child Health Practice. Churchill Livingstone, Edinburgh.

National Institute for Health and Clinical Excellence, 2006 (updated 2010). Nutritional support in adults. Clinical guidance 32. Online. Available: www.nice.org.uk September 2012.

National Institute for Health and Clinical Excellence, 2008. Improving the Nutrition of Pregnant and Breast-feeding mothers and children in low-income households. Public health guidance PH11. Online. Available: www.nice.org.uk September 2012.

National Institute for Health and Clinical Excellence, 2011. Alcohol-use disorders. Clinical guidance CG115. Online. Available: www.nice.org.uk September 2012.

National Institute for Health and Clinical Excellence, 2011. Food allergy in children and young people. Clinical guidance CG116. Online. Available: www.nice.org.uk September 2012.

NHS Choices, 2011. Your baby's first solid food. Online. Available: www.nhs.uk/conditions/pregnancy-and-baby/pages/solid-foods-weaning.aspx September 2012.

NHS Education for Scotland, 2006. A multi-faith resource for healthcare staff. NES, Edinburgh. Online. Available: http://www.nes.scot.nhs.uk/media/3720/march07finalversions.pdf.pdf August 2012.

Nicol, M., Bavin, C., Cronin, P., et al., 2012. Essential nursing skills, fourth ed. Mosby, Edinburgh.

Russell, C.A., Elia, M., 2011. Nutritional screening survey in the UK and Republic of Ireland in 2010. BAPEN. Online. Available: www.bapen.org.uk/pdfs/nsw/nsw10/nsw10-report.pdf September 2012.

Townsend, E., Pitchford, N.J., 2012. Baby knows best? The impact of weaning style on food preferences and body mass index in early childhood in a case-controlled sample. BMJ Open 2, e000298 doi:10.1136/bmjopen-2011-000298 September 2012.

Elimination of urine: care and promoting continence

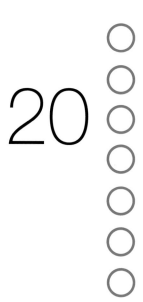

20

Martin Steggall

LEARNING OUTCOMES

This chapter will help you:

- Outline the anatomy and physiology of the urinary system and normal micturition
- Understand the common problems with micturition across the lifespan
- Outline the rationale for assessment of urine and micturition
- Describe the composition and characteristics of urine
- Outline the nursing interventions associated with micturition including cultural aspects
- Describe the measures taken to promote continence
- Define the different types of incontinence and the potential management of each
- Outline the care needed for a person who has an indwelling urinary catheter.

Introduction

Benchmarks for Bladder, Bowel and Continence Care form one of the 12 *Essence of Care 2010* Benchmarks for the Fundamental Aspects of Care (Department of Health, DH, 2010).

The *Essence of Care* aims to improve quality in care and has therefore been designed to share good practice among health providers, identifying best practice and remedying poor practice, effectively improving the quality of care that people receive.

Central to this theme, or any that aims to improve care, is a sound understanding of the issues, in this instance related to continence and incontinence. Even though some nurses may not do 'hands-on' care, they must understand the processes involved because they are accountable for delegated care (see Chs 6, 7). It is essential therefore to have a thorough grounding in the anatomy and physiology of the urinary system.

Two of the most commonly seen problems associated with urinary elimination are urinary tract infections (UTIs) and loss of continence. The importance of promoting continence cannot be overstated. The report *National Audit of Continence Care* (Royal College of Physicians, RCP 2010) found variability in adherence to national guidance. The overall findings were that 'People of all ages, and vulnerable groups in particular (frail older people, younger people with learning disability) continue to suffer unnecessarily and often in silence, with a 'life sentence' of bladder and/or bowel incontinence' (RCP 2010, p 6).

The urinary system is vital for homeostatic balance, ensuring that there is excretion of unwanted waste products, water balance and assisting with the control of blood pressure, to name a few examples. An understanding of the normal physiology of the urinary system will enable the nurse to care for the patient by anticipating potential problems and understanding the rationale for managing actual problems.

Elimination of urine crosses several traditional specialty boundaries, i.e. renal, urology, continence and gynaecology nursing; an understanding of how this system works is essential for nurses working in all fields of practice, so that safe and appropriate nursing care can be offered.

Overview – anatomy and physiology of the urinary system

The urinary system comprises the kidneys (2), ureters (2), bladder and urethra (Fig. 20.1). Readers should consult their own anatomy and physiology books for further details.

The kidneys

The kidneys are paired organs that lie against the back (dorsal) body wall behind the parietal peritoneum (retroperitoneal) in the superior lumbar region, i.e. they are either side of the spinal

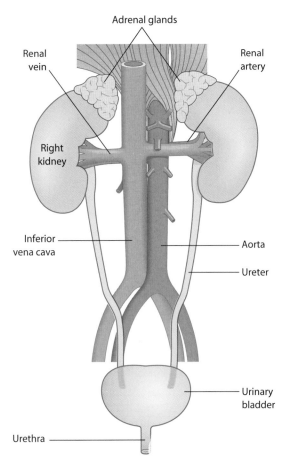

Fig. 20.1 • Urinary tract. (Reproduced with permission from Brooker, C., Nicol, M. (Eds.), 2003. Nursing adults. The practice of caring. Mosby, Edinburgh.)

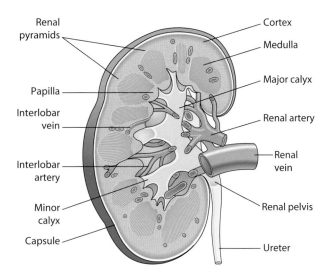

Fig. 20.2 • Longitudinal section through a kidney. (Reproduced with permission from Brooker, C., Nicol, M. (Eds.), 2003. Nursing adults. The practice of caring. Mosby, Edinburgh.)

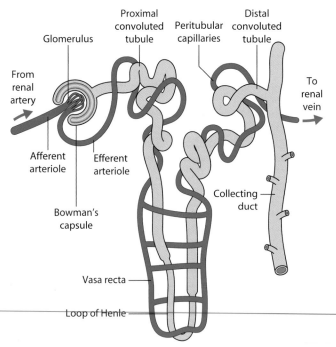

Fig. 20.3 • A nephron and blood vessels (simplified).

column at about the level of the lower ribs, but lying towards the back. When a kidney is cut longitudinally three distinct areas can be seen with the naked eye (Fig. 20.2):

- An outer fibrous capsule
- A cortex
- A medulla, comprising the tissue of the renal pyramids.

The kidneys are key organs with the functions that include:

- Production of urine by filtration of the blood contents, reabsorption of substances that are useful to the body and secretion of waste products
- Control and maintenance of fluid balance (see Ch. 19)
- Maintenance of acid–base balance (see Ch. 19)
- Control and maintenance of electrolyte balance (see Ch. 19)
- Renin production – an enzyme involved with the control of blood pressure
- Control of calcium absorption and activation of vitamin D
- Erythropoietin production – a hormone that stimulates red blood cell production.

In adults, each kidney receives approximately 625 mL of blood/minute from branches of the renal artery. A high volume of blood supply to the kidneys is required to maintain glomerular filtration rates (GFR) (see below) and to supply oxygen to active cells.

Nephron

Each kidney is composed of approximately 1 million microscopic functional units, the nephrons, and a system of collecting ducts that carry urine through the renal pyramids into the calyces and renal pelvis and hence to the ureter.

A nephron has a glomerulus (a knot of arterial capillaries) and a renal tubule that consists of a glomerular (Bowman's) capsule enclosing the glomerulus, a proximal convoluted tubule (PCT), loop of Henle, distal convoluted tubule (DCT) and the accompanying blood vessels (Fig. 20.3).

Blood enters the glomerulus from the afferent arteriole, but this is dependent on blood pressure. Small holes (fenestrations) in the lining of the capillary allow small molecules such as glucose to pass through into the renal tubule. However, larger molecules such as proteins cannot normally pass through the glomerular filtration barrier.

Blood leaves the glomerulus in the efferent arteriole, which forms a second capillary network around the renal tubule, the peritubular capillaries and more specialized capillaries called the vasa recta (see Fig. 20.3). The peritubular capillaries form larger and larger veins that carry blood to the renal vein.

The filtration membrane allows large quantities of fluid and small particles such as sodium and glucose to leave the blood and enter the tubule. At this stage, the fluid is called filtrate; it will become urine as it passes down the tubule. Substances needed by the body such as glucose are reabsorbed in the PCT and returned to the blood.

Control of blood flow into the glomerulus

The glomerular filtration rate (GFR) is the volume of plasma filtered through the glomerulus in 1 minute; the adult GFR is about 120 mL/min. Although GFR changes with age, all age groups need to maintain GFR to excrete waste products and balance the amount of water in the body (Box 20.1).

> **Glomerular filtration rate at the extremes of the lifespan**   Box 20.1
>
> Newborn babies have a low GFR and are therefore vulnerable to fluid overload. Children reach adult GFRs between the 1st and 2nd years of life. Older people usually have a decreased GFR, and also total body water, and are therefore at increased risk of having adverse drug reactions if a drug, e.g. the heart drug digoxin, accumulates in the body because it is not excreted quickly enough.

GFR can be controlled to ensure that a constant supply of blood is received at the correct pressure, ensuring that urine is constantly produced. This control is achieved by changing the diameter of the renal arteries and afferent and efferent arterioles by various processes that include:

- The renin-angiotensin-aldosterone mechanism/system, that results in vasoconstriction
- Chemicals, e.g. prostaglandins and nitric oxide, which can widen the diameter of the arterioles, resulting in vasodilation.

The amount of urine output is therefore a guide for whether the kidneys are receiving blood at the correct volume and pressure. The minimum urine output, i.e. the smallest volume that will allow the body to excrete waste products, is 0.5 mL/kg/h in both children and adults, although there are exceptions to this rule.

Control of blood volume

The amount of fluid in the body is carefully controlled by many organ systems (see Ch. 19). Several substances help to balance the volume of fluid in the body, particularly antidiuretic hormone (ADH).

ADH, or vasopressin, is released from the brain (stored in the posterior pituitary gland) when blood fluid volumes fall, e.g. as may occur from blood loss. ADH increases the permeability of the renal tubule, increasing water reabsorption. When plasma ADH levels are low, a large volume of urine is excreted (diuresis), and the urine is dilute. When plasma levels are high, a small volume of urine is excreted (antidiuresis), and the urine is concentrated.

Alcohol inhibits the release of ADH and therefore should be avoided when dehydrated (see Ch. 19). Caffeine also acts as a diuretic, i.e. making people pass urine more frequently, by increasing the GFR and inhibiting sodium reabsorption.

Urine production in the nephron

There are three processes involved in the production of urine: filtration (see above), reabsorption and secretion. The sections of the nephron include:

- Proximal convoluted tubule – the main site of reabsorption
- Loop of Henle – the main site of water balance
- Distal convoluted tubule – the site of sodium control
- Collecting duct –maintains a role in acid/base balance and some water reabsorption.

Lower urinary tract

The lower urinary tract comprises the two ureters, the urinary bladder and urethra (see Fig. 20.1).

Ureters

The ureters are hollow tubes that convey urine from the renal pelvis to the bladder. They are approximately 30 cm in length and implant into the posterior bladder at the ureteric orifices. Urine moves down the ureters by peristalsis, rhythmic contraction of the smooth muscle layer in the wall of the ureters.

Bladder

The bladder is a temporary reservoir for urine. It is a muscular sac lined with transitional epithelial cells (urothelium). When the bladder is empty the lining is arranged in folds called rugae. These folds disappear when urine fills the bladder. The smooth muscle layer is called the detrusor and is an exceptionally strong muscle that contracts to empty the bladder. The three openings in the bladder wall – two ureteric orifices and the urethra – form a triangle called the trigone. The organs associated with the bladder in women and men are illustrated in Figure 20.4.

The bladder is able to distend but when the adult bladder contains around 300–400 mL of urine, the urge to pass urine occurs. The volume is much less in infants and toddlers and depends on size and age, but the bladder wall becomes stretched when sufficient volume of urine is in the bladder (see p. 495), although this will be dependent on the infant's feeding regimen, with urine volumes increasing as the child's urinary system matures.

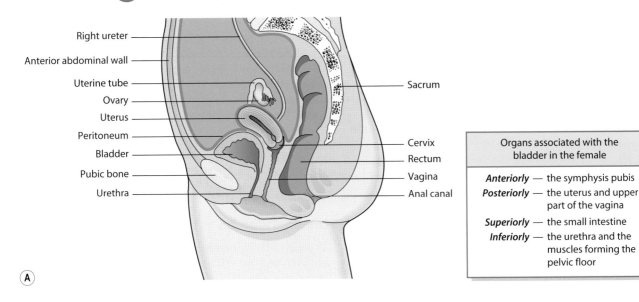

Organs associated with the bladder in the female	
Anteriorly —	the symphysis pubis
Posteriorly —	the uterus and upper part of the vagina
Superiorly —	the small intestine
Inferiorly —	the urethra and the muscles forming the pelvic floor

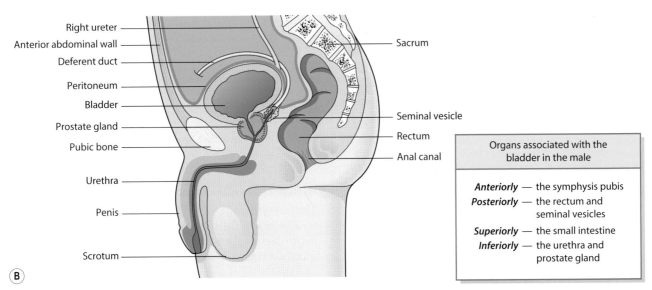

Organs associated with the bladder in the male	
Anteriorly —	the symphysis pubis
Posteriorly —	the rectum and seminal vesicles
Superiorly —	the small intestine
Inferiorly —	the urethra and prostate gland

Fig. 20.4 ● Organs associated with the bladder: (A) The female. (B) The male. (Reproduced with permission from Waugh, A., Grant, A., 2001. Ross and Wilson anatomy and physiology, ninth ed. Churchill Livingstone, Edinburgh.)

The main defences against infection in the urinary system are the flow of urine, the acidity of urine and, in males, the length of the urethra. Urine is normally acidic (see p. 499), which inhibits bacterial growth.

Urethra

The urethra carries urine from the bladder to the outside. In males, the urethra is around 20–25 cm in length, has several curves and passes through the prostate gland. In addition to carrying urine, the male urethra also conveys semen. The female urethra is approximately 3–5 cm in length, is straight and not involved in reproduction. The shorter female urethra, the moist perineal environment and the nearness to the anus all increase the risk of UTI (Waugh & Grant 2010).

The urethra passes through the muscular pelvic floor where internal and external urethral sphincters are located. The external sphincter is under voluntary control or, more accurately, the external control develops during childhood. Normally, the sphincters keep the urethra closed so that urine does not leak from the bladder.

Urinary elimination

Micturition, voiding and urination all refer to the process of passing urine. It is an extremely complex process that involves nerve impulses, coordinated muscle contraction and relaxation of the internal and external urethral sphincters. This process develops over the first few years of life, which explains why infants and toddlers are not continent. The nerve supply from the bladder to the spinal cord is incomplete until the age of around 2 years when the toddler gradually learns that the sensation in the bladder means that they need to pass urine.

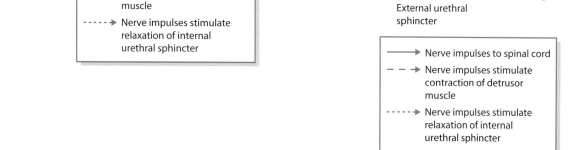

Fig. 20.5 • Control of micturition: (A) Simple reflex control when conscious effort cannot override the spinal reflex. (B) Control of micturition when conscious override is possible. (Adapted with permission from Waugh, A., Grant, A., 2001. Ross and Wilson anatomy and physiology, ninth ed. Churchill Livingstone, Edinburgh.)

When the infant's bladder fills with urine the bladder wall is stretched and nerve impulses pass to the spinal cord. This initiates a spinal reflex that causes detrusor muscle contraction, internal sphincter relaxation and the infant voids urine (Fig. 20.5A).

When development is complete and continence is achieved, the urethral sphincters and the bladder are controlled by a more complex nervous system (Fig. 20.5B). As before, the bladder fills with urine and the bladder walls are stretched, resulting in a nerve impulse being sent to the spinal cord. Now, however, the nerve impulse is directed upwards to the cerebral cortex of the brain, where the impulse is interpreted as the desire to pass urine. This usually results in a behavioural response, i.e. going into the lavatory or asking for a bedpan. Conscious inhibition of reflex bladder contraction and sphincter relaxation is possible for a short time when it is not convenient to pass urine such as driving on a motorway until the service station is reached.

The cerebral cortex sends another nerve impulse to the spinal cord, and then on to the bladder and internal urethral sphincter. As the detrusor muscle contracts there is reflex relaxation of the internal sphincter and voluntary relaxation of the external sphincter, allowing urine to pass through the urethra. Once the bladder is empty the nerve impulses stop, the detrusor muscle stops contracting and the sphincters close.

Micturition can be aided by increasing pelvic pressure through contracting the abdominal muscles and lowering the diaphragm (Valsalva manoeuvre).

Factors affecting micturition

There are multiple factors affecting micturition (Box 20.2).

Micturition is usually under a degree of conscious control. Usually an adult or older child passes urine alone, at a time determined by them and in surroundings that are usually comfortable and known to them. Hospitalization therefore can be a contributory factor affecting micturition. People can become disorientated or positioned too far from the lavatory, which can cause loss of continence. Furthermore, a person's normal urinary habits can be altered by anxiety, following surgery or

Factors affecting micturition — Box 20.2

- Developmental stage (see Ch. 8)
- Lack of privacy
- Anxiety (see Ch. 11)
- Lack of suitable facilities
- Weather
- Mobility (see Ch. 18)
- Constipation (see Ch. 21)
- Medication
- Fluid intake (see Ch. 19)
- Disease or injury, e.g. UTIs, prostate enlargement, kidney failure, diabetes mellitus, stroke, spinal injury.

Urinary tract infection — Box 20.4

UTIs are more common in females than in males, except in infants under 1 year due to periurethral colonization, breast-feeding or an immature immune system (O'Brien et al 2011). The site of the infection determines the term used to describe the infection:

- Acute pyelonephritis is an infection in the kidney
- Cystitis is an infection in the bladder.

Urinary tract infections are caused by bacterial invasion, e.g. *Escherichia coli.* Normally, the urine does not contain bacteria; the presence of bacteria in the urine is termed bacteriuria. Bacteriuria can be symptomatic, e.g. painful voiding or dysuria, or asymptomatic. Pyuria is the presence of white blood cells (WBCs) in the urine, indicating inflammation of the bladder lining. Bacteriuria without pyuria suggests bacterial colonization, not infection (see Ch. 15).

In children, UTIs tend to be classified into initial infections and recurrent infections. Sometimes the cause of infection can be linked to a congenital abnormality that results in vesicoureteric reflux (VUR) or backflow of urine from the bladder into the ureters or kidney. It is essential to identify the presence of UTI in children so it can be investigated and the cause treated to prevent later renal damage. UTI in young children can be particularly difficult to diagnose because of several non-specific signs such as poor feeding, fever, vomiting or failure to thrive, as well as the development of language and children's concepts of health and ill health. This may also be the case in some people with a learning disability.

UTIs in older people are common. The symptoms can range from asymptomatic bacteriuria to life-threatening sepsis. The majority of older people with bacteriuria remain asymptomatic, although symptoms such as lethargy, confusion, anorexia and incontinence may be caused by bacteriuria.

---

illness, through constipation or dehydration, and these factors should be considered when caring for people irrespective of age. Obesity is associated with some types of incontinence (see pp. 505–506) in women but not in men.

Many drugs can also affect the person's ability to urinate normally, from diuretics (e.g. furosemide), which increase urinary volume and frequency, to analgesics that can cause confusion and disorientation. Caffeine, found in tea, coffee and cola-type drinks, as well as performance-enhancing drinks, can have an excitatory effect on the bladder muscle, causing urgency and frequency, as well as being a diuretic. Alcohol acts as a diuretic by affecting ADH release, irrespective of overall hydration. Box 20.3 provides an opportunity to consider how micturition may be affected.

Reflective practice — Box 20.3

Changes to micturition

Think about a situation in which your own micturition was affected, such as being anxious about a new placement, or having a full bladder and being unable to find a public lavatory, or perhaps you needed to pass urine where another person could hear or see you.

Student activities

- Think about how you felt and consider reasons for this.
- Now consider an occasion when a client's/patient's normal pattern of micturition was affected by one of the factors in Box 20.2.
- Discuss with your mentor the nursing interventions used to minimize the disruption.

Common urinary disorders

Urinary tract infection (UTI) and loss of continence (incontinence) are very common. These and other conditions that affect the normal urinary elimination are outlined in Table 20.1. Further detail about UTIs is provided in Box 20.4. (See also Further reading, below, e.g. Cotton & Steggall (2011); Steggall (2011). Some patient groups also provide useful information, see Useful websites, below.)

Assessment and observation of urine and urinary elimination

Before taking a urine sample, it is essential to ask the person about any problems with micturition and urinary symptoms (Box 20.5). The key features are the type of symptoms, duration of the problem, what makes it better or worse, and any other circumstances that could exacerbate the problem, e.g. the lavatory is upstairs so the person cannot get to it quickly enough due to arthritis. Bowel habit is also important to assess, since constipation can cause pressure on the urethra/bladder, thereby resulting in urinary symptoms (see Ch. 21).

As well as the focused assessment, the nurse should note how mobile and dextrous the person is. Part of the assessment is gaining a picture of the person and their abilities; this will help guide nursing management and what continence products/support they will need.

Measuring urine output and observing voiding patterns

This can involve the use of a fluid balance chart, weighing nappies, weighing patients daily and completing frequency-

Table 20.1 Common urinary disorders

Disorder	Description
Benign prostatic enlargement (BPE)	An enlarged prostate gland caused by increased cell size or growth of new cells occurring mainly in older men Leads to urinary problems such as poor stream, dribbling, frequency and retention (see Box 20.5)
Cancer	Cancer may affect the kidney, ureter, bladder and prostate gland A cancer affecting the kidney, known as a nephroblastoma (Wilms' tumour), is common during childhood Bladder cancer can cause painless haematuria (blood in the urine) Cancer of the prostate gland is a common male cancer, which can cause symptoms similar to those of BPE
Diabetic nephropathy (kidney disease)	Progressive kidney disease associated with diabetes Caused by damage to the renal blood vessels, loss of glomeruli and renal failure
Glomerulonephritis	Inflammation of the glomerulus (of the nephron), of which there are many different types
Incontinence of urine	An inability to control the voiding of urine The main types are outlined on pages 505–506
Reflux nephropathy (chronic pyelonephritis)	Kidney damage caused by the backflow of infected urine from the bladder up the ureters (vesicoureteric reflux – VUR) (see Box 20.4)
Renal (kidney) failure	Renal failure can be acute or chronic: • *Acute renal failure* (ARF) occurs when previously healthy kidneys suddenly fail because of reduced blood supply, e.g. severe haemorrhage; it is potentially reversible • *Chronic renal failure* (CRF) occurs when irreversible and progressive damage, such as from diabetic nephropathy, leads to end stage renal disease (ESRD)
Renal stones (calculi)	Stones can form in the kidney They may move down the ureters to cause intense pain (renal colic), obstruct the flow of urine from the kidney, predispose to infection and may cause renal damage
Urinary tract infection (UTI)	Infection affecting the urinary tract is common across the lifespan (see Box 20.4)

Problems with micturition and urinary symptoms	Box 20.5

- *Dribbling:* Occurs with bladder outflow obstruction such as benign prostatic enlargement (BPE) or damage to the pelvic floor (more common in women who have had children)
- *Dysuria:* Pain on passing urine. Often a feature of UTI
- *Enuresis:* Incontinence of urine (see pp. 505–506)
- *Frequency:* The need to pass urine more often than is usual or acceptable for the person. Usually small amounts of urine are passed. Often associated with UTI but can be due to anxiety, bladder outflow obstruction or bladder irritability caused by infection or injury
- *Hesitancy:* A delay in starting to pass urine. Could be a result of bladder outflow obstruction, hypersensitivity or instability
- *Incomplete emptying:* Indicates a failure of the bladder to empty completely; results in acute urinary retention
- *Poor urinary flow:* May be due to bladder outflow obstruction
- *Retention:* Inability to pass urine due to obstruction or bladder failure such as BPE
- *Strangury:* Frequent painful desire to void small amounts of urine, due to muscle spasm associated with irritation or inflammation such as UTI
- *Urgency:* Strong desire to pass urine, which, if not acted upon immediately, may lead to urge incontinence. Associated with detrusor instability or UTI.

volume charts. In addition, assessment of the skin and mucous membranes and blood pressure monitoring will also enable assessment of hydration (see Chs 17, 19).

Fluid balance chart

Urinary output must be recorded on a 24-hour input and output chart (see Ch. 19) if there are concerns about the elimination of urine or renal function. Frequent measurements of urinary output, e.g. hourly, may be used to monitor critically ill patients (see Ch. 14).

The minimum amount of urine needed to excrete waste from the body was discussed on page 493, i.e. 0.5 mL/kg per hour in both children and adults.

Therefore, an infant weighing 5 kg must produce 2.5 mL/h (60 mL in 24 hours), whereas an adult weighing 55 kg must produce 27.5 mL/h (660 mL in 24 hours). Obviously these are minimum amounts and people produce much larger volumes of urine under everyday conditions, approximately 1 mL/kg per hour but up to 2 mL/kg per hour (Box 20.6). The volume of urine produced depends on many factors, including fluid intake, fluid loss and renal function, but a healthy adult should aim to pass more than 1000 mL daily, with an 'ideal' urinary volume of 2000 mL. This ensures that the kidney and lower urinary tract are 'flushed' regularly, thus reducing the risk of UTI.

? Critical thinking   Box 20.6

Variations in urinary volume

Measure your own urine output for 24 hours and calculate the mL/kg per hour.

Student activities

• Think about the factors that might have influenced the volume on that particular day.

• When you are next helping to care for a person who is having their fluid intake and output measured, calculate how much urine they are producing per kg per hour. Try to do this for a child and an adult.

• Discuss the findings and factors affecting them with your mentor.

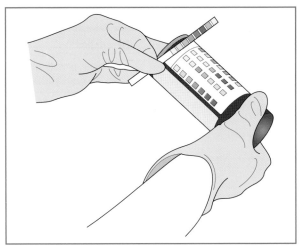

Fig. 20.6 • Urine testing. (Reproduced with permission from Nicol, M., Bavin, C., Cronin, P., et al., 2008. Essential nursing skills, third ed. Mosby, Edinburgh.)

Weighing nappies

Accurate measurement of urine volume in infants and young children is more difficult but can be achieved by weighing wet nappies. The known dry weight of the nappy is subtracted from the weight of the nappy after the infant or child has passed urine. The difference in weight in grams approximately corresponds to millilitres of urine voided.

Frequency–volume charts

Frequency–volume charts can be completed by the person or carer at home and brought to the clinic to be assessed. They are particularly helpful in gaining an insight into voiding patterns. The volume of fluid taken in, the urine output and occasions when the person had an episode of incontinence should all be recorded. Although frequency–volume charts are widely advocated for assessing urinary incontinence (see p. 505), they can focus the person's attention on their urinary symptoms, leading to inaccuracies and additional distress. To minimize this, the charts should be completed for at least 5 days, and when the person is seen again, time should be taken to discuss how they feel about their condition.

Observation of urine and urinalysis

Observation of urine and routine urinalysis by the nurse are both important in the routine screening for abnormalities and possible disease. 'Urinalysis is an important part of patient assessment and could potentially indicate the presence of a serious disease' (Steggall 2007, p 42). Any abnormal findings should prompt further urinary analysis by the laboratory, e.g. by sending a midstream specimen of urine (MSU) (see p. 501). Urine normally contains:

• Water (96%)

• Electrolytes (2%)

• Waste (2%) – urea, creatinine, uric acid, drug and food residues and small amounts of urobilinogen (note that both a reduction in or excessive amounts of urobilinogen are abnormal).

The urine used for routine urinalysis should be a fresh 'midstream' sample. This can pose problems for people who are unable to stop and start their urine and 'catch' the middle part of the flow. People can be assisted in catching the stream by use of a clean funnel. A 'clean catch' sample may be the best alternative in infants, small children, some adults with dementia and some people with learning disabilities. Urine samples should not be the first void of the day unless the urine is being tested for renal tuberculosis (TB). Before performing the urinalysis, the nurse should always observe the sample for colour, clarity and odour (Table 20.2), as these physical characteristics can give valuable clues about potential abnormalities.

Urinalysis using a reagent test strip is a quick and simple test for assessment of renal function, hydration and nutritional state (Fig. 20.6). Urine reagent sticks usually test for the following:

• Specific gravity (SG)

• pH

• Protein

• Blood

• Glucose

• Ketones

• Urobilinogen

• Bilirubin.

Some reagent sticks also include a test for nitrites and leucocytes (white blood cells), the presence of which might indicate bacteriuria and UTI, respectively. Since the kidneys excrete waste, the presence of substances not normally excreted, e.g. protein, glucose, can help with diagnosis of renal disease, diabetes mellitus, infection, etc. (Table 20.2).

This test is relatively simple and accurate to use, although nurses should be familiar with the manufacturer's recommendations for use (Box 20.7, p. 500). Care should be exercised to avoid contaminating samples, e.g. from menstrual blood that could give rise to inaccurate results.

Collection of urine samples for the laboratory

When a urine sample is required, the person or parents/carers of children should be advised why that sample is necessary, e.g.

Table 20.2 Normal characteristics of urine and the significance of abnormalities

Physical and chemical characteristics	Normal findings – observation and urinalysis	Possible significance of abnormal findings
Colour	Pale straw colour to deep amber depending on the concentration	Dark urine may indicate dehydration Blood in the urine (haematuria) can be bright red or can give the urine a smoky appearance Bilirubin turns the urine a brown/green colour or the urine may even be frothy Certain foods or drugs may also influence colour: eating red beet (beetroot) can produce 'pinkish' urine; the drug rifampicin can cause orange/red urine
Clarity (need urine in a clear container)	Usually clear with possible turbidity caused by mucus	Cloudiness or debris can indicate material, such as pus, that needs further investigation
Odour	Freshly voided urine may have a slight aromatic odour but does not usually smell, whereas stale urine can smell of ammonia	A 'fishy' smell would indicate an infection and a 'pear-drop' smell indicates ketones in the urine Certain foods can change the odour
Specific gravity (SG)	The normal SG range of urine is 1.001–1.035, depending on the solids contained in the urine, i.e. a high SG indicates a high level of solids Infants and small children tend to have a relatively fixed SG of 1.008. Their renal system is relatively immature and the kidneys are unable to concentrate or dilute urine (Wilson 2011)	A high SG is found if the urine is concentrated; this may indicate that the person is dehydrated (see Ch. 19) Conversely, dilute urine will have a low SG, which occurs normally when the fluid intake is increased, but can occur during a stage of renal failure When assessing SG, ambient or environmental temperatures should be considered; dehydration can occur quicker in hot conditions
pH	The pH of urine is normally acidic, but within the pH range of 5–8 urine is considered normal Urinary pH is influenced by dietary intake	Very acidic urine may suggest urinary stone formation, whereas alkaline urine suggests an infection with certain types of bacteria such as *Proteus mirabilis*
Protein	Negative	Proteinuria can indicate glomerular/renal damage, although a UTI can cause this Transient proteinuria can occur in children during febrile illnesses or exercise; persistent proteinuria would necessitate a 24-hour urine collection
Blood	Negative	Blood in the urine is called *haematuria* Haematuria usually indicates problems somewhere in the urinary tract, e.g. cancers, renal damage, stones, or it can be due to causes outside the urinary tract, e.g. as a side-effect of anticoagulant drugs or a blood clotting problem Haematuria can be 'frank', i.e. the urine clearly contains blood, or microscopic It is important to eliminate the possibility that haematuria is due to contamination with menstrual blood
Glucose	Negative	Glucose in the urine is termed *glycosuria* Glycosuria can indicate diabetes mellitus but also can occur during pregnancy, in physiological stress and in people taking corticosteroids Glycosuria can be accompanied by a high urine output, because the glucose molecules draw water with it, resulting in high volume urine output and subsequent dehydration
Ketones	Negative	The presence of ketones in the urine is called *ketonuria* Ketones are formed during the abnormal breakdown of fat and can be seen after prolonged vomiting, fasting, starvation and poorly controlled diabetes mellitus

Continued

Table 20.2 Normal characteristics of urine and the significance of abnormalities—cont'd

Physical and chemical characteristics	Normal findings – observation and urinalysis	Possible significance of abnormal findings
Urobilinogen	Small amounts of urobilinogen are normally found in the urine	Elevated levels may indicate liver damage or abnormal breakdown of red blood cells (haemolysis) A reduction or absence occurs in biliary obstruction, i.e. when bile does not reach the intestine
Bilirubin	Negative	The presence of bilirubin can indicate liver disease or biliary obstruction
White blood cells	None	The presence of white cells is associated with UTI, but may indicate more severe renal problems
Nitrites	Negative	A positive test for nitrite is associated with bacteriuria (see p. 496)

Note: All abnormal findings must be reported.

Nursing skills — Box 20.7

Testing urine

Equipment

- Lavatory, urinal or bedpan
- Urine in a clean disposable container or a wet nappy
- Reagent test sticks in original container
- Watch with a second hand.

Preparation

Explain the procedure and seek verbal consent; maintain respect and dignity at all times. The nurse washes and dries hands and puts on non-sterile gloves, plus plastic apron if assisting the person to collect the sample.

Procedure

- Check the expiry date on the container of reagent strips and make sure that the container has not been left open (to prevent contamination)
- Dip the reagent strip into the urine, so that all the reagents are covered with urine. Remove the test strip from the urine. Remove excess urine by tapping the stick against the inside of the urine container
- Check the time on your watch as accurate timing is imperative
- Wait for the recommended time before reading the test strip against the reference guide on the outside of the container without it touching the container. Remember the results
- Put the used stick in the clinical waste and dispose of the urine safely in the sluice or lavatory
- Discard the disposable container as per local policy
- Remove gloves and wash hands (see Ch. 15)
- Record the results on the nursing observation chart and in the nursing notes. This is an important part of the process of urinalysis because it forms an integral component of holistic care. If any abnormalities are detected, refer to the registered nurse for advice. The registered nurse will discuss the result with the person as appropriate.

Note: Some hospital units or GP centres have automatic urine testing machines. It is essential to gain training in how to use these machines to ensure that accurate results are obtained. See Steggall (2007).

to confirm an infection, etc. The accuracy of any test and subsequent diagnosis of urinary tract abnormality can be influenced by many factors, e.g. the amount of bacterial contamination when the urine is collected (see Ch. 15).

The options for urine collection from infants and young children are outlined (Box 20.8).

Collecting urine samples from infants and young children — Box 20.8

Urinary specimens are the main method used to diagnose UTI, but it is particularly difficult to obtain an uncontaminated sample from children, and the reliability of the test is related to the quality of the urine sample collected. The four ways in which to obtain a urine sample in children are:

- A 'bagged' sample obtained by attaching the correct size plastic bag to the perineum
- A 'clean catch'
- A midstream void
- Suprapubic bladder aspiration.

The plastic bag specimen is least favoured because of the high degree of contamination of the sample from the perineum and rectum. For non-emergency urinary specimens the infant or child can be seated over a sterile receptacle and the urine collected and tested. This is referred to as a 'clean catch'. The midstream urine sample is the most reliable but not always possible in young children. Girls must be encouraged to part the labia and in older boys the foreskin should be retracted to prevent contamination.

Suprapubic bladder aspiration is only performed when the sample is needed urgently in children less than 2 years of age. It is an advanced role undertaken by specially trained nurses who have demonstrated competence in this technique.

Resource

Trigg, E., Mohammed, T.A., 2010. Practices in children's nursing, third ed. Churchill Livingstone, Edinburgh, pp. 310, 348–350.

In adults, most samples are voided midstream urine (MSU) (Box 20.9) or a catheter specimen of urine (CSU) (see p. 512). In order to identify infection, urine is sent to the laboratory for microscopy, culture and sensitivity (MC&S).

Nursing skills Box 20.9

Collecting a midstream specimen of urine

Equipment

- Lavatory, urinal or bedpan
- Sterile specimen pot
- Soap and water
- Paper towels
- Gauze swabs.

Preparation

Explain what you are going to do and seek verbal consent; maintain respect and dignity at all times. The nurse washes and dries hands and puts on non-sterile gloves, plus plastic apron if assisting the person to collect the sample.

Procedure

- The person should clean around the external urethral meatus with the warm soapy water. In older boys and adult males, the foreskin (if present) should be retracted, and the glans cleaned with the swab, using each swab once only. In females, the swabs should also be used singly, and the perineal area should be cleaned from front to back (see Ch. 16)
- The person should start to pass urine, directing the middle part of the stream into the sterile pot
- After the sample has been obtained, the person should be offered handwashing facilities
- The specimen should be labelled with the person's details, put into the plastic specimen bag along with the laboratory request form and placed in the specimen fridge ready for transporting to the laboratory (Fig. 20.7). If a red-topped specimen bottle is used the specimen can be stored at room temperature until it is taken to the laboratory.
- Finally, the date, time and type of sample taken should be documented in the nursing notes.

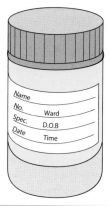

Fig. 20.7 • Urine specimen and request form. (Reproduced with permission from Nicol, M., Bavin, C., Bedford-Turner, S., et al., 2004. Essential nursing skills, second ed. Mosby, Edinburgh.)

The scientist will confirm the presence of microorganisms on microscopy; these will be grown on an appropriate culture medium and sensitivity tests will determine the most effective antibiotic to treat the infection. Urine may also be collected for cytology, looking for abnormal cells, such as cancer cells from the urinary system, that are passed in the urine. Urine samples, often collected over 24 hours, may be analysed for electrolyte levels, protein and various hormones and other chemicals (see Further reading, below, e.g. Nicol et al 2012).

Voided urine specimens are the most acceptable and simplest form of collection for people. A midstream sample is used because it does not contain any debris that may be in the urethra, thus preventing a false result. It is essential for the external urethral meatus to be cleaned before collection of the sample. This helps to reduce the amount of contaminants in the sample.

Common urinary investigations

The following investigations may be used to diagnose or evaluate treatment for disorders of the urinary tract and elimination:

- *Urine tests:* Urinalysis, midstream urine for MC&S, cytology, 24-hour collection for protein, electrolytes, hormones and other chemicals
- *Blood tests:* Full blood count, urea and electrolytes (U&Es), creatinine, prostate specific antigen (PSA)
- *Endoscopy:* Flexible cystoscopy
- *Ultrasound:* Urinary tract (kidneys, ureters and bladder, KUB), renal ultrasound, post-void residual volume
- *Biopsy:* Renal, bladder (during cystoscopy)
- *X-rays:* Intravenous urogram (IVU), cystogram (or cystourethrogram), angiography
- Computed tomography (CT scan)
- Magnetic resonance imaging (MRI)
- *Urodynamic tests:* Cystometry, uroflowmetry to evaluate voiding pattern
- *Pad testing* to assess whether urine is voided or assess leaking.

Simple explanations of some these investigations are provided on the NHS choices website (see Useful websites, below) and will help you provide patient information (Box 20.10); more detailed nursing explanations can be found in Further reading, below, e.g. Cotton & Steggall (2011); Steggall (2011); Walker (2011).

Intravenous urogram

Brian is 22 years old and has a mild learning disability. He lives at home with his parents and his younger sister. Brian has had several UTIs and is to have an intravenous urogram (IVU) in order to identify any abnormalities of his urinary tract.

Student activities

- Find out about what happens before, during and after an IVU.
- Identify the key information needed by Brian so that he is well prepared psychologically and physically for the IVU.
- Consider how to provide Brian with information that meets his needs.
- Find out if there is a learning disabilities liaison nurse in your area.

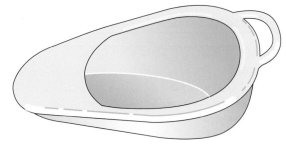

Fig. 20.8 • Slipper bedpan. (Reproduced with permission from Nicol, M., Bavin, C., Bedford-Turner, S., et al., 2004. Essential nursing skills, second ed. Mosby, Edinburgh.)

Nursing interventions – micturition

Assisting people with urinary elimination starts with ensuring that adequate hydration has been provided (see Ch. 19). For many people, their fluid requirements are higher when hospitalized than at home, e.g. people may be sweating, vomiting, have diarrhoea, blood loss, etc., all of which lead to fluid loss from the body.

People may also be weakened by their condition or treatment and may well require assistance in meeting their elimination needs. Many people will feel more comfortable using the lavatory on the ward rather than a urinal, commode or bedpan, and should be escorted or assisted to the lavatory by the nursing staff, to assess their mobility and maintain safety (see Chs 13, 18). For those unable to use the lavatory, a urinal, bedpan, potty or commode will need to be provided. This should be provided quickly and efficiently to limit any embarrassment that the person may have. The nurse should ensure privacy and maintain the person's dignity at all times. The nurse must consider cultural needs, e.g. Hindus and Muslims require that nurses of the same sex meet their intimate care needs (see Ch. 16).

Use of urinal, bedpan and commode

Passing urine is usually private and therefore asking people to pass urine in an out-patient department or ward can put them under considerable pressure, especially when they have a long-standing continence problem. The person should be assured that there will be a bedpan/urinal/commode or a lavatory available for them, that they will not be interrupted, and that the nurse will assist them as much as they want, provided that their safety can be maintained.

If the person is unable to walk to or be taken to the lavatory, a commode/bedpan (see Ch. 21) or urinal will be required. Respect and dignity need to be maintained by ensuring the curtains are completely closed round the bed space and the person allowed time to pass urine without interruption. It is also important to ensure that other members of staff and visitors are aware that the person requires privacy.

For males, using a urinal is relatively simple, provided they are able to sit up. Some men find it difficult to pass urine unless they are standing. It may be necessary to help the person position the penis and hold the urinal. Once completed, the urinal should be covered with a paper towel and removed. The person should then be provided with handwashing facilities. Some cultures, e.g. Muslims, wash their genitalia using running water after passing urine or faeces. A jug of water for washing is provided if the person is confined to bed.

The use of a slipper bedpan (Fig. 20.8) for women is easier and more comfortable to use, since it can be inserted from the side. If the woman is immobile, assistance with mobilizing will require additional staff and handling aids (see Chs 13, 18).

Tissues/lavatory roll is provided but should not be placed in the bedpan if the person's fluid intake and output is being recorded because this will give an inaccurate result. Used tissue should be placed in a separate disposable receptacle; the used tissue is disposed of by flushing it down the sluice. The use of an incontinence pad will catch any urine that accidentally spills from the bedpan, but should not be left under the person once they have been assisted off the bedpan because 'inco' pads can contribute to the development of pressure ulcers (see Ch. 25) and are uncomfortable to sit on.

Again, the person should be allowed privacy and time to pass urine. The person is provided with handwashing facilities and the necessary assistance to clean and dry the perianal area to remove urine, which can contribute to the development of pressure ulcers (see Ch. 25).

If the person is able to use a commode, this can often assist with passing urine. For most people, voiding when lying flat is extremely difficult (Box 20.11). Using the commode can help

 Reflective practice Box 20.11

Position for passing urine

Think about a person you have helped to care for who had difficulty passing urine because of their position or lack of mobility.

Student activities

- What made the position difficult?
- Discuss with your mentor the measures taken to minimize the problem.

the person by returning a degree of 'normality' to passing urine. Before providing the commode, it must be thoroughly cleaned with soap and warm water and carefully dried (see Ch. 15). Attention should be paid to safety, ensuring the bed space is free from obstruction. The wheel brakes on the commode should be in working order and applied to maintain the person's safety. Lavatory tissue must be provided in a separate receptacle for the person to use.

In all instances, the nurse call bell must be left within easy reach of the person. If a fluid balance chart is being kept, do not assess the volume of urine at the bedside, but make a note of the volume in the sluice room before discarding. The nurse must dispose of gloves and wash their hands before recording the voided volume on the person's chart. See Further reading, below, e.g. Nicol et al (2012) for information about helping people who require bedpans, urinals or commodes for urinary elimination.

Promoting continence

Loss of continence affects all age groups and includes school-aged children, postpartum women, postmenopausal women, older men with prostate problems, etc. Urinary incontinence is not uncommon, particularly in women; '32% of the female population experience it compared to 13% of the male population' (NHS Choices 2010).

Loss of continence is often preventable, and can be improved in many cases. However, maintaining continence is always the preferred option and nursing care should be individualized to meet the person's needs, in accordance with the *Essence of Care 2010* benchmarking statements (DH 2010).

In a review of descriptive studies of incontinence in older people in care homes, Roe et al (2011) report that the most common approach used was incontinence pads and toileting programmes. Moreover, they did not identify any studies that tried to maintain continence in care homes residents.

When assessing the person using a model of nursing, elimination must be included. As discussed above, there are many factors that can affect micturition, but nurses themselves cause some of these. People should feel confident that their request for a commode, urinal or bedpan will be promptly met, or that assistance in getting to the lavatory will be swiftly provided so that their anxiety about hospitalization is not worsened.

Consideration should also be given to the proximity of the lavatory to the person's bed space, i.e. a person who has difficulty in mobilizing should not be situated at the end of a ward. Accessibility of the lavatory is also important at home. A commode may be used at home if the person is unable to climb stairs to the lavatory. Adaptations to the lavatory, such as a raised seat and handrails, can increase independence and help to maintain continence (see Fig. 21.5, p. 525).

Making appropriate choices or small changes to clothing can help people to remain continent. For example, a woman with poor manual dexterity may be unable to remove trousers, tights and pants in time but a wraparound skirt allows her to use the lavatory (Fig. 20.9). The use of Velcro® fastenings instead of buttons and zips can also be helpful.

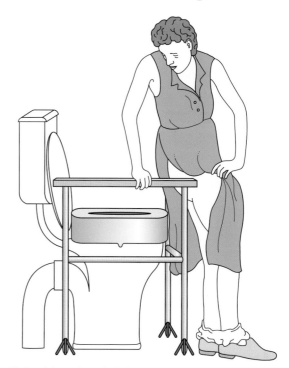

Fig. 20.9 • Adaptation of clothing. (Adapted with permission from Jamieson, E.M., McCall, J.M., Whyte, L.A., 2002. Clinical nursing practice, fourth ed. Churchill Livingstone, Edinburgh.)

Furthermore, the nurse should consider the effects of medication on elimination. Many drugs can affect the ability to urinate normally, from diuretics ('water tablets') that increase urinary volume and frequency, to analgesics and sedatives that can cause confusion and disorientation.

Box 20.12 outlines some factors that affect the person's ability to maintain continence. Many of these factors can cause urinary incontinence (involuntary loss of urine).

Normal voiding habits

Essentially there is no 'normal' pattern of voiding; however, there are clearly abnormal patterns. Between the ages of 18 months and 3 years, children become aware of the sensations to pass urine as their nervous system develops. It would still be within the range of 'normal' for children to wet the bed until the age of 5 years. Daytime wetting decreases as the child ages and the majority of children over 5 should be continent during the daytime. Only 1% of girls and 0.8% of boys wet during the day.

As the child ages, voiding volumes increase, estimated to be:

$$\text{Age in years} \times 30 + 30 = \text{volume in mL}$$

until they reach the adult range of around 400 mL every 4–6 hours or so.

The main feature, however, is that the amount voided is dependent on the amount of fluid consumed and whether the kidneys are functioning properly. People with voiding problems often reduce their fluid intake, which almost universally worsens the situation by increasing the risk of UTI and reducing the benefits of flushing the urinary system.

Factors affecting ability to maintain continence   Box 20.12

- Caffeine in tea, coffee and 'cola' drinks has an excitatory effect on the bladder muscle, causing urgency and frequency, as well as being mildly diuretic
- Alcohol has sedative and diuretic properties
- Medication side-effects, e.g. diuretics, antipsychotics, anticholinergics, analgesics, sedatives, can affect continence by causing retention of urine, or changes in behaviours that can affect continence. Diuretics – particularly loop diuretics, e.g. furosemide – can cause frequency or urgency, or worsen incontinence
- Older people often take many prescribed medicines (polypharmacy), including diuretics that increase urine volume and therefore can affect continence
- Obesity is associated with stress and urge incontinence (see p. 506)
- Constipation, faecal impaction
- Lack of mobility
- Lack of accessible facilities, e.g. lavatory upstairs
- Inability to remove/undo clothing
- Cognitive impairment such as dementia
- Pregnancy and childbirth (mainly stress incontinence) that may be caused by a hormone imbalance, but usually resolves postnatally (Getliffe & Dolman 2008)
- After the menopause due to oestrogen deficiency causing loss of collagen, and to previous damage to the pelvic floor
- Neurological conditions, e.g. stroke, multiple sclerosis, Parkinson's disease, spinal cord damage, affect the central inhibition of micturition (see pp. 496, 506)
- Diabetes causing autonomic nerve damage
- Urinary tract problems – UTI, prostate enlargement, bladder stones, bladder cancer.

Achieving urinary continence during childhood

Continence is achieved by socialization of the child and development of the nervous system. Some children aged 2 years will be dry in the daytime, around 90% of 3 year olds will be dry during the day and most 4-year-old children will be reliably dry (NHS Choices 2009). For a child to develop continence, they must:

- Be aware that they are wetting
- Be getting a sensation to void
- Understand that they must tell someone when they want the potty or to go to the lavatory (this can be quite difficult if the child is enjoying playing or is 'busy' with activities)
- Be able to release the urine when they are using the lavatory.

Introducing the child to the potty at a time when a routine is often already established, e.g. before a bath at bedtime, can facilitate this learning. The child is encouraged to sit on the potty. It can be helpful to bring a book to read with the child, so that their concentration can be maintained. Once the child has passed urine (or faeces) it is essential to reward them in the form of praise. This helps the child to understand what the potty is for, and that passing urine/faeces in the potty is

'good'. The 'right' time to start potty training depends on each child, but once the child notices that they are wet or soiled is an indication of maturity and therefore a good time to start. Children can control their bowels before their bladders. It may take a long time, many months, before the child notices the desire to void, but a toileting routine will help in establishing some patterns that will promote continence (Box 20.13).

Nursing skills   Box 20.13

Potty training

- Make sure the potty is in a prominent position so the child notices it and gets to know what it is for
- Try to potty train at the same time every day. If, for example, the child is soiled immediately after mealtimes, start potty training immediately after the meal and suggest they try the potty. If they do not, postpone potty training for a few weeks
- If they void in the potty, praise them (verbally – not by using sweets)
- Eventually the child will ask for the potty. Consider having at least two potties (one downstairs and one upstairs) to help avoid accidents
- Try to instil a toileting regimen, e.g. after meals. This will help in establishing a set routine and overcome problems in encouraging the child to use the potty when they are busy playing
- Finally, encourage the child to wash their hands after each use of the potty.

Boys need to learn to stand to pass urine, that it is acceptable to pass urine in front of other males, but not females, and that the whole process is usually conducted behind closed doors. This will take some time; the essential element is not to make this too stressful or put too much pressure on the child, since they will not cope with the extra demand. In addition, children need to be able to undo clothes, pull down pants or tights, wipe or wash themselves afterwards and flush the lavatory.

'Accidents' should be anticipated until the age of 5 years or so. These include episodes when the child is too engrossed in playing, e.g. to pay attention to the signals from the bladder, or not sure where the lavatory is located and changes in their lives such as a new baby arriving or just starting school.

Enuresis is leakage of urine occurring on a regular basis (at least once per week). It is important to check physical causes, such as proximity to a lavatory, as well as physical disabilities that may interfere with manual dexterity or movement.

Nocturnal enuresis (bedwetting) is the passing of urine involuntarily at nighttime. Again, for a diagnosis, the child will be older than 5 years and not have any congenital abnormality that may affect the nervous or urinary system, e.g. spina bifida.

The causes of bedwetting are not fully understood. Bedwetting can be considered to be a symptom that may result from a combination of different predisposing factors. There are a number of different disturbances of physiology that may be associated with bedwetting. These disturbances may be categorised as sleep arousal difficulties, polyuria and bladder dysfunction.

(National Institute for Health and Clinical Excellence, NICE 2010, p 5).

Note: polyuria is the excretion of an excessive amount of urine. Enuresis is often subdivided into types, which include diurnal enuresis, true or 'giggle' incontinence and functional incontinence (Box 20.14).

Enuresis   Box 20.14

The aetiology of enuresis is complex, but includes problems with bladder structure and function, UTI and sleep patterns. There is also thought to be a behavioural/emotional component to some types of enuresis. Separation from the family or family tension, such as a new sibling, may provoke or maintain enuresis; furthermore, poor self-esteem in the child will exacerbate bedwetting.

Types

- Diurnal enuresis, or day and night wetting, can be caused by lack of attention to the sensation to void
- Nocturnal enuresis is nighttime bedwetting. In some children, there is delay in learning to control emptying of the bladder and this may be associated with unusually deep sleep
- 'Giggle' incontinence is uncommon, but characterized by complete bladder emptying when the child laughs or giggles, and this can persist into adulthood. There is usually normal function of the bladder and sphincters
- Functional incontinence results from a problem with the urinary sphincter or bladder (or both).

Management

The management of enuresis is aimed at keeping the child dry throughout the day and night, and is often achieved through change in behaviours (Box 20.15).

Devices can be used that sense when urine has leaked which then sound an alarm that wakes the child. On waking, the urinary sphincters tend to close, which allows the child to empty their bladder in the lavatory or potty. It can take time for the child to get used to these devices.

Nurses should support parents or carers by providing information about treatment and support groups (see Useful websites, below).

Pelvic floor awareness and exercise

Pelvic floor exercises are designed to 'strengthen' weakened pelvic floor muscles caused for example by childbirth, chronic cough, heavy lifting, prostate/pelvic surgery, etc. (Chartered Society of Physiotherapy 2011). They are useful in men and women with bladder/continence problems. The exercises involve contracting the pelvic floor to strengthen it, therefore strengthening the muscles that surround the internal and external urinary sphincters (Box 20.16).

Use of frequency–volume charts

Frequency–volume charts can assist in the promotion of continence (see p. 498). The chart can be used to prompt the person to attempt to void every couple of hours to prevent 'accidents', then gradually increase the time between voids. This timing would need to be titrated to the fluid input; a high

---

 ### Health promotion   Box 20.15

Behavioural programme for enuresis

As with any behavioural programme, it is essential to establish a baseline from which to compare change. A chart could be used to record episodes of bedwetting and rewards given for goals achieved, e.g. using a potty, or keeping dry overnight.

The child is taught how to sit on the lavatory, with feet flat on the floor to promote a relaxed position that limits abdominal straining. This allows the detrusor muscle to work properly. The child should be encouraged to pass their urine in one go, not to stop and start the flow. Occasionally, the child cannot completely empty their bladder. They should be encouraged to pass urine, then wait for a few minutes, and then try again. Fluids are encouraged because reducing fluid intake can lead to infections and dehydration.

Finally, it is essential to reward the child, e.g. by making a chart and affixing self-adhesive stars to it, to show how the child is progressing. In addition, positive rewarding, such as simple praise, can also help the child.

Resource

Rogers, J., 2002. Managing daytime and nighttime enuresis. Nursing Standard 16 (32), 45–52.

 ### Health promotion   Box 20.16

Pelvic floor awareness and exercises

Pelvic floor awareness and exercise training are useful for both men and women who suffer continence problems from a variety of causes.

Student activities

- Access the Chartered Society of Physiotherapy 2011 *Personal training for your pelvic floor muscles* resource at: www.csp.org.uk/sites/files/csp/secure/Pesonal-training-pelvic-floor.pdf September 2012.
- What are the symptoms of weak pelvic floor muscles?
- How can people find their pelvic floor muscles?
- What exercises are suggested?
- Discuss with your mentor how you could use the information in your own practice.

---

fluid input will result in increased urine output if renal function is normal, so more voids would be required.

Types of urinary incontinence

There are several types of incontinence, each with different causes (Table 20.3) (see also Box 20.14).

Common findings of the effects of incontinence can include isolation and feelings of loneliness and shame, threatening self-image and disrupting usual activities of living. However, for some, accessing healthcare can be problematic, especially if English is not their first language. Doshani et al (2007) state that the true prevalence of incontinence is hard to establish in certain groups such as ethnic minority populations. South Asian Indian women in the study normalized the symptoms of

Table 20.3 Types and causes of incontinence

Type of incontinence	Causes
Enuresis	See Box 20.14
Stress incontinence – leaking when coughing, laughing, sneezing or during physical activity (increases intra-abdominal pressure)	More common in women and is associated with damage to the pelvic floor following childbirth Symptoms of stress incontinence worsen with age and are aggravated by obesity Stress incontinence rarely occurs in men, but may occur following prostate surgery
Urge incontinence (overactive bladder/detrusor instability) – rushing to the lavatory, frequency, leaking urine	More common in women, due to anatomical changes related to childbirth, but also because of the shorter urethra and weaker pelvic floor, compared to men Neurological conditions Commonest type of incontinence in older people
Voiding difficulties (inefficiency) – incomplete bladder emptying, hesitancy	Commonly occurs in neurological conditions such as stroke, multiple sclerosis, etc. Occurs in women with a cervicovaginal prolapse and men with prostatic enlargement
Overflow incontinence – involuntary leak of urine from an overdistended bladder	Occurs in men and women (less common) Causes include obstruction of the urethra or bladder outlet, e.g. BPE Can occur in women with pelvic prolapse or as a complication of surgery to correct the prolapse Can be caused by underactive detrusor muscle that is associated with conditions such as multiple sclerosis, strokes or as a side-effect of some medicines
Reflex incontinence – incontinence without warning	Can be caused by urethral strictures (narrowing) or an enlarged prostate
Functional incontinence – as an impairment of physical or mental ability	Causes include spina bifida, muscular dystrophy, etc.
Mixed with both urge and stress	Common in postmenopausal women

incontinence and ascribed them to child-bearing and ageing; they felt embarrassed to talk to a male health professional and reported a lack of culturally sensitive material (Doshani, 2007). The provision and promotion of culturally-sensitive continence services in relevant areas is vital in attracting those people who need help.

Management of urinary incontinence

The aim of management is to promote continence, ideally without surgical means. Simple interventions include the following:

- The first therapy in assisting an individual in becoming continent is to adopt a behavioural programme. Behavioural changes start with the reduction of dietary irritants, e.g. caffeine drinks, and an increase in water intake, i.e. up to 1500 mL/day. People should be encouraged to build up the volume input over time (i.e. weeks), but must drink enough to avoid urine concentration that may predispose to UTI. Additional strategies include drinking less fluid before retiring to bed.
- Prevent constipation
- Pelvic floor exercises (see p. 505)
- Keeping a voiding diary or charting fluid input/output may help in reminding people to void, thereby achieving regular bladder emptying, resulting in fewer episodes of incontinence
- Passing urine just before retiring to bed

Information about other treatment options such as bladder retraining, biofeedback, electrical stimulation, medication, e.g. trospium, solifenacin, duloxetine, etc. and surgery can be found in Further reading, below, e.g. Fillingham & Douglas 2004; Walker 2011.

Continence nurse specialist

The management of urinary incontinence requires a multidisciplinary approach to care, i.e. specialist continence nurse, doctor (hospital doctor or GP), physiotherapist and pharmacist. An accurate diagnosis of the type of incontinence is essential. A registered practitioner should prescribe pharmacologic management options and a multidisciplinary plan devised for each person.

The specialist nurse will coordinate and manage these approaches, forming longstanding links with the person (Boxes 20.17 and 20.18).

Continence aids (devices)

When the person, despite every effort, cannot achieve continence, the use of appropriate pads and other devices may be indicated. Devices can either be to contain the urine, e.g. with a pad that absorbs the urine, or devices that carry the urine away from the body, e.g. urinary sheaths (Conveen®) or a pubic pressure urinal, catheters (see pp. 508–514), urological stomas (see p. 514) or other surgical solutions.

Pads

Protective pads to keep clothing or bed linen dry decrease the person's embarrassment, the risk of pressure ulcers (see

Reflective practice   Box 20.17

Specialist continence services

Think about a person you have met on placement who was unable to achieve continence.

Student activities

- Did the specialist nurse see them?
- If yes, what interventions did the specialist nurse suggest?
- Find out what specialist continence services are available in your area (community and hospital)
- Discuss the role of the continence specialist nurse in promoting continence with your mentor.

Resources

Royal College of Nursing, 2002. (revised 2006) Improving continence care for patients. The role of the nurse. Online. Available: www.rcn.org.uk/__data/assets/pdf_file/0003/78555/001952.pdf September 2012.

Scottish Intercollegiate Guidelines Network (SIGN), 2005. (updated) Management of urinary incontinence in primary care. A national clinical guideline. Online. Available: http://sign.ac.uk/pdf/sign79.pdf September 2012.

(?) Critical thinking   Box 20.18

Mrs Malak

Mrs Malak is a 55-year-old woman who has had five children. She attends the out-patient clinic and gives a history of incontinence when she coughs or sneezes and when she holds on to her urine for too long. This has been getting worse for several years, and she admits to staying at home rather than risk incontinence. She is distressed and extremely embarrassed. Her relationship with her husband has also deteriorated.

Student activities

- What type of incontinence do you think Mrs Malak has?
- What practical interventions might be helpful for Mrs Malak?
- What are the likely tests and investigations that she may need to undergo?
- What other issues may there be for Mrs Malak's care? Consider the modesty issues, possible need for interpreter/female staff/special hygiene requirement? She will need to pray five times a day and may choose to fast during Ramadan (see Ch. 19). Will this affect her ability to try behavioural changes?
- Which members of the multidisciplinary team will support her?

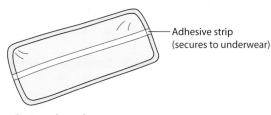
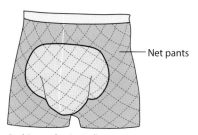
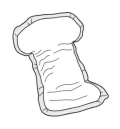
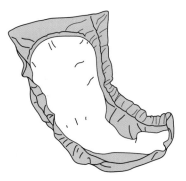

Small shaped pad (elasticated)   Full shaped pad (elasticated)

Fig. 20.10 • Disposable pads.

Ch. 25) and the amount of laundry needed. It is important to select the most suitable pad for the person. A woman who only has stress incontinence when she exercises can often manage with a slim pad worn inside her normal underwear, whereas a person who is incontinent of all urine may need to wear a body pad (similar in shape to a nappy) that will absorb more urine (Fig. 20.10).

If pads are worn, particular attention should be paid to skin care. It is better to protect the skin rather than treat sore or damaged skin (Sanders 2002); this is particularly problematic

in children. The perianal region is the site most commonly affected, along with the thighs and legs. To limit damage to the skin, personal hygiene should be considered a priority and advice sought from the tissue viability nurse specialist (see Chs 16, 25).

Urinary sheath

A urinary sheath (also called external catheter or condom catheter) is a sleeve of latex or silicone that fits over the penis

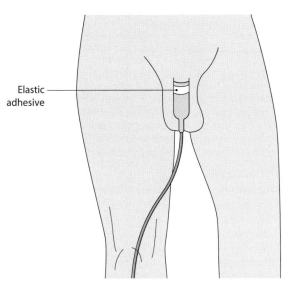

Elastic adhesive

Fig. 20.11 ● Urinary sheath. (Reproduced with permission from Nicol, M., Bavin, C., Bedford-Turner, S., et al., 2004. Essential nursing skills, second ed. Mosby, Edinburgh.)

and is attached to a night drainage or, preferably, a leg drainage bag to aid mobility. They can remain on the penis for between 24 and 48 hours and are used to promote continence where the use of pads is unwanted.

The urinary sheath is similar to a condom except that there is a short tube on the tip that allows urine to flow into a tube connected to a drainage bag (Fig. 20.11). Like most devices, urinary sheaths come in varying sizes (based on the diameter of the flaccid penis) and it is essential that the correct size be used to allow some natural movement in the penis, but not too loose that the sheath becomes detached or leaks urine (Box 20.19). Most manufacturers of sheaths provide a 'size' guide to assist in correct selection of the sheath but they do not suit all men. Common problems encountered include urine leakage, detachment and skin soreness from prolonged contact with urine or adhesive damage. 'Skin soreness or breakdown … can be caused by poor hygiene, latex allergies and pulling or rough handling of the sheath' (Nicol et al 2012, p 241).

Care of people with a urinary catheter

Catheterization is common and all nurses will care for a person who has a catheter. Therefore this section will deal, in some depth, with the care involved. There are many reasons why a person would require catheterization, but the most common are to:

- Relieve retention of urine
- Determine residual volume of urine
- Accurately measure urine output in critically ill people
- Bypass obstruction
- Introduce drugs, e.g. cytotoxic drugs
- Enable bladder function tests to be performed, e.g. urodynamics
- Allow irrigation of the bladder
- Manage incontinence – as a last resort.

 Nursing skills Box 20.19

Application of a urinary sheath
Equipment
- Penile sheath with adhesive
- Measuring disc
- Catheter bag (night drainage or a leg bag)
- Warm water, soap, disposable cloth and towel.

Preparation
Explain what you are going to do and seek verbal consent – maintain respect and dignity at all times. Ask if he has a latex allergy. The nurse washes and dries hands, then puts on non-sterile gloves and plastic apron.

All equipment should be taken to the bedside. Curtains must be drawn to maintain dignity. Assist the man into a sitting position.

Procedure
- The glans penis needs to be socially clean, as does the shaft of the penis before the sheath is applied. Avoid using creams, sprays or powder on the penis since this may affect adhesion of the device. The foreskin should be returned to its normal position after washing. Pubic hair needs to be away from the site of attachment and may need to be trimmed so that the hair does not interfere with the adhesive
- Using the size guide provided, assess the diameter of the penis. This will ensure that the correct size of sheath is used. The correct size is important to avoid problems with urine leaking and skin irritation
- To apply the sheath, hold the penis and roll the sheath down the shaft of the penis. Some sheaths come with applicators which should be used
- At the base of the penis, the sheath should be secured. This depends on the type of sheath
- The sheath should be attached to a leg bag during the day (to promote mobility) and a night drainage bag overnight, making sure that the tube does not become twisted
- Once the sheath is attached, maintain comfort and dignity by replacing loose clothing or bedding
- Dispose of clinical material in the clinical waste bins, remove gloves and wash and dry your hands, then document your actions in the nursing notes
- A care plan should be prepared to ensure that signs of infection, irritation, discomfort, pain or failure of the device are noted immediately. The sheath should be checked twice a day, but must be removed after 24–48 hours.

The introduction of infection (see p. 496), thereby causing harm to the person, is a potentially serious problem that can occur whenever a person is catheterized. Approximately 20% of healthcare associated infections (HCAIs) are UTIs and 80–95% of these originate from an indwelling urinary catheter (Prieto & Kilpatrick 2011). For these reasons, catheterization should never be undertaken without consideration of the potential risks and alternatives to catheterization. Hospital-acquired UTI leads to prolonged hospital stay and increased treatment costs. Once the catheter is in the bladder, the person should be encouraged to drink as much as they can, if possible more than 2 L/day. This will help to 'flush' the urinary tract and limit the chances of UTI. The catheter should be removed as soon as possible; the longer it remains *in situ* the greater the risk of UTI.

Catheters are hollow tubes that are usually inserted through the urethra into the urinary bladder, and are normally used to let urine drain from the bladder as part of medical treatment or instilling fluids.

Occasionally, a catheter will be inserted suprapubically through an artificial tract in the abdominal wall, above the pubic bone, into the bladder. The insertion of a suprapubic catheter tends to be completed by medical staff, although some senior nurses have been trained in this procedure.

Clean intermittent self-catheterization (ISC) is another method of draining urine from the bladder (Box 20.20).

In general, catheterization is an aseptic technique (see Ch. 15), although ISC may be a clean procedure. Catheterization of females is a basic nursing skill. Before nurses can perform female catheterization they must have training and supervised practice and be assessed as competent. Once assessed as competent, then female catheterization can be performed as a student nurse (Box 20.21). Male urethral catheterization is a skill that requires further training after registration. This is due

| Intermittent self-catheterization | Box 20.20 |

The person or their carer passes a catheter into the bladder to drain residual urine, preventing damage to the bladder by overstretching (distension), reducing infection and minimizing incontinence (Newman & Willson 2011). ISC can be used for people with, e.g. multiple sclerosis, spina bifida or spinal injury.

ISC can enhance independence, since there are no obvious signs of a urinary catheter and the person can 'control' when they void (of great benefit to children and adults who wish to remain active), but the major advantage of ISC from a clinical perspective is that the incidence of UTI is reduced compared to indwelling urethral catheters. Additional benefits of ISC (for adults) include maintenance of sexual activity (Newman & Willson 2011).

The frequency of ISC is dependent on the person's needs, although it is important that the amount of urine drained from the bladder does not exceed 400–500 mL because this can cause nerve damage from overstretching (Newman & Willson 2011).

 ## Nursing skills
Box 20.21

Female catheterization

Equipment
- Catheterization pack
- Sterile local anaesthetic (6 mL)
- 1 pair of sterile gloves, 1 pair of non-sterile gloves
- Sachet of sodium chloride 0.9% (normal saline) for cleansing
- A good light source
- A clinical waste bag
- A sterile 10 mL syringe and 10 mL sterile water for injection
- Two catheters (in case one becomes contaminated) of the correct size and for the correct duration of use
- Catheter bag and catheter bag stand
- Absorbent sheet
- Plastic apron.

Preparation
Explain what you are going to do and seek verbal consent; maintain respect and dignity at all times. Ask the woman to wash and dry genitalia, assist as necessary. The nurse washes and dries hands.

Procedure
- Assist the woman into a recumbent (lying down on her back) position
- Place the absorbent sheet underneath the woman's buttocks. This will help to protect the bedding and therefore avoid unnecessary moving of the woman
- Wash hands and, using aseptic technique (see Ch. 15), open the sterile catheterization pack, remove the sterile drape and put the normal saline in the sterile pot inside the pack
- Cover the woman with the sterile drape that is found in the catheterization pack
- Put on non-sterile gloves and apron. The woman should bend her knees and open (abduct) her hips to allow thorough cleaning of the vulval area with normal saline. The vulva should be cleaned from the labia minora then the vestibule (and wiped from front to back). Dispose of gauze swabs used to clean the vulva into the contaminated waste bag

- Apply the local anaesthetic to the urethra and wait 3–5 minutes, allowing the anaesthetic time to work
- Remove non-sterile gloves, wash hands or use alcohol hand-rub
- Open all sterile equipment onto sterile field. Draw up the 10 mL of water into the syringe. Open the sterile catheter bag. Remove the catheter from the outer packet. Note that catheters come with two covers; the outer cover should be discarded. Put on sterile gloves (see Ch. 15)
- Open the catheter along the perforations, making sure that you do not touch the catheter itself. Using your non-dominant hand, part the labia minora using a piece of sterile gauze or your gloved fingers (Fig. 20.12)
- Insert the tip of the catheter into the urethral opening. Gently continue to insert the catheter into the urethra. This is a difficult skill and will need practice. Do not touch the catheter, but as the catheter goes into the urethra, remove the outer sterile covering of the catheter (see Fig. 20.12)
- The catheter should be inserted to the fullest extent, i.e. the 'y' junction. Urine should flow from the catheter. This can be collected in the kidney tray that is in the catheterization pack
- Once the catheter is fully in, inflate the balloon using the sterile syringe and inflation port (Fig. 20.13)
- Once inflated, gently pull the catheter back until resistance is felt. This confirms that that catheter is in the correct place
- Attach the catheter bag to the catheter, then to the catheter stand
- Clear away all equipment and make sure that the woman is comfortable
- Consider obtaining a urine sample from the collection port
- Record the insertion date, size of the catheter, balloon volume and the volume of sterile water used to inflate the balloon, reason for catheterization and amount of anaesthetic used in the medical and nursing notes. Make sure that the catheter does not remain in the bladder for longer than the recommended time.

to the potential harm, i.e. damage to the urethra or prostate gland, that can occur when catheterizing a male.

Types of catheter

Selection of the catheter needs to be based on the indications for catheterization and the length of time it will be *in situ* – this will determine whether an intermittent, short- or long-term self-retaining catheter will be used. Self-retaining Foley catheters have a balloon at the end of the catheter that is inflated after it has been inserted (Fig. 20.14). The balloon stops the catheter from falling out.

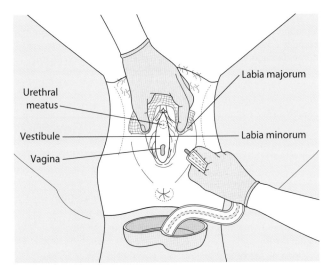

Fig. 20.12 • Female catheterization. (Reproduced with permission from Nicol, M., Bavin, C., Bedford-Turner, S., et al., 2004. Essential nursing skills, second ed. Mosby, Edinburgh.)

The types of catheter and their uses are:

- *Intermittent:* Balloon-less, very small and used for insertion of drugs or to release urine stored in the bladder
- *Short-term self-retaining:* Typically used in hospital for assessment of postoperative urine output
- *Long-term self-retaining:* Used for people who need to have a catheter *in situ* for more than 2 weeks.

Catheter length

Catheters come in different lengths for men and women. The 'male' length catheter is almost twice as long as the 'female' length catheter. No attempt should be made to insert a female length catheter into a male.

Catheter materials

The length of time that a catheter can remain *in situ* is dependent on the material that it is made from, e.g. latex catheters can remain *in situ* for up to 14 days, whereas silicone or hydrogel-coated catheters can remain *in situ* for up to 3 months.

The 'short-term' catheters easily become encrusted or coated with the debris from the urine in the bladder. Longer-term catheters, e.g. the silicone-or hydrogel-coated catheters, tend to encrust at much slower rates than short-term catheters, and are therefore used for people who need a catheter *in situ* for more than 2 weeks.

Catheter lumen size

Each type of catheter is produced in different sizes. The size of the internal diameter is measured in Charrière scale (Ch) or French Gauge (FG). One Ch or FG equals 0.3 mm, so a 12 Ch catheter is approximately 4 mm in diameter. The important point here is that the larger the Ch/FG size, the

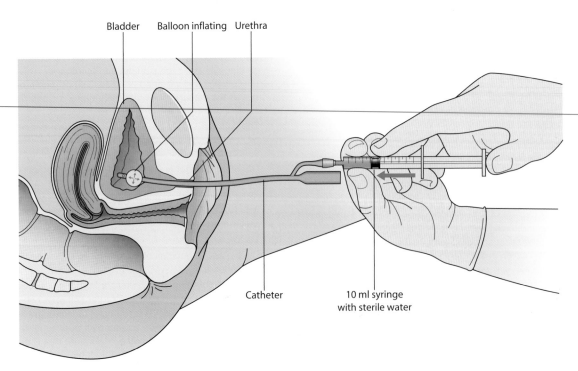

Fig. 20.13 • Inflating the catheter balloon.

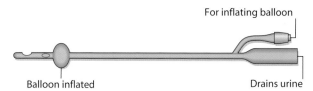

Fig. 20.14 • Self-retaining catheter (double-lumen Foley).

more the urethra will be dilated or stretched when a catheter is *in situ*.

The 'golden rule' for catheterization is always to select the smallest size catheter to do the job. Examples include:

- For retention of urine, a catheter between Ch/FG 10–12 is used for women, and 12–14 for men
- If haematuria is evident, a large bore catheter or an irrigation catheter will be required, at a size of Ch/FG 18–30
- For infants and children, a size Ch/FG 6–8 would normally be used, but again depends on the reason for catheterization and the age and size of the child.

Balloon size

A self-retaining catheter will come with instructions of how much to inflate the balloon once it is in situ. It is normally inflated with 10 mL of sterile water, but there is a chance that, over time, some of this fluid will leech out. The importance of filling the balloon with the correct volume is that the drainage ports in the catheter should be level; underfilling of the balloon results in a leaning over of the catheter tip, preventing drainage.

Overfilling the balloon can worsen detrusor muscle instability or cause urine to bypass around the catheter. In addition, the added volume will put pressure onto the bladder neck that can result in necrosis of the bladder neck and incontinence.

Drainage systems

The selection of a closed drainage system should be on an individual basis, but the main consideration should be whether the person is mobile or not, or whether the urine volume needs to be accurately recorded, in which case a urometer is needed. Leg bags are available in 350, 500 and 700 mL sizes, and should be worn where it is most comfortable for the patient, and secured in accordance with the manufacturer's instructions. Irrespective of leg bag size or location used, it is important to make sure the tubing does not become kinked, because this will prevent drainage. Dragging on the catheter, which can cause injury to the urethra and external urethral opening, must be avoided by securing the bag.

If a person is mobile, they should not be encumbered by carrying a catheter bag round with them which limits their ability to mobilize safely (see Chs 13, 18). A leg bag *must* be used. This allows the person to have both hands free to assist them with mobility. It also confers dignity since a leg bag is relatively discreet. Immobile or non-ambulatory people would normally use a 2 L 'night-bag', which must be attached directly

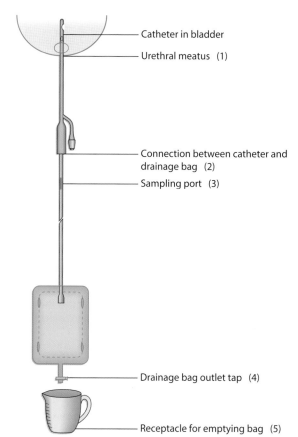

Fig. 20.15 • Closed drainage system showing potential entry points (1–5) for pathogenic microorganisms.

to a catheter stand to prevent dragging on the urethra and cross-infection from the floor.

All catheter drainage bags are a 'closed system' and should be carefully looked after in order to minimize infection. Each time the bag is opened or drained, the potential for infection increases. Figure 20.15 illustrates the points in the 'closed system' at which pathogenic microorganisms can gain entry.

If the person is using a 2 L drainage bag at night, they could use a 500 mL drainage bag during the day. The 2 L night bag is capped using a single-use sterile spigot (bung) and not allowed to touch the floor, as this is a potential source of infection. At all times the urine bag should be kept below the level of the bladder to prevent urine from tracking back into the bladder and causing infection. Although the catheter bags have one-way filters to prevent backflow of urine, they should be changed weekly (Drug Tariff 2003) to prevent harbouring bacteria that could cause UTI. The simplest way to ensure that this is completed is to put the date that the bag was opened on the drainage bag and record the date in the nursing notes; alternatively, the date that the bag needs to be changed can be recorded on the bag itself. Essentially, the most important aspect is that the bag is changed once per week if the individual is in hospital.

As emptying the drainage bag breaches the 'closed' system and increases the infection risk, it must be done carefully (Box 20.22).

Nursing skills   Box 20.22

Emptying the catheter bag

Equipment

- Disposable measuring jug or a sterile jug that is used *only* once
- Cover or paper towel
- Alcohol swab.

Preparation

Explain what you are going to do and seek verbal consent – maintain respect and dignity at all times. The nurse washes and dries hands, then puts on non-sterile gloves and plastic apron.

Procedure

All equipment should be taken to the bedside. If the drainage bag is a 2 L bag, then it should already be attached to a catheter bag stand. The bag will not need to be removed.

- Hold the bag over the disposable jug, making sure the drainage port does not touch the jug. Open the drainage port and allow the urine to flow into the jug. Do not let the jug become more than three-quarters full to minimize the risk of spillage (Fig. 20.16)
- When the urine bag is empty, wipe the drainage port with the alcohol swab to stop urine from dropping onto the floor
- Reposition the catheter bag, making sure that the catheter tube has not become kinked or tangled
- The jug should then be covered and taken to the sluice. The amount of urine should be measured then disposed of in the sluice. According to local policy the disposable jug is discarded and a non-disposable jug is resterilized by the sterile supplies department
- Gloves and aprons are removed and the hands thoroughly cleaned and dried before attending to the next person
- Fluid balance charts are completed as necessary.

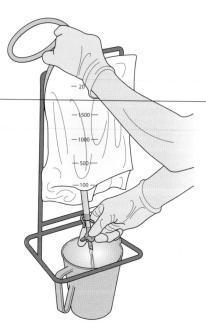

Fig. 20.16 • Emptying the catheter bag. (Reproduced with permission from Nicol, M., Bavin, C., Cronin, P., et al., 2008. Essential nursing skills, third ed. Mosby, Edinburgh.)

Collecting a catheter specimen of urine

A catheter specimen of urine (CSU) for bacteriological investigation is obtained from the sampling port on the drainage tubing using a sterile syringe (Box 20.23).

Nursing skills   Box 20.23

Collecting a catheter specimen of urine

Equipment

- 10 mL sterile syringe
- Sterile specimen container with screw-top lid
- Alcohol swab.

Preparation

Explain what you are going to do and seek verbal consent; maintain respect and dignity at all times. The nurse washes and dries hands, then puts on non-sterile gloves and plastic apron.

Procedure

- Draw the curtains round the bed space to maintain the person's privacy
- Expose the section of the catheter bag tubing with the sampling port. Swab the port with the alcohol swab and wait 30 seconds for the alcohol to dry. If there is no urine in the tubing, the catheter bag tube can be clamped to allow collection of urine
- Insert the syringe into the port; if a needle is used, make sure it does not perforate the catheter tubing. Withdraw approximately 10 mL of urine from the catheter tubing. Remove the syringe. Unscrew the sterile specimen container and transfer the contents of the syringe into the container slowly to prevent spillage. Screw the top back onto the container, and then write the person's details on the container. Replace bedding before opening the curtains
- Take the specimen to the sluice; remove gloves and wash hands before putting the sample into a plastic specimen bag. The specimen should be placed in the specimen fridge, along with the laboratory request form ready for transport to the laboratory as soon as possible. If a red-topped specimen bottle is used the specimen can be stored at room temperature until it is taken to the laboratory
- Finally, the date, time and type of sample taken should be documented in the nursing notes.

Catheter hygiene

The body's normal protective measures, e.g. closed urethra, are bypassed when a catheter is *in situ*. The epic2 evidence-based guidelines state that normal daily hygiene, including bathing or showering is effective for meatal hygiene (Pratt et al 2007).

In some situations, such as faecal incontinence, catheter hygiene may be required more frequently in order to limit the chance of infection. For example, twice daily catheter hygiene may be completed in the morning and before going to bed. The person who is able to use their hands and see the catheter can be taught to carry out their own catheter hygiene.

Warm soapy water should be used to clean around the catheter where it enters the urethra. In uncircumcised males, this also involves retracting the foreskin, cleaning the glans penis and replacing the foreskin. This should be completed at frequent enough intervals to prevent encrustation around the urethral meatus; thus removing a potential source of infection.

If the person wants a bath, it is important to ensure that all wounds have completely healed so that infection is not introduced or spread. 'Patients may take a bath or a shower with the catheter and drainage bag in place' (Turner & Dickens 2011, p 55). It is important to ensure that the catheter bag does not touch the floor while the person is having their bath, as this would allow bacteria to enter the bag and become a potential cause of infection.

The principles of care of a person with a catheter in situ are summarized in Box 20.24.

Removal of a self-retaining catheter

A registered nurse or doctor will decide on the removal of a self-retaining catheter. They will also decide if a catheter specimen of urine is required. If a specimen is required, collect a CSU before removing the catheter. The technique for removal is clean rather than aseptic but sterile syringes must be used. As with all procedures, the nurse must wash their hands and prepare their equipment before attempting the procedure.

All catheters should have the balloon deflated before removing the catheter. It is essential to check the medical/nursing notes to see how much water was used to inflate the balloon. Although the catheter itself indicates how much water should be inserted, the correct amount is not always used. Usually, when the syringe is attached to the inflation/deflation port, the pressure in the balloon means that the syringe will automatically fill with the fluid in the balloon. If the balloon does not deflate, then report this to the registered nurse.

Depending on how long the catheter has been *in situ*, there will be a period of time before bladder function returns to normal. People should be encouraged to drink plenty (2–3 L) of fluid per day and to use a measuring jug to check how much urine has been voided at each attempt. Although the amount of urine voided varies according to age, adults should not be discharged home until they are voiding a minimum of 150 mL. The catheter can cause localized trauma or damage to the urethra and bladder. The effect of this trauma can be haematuria, but this should be minimal and resolve after a few days. People should be encouraged to seek advice from a nurse or doctor if they have any deterioration in their urinary function or if haematuria persists for more than a couple of days.

Sexual activity and urethral catheterization

There is no reason why people should abstain from sexual activity if they have a catheter *in situ*. The key point is that sexual activity does not have to end if one partner has been catheterized. As people will not be sure how to broach this issue with the nurses caring for them, the registered nurse should adopt a proactive approach. A simple statement such as, 'Some people feel their sex lives change once they are catheterized, but this does not need to be the case. If you would like to discuss this, let me know and I can go through

---

Care of a person with a catheter *in situ*   Box 20.24

Problem

A catheter is *in situ* for whatever reason.

Goal

To reduce the risk of infection, blockage (i.e. urine not flowing, low abdominal pain, spraying of urine from the urethra), trauma and discomfort.

Nursing actions

- Record urine output and perform dipstick urinalysis a minimum of once per week. Ensure that urine output is greater than 0.5 mL/kg per hour. If there are any positive indicators on urinalysis, such as blood, protein, leucocytes, nitrites, etc., a catheter specimen of urine should be sent for MC&S if it is a short-term catheter. If long term, refer to the district nurse/GP
- Encourage fluid intake of between 2 and 3 L/day. If oral fluids cannot be taken, or are taken in insufficient quantity, consider other routes (see Ch. 19)
- Check temperature, pulse, BP and respiratory rate as condition dictates (for those in hospital)
- Observe for signs of infection, i.e. pyrexia, but also sepsis, i.e. hypotension, increase in pulse and respiratory rates, and pyrexia. Smelly, cloudy or bloody urine will indicate an infection. Seek advice from the senior nurse/doctor immediately
- Catheter hygiene requires daily urethral meatal cleansing with warm soapy water (see p. 512)
- Encourage the use of leg bags during the day to promote mobility
- Only empty the catheter bag when three-quarters full
- Keep the urine drainage bag below the level of the bladder. Use a stand to ensure that the drainage tap does not touch the floor
- Encourage a high fibre diet to minimize constipation; administer prescribed aperients where necessary. Impacted faeces can block the outflow of urine, causing urinary retention
- Bladder washouts may be required to remove clots after urological surgery. '… commercially prepared catheter maintenance solutions (CMS), are sometimes used in the management of long-term urethral catheters to dissolve encrustations' (Nicol et al 2012, p. 269). The catheter may need to be changed
- If the person is going home with a catheter *in situ*, ensure that the catheter is a long-term catheter and provide a district nurse referral after assessing the person's/carer's ability to self-care. Educate the person about the importance of handwashing before and after catheter care or emptying or changing the bag
- Arrangements for emergency changes of the catheter should be prearranged via the district nursing team/GP, or the local policy may be to refer directly to the local Emergency Department
- With regard to sexual activity, drainage bags should be capped off. Men can use a condom to secure the catheter along the underside of the penis. Women can tape the catheter to the abdomen.

(See Further reading, below, e.g. Dougherty & Lister 2011.)

Table 20.4 Complications of catheterization

Complication	Cause	Solution
Infection	Incorrect insertion, size, poor technique	Only undertake catheterization when assessed as competent Use strict aseptic technique Observe the urine for signs of infection Change the catheter in accordance with manufacturer's instructions Change the catheter bag weekly, or more frequently if the person's condition dictates
Pain	Detrusor spasm due to irritation; irritation to urethra/external meatus	Ensure the correct size catheter is used – large catheters will cause more pain Make sure the catheter has not been in too long Provide analgesia as prescribed and note efficacy Medication to reduce detrusor spasm, e.g. oxybutynin Local anaesthetic gel may be applied on the glans or external urethral meatus to reduce irritation
Blockage	Debris, e.g. blood clots, bladder tissue; catheter tubing may be kinked or the catheter bag blocked	Ensure that the catheter or drainage tube is not twisted or caught up with any equipment Make sure the catheter has not been in too long Observe the urine for blood or debris The catheter may need to be 'flushed' or a bladder washout performed If these measures fail, the catheter will need to be changed
Bypassing	Detrusor instability	Make sure the catheter has not been in too long If possible, put in a smaller size catheter Detrusor muscle relaxants, e.g. oxybutynin
Urethral strictures	Damage to the urethra	Medical management or either surgery or dilatation of the urethra, followed by a period of intermittent self-catheterization to keep the urethra open
Trauma to urethra	Can occur when the catheter and catheter bag are not secured properly Causes tension on the catheter by weight of urine in the bag, resulting in damage to the bladder, urethra and external urethral meatus	Ensure that the catheter is correctly secured to either a catheter bag stand or the person's leg
Encrustation	Leaving the catheter in the urinary bladder for longer than the manufacturer's instructions	Change catheter as per manufacturer's instructions

the options with you', can help in broaching the subject, although any discussion should be with your mentor initially.

Complications of catheterization

The complications of catheterization are outlined in Table 20.4.

Urinary stomas

Urinary stomas are openings in the skin that drain urine from the urinary system. Some people may have had their bladders removed (cystectomy) or find that the bladder muscle does not work, resulting in potential harm to the kidneys. For these people, the urine needs to be diverted, or a passageway (conduit) formed, to help drain the urine from the urinary system. The main reasons for urinary diversion include cancers in the urinary system, congenital abnormalities, e.g. spina bifida, and complete bladder failure.

There are many different ways in which urine can be diverted from the bladder; collectively they are called 'urostomies' (see Further reading, below, e.g. Fillingham & Douglas 2004).

SUMMARY

- This chapter covers basic but essential aspects of nursing interventions in relation to promoting continence and urinary elimination.
- The *Essence of Care 2010* Benchmarks for Bladder, Bowel and Continence Care is included and used to underpin the nursing practices that you will see during placements.
- The nurse's role in preventing incontinence is discussed, especially the assessment of urinary function across the lifespan, and the subsequent effects that incontinence can cause.
- Nursing interventions for people with problems associated with incontinence have been considered. The emphasis has been on simple nursing interventions such as ensuring that people can access the lavatory easily, but more complex interventions have been outlined.
- The partnership between the person/parents/carers and the MDT is stressed.
- The importance of promoting continence cannot be overstated; the nurse's role is central in ensuring that people in their care receive sufficient assistance in maintaining continence/promoting continence. UTIs are common and are encountered in all areas of practice.

KEY WORDS AND PHRASES FOR LITERATURE SEARCHING

Catheters
Continence
Elimination
Urinary
Urinary tract infection

 Useful websites

Bladder and Bowel Foundation http://bladderandbowelfoundation.org
British Association of Urological Nurses (BAUN) www.baun.co.uk/guidelines.html
Education and Resources for Improving childhood Continence (ERIC) www.eric.org.uk
National Institute for Health and Clinical Excellence (NICE) www.nice.org.uk
NHS choices www.nhs.uk/Pages/HomePage.aspx
Scottish Intercollegiate Guidelines Network (SIGN) http://sign.ac.uk
All websites accessed September 2012.

References

Chartered Society of Physiotherapy, 2011. Personal training for your pelvic floor muscles. Online. Available: www.csp.org.uk/sites/files/csp/secure/Pesonal-training-pelvic-floor.pdf September 2012.

Department of Health, 2010. Essence of care 2010. Benchmarks for bladder, bowel and continence care. Online. Available: www.dh.gov.uk/ September 2012.

Doshani, A., Pitchforth, E., Mayne, C.J., et al., 2007. Culturally sensitive continence care: a qualitative study among South Asian Indian women in Leicester. Family Practice 24 (6), 585–593.

Drug Tariff, 2003. Part 1xb. Department of Health, National Assembly for Wales. TSO, London, in Association for Continence Advice: Notes on good practice.

Getliffe, K., Dolman, M., 2008. Incontinence in perspective. In: Getliffe, K., Dolman, M. (Eds.), Promoting continence: a clinical research resource, third ed. Baillière Tindall, Edinburgh.

National Institute for Health and Clinical Excellence, 2010. Nocturnal enuresis. Clinical Guideline CG111. Online. Available: http://guidance.nice.org.uk/CG111/Guidance/pdf/English September 2012.

NHS choices, 2009. How to potty train. Online. Available: www.nhs.uk/Planners/birthtofive/Pages/Pottytrainingtips.aspx September 2012.

NHS choices, 2010. The taboo of incontinence. Online. Available: www.nhs.uk/Livewell/incontinence/Pages/Breakingthetaboo.aspx September 2012.

Newman, D.K., Willson, M.M., 2011. Review of intermittent catheterization and current best practices. Urologic Nursing 31 (1), 12–48.

Nicol, M., Bavin, C., Cronin, P., et al., 2012. Essential nursing skills, fourth ed. Mosby, Edinburgh.

O'Brien, K., Stanton, N., Edwards, A., et al., 2011. Prevalence of urinary tract infection (UTI) in sequential acutely unwell children presenting in primary care: Exploratory study. Scandinavian Journal of Primary Health Care 29 (1), 19–22.

Pratt, R.J., Pellowe, C.M., Wilson, J.A., et al., 2007. epic2 National evidence-based guidelines for preventing healthcare-associated infections in NHS hospitals in England. Journal of Hospital Infection 65 (Supplement 1), S1–S64.

Prieto, J., Kilpatrick, C., 2011. Infection prevention and control. In: Brooker, C., Nicol, M. (Eds.), Alexander's nursing practice, fourth ed. Churchill Livingstone, Edinburgh.

Roe, B., Flanagan, L., Jack, B., et al., 2011. Systematic review of the management of incontinence and promotion of continence in older people in care homes: descriptive studies with urinary incontinence as primary focus. Journal of Advanced Nursing 67 (2), 228–250.

Royal College of Physicians, 2010. National Audit of Continence Care. Combined Organisational and Clinical report. Online. Available: www.rcplondon.ac.uk/resources/national-audit-continence-care August 2011.

Sanders, C., 2002. Choosing continence products for children. Nursing Standard 16 (32), 39–43.

Steggall, M.J., 2007. Urine samples and urinalysis. Nursing Standard 22 (14), 42–45.

Turner, B., Dickens, N., 2011. Long-term urethral catheterisation. Nursing Standard 25 (24), 49–56.

Waugh, A., Grant, A., 2010. Ross and Wilson anatomy and physiology in health and illness, eleventh ed. Churchill Livingstone, Edinburgh.

Wilson, D., 2011. Balance and imbalance of body fluids. In: Hockenberry MJ, Wilson D (Eds.), Wong's nursing care of infants and children, ninth ed. Mosby, St Louis.

Further reading

Cotton, J., Steggall, M.J., 2011. Nursing patients with disorders of the reproductive systems (Part 1). In: Brooker, C., Nicol, M. (Eds.), Alexander's nursing practice, fourth ed. Churchill Livingstone, Edinburgh.

Dougherty, L., Lister, S. (Eds.), 2011. The Royal Marsden Hospital Manual of clinical nursing procedures, eighth ed. Wiley-Blackwell, Oxford.

Fillingham, S., Douglas, J., 2004. Urological nursing, third ed. Baillière Tindall, Edinburgh.

National Institute of Health and Clinical Excellence, 2006. Urinary incontinence: The management of urinary incontinence in women. Clinical Guideline CG40. Online. Available: http://guidance.nice.org.uk/CG40 September 2012.

Nicol, M., Bavin, C., Cronin, P., et al., 2012. Essential nursing skills, fourth ed. Mosby, Edinburgh.

Rogers, J., 2008. Mainly children. In: Getliffe K, Dolman M (Eds.), Promoting continence: a clinical research resource, third ed. Baillière Tindall, Edinburgh.

Steggall, M.J., 2011. Nursing patients with urinary disorders. In: Brooker, C., Nicol, M. (Eds.), Alexander's nursing practice, fourth ed. Churchill Livingstone, Edinburgh.

Walker, S., 2011. Maintaining continence. In: Brooker, C., Nicol, M. (Eds.), Alexander's nursing practice, fourth ed. Churchill Livingstone, Edinburgh.

Waugh, A., Grant, A., 2010. Ross and Wilson anatomy and physiology in health and illness, eleventh ed. Churchill Livingstone, Edinburgh.

Elimination of faeces: care and promoting continence

21

Susan H. Walker

LEARNING OUTCOMES

This chapter will help you:

- Understand the structure and function of the large intestine, rectum and the anal canal
- Describe normal defecation in the child and the adult
- Outline factors which affect bowel habit
- Demonstrate an awareness of holistic assessment and history-taking
- Outline the *Essence of Care* 2010 (Department of Health 2010) best practice benchmarks concerned with bowel and continence care
- Describe nursing interventions that maintain or restore normal defecation
- Outline some common conditions affecting the large intestine, rectum and the anal canal
- Outline some common diagnostic procedures
- Develop an understanding of the assessment and nursing management of constipation, diarrhoea and faecal incontinence.

Introduction

The elimination of faeces (defecation), which requires proper functioning of the gastrointestinal (GI) tract, is vital in the maintenance of homeostasis. When defecation is disrupted, it can adversely affect the person's quality of life and ultimately their health. Unfortunately, many people still choose to ignore symptoms that may be indicative of disease because they are too embarrassed to discuss their bowel habit or fear the prospect of undergoing physical examination.

Meeting patients' bowel needs was included in the original *Essence of Care* document in 2001, which detailed patient-focused benchmarks to assist health professionals in raising standards for basic but essential aspects of care. Bowel care continues to be prominent in the *Essence of Care 2010: Benchmarks for Bladder, Bowel and Continence Care* (Department of Health, DH 2010). This chapter contributes to the attainment of those standards for patients/clients who require assistance with bowel care and defecation.

The chapter outlines the anatomy and physiology of normal defecation and the factors that affect it. The nursing interventions needed to assist patients with defecation, including relevant health promotion, are discussed in detail. The importance of a holistic approach to care, that is person centered, is illustrated in the section dealing with patients/clients who experience a range of problems with defecation. The nurse's knowledge and skill is fundamental in the assessment of bowel habit and the delivery of holistic care based on best evidence.

The nurse must work in partnership with the patient/client/carers and parents and other health and social care professionals in the multidisciplinary team (MDT), to achieve independence of faecal elimination for the patient/client wherever possible, and to promote personal dignity when assistance is required. Integrated throughout this chapter will be the competencies which form part of the relevant NMC Essential Skill Clusters (ESC) in care, compassion and communication and organizational aspects of care (Nursing and Midwifery Council, NMC 2010).

An overview of defecation

This section covers the anatomy and physiology of the large intestine and defecation and the factors that affect it. Holistic assessment of faecal elimination is explored and an outline of common conditions and investigations is provided.

An inability to excrete waste leads to loss of homeostasis and disruption of cellular function. In the body, the large intestine (bowel) plays the major role in the elimination of solid waste (faeces).

The gastrointestinal (GI) tract is a coiled muscular tube which comprises:

- Mouth
- Pharynx
- Oesophagus

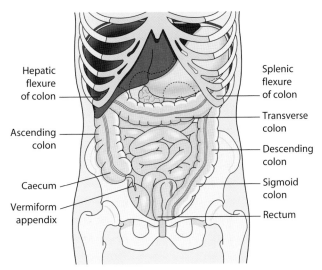

Fig. 21.1 • Parts of the large intestine and their positions. (Reproduced with permission from Waugh, A., Grant, A. (Eds.), 2010. Ross and Wilson anatomy and physiology, eleventh ed. Churchill Livingstone, Edinburgh.)

- Stomach
- Small intestine (duodenum, jejunum and ileum)
- Large intestine (caecum, colon, rectum and anal canal) (Fig. 21.1).

(See Chs 16, 19 and your anatomy and physiology book.)

Large intestine, rectum and anal canal

Most absorption of nutrients occurs within the small intestine (see Ch. 19). Remaining waste material passes into the large intestine where it gradually solidifies, as water is reabsorbed into the bloodstream through the bowel mucosa. The resultant material, faeces, is a semi-solid brown mass. Despite absorption of water, 60–70% of the weight of faeces is water. Faeces contains undigested fibre residues and mucus, which help lubricate the faeces or stool, aiding defecation.

Structure

Four layers of tissue form the walls of the large intestine:

- Adventitia – serous outer layer
- Muscle layer – longitudinal and circular muscle fibres concerned with moving intestinal contents by peristalsis (rhythmic wave-like contraction and dilatation)
- Submucosal layer
- Mucosal lining.

Two folds of the circular muscle layer form the ileocaecal valve, which controls the passage of material from the ileum to the caecum (first part of the large intestine). The circular muscle layer also forms the anal sphincters (see Fig. 21.2). The longitudinal muscle layer in the colon consists of three bands called taeniae coli (Fig. 21.2). The bands are shorter than the colon, producing a sacculated appearance, referred to as haustrations. The rectum and anal canal are surrounded by longitudinal muscle fibres, without haustrations.

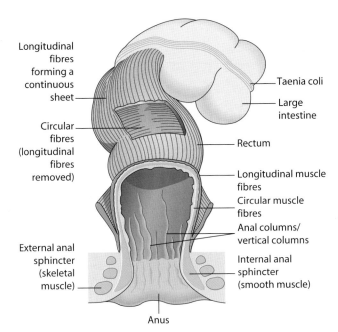

Fig. 21.2 • Rectum and anus. (Reproduced with permission from Waugh, A., Grant, A. (Eds.), 2010. Ross and Wilson anatomy and physiology, eleventh ed. Churchill Livingstone, Edinburgh.)

The submucosal layer contains lymphoid tissue, providing defence from microbes. Mucus-secreting cells line the colon and upper part of the rectum. The mucosa in the upper part of the anal canal is arranged in vertical folds, known as vertical columns (see Fig. 21.2). Each column contains a terminal branch of the superior rectal vein and artery. Stratified squamous epithelium lines the anus, which is continuous with the rectal mucosa, merging with the perianal skin outside the external sphincter.

The large intestine is about 1.5 metres in length, comprising the caecum, colon (ascending, transverse, descending and sigmoid), rectum and anal canal (see Fig. 21.1).

The caecum has a vermiform appendix. There is a T-junction where the ileocaecal valve opens into it. The ascending, transverse, and descending colon is named in relation to its anatomical position (see Fig. 21.1). At the pelvis, the descending colon becomes the sigmoid colon and then the rectum. The rectum is about 3 cm long in infants, growing to 13 cm in adults, terminating at the anal canal. The anal canal leads from the rectum to the exterior. It has two muscular sphincters: one internal (involuntary muscle); one external (voluntary skeletal muscle), which are involved in the process of defecation (see Fig. 21.2).

Functions

Functions of the large intestine, rectum and anal canal include:

- Microbial activity
- Absorption
- Mass movement of faeces.

Waste material remains in the large intestine for 12–24 hours before expulsion from the body as faeces. Bacteria that colonize the large intestine include *Escherichia coli*, *Enterobacter aerogenes*, *Streptococcus faecalis* and *Clostridium perfringens*, which digest waste products. Colonic bacteria can become pathogens if transferred to another part of the body (see Ch. 15). The bacteria metabolize remaining carbohydrates and amino acids, releasing gases, which contribute to faecal odour. Gas is expelled from the anus as flatus. In Western society, the passing of flatus is considered a natural bodily function, but offensive and unacceptable in public. Absorption in the large intestine is mostly of vitamins K and B group produced by microbial action, some electrolytes and water. Mass movements, long, slow, powerful contractile waves move over the colon during or after eating, propelling faeces towards the rectum.

Normal process of defecation

Involuntary, reflex or automatic defecation occurs in infancy because the infant has not yet developed voluntary control of their external anal sphincter. By the 2nd or 3rd year of life, a child usually has the ability to override the defecation reflex (see below). The rectum is normally empty, and the defecation reflex is initiated when faeces moves into it, causing stretching of the rectal walls. The defecation reflex is mediated through the spinal cord and causes the walls of the sigmoid colon and the rectum to contract and the anal sphincter to relax, allowing faeces to pass into the anal canal. These contractions bring with them a feeling of fullness. Once control has been achieved it is usually possible to delay the opening of the external anal sphincter (controlled through the pudendal nerve). Defecation is aided by voluntary contraction of the diaphragm and abdominal muscles to increase intra-abdominal pressure and force faeces down. This is achieved by the Valsalva manoeuvre – a forced expiration against a closed glottis (opening between the vocal cords).

Reflex defecation may occur after a stroke, with sacral spinal cord damage or damage to the pudendal nerve.

Factors affecting defecation

Many psychological, social, cultural and physical factors can affect defecation and bowel habit (Box 21.1).

Faecal elimination is a normal bodily function, but it carries a taboo. Many people isolate themselves when continence

---

Factors that affect defecation and bowel habit	Box 21.1

Physical factors

- Age – particularly at the extremes of age (see p. 520)
- Ignoring the urge to defecate – leads to constipation (alteration in normal bowel movements, resulting in the less frequent and uncomfortable passage of hard stools)
- Reduced physical activity/immobility – leading to constipation
- Mobility – lack of mobility can prevent the person accessing the lavatory
- Diet/type, amount of food, eating habits – lack of fibre causes constipation; some foods in excess, e.g. fruit, lead to diarrhoea (a loose watery stool that occurs frequently)
- Fluid intake – dehydration (see Ch. 19) causes constipation
- Hormones – constipation can occur during pregnancy.

Emotional/psychological factors

- Anxiety and stress – cause diarrhoea
- Low mood, depression and dementia – leading to constipation
- Life events such as bereavement or new sibling, etc. can affect bowel habit.

Facilities and environment

- Poor facilities (cold, dirty, dark, too many stairs, too far away)
- Lack of privacy
- Admission to hospital and use of a bedpan/commode.

All the above can cause people to ignore the urge to defecate, leading to constipation.

Bowel conditions

Congenital and acquired bowel conditions (see p. 524) both affect defecation and include:

- Gastroenteritis – causes diarrhoea
- Inflammatory bowel disease (IBD) – causes diarrhoea
- Intestinal obstruction – causes constipation
- Diverticular disease – causes constipation

- Colorectal cancer – causes a change in bowel habit (alternating diarrhoea/constipation)
- Painful anorectal conditions, e.g. haemorrhoids, cause people to 'put off' defecation.

Neurological conditions

Many neurological conditions can affect the bowel or sphincter control, e.g. multiple sclerosis, paraplegia or stroke. Multiple sclerosis and paraplegia can cause constipation.

Systemic conditions

- Underactive thyroid gland – causes constipation
- Overactive thyroid gland – causes diarrhoea
- Electrolyte imbalance (see Ch. 19), e.g. low potassium level in the blood (hypokalaemia) – causes constipation
- Food sensitivities and intolerance – cause diarrhoea
- Infection – causes diarrhoea.

Medication

- Opioids, e.g. morphine, codeine (see Ch. 23) – cause constipation
- Antibiotics – cause diarrhoea
- Laxatives (drugs that stimulate or increase evacuation of faeces from the bowel) – cause diarrhoea, especially if misused such as in eating disorders, or paradoxically constipation when overused
- Diuretics (see Ch. 20) can lead to excess fluid and potassium loss and cause constipation
- Antidepressants, e.g. amitriptyline, can cause constipation; fluoxetine can cause change in bowel habit
- Iron – causes altered bowel habit (constipation or diarrhoea)
- Antimuscarinics (anticholinergics), e.g. oxybutynin, causes constipation.

problems occur, due to feelings of shame, personal dirtiness and smells. In Western society, this can be related to sociocultural factors, where both the anal region and defecation are 'private'.

Age and defecation

In infants, defecation occurs involuntarily. Milk-fed infants normally have yellowish, malodorous faeces. Infants have small stomachs, and material moves rapidly through the GI tract. Four to six soiled nappies in 24 hours is not uncommon. Faecal soiling requires prompt cleansing to reduce discomfort. The infant is dependent upon parents/carers to attend to their elimination needs until they reach the stage of psychosocial and motor development that allows them to gain control over defecation. Potty training normally commences when the child is between 18 months and 2 years of age (Box 21.2). However, for some children with a physical or learning disability, this may not be possible (Box 21.3).

Developing control of defecation in healthy children	Box 21.2

In order to control defecation a child needs to:

- Have control over the anal sphincter
- Recognize the sensation to defecate and associate this with feeling clean, dry and comfortable
- Have the motor skills needed for sitting on a 'potty' or lavatory
- Have the ability to convey the need to defecate so the child can be provided with a potty or taken to the lavatory. The lavatory then becomes recognized and associated with defecation
- Associate the positive feedback of parents/carers with the activity of successful defecation.

This is assessed by an ability to convey the need to defecate, recognize an appropriate place, maintain a position for successful defecation and associate this with a positive response from grown-ups and the comfortable feeling of being clean and dry.

Reflective practice	Box 21.3

Children with a learning disability – development in relation to defecation

Think about how this aspect of development in children with a learning disability may be different from that in other children.

Student activity

- Find out what services are available in your area to support parents/carers of children with learning disabilities with this aspect of motor and psychosocial development.

Potty training is seen as a normal stage of development and parents will often produce a potty for the child to use in communal areas of the home (see also Ch. 20), encouraging the child to 'perform' in front of visitors, and positively praising the successful result when the potty is used. Parents/carers often take great pride in their child's successful potty training. When potty training is achieved, the child will progress to the

lavatory and suddenly asking to use a potty or removing underwear in front of others results in a reprimand, as this behaviour is now unacceptable. Elimination has become a private function. Behaviours learned as a child will influence attitudes and behaviours related to defecation throughout life.

Early experiences associated with defecation can influence toilet habits. A child may refuse to use a school lavatory, or develop a fear of a dark lavatory, which may lead to regression (see Ch. 11), resulting in soiling underclothes with urine and faeces as an alternative to visiting the lavatory. Constipation (see pp. 527–532) can develop if a child does not respond to the urge to defecate during school hours, retaining faeces until they can reach their own lavatory. In a young child, control over the bladder and bowel may be lost if the child is engrossed in a game, greatly excited or experiences great fear.

The lifestyle choices adopted during childhood and adolescence, such as poor diet and inactivity can persist into adulthood to affect defecation and health.

Age changes can affect defecation. A reduction in muscle strength and mobility makes older people susceptible to problems associated with elimination, e.g. constipation. The external sphincter may weaken or people can have reduced sensation, which may give rise to faecal soiling, e.g. when passing flatus. Older people are also more likely to take medications that affect bowel habit, e.g. non-steroidal anti-inflammatory drugs (NSAIDs) can cause diarrhoea, which may result in loss of continence.

There is also a greater risk of developing bowel (colorectal) cancer in those over 50 years of age (see pp. 523–524). An older person may be reluctant to seek help, due to embarrassment or concern about a cancer diagnosis.

Holistic assessment of defecation

Nurses are expected to show attentiveness, kindness and sensitivity (NMC 2010). Many patients are embarrassed to discuss elimination difficulties and the assessment interview requires privacy and a sensitive and skilled approach. Age-appropriate language should be used, e.g. a child or indeed some adults with learning disabilities may have special names for faeces (e.g. 'number 2' or 'poo'). The nurse should ask the parents/carers for this information.

It is important to work in partnership with patients/carers during the holistic assessment in order to develop a mutually agreed personal plan of care. Nurses will need to apply knowledge of age changes, developmental factors (see Ch. 8), related anatomy and physiology and bowel conditions.

Assessing normal bowel habit – patterns of defecation and characteristics of faeces

Normal bowel habit varies from person to person and changes during the lifespan. The normal stool frequency is between three per week and three per day (Walter et al 2010). Defining normal bowel habit is important when evaluating diarrhoea, constipation and other conditions affecting defecation, e.g. irritable bowel syndrome (IBS) (Walter et al 2010).

The assessment of stool type can be enhanced by the use of a pictorial assessment tool such as the Bristol Stool Form Scale

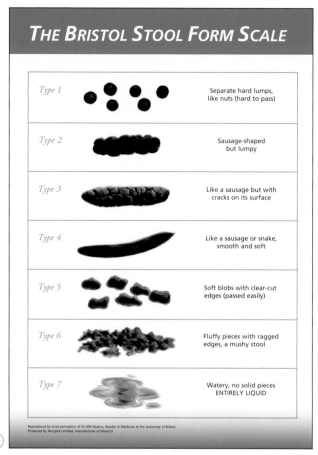

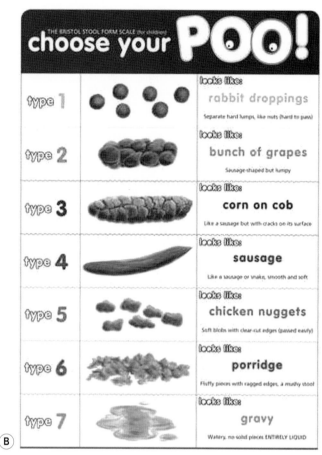

Fig. 21.3 • (A) Bristol Stool Form Scale. (Reproduced by kind permission of Dr KW Heaton, Reader in Medicine at the University of Bristol. ©2000, Norgine Ltd). (B) Children's Bristol Stool Form Scale (Concept by Professor DCA Candy and Emma Davey, based on the Bristol Stool Form Scale by Dr KW Heaton, Reader in Medicine at the University of Bristol. ©2005 Norgine Ltd.) For further copies of the Bristol Stool Form Scales, Freephone Norgine on 0800 269865 or e-mail mss@norgine.com.

(Fig. 21.3A) or the Children's Bristol Stool Form Scale, which uses child-friendly language to describe stool type (Fig. 21.3B). The nurse should measure fluid stools and record the volume lost on the fluid intake and output chart (see Ch. 19). Table 21.1 outlines the normal characteristics of faeces and defecation and some abnormalities.

Nursing history

When assessing and taking a history of a person's bowel habit, the nurse must ask about normal bowel habit, changes that have occurred, noting when they first occurred and how long they have been present. Unexplained changes may indicate diseases such as cancer. The nursing history typically includes information about the following:

- Usual bowel habit: how often, time of day, relation to mealtimes/hot drinks
- Does the person feel that their bowel habit is normal?
- Measures taken to promote defecation such as trying at the same time, after breakfast/hot drink, eating specific foods (e.g. dried apricots), avoiding foods that affect bowel habit, laxatives (see pp. 528–529)
- Does the person always respond to the urge for defecation
- The normal/usual stool colour, shape and consistency

- Usual fluid intake, types of food and preferences, amount of fibre, meal frequency and when main meal taken (see Ch. 19)
- How emotions affect defecation, e.g. anxiety about using a public lavatory
- Oral health, own teeth; if dentures are used are they well fitting? (see Ch. 16)
- Usual level of mobility, manual dexterity and exercise pattern
- Whether they use the lavatory, commode, bedpan or potty
- Is the person's lavatory modified, e.g. handrails or raised seat?
- Is the person independent for bowel care or do they need help?
- History of faecal soiling/incontinence
- Usual medication (over-the-counter and prescribed) and use of illegal drugs
- History of conditions, e.g. IBS, spinal injury, or surgery that might affect defecation
- The presence of a stoma that discharges faeces and, if so, the frequency and nature of discharge. Is the person self-caring?

Table 21.1 Characteristics of faeces and defecation

Characteristic	Normal	Abnormal
Frequency	Infants vary: breast milk 4–6 times/day or less; formula milk 1–3 times/day Adults: daily to 3 times/week	More than 6 times/day or less than once every 1–2 days More than 3 times/day or less than 3 times a week
Consistency (see Fig. 21.3)	Soft, formed	A range between the two extremes of: • Separate hard lumps in constipation • Completely liquid in diarrhoea
Amount	Adults: depends on fibre intake, stool weight is lighter for those with refined/processed diets than those with a vegetarian mixed diet.	Reduced volume with frequent stools
Colour	Infant: yellow Adult: brown	Clay/putty colour – absence of bile Green – gastroenteritis Red – eating beetroot Blood: • Bright red if lower GI bleeding • Melaena – characteristic offensive odour, black and tarry if bleeding from upper GI tract Black/grey with oral iron Pale if contains undigested fat
Shape	Resembles rectal diameter	Narrow 'ribbon stools' such as with increased peristalsis
Odour	Characteristic – depends on diet	Offensive if pus, fat or blood is present
Constituents	Water Intestinal epithelial cells Mucus Microorganisms Undigested fibre (non-starch polysaccharide (NSP)) Electrolytes Fat Stercobilin – pigment that colours faeces Various chemicals	Less water in constipation More water in diarrhoea Excess mucus and pus with inflammatory bowel disease (IBD) Blood – see above Foreign bodies Parasites, e.g. threadworms (Box 21.4), tapeworm segments
Flatus	Depends on diet, e.g. increases after beans, onions, etc.	May be reduced if the bowel is obstructed
Pain/discomfort on defecation (dyschezia)	Normally no pain or straining	Abdominal pain relieved by defecation Pain in the rectum (proctalgia) and anus during defecation Straining with constipation

- Changes in behaviour, e.g. a child who develops faecal incontinence after the birth of a sibling
- Increasing confusion or aggression in an older adult with dementia
- Change of environment such as moving into a care home
- Changes to routine or elimination habits
- Change in the mode of eliminating, e.g. frequency, pain, straining, increased flatus, etc.
- Changes to colour, consistency, shape or amount of faeces
- Have dietary habits altered? If so, how?
- Recent changes in health status.

A holistic assessment will ascertain how culture, beliefs and religious practices influence defecation (see p. 526). Acknowledging this individuality will ensure that the person's needs are met.

 Health promotion   **Box 21.4**

Threadworms

You have been asked by your mentor to help prepare an information sheet about threadworms (*Enterobius vermicularis*) for parents/carers.

Student activity

- Access the website below and prepare a summary of the main points concerning threadworm infestation in children and preventing reinfestation.

Resource

NHS Choices, 2011. Threadworms. Online. Available: www.nhs.uk/conditions/threadworms/Pages/Introduction.aspx September 2012.

Name: Hospital number:			Department/ward:			Consultant:			
Date	Time	Amount	Colour	Consistency (Bristol Scale 1–7)	Blood	Mucus	Comments, e.g. pain, flatus, straining, etc	Nurse's signature

Fig. 21.4 • Stool record chart.

Some people will resist the urge to defecate if this means using a lavatory other than their own and individual bowel assessment must incorporate any psychological and environmental factors affecting bowel habit.

It can be helpful for patients/parents to keep a diary of bowel actions to establish a pattern; this is particularly helpful when bowel-training programmes are in progress. Nurses should record bowel actions in the nursing notes and on the appropriate charts, e.g. a stool record chart (Fig. 21.4) and episodes of diarrhoea are measured and recorded on the fluid intake and output chart.

Common bowel conditions

Some knowledge of congenital and acquired conditions will assist patient assessment (Table 21.2).

Common investigations

There are many different investigations used to identify disorders affecting the large bowel and elimination of faeces (see also Ch. 19). These include:

- Blood tests – full blood count, urea and electrolytes
- X-rays – plain abdominal X-ray, barium enema
- Digital rectal examination (DRE)
- Stool/faecal samples – for microscopy, culture and sensitivity for infection, faecal occult blood (FOB, screening – see Box 21.5); fat content (3–5 day sample) and parasites

- Endoscopy including biopsy and treatments – rigid or flexible sigmoidoscopy (screening test), colonoscopy. Both sigmoidoscopy and colonoscopy involve the insertion of a long thin tube, with a camera, into the rectum and colon to observe the inside of the bowel. This allows the recording of images, biopsies of abnormal findings in the bowel lining, removal of polyps and other treatments (Box 21.6).
- Ultrasound scan (USS), computed tomography (CT), magnetic resonance imaging (MRI)
- Adhesive tape slides for threadworms.

Accessing the simple explanations of some of these investigations on the NHS choices website (see Useful websites, below) will help you provide patients with information.

Nursing interventions to promote defecation

Nurses can assist people by promoting normal defecation (Box 21.7), providing a suitable environment and facilities, preventing or dealing effectively with alterations such as constipation or diarrhoea and ensuring that privacy and dignity are maintained.

Alterations in defecation can include changes in frequency or consistency, loss of continence and the care needed following the formation of a stoma. Many alterations can be anticipated by the nurse and either prevented or at least minimized, such as being aware that people who have to use

Table 21.2 Common bowel conditions

Condition	Description
Appendicitis	Inflammation of the appendix
Irritable bowel syndrome (IBS)	A common condition of bowel dysfunction for which no organic cause can be found There is pain and passage of mucus rectally, with alternating diarrhoea and constipation
Inflammatory bowel disease (IBD): Crohn's disease and ulcerative colitis	Depending on the type and severity there is pain, diarrhoea, blood and mucus passed rectally, malabsorption, anaemia, weight loss and fever Complications include bowel obstruction and perforation, toxic dilatation, fluid and electrolyte disturbances (see Ch. 19) and colorectal cancer
Diverticular disease	The presence of sacs (diverticula) in the wall of the colon increases with age May be asymptomatic, may bleed, or become inflamed to cause diverticulitis, or perforate
Cancer of the colon or rectum (colorectal)	A common cancer in the UK (Box 21.5)
Rectal prolapse	The rectum is displaced downward and the mucosa may be visible outside the anus. Associated with chronic constipation and straining to defecate
Haemorrhoids (piles)	Varicosities in the rectum/anus; may be internal or external May occur with chronic constipation and straining May be itching, burning, pain and bleeding during defecation
Anal fissure	Break in the skin or anal mucosa, associated with constipation Causes pain/bleeding when passing faeces
Imperforate anus	Congenital anomaly where an infant does not have a patent anal opening or the anus does not communicate with the bowel above Corrected surgically
Hirschsprung's disease (congenital megacolon)	Defective nerve supply to the terminal colon leads to defective peristalsis, build-up of faeces, massive dilatation and bowel obstruction

Health promotion   Box 21.5

Colorectal cancer – early detection

A total of 39 991 people in the UK were diagnosed with colorectal cancer in 2008 (Cancer Research UK 2011). It is essential to seek professional advice early if any of the following occur:

- A change in bowel habit, diarrhoea or looser faeces lasting longer than 6 weeks, or constipation
- Bleeding from the rectum or blood and mucus passed with faeces
- A mass in the abdomen (right side), or in the rectum
- Feeling of incomplete emptying after defecation
- Pain in the rectum or abdomen

Plus less specific signs and symptoms, e.g. unplanned weight loss, signs/symptoms of anaemia such as tiredness.

A screening programme for colorectal cancer, using faecal occult blood (FOB) samples, is available throughout the UK. All people aged 60–75 years are invited for screening every 2 years. People aged 75 years or over can request screening.

At the time of writing, the NHS in England is planning to introduce a 'one-off' flexible sigmoidoscopy when people reach 55 years of age. People will be able to request the investigation up to their 60th birthday. Thereafter, people will be offered the FOB test described above.

Resource

NHS Cancer Screening Programmes:
www.cancerscreening.nhs.uk/ September 2012.

Critical thinking   Box 21.6

Mary – preparation for colonoscopy

Mary noticed blood on the tissue after defecation and eventually plucked up courage to see her GP who referred Mary to the hospital for a colonoscopy.

Student activities

- Find out what happens during a colonoscopy.
- Obtain a copy of the local patient information sheet about bowel preparation prior to colonoscopy, other bowel investigations and surgery.
- Identify the information needed by Mary so that she is physically and mentally well prepared for her investigation.

Resource

Cancer Research UK, 2011. Bowel cancer tests. Online. Available: http://cancerhelp.cancerresearchuk.org/type/bowel-cancer/diagnosis/bowel-cancer-tests September 2012.

a bedpan or commode (see pp. 526–527) are more likely to become constipated.

Many patients will require assistance with their faecal elimination needs. Nurses must give full explanations and obtain informed consent prior to interventions. Most people will want to use the lavatory. For those unable to do so, a bedpan, potty or commode will need to be provided promptly and efficiently to limit worries about 'accidents' and any embarrassment that the person may have. Where there is embarrassment about malodorous stools, the nurse can provide an air freshener to

Promoting normal defecation — Box 21.7

- Assessment of bowel habit and reassessment as required (see pp. 520–523)
- Encouraging regular habits, e.g. responding to the urge to defecate (Box 21.8)
- Promoting exercise and mobility (see Ch. 18); involve the MDT
- Encouraging a balanced, high-fibre diet (see Ch. 19)
- Maintaining or increasing fluid intake (see Ch. 19)
- Reviewing medication that may affect defecation (see Chs 12, 22 and 23)
- Relieving pain associated with defecation (see Ch. 23)
- Minimizing patient embarrassment through interpersonal skills (see Ch. 9)
- Providing suitable facilities for defecation
- Meeting privacy and dignity needs
- Being aware that the nurse's attitudes (comments or facial expressions when dealing with faeces) can affect a patient's bowel habit
- Meeting cultural or religious needs
- Anticipating and, where possible, preventing problems such as constipation
- Maintaining faecal continence
- Ensuring that nursing interventions are evidence-based (see Ch. 5)
- Contributing to a multiprofessional approach to patient management.

Health promotion — Box 21.8

Promoting good habits in children

Children should be encouraged to use the lavatory after breakfast prior to leaving home for school. They should be encouraged to use the school lavatory during play and lunch times but to always respond to the urge to defecate by asking to be excused if it occurs during class time. However, some children may be reluctant to defecate in the school lavatory.

Student activities

- Make a list of factors that might make a child reluctant to use the school lavatory.
- Select one of the factors and think about how the problem might be solved.

keep in the locker, which can be discreetly sprayed following the use of the bedpan/commode or carried to the lavatory in a dressing gown pocket. However, the nurse must first check that the patient and those close by have no breathing difficulties or allergies.

Environment and facilities

The importance of a suitable environment for bowel care is illustrated by it being a benchmark of best practice in the *Essence of Care 2010* (DH 2010) (Box 21.9).

Reflective practice — Box 21.9

Benchmarks for Bladder, Bowel and Continence Care

'All bladder and bowel care is given in an environment appropriate to *people's* needs and preferences' (DH 2010, p 19).

Student activities

- Think about an experience from a recent placement or when you were a patient and compare the care given against the benchmark above.
- Discuss with your mentor how this aspect of bowel care could be improved.

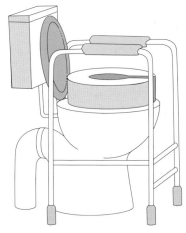

Fig. 21.5 • Use of raised seat and hand rails to promote independence at home. (From Jamieson, et al., 2007. Clinical Nursing Practices, fifth ed. Churchill Livingstone, Edinburgh.)

Patients/clients must be informed where the lavatory facilities are located. The nurse must show them and assess whether they need help to access the lavatory. A nurse call system/bell must be available.

The environment for elimination must be suitable for the purpose. The lavatory area must be clean, warm, dry, comfortable and private, with handwashing facilities to reduce the risk of infection (see Ch. 15). Lavatory tissue must be available and, for some people, running water to wash the perianal area. Adequate ventilation and/or air fresheners can reduce potential embarrassment regarding odour.

The normal position for defecation is sitting or squatting, leaning slightly forward to increase the intra-abdominal pressure with the Valsalva manoeuvre (see p. 519). A footstool may aid height and hip flexion for a child. A higher lavatory seat can aid people with reduced mobility as rising from a low lavatory will be difficult; again a footstool will aid correct positioning for defecation. The provision of a higher seat and handrails can maintain independence for many people (Fig. 21.5).

Space is essential for a person with a disability, to aid transfer to and from the lavatory. Handles fixed to the lavatory wall are an effective means of assisting with transfer. A change in environment, e.g. change in diet, new surroundings, can compromise bowel habit, particularly if accompanied by a change in the person's level of dependence. Some people will need assistance to use the lavatory (Box 21.10). People may need assistance to manipulate clothing due to lack of mobility or dexterity, or lack of understanding. Various adaptations to clothing may need to be considered in order to maintain the person's independence and dignity (Box 21.11).

 ### Nursing skills   Box 21.10

Taking a patient to the lavatory

- Respond immediately to the patient's request
- Put on plastic apron and non-sterile gloves if help is needed with personal hygiene
- Ascertain whether a stool specimen is required (see p. 533)
- Assist the patient from the bed or chair as required (see Ch. 18)
- Ensure the patient is wearing slippers and dressing gown to promote a safe environment and dignity
- Collect any personal items such as toiletries, sanitary towels, fresh underwear
- Guide to the lavatory cubicle or take in a wheelchair
- Offer assistance with clothing if required
- Remain in the immediate vicinity if the patient requests/ requires and maintain privacy
- Once the patient has defecated, offer assistance with personal hygiene, ensuring perianal area is clean and dry, and help with clothing. Consider cultural preferences for running water for hygiene purposes. When assisting females with personal hygiene, wipe from front to back to avoid bacterial contamination of the urethra (see Chs 16, 20)
- Offer handwashing facilities to the patient
- Remove gloves if you have assisted with personal hygiene and wash your hands
- Escort back to bed/chair, make sure that the patient is comfortable and has everything they need, e.g. call bell, drink, within reach
- Document bowel movement in patient records.

Reflective practice   Box 21.11

Adaptation to clothing

Think about a person who had difficulty removing clothing in order to use the lavatory. They may have had a learning disability or dementia, or had poor dexterity following a stroke, etc.

Student activities

- What particular difficulties did they experience?
- Research adaptations that might have helped.

Resource

Disabled Living Foundation. Clothing and footwear. Online. Available: www.livingmadeeasy.org.uk September 2012.

Cultural needs

Nurses must be able to provide sensitive, antidiscriminatory care that demonstrates an understanding of cultural, religious, gender and sexuality needs. For example, Sikhs, Hindus and Muslims require that nurses of the same gender meet their intimate hygiene needs (see Ch. 16). Personal hygiene is very important and washing with water after using the lavatory is normal practice for many groups. In Islam a cleansing ritual is performed before prayers and this becomes void after urination, defecation, passing flatus or vomiting and needs to be repeated (Akhtar 2002). Muslims also prefer to wash their genitalia and perianal area with running water after using the lavatory. Offering a jug of water following elimination will meet this need. The left hand is used for personal cleansing.

Bedpans and commodes

Some patients will need to use a bedpan or commode (Fig. 21.6). Many patients worry about spillages and offensive sounds and smells in the ward. Nurses must ensure that privacy and dignity are maintained and that care is culturally sensitive. Assisting a patient onto a bedpan or commode requires the nurse to complete an appropriate risk assessment for moving and handling (see Chs 13, 18). Box 21.12 outlines how the

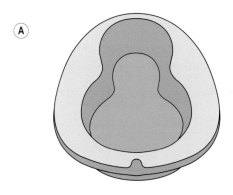

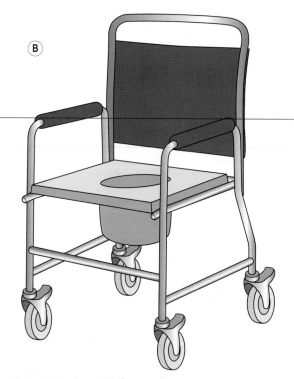

Fig. 21.6 • (A) Bedpan. (B) Commode.

Providing a bedpan or commode

- Respond immediately to request
- Put on plastic apron and non-sterile gloves (Ch. 15)
- Collect either the clean bedpan and a bedpan cover, or the commode from the sluice. The commode is first checked to ensure that the brakes are in working order and the commode is clean
- Take the bedpan or commode to the bedside; if using the commode, position and apply the brakes
- Draw curtains around the bed to promote privacy and dignity
- Ensure wipes and tissues are readily available
- Assist the patient onto the bedpan, if possible well supported in an upright position. Offer assistance if needed to remove/move clothing. Placing a disposable incontinence sheet under the bedpan will aid personal cleansing following defecation.

If a commode is used, ensure that slippers are worn by the patient to prevent slipping. Assist the patient from the bed to the commode, offering assistance to remove/move clothing. Once the patient is safely seated on the commode cover their knees with a blanket to promote dignity and maintain comfort

- Once the patient is safely seated on the bedpan or commode ensure support with balance is offered as required
- Instruct the patient not to remove themselves from the bedpan unaided as this may lead to injury or spillage of contents, or not to attempt to transfer themselves from commode to bed unaided
- Stay with the patient if they wish or require constant supervision, or ensure that the patient can reach the call bell to indicate they have finished
- Remove the commode or bedpan and ensure that the protective sheet is in place
- Offer assistance with personal cleansing as required and remove the incontinence sheet from beneath the patient. When assisting females, wipe from front to back to avoid bacterial contamination of the urethra (see Chs 16, 20)
- Remove the commode or covered bedpan with protective sheet to the sluice
- Observe the colour, amount and consistency of the stool passed (see p. 522)
- Take any required samples before disposing of the stool (see p. 533)
- Wash/sterilize/dispose of the bedpan, or clean the commode according to local policy (see Ch. 15)
- Remove and dispose of apron and gloves and wash hands (see Ch. 15)
- Return to the patient to offer handwashing equipment: wet and dry wipes, or a bowl, jug of water and hand towels (see Ch. 15). Respect cultural preferences
- Ensure that the patient is comfortable and has everything they need, e.g. call bell, drink, within reach
- Make sure the immediate environment is tidy, use air-freshener as necessary and open the curtains
- Document bowel action in patient records and report any abnormalities.

nurse can provide a bedpan or commode safely, while maintaining privacy and dignity.

Commodes provide a more normal position for defecation and can be used in the lavatory for greater privacy. The commode can be used beside the bed, if privacy and dignity can be ensured. A patient may be transferred from the bed to a wheelchair, taken to the lavatory and there transferred to the commode, which can be moved over the lavatory. The commode should never be used for transport between the bed and lavatory due to the risk of cross-infection.

Constipation

A precise definition for constipation can be difficult given the normal variation in bowel habit. Useful definitions may be:

- Bowel movements less than three times a week
- Needing to strain during defecation on more that 25% of times
- Passing pellet-like or hard faeces on more than 25% of times (NHS choices 2010)

(see Further reading, below, e.g. Rome Foundation criteria). A person's perception of their own constipation may be the most accurate (Kyle 2008).

Constipation is usually temporary and not life-threatening. People often treat it with over-the-counter (OTC) laxatives without advice from a healthcare professional. This can lead to recurrence however, and a key part in the management of constipation is education for prevention (see Box 21.7, p. 525). When there is no underlying medical cause for recurrent episodes of constipation, the term chronic idiopathic constipation is used. Many people do seek medical advice and in the UK, several million pounds are spent each year on prescriptions for constipation and OTC laxatives.

Constipation may be secondary to systemic or bowel disease and a thorough assessment on presentation is undertaken to ensure that underlying disease is detected.

Contributing factors and causes of constipation

The dry, hard stools of constipation occur when the colon absorbs too much water. This happens when the muscular contractions of the colon are sluggish, and movement of the stool through the colon is slow. Lack of fibre in the diet reduces bulk, slowing down motility. Most people will experience an episode of constipation at some time or another such as during pregnancy, following childbirth or surgery.

Constipation affects all age groups. It is most common in the very young and older adults. Constipation in children has a prevalence of between 5–30% (National Institute for Health and Clinical Excellence, NICE 2010). Constipation is not an inevitable consequence of ageing, it is usually due to factors such as lack of exercise and a reduction in the consumption of fruit, vegetables, bread and reduced fluid intake. Older people may drink less in an attempt to control urinary incontinence (see Ch. 20), particularly if mobility is poor and assistance with reaching the lavatory is required. Fibre intake is positively associated with increased frequency of bowel movement and faecal mass.

Box 21.1 (p. 519) outlines factors that affect defecation and bowel habit, including those that cause constipation. Nurses should always be aware of situations, such as during pregnancy

Box 21.13 Preventing constipation and promoting continence in pregnancy and following childbirth

Approximately 40% of women experience constipation during their pregnancy (NHS choices 2010). Lifestyle advice by midwives and general practitioners (GPs) to prevent/treat constipation includes increasing dietary fibre, fluid intake and appropriate exercise. The taking of laxatives may be necessary if constipation persists. Poorly absorbed laxatives such as bulk forming types, e.g. bran, should initially be prescribed for pregnant women (*British National Formulary*, BNF 2012). However, it may be necessary for the GP or other prescriber to prescribe an osmotic laxative, e.g. lactulose, or a stimulant laxative, e.g. senna (BNF 2012).

Pain may be experienced during elimination, stinging when passing urine and pain due to the increased abdominal pressure required to force faeces downwards during defecation. Women may avoid/limit elimination to avoid pain, leading to urinary tract infection (see Ch. 20) and constipation.

Damage to the anal sphincters is not uncommon during a woman's first vaginal delivery. After delivery women many experience difficulties with elimination following episiotomy (a perineal incision to enlarge the vaginal outlet) or perineal tear, due to the wound, sutures and bruising. Women who experience a third degree tear may develop faecal incontinence, despite surgical repair.

While encouragement with diet, fluids, movement and personal hygiene to aid healing are offered, keeping the pelvic floor muscles strong to provide support to the bladder, bowel and the uterus in pregnant women is also essential. Pelvic floor exercises are encouraged both during pregnancy and following the birth, to maintain a healthy pelvic floor, and to promote continence. While there are different pelvic floor exercises for different muscles, pelvic floor exercises usually require the muscles around the rectum to be tightened (lifting the perineum), and the tightness maintained for as long as possible, relaxing and repeating the exercise. Physiotherapists support midwives in teaching and encouraging women to do these exercises during pregnancy and after the birth of their baby. Women with a history of continence difficulties will require referral to a continence nurse specialist, for assessment and a plan of treatment.

Resource

Chartered Society of Physiotherapists (CSP), 2009. Personal training for your pelvic floor muscles: www.csp.org.uk/sites/files/csp/secure/Pesonal-training-pelvic-floor.pdf.

(Box 21.13), when constipation is likely to occur and anticipate the need for interventions, e.g. laxatives when opioid drugs are used for pain relief (see Ch. 23).

Effects of constipation

The effects of constipation include:

- Abdominal colic
- Flatulence, bloating
- Lethargy and feeling generally unwell
- Irritability and fretfulness in children, e.g. no interest in play
- Excessive straining during defecation
- Headache
- Nausea
- Halitosis ('bad breath')
- Faecal impaction with overflow diarrhoea (spurious). This may be mistakenly diagnosed as diarrhoea. Antidiarrhoeal drugs should never be prescribed, this will exacerbate the constipation
- An abdominal mass
- Increased confusion in people with dementia
- Changes in behaviour and distress in people with a learning disability
- Sudden or worsening urinary incontinence due to hard faeces pressing on the bladder or urethra.

Assessment of constipation

A thorough and complete assessment and history are essential to determine the normal bowel habit for the person (see pp. 520–523) and to identify contributing factors or causes for constipation (see Box 21.1). Constipation can be a chronic problem.

Self-assessment of bowel habit is helpful and the person/parent can be taught the use of the Bristol Stool Form Scale (see Fig. 21.3). They may be asked to log their dietary and fluid intake and keep a record of daily exercise.

A doctor or a registered nurse who is appropriately trained and competent will perform a physical examination. This will include:

- Abdominal palpation, which may reveal the presence of a faecal mass
- DRE involving the insertion of a lubricated gloved finger into the rectum. It can be performed to assess tone of the anal sphincter and rectal contents. Normally, the rectum is empty but can often contain hard stools in constipation. Explicit informed consent must be obtained from the patient/parent, and documented in nursing and medical records (Royal College of Nursing, RCN 2008).

Management of constipation

Most people who experience constipation will not require extensive investigation and can be successfully treated with lifestyle changes that include increasing fluid intake, exercise and fibre content of the diet (see Ch 19).

Laxatives may be prescribed. They are only used if the person is constipated and the cause is not an undiagnosed condition such as intestinal obstruction. Laxatives (also known as aperients) are drugs that cause the bowel to empty in a variety of ways. There are several types of laxatives; most commonly used are four basic types (below), plus bowel cleansing solutions (Table 21.3):

- Bulking agents
- Faecal softeners
- Stimulants
- Osmotic.

Laxatives can be administered orally, rectally as suppositories or as an enema. Many patients will self-administer enemas or suppositories and parents/carers can also be shown how to do this. A degree of mobility and manual dexterity is required.

Table 21.3 Laxatives – oral and rectal

Type	Examples and routes	Action/comments
Bulking agents	Bran, ispaghula, sterculia and methylcellulose (also a faecal softener) – oral	Increase fibre in the stool, thereby increasing the water absorption by the stool Produces softer, bulkier stool, which stimulates peristalsis and is easier to pass *Note:* Sufficient oral fluids are required to prevent intestinal obstruction
Faecal softeners	Arachis oil retention enema *Note:* Rectal arachis oil is obtained from peanut/groundnut oil and must never be administered to a person with peanut allergy	Softens the stool and also lubricates the hard stool, making it easier to pass
Stimulants	Senna – oral Bisacodyl – oral and rectal (suppositories) Docusate sodium (also a softener) – oral and rectal (micro-enema) Dantron – oral Glycerol suppositories – rectal Sodium picosulfate (Picolax®) – oral	Stimulate the nerves in the colon and increase intestinal motility Used for bowel cleansing (see below)
Osmotic laxatives	Lactulose – oral Phosphate and sodium citrate enemas, e.g. Fleet® Ready-to-use Enema, Micralax® Micro enema® – rectal Macrogols, e.g. macrogol, Movicol® – oral	Act by drawing water into the colon or retaining water in the colon by osmosis, thus distending the colon and stimulating peristalsis
Bowel cleansing solutions	Various preparations, e.g. macrogol oral powder (non-proprietary), Fleet Phospho-soda®, Picolax®	Used before colonoscopy examination, barium enema or bowel surgery
Peripheral opioid-receptor antagonists	Methylnaltrexone	Use in palliative care to treat constipation associated with opioid analgesics
5HT$_4$-receptor agonists	Prucalopride	Can be used for women with chronic constipation unrelieved by other laxatives

People who self-administer should be directed to the manufacturer's instructions and advised to contact their practice nurse or GP if problems arise.

Bowel cleansing solutions are used to empty the lower bowel before investigations that include colonoscopy and barium enema X-ray (see Box 21.6 and p. 523) and before bowel surgery. Laxatives are also prescribed to prevent constipation, e.g. when people are receiving opioid drugs to relieve pain (BNF 2012).

Enemas

An enema (evacuant or retention) is the introduction of fluid into the rectum or lower bowel for the purpose of producing a bowel movement or instilling medication. The drugs administered rectally include corticosteroids used in inflammatory bowel disease (IBD), etc. (see Ch. 22).

• *Evacuant*, e.g. phosphate enemas supplied in single dose packs with a standard or long rectal tube, or sodium citrate micro enema (Fig. 21.7). These are used to evacuate the rectum and lower colon of flatus and faecal matter. The enema solution is retained for a short time only (always follow the manufacturer's recommendations and local policy) and is then expelled from the bowel along with faeces and flatus
• *Retention*, e.g. single-dose arachis oil enema (see Fig. 21.7). Retention enemas are usually retained in the

bowel for longer than an evacuant enema in order to soften and lubricate impacted faeces, making it easier to pass.

Informed patient/parent consent must be obtained. The patient must understand what an enema involves, and what is required of them, i.e. retention of the enema solution. The patient must understand the benefits and risks of the intervention in relation to symptom relief, and that this will be short term. A nurse of the same gender as the patient may minimize embarrassment during administration of the enema. Contraindications include:

• Intestinal obstruction
• Paralytic ileus – lack of peristalsis, common after surgery when the bowel has been handled
• Where there is risk of circulatory overload (see Ch. 19)
• Following certain types of gastrointestinal or gynaecological surgery unless written medical consent is given
• IBD.

The enema must be prescribed by an appropriately qualified practitioner and local policy followed regarding checks on medication and patient identity for the administration of medicines (see Ch. 22). Box 21.14 outlines how the nurse can administer an enema safely and effectively while maintaining privacy and dignity.

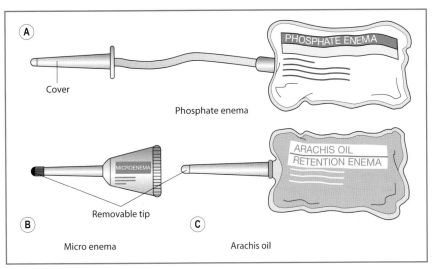

Fig. 21.7 • Types of enema. (From Nicol, et al., 2008. Essential nursing skills, third ed. Mosby, Edinburgh.)

 Nursing skills

Box 21.14

Enema administration – adults

Equipment

- Incontinence pads to protect bed/trolley
- Disposable gloves and apron
- Disposable wipes and tissues
- Prescribed enema/prescription chart
- Jug of water at required temperature, bath thermometer
- Lubricating gel
- Commode or bedpan and tissue, or access to a lavatory.

Preparation

- Explain the procedure to ensure informed consent
- Check that patient does not have a peanut/groundnut allergy before giving an arachis oil enema
- Ensure privacy by using a treatment room or pull curtains around the bed. Ask other staff to avoid interruptions
- Some enemas need to be warmed 'in a jug of water to a hand-hot temperature' (Kyle 2007, p 27). Always follow the manufacturer's recommendations for single, pre-prepared products
- Assist the patient into the left lateral position, with knees flexed (Fig. 21.8). This allows the nozzle or tubing of the enema to follow the natural anatomy of the rectum (Nicol et al 2008)
- Place an incontinence pad/sheets under the patient's hips and buttocks to protect the bedding and relieve potential distress if fluid is expelled from the anus
- Cover the lower body with a blanket to maintain dignity
- Put on a protective apron, wash hands and put on non-sterile gloves (see Ch. 15).

Procedure

- Lubricate the enema nozzle to minimize anal/rectal trauma
- Separate the patient's buttocks and observe for soreness or other abnormalities
- Introduce the nozzle into the anal canal, which is approximately 3.8 cm in length in adults, and then advance to approximately 10 cm to ensure the tip reaches the rectum. This is normally the full length of the nozzle for pre-prepared enemas

- To administer an evacuant enema, roll the packaging slowly from bottom to top to prevent backflow of the solution into the packet
- Remove the nozzle slowly while still keeping the bag rolled, and encourage the patient to hold onto the solution for as long as possible; however, the effect can be rapid and the patient should not be left without easy access to a nurse call bell
- A retention enema should also be introduced slowly. Again the patient is encouraged to hold onto the solution for as long as prescribed. If possible, this may be aided by raising the foot of the bed against gravity
- Wipe the patient's perianal/perineal area and leave them clean and dry. Cover the patient
- Ensure access to a nurse call bell, a bedpan, a commode or lavatory. When called, give any assistance required (see Box 21.12)
- Take the commode or covered bedpan with protective sheet to the sluice
- Observe the colour, amount and consistency of the stool passed (see p. 522)
- Collect faecal specimen if required (see Box 21.16)
- Wash/sterilize/dispose of the bedpan, or clean the commode according to local policy (see Ch. 15)
- Remove and dispose of apron and gloves and wash hands (see Ch. 15)
- Return to the patient to offer facilities for personal hygiene and handwashing: wet and dry wipes, or a bowl, jug of water and hand towels. Respect cultural preferences
- Ensure that the patient is comfortable and has everything they need, e.g. call bell, drink, within reach
- Make sure the immediate environment is tidy, use air-freshener as necessary and open the curtains
- Document the type of enema given, the resultant bowel action and any specimens collected in patient records and report any abnormalities
- Continue to monitor bowel function, along with reassessment and evaluation of the patient's presenting symptoms.

Suppositories

Rectal suppositories, like enemas, are used to evacuate the lower bowel. They are also used to administer prescribed medications, e.g. bronchodilators, antibiotics and analgesics (see Chs 22, 23). More commonly, they are used to relieve consti-

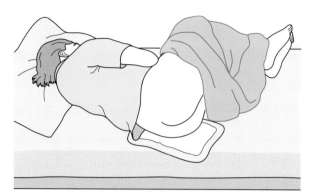

Fig. 21.8 • Left lateral position for administration of enemas and suppositories.

pation. Lubricant suppositories such as glycerol can be purchased without prescription (see Table 21.3).

The procedure for administering suppositories is similar to that for an enema (Box 21.15). If administering a medicated suppository, the patient should first empty their bowel if possible, this enables better suppository retention and drug absorption. Contraindications include:

- Intestinal obstruction
- Paralytic ileus
- Following certain types of gynaecological or gastrointestinal surgery unless written medical consent is given.

Manual faecal evacuation

Patients with chronic constipation may require manual faecal evacuation. This must only be undertaken by a registered practitioner who is trained and competent in the procedure and has obtained the person's informed consent. Prior to this procedure, the patient's pulse rate is recorded, noting rhythm, regularity and strength as well as rate (see Chs 14,

---

 Nursing skills Box 21.15

Administration of suppositories

Equipment

- Incontinence pads to protect bed/trolley
- Disposable gloves and apron
- Disposable wipes and tissues
- Prescribed suppositories/prescription chart
- Lubricating gel
- Commode or bedpan and lavatory tissue, or easy access to a lavatory.

Preparation

- Explain the procedure to ensure informed consent
- Ensure privacy by using a treatment room or pull curtains around the bed. Ask other staff to avoid interruptions
- Assist the patient into the left lateral position, with knees flexed (see Fig. 21.8)
- Place an incontinence pad/sheets under the patient's hips and buttocks to protect the bedding and relieve potential distress if fluid is expelled from the anus
- Cover the lower body with a blanket to maintain dignity
- Put on a protective apron, wash hands and put on non-sterile gloves (see Ch. 15).

Procedure

- Follow manufacturer's recommendations. Lubricate the apex (pointed) end of the suppository.

Note: There is continuing debate regarding whether suppositories should be inserted apex or base (blunt-end) foremost. Manufacturers generally advise apex foremost insertion. Bradshaw and Price (2007) consider the reliability of the evidence which highlights the requirement for further studies in order to supply reliable evidence.

- Separate the patient's buttocks and insert the suppository (Fig. 21.9), using your index finger to advance the suppository. Repeat for a second suppository.

- Wipe the patient's perianal/perineal area and leave them clean and dry. Cover the patient
- Ask the patient to retain the suppositories for as long as possible, up to 20 minutes, for evacuant suppositories to melt and soften the stool, making it easier to pass
- Ensure access to a nurse call bell, a bedpan, a commode or lavatory. Give assistance as required (see Box 21.12)
- Remove commode or covered bedpan with protective sheet to the sluice
- Observe the colour, amount and consistency of the stool passed (see p. 522)
- Collect faecal specimen if required (see Box 21.16)
- Wash/sterilize/dispose of the bedpan, or clean the commode according to local policy (see Ch. 15)
- Remove and dispose of apron and gloves and wash hands (see Ch. 15)
- Return to the patient to offer facilities for personal hygiene and handwashing: wet and dry wipes, or a bowl, jug of water and hand towels. Respect cultural preferences
- Ensure that the patient is comfortable and has everything they need, e.g. call bell, drink, within reach
- Make sure the immediate environment is tidy, use air-freshener as necessary and open the curtains
- Document the type of suppositories given, the resultant bowel action and any specimens obtained in patient records and report any abnormalities
- Continue to monitor bowel function, along with reassessment and evaluation of the patient's presenting symptoms

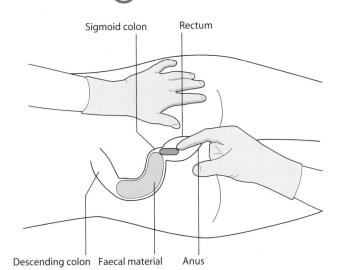

Fig. 21.9 • Insertion of a rectal suppository. (From Jamieson, et al., 2007. Clinical nursing practices, fifth ed. Churchill Livingstone, Edinburgh.)

17). This will serve as a baseline, as it is important to respond to changes in the patient's condition during this procedure, as manual evacuation can cause vagal stimulation and slow the heart rate. A second nurse present is able to constantly monitor and reassure the patient. Privacy and dignity for the patient must be maintained at all times (Royal College of Nursing 2008).

Diarrhoea

Diarrhoea, like constipation, is difficult to define. Spiller and Thompson (2010) refer to diarrhoea as the urgent passage of liquid stools, eight times per day. Diarrhoea occurs in many acute and chronic gastrointestinal disturbances. Transit through the bowel is rapid, and loose stools indicate that the bowel mucosa is irritated and is not absorbing enough water from the stool.

Contributing factors and causes of diarrhoea

Chronic diarrhoea may be associated with underlying pathology such as IBD (see Table 21.2, p. 524) or malabsorption due to lactose intolerance. Causes of acute diarrhoea include:

- Side-effects of treatment (e.g. radiotherapy), medication (e.g. antibiotics) or enteral feeding via a nasogastric tube (see Ch. 19)
- Infections, e.g. bacterial or viral gastroenteritis, which are a common cause of diarrhoea in infants and small children (see Ch. 15)
- The use of broad-spectrum antibiotics which can predispose to superinfection with the bacterium *Clostridium difficile;* this leads to pseudomembranous colitis and is responsible for outbreaks of diarrhoea in many clinical areas and care settings
- Food intolerance or allergic reaction

- Stress and anxiety
- Change in diet or excesses, e.g. alcohol or fatty food.

(See Box 21.1, p. 519.)

Effects of diarrhoea

The effects of diarrhoea include:

- Foul smelling, watery stools with loss of nutrients
- Increased frequency
- Loss of fluid and electrolytes – potentially life-threatening, e.g. in infants, children and frail older people (see Ch. 19)
- Perianal soreness
- Flatulence and faecal soiling
- Abdominal pains and cramps
- Nausea/vomiting, and pyrexia, e.g. with infective diarrhoea
- Poor appetite
- Headache
- Embarrassment and urgency to access a lavatory
- Loss of continence.

Note: It is vital to exclude faecal impaction with faecal leakage (spurious diarrhoea) (see p. 528).

Assessment of diarrhoea

A thorough and complete assessment and history are essential to determine the normal bowel habit for the person (see pp. 520–523) and to identify any contributing factors or causes for the diarrhoea (see Box 21.1, p. 519).

Episodes of diarrhoea are recorded on a stool chart (see Fig. 21.4, p. 523). Frequent, loose watery stools should be measured and recorded on the fluid intake/output chart in order to assess fluid loss. Self-assessment of bowel habit using, e.g. the Bristol Stool Form Scale (see Fig. 21.3, p. 521) can be helpful. Dietary intake should be recorded.

Management of diarrhoea

Management depends on whether the diarrhoea is acute or chronic. Dehydration must be prevented. Adults and children are advised to take frequent sips of water (NHS choices 2011). Oral dehydration salts can be purchased OTC following advice from the pharmacist (see Ch. 19).

Adults should eat solid food if they feel well enough and if children are not dehydrated, they can be offered their normal solid food (NHS choices 2011). Where people do not feel like eating, they should continue to drink and try to eat when they feel able.

Infants with diarrhoea should be fed as normal if they will breast-feed or take formula milk. The formula feed should be of usual strength. If oral rehydration preparations are used, breast or formula milk should continue to be offered between oral rehydration fluids (BNF 2012).

Adults may use antidiarrhoeal drugs, e.g. loperamide. The presence of a high temperature, or blood or mucus in their stool, means medical advice should be sought. Parents and carers should not give OTC antidiarrhoeal drugs to children. Nursing interventions include those to:

Nursing skills   Box 21.16

Collection of stool/faecal sample

The patient or parent/carer often collects the sample at home and should follow the instructions provided with the sample container. Stool samples are also collected for faecal occult blood testing and for the presence of parasites.

Equipment

- Disposable gloves and apron
- Bedpan or commode
- Sterile stool sample container (with integral spatula) and specimen bag
- Request form for microbiology.

Preparation

- Explain the procedure to the patient to ensure informed consent
- Collect the specimen container, request form and transport bag
- Put on plastic apron and non-sterile gloves (see Ch. 15)
- Ensure privacy. Where possible the person should go to the lavatory to produce a sample; where this is not possible the person is offered a bedpan or the commode
- Ensure that a nurse call bell is available and assist as required
- Place a clinically clean bedpan beneath the lavatory seat
- Ideally the person should void urine separately, but if this is not possible lavatory tissue in the bedpan will absorb most of the urine
- The bedpan/commode is removed to the sluice and the stool examined for colour and consistency, and evidence of parasites (see p. 522)
- Open the faecal sample container and use the integral spatula (fixed in the lid) to collect a small amount of faeces from the bedpan and place the faeces and spatula in the container. Make sure that the sample container lid is securely closed
- Dispose of the remaining excreta in line with local policy
- Wash/sterilize/dispose of the bedpan, or clean the commode according to local policy (see Ch. 15)
- Assist with hygiene needs if required
- Remove gloves and apron and wash hands
- Label the specimen container with the correct patient information and enclose in a specimen bag with the completed request form
- Arrange for transfer to the laboratory
- Document the observation made of the faecal matter on the stool chart
- Record date and time the specimen was collected in patient records.

- Ensure that the person is located close to the lavatory, has an en-suite side ward or a bedpan/commode readily available
- Provide adequate ventilation and/or air fresheners to minimize embarrassment
- Provide soft tissue or wet wipes or use of a bidet
- Provide assistance with perianal hygiene and change pads or napkins promptly to prevent skin damage, observing for soreness and applying barrier cream

- Provide clean clothes and bed linen
- Observe for signs of fluid depletion (see Ch. 19)
- Ensure adequate fluid replacement (see Ch. 19)
- Implement infection prevention and control measures such as handwashing and seek advice from Infection Control Nurses (see Ch. 15)
- Collect a faecal sample for microbiological examination (Box 21.16)
- Provide appropriate dietary and food hygiene advice (Box 21.17).

Health promotion   Box 21.17

Preventing travellers' diarrhoea

Travellers' diarrhoea is usually caused by viruses and as such does not respond to antibiotics. However, some types are bacterial. The source is often the water supply in areas where sanitation and general hygiene are poor.
Advice to travellers about preventing diarrhoea includes:

- Using bottled water (sealed bottles) for drinking and teeth cleaning
- Avoiding ice cubes in cold drinks
- Avoiding salads and uncooked foods
- Washing hands after using the lavatory and before eating
- Obtaining necessary vaccinations before travelling
- Carrying a supply of antidiarrhoeal drugs and oral rehydration salts.

Resource

NHS Choices, 2011. Travellers' diarrhoea – prevention: www.nhs.uk/conditions/travellersdiarrhoea/pages/whileyoureaway.aspx September 2012.

Faecal incontinence

Faecal incontinence, is described as the recurrent and uncontrolled passage of liquid or solid faeces (Bharucha and Wald 2010). The defining characteristics for faecal incontinence include:

- Faecal soiling
- Involuntary passage of faeces (in a socially inappropriate place)
- Lack of awareness of the urge to defecate, or muddling the sense with that of passing flatus.

Faecal incontinence is a taboo subject with a high degree of social stigma; it is often associated with regression and lack of control.

Current epidemiological information shows that between 1% and 10% of adults are affected with faecal incontinence, depending on the definition and frequency of faecal incontinence used. It is likely that 0.5–1.0% of adults experience regular faecal incontinence that affects their quality of life.

(NICE 2007, p 1).

However, faecal incontinence tends to be underreported because people find it repugnant and are often reluctant to seek help, meaning its prevalence is underestimated.

Faecal incontinence in children is referred to as encopresis, defined as repeated involuntary or voluntary faecal soiling of clothing by a child over 4 years of age (see p. 535).

Continence services are available, and need to be accessible for all and this is made clear in the benchmark of best practice: 'People and carers have direct access to staff who can advise them on continence management' (DH 2010, p 8). Integrated continence services span both primary and secondary care settings, focusing on healthy living and ensuring specialist continence advice for maintaining both faecal and urinary continence and care if continence is lost (Box 21.18). The philosophy underpinning such services is that promoting continence will reduce the incidence of incontinence.

Reflective practice Box 21.18

Continence services

Think about a patient/client or a relative who had faecal incontinence.

Student activities

- Did this person have support from the continence service?
- Is there an integrated continence service with a specialist continence nurse available in your area?

Causes of faecal incontinence

The causes of faecal incontinence include:

- Constipation – among the commonest causes in older people
- Diarrhoea – such as with IBD
- Pelvic floor problems, including loss of sensation, weak muscles or rectal prolapse in older people. May be caused by damage during childbirth many decades earlier
- Loss of sensation caused by damage to nerves controlling sphincter/rectum, e.g. long-term straining to defecate, stroke, spina bifida and conditions such as multiple sclerosis
- Sphincter abnormalities or damage, e.g. after haemorrhoid surgery, or reduced rectal capacity caused by chronic inflammation, surgery, etc.

Factors that contribute to faecal incontinence include dementia, lack of facilities or poor access, immobility and poor manual dexterity.

Box 21.1 (p. 519) outlines factors that affect bowel habit, many of which can lead to loss of continence, e.g. faecal impaction with overflow (spurious) diarrhoea.

Effects of faecal incontinence

The effects of faecal incontinence include:

- Embarrassment caused by odour and noisy/explosive defecation

- Low self-esteem
- Urgency to defecate
- Perianal soreness
- Risk of pressure ulcer development (see Ch. 25)
- Behaviours to conceal problem, e.g. hiding soiled underwear
- Financial – clothing/pads/laundry
- Social – isolation and loneliness, need for proximity to lavatory.

Access to a lavatory is a major concern for people who experience urgency to defecate, particularly those with IBD who have bowel actions that are explosive, noisy and malodorous (Box 21.19).

Reflective practice Box 21.19

Urgency and defecation

23-year-old Rosa has IBD and needs to plan any outings very carefully because if she is unable to respond at once to the urge to defecate she will soil her underwear. She needs to know the location of every public lavatory and always has clean underwear, a bag for soiled pants and wet wipes in her bag.

Student activities

- Consider with another student the psychological and social impact of the potential for faecal incontinence on this young woman's life.
- How would you feel about the possibility of being 'caught short' in a public place?

Assessment of faecal incontinence

When a person with faecal incontinence has the confidence to seek help, it is important that the nurse empowers the person/carer to be involved in the assessment and care planning process, maximizing comfort and dignity. Consideration for the person affected and their and the carers' ability to cope is important. The nurse should promote self-caring where appropriate or assist/make provision for those unable to maintain their own continence.

A full patient history and physical assessment, will determine a person's normal bowel habit (see pp. 520–523), identifying contributing factors/causes for faecal incontinence and quality of life issues (see Box 21.1, p. 519). Assessment should also include a DRE (with consent) by a trained and competent health professional, unfortunately this is not always performed, for example only 15% of older people in care homes had this examination (Royal College of Physicians 2010). Mobility and manual dexterity, and access to appropriate facilities for defecation must be assessed, along with factors including cognition and motivation. Those with dementia or learning disability should be afforded the same care and treatment during assessment and management of faecal incontinence as other people (NICE 2007).

Episodes of incontinence can be recorded on a stool chart (see Fig. 21.4, p. 523) and self-assessment of bowel habit using, e.g. the Bristol Stool Form Scale (see Fig. 21.3, p. 521) can be helpful. Keeping a diary of food and fluid intake and regular exercise pattern is also helpful.

Managing faecal incontinence

Management depends on the cause. It is often secondary to constipation and may be resolved through the following:

- Laxatives (oral or rectal) (see pp. 528–531)
- Increased fibre and fluid intake
- Regular meal times
- Increased exercise (stimulates gastrointestinal motility)
- Immediate response to the urge to defecate when normal sensation/sphincter muscle function is present.

Toileting programmes that follow the person's previous normal bowel habit, such as sitting on the lavatory after breakfast, are helpful. For patients requiring assistance to the lavatory, an immediate response from the nurse to the patient's request is essential before the gastrocolic reflex subsides.

When patients have impairment of both sensation and sphincter control, as in conditions such as multiple sclerosis, the bowel is usually emptied by routine administration of enemas or suppositories (see pp. 531, 532).

Antidiarrhoeal drugs such as loperamide may be used to produce a more formed stool if the faecal incontinence is due to a very liquid stool.

Advanced methods such as biofeedback are used by specialist nurses and physiotherapists to retrain the anal sphincter muscles that control release of faeces. Other methods may be more radical and involve surgery; these interventions will be specific to the cause, i.e. rectal prolapse.

Continence may not be achievable and nurses will need to plan care that minimizes the effects while continuing to promote continence. This care includes:

- Maintaining dignity and privacy
- Advice regarding suitable underwear, e.g. for use with small pads
- Providing appropriate pads
- Protection for bedding/chairs
- Skin care, cleanliness and use of barrier cream
- Checking for skin damage (see Ch. 25)
- Education about safe disposal of pads, etc.
- Ensuring that patients are aware of entitlement to benefits, e.g. attendance allowance
- Providing contact details of support groups (see Useful websites, below).

Encopresis

There is sometimes confusion caused in diagnosis of encopresis and faecal soiling with other childhood problems. Fear associated with using the lavatory may lead to a child soiling their clothes. Children who are isolated and lonely may smear faeces; however, this is different from encopresis, as they have bowel control and their behaviour is a sign of an emotional disorder (Heins & Ritchie 1985).

In most cases of encopresis, prolonged constipation and faecal impaction is the likeliest cause. Stretch receptors in the rectum are continually stimulated because the rectum is full of faeces. This leads to the prohibition of signals and loss of the normal response of muscle contraction. It can take some months for an overstretched rectum to return to normal functioning.

For a school-age child, social acceptance, and a feeling of belonging and peer inclusion aids development of self-esteem and confidence (Gross 2010). A child with encopresis is likely to experience difficulties (Box 21.20). The child may be unable to wash/change in privacy after faecal soiling and this may lead to 'being smelly' and a focus of fun for other children or bullying. The child/family may avoid activities where there is a need to undress in public, and decline school trips and sleep-overs to avoid embarrassing situations. Family support is vital; reprisal and rejection from constant criticism and telling off will only lead to further isolation and lowering of self-esteem (Gross 2010).

 Reflective practice   **Box 21.20**

Encopresis – the emotional and social effects

Sam is 8 years old and attends primary school. Over the last few months Sam has developed faecal soiling.

Student activities

- Consider some of the emotional and social difficulties Sam may experience.
- Discuss with your mentor how these difficulties may affect Sam's relationships with his classmates and his ability to fully engage in school and social activities.

The MDT will be involved in planning strategies and supporting the child and family in resolving the problem. The team will include the specialist continence nurse, GP, psychologist, school nurse, community nurse and dietitian.

Strategies used to resolve encopresis will include dealing with constipation and education (see pp. 527–528) about increasing dietary fibre, fluids and exercise.

The bowel must regain the ability to respond to stretch receptor signals, and to contract and relax to expel faeces from the bowel. Recording times faecal soiling occurs and encouraging a visit to the lavatory, usually 20 minutes after eating, when the bowel muscles begin to respond to the feeling of fullness, may help.

A breakfast comprising a high-fibre cereal, e.g. porridge, will help but a laxative may be necessary. Choosing high-fibre options, e.g. fruit and vegetables from school dinner menus or granary bread sandwiches with salad and a fruit, plus sufficient water for the day, is essential. Again, visiting the lavatory after meals when the bowel muscles begin to respond to the feeling of fullness is important. Informing teachers of the need to access lavatory facilities, even although this may disrupt lessons, is important, as is access to somewhere private to change for physical education lessons.

Caring for a person with a stoma

A stoma is an artificial opening of an internal organ, such as the bowel discharging faeces onto the surface of the body (Fig. 21.10). Types of stomas include:

- Colostomy – the colon opens onto the abdominal wall
- Ileostomy – the ileum opens onto the abdominal wall
- Urostomy – a stoma that drains urine (see Ch. 20).

Colostomy patients form the largest proportion of patients requiring a stoma. A colostomy may be performed as a temporary measure to divert faeces away from a healing anastomosis (join) or diseased area, allowing bowel continuity to be restored at a later date. When this is not possible the colostomy will be permanent. The anatomical position of the stoma will determine the faecal consistency. An ascending colostomy will produce soft/liquid stool, while transverse and descending colostomies produce an increasingly formed stool because a greater length of colon absorbs more water from the faeces (see Fig. 21.1, p. 518). The stool from an ileostomy will be more fluid. A stoma may be formed for a variety of reasons including:

- Colorectal cancer
- Trauma
- Bowel ischaemia (poor blood supply)
- Congenital bowel malformations
- Hirschsprung's disease
- Diverticular disease
- IBD
- Faecal incontinence
- Intestinal obstruction
- Intestinal inflammation following irradiation.

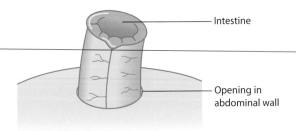

Intestine is folded over on itself and joined to the abdominal wall with sutures

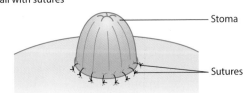

Fig. 21.10 • Stoma formation.

Specific care for patients having a stoma

Preparation for stoma formation will depend on the reason for surgery, and whether it is planned or undertaken as an emergency. Readers are directed to Further reading, below, e.g. Vujnovich 2008 and Ch. 24 for details of general pre- and postoperative care.

Preoperatively, physical and psychological preparation should include:

- Dietary modification – normal diet up to 24 hours before surgery then clear fluids only. A bowel cleansing solution such as sodium picosulfate (Picolax®) may also be administered to clear the bowel and aid visibility for the surgeon and reduce the risk of infection
- Prophylactic antibiotic therapy will be prescribed
- A full explanation of all aspects of the surgery, the immediate aftercare, e.g. intravenous fluids, nasogastric tube for aspiration, drains, etc., and gradual reintroduction of oral fluids and diet
- Specific information about the positioning of the stoma, the type of discharge from it (loose or semi formed stool), as this will influence the appliance (pouch /bag) chosen. The presence of allergies also needs to be considered, as most stoma appliances have a flange that adheres directly to the skin. The patient needs to see and reach the stoma, and have sufficient manual dexterity to manage it. The patient/carer surgeon and stoma care nurse will plan stoma position
- The opportunity for the patient/family/carers to talk about issues of altered body image, relationships and resumption of activities such as sport and work is essential. The specialist stoma care nurse will provide information, education and support to the patient, family and the nursing team. Some patients may benefit from meeting and talking with a person who has a stoma.

Specific postoperative care will include:

- Ensuring that intravenous fluids are maintained until oral fluids and diet can be reintroduced. Following bowel surgery, peristalsis is reduced (paralytic ileus), normally returning after 48 hours. Small amounts of oral fluid are then introduced, increasing in amount if tolerated, and progressing to a light diet, usually within 5 days if the stoma begins to function. The amount of observed flatus and audible bowel sounds give an indication that the stoma is starting to work.
- Ensuring that the nasogastric tube is draining or gastric contents are aspirated by syringe at regular intervals to reduce the risk of nausea and vomiting until peristalsis returns
- Administration of prophylactic antibiotics
- Observation of the stoma to include colour, length, location, size, etc. Colour is very important; normally the stoma is red and moist and signs of a poor blood supply such as a dark red or dusky appearance must be reported at once and recorded in the nursing notes. Failure to deal with this can lead to bowel necrosis
- Further opportunities for patient/family/carers to talk about issues of altered body image (see below).

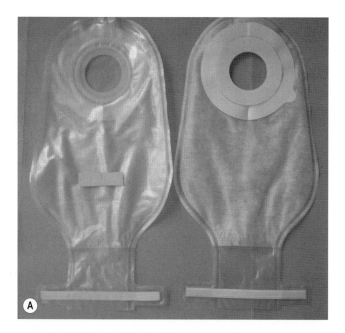

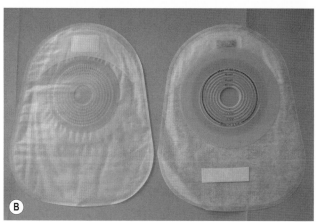

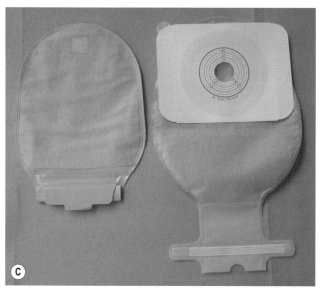

Fig. 21.11 • Selection of stoma pouches/bags – front and back views: (A) Drainable pouch/bag. (B) Sealed pouch/bag. (C) Opaque pouch/bag (drainable).

Appliances and skin care

Usually 48 hours postoperatively, the drainable appliance put on in theatre is changed for the first time. A clear plastic pouch is usually used when in hospital, as this allows the nurses to observe the stoma and any output directly. Patients are initially distressed by the odour produced when the pouch is emptied or changed, but should be reassured that this will decrease as diet is reintroduced and later, they will identify for themselves which foodstuffs produce most odour. Opaque pouches with flatus filters and charcoal to reduce odour can be introduced later should they be required.

Appliances may be either one-or two-piece, with a flange, sealed or drainable (Fig. 21.11). A two-piece appliance allows the flange to remain in contact with the skin while the pouch is emptied/changed. The flange is usually changed every 2–3 days. Sealed pouches are often used with a colostomy. Patients with an ileostomy generally use a drainable pouch. Skin must be kept in optimum condition to tolerate the stoma appliance.

Karaya, a natural absorbent rubber, revolutionized stoma care in the 1950s. In 1972, Stomahesive® was introduced. It is a flat wafer that is resistant to temperature, perspiration and the gastrointestinal fluids which come into direct contact with it. Stomahesive can be tolerated by inflamed and weepy skin and can be left in place for up to 15 days without requiring change.

If skin is prone to inflammation the longer the wafer can remain in situ the better. Skin should be cleansed and dried when appliances are changed.

The therapeutic relationship between the patient and the healthcare team is important in assisting acceptance of the stoma. Seeing the nurses at ease providing early stoma care, patients/parents and carers are more likely to accept the changes to their physical appearance. Box 21.21 outlines changing a stoma pouch.

Continuing stoma care – advice and support for patients

Various designs and colours of pouches are available, including some designed specifically for children. Pouches and appliances are designed to lie flat, be odour-free, rustle-free and to be unnoticeable under clothing. Appliances can be left in place or removed during bathing/showering. Once the patient has found a suitable appliance, the stoma care nurse will advise them about obtaining supplies after discharge.

On discharge, patients receive sufficient appliances for a week, and are provided with contact numbers/email address for the stoma care nurse. The district nurse or GP will provide prescriptions for further appliances. Supplies may be sourced direct from the manufacturer or the local pharmacy. The GP, district nurse and the stoma care nurse will assist the patient/parent to prevent or overcome any problems. The dietitian may also provide advice, promoting a balanced diet (see Ch. 19). The health visitor and school nurses will provide ongoing care for children.

Clothing which has some stretch provides most comfort by avoiding the restrictions of waistbands and belts.

Nursing skills

Box 21.21

Changing a stoma pouch

A planned teaching programme ensures that the patient does not feel rushed and has the opportunity to develop confidence and dexterity with the procedure. Initially, pouch changes are managed by the bedside but the aim is for the patient to change the appliance in the bathroom. This will increase confidence for coping at home. In the case of a child, the parents/carers will be taught to care for the stoma until the child is able to self-care.

Equipment

- Bowl of warm water
- Gauze wipes
- Barrier cream
- Clean stoma appliance – one- or two-piece
- Stoma template/measurement tool (Fig. 21.12)
- Scissors and a pen if a new flange for a two-piece appliance is required or to customize a one-piece appliance to the patient's stoma
- Clinical waste disposal bag
- Protective sheet
- Disposable gloves and apron
- Disposable jug for the used appliance or the faecal drainage from a drainable bag. If supporting a patient/client in the bathroom the contents of a drainable bag may be emptied directly into the lavatory.

Preparation

- Prepare the patient for the procedure, remembering that many patients will be anxious and distressed about seeing the stoma
- Explain the procedure to the patient to ensure informed consent
- Wash and dry hands and put on protective gloves and apron
- Ensure privacy
- Protect the bedding

- Empty contents from a drainable appliance bag
- Gently remove the used pouch from top to bottom. Support the surrounding skin to avoid pulling and discomfort
- Use the soft gauze to wash the skin around the stoma and dry thoroughly. Dispose of used wipes in the clinical waste bag
- Observe skin condition for redness or excoriation
- If necessary, measure the stoma by placing the curved edges of the measurement tool around the stoma until an exact measurement is achieved. This provides a template for cutting the flange in the new appliance to the correct size, ensuring a good fit to prevent excoriation of the surrounding skin by contact with faecal material
- When applying the new flange, ensure the lower edge fits with the bottom of the stoma, folding the top half over the stoma and pressing firmly to the skin. Attach the new pouch, remembering to apply clip if appropriate (Fig. 21.13)
- Remove equipment to the sluice. Measure the faecal material if fluid output is being recorded. The used pouch or disposable jug should be emptied into the sluice or lavatory. The pouch and disposable jug are disposed of in the clinical waste
- Remove protective gloves and apron and wash hands (see Ch. 15)
- Return to the patient to offer handwashing facilities if the patient assisted with the pouch change. Respect cultural preferences
- Ensure that the patient is comfortable and has everything they need, e.g. call bell, drink, within reach
- Make sure the immediate environment is tidy, use air-freshener as necessary and open the curtains
- Document the procedure in the nursing notes, including the appearance of the stoma, skin condition and the faecal matter produced. Record output as appropriate.

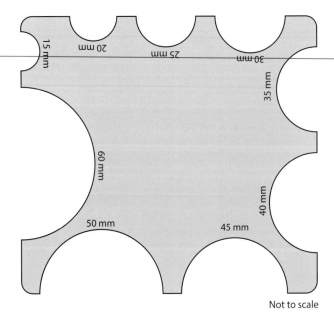

Not to scale

Fig. 21.12 • Stoma measurement tool.

Most patients will quickly discover any food/drink that affects stoma function, e.g. changes in stool consistency, odour, blockage or excess flatus. However, they should be given advice regarding eating a balanced diet (see Ch. 19) and informed about food and drink that are known to cause problems. For example, beer and onions can cause flatus, and eggs and onions are associated with odour.

Support groups are very useful sources of information and support (see Useful websites, below).

Living with a stoma: psychological and social impact

Brown and Randall (2005) undertook a systematic review of the psychological and social impact of stoma surgery on people's lives. The review demonstrated that nurses play a part in helping patients come to terms with their diagnosis, prognosis, adapting to life with a stoma, teaching practical caring skills, addressing family and support networks, employment, body image and sexuality. Adaptation to changes in body image is often associated with the grieving process and recovery time is

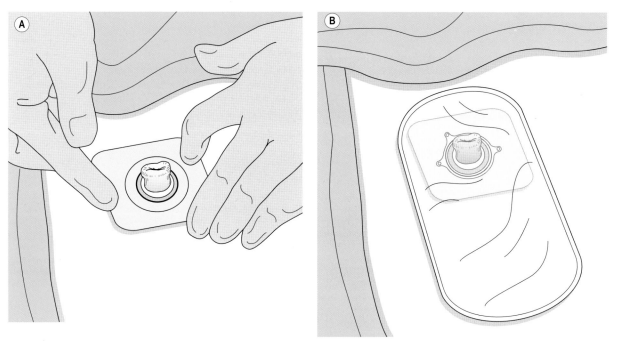

Fig. 21.13 • Changing a stoma pouch/bag: (A) Fitting the flange. (B) Stoma pouch/bag in place. (Reproduced with permission from Nicol, M., Bavin, C., Cronin, P., et al., 2008. Essential nursing skills, third ed. Mosby, Edinburgh.)

individual. Some patients with a stoma may initially feel repulsed and embarrassed, believing their stoma reduces their sexual attractiveness. This can impact on both personal relationships and social activities, such as confidence to return to work. Workplace facilities are important, particularly a private lavatory and washing area such as a toilet cubicle with a wash basin within the cubicle.

Brown and Randall (2005) found that while most patients experience negative feelings after stoma formation, this is dependent on the purpose for the stoma, and that patients react differently, with their reactions often changing over time. Nurses should encourage patients to express their feelings, and where appropriate, counselling should be provided by specialist stoma nurses.

Effective pre- and postoperative nursing care and seamless care between hospital and home affords patients the best physical and psychological care and support available. This is required in order for them to manage their changed continence status and to improve, maintain and/or recover their physical and psychological health and well-being.

achievable goals, in any care setting. Thorough bowel habit assessment will enable care to be planned and implemented that takes into account individual lifestyle, culture, beliefs and behaviours.

♦ Promoting the reporting of changes in bowel habit is an essential nursing role.

♦ Bowel care is far from basic; it requires a skilled and knowledgeable practitioner.

♦ Bowel care is essential care. For those individuals who recognize a persistent change in bowel habit, and actively seek help and advice, much can be done to resolve distressing symptoms.

♦ The nurse requires knowledge of common bowel conditions and their management, based on best evidence.

♦ Skill is required in eliciting information, as many patients will be inhibited in this process. Tact is vital, as is the need to provide privacy and promote dignity during any nursing interventions.

♦ Equity in access to services ensures individuals receive the best advice and support available to promote independence in faecal elimination wherever possible, and to promote personal dignity when assistance with faecal elimination is required.

SUMMARY

♦ Defecation is a normal bodily function, yet it carries great taboo.

♦ The inability to defecate normally can impact on the person's physical, psychological, social, spiritual and emotional well-being.

♦ Symptoms of disease are often ignored due to the embarrassment and fear of cancer and physical examination.

♦ Holistic assessment is necessary to ensure that health professionals work together in partnership with patients, setting

KEY WORDS AND PHRASES FOR LITERATURE SEARCHING

Bowel care

Constipation

Diarrhoea

Faecal incontinence

Stoma care

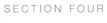

Useful websites

BBC www.bbc.co.uk/health

Colostomy Association www.colostomyassociation.org.uk

Crohn's and Colitis UK www.nacc.org.uk/content/home.asp

Ileostomy and Internal Pouch Support Group www.the-ia.org.uk

National Digestive Diseases Information Clearing House (US site) http://digestive.niddk.nih.gov

NHS Choices www.nhs.uk/Pages/HomePage.aspx

NHS Evidence www.evidence.nhs.uk/topics

The Bladder and Bowel Foundation (formally the Continence Foundation) www.bladderandbowelfoundation.org

All websites accessed September 2012.

References

Akhtar, S..G., 2002. Nursing with dignity – Islam. Nursing Times 98 (16), 40.

Bharucha, A.E., Wald, A.M., 2010. Anorectal disorders. American Journal of Gastroenterology 105 (4), 786–794.

Bradshaw, A., Price, L., 2007. Rectal suppository insertion: the reliability of the evidence as a basis for nursing practice. Journal of Clinical Nursing 16 (1), 98–103.

British National Formulary, 2012. Online. Available: http://bnf.org/bnf/index.htm September 2012.

Brown, H., Randall, J., 2005. Living with a stoma – a review of the literature. Journal of Clinical Nursing 14, 74–81.

Cancer Research UK, 2011. Bowel (colorectal) cancer – UK incidence statistics. Online. Available: http://info.cancerresearchuk.org/cancerstats/types/bowel/incidence/ September 2012.

Department of Health (DH), 2010. Essence of care 2010 Benchmarks for bladder, bowel and continence care. Online. Available: www.dh.gov.uk/en/Publicationsandstatistics/Publications/PublicationsPolicyAndGuidance/DH_119969 September 2012.

Gross, R.D., 2010. Psychology: the science of mind and behaviour, sixth ed. Hodder and Stoughton, London.

Heins, T., Ritchie, K., 1985. Beating sneaky poo. ACT Health Authority, Canberra Publishing, Canberra.

Kyle, G., 2007. Bowel Care, Part 4 – Administering an enema. Nursing Times 103 (45), 26–27.

Kyle, G., 2008. Constipation: An examination of the current evidence. Continence UK 2 (3), 61–67.

National Institute for Health and Clinical Excellence, 2007. Faecal incontinence: the management of faecal incontinence in adults. Clinical guideline CG49. Online. Available: www.nice.org.uk/nicemedia/live/11012/30548/30548.pdf September 2012.

National Institute for Health and Clinical Excellence, 2010. Constipation in children and young people. Clinical guideline CG99. Online. Available: www.nice.org.uk/nicemedia/live/12993/48741/48741.pdf September 2012.

NHS choices, 2010. Constipation. Online. Available: www.nhs.uk/conditions/constipation/pages/introduction.aspx September 2012.

NHS choices, 2011. Diarrhoea – treatment. Online. Available: www.nhs.uk/Conditions/Diarrhoea/Pages/Treatment.aspx September 2012.

Nicol, M., Bavin, C., Cronin, P., et al., 2008. Essential nursing skills, third ed. Mosby, Edinburgh.

Nursing and Midwifery Council, 2010. Standards for pre-registration nursing education – Annexe 3. Online. Available: http://standards.nmc-uk.org/Documents/Annexe3_%20ESCs_16092010.pdf September 2012.

Royal College of Nursing, 2008. Bowel care, including digital rectal examination and manual removal of faeces. Royal College of Nursing, London.

Royal College of Physicians, 2010. National Audit of Continence Care. Combined Organisational and Clinical report. Online. Available: www.rcplondon.ac.uk/resources/national-audit-continence-care September 2012.

Spiller, R.C., Thompson, W.G., 2010. Bowel Disorders American. Journal of Gastroenterology 105 (4), 775–778.

Walter, S.A., Kjellstrom, L., Hyhlin, H., et al., 2010. Assessment of normal bowel habits in the general adult population: the Popcol study. Scandinavian Journal of Gastroenterology 45 (5), 556–566.

Further reading

Dougherty, L., Lister, S. (Eds.), 2011. The Royal Marsden Hospital Manual of clinical nursing procedures, eighth ed. Wiley-Blackwell, Oxford.

Getliffe, K., Dolman, D., 2008. Promoting continence, third ed. Baillière Tindall, Edinburgh.

Jooton, D., 2002. Nursing with dignity – Hinduism. Nursing Times 98 (15), 38.

Kaur Gill, B., 2002. Nursing with dignity – Sikhism. Nursing Times 98 (14), 39–41.

Nicol, M., Bavin, C., Cronin, P., et al., 2012. Essential nursing skills, fourth ed. Mosby, Edinburgh.

Rome Foundation, 2006. Appendix A: Rome III diagnostic criteria for functional gastrointestinal disorders. Functional constipation. Online. Available: www.romecriteria.org/criteria September 2012.

Vujnovich, A., 2008. Pre and post-operative assessment of patients with a stoma. Nursing Standard 22 (19), 50–56.

Walker, S., 2009. Continence, bowel and bladder care. In: Iggulden, H., Macdonald, C., Staniland, K. (Eds.), Clinical skills: the essence of caring. Open University Press/McGraw-Hill Education, Maidenhead.

Walker, S., 2011. Maintaining continence. In: Brooker, C., Nicol, M. (Eds.), Alexander's nursing practice, fourth ed. Churchill Livingstone, Edinburgh.

Waugh, A., Grant, A. (Eds.), 2010. Ross and Wilson anatomy and physiology, eleventh ed. Churchill Livingstone, Edinburgh.

Promoting the safe administration of medicines

22

Jayne Donaldson

LEARNING OUTCOMES

This chapter will help you:

- Outline the legal and professional principles governing the use of medicines
- Explain how medicines must be stored, ordered and prescribed in hospital and community settings
- Outline common groups of drugs and their actions
- Explain the nurse's role in the safe administration of prescribed drugs
- Describe the nursing skills used to administer drugs by commonly used routes
- Discuss the nurse's role in promoting medicines adherence
- Describe factors that contribute to drug errors and how such incidents are handled.

Introduction

Safe administration of medicines is of paramount importance to ensure patient/client safety. The legislation and professional guidance (Nursing and Midwifery Council, NMC 2008, 2010a) that should enable this are explored at the beginning of this chapter. The requirements for safe storage, ordering and prescribing of medicines in hospital and community settings are then reviewed.

In order to understand how drugs act, some pharmacological principles are explained and their implications for nursing practice are illustrated. Commonly used groups of drugs and their effects are listed. Adverse drug reactions or side-effects, and the safeguards that apply to newly marketed medicines are considered. Medications come in several forms and are administered by a variety of routes, several of which are described later in this chapter.

This chapter discusses the essential checks that must be carried out before administering medicines and how to obtain valid consent. An overview of calculating drug doses is provided. The nursing skills needed to administer medication by several common routes are explained in detail using an

evidence-based approach. Towards the end of the chapter, polypharmacy and the nurse's role in maximizing medicines adherence is explored. This is important in maintaining patient/client safety and maximizing effective use of NHS financial resources. Finally, drug errors, the factors that may predispose to these incidents and how they are dealt with are considered.

Legislation concerning medicines

All medicines are potentially harmful and nurses must be fully aware of the importance of safe storage, ordering and prescribing of drugs, which are explained later in this section. The manufacture, safe storage, prescription and sales of medicines within the UK are subject to Acts of Parliament and guiding regulations, with which every nurse should be familiar:

- The Medicines Act 1968
- The Misuse of Drugs Act 1971
- The Misuse of Drugs Regulations 1985.

Additional legislation governs prescribing by appropriately qualified registered nurses. Nurses also need to be familiar with the professional guidance from the NMC.

The Medicines Act 1968

This act protects manufacturers, prescribers and recipients of medicines. It controls licensing, manufacturing and distribution of medicines, the registration of retail pharmacists and identifies three classes of medicinal products:

- Prescription only medicines (PoMs) – potent medicines that can be sold or supplied on prescription only, e.g. antibiotics
- Pharmacy only medicines (P) – may only be sold under the supervision of a pharmacist, e.g. bronchodilators
- General sales list medicines (GSL) – can be sold in any retail outlet, e.g. supermarkets. Examples include aspirin and paracetamol.

The Act stipulated that only doctors, dentists and veterinary surgeons could prescribe medicines; however, later legislation has since extended prescribing to appropriately qualified registered nurses (RNs) (see below) and other healthcare professionals such as some pharmacists. The Act outlines:

- How drugs should be labelled
- The types of container to be used to contain drugs between the factory and the patient/client
- Controls that govern the writing of prescriptions (see Box 22.3, p. 545).

Many medicinal products not governed by legislation are widely available, e.g. homeopathic and herbal preparations. In addition, GSL medicines – often referred to as 'over-the-counter (OTC) drugs', such as aspirin and medicines for indigestion – are widely believed to be safe. However, they can have serious side-effects and may interact with each other and with prescribed medicines. Additionally, the use of alcohol and recreational drugs can have harmful effects and they too can interact with prescribed medication.

The Misuse of Drugs Act 1971

This Act identified controlled drugs that are likely to cause dependence and other harmful effects if misused. It aims to prevent the misuse of these drugs and protects public safety by controlling their importation, exportation, supply and possession. Controlled drugs are widely known as CDs and were previously known as 'dangerous drugs of addiction'. The Act classifies CDs according to the harm they may cause if misused.

- *Class A* (most harm) includes cocaine, diamorphine (heroin), methadone, morphine, ecstasy and lysergide (LSD) and also injectable forms of Class B drugs
- *Class B* (intermediate harm) includes cannabis, oral amphetamines, barbiturates and codeine
- *Class C* (least harm) includes most benzodiazepines, androgenic and anabolic steroids, and growth hormone.

The Misuse of Drugs Regulations 1985

This divides controlled drugs into five schedules, which have specific requirements regarding their supply, possession, prescribing and record-keeping. There is a legal requirement to keep a controlled drug register for drugs in Schedule 2, which includes the most addictive drugs used in practice such as morphine and pethidine. Further information can be found in the *British National Formulary* (BNF; see Useful websites, p. 562). Storage, ordering, prescribing and administration of CDs are described later.

Non-medical prescribing

The Medicinal Products: Prescription by Nurses Act 1992 and The Health and Social Care Act 2001 contain the primary legislation that allows nurse prescribing and its subsequent extension to 'non-medical prescribing'. Since the publication of the Crown Report, *Review of prescribing, supply and administration of medicines* in 1999, many legislative changes have taken place to implement the government's policy of extending prescribing responsibilities to non-medical professions. According to the National Prescribing Centre (2010), the aims of non-medical prescribing are:

- To make more effective use of the skills and expertise of groups of professions
- To improve patients' access to treatment and advice
- To improve patient choice and convenience
- To contribute to more flexible team working across the NHS.

Currently, nurses, pharmacists, optometrists, physiotherapists, podiatrists and radiographers can train to prescribe within their clinical competence (National Prescribing Centre 2010). Members of these professions can train to become supplementary prescribers, prescribing in partnership with a doctor or dentist in accordance with a patient-specific clinical management plan. Nurses and pharmacists can now prescribe all controlled drugs, and physiotherapists and podiatrists will be independently prescribing by late 2013.

Patient Group Directions (PGD)

PGDs are written instructions for the supply or administration of named medicines to specific groups of patients who may not be individually identified before presenting for treatment. Guidance, and the legal standing, on the use of PGDs are contained within Department of Health (2000), *Health Service Circular (HSC) 2000/026*. (*Note*: In Wales: WHC 2000/116; separate guidance has also been issued in Scotland and Northern Ireland). It is vital that anyone involved in the delivery of care within a PGD is aware of the legal requirements (National Prescribing Centre 2009). It is not a form of prescribing. Students cannot supply or administer under a PGD but would be expected to understand the principles and be involved in these processes under supervision (NMC 2010b,c).

Professional advice that affects nurses

In relation to the administration and prescribing of medicines, nurses are not only constrained by the legislation above but also by *Standards for medicines management* (NMC 2010b). These outline nurses' professional accountability (see Ch. 7) in relation to knowledge of drugs and their actions, and the safe administration of medicines. Nurses must also be familiar with the *The code: Standards of conduct, performance and ethics for nurses and midwives* (NMC 2008); *Guidance on professional conduct for nursing and midwifery students* (NMC 2010a) and *Record keeping: guidance for nurses and midwives* (NMC 2009).

The NMC (2010b) recommend that only RNs, midwives and specialist community public health nurses should be involved in the administration of medicines. Practitioners must always be aware of local policy, as it may vary regarding the number of practitioners involved. For example, in some placements, the second checker will also require to be a registered practitioner, whereas in others, this may be a student nurse.

The *Standards for pre-registration nursing education* (NMC 2010c) state that student nurses must be able to demonstrate competence in essential skills including administration of medicines. Student nurses undertaking administration of medicines must do so only under the direct supervision of an RN. The RN must countersign the signature of a student who administers any prescription (NMC 2010b).

Storage of medicines

In clinical settings, all drugs, not just CDs and including GSL medicines, are 'controlled' by the legislation outlined above. Storage depends on the type of drug and the setting involved.

Storage of non-controlled medicines in hospitals and nursing homes

The *Duthie report* (Department of Health, DH 1988) set out precautions concerning the storage of medicines in hospitals to safeguard staff and patients/clients. The nurse in charge of a clinical area is responsible for the safe storage of all medicines (Box 22.1). Safe storage requires that:

1. Medicines are always stored in:
   - A locked cupboard
   - A locked medicine trolley (Fig. 22.1A)
   - A locked section of the patient's/client's bedside locker (Fig. 22.1B), or
   - A locked refrigerator that is only used for drugs
2. Some medicines are stored at room temperature (between 15° and 25°C), others require to be kept in a cool dark cupboard and some are stored in a refrigerator (between 1° and 4°C), e.g. vaccines and reconstituted antibiotics
3. Disinfectants/antiseptics such as chlorhexidine, intravenous (i.v.) fluids such as 0.9% sodium chloride, clinical reagents such as urine testing materials and topical substances, including creams and ointments, should be stored in locked cupboards and separately from other medicines
4. Medicines should always be kept in their original packaging, e.g. blister packaging is designed to reduce decomposition of the drugs by moisture.

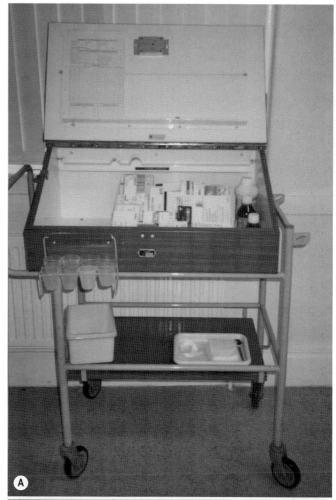

 Reflective practice　　　　　　**Box 22.1**

Storage of medicinal products

Medicinal products are stored in different parts of placements and under different conditions.

Student activities

1. In your placement, identify at least one medicine that is stored:
   - At room temperature
   - In the drugs refrigerator.
2. Find out where the following are stored:
   - Disinfectants
   - Urine testing materials
   - Creams and ointments
   - i.v. fluids.

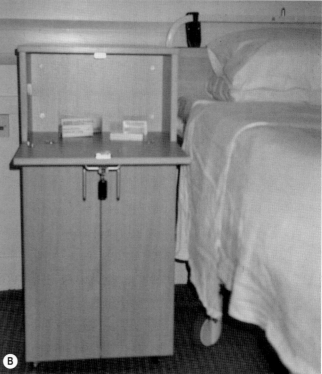

Fig. 22.1 • Storage of medicines: (A) Medicine trolley. (B) Locked section of bedside locker.

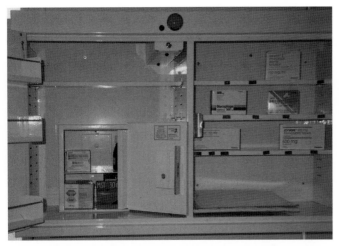

Fig. 22.2 • Drug cupboard with an inner controlled drugs cupboard.

Ordering controlled drugs	Box 22.2

- A specific controlled drug order book with carbonized order sheets is used
- Qualified practitioners sign the controlled drugs ordering book using a separate page for each drug
- This is sent to pharmacy in the normal way unless it is non-stock or needed urgently, in which case a member of staff may take the controlled drug order book to the pharmacy
- A pharmacist dispenses controlled drugs
- The signature of the member of staff responsible for their safe delivery to the ward/department is required before leaving the pharmacy
- They are transported to the ward/department in a sealed package
- Controlled drugs are accepted on the ward/department by an RN and the package is checked to ensure that it is still intact
- Two RNs or one RN and the pharmacist check the drug packaging
- The drug is checked against the order form
- The total number of tablets, ampoules of the drug or volume of liquid is checked and added to the stock in the controlled drug register.

Storage of controlled drugs in hospitals and nursing homes

Because of their potential to cause harm if misused, there are specific legal requirements concerning the ordering, storage and dispensing of controlled drugs. Controlled drugs are the responsibility of the charge nurse. They are kept locked in an inner cupboard within a cupboard (Fig. 22.2). The keys for both cupboards are held in the sole custody of the charge nurse or a designated RN or other healthcare professional. The contents of the cupboard and the controlled drug register are checked regularly according to local policy. This may be at each change of shift, daily or weekly. The controlled drug register is kept as an accurate record of the contents of the controlled drugs cupboard. Once completed, the registers are kept in the clinical area for 2 years.

Good practice in relation to prescriptions	Box 22.3

As the RN administering medicines, you need to ensure that the prescription is:

- not for a substance to which the patient is known to be allergic or otherwise unable to tolerate
- based, whenever possible, on the patient's informed consent and awareness of the purpose of the treatment
- clearly written, typed or computer-generated and indelible
- specifies the substance to be administered, using its generic or brand name where appropriate and its stated form, together with the strength, dosage, timing, frequency of administration, start and finish dates, and route of administration
- is signed and dated by the authorized prescriber
- in the case of controlled drugs, specifies the dosage and the number of dosage units or total course; and is signed and dated by the prescriber using relevant documentation as introduced, for example, patient drug record cards

And that you have:

- clearly identified the patient for whom the medication is intended
- recorded the weight of the patient on the prescription sheet for all children, and where the dosage of medication is related to weight or surface area (e.g. cytotoxics) or where clinical condition dictates recording the patient's weight.

Accepted abbreviations for drug routes

- i.m. – intramuscular
- INHAL – inhalation
- i.v. – intravenous
- p.r. – per rectum
- p.v. – per vaginam
- s.c. – subcutaneous
- s.l. – sublingual
- TOP – topical

Notes: depending on local policy, abbreviations may also be written in upper case letters without punctuation, e.g. IM, IV, SC, etc.

Units

SI units are normally used in prescriptions avoiding the use of decimal points:

- *Mass:* 1 kilogram (kg) = 1000 grams; 1 gram (g) = 1000 milligrams; 1 milligram (mg) = 1000 micrograms[a]
- *Volume:* 1 litre (L) = 1000 millilitres; 1 millilitre (mL) = 1000 microlitres[a]

International units (IU) are used for some preparations, e.g. heparin, insulin (see Table 22.1).

[a]This must not be abbreviated.

Storage of medicines in the home

The strict regulations used in hospitals cannot be maintained in people's homes. A family member may collect any medicine if the person for whom the drug is prescribed is unable to do so. In general, patients/clients should be advised to:

- Check the manufacturer's instructions concerning storage
- Keep medicines that require refrigeration away from raw food
- Keep medicines out of reach of children.

PRESCRIPTION AND ADMINISTRATION RECORD
Standard Chart

Hospital/Ward: 17	**Consultant:** DR BROWN	**Name of Patient:** DAVID BURTON
Weight: 72Kg	**Height:**	**Patient Number:** 01234567
If re-written, date:		**D.O.B.** 13/12/45
DISCHARGE PRESCRIPTION		
Date completed:-	**Completed by:-**	(Attach printed label here)

ONCE ONLY

Date	Time	Medicine (Approved Name)	Dose	Route	Prescriber - Sign + Print	Time Given	Given By
13/03/07	11:10	PETHIDINE	50mg	I.M	RaReid R.A.REID	11:20	CB

REGULAR THERAPY

PRESCRIPTION		Patient's Own Medicine	Date → Time ↴	06/03	07/03	08/03	09/03	10/03	11/03	12/03	13/03	14/03				
Medicine (Approved Name) DIGOXIN		For use	6													
			(8)		HB	CB	HB	HB	HR	CB	HR	HB	CB				
Dose 125 MICROGRAMS	Route ORAL	Quantity	12													
Notes	Start Date 06/03/07	Date	14													
			18													
Prescriber - sign + print RaReid R.A.REID	Pharmacy SK		22													
Medicine (Approved Name) FUROSEMIDE		For use	6													
			(8)		HB	CB	HB	HB	HR	CB	HC	HB	CB				
Dose 40mg	Route ORAL	Quantity	12													
Notes	Start Date 06/03/07	Date	14													
			18													
Prescriber - sign + print RaReid R.A.REID	Pharmacy SK		22													

AS REQUIRED THERAPY

PRESCRIPTION		Patient's Own Medicine													
Medicine (Approved Name) SALBUTAMOL		For use	Date	07/03	11/03	14/03									
			Time	08:05	18:35	21:10									
Dose 2 PUFFS	Route INHAL	Quantity	Dose	2 puffs	2 puffs	2 puffs									
			Initials	CB	CB	CB									
Notes For breathlessness MAX ~ 4 × dose/per day	Start Date 07/03/07	Date	Date												
			Time												
Prescriber - sign + print RaReid R.A.REID	Pharmacy SK		Dose												
			Initials												

Fig. 22.3 • Prescription chart. (Reproduced with permission from NHS Lothian 2005.)

Controlled drugs are dispensed from the pharmacy in the normal way. However, the pharmacist keeps a register of controlled drugs ordered, the amount delivered to the pharmacy and the volume or amount dispensed.

Ordering drugs in hospitals

This depends on the type of drug to be ordered.

Controlled drugs

In hospitals, qualified practitioners order controlled drugs in a specific way (Box 22.2).

Non-controlled drugs

In hospitals, this is usually the responsibility of the RN and/or pharmacist. Upon receipt, the order sheet is checked by an RN to ensure that the correct medicines have been supplied.

Principles of prescribing

It is essential to ensure that the prescription meets the principles laid down in the *Standards for medicines management* (NMC 2010b). In order to safeguard both the public and practitioners, specific guidelines govern the prescribing of medicines (Box 22.3). Drugs may be prescribed:

- Regularly, i.e. for administration at particular times each day
- 'As required', e.g. painkillers, when the dose interval, maximum number of daily doses and reason for administration must be included
- Once only, e.g. for preoperative medication.

If the prescription does not meet the required standards for safe practice, the nurse should contact the prescriber to amend their prescription before proceeding further. An example of a prescription sheet is provided in Figure 22.3.

Introduction to pharmacology

Pharmacology is the science of chemical substances, e.g. drugs, medications and other substances such as herbal and homeopathic preparations (see Ch. 10) that interact with the body. These interactions are divided into:

- *Pharmacodynamics*, which considers the effect of drugs on the body or 'what the drug does to the body'
- *Pharmacokinetics*, which explains how the body affects a drug with time, i.e. 'what the body does to the drug'.

This section provides an overview of important processes; further information can be found in Further reading suggestions, p. 562.

Pharmacodynamics

Receptors on cell membranes often act as recognition sites for substances produced by the body to regulate or mediate specific functions. Substances that act on cell membrane receptors include hormones and neurotransmitters – chemicals that transmit nerve impulses across the tiny gaps (synapses) between nerve cells. Many drugs produce their effects because they are structurally similar to the naturally occurring substances that act on receptors (Fig. 22.4A). Drugs that act on receptor sites in a similar way to natural body substances are known as agonists, whereas those that prevent (block) their normal action are known as antagonists. Therefore, by attaching to specific receptor sites on target cells, some drugs act by stimulating or blocking the storage, manufacture or release of naturally produced substances.

However, not all drugs act on receptor sites, e.g. antacids reduce indigestion by neutralizing gastric acid. Many other drugs act by inhibiting the actions of enzymes (Fig. 22.4B), e.g. non-steroidal anti-inflammatory drugs (NSAIDs), or by blocking ion channels in cell membranes (Fig. 22.4C), e.g. local anaesthetics.

Pharmacokinetics

Important processes influence plasma levels of a drug within the body, in particular absorption, distribution, metabolism and excretion (Fig. 22.5). Knowledge of pharmacokinetic principles is useful when considering factors that determine how much of a drug is needed to maintain appropriate (therapeutic) blood levels.

Absorption

The oral route is most commonly used for administration of drugs (see p. 550). In order to exert its action at the desired site, the drug must be absorbed from the digestive tract into the blood, which then travels through the liver before entering the systemic circulation (see First pass metabolism, below). The rate of absorption can be affected by several factors, including the presence or absence of food in the stomach. It is recommended that some drugs are taken half an hour before meals, e.g. some antibiotics are absorbed more effectively on an empty stomach.

First pass metabolism

Drugs taken orally are usually absorbed in the small intestine and then transported to the liver via the hepatic portal vein before reaching the systemic circulation. Many drugs are broken down, or metabolized, as they pass through the liver and when this is extensive, only a small amount enters the systemic circulation and even less reaches the site of action. This effect is called first pass metabolism.

Glyceryl trinitrate, which is given to provide very rapid relief from cardiac pain in angina, is almost completely broken down in the liver. It is administered sublingually (placed under the tongue) or as a spray to the oral mucosa. The oral mucosa has an extensive blood supply that facilitates rapid absorption and therefore the action of glyceryl trinitrate is also very rapid. The blood from the oral mucosa enters the systemic circulation, thus allowing the drug to relax the smooth muscle, including the vascular smooth muscle, within minutes of being

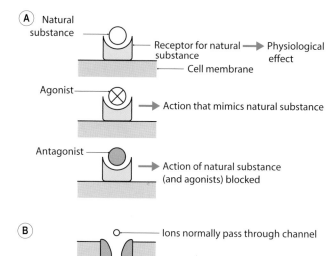

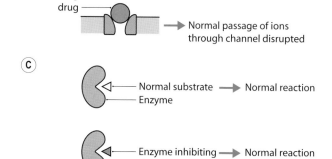

Fig. 22.4 • Sites of drug action: (A) Receptors. (B) Ion channels. (C) Enzymes. (Adapted with permission from Rang, H.P., Dale, M.M., Ritter, J., et al., 2003. Pharmacology, fifth ed. Churchill Livingstone, Edinburgh.)

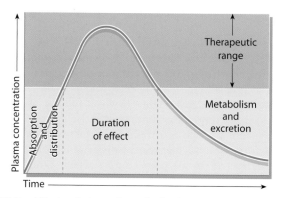

Fig. 22.5 • Effects of absorption, distribution, metabolism and excretion on the plasma concentrations of an administered drug. (Reproduced with permission from Downie, G., Mackenzie, J., Williams, A., 2003. Pharmacology and medicines management for nurses, third ed. Churchill Livingstone, Edinburgh.)

administered. This rapidly relieves the pain of angina and also avoids first pass metabolism.

Other drugs are given by injection or as transdermal patches (see p. 558 and Fig. 22.14) to avoid first pass metabolism. In people suffering from liver disorders, first pass metabolism is reduced, and therefore drug doses must be reduced to take this into account.

Distribution

After entering the bloodstream, the drug is transported throughout the body. In the capillaries drugs diffuse out of the bloodstream to reach their site(s) of action. Movement from the bloodstream into the tissues may be influenced by several factors such as the extent of plasma binding (see below), the quality and quantity of plasma proteins and blood flow. Where there is good systemic blood flow, drugs are transported more rapidly into the tissues. In some cardiac conditions, where the cardiac output is reduced (see Ch. 17), drug distribution will also be reduced. Many drugs cross the placenta, causing abnormal fetal development, and must therefore be avoided during pregnancy.

Plasma binding

Many drugs bind to plasma proteins in the blood. Some of the drug is bound and the remainder is unbound; however, only the unbound form is active. People who have a liver disorder or malnutrition have fewer plasma proteins available for binding and therefore more of the drug remains unbound and is available to act. In such situations, the dosage must be reduced to avoid excessive plasma levels, e.g. warfarin (see Table 22.1), which may cause severe bleeding.

Metabolism

Metabolism includes processes that often involve specific enzymes which may break down the drug, combine it with another chemical (conjugation) or increase its solubility in water. In these states, drugs are usually more active and can be easily eliminated by the kidneys. Some drugs are already water soluble and so do not require to be metabolized. Most drugs are metabolized in the liver.

Half-life

This is also referred to as $t_{1/2}$ and is the time taken for the concentration of a drug in the bloodstream to fall by half of its original value. The half-life determines the length of time a drug is available within the body and the intensity of its action. The plasma concentration of a drug at one half-life is 50%, at two half-lives it is 25%, etc. By five half-lives, most of the drug will have been eliminated from the body regardless of the dose or route of administration. The half-life is therefore used to determine the number of daily doses required for drug plasma levels to remain within the therapeutic range (see Fig. 22.5). It can also be useful when estimating how long it will take for a drug to be cleared from the body, e.g. in overdosage.

Excretion

The kidneys excrete most drugs from the body. The more water soluble the substance, the more easily it is excreted by the kidneys. People with kidney failure or impaired renal function may suffer toxic effects as elimination of drugs is reduced. Digoxin is a commonly used cardiac drug that can be toxic in older adults because kidney function is often reduced in this age group. The kidneys can reabsorb those drugs that are lipid soluble, making them available within the body for longer.

Some drugs are excreted by the lungs or from the digestive tract.

Therapeutic range

To achieve optimal concentrations at the target tissue the correct dose must be given. If this is too low, drug action will be ineffective; if too much is administered it may produce side-effects that might be toxic. The therapeutic range refers to the plasma levels of a drug that must be maintained so that it can exert its optimal response without producing side-effects (Fig. 22.6). Some drugs have a narrow therapeutic range while for others this is wider. Nurses need to recognize the implications of this in relation to drug administration, i.e. if drugs are omitted or given at times other than those prescribed, plasma drug levels will not be maintained in the therapeutic range.

Measurement of plasma drug levels is carried out when drugs with a narrow therapeutic range are used, e.g. gentamicin (an antibiotic) causes irreversible kidney damage and hearing impairment when therapeutic levels are exceeded. Children, until their liver and kidneys are fully mature, older adults whose kidney and liver function may be declining and people with a liver or kidney disorder are at greatest risk of toxicity.

Adverse drug reactions

All medicines have the potential to cause harm including over-the-counter medication. Interactions increase with the number of drugs used, including homeopathic and herbal preparations, recreational drugs and alcohol. It is important, therefore, that nurses know about and can recognize potential adverse effects of drugs they administer. Adverse drug reactions (ADRs) include any unwanted effects of drugs, which range from minor side-effects to those that are harmful, serious and sometimes fatal. They can be classified into five groups, of which the two outlined below are the most common (Medicine and Healthcare products Regulatory Agency, MHRA 2010).

Type A

These are predictable, dose dependent and can be anticipated. They are related to the physiological effects of the drug, e.g. that constipation occurs in people receiving morphine.

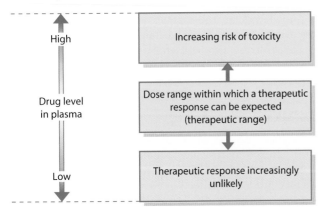

Fig. 22.6 • Therapeutic range. (Reproduced with permission from Hopkins, S.J., Kelly, J.C., 1999. Drugs and pharmacology for nurses, thirteenth ed. Churchill Livingstone, Edinburgh.)

Type B

These types are bizarre or idiosyncratic, unexpected and rare reactions, which are not dose related. However, they are generally severe, causing serious and sometimes fatal consequences such as severe allergic responses. Genetic, host and environmental factors are thought to contribute to their occurrence.

Surveillance for ADRs

Potential new drugs must undergo approved and staged clinical trials that report to the Committee on Safety of Medicines to ensure that they are as safe as possible before being granted a product licence. Once marketed, they become more widely available and the Committee on Safety of Medicines keeps them under surveillance so that the occurrence and incidence of ADRs can be monitored. Drugs under surveillance have the symbol ▼ in their BNF listing (see Useful websites, p. 562).

As a RN, if a patient experiences an adverse drug reaction to a medication, you must take any action to remedy harm caused by the reaction. You must record this in the patient's notes, notify the prescriber and notify the occurrence immediately via the Yellow Card Scheme.

Naming of drugs and common groups

Drugs that have similar functions are classified into groups and there is more than one name for each drug. Some names reflect drug actions more clearly than others.

Naming of drugs

The recommended International Non-proprietary Name (rINN) of a drug is also referred to as the generic, non-proprietary or British Approved Name (BAN). This name may start with a lower case letter, e.g. 'p' in paracetamol.

The manufacturer gives the trade or proprietary name to a particular preparation. This is recognized by the symbol ® denoting its registered trademark, which follows its name on the packaging. Proprietary names start with a capital letter, e.g. 'P' in Panadol®, which is a trade name for paracetamol. The manufacturer who has registered a drug has exclusive marketing rights for up to 10 years, during which time they can recover the development costs. Different drug companies often manufacture similar or identical generic preparations and may give them similar names.

To avoid errors, and because manufacturers price drugs differently, the Department of Health (1999) recommended that drugs be prescribed by their generic name (e.g. paracetamol) and that trade names (e.g. Panadol®) should only be specified if a particular manufacturer's drug has different effects. Lists of drugs can be found in the BNF.

Common groups of drugs and their actions

Common drug groups are listed in Table 22.1 together with their effects and examples. Nurses must understand how

Table 22.1 Common drug groups and their actions

Group	Effect	Common examples (generic names)
Analgesics: 　Opioids 　Non-opioids 　(see also NSAIDs and Ch. 23)	Reduce or prevent pain	Morphine Aspirin, paracetamol
Antacids	Counteract gastric acidity in indigestion	Aluminium hydroxide, magnesium trisilicate
Antibiotics (antibacterials)	Kill bacteria (bactericidal) or arrest their growth (bacteriostatic)	Ampicillin, erythromycin, gentamicin
Anticoagulants	Prevent and/or break down blood clots in the circulation	Warfarin (oral), heparin (parenteral)
Anticonvulsants (antiepileptic)	Control and prevent seizures	Phenytoin, sodium valproate
Antidepressants: 　Monoamine oxidase inhibitors (MAOIs) 　Selective serotonin reuptake inhibitors (SSRIs) 　Tricyclic antidepressants	Improve low mood	Phenelzine Fluoxetine Amitriptyline
Antidiarrhoeals	Reduce intestinal motility	Codeine phosphate, loperamide
Antiemetics	Alleviate nausea and/or vomiting	Metoclopramide, cyclizine
Antifungals	Combat fungal infection	Nystatin, fluconazole
Antihistamines	Treat and prevent allergic reactions	Chlorphenamine (chlorpheniramine)
Antihypertensives	Several groups that act in different ways to reduce high blood pressure, e.g.: 　　Beta-blockers 　　Angiotensin converting enzyme (ACE) inhibitors	Atenolol, propranolol Captopril, enalapril
Antipsychotics (neuroleptics): 　Typical 　Atypical	Alleviate symptoms of psychotic illness	Haloperidol Clozapine
Antipyretics	Lower raised body temperature	Paracetamol, aspirin
Anxiolytics	Alleviate anxiety and related symptoms	Diazepam
Aperients, laxatives	Promote emptying/evacuation of the bowel	Lactulose, bisacodyl
Bronchodilators	Relax bronchial smooth muscle, thus increasing air entry to lungs	Salbutamol
Diuretics	Groups of drugs that increase production of urine	Bendroflumethiazide, furosemide (frusemide)
Hypoglycaemic agents (antidiabetic): 　Oral 　Parenteral, usually given by subcutaneous injection (see p. 557)	Lower raised blood glucose levels in diabetes mellitus	Metformin, glipizide Insulin – short-, intermediate- and long-acting preparations
Hypnotics	Promote sleep	Zopiclone
Non-steroidal anti-inflammatory drugs (NSAIDs)	Reduce inflammation (see Ch. 23)	Ibuprofen, aspirin
Thrombolytics ('clot busting' drugs)	Disintegrate blood clots in, e.g. myocardial infarction, deep vein thrombosis (DVT), pulmonary embolism	Streptokinase, alteplase

commonly used drugs in their practice area act and be familiar with their side-effects and contraindications in order to maintain patient/client safety (Box 22.4). This information can be found in the BNF/Children's BNF.

(?) Critical thinking   **Box 22.4**

Drug groups, their actions and routes of administration

Under the supervision of your mentor, you are to be involved in drug administration. In order to do this safely, preparation is required.

Student activities

1. Within your placement:
   - Identify commonly used drugs and the groups to which they belong (see Table 22.1).
   - For these drugs, consider their intended effects and relate them to the patient's/client's clinical condition.
   - Find out about the side-effects of each drug.
2. There are many different routes used to administer medicines. Find out:
   - What routes are used.
   - If there is more than one route that could be used for administering any of the drugs identified above.

Medicinal preparations and routes of administration

Medicines are manufactured in different forms for administration by particular routes. The different forms and their characteristics are summarized in Table 22.2. The prescribed route is determined by which will provide the optimal effect and minimize side-effects, and the preparations available.

Routes of administration can be divided into two categories: systemic and local (Table 22.3). Following systemic administration, the drug circulates throughout the whole body. Use of local routes, e.g. inhalation or per vagina, involves giving lower doses directly to the site of action. As a result, the amount of the drug elsewhere in the body is relatively low and side-effects are less likely. The term 'parenteral' includes all routes of administration except the oral route.

Oral medication

Once swallowed, drugs are usually absorbed from the small intestine. Oral preparations include tablets, capsules and liquids (see Table 22.2). Some tablets are manufactured to exert their effect over long periods and are described as 'slow release' (SR) or 'extended release' (XR). Other tablets are covered in an enteric coating (e/c). For example, NSAIDs are

---

Table 22.2 Drug preparations for administration by specific routes

Type	Characteristics
Oral preparations	
Tablets	Powdered substances compressed or moulded into solid forms Many are covered or sugar-coated to assist swallowing or to prevent them dissolving in the stomach, which may result in release or disintegration of the drug causing gastric irritation Some tablets should be swallowed when fully dissolved in water and are labelled: soluble, dispersible or effervescent
Capsules	Medication contained within a soluble shell, usually made of gelatin to aid swallowing and which carries the drug to the small intestine where it is absorbed
Lozenges	A solid form intended for sucking until fully dissolved; absorption is through the oral mucosa
Solutions	Medication is dissolved in a solvent, usually water
Suspensions	Contain solid particles that are dispersed in a liquid, not necessarily water
Syrup	A thick concentrated solution of medication that may include sugar (see Box 22.6) and flavouring
Emulsion	Minute globules of one liquid dispersed through another liquid
Preparations administered by other routes	
Pessaries	Moulded or compressed form of medication inserted into the vagina
Suppositories	Medicated solid bodies inserted into the rectum
Enemas	Medicated suspensions, oils or foam solutions administered into the rectum
Nebulized solutions	Minute liquid particles inhaled into the lungs as a vapour using a nebulizer (see Ch. 17)
Dry powder inhaler	A solid that is converted into minute particles, which are inhaled
Metered dose inhaler	A pressurized device that delivers a preset dose of tiny medicated particles into the lungs

Table 22.3 Common routes of drug administration

Route	Systemic/local	Site of administration
Oral	Systemic	Taken by mouth and swallowed, or given via a nasogastric tube (see Ch. 19)
Sublingual	Systemic	Sprayed into the mouth or allowed to dissolve under the tongue or in the cheek
Topical	Can be local and/or systemic	Applied onto the skin, e.g. ointments, creams (local, see p. 558), transdermal patches (systemic, see p. 558) or mucous membranes, e.g. eyes (local), ears (local)
Vaginal	Can be local and/or systemic	Vaginal preparations can be in the form of creams, pessaries, aerosol foams, gels and tablets
Rectal	Can be local and/or systemic	Rectal preparations can be in the form of suppositories or enemas
Inhalation	Local	Inhaled into the lungs, e.g. metered-dose inhalers (with or without a spacer device), nebulizers, steam inhalations
Injections:	Systemic	
Intradermal		Into the skin
Subcutaneous (s.c.)		Into the subcutaneous tissue under the skin (see Fig. 22.9A)
Intramuscular (i.m.)		Into a skeletal muscle (see Fig. 22.9B)
Intravenous (i.v.)		Into a vein by a trained registered practitioner
Intraosseous		Into a bone by a trained registered practitioner
Intrathecal		Into the subarachnoid space (within the meninges) via a lumbar puncture by a trained registered practitioner

potential gastric irritants and are enteric coated so that they travel through the stomach unchanged before entering the small intestine where they are absorbed, thus avoiding gastric irritation. People should therefore swallow these tablets whole and not crush or chew them, so that the enteric coating and/or extended release action is maintained. Crushing tablets increases the risk of adverse drug reactions and toxicity. When controlled/slow release tablets are crushed, the whole dose may be released within a few minutes instead of over the longer period intended. Manufacturers' instructions usually warn against the crushing of tablets or opening of capsules as this is outwith the marketing licence and this option should be discussed with the prescriber first. When available, it is safer to use liquid preparations when swallowing tablets is difficult or impossible.

Sublingual route

Some preparations put into the mouth are not intended for swallowing, including those for sublingual administration, which avoids first pass metabolism (see p. 545), e.g. glyceryl trinitrate. Sublingual tablets are placed under the tongue and allowed to dissolve slowly.

Parenteral medication

Parenteral medication includes those given by any route other than the alimentary tract. This includes preparations that are:

• Given by injection (see p. 554)
• Inserted into body orifices, e.g. pessaries and suppositories (see Table 22.3)
• Instilled, e.g. into the eye, nose or ear
• Inhaled through the mouth (see Ch. 17) or nasal passages, e.g. bronchodilators or nasal decongestants.

Administering prescribed medication

Nurses should exercise professional judgement when administering medicines (NMC 2010b) and bear in mind that they are accountable when carrying out medical instructions (NMC 2008; see also Ch. 7). Medicines must always be administered in accordance with legislation (see p. 541) and local policies. It is every nurse's duty to be familiar with these policies and student nurses should refer to these in each new placement (NMC 2010a,b). The importance of gaining consent and situations in which covert administration may be appropriate are considered below; calculation of drug doses is explained. The later parts of this section explain how nurses administer drugs by a number of routes.

Consent

It is important that healthcare professionals are aware of the individual's right to refuse treatment, including medication, and must always respect their decisions (NMC 2010b). Adults must always be presumed to have the mental capacity (see Ch. 6) to consent to, or refuse, treatment, including taking medication, and no medication should be given without their agreement.

However, there are certain situations when people may not be capable of providing informed consent. People with mental health problems, including dementia or a learning disability may lack the capacity to make the decision whether or not to take medication (Box 22.5). When patients/clients are incapable of providing consent, or their wishes are contrary to their best interests (see Ch. 6), a registered practitioner should consult relevant people such as the family, carers or members of the multidisciplinary team (MDT). Assessment of capacity is primarily a matter for the treating clinicians

┌───┐
│ **(?) Critical thinking**   **Box 22.5** │
│   │
│ **Drug administration policies and obtaining consent** │
│ Drug administration policies may vary between care settings. │
│   │
│ **Student activities**   │
│ 1. Within your placement, locate and read the local drug │
│   administration policy and identify: │
│   • Who must be involved in administration of controlled drugs. │
│   • Who must be involved in administration of non-controlled │
│   drugs.   │
│ 2. Bana is a client with a moderate learning disability who │
│   attends a day centre on weekdays. She receives regular │
│   medication to prevent seizures.   │
│   • Think about how you would explain a change in the dose │
│   of Bana's medication to her.   │
│   • Discuss with your mentor the ways in which you could gain │
│   informed consent from Bana before administering her │
│   medication.   │
└───┘

but nurses as members of the MDT should be involved in such discussions.

For people detained under mental health legislation, the principles of consent still apply to medications prescribed for other conditions. In other words, only medicines prescribed for mental health problems can be administered without the client's consent.

The Children Act 2004 ensures that children's wishes and feelings are taken into account, that they should always be consulted (subject to age and understanding) and kept informed about what is planned (see Ch. 6).

Covert administration of medicines

The NMC (2007) states that:

> … disguising medication in the absence of informed consent may be regarded as deception. However, a clear distinction should always be made between those patients/clients who have the capacity to refuse medication and whose refusal should be respected, and those who lack this capacity. Among those who lack this capacity, a further distinction should be made between those for whom no disguising is necessary because they are unaware that they are receiving medication and others who would be aware if they were not deceived into thinking otherwise.

The NMC (2007) recognizes that there may be certain exceptional circumstances in which covert administration may be considered, to prevent a patient/client from missing out on essential treatment. In such circumstances and in the absence of informed consent, the following considerations may apply:

- The best interests of the patient/client must be considered at all times
- The medication must be considered essential for the patient's/client's health and well-being or for the safety of others
- The decision to administer a medication covertly should not be considered routine, and should be a contingency measure. Any decision to do so must be reached after assessing the care needs of the patient/client individually.

This should be patient/client-specific, in order to avoid the ritualized administration of medication in this way

- There should be broad and open discussion among the multiprofessional clinical team and the supporters of the patient/client, and agreement that this approach is required in the circumstances. Those involved should include carers, relatives, advocates and the multidisciplinary team (especially the pharmacist). Family involvement in the care process should be positively encouraged. The method of administration of the medicines should be agreed with the pharmacist
- The decision and the action taken, including the names of all parties concerned, should be documented in the care plan and reviewed at appropriate intervals.

Regular attempts should still be made to encourage the patient/client to take their medication.

Calculation of drug doses

The units used for drug doses and accepted abbreviations are shown in Box 22.3 (p. 544). Most drugs are manufactured in a form that enables straightforward administration, and some are found in a variety of strengths. This helps to ensure that the prescribed dose can be provided accurately and is easily calculated.

Accurate calculation of drug doses requires practice. Student nurses must always have their drug calculations checked by a RN.

Tablets and capsules

In order to calculate the number of tablets or capsules required, the nurse needs to know the dose prescribed and the strength of tablets/capsules available. The following formula is then used:

$$\frac{\text{dose prescribed}}{\text{dose available}} = \text{number of tablets or capsules to be given}$$

For example: An adult is prescribed 1 g of paracetamol, for which 500 mg tablets are available.
Using the above formula:

$$\frac{1000 \text{ mg (or 1 g)}}{500 \text{ mg}} = 2 \text{ tablets.}$$

If the calculation reveals that a tablet requires to be halved, a scored tablet is halved using a tablet splitter. Only scored tablets must be split to provide the correct dose and prevent potentially serious consequences. If the tablet cannot be halved, the medication should be withheld and advice should be sought from the prescriber and/or pharmacist.

Liquid preparations

In the case of liquid preparations, the nurse needs to know the prescribed dose and the amount or weight of drug in a given amount of solution.

The following formula is used:

$$\frac{\text{dose prescribed} \times \text{volume available}}{\text{dose available}} = \text{volume to be given (mL)}$$

For example: An adult is prescribed 500 mg of penicillin. The stock is syrup containing 125 mg/5 mL.
Using the above formula:

$$\frac{500 \text{ mg} \times 5}{125 \text{ mg}} = 20 \text{ mL of syrup to be given}$$

Calculations based on body weight or surface area

These are used for some drugs in adults, e.g. chemotherapy treatment for cancer, and also in children.

Body weight

Body weight is often used for calculating doses for children and also for older adults. The following formula is used:

$$\frac{\text{Weight (kg)} \times \text{dosage per day}}{\text{Number of doses per day}} = \text{mg per dose}$$

For example: A child weighing 16 kg is prescribed intravenous erythromycin for a severe infection. The dosage is 50 mg/kg per day in four doses.
Using the above formula:

$$\frac{16 \text{ kg} \times 50 \text{ mg/kg/day}}{4 \text{ doses/day}} = 200 \text{ mg/dose}$$

In other words, a 200 mg injection would be administered every 6 hours.

Surface area

Doses are calculated according to body surface area, which is estimated in square metres (m^2) using a nomogram (a graph that determines surface area from measurements of height and weight). This may be used for chemotherapy in people of all ages. Drug doses are calculated using the following formula:

$$\text{surface area} \times \text{prescribed dosage} = \text{dose required}$$

For example: A child is prescribed cytarabine. The recommended dosage is 120 mg/m^2 and their surface area is 0.5 m^2.
Using the above formula:

$$0.5 \text{ m}^2 \times 120 \text{ mg/m}^2 = 60 \text{ mg}$$

For more examples of drug calculations, see Gatford & Phillips 2011.

Preparation for the administration of medications

Nurses must be familiar with both the procedure and the drugs(s) to be given in order to answer any questions the patient/client may ask about their medication and to

administer it safely. It is important to explain to the patient/client how the drug works and how it is to be administered. Explanation may be either verbal, using language appropriate to the individual, and/or in writing, and must include the reason why the drug has been prescribed. Before receiving a new medicine, people may feel anxious about its administration and/or their reaction to it.

It is essential to ensure that any allergies are written in the medical/nursing notes and on the prescription sheet to ensure that people are not given drugs to which they are allergic.

There are several additional and specific precautions that must be adhered to when prescribing and administering drugs to children and also points of good practice (Box 22.6).

Administering medicines to children — **Box 22.6**

Specific precautions for children

- In both hospital and community settings, medications must always be kept out of reach of children
- Most paediatric drug dosages, which includes children under 50 kg or before puberty, are prescribed according to age, body weight, body surface area or a combination of these parameters
- Student nurses must always have their calculations checked by an RN
- When calculating any dose for children, an RN must also have their calculations checked by another RN as accurate doses are very important since even small discrepancies can be dangerous and overdosage fatal.

Points of good practice

- As children may experience difficulty in swallowing solid medications, transdermal patches (see p. 558) or liquid forms may be prescribed
- Some liquid preparations contain sugar to make them more palatable. Where a liquid preparation is required over a long period, a sugar-free version should be prescribed to reduce the incidence of dental caries. This is also important in children with diabetes
- If the dose is less than 1 mL, oral syringes should be used. This avoids the possibility of the preparation being injected and allows accurate dose measurement
- Medications should not be diluted in bottle feeds or other liquids as the drug may interact with milk or other liquid and the dose cannot be guaranteed if the drink is not completely finished
- Injections should be avoided whenever possible. Guidance on injection techniques in children can be found in the *Position Statement on Injection Technique* (Royal College of Paediatrics and Child Health 2002; see also p. 555).

Checks are carried out to ensure that the correct patient/client is given the right medication (correct dose via the right route and the correct preparation) at the right time and that the correct documentation is accurately completed afterwards. It is essential to adopt a systematic approach to ensure that medicines are administered safely (Box 22.7).

Nursing skills Box 22.7

Principles of drug administration

- If administering medicines to a group of patients/clients the medicine round should begin with the first individual and move on to the next in order
- Accurate identification of the person to whom the medicine is to be administered is paramount. Local policy regarding identification of patients/clients, especially for children, older adults, people with mental health problems or a learning disability and those who are unconscious, must be followed
- The prescription chart (see Fig. 22.3) is checked carefully and if there are any doubts about its accuracy, the procedure must be stopped and clarification sought
- The medication is checked against the written prescription and the expiry date checked to ensure it is in date
- The recording section of the prescription chart is checked to ensure that the medication has not already been administered
- The medicine is selected and carefully checked against the prescription
- This procedure is repeated for all medicines to be administered together. Care must be taken to ensure that medications given together are compatible, i.e. they will not interact with one another, using the BNF if necessary
- Immediately after administration, the recording section on the prescription chart is initialled.

Administration of oral medications

When possible, the patient/client is assisted to sit upright, as this makes swallowing easier. The person should be offered a glass of water, which moistens the mouth, prevents tablets or capsules sticking to the oral or oesophageal mucosa and aids their transport to the stomach. Principles for administering oral preparations are shown in Box 22.8. Some medications should be given at specific times. For example, nystatin pastilles given to treat an oral fungal infection should be taken after food as the drug would be removed by food and drink.

 Nursing skills Box 22.8

Administration of oral preparations

- Medication is dispensed directly from its original packaging without touching it (Fig. 22.7)
- All tablets and capsules are dispensed into medicine containers
- Liquid medication is dispensed into separate containers
- Medicine containers are placed on a tray and taken to the patient/client
- The person's identity is confirmed according to local policy and they are consulted as to how they wish to take their medication: some people prefer to swallow tablets or capsules from the container, some like to lift them out of the container and others prefer the tablets placed into their hand to swallow either all together or one by one. If a person is unable to manipulate the medications then they are delivered into their mouth using a spoon to avoid cross-infection
- Immediately after administration, each medicine is signed as given on the recording sheet.

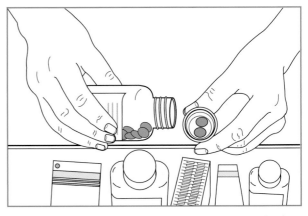

Fig. 22.7 • Non-touch technique for dispensing oral medication. (Reproduced with permission from Nicol, M., Bavin, C., Bedford-Turner, S., et al., 2004. Essential nursing skills, second ed. Mosby, Edinburgh.)

Nurses administering medicines should be aware of specific instructions.

Injections

Injections are considered the appropriate route of administration when:

- Fast onset of action is required
- Fasting is required
- Digestive enzymes would inactivate the drug, e.g. insulin
- Long-term release of the drug is necessary, e.g. depot injections (see Z-track technique, pp. 556–557 and Fig. 22.12).

Injections can be given via the intradermal, subcutaneous, intramuscular, intravenous, intraosseous and intrathecal routes (see Table 22.3). Student nurses are normally only involved in administering injections by the subcutaneous and intramuscular routes.

Preparing and giving injections

Preparation of injections is carried out in accordance with local policies and the *Good Practice Statement* (Clinical Resource and Audit Group 2002; Dougherty and Lister 2011). Box 22.9 outlines the steps in preparing or 'drawing up' injections. This section also considers intramuscular (i.m.) and subcutaneous (s.c.) injections, and the sites used. As i.m. injections are given into muscles and s.c. injections into the more superficial subcutaneous tissue, the depth of these injections is different.

Skin cleansing prior to injections

There is some controversy about the need to cleanse the skin prior to injections. The skin should be cleansed using an alcohol wipe only if local policy recommends this. Some local policies state that if the patient is physically clean, and the nurse follows local hand hygiene policy and uses a non-touch technique during the procedure (see Ch. 15), skin cleansing with an alcohol-impregnated wipe is not required. If used, the skin should be cleansed for 30 seconds and then allowed to dry for

Drawing up injections

- Collect the equipment required, i.e. a suitable tray to hold the materials, an appropriately sized syringe, two appropriately sized needles, an alcohol-impregnated wipe and the ampoules(s) containing the correct medication
- Clean the work surface where preparation will take place according to local policy
- The hands are thoroughly washed and dried, and gloves worn as per local policy
- The prescription is checked
- The integrity of the needle and syringe packaging and their expiry dates are checked
- Peel apart the packaging as directed by the manufacturer to expose the plunger end of the syringe
- Lift the syringe out by the barrel taking care to ensure that the nozzle does not become contaminated
- Peel apart the packaging to expose the hub of the needle
- Assemble the needle and syringe, and place in the tray
- Open the ampoule according to the manufacturer's instructions
- If an ampoule with a rubber or plastic top is used then the top is cleansed with the alcohol-impregnated wipe for 30 seconds and allowed to air dry for 30 seconds
- After removing the sheath, the needle is carefully inserted into the ampoule at a 45° angle. The prescribed dose is carefully withdrawn using a non-touch technique (Fig. 22.8). Care must be taken to ensure that the needle does not hit the bottom of the ampoule as this would blunt the tip
- Gently tap the syringe barrel to encourage any air bubbles to rise towards the air space (NPSA 2007b)
- Push the barrel slowly upwards, expelling any air from the syringe; this is complete when droplets of liquid are seen at the top of the needle. The syringe is now primed ready for use
- At this point the unsheathed needle is discarded and a second sheathed needle is fitted to reduce the risk of needlestick injuries (see local policy)
- The tray containing the drawn-up injection and empty ampoule, and the prescription chart are taken to the patient/client.

another 30 seconds in order that adequate skin disinfection is achieved (Workman 1999).

The intramuscular route

Intramuscular injections are delivered into the muscles below the skin. Figure 22.9B shows the needle angle used to access the muscle layer. There are several sites that can be used for i.m. injections. The person's general health and age are considered before deciding upon the most appropriate site. Older and emaciated people are likely to have less muscle than those who are young and active. The proposed site should be inspected for signs of swelling, inflammation, infection and skin lesions; affected areas should be avoided.

Deltoid muscle

The deltoid muscle is commonly used for vaccinations and for older children (Royal College of Paediatrics and Child Health 2002) (Fig. 22.10C).

Dorsogluteal site

The dorsogluteal site, also known as 'the upper outer quadrant' of the buttock, uses the gluteus maximus muscle (Fig. 22.10A). Studies have shown that there is relatively slow uptake of medication from this site (Rodger & King 2000). This is due to the large amount of adipose tissue located there, even in mildly obese patients, and means that the medication often ends up in the adipose tissue rather than the muscle (Workman 1999). The nurse must therefore choose an appropriate length of needle depending on the size of the adult. There is also a risk of damaging the sciatic nerve if the site is not carefully located.

Ventrogluteal site

The ventrogluteal site accesses the gluteus medius muscle (Fig. 22.10D). Following an extensive literature review, Beyea and Nicoll (1995) promote the use of this site as it avoids potential sciatic nerve damage and the adipose tissue in the area is of

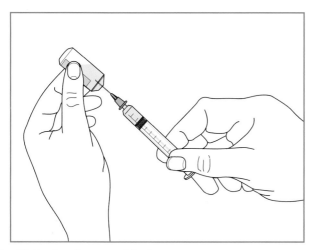

Fig. 22.8 • Drawing up an injection. (Reproduced with permission from Nicol, M., Bavin, C., Bedford-Turner, S., et al., 2004. Essential nursing skills, second ed. Mosby, Edinburgh.)

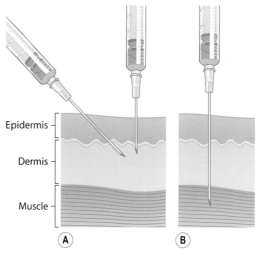

Fig. 22.9 • Skin layers and needle insertion for injections: (A) Subcutaneous. (B) Intramuscular. (Reproduced with permission from Downie, G., Mackenzie, J., Williams, A., 2003. Pharmacology and medicines management for nurses, third ed. Churchill Livingstone, Edinburgh.)

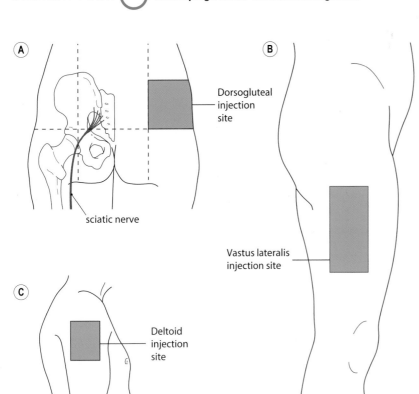

Fig. 22.10 • Intramuscular injection sites. (A,B,C reproduced with permission from Nicol, M., Bavin, C., Bedford-Turner, S., et al., 2004. Essential nursing skills, second ed. Mosby, Edinburgh. D, reproduced with permission from Wong, D.L., Hockenberry-Eaton, M., 2001. Wong's essentials of pediatric nursing, sixth ed. Mosby, St Louis.)

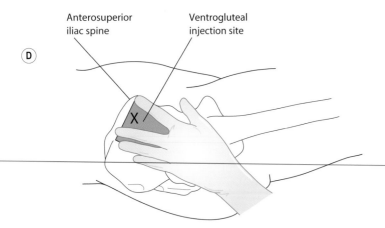

relatively consistent thickness, thus ensuring the medication is administered into the muscle tissue (Greenway 2004). Workman (1999) suggests that a standard 21G (green) needle could be used in most adults of any size due to the consistent thickness of adipose tissue over this site.

Vastus lateralis muscle

This muscle is on the outer aspect of the thigh (Fig. 22.10B) and can be used for children, including infants (Royal College of Paediatrics and Child Health 2002). However, Beyea and Nicoll (1996) suggest that, after 7 months of age, the ventrogluteal site should be the site of choice.

Rectus femoris

The rectus femoris is the anterior quadriceps muscle of the thigh. This is rarely used in adults, but can be easily accessed for self-administration or for infants (Workman 1999).

Administering intramuscular injections

The principles of administering i.m. injections are shown in Box 22.10.

The Z-track technique, formerly used exclusively for medications that stain the skin, is now widely recommended for all i.m. injections, as it is believed to reduce pain and leakage of medicine from the injection site. This technique involves

Nursing skills   Box 22.10

Administration of intramuscular injections

Principles

- The technique is explained to the person and their agreement is sought
- Handwashing is carried out according to local policy and gloves worn
- The injection is drawn up as outlined in Box 22.9
- Privacy is ensured and the injection site exposed
- The skin is cleaned according to local policy
- The normal needle size for adults is 21G (green) (Nicol et al 2012). Local policy may recommend the use of smaller needles (23G blue) for e.g. very thin individuals or children
- The skin is stretched or pulled (Fig. 22.11) using the non-dominant hand. Alternatively, the Z-track technique (Fig. 22.12) should be used
- The syringe barrel is held like a dart or pencil in the dominant hand
- The patient/client is informed and the needle inserted swiftly and firmly into the skin at an angle of 90° (see Fig. 22.11). The needle is inserted until about only 0.5 to 1 cm is showing (Nicol et al 2012)
- The plunger is withdrawn slightly to check that the needle is not in a blood vessel. Nicol et al (2012) recommend that if blood is present at this stage, the needle should be withdrawn, the needle and syringe discarded and the injection drawn up again using fresh equipment
- The plunger is then firmly and steadily depressed until all the fluid has been expelled
- The syringe is quickly removed and the alcohol-impregnated wipe held firmly over the puncture site until any bleeding stops
- The syringe and unsheathed needle are disposed of immediately into the designated sharps bin
- The remaining equipment is discarded
- Handwashing is carried out according to local policy
- The recording sheet is signed.

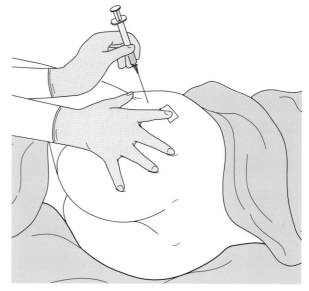

Fig. 22.11 • Intramuscular injection technique. (Reproduced with permission from Nicol, M., Bavin, C., Bedford-Turner, S., et al., 2004. Essential nursing skills, second ed. Mosby, Edinburgh.)

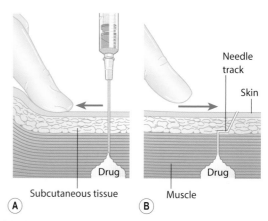

Fig. 22.12 • Administering a Z-track injection. (Reproduced with permission from Downie, G., Mackenzie, J., Williams, A., 2003. Pharmacology and medicines management for nurses, third ed. Churchill Livingstone, Edinburgh.)

gently pulling the skin and subcutaneous tissue so that it is no longer directly over the underlying muscle before carrying out the injection (Fig. 22.12) (Workman 1999). This is widely used for depot injections, commonly given to people with mental health problems.

Subcutaneous injections

These are given into the subcutaneous fat or connective tissue that lies between the muscles and the skin (see Fig. 22.9A). A short fine needle is used, e.g. 25G (orange) (Workman 1999). This route is suitable for drugs such as insulin that require slow and steady release. If a needle longer than 9 mm (25G orange) is used, an angle of 45° is recommended. When a shorter needle is required, e.g. for the administration of insulin, an angle of 90° is recommended (Workman 1999).

Some s.c. injections are pre-filled with the drug (such as heparin, given to prevent deep venous thrombosis), which means that there is no need to draw up the injection and therefore reduces the risk of needlestick injury. When using a shorter needle, it is not necessary to aspirate before injecting (Peragallo-Dittko 1997).

Figure 22.13 shows the sites that can be used for s.c. injections. People who require frequent s.c. injections, e.g. those with diabetes, should rotate injection sites and avoid using alcohol-impregnated wipes, which harden the skin. The principles of giving s.c. injections are shown in Box 22.11.

Rectal administration

This route is selected when:

- A person is unable to swallow oral preparations or during nausea and/or vomiting
- Medication may cause irritation of the upper gastrointestinal tract
- Drug delivery is required near to a diseased site, e.g. corticosteroids for inflammatory bowel disease
- Evacuation of the rectum is required, i.e. a laxative effect.

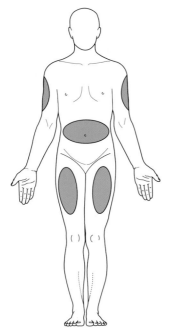

○ **Nursing skills** Box 22.11

Administering subcutaneous injections

Principles

- The technique is explained to the person and their agreement is sought
- Privacy is ensured by, e.g. closing the cubicle door or pulling the screens
- Handwashing is carried out according to local policy and gloves worn
- The injection is drawn up as outlined in Box 22.9
- Select a suitable site
- Skin cleansing is not usually required if the skin is clean
- The site is exposed and the skin fold pinched
- The drug is injected using the desired angle (see Fig. 22.9A). For a 90° angle, the syringe is held in a 'pencil' grip and the needle is stabbed through the skin. For a 45° angle, the syringe is cradled across all four fingers, steadied with the thumb and, with the needle bevel uppermost, is pushed gently through the skin
- The syringe and unsheathed needle are disposed of immediately into the designated sharps bin
- The remaining equipment is discarded
- Handwashing is carried out according to local policy
- The recording sheet is signed.

Medication can be inserted into the rectum as suppositories and enemas (see Ch. 21). When this route is used for therapeutic drug administration (rather than for evacuation of the rectum), it must be explained that the medication should be retained, as many people associate suppositories and enemas with evacuation of the bowel. Ready access to lavatory facilities is necessary following administration of evacuant medication.

Inhaled medication

Medications can be introduced directly into the airways for local action (e.g. bronchodilators to relieve bronchospasm, corticosteroids to reduce inflammation) in respiratory conditions such as asthma and chronic bronchitis. Action via this route is fast and high concentrations can be delivered quickly to the site of action. There are different types of inhaler devices and their use is explained in Chapter 17. These include:

- Metered dose inhalers
- Dry powder inhalers
- Nebulizers.

Administration of topical medication

The patient should be prepared to receive medication following the principles outlined in Box 22.7 (p. 554) Box 22.12 provides the principles involved in administering topical creams, ointments or lotions that are usually prescribed for skin conditions.

○ **Nursing skills** Box 22.12

Administration of creams, ointments and lotions
Principles

- The technique is explained to the person and their agreement is sought
- Handwashing is carried out according to local policy
- An apron and gloves (to prevent absorption through the skin) are worn
- Creams, ointments or lotions are applied to clean, dry skin and gently rubbed in using sterile, strand-free gauze (Nicol et al 2012)
- Handwashing is carried out according to local policy
- The skin and/or any lesions are assessed and changes documented in the nursing notes.

Transdermal patches

Transdermal patches are used to deliver medication such as hormones, opioids and nicotine replacement therapy (Fig. 22.14). In these situations, topical application is used to provide systemic effects, usually for a prolonged period. The old patch is removed, the skin cleaned and a new patch is applied, usually to a different area. The skin is observed for redness, soreness and other signs of a reaction to either the drug or the adhesive. Patches are placed on non-hairy areas according to the prescription and the manufacturer's instructions.

Other routes

Less frequently, nurses administer medication in other ways, e.g. instillation of drops into the eyes, ears or nose or insertion of pessaries into the vagina. Principles of patient preparation are the same irrespective of the route, but detailed discussion of these is beyond the scope of this book and can be found in Nicol et al (2012).

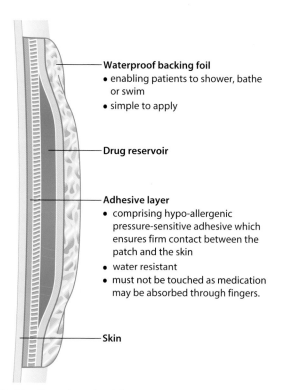

Waterproof backing foil
- enabling patients to shower, bathe or swim
- simple to apply

Drug reservoir

Adhesive layer
- comprising hypo-allergenic pressure-sensitive adhesive which ensures firm contact between the patch and the skin
- water resistant
- must not be touched as medication may be absorbed through fingers.

Skin

Fig. 22.14 • Transdermal patch. (Reproduced with permission from Downie, G., Mackenzie, J., Williams, A., 2003. Pharmacology and medicines management for nurses, third ed. Churchill Livingstone, Edinburgh.)

Post-drug administration measures

After administration of any medication, the nurse must always ensure that:

- The patient/client is comfortable
- Any equipment is removed and disposed of appropriately
- Administration has been recorded in line with professional and legal requirements (NMC 2010b) and local policy.

The nurse must ensure that the patient/client knows:

- Why the medication has been given
- When the medicine should take effect, e.g. around 20 minutes for i.m. injections
- Any potential side-effects and to report these if they occur.

The RN must check that:

- The prescription chart has been signed/initialled according to local policy if the medicine has been administered. If medication has not been administered, the reason for this must be documented
- The controlled drugs register has been completed, where appropriate, in accordance with local policy
- Medicines administered by student nurses have been countersigned
- Any adverse drug reactions are reported to the prescriber and/or charge nurse.

It should be noted that if the patient has been unable to swallow medicines, this should be reported immediately to the

pharmacist and prescriber. A suitable alternative may be prescribed and dispensed.

Adherence and polypharmacy

The success of any medication regimen is most likely when it is completed according to the prescription. In this section, adherence and polypharmacy, and links between the two are considered.

Adherence

In order that medication can achieve its intended benefit it is important that people adhere to and complete the prescribed course or continue to take it when a chronic condition is present. Between one-third and one-half of medicines prescribed for long-term conditions are not used as recommended, which means that many patients are not receiving their prescribed medication and its associated health benefits; this also represents significant wastage of NHS resources (National Institute for Health and Clinical Excellence, NICE 2009).

Adherence (NICE 2009) is a patient-centred approach to treatment, such as taking medicines, where an agreement between a patient/client and a healthcare professional is negotiated. This approach may also be referred to as concordance. This person-centred approach to medicines management is supported by NICE guidelines (2009), where an individual's beliefs and wishes about taking medication are central to any consideration of treatment options. Adherence is maximized when:

- An open no-blame approach that encourages frank discussion about any doubts is used
- A patient-centred approach is adopted
- The individual's perceptions and any practical barriers to adherence are regularly reviewed.

The key to adherence is effective patient/client education. It is important to openly discuss issues and confirm that the individual understands:

- Why the medication is necessary
- What benefits the medication should have
- Side-effects that may be experienced
- How and when to take the medication
- Who to contact if they have any questions to ask.

Written information must also be provided by including patient information leaflets (PILs) with medication unless all the necessary information can be included on the label. This will reinforce verbal information provided by healthcare professionals. However, it cannot be assumed that people will be able to read or understand the PILs and for this reason nurses should confirm peoples' understanding of medicines they take when assessing medicines adherence.

Non-adherence

Non-adherence is common and may be:

- Intentional – when the patient/client chooses not to follow the recommended treatment, usually due to their beliefs and concerns. When this is the case, the patient's/client's wishes must be respected (NMC 2008) and alternatives should be considered

- Non-intentional – where the individual wishes to follow the prescription but has practical difficulties in doing so (see below).

Polypharmacy

The Department of Health (2001) define polypharmacy as being prescribed four or more drugs simultaneously. This is associated with more adverse drug reactions, predisposes to readmission of older adults following discharge from hospital and increases non-adherence. The National Patient Safety Association (NPSA 2007a) reported that 6.5% of all non-elective admissions were related to adverse drug reactions (ADRs), of which 72% were judged to be avoidable. The Department of Health (2001) reviewed medicine-related aspects in the care of older adults and highlighted that medicine use increases with age:

- 80% of people over 75 years of age took at least one prescribed drug
- 36% took more than four medications.

People may forget to mention any over-the-counter medicines that they take regularly, assuming that they are not 'real' medications, and the nurse should therefore specifically ask patients/clients about these products when discussing patient's/client's medicines, as their use is widespread.

Nurses should be aware that both under- and over-medication can arise from personal beliefs, forgetfulness, improvement in a person's condition, lack of knowledge and/or misunderstanding about the drugs and that these should be considered when assessing adherence and monitoring response to treatment.

Improving medicines adherence

Many people will require support to maximize medicines adherence. Nurses must consider physical and psychological factors when explaining, demonstrating and teaching people about medication (Box 22.13). Relatives and carers may also become involved in education about drug treatment in, for example, children and people with a learning disability.

Older adults often have several conditions needing treatment with medicines which frequently leads to polypharmacy and confusing medicine regimens. Medicines adherence is lower when complicated drug regimens are prescribed.

There are also many other reasons why a person may not or cannot take their medication as prescribed. Physical factors include difficulty getting to the pharmacy to collect medication or difficulty with swallowing. Individuals who lack manual dexterity and are unable to open the packaging may require medications to be organized in a Dosette box or supplied in easy-to-open containers. For those with visual impairment, large-print labels help. People's religious or cultural beliefs may affect adherence; for example, vegetarians and people who do not eat beef (e.g. Hindus) may refuse to take gelatin capsules. For patients/clients who have difficulty in remembering when to take the medicine

---

Health promotion	Box 22.13

Medication in older adults

Mary is 79 years old and was admitted to hospital in a confused state. Investigations revealed she had a chest infection. She takes regular medication for high blood pressure and arthritis and has been prescribed antibiotics for her chest infection.

Student activities

Looking at the factors that may influence a person's medicines adherence with their drug regimen, think about those that may apply to Mary:

1. Identify the nursing interventions that will help maximize adherence and concordance after Mary is discharged.
2. Find out from the pharmacist what aids to adherence are available in your placement.
3. Speak to some patients/clients in your placement and find out:
   - How much they know about drugs they take regularly
   - The likely extent to which they comply with prescribed treatment
   - What medications they often buy for themselves in a shop or pharmacy.

---

or if they have taken it, keeping a chart and ticking this when medicines have been taken may be used. Other people may stop taking their medication when their symptoms are alleviated or if side-effects (actual or perceived) occur.

Using a person-centred approach to identify and overcome factors that may predispose to poor medicines adherence forms the basis of enabling people to better follow their drug treatment.

Dosette boxes

These contain sections for each day of the week, which are further divided to correspond with the times of day when the patient/client takes their medication, e.g. '8 am, 12 midday, 6 pm, 10 pm'. Each daily column has a sliding lid that can be opened to expose only the drugs to be taken at a particular time (Fig. 22.15). Individuals, carers, pharmacists or other health-care professionals can fill these boxes with the appropriate prescribed medications. There may, however, be a loss of efficacy if tablets are removed from blister packs and put into these boxes.

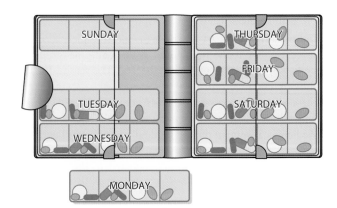

Fig. 22.15 • Dosette box.

Self-medication

People take their own medicines at home and self-medication before discharge is good preparation for this; self-medication is associated with improved adherence. Since the introduction of lockable medicine cabinets (see Fig. 22.1B) at each hospital bedside, self-administration has become more widespread in hospitals. As an RN you are responsible for the initial and continued assessment of patients who are self-administering, and have continuing responsibility for recognising and acting upon changes in a patient's condition with regards to safety of the patient and others (NMC 2010b). RNs should assess the patient's suitability to self-administer medicinal products both in the hospital and primary care settings, and nurses should be aware of their professional responsibility and accountability in relation to medicines management (NMC 2010b).

Drug administration errors

Much has been done to make drug administration safe and yet errors do still sometimes occur. The extent of drug errors has been the subject of much attention from the government, hospital management, pharmacists and healthcare professionals, all of whom consider the safe administration of medicines to be an essential nursing skill.

Following studies into how errors occur, changes to drug administration policies have been made in an effort to make this as safe as possible. Student nurses are taught how to administer drugs safely in university, then supervised carrying this out in practice, and later assessed as competent before gaining registration. Thereafter, nurses are expected to continually update their knowledge of the drugs they administer. In spite of this, errors sometimes still occur and the consequences for a patient/client can be fatal. The consequences for nurses can result in disciplinary action, an investigation of professional misconduct, criminal charges or a civil case for negligence (see Ch. 6). Most importantly, however, being involved in drug errors significantly reduces their confidence as practitioners.

Minimizing errors

There are many models aimed at minimizing the occurrence of drug errors. NPSA (2009) suggested a model to safeguard the recipient, the nurse (administrator), the pharmacist (dispenser) and the prescriber. All involved should know:

- The patient/client
- The drugs
- How to communicate clearly (see Ch. 9)
- Drug names that look and/or sound alike.

The storage and distribution of drugs should be restricted and standardized, and any drug delivery systems should be assessed for safety and be user-friendly. The care environment should be conducive to safe working practices that include nurses having appropriate education and sufficient practice before being assessed as competent to administer drugs safely. In order to reduce drug errors, emphasis is placed on drug administration processes rather than the practitioners involved.

Over 90% of medicines incidents reported to the NPSA are associated with no harm or low harm; in 2007, some 70 000 medications incidents were reported (NPSA 2009). The key findings were that:

- Injectable medicines represented 62% of all reported incidents that led to death or severe patient harm
- Three types of medicines errors accounted for 71% of the most serious incidents (deaths and cases of severe patient harm), namely:
  - ○ Unclear/wrong dose or frequency
  - ○ Administration of the wrong medicine
  - ○ Omission or delay in administering medicines
- The types of medicines most frequently associated with severe patient harm and fatalities were: cardiovascular drugs, anti-infective agents, opioids, anticoagulants and anti-platelet drugs.

Contributing factors identified in nurses and nursing practices that have been implicated in drug errors include:

- Poor mathematical skills
- Lack of knowledge of medications
- Tiredness caused by, e.g. long shifts and shift patterns
- High workload
- Interruptions during drug administration.

In some areas, nurses wear red tabards when undertaking medicine rounds as a signal to others around that they are not to be disturbed; NPSA (2007a) reported that one such programme had reduced drug administration errors.

Dealing with drug errors

As an RN, if you make an error, you must take any action to prevent any potential harm to the patient and report this as soon as possible to the prescriber, your line manager or employer (according to local policy) and document your actions.

SUMMARY

- ◆ Nursing practice is underpinned by legislation that governs the safe storage, ordering and prescribing of medicines.
- ◆ Pharmacodynamic principles are used to explain 'what drugs do to the body'.
- ◆ Pharmacokinetic principles help to explain 'what the body does to drugs'.
- ◆ Nurses must be familiar with actions and side-effects of drugs commonly used in each placement.
- ◆ Safe administration of medicines requires a methodical approach that follows local policies.
- ◆ Nurses need to be familiar with a range of routes used for drug administration.
- ◆ Patient/client education about prescribed drugs is important.
- ◆ Polypharmacy is the prescribing of more than four drugs simultaneously and is associated with poorer medicines adherence.
- ◆ Awareness of predisposing factors may reduce drug administration errors.
- ◆ Drug errors should be approached using a 'no blame' culture.

KEY WORDS AND PHRASES FOR LITERATURE SEARCHING

Drug administration

Drug calculations

Injections

Medicines

Prescribing

Self-medication

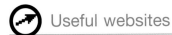 Useful websites

British National Formulary and *British National Formulary for Children* www.bnf.org/bnf
Medicines and Healthcare Products Regulatory Agency
   www.mhra.gov.uk/index.htm
National Patient Safety Agency www.npsa.nhs.uk
All websites accessed September 2012.

References

Beyea, S., Nicoll, L., 1995. Administration of medications via the intramuscular route: an integrative review of the literature and research-based protocol for the procedure. Applied Nursing Research 8 (1), 23–33.

Beyea, S., Nicoll, L., 1996. Administering IM injections the right way. American Journal of Nursing 96 (1), 34–37.

Clinical Resource and Audit Group, 2002. Good practice statement for the preparation of injections in near-patient areas, including clinical and home environments. Online. Available: www.scotland.gov.uk/Publications/2002/12/16049/15922 September 2012.

Department of Health, 1988. Guidelines for the safe and secure handling of medicines (The Duthie Report). HMSO, London.

Department of Health, 1999. Review of prescribing: supply and administration of medicines. TSO, London.

Department of Health, 2000. Health Service Circular 2000/026 Online. Available: www.dh.gov.uk/en/Publicationsandstatistics/Lettersandcirculars/Healthservicecirculars/DH_4004179 September 2012.

Department of Health, 2001. Medicines and older people: implementing medicine-related aspects of the National Service Framework. TSO, London.

Dougherty, L., Lister, S. (Eds.), 2011. The Royal Marsden Hospital manual of clinical nursing procedures, eighth ed. Wiley Blackwell, West-Sussex.

Gatford, J.D., Phillips, N., 2011. Nursing calculations, eighth ed. Churchill Livingstone, Edinburgh.

Greenway, K., 2004. Using the ventrogluteal site for intramuscular injection. Nursing Standard 18 (25), 39–42.

Medicine and Healthcare products Regulatory Agency (MHRA), 2010. Healthcare Professional Reporting: Adverse Drug Reactions. Online. Available: www.mhra.gov.uk/Safetyinformation/Reportingsafetyproblems/Reportingsuspectedadversedrugreactions/Healthcareprofessionalreporting/Adversedrugreactions/index.htm September 2012.

National Patient Safety Agency, 2007a. Safety in doses: medication safety incidents in the NHS. Online. Available: www.nrls.npsa.nhs.uk/EasySiteWeb/getresource.axd?AssetID=61392 September 2012.

National Patient Safety Agency, 2007b. Promoting safer use of injectable medicines. Alert No. 2007/20. Online. Available: www.nrls.npsa.nhs.uk/resources/?entryid45=59812 September 2012.

National Patient Safety Agency, 2009. Safety in doses: improving the use of medicines in the NHS. Online. Available: www.nrls.npsa.nhs.uk/resources/patient-safety-topics/medication-safety/?entryid45=61625 September 2012.

National Institute for Health and Clinical Excellence, 2009. Medicines adherence: involving patients in decisions about prescribed medicines and supporting adherence. Quick reference guide. Online. Available: www.nice.org.uk/nicemedia/live/11766/42891/42891.PDF September 2012.

National Prescribing Centre, 2009. Patient group directions. Online. Available: www.npc.nhs.uk/non_medical/resources/patient_group_directions.pdf September 2012.

National Prescribing Centre, 2010. Non-medical prescribing. Online. Available: www.npc.nhs.uk/non_medical September 2012.

Nicol, M., Bavin, C., Cronin, P. et al., 2012. Essential nursing skills, fourth ed. Mosby, Edinburgh.

Nursing and Midwifery Council, 2007. Covert administration of medicines: Disguising medicine in food and drink. Online. Available: http://www.nmc-uk.org/Nurses-and-midwives/Regulation-in-practice/Medicines-management-and-prescribing/Covert-administration-of-medicines/ October 2012.

Nursing and Midwifery Council, 2008. The code: Standards of conduct, performance and ethics for nurses and midwives. Online. Available: http://www.nmc-uk.org/Nurses-and-midwives/Standards-and-guidance1/The-code/The-code-in-full/ October 2012.

Nursing and Midwifery Council, 2009. Record keeping: Guidance for nurses and midwives. Online. Available: http://www.nmc-uk.org/Documents/NMC-Publications/NMC-Record-Keeping-Guidance.pdf October 2012.

Nursing and Midwifery Council, 2010a. Guidance on professional conduct for nursing and midwifery students. Online. Available: http://www.nmc-uk.org/Documents/NMC-Publications/NMC-Guidance-on-professional-conduct.pdf October 2012.

Nursing and Midwifery Council, 2010b. Standards for medicines management. Online. Available: http://www.nmc-uk.org/Documents/NMC-Publications/NMC-Standards-for-medicines-management.pdf October 2012.

Nursing and Midwifery Council, 2010c. Standards for pre-registration nursing education. Online. Available: http://standards.nmc-uk.org/PreRegNursing/statutory/background/Pages/introduction.aspx October 2012.

Peragallo-Dittko, V., 1997. Re-thinking subcutaneous injection technique. American Journal of Nursing 97 (5), 71–72.

Rodger, M.A., King, L., 2000. Drawing up and administering intramuscular injections: a review of the literature. Journal of Advanced Nursing 31 (3), 574–582.

Royal College of Paediatrics and Child Health, 2002. Position statement on injection technique. Online. Available: www.rcpch.ac.uk September 2012.

Workman, B., 1999. Safe injection technique. Nursing Standard 13 (39), 47–53.

Further reading

Greenstein, B., Gould, D., 2009. Trounce's clinical pharmacology for nurses, eighteenth ed. Churchill Livingstone, Edinburgh.

McGavock, H., 2011. How drugs work: basic pharmacology for healthcare professionals, third ed. Radcliffe, Oxford.

Pain management – minimizing the pain experience

23

Carol Chamley   Gay James

LEARNING OUTCOMES

This chapter will help you:

- Explain the biopsychosocial effects of pain on people throughout the lifespan
- Outline different types of pain
- Explore the subjective and individual impact of pain on people
- Discuss how the gate control theory of pain influences nursing management of pain
- Demonstrate an awareness of holistic pain assessment
- Describe the principles of pharmacological management of pain
- Outline non-pharmacological approaches to pain management.

Introduction

Pain is a common experience throughout life. It may be argued that people start life with acute pain following birth, though this may only recently have been acknowledged. As people age, degenerative disorders often lead them to accept pain as a natural consequence of ageing. This acceptance can limit quality of life, an important issue in the ageing population. Over the past 50 years, advances in pain management have been possible due to an improved understanding of the multidimensional nature of pain and subsequent advances in treatments.

Pain is recognized as an indicator of tissue damage and, from childhood, pain is associated with injury. The pain experience is not just a sensory signal; pain triggers complex physiological, emotional and social responses. These are influenced by many factors that include pain type, age, past experiences, emotional state, environment, culture and cognitive appraisal.

Pain is often a warning of tissue injury; allowing people to respond to external or internal triggers, it may also cause physiological stress and emotional distress, which can harm the individual if unrelieved. Though trauma may not initially be associated with pain at the time of injury; often a sports injury is not recognized until the game is over.

Poor pain management can lead to physical and emotional problems; postoperatively, it is linked to complications and delayed recovery. In children, pain may lead to regression (Ch. 11); ineffective management can have serious implications for future contact with healthcare in adult life.

Nurses are frequently key workers in the management of pain. Pain recognition and prioritization are vital aspects of patient/client care. Pain is a common experience across all care settings. The importance of preventing and managing pain is highlighted in the Essence of Care 2010 (Department of Health, DH 2010). An elementary understanding of pain and its management is relevant to foundation studies and central to all fields of nursing.

The Nursing and Midwifery Council (NMC 2010) have identified five *Essential Skills Clusters* (ESCs) and competencies required for registration. Many of these apply to pain management, and will be explored in this chapter.

The nature of pain

This part of the chapter outlines the different types of pain, gate control theory, pain physiology and psychological and cultural aspects of pain.

Pain is a subjective, complex and multidimensional experience that has physical, psychosocial, emotional and spiritual elements. Due to its complexity, a simple agreed definition for pain is elusive. The International Association for the Study of Pain (IASP) (Merskey & Bogduk 1994) defines pain as 'an unpleasant sensory and emotional experience associated with actual or potential tissue damage, or described in terms of such damage'. In 1968, McCaffery proposed a simple statement which is widely accepted in nursing as it emphasizes the individual nature of pain and the patient is clearly identified as the key person in pain assessment – 'Pain is: whatever the experiencing person says it is, existing whenever he says it does' (McCaffery & Pasero 1999).

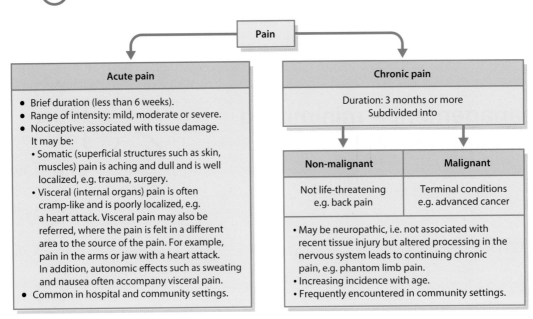

Fig. 23.1 • Types of pain.

Types and characteristics of pain

Distinctions between types may not be possible (McCaffery & Pasero 1999). One category is acute or chronic, which classifies pain according to a timescale (Fig. 23.1). This chapter concentrates on acute and chronic pain; however, pain can be categorized in other ways that include:

- Cause related to pathology
- Nociceptive or neuropathic
- Clinical specialty/client group.

In order to provide appropriate care, nurses need to appreciate the type of pain experienced, as this influences assessment and suitability of pharmacological and non-pharmacological interventions.

Acute pain

Acute pain (Fig. 23.1) is usually of brief duration (<6 weeks) and is commonly nociceptive, associated with tissue injury which subsides as healing takes place (Box 23.1). Acute pain is very common; it ranges in intensity from transitory pain felt after a minor bump to severe pain associated with trauma or disease, e.g. fractures or heart attack. Mild acute pain may be

---

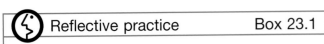

◯ Reflective practice	Box 23.1

Acute pain

Think about a recent minor injury you had, such as a cut or a bruise.

Student activities

- Reflect on the intensity of pain you experienced at the time.
- How long was it before the pain subsided to soreness/ache and when did it cease?

---

managed successfully with patient/parent-initiated interventions at home. However, the pain may also indicate problems and motivate the person to seek medical advice.

Acute nociceptive pain may be referred; this is when pain arises in internal organs (viscera) but is experienced some distance from the source of the pain. For example, a heart attack frequently causes pain down the left arm and up the neck and jaw, despite there being no tissue injury in those areas. Sensory impulses from the left arm and heart enter the spinal cord at the same level. Normally, few sensory impulses are processed from the heart so when more impulses are received for processing, this results in perception of pain arising from the arm. Another example of referred pain is the initial pain of acute appendicitis, which is felt around the umbilicus (Fig. 23.2).

Chronic pain

When pain does not resolve and becomes chronic (Fig. 23.1) (usually lasting longer than 3 months) the effect on a person's quality of life can lead to depression and social isolation. For children, this may seriously influence their education and their future potential as adults. For adults, it can cause relationship problems, isolation and financial difficulties and it may lead to mental health problems, including suicidal ideation. Chronic pain is further subdivided into non-malignant and malignant (life-threatening) pain.

Chronic non-malignant pain

Chronic non-malignant pain is not life-threatening and may be due to continuing tissue injury, e.g. rheumatoid arthritis, where degeneration may continue for life. Chronic non-malignant pain can involve alterations in pain processing by the nervous system, which results in pain memories. This is known as neuropathic pain, e.g. phantom limb pain where pain is perceived as coming from the amputated part, or the nerve pain (neuralgia) after shingles (Box 23.2). Neuropathic pain may

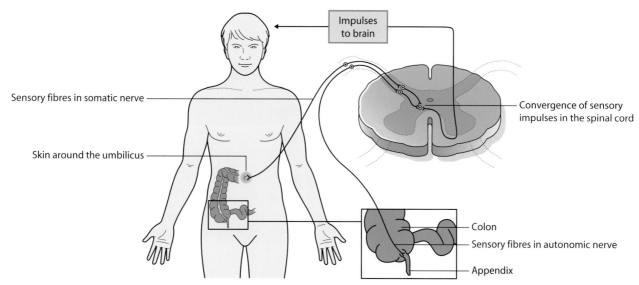

Fig. 23.2 • Referred pain – acute appendicitis. (Adapted with permission from Rutishauser, S., 1994. Physiology and anatomy. Churchill Livingstone, Edinburgh.)

Neuropathic pain after shingles	Box 23.2

The acute pain of shingles (herpes zoster) can also lead to chronic pain known as postherpetic neuralgia if the pain is not well managed. The chronic continuing pain becomes typical of neuralgia with:
- Abnormal skin sensitivity in the area (allodynia)
- Continuous burning or aching pain with additional shooting pain.

This can have serious effects on quality of life, affecting sleep, mobility and social interaction, particularly a concern in older people. The aggressive management of the acute pain with appropriate drugs reduces the risk of postherpetic neuralgia developing.

---

exist without any identifiable tissue damage, it is difficult to treat and can be particularly baffling for patients and carers, as it does not follow the more familiar acute pain pattern and may continue for many years. It is now recognized that all pain involves psychological and physiological factors, and that the role of psychological factors increases when the condition is long lasting (Sarafino 2008).

The Pain in Europe study identifies the most common reasons for chronic pain as back pain in all age groups, and arthritis; individuals were living with chronic pain for an average of 7 years (Fricker 2003). Some 49% of chronic pain sufferers have diagnosed depression (Chronic Pain Policy Coalition, CPPC 2007). This has implications for community support required by this group. Chronic pain can impact on the following:

- Person's behaviour causing disability
- Psychological state causing emotional distress
- Social interaction (loss of confidence).

This can be destructive to normal quality of life for the individual and carers, and management should focus on all areas to provide holistic care (James 2011). Many people with chronic pain are in community settings and may require support from the primary care team with referral to specialist multi-disciplinary teams (MDT) (see p. 575) to achieve the best pain management.

Chronic malignant pain

Chronic malignant pain is associated with life-limiting conditions, often linked to cancer, where the progression and spread of disease cause pain. However, pain is rarely a presenting symptom of cancer. Initially, the 'cancer journey' involves acute pain (nociceptive) associated with diagnostic procedures and treatments. If the cancer spreads, pain can then become chronic and more complex, involving nociceptive, neuropathic and psychological components that require regular review and adjustment of treatment to meet the person's needs (Ch. 12). This is recognized as 'total pain' and requires skills across the MDT (Paz & Seymour 2008). However, people with cancer pain can also suffer acute pain, e.g. pain following a pathological fracture.

Gate control theory

Melzack and Wall's (1965) gate control theory proposed that active processing of nerve impulses (modulation) occurs in the spinal cord, where the pain sensation first enters the central nervous system (CNS). The gate is opened or closed depending on the combination of sensory ascending impulses from the periphery or descending impulses from the brain. Pain will only be appreciated if the gate is open. This recognized the psychological influences on pain such as anxiety and provided an explanation for clinical observations of pain perception. The theory is proving to be robust and has been refined by further research. The subsequent discovery of endogenous opioids enabled the actual mechanism of modulation to be understood in more detail. The gate control theory

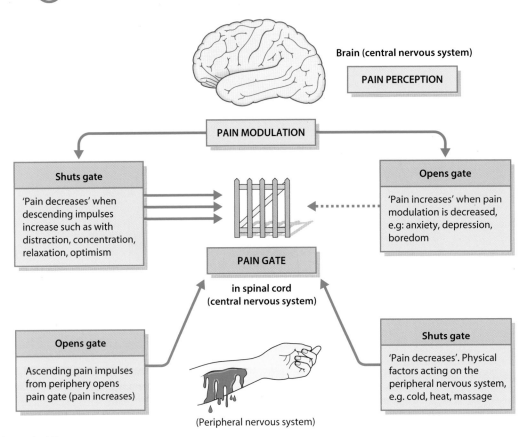

Fig. 23.3 • Gate control theory.

is acknowledged as providing a good theoretical basis for understanding pain perception in individuals as it recognizes factors that open or close the gate and guides approaches to managing pain (Fig. 23.3).

The theory recognizes the multidimensional nature of pain and explains many aspects of pain that are known to influence pain perception and can be used in pain management. As psychological (emotional) and cognitive (evaluative) aspects appear to influence the opening and closing of the 'pain gate', it encourages nurses to take holistic approaches to pain management, which acknowledges these components. This supports the unique nature of a person's pain experience; even when pain physiology appears to be closely matched, the emotional state and cognitive appraisal (past experience and meaning) of the experience can result in different pain perception by individuals. Table 23.1 summarizes the factors known to influence the 'pain gate'. Influences on a person's perception of pain (Box 23.3) and effects of chronic pain (Box 23.4) are provided.

Physiology of pain

The experience of pain results from integrated processes involving chemicals, sensory receptors, nerve fibres, and CNS processing. Knowledge of pain physiology enables nurses to understand how interventions can relieve pain. Acute (nociceptive) pain is described as involving four processes (Fig. 23.4):

- Transduction
- Transmission
- Modulation
- Perception.

Transduction

Injury causes the release of inflammatory chemicals that form an 'algesic soup' (meaning pain-causing). These chemicals

Table 23.1 Factors known to influence the 'pain gate'

Conditions	Conditions which may open the gate *'Make the pain worse'*	Conditions which may close the gate *'Make the pain better'*
Physical	Extent of injury Inappropriate activity Fatigue	Medication Heat, cold, massage, transcutaneous electrical nerve stimulation (TENS)
Emotional	Anxiety Depression	Positive emotions (feeling happy or optimistic) Relaxation, rest
Mental	Boredom Focusing on pain	Intense concentration Distraction

(Summarized from Sarafino 2008.)

Reflective practice Box 23.3

Influences on pain perception

Pain is influenced by a number of factors such as knowing the cause or not. Consider the following:

- Pain of known cause such as a migraine compared with sudden chest pain
- Pain after planned, curative surgery compared with pain following emergency surgery or trauma.

Student activities

- How might knowing the cause of pain influence perception?
- Think about how reasons for surgery can influence pain perception.
- Discuss with your mentor how these events can be explained by the 'pain gate' control theory?

Reflective practice Box 23.4

Chronic pain – biopsychosocial perspective

Think about a patient, client or someone you know who has chronic pain, e.g. back pain.

Student activities

- Reflect on how the person might feel about having no identifiable reason for the pain
- How may emotions affect the 'pain gate' for chronic pain?
- How much empathy and support do you think the person received from health professionals and family?
- Discuss with another student the impact of chronic pain on the normal activities of daily living.

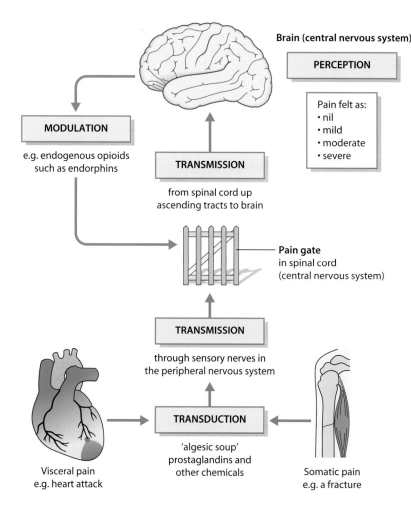

Fig. 23.4 • Pain physiology.

stimulate nociceptors (receptors responding to stimuli that are harmful and cause pain) on sensory nerves, which transmit impulses from somatic areas (skin, joints, bone) and the viscera (internal organs). Prostaglandins are among the key chemicals released by damaged tissues. Non-steroidal anti-inflammatory drugs (NSAIDs) relieve pain by inhibiting prostaglandin production.

Transmission

Transmission is the spread of pain impulses through sensory nerves in the peripheral nervous system (PNS) to the spinal cord and pain gate region up the ascending tracts to the brain.

The nerve impulses are processed in the 'pain gates' in the spinal cord. Further transmission can be influenced by fast peripheral non-pain sensation (touch, pressure) activity, which can inhibit further transmission so shuts the gate, or non-activity leaves the gate open (Fig. 23.3).

This is the basis for the use of local pressure, massage and other non-pharmacological coping strategies used to help shut the 'pain gate' (see pp. 582–585).

Many of the pharmacological treatments for pain act by interfering with the transmission of pain impulses along the pathway between the tissue injury and the brain (cortex).

Modulation

Modulation describes the inhibition of pain impulses by neural and chemical influences on the 'pain gate'. Nerves that descend from the brain stem to the spinal cord close the gate by releasing endogenous opioids, e.g. endorphins (Box 23.5). Endogenous opioid modulation may also explain the variation in pain perception in clinical practice. Some individuals have more effective modulation than others (McCaffery & Pasero 1999). Pain modulation allows the psychological influences on pain perception to be explained. For example, negative or positive past experiences – anxiety/fear and depression, or relaxation and optimism – all influence pain modulation, either opening or closing the 'pain gate'. Modulation may also be influenced by genetic factors, age and pain type, which could influence the endogenous opioid mechanisms.

Endogenous opioids	Box 23.5

- From animal studies it appears that the endogenous opioid system develops after birth and declines with age. This could have implications for human subjects, particularly infants and older people
- Individual variations in pain tolerance and opioid analgesia response may indicate differences in endogenous opioid activity
- Opioids are released in response to extended physical exertion, e.g. 'runners high'
- Acupuncture appears to stimulate the endogenous opioid system (Ch. 10)
- Major trauma is accompanied by release of endogenous opioids, which may explain the initial absence of pain in some people at the time of trauma
- Endorphin levels are lower in some people with chronic pain. This may explain why their pain worsens and why they are highly sensitive to acute pain.

Perception

There is no central pain centre within the brain but opioid-binding sites involved in pain perception have been found in several areas in the brain. Pain perception is a complex process involving sensory impulses from the 'pain gates' and activation of responses via the limbic ('primitive' brain area influencing emotions) and autonomic nervous system (ANS) to develop a pain experience that includes emotional and subjective sensory components. Immediate responses associated with acute pain and activation of the sympathetic nervous system include heightened awareness and anxiety. Longer-term responses to chronic pain involve behavioural adaptations, and psychological and social changes.

Psychological factors influence pain perception, e.g. emotional distress, anxiety and helplessness are recognized as increasing the pain experience and are significant clinically. Sarafino (2008) notes the importance of psychological, social and behavioural factors that become more dominant in chronic pain. Cognitive behavioural therapy (Field & Swarm 2008) may be used in chronic pain to change people's thoughts and behaviour and to enhance coping skills, so improving quality of life.

Individual pain responses are influenced by appraisal and past experiences. Responses are also modified by culture and social conditions and children learn about acceptable pain behaviour for their social group. McCaffery and Pasero (1999) note that some societies value a stoic response to pain, probably closely aligned with valuing high pain tolerance. This can lead to judgemental, negative attitudes to less stoic histrionic expression of pain. This is why the person's direct communication of their pain experience is vital, as it is the most valid assessment. Individual differences lead to great variations in the pain experienced and in how it is expressed by similar pain-provoking stimuli. An individual's pain cannot be predicted with accuracy.

Pain threshold and pain tolerance

Pain threshold (pain perception), is described as the lowest intensity at which a stimulus is experienced as pain. This relates to the point at which the painful stimulus is first acknowledged. The pain perception threshold is relatively constant and not, as is commonly thought, something that varies widely between individuals and cultures (Chamley 2011).

Pain tolerance relates to intensity or duration of pain and the maximum amount of pain that an individual can cope with. Pain tolerance may vary between and within individuals at different times, and may be influenced by emotional and cultural factors; pain tolerance is often referred to as being high or low (Box 23.6). Thus, an individual with high pain tolerance can withstand intense or protracted pain before requiring pain relief. Conversely the opposite is likely for those individuals with low pain tolerance. There is little evidence to suggest that children have different pain tolerance from adults although there may be a link between the age of the child and their pain threshold. Guidelines for pain assessment in older people note that stoicism and reticence can hinder self-reporting (British Pain Society, BPS 2007).

Reflective practice	Box 23.6

Pain tolerance

Think about a client or patient who experiences chronic pain.

Student activities

- Is their pain tolerance always the same?
- Do they need the same amount of medication each day?
- If there are differences, what factors might affect tolerance?

Pain psychology – personal and sociocultural influences

The pain experience is the end result of a number of dynamic interrelated factors. Recent thinking has moved away from personality and overt pain behaviours to focus on mental processes, e.g. comprehension and memory, that mediate pain behaviours. It is now recognized that children can and do remember pain experiences and learn from modifying their responses to future episodes, e.g. injections, dental treatments. There has been a view that neonates did not remember pain; studies have established that infants do remember painful events (Kennedy et al 2008). Furthermore, the interrelationship between pain, fear and anxiety has been extensively investigated over time and evidence suggests that anxiety and fear undoubtedly magnify pain perceptions, particularly in children. Studies have included other variables including memory, locus of control, self-efficacy, coping mechanisms/styles and depression (Box 23.7).

Evidence-based practice   Box 23.7

Depression and chronic pain

Raftery et al (2011) report that chronic pain affects about a third of people in Ireland, and depressive symptoms occur five times more often than in people without chronic pain.

Student activities

- Access the study by Raftery et al (2011).
- Discuss their findings with your mentor in relation to the management of chronic pain in your area.

Resource

Raftery, M.N., Sarma, K., Murphy, A.W., et al., 2011. Chronic pain in the Republic of Ireland – Community prevalence, psychosocial profile and predictors of pain-related disability: Results from the Prevalence, Impact and Cost of Chronic Pain (PRIME) Study, Part 1. Pain 152 (5), 1096–1103.

Cultural influence on the perception of pain has been extensively documented. It appears that pain and culture are closely linked, especially when responses and behaviours are closely aligned to culturally specific traditions, rules and rites of passage associated with a particular culture. For example, in Africa, the men of the Kikuya or Masai tribes are expected to respond to pain with dignity and composure, whereas it is acceptable for the women to wail and cry. There is some evidence to suggest that the further that an individual is away from the original immigrant population, the less culturally specific the behaviours become. Therefore, a pain response may be modified or diluted according to the multicultural society in which the person lives. An action enquiry by Lovering (2006) explored cultural attitudes towards pain in diverse groups of females (Filipino, Saudi, Irish and south African cultures of Asian, Afrikaans and Tswana), in a non-Western setting to explore 'cultural attitudes towards pain'. There were similarities and differences across cultures. The differences give support to the view that cultural background influences how pain is experienced and expressed to others. Afrikaans and Tswana are stoic and deny having physical pain. Asian, Filipino, Saudi and Irish were more likely to verbalize pain. Dalton (1989) reported that nurses' own cultural beliefs would influence assessment and management of their patients' pain. Studies related to children, culture and pain found similar features to those found in adults. However, nurses view the child and family as part of a sociocultural group and a multicultural approach to pain management is crucial to manage the child's pain experience effectively. Of equal importance are the implications of culture and ethnicity for nurses who will all have their own values, attitudes, beliefs and explanatory models of health and illness (Ch. 1) (Box 23.8).

Reflective practice   Box 23.8

Values, beliefs and attitudes towards pain

Think about your own values, beliefs and attitudes towards pain and the episodes that formed these.

Student activity

- Reflect on how your attitudes towards pain might influence your response to a patient/client who reports having unbearable pain.

Pain – myths, misconceptions and facts

Pain is complex, making it difficult to define, describe, explain and measure, thus increasing the likelihood that pain is underdetermined and undertreated. Some believe that complete pain relief is not achievable or necessarily desirable, especially after minor injury where low intensity pain limits overexertion. Moreover, pain is a valuable diagnostic tool and can be a learning mechanism. However, pain that is severe and prolonged, or which limits activity and movement, can be detrimental to recovery and general well-being (Box 23.9).

Moreover, enduring myths and misconceptions relating to pain all reflect prejudice, outmoded beliefs and poor knowledge and understanding. Collectively, these present healthcare professionals with challenges to manage pain effectively, as knowledge and beliefs relating to pain and its subsequent management are the foundations upon which healthcare professionals make judgements and decisions.

Myths and misconceptions flourish, despite these having been disproved by sound evidence. In particular, two such myths that continue to perpetuate the undertreatment of pain relate to fears about respiratory depression and addiction from the use of strong opioid analgesics, e.g. morphine. Box 23.10 outlines some pain myths and facts.

In order to dispel myths and misconceptions, nurses need to attain and maintain up-to-date evidence-based knowledge about pain and practical experience of relating this knowledge to preventing and managing pain. This knowledge includes:

- 'causes of pain and major influences on pain
- effects of unalleviated pain
- appropriate methods of assessing pain
- pharmacological interventions according to individual needs

○ potential complications of pain-relieving interventions and monitoring, preventing and treating them
○ appropriate non-pharmacological interventions'

(Davies & Taylor 2003, p 118).

Pain assessment

There are several good reasons why objective and systematic assessment of pain is necessary. Article 3 of the Human Rights Act (1998) states that 'no one shall be subjected to torture or to inhuman or degrading treatment or punishment'. This part of the chapter provides an outline of pain assessment. The CPPC (2007) have campaigned that pain should be considered as the 5th vital sign to improve awareness and recognition.

McCaffery and Pasero (1999) summarize the essential message about pain assessment as:

Detrimental effects of pain	Box 23.9

Respiratory effects (Ch. 17)
- Reduced lung capacity and ineffective coughing, leading to retention of secretions and chest infections
- Reduced oxygen to the tissues and respiratory failure.

Cardiovascular effects (Ch. 17)
- Rapid heart rate and high blood pressure may reduce the blood supply (ischaemia) to the heart muscle, leading to a heart attack.

Gastrointestinal effects
- Decreased bowel motility leading to constipation, nausea and vomiting and prolonged need for intravenous fluids (Chs 19, 21)
- Nausea caused by inappropriate analgesia leading to dehydration and poor nutritional intake.

Nervous system and hormones
- Increased secretion of catecholamines such as adrenaline (epinephrine) and stress hormones, e.g. corticosteroids, which in turn increase metabolism and oxygen consumption and promote sodium and water retention (Chs 17, 19). These changes are not caused exclusively by pain, but unrelieved pain may increase the extent of the changes.

Poor/reduced mobility (Ch. 18)
- Deep vein thrombosis (Chs 18, 24)
- Reduced musculoskeletal function (Ch. 18), e.g. joint stiffness
- Pressure ulcers (Ch. 25).

Psychological effects (Ch. 11)
- Fear and anxiety
- Helplessness
- Depression
- Fatigue.

Social effects
- Isolation and withdrawal from family/friends
- Inability to function within the family unit or maintain normal roles.

(Based on Davies & Taylor 2003).

- Ask the patient about their pain
- Accept and respect what they have to say
- Intervene to relieve their pain
- Ask them again about their pain.

Pain assessment is cyclical, involving assessment, intervention and reassessment.

Pain assessment therefore sets the tone for the therapeutic relationship formed with the patient/client/family in the assessment and treatment process, and underpins the respect and concern of the healthcare team. Furthermore, assessment is the foundation for therapeutic pain management. In acute pain, the objective of assessment might be to evaluate the need for and effectiveness of medication, whereas in chronic pain the focus is on how the pain affects the person's ability to function normally. One of the purposes of assessment is to facilitate objective clinical decision-making in pain management.

Pain is multidimensional and a holistic assessment must address all aspects of the pain experience, the critical components of which are:

- Physiological – primarily concerned with (cause), acute or chronic
- Sensory – how the pain feels, its characteristics, e.g. location, intensity and quality
- Affective – how the pain makes the individual feel; mood

Some pain myths – fact or fiction?	Box 23.10

Myths (false)
1. Older adults may believe that chronic pain is inevitable during ageing, that nothing can be done, and it is a sign of serious illness or impending death.
   False: but this myth is firmly embedded in sociocultural beliefs and poses significant barriers to pain relief for older people.
2. Infants and children experience less pain than adults.
   False: younger children may perceive a greater intensity of pain than older children and adults.
3. Behaviour accurately reflects pain.
   False: children and adults who are sleeping, or are active, playing, reading, etc., may still have pain but are coping.
4. Psychological dependence and respiratory depression are common side-effects of opioid analgesics.
   False: these are uncommon, but fear of them by nurses and patients can hamper effective pain management.

Facts (true)
1. People with severe motor problems or a learning disability are particularly prone to pain, e.g. earache, muscle spasm, and may be unable to articulate their pain clearly.
   True.
2. Treating depression improves pain in older people.
   True: treating depression in older people helps them cope with the pain of chronic conditions and improves quality of life.
3. Complementary and alternative medicine (CAM) therapies have an important role in pain management.
   True: various techniques are available to patients/clients as coping strategies for managing pain (see Ch. 10).

- Cognitive – the manner in which the pain affects the person's thought processes, embraces values, beliefs and coping strategies
- Behavioural – behaviours may be adopted in order to reduce pain related to rest and activity, medication and treatments. Behaviours may be adopted because the person cannot communicate to others that they are in pain
- Sociocultural – relates to age/gender, culture, folklore, spiritual and other factors.

Holistic pain assessment

Determining the level of pain experienced by an individual is one of the most challenging activities that nurses undertake. However, it is important to distinguish between pain measurement and holistic pain assessment. Pain measurement utilizes an intensity scale which is unidimensional without consideration of other pain components. In contrast, pain assessment is multidimensional and requires different knowledge and skills, including pain measurement.

When assessing pain, nurses should be measuring not only the severity of the pain but also what the experience means to that person. However, it is notable that there is a difference between pain measurement and assessment, and when these definitions are applied to human suffering it requires the nurse to evaluate the whole experience and what it means to the person. Melzack and Katz (1994) proposed that the main aims of pain assessment are to:

- Determine the intensity, quality and duration
- Aid diagnosis
- Determine the most appropriate therapy
- Evaluate the relative effectiveness of different therapies
- Monitor standards of clinical practice.

Pain assessment is important because it provides the person with the opportunity to verbalize their pain (if able), includes the personal pain experience (Davies & Taylor 2003) and engages the person and/or their family with healthcare systems.

The 'gold standard' is always to ask the person about their pain experience. Assessment will be influenced by the person's ability to respond and the type of pain will also influence assessment priorities, e.g. priorities will be different in the acute pain after a heart attack to those in chronic back pain.

Communication skills are essential for effective pain assessment; the person needs to be encouraged to report pain (Ch. 9). If the person's condition allows, use open questions that allow them to elaborate upon their pain.

- How would you describe your pain/discomfort? (see Pain language, below)
- When did you first feel the pain?
- Is there anything that makes the pain worse or better?
- How does the pain affect your daily activities?

For children and young people, Sepion (2009) explains that developmental age, environment and circumstances are important considerations for pain assessment. The BPS (2007) indicate that reticence and stoicism may be barriers to

self-reporting and advocate a multidimensional approach including the use of observation, e.g. facial expression and behaviour, and also that they may use words other than 'pain' for assessment in the older client.

The potential barriers and differences in pain expression, e.g. due to culture, age, personality, gender and cognitive ability, must be acknowledged by the nurse. However, for some people, verbal communication may be difficult, absent or not yet developed. Furthermore, cultural and language difficulties may hamper the assessment process. Recently a position statement addressing five patient populations who may be unable to self-report has been published to guide assessment in these more challenging groups (older adults with advanced dementia, infants and preverbal toddlers, critically ill/unconscious patients, patients with intellectual disabilities, and end-of-life care). Nurses are identified by the authors Herr et al (2011) as integral to ensuring assessment and treatment of these vulnerable groups.

Behavioural responses to pain

Behavioural responses to pain are important in the assessment of all patients/clients but can be especially relevant when people are unable to verbalize their pain. Although there are only limited pain assessment tools available for vulnerable groups, it is important to understand that people with special needs experience pain the same as everyone else. It is vital that nurses recognize that they may be unable to verbalize their pain or explain it clearly. Vulnerable people include the following:

- Cognitive impairment, e.g. confusion, dementia
- Mental distress
- Severe physical and/or learning disability
- Speech problems, e.g. stroke
- Altered consciousness
- Pre-verbal children
- Older people
- People not fluent in the language used.

Certain behaviours are useful for identifying patients/clients who may be experiencing pain, e.g. agitation, rocking, being quiet. In situations where verbal communication is limited or impossible, observations of behaviour alone can be used. Abbey et al (2004) recommend that the pain scale for dementia should be used as a patient activity based assessment to improve reliability; it relies upon observation of behaviour, body language and facial expression (Box 23.11).

In addition to the limited availability of assessment tools for vulnerable groups, there may also be a culture where lack of assessment hampers effective evaluation of pain management. Furthermore, pain assessment can fail if there is poor communication between the nurse and the patient/client or family.

Pain language

There are many words used to describe pain (Box 23.12). Numerous people develop their own pain language and behaviours that communicate pain. Instead of the word pain, depending upon the age and stage of development, children may use special words such as 'bad'. Older people may use 'sore', 'hurt',

? Critical thinking   Box 23.11

Abbey Pain Scale

The Abbey Pain Scale (Abbey et al 2004) assists pain assessment in people with dementia who cannot verbalise. It is a patient activity based assessment to enhance accuracy. Staff should observe for key areas then repeat one hour after interventions to determine effectiveness.
Key areas include:

- Vocalization, e.g. whimpering, groaning, crying
- Facial expression, e.g. tense, frowning, grimacing, etc.
- Change in body language, e.g. fidgeting, rocking, etc.
- Behavioural change, e.g. increased confusion, food refusal, altered patterns
- Physiological change and note physical changes, e.g. vital signs, perspiring, pallor, flushing
- Physical changes, e.g. skin tears, contractures.

(each is scored from 0=absence , 1=mild, 2=moderate, 3=severe)

Student activities

- Discuss with another student how you would record behaviours which may indicate pain.
- How would you discover the person's normal behaviour pattern?

⟳ Reflective practice   Box 23.12

Some words used to describe pain

Aching, burning, cramping/crampy, cruel, dragging, exhausting/tiring, gnawing, heavy, pounding, punishing, sharp, tiring, throbbing.

Student activity

- Reflect on your own pain language. How could it influence your response to a patient's description of pain?

'aching' (BPS 2007). Descriptions of pain expressions may have little or no meaning outside the family and reinforce the need for partnerships, and child- and family-centred care in pain management with infants, children and others with communication difficulties. Therefore, identifying pain language in all patients/clients is important for the delivery of high quality care and also informs the assessment process.

Assessing children's pain

Until recently, pain in children was not recognized or prioritized, resulting in poor pain management (Twycross et al 2009). Infants and children have the right to careful consideration, as they may experience pain differently from adults. The child's experience of pain is often separate from their experience of their illness or disease. As with adults, children have different experiences and reactions to pain from the same stimulus, and the relationship between the pain stimulus and the response is neither direct nor simple.

Knowing how children develop their understanding of health and illness will enhance the quality of care offered to each child. Evidence suggests that most health professionals do not approach children according to their developmental level but rather address all children according to Piaget's concrete operational stage of development (Ch. 8). Knowledge about a child's understanding of illness will ensure that nurses provide age-specific explanations for each child, thus reducing the anxiety and distress occurring during hospitalization (Twycross et al 2009). A child's developmental stage affects their perception and ability to adequately report or express the pain they feel.

Children are entitled to feel secure and to be nursed in an atmosphere where compassion, trust and caring are central to all decisions. These principles must underpin the child's pain assessment and management, with the child central to all considerations and decisions.

The QUESTT model (Baker & Wong 1987) encompasses many important features of assessment and involves:

- Questioning the child (where appropriate)
- Using pain rating scales (see below and pp. 573–574)
- Evaluating behaviour and physiological changes
- Parental involvement
- Taking the cause of pain into account
- Taking action and evaluating the results.

This provides a comprehensive overview of the child's pain and informs management.

Pain history

Establishing a pain history is important as it will not only identify previous pain experiences, but may also offer insights into how the person's knowledge and perception have determined coping strategies, and how this may influence the current situation. This is particularly important for vulnerable groups (see above). Children can be better prepared for painful procedures by comparing previous experiences with the new experience and often children develop strategies that compare one situation with another. Furthermore, pain behaviours may be an integral part of the pain history and behavioural cues may be important pain indicators. Being sensitive to pain indicators mean that practitioners can intervene at an early stage before pain is fully established. It is also useful to establish if there are separate behaviours relating to sudden acute pain and chronic pain. Again this is important in patients/clients who have difficulties in articulating pain.

Pain diaries

These are useful for the assessment of chronic pain and a means of reflecting upon the many components of pain, e.g. physical, emotional, social. They can also include numerical ratings and pain descriptions (see Box 23.12).

Pain maps

The patient, if able, is asked to identify, mark or sketch areas on a body outline or 'body map' that reflects the area(s) of pain (see p. 576). Pain maps are used increasingly as part of assessment, especially for patients with complex chronic pain. Pain maps can empower the patient during the assessment; they can be used across the lifespan and are important tools for informing decisions about pain management and providing a basis for evaluating the effectiveness of treatment.

Pain assessment tools

Pain assessment tools must be reliable and valid. Reliability relates to issues of consistency, stability and the repeatability of measurements made by different nurses; validity refers to the appropriateness, applicability and the representativeness of measurements made as true findings of an individual's pain at any given time. Different types of pain assessment tools can be classified as follows:

- Self-report scales – what people say
- Observation techniques – what people do
- Physiological measurements such as heart rate.

There are wide variations in the levels of sophistication of these tools and also between approaches to pain assessment. Pain assessment tool selection must be based on the patient's age and ability, a child's developmental stage, patient preferences, amount of time available to teach the patient about the scale and the nurse's knowledge (Box 23.13).

Evidence-based practice   Box 23.13

Choosing the most appropriate pain assessment tool

Studies have identified that patient preference is important with practical acceptability of tools.

- Visual impairment in older people may limit practicality for self-report scales. Herr and Mobily (1993) recommended a bold Arial font on buff-coloured paper to overcome visual difficulties
- The pain 'thermometer'(0–10/100) scale (picture of a thermometer) has been well received by older people (Benesh et al 1997)
- Within pain assessment, the nurse should evaluate patient fears/concerns regarding analgesics since this may be an important issue in successful pain management. Fear of analgesic drugs and their side-effects or acceptance of pain as inevitable can be barriers to effective pain management
- Self-expression may be limited, thus requiring the nurse to use alternative aspects such as behavioural indicators. Observing the facial expressions and vocalizations of people with advanced dementia is an accurate means for assessing the presence of pain, but not its intensity (BPS 2007; Abbey et al 2004).

Student activity

- Access either BPS (2007) or Abbey et al (2004) and discuss with your mentor how the findings could be used effectively with your patient/client group.

Self-report scales

Self-report assessment scales include visual analogue scales (VAS), verbal numerical rating scales and categorical verbal rating scales but can also include pain interviews or questionnaires that incorporate variables such as coping skills (Fig. 23.5). Self-report scales can be modified, e.g. the pain

'thermometer' scale or by using a child's own words on the scale, e.g. 'worst hurt' (Box 23.14). They can also be used with pain maps or pain diaries.

Reflective practice   Box 23.14

Using self-report pain scales

Think about the self-report scales you have seen in use.

Student activities

- Were the scales in use suitable for all patients/clients?
- Were existing scales modified to increase their suitability?
- Discuss with your mentor how sociocultural factors may influence how a person uses a scale.

The BPS (2006) provides a self-administered pain rating scale, which considers pain intensity, distress and interference on activities, in addition to considered relief from treatment and is produced in several languages.

Visual analogue scale

The visual analogue scale (VAS) is a 10 cm horizontal line with indicators of severity such as 'no pain' at one end to 'worst pain possible' at the other end (Fig. 23.5A). Patients mark the position on the scale that best reflects their current pain. This is also a useful tool for children, but the child needs the ability to translate their experience into an analogue format and to be able to understand proportions (from 9 or 10 years).

Verbal numerical rating scales

Verbal numerical rating scales are based upon the VAS but use a scale where 0 is 'no pain' and 10 is 'worst possible pain' (Fig. 23.5B). These usually provide a more reliable means of measuring pain and can be used with descriptions as well as numbers.

Categorical rating scale

One of the most commonly used tools postoperatively, it offers the patient a series of terms that best describes their pain (Fig. 23.5C). It is simple and effective to use in clinical practice and can be incorporated into an observation chart. Pain on movement rather than at rest is important to assess. Pain intensity at rest is not a reliable indicator of effective pain management, especially postoperative pain.

Self-report scales for children

Self-report scales for children include:

- 'Faces' scale (from 3 years) – series of faces depicting a smile through neutral to total misery (Fig. 23.5D)
- Pain thermometer
- Colour scale (4–10 years) – used with a body map it provides information about pain intensity and location. It has a series of colours from which the child chooses the colour that best represents their pain to create a 'key'. Once the key has been created the child is encouraged to colour in the outline of where it hurts

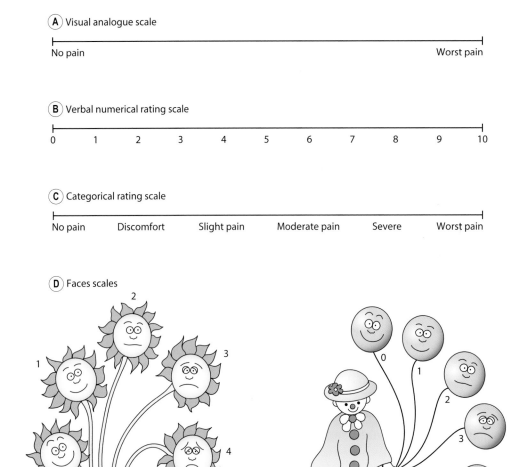

Fig. 23.5 • Self-report pain scales: (A) Visual analogue scale. (B) Verbal numerical rating scale. (C) Categorical rating scale. (D) Faces scales.

• Poker chip (4–8 years) – the child rates their pain in a concrete manner using the chips that are described as 'pieces of hurt'.

Hockenberry and Wilson (2011) in Further reading, below, provides comprehensive information on pain assessment tools for infants, children and young people.

Observation techniques

This involves recording variables including:

• Sleep patterns
• Rest periods
• Pain behaviours
• Verbal and motor responses.

Observational tools for adult pain assessment and measurement show potential when used by trained observers and there are clearly defined terms and boundaries. A number of observational tools have been developed to assess pain in children aged 0–5 years, who are unable or less able to use self-report scales. Observation may also be useful in cases where self-report tools may be unreliable or unsuitable, as with people with a learning disability and those with communication/language difficulties.

Physiological measurements

The quest for objectivity in pain assessment has led some to measure such factors as increased heart rate, feeling faint, etc. or disease activity as equivalents for the experience of pain.

Physiological measurements such as respiratory rate, blood pressure, heart rate and oxygen saturation (Ch. 17) have their limitations. However, they are used in critical care situations and advanced dementia (Abbey et al 2004), and also in neonatal pain assessment, because there are few comprehensive neonatal assessment tools available.

Multimethod approaches to pain assessment

These approaches give richer information regarding the pain experience of the patient/client and often pain assessment tools combine quantitative and qualitative elements (Ch. 5). One such tool is the Pain Anxiety Symptoms Scale (PASS) which incorporates three modes: cognitive, overt behaviour and physiological, including reports of changes, e.g. sweating, feeling faint and dizzy, etc. Various multimethod approaches exist for assessing pain in infants, children and young people; the Royal College of Nursing (RCN 2009) has evaluated the validity and reliability of a range of these tools.

Assessment for different types of pain

The choice of assessment method must be appropriate for the person and the pain type. In acute pain, a unidimensional intensity self-report scale, e.g. the categorical rating scale, is sufficient for evaluation of interventions, especially if there is a single pain location.

However, with chronic pain, a body map is frequently required to improve recognition and communication of pain location and pattern. For patients with cancer-related pain, a body map is essential because, as the cancer advances, several pain locations may develop (Ch. 12). The different pain locations require regular reassessment as the disease progresses. In addition, the impact of the pain on mood and behaviour are important considerations which are missed if a unidimensional intensity scale is used.

Questions that explore quality of sleep and the impact of pain on mobility and social interaction are valuable (Chs 10, 18). Patients are asked about what makes the pain better or worse, thus helping to identify characteristics that may help in evaluating treatment options and coping skills that people have developed. The quality and character of pain may guide pharmacological management, e.g. a pain described as 'shooting' may be neuropathic such as after shingles (see pp. 564–565). Neuropathic chronic pain can be particularly difficult for patients to express. Mann (2008) advocates that nurses should become more aware of neuropathic pain assessment. The medical term allodynia is used to describe people experiencing pain from stimuli that are not usually painful such as touch. This is especially difficult for patients to communicate.

Pain clinics and specialist nurse practitioners use detailed tools and may request pain diaries in order to evaluate the pain experience comprehensively.

An example of a more comprehensive assessment tool that combines a body map, self-report scale, pain description with factors increasing or decreasing pain is shown in Figure 23.6 (p. 576).

Pain management

This section outlines holistic pain management, pharmacological pain relief and a variety of non-pharmacological approaches used to enhance coping strategies.

Effective pain management is complex and requires a holistic approach, starting with a thorough assessment (see pp. 570–575). The type of pain and the person's response are important factors to consider when planning strategies for pain management. Pain may be a primary reason for care or it may be a longstanding problem. Pain management usually involves a combination of pharmacological and non-pharmacological measures.

Mild acute pain following minor injury may be easy to resolve with simple painkillers, an ice pack and sympathetic listening, information and support from the nurse. Many hospitals now have acute pain teams to support pain management following surgery and act as a resource to clinical staff.

However, for chronic pain, a multidisciplinary approach is most effective, with management taking place in the community and hospital. MDTs may include pain specialist consultants, pain nurse specialists, physiotherapists, occupational therapists, clinical psychologists and pharmacists. Support for patients with chronic pain depends on the cause of the pain, but advice and help are available from palliative care specialists (Ch. 12) and specialist pain clinics.

Pharmacological management

Depending on the pain type, patient's age and setting, there are a range of pharmacological approaches available, including the use of analgesics (widely described as painkillers). The nurse has a key role in teaching patients and family about the safe management of drugs including analgesics (Box 23.15, Ch. 22). Nurses advising patients/clients about self management of pain following trauma, surgery, etc., must be aware of concerns around over-the-counter (OTC) analgesics and risks of polypharmacology. The variability in individual responses to analgesics presents nurses with a key responsibility in monitoring effects and side-effects in order to achieve successful pain management.

 Health promotion   **Box 23.15**

Aspirin and Reye syndrome

A friend asks you why he should not give aspirin to his 8-year-old son. He has heard someone talking about a serious side-effect and is confused about which over-the-counter painkillers are safe for children. He wants to know some basic facts and where to get information.

Student activities

- Access the *British National Formulary for Children* (www.bnf.org/bnf) and find some basic facts about aspirin and Reye syndrome.
- What is the advice about when young people can take aspirin?
- Find out where your friend can get information about painkillers for children.

Registered nurses (RNs) who have completed additional training are able to prescribe analgesics from the *Nurse Prescribers' Formulary for Community Practitioners* and qualified Nurse Independent Prescribers are able to prescribe any

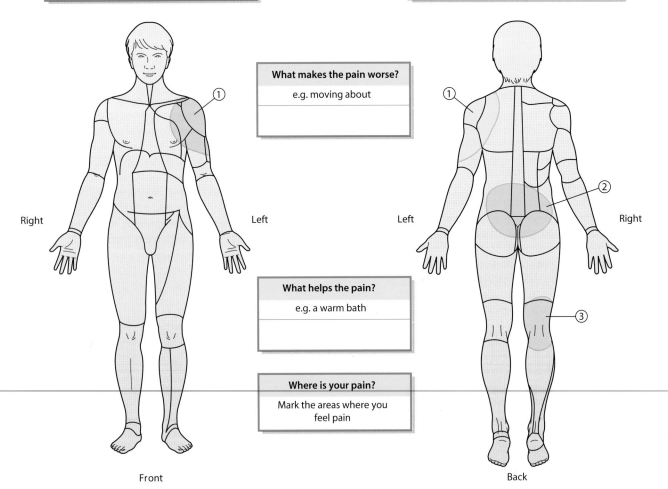

Patient's details:

Dept/Ward: ....

Consultant: ....

4 ——— Unbearable pain	
3 ——— Severe pain	
2 ——— Moderate pain	
1 ——— Slight pain	
0 ——— No pain	

AC – Aching	SO – Sore
BU – Burning	SP – Sharp
DU – Dull	ST – Stabbing
GN – Gnawing	TE – Tender
PN – Pins and needles	TH – Throbbing
SH – Shooting	TI – Tingling

What makes the pain worse?

e.g. moving about

What helps the pain?

e.g. a warm bath

Where is your pain?

Mark the areas where you feel pain

Right   Left   Left   Right

Front   Back

Fig. 23.6 • Pain assessment tool. (Reproduced with permission from Brooker, C., Nicol, M. (Eds.), 2003. Nursing adults. The practice of caring. Mosby, Edinburgh.)

medicine for any medical condition within their competence, including controlled drugs (British National Formulary, BNF 2012).

Communication between members of the MDT, which includes the patient and family, is essential. Nurses may need to act as advocate for patients to ensure any adjustment to analgesic prescription required to achieve acceptable pain management.

Age and analgesic drugs

The patient's age is an important consideration when analgesics are chosen: the drug type, dose required and the most suitable administration route. Infants, children, adults and older people have different body compositions (water as a percentage of body weight decreases during the lifespan, Ch. 19) and the metabolism and elimination of drugs are affected by the developmental stage.

Infants and children metabolize and eliminate drugs differently from adults and this must be considered in the dose calculations. For example, neonates and pre-term infants are particularly vulnerable to the harmful effects of drugs because liver enzyme systems and kidney function are immature and plasma protein concentrations are low. Weight, height and age are important in calculating children's drug doses (Ch. 22).

There are also important considerations for the older person as reduced metabolism and excretion of drugs can result in accumulated effect and reduced doses may be required. In addition, polypharmacy causes concern with drug interactions. Poor pain management can significantly reduce quality of life, particularly in chronic pain, therefore effective pain management is essential in maintaining optimum independence and mobility in older people. This is a particular concern for people with dementia who are more likely to suffer chronic pain but be unable to express their pain.

Pregnancy and analgesic drugs

The use of analgesics (prescribed and OTC), and indeed any drug or herbal remedy, when 'trying for a baby' and during pregnancy may pose a risk to the fetus. Similarly there are potential risks for breast fed babies with maternal analgesic use. This is of concern and nurses should advise women to seek guidance about any drug including analgesic use from reliable sources, e.g. midwife, GP, pharmacist (see NHS Choices 2011, in Further reading, below).

Drugs used in pain management

These can be divided into three groups: non-opioids, opioids and adjuvants (Table 23.2).

Nurses need to develop an adequate knowledge of analgesic action and potential side-effects (Box 23.16). Unfortunately, there are no perfect analgesics; all drugs that relieve pain also have side-effects. These range from mild light-headedness to

---

? Critical thinking   Box 23.16

Side-effects of analgesic drugs

Select an example from each group: non-opioids, opioids and adjuvants.

Student activities

- Use the *British National Formulary* to learn about the side-effects of the drugs chosen.
- Consider any side-effects encountered in placements.

---

more troublesome problems that occur with opioids that include constipation, nausea and sedation, up to life-threatening respiratory depression, or NSAID-induced gastric ulceration or kidney failure. The nurse is responsible not only for the evaluation of pain reduction but also the occurrence of side-effects. Of concern NSAIDS are the most widely self administered OTC analgesics so public awareness of possible harmful effects is essential.

Mild sedation can be a useful side-effect in the management of acute pain, e.g. following major trauma, as it will reduce anxiety and distress. However, for chronic pain management, independence with minimum disruption to daily living is important; frequent administration is therefore undesirable and side-effect management is essential.

With opioid analgesics such as morphine, the higher the dose, the greater the risk of side-effects. The dose is therefore increased in graduated amounts known as titration, which allows optimum pain relief without adverse side-effects (Fig. 23.7). However, knowledge of likely side-effects allows pre-emptive action to be taken, e.g. laxatives are always prescribed for patients having codeine or morphine.

When an adjuvant drug, e.g. amitriptyline, is prescribed, it may take days or weeks before there is a therapeutic effect. This must be explained, as patients may expect a prompt

---

Table 23.2 Drug groups used in pain management

Drug group	Examples	Details
Non-opioid	Aspirin, paracetamol, NSAIDs, e.g. ibuprofen, diclofenac, and local anaesthetics, e.g. lidocaine	Non-opioids work in a variety of ways, e.g. NSAIDs inhibit the production of 'algesic' chemicals such as prostaglandins that stimulate the pain-sensitive nociceptors which mediate the inflammatory response.
Opioid	Buprenorphine, codeine, dihydrocodeine, diamorphine, fentanyl, methadone, morphine, pethidine, tramadol	A group of naturally occurring (from opium poppies) and synthetic analgesics. They act on opioid receptors in the central nervous system and block pain transmission by mimicking the effects of naturally occurring endorphins at the receptors, thus lessening pain. They range in strength and efficacy from the weak opioid codeine to morphine.
Adjuvant	These include: • Anticonvulsants, e.g. gabapentin • Antidepressants, e.g. amitriptyline • Antispasmodics, e.g. hyoscine butylbromide • Capsaicin (derived from chillies) • Corticosteroids, e.g. dexamethasone	Adjuvants act to enhance the action of analgesics, e.g. amitriptyline enhances pain modulation and is useful for neuropathic pain.

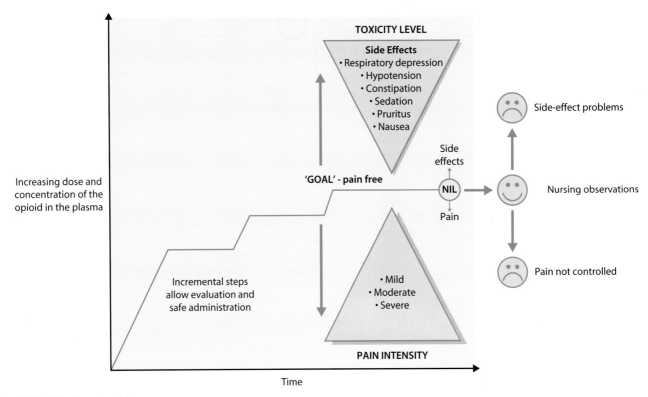

Fig. 23.7 • Titration of opioids.

response and may therefore discontinue the therapy. Starting adjuvants at a low dose and gradually increasing the dose helps to reduce side-effects and improves patient tolerance.

Routes of administration

The routes used for the administration of analgesic drugs include:

- Oral (p.o.) – either swallowed or mucosal absorption
- Intranasal sprays
- Topical/transdermal as creams, gels or patches
- Rectal
- Subcutaneous (s.c.)
- Intramuscular (i.m.)
- Intravenous (i.v.)
- Inhalation
- Epidural
- Nerve blocks using local anaesthetics, e.g. bupivacaine
- Intraspinal drug delivery via an intraspinal catheter and a pump.

Nurses need to know about different routes of administration and be familiar with relative advantages and disadvantages of each route (Ch. 22). Analgesic administration may be low technology, e.g. oral self-administration at home, where the nurse's role is educational; or invasive, high technology approaches where drugs are introduced into the epidural space (Fig. 23.8), used to manage severe pain with additional staff training and support from pain teams. In general, the analgesic approach should be appropriate for the pain type and intensity, and should suit the person concerned.

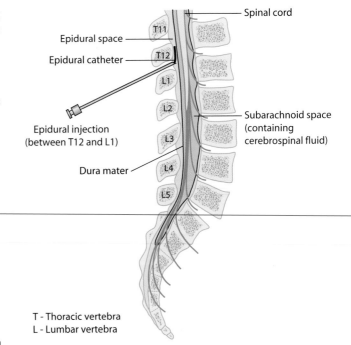

Fig. 23.8 • Epidural analgesia.

An important consideration is the flexibility and availability provided by different routes of administration. In acute severe pain, the route needs to be fast-acting and the dose easily adjustable to allow optimum effect without development of adverse side-effects. The most widely available routes for adults are i.m. and s.c. opioid administration; the effectiveness of these routes has been greatly improved by the use of algorithms by RNs to provide greater flexibility to meet individual patient's needs.

Opioids may be required for chronic severe pain, e.g. modified release morphine given twice daily or transdermal fentanyl (patch). Transdermal fentanyl takes 12 hours to reach therapeutic levels but lasts 3 days, thereby avoiding the inconvenience of frequent administration and allowing the patient to get on with activities of living.

The most common routes of administration (p.o., i.m., i.v.) rely upon sufficient quantity of the drug reaching the circulation to achieve therapeutic effect. An injection is not necessarily more powerful than an oral drug, a common misconception; the analgesic should be matched to pain intensity and a suitable route chosen. The i.v. route allows for rapid therapeutic effect to be achieved within 5 minutes, which makes patient-controlled i.v. administration a fast and flexible method of managing acute pain. Intramuscular and s.c. routes have a delayed onset as the drug has to be absorbed from the muscle or fat before it can reach the circulation.

The oral route can be as fast as i.m. if the drug is designed for rapid absorption. Avoidance of painful injection is essential in children and often desirable in adults because treating pain with injections can lead to reluctance to report pain. It is important to note that oral morphine is subject to first pass effect/metabolism in the liver (Ch. 22), thus explaining why the oral route requires a dose higher than that given by i.v. or i.m. injection. This has important safety issues for the nurse.

Nurses need to be especially aware of potential benefits and reduced side-effects linked with different routes for administration of NSAID analgesics for older people, many of whom will be taking prescribed medication or OTC drugs (Box 23.17). Topical applications of NSAIDs can be effective without the added risks associated with systemic oral adverse effects e.g. gastric ulceration and complications of drug compatibility with polypharmacology (Greener 2009).

Patient-controlled analgesia

Patient-controlled analgesia (PCA) usually means i.v. administration but also includes oral, inhaled nitrous oxide and oxygen (Entonox®), and s.c. or epidural administration (Ch. 24). Specialized equipment is needed for safe administration of analgesics by these routes and PCA requires patient education and

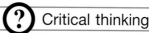

> **? Critical thinking**   Box 23.17
>
> **Over-the-counter and prescribed medicines**
>
> Gwen, aged 72 years, visits the practice nurse for medication review; she has hypertension (prescribed a diuretic and ACE inhibitor) and osteoarthritis of both knees which limits mobility.
>
> Gwen reports buying her own analgesics (ibuprofen) and now takes glucosamine for her knees.
>
> **Student activities**
>
> - Use a pharmacology resource to identify why the practice nurse raises concerns about using NSAIDs with her current antihypertensive medication.
> - The nurse also indicates that glucosamine is not advisable. Why?

reassurance. Children can safely self-administer inhalation, i.v. or s.c. PCA.

Because PCA administration relies on the fact that a sedated patient will not be able to administer more analgesia, and therefore cannot overdose, carers and staff must understand they should not administer for the patient.

Regular assessment and management of nausea, a common side-effect of opioids, is important. This is particularly so with i.v. PCA, as the patient is unlikely to use it effectively if they feel sick every time they press the dosing button. It is important that there is regular assessment of postoperative nausea and vomiting (Ch. 24). (See Chamley (2011) for more information.)

Administration of analgesic drugs

Analgesics with a fast onset and short duration of action need to be administered frequently to maintain therapeutic effect and prevent pain, e.g. oral morphine liquid 4-hourly. This is why the 'as required' (p.r.n.) approach to pain management, which relies on patients reporting pain, is criticized; the intermittent administration results in regular pain with periods of relief. Good pain management requires regular administration of a suitable analgesic to avoid pain (Fig. 23.9). Regular administration 'by the clock', or techniques which allow the patient to administer as soon as pain is present, e.g. by using i.v. PCA,

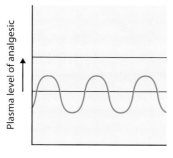
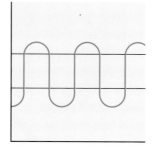
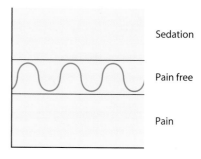

- Dose too small
- Intermittent pain

- Dose too large and too widely spaced
- Intermittent pain and drowsiness

- Timing and dose correct
- No pain

Sedation

Pain free

Pain

Fig. 23.9 • Adjusting the dose to keep the patient pain-free. (Reproduced with permission from Greenstein, B., Gould, D., 2004. Trounce's clinical pharmacology for nurses, seventeenth ed. Churchill Livingstone, Edinburgh.)

have greatly improved pain management. Many patients manage pain at home following early discharge or day case surgery. Advice is required about taking painkillers regularly to avoid pain at first and how to step down the 'analgesic ladder' (see below) to milder analgesics as the pain subsides. Advice regarding avoidance of constipation (Ch. 21) should also be included if opioids are prescribed.

Analgesic potency

Pain management is achieved by administering the most suitable analgesic drug combination. The pain type (acute or chronic) and intensity (mild, moderate or severe), the patient's age and individual sensitivities are all important considerations. A useful tool when considering the choice of analgesic is the 'analgesic ladder' (World Health Organization, WHO 2005), which groups drugs into categories that match analgesic potency with pain intensity (Fig. 23.10; Ch. 12):

- *Mild pain:* Drugs at the bottom of the analgesic ladder are useful for mild pain; these include the non-opioids, e.g. paracetamol and adjuvants
- *Moderate pain:* Step 1 drugs are administered at the correct dose and interval; if pain is not controlled, then a drug from the Step 2 is considered, e.g. co-codamol (paracetamol + the weak opioid codeine)

- *Severe pain:* When pain is not relieved by Step 2 drugs, then a strong opioid, e.g. morphine, is recommended in combination with non-opioid and adjuvant drugs.

This ladder was first proposed for use by the World Health Organization in the management of cancer pain in the 1980s; however, it is considered useful for other pain types. It can be used to guide analgesic prescribing in various settings, e.g. community, Emergency Department and hospital. Postoperative pain relief often starts at the top of the ladder and steps down as pain subsides. In contrast, for chronic malignant cancer pain, the analgesia will be adjusted as pain intensity increases with advancing disease; for many patients this approach has been successful in achieving good pain control (Ch. 12).

A study by Moore et al (2003) compared analgesic effectiveness in acute pain (Box 23.18).

A combination of analgesic drugs, known as the balanced or multimodal approach, is recommended for effective pain management. In combination, the drugs target different areas involved in pain physiology (see pp. 566–568), which appears to improve the analgesic effect.

This can enhance pain management because less opioid is required (opioid sparing) when given in combination, and this reduces side-effects (Parsons & Preece 2010). Examples include oral co-codamol (paracetamol and codeine) and epidural administration of an opioid with local anaesthetic.

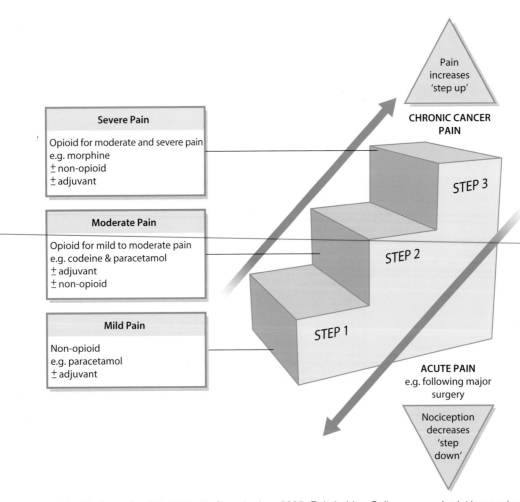

Fig. 23.10 • Analgesic ladder (based on World Health Organization, 2005. Pain ladder. Online: www.who.int/cancer/palliative/painladder/en).

Pre-emptive and procedural pain management

The principle of providing analgesia before tissue injury to minimize pain is generally accepted as good practice. Some patients require repeat procedures and previous poor pain management can make patients fearful and reluctant to participate again. This is a particularly important issue for children and leads to further distress. Furthermore, poorly managed procedural pain is thought to contribute to physiological changes, which in some patients have been linked to chronic pain development (Mann & Carr 2009). Certain procedures in clinical practice, e.g. taking blood samples, cannulation, painful dressings and postoperative physiotherapy, are recognized as causing pain, and planning care to minimize this is essential. Both pharmacological treatment and psychological support are required. The management of procedural or transitory pain can be achieved by a variety of techniques:

1. Blocking pain transmission with local anaesthetics:
   - Topical application of creams containing a eutectic mixture of local anaesthetics (EMLA), e.g. lidocaine with prilocaine prior to venepuncture, etc. (Box 23.19)
   - Instillation of lidocaine gel into the urethra prior to catheterization (Ch. 20)
   - Subcutaneous infiltration of lidocaine prior to wound suturing in the Emergency Department.
2. Nitrous oxide 50% + oxygen 50% (Entonox®) inhalation by self-administration, e.g. during a painful dressing. Note that it is widely used during labour.
3. Administration of a short-acting strong opioid, which allows for rapid recovery.

Drug tolerance and dependence

The use of analgesics is influenced by drug tolerance, dependence and addiction. A common misperception that opioid analgesics lead to addiction has a negative influence on pain management. Several authors (Mann & Carr 2009; Mann 2003) identify that nurses and patients have exaggerated fears about addiction risk with opioids. This affects drug prescribing by medical staff, pain reporting by patients and drug administration by nurses leading to unrelieved pain.

- Physiological tolerance occurs when a patient becomes used to a drug and may require larger doses for the same effect. Tolerance to some side-effects of opioids is a useful adaptation. Initially, central side-effects such as sedation and nausea and vomiting occur, but tolerance to these side-effects develops with time. Unfortunately, tolerance to peripheral side-effects, e.g. constipation, does not occur and so must be prevented.
- Physical dependence is described as an adaptive state (Mann 2003). Physical disturbance with 'withdrawal symptoms' occurs in a physically dependent person if opioids are suddenly stopped (Mann & Carr 2009); opioids are therefore gradually reduced.
- Addiction is a disorder of psychological dependence and craving when the person is not using the drug for analgesia. The risk of addiction with the use of opioids for pain relief is below 1% (Mann & Carr 2009). Use for acute pain has minimal risk. Evidence from the management of chronic malignant pain shows that people can maintain normal activities without demonstrating features of addiction. Increasingly, opioids are being used for severe chronic non-malignant pain. Fricker (2003) identified that 50% of chronic pain patients in the UK were prescribed weak opioids (codeine, dihydrocodeine, tramadol) and 12% required strong opioids (morphine-modified release or fentanyl patch). The British Pain Society (2010a,b) provides recommendations for professionals and patients about the appropriate use of opioids which includes education regarding long-term side-effects.

The management of pain in people who misuse drugs often requires support from the acute pain team, as drug tolerance means that larger doses will be needed. The route of administration also requires careful consideration: for example, regular i.m. administration would not be desirable, as it encourages dependence on an invasive approach (Box 23.20).

Critical thinking   Box 23.20

Opioid misuse and pain relief

Leo is having major surgery but providing postoperative pain relief is complicated by his misuse of heroin. The acute pain team is able to prescribe an analgesic regimen to relieve his pain. Although the focus of immediate care remains effective pain management, rehabilitation will become a future goal. Drug rehabilitation requires skilled specialist support.

Student activities

- Discuss with your mentor the role of the acute pain team in the care of people who misuse opioids.
- Which services are available locally for community-based drug rehabilitation, e.g. Community Alcohol and Drug Service.

Non-pharmacological methods of pain control

Over recent years non-pharmacological methods of pain control such as massage and the use of essential oils have become more widely accepted within conventional healthcare systems, although many still lack robust evidence of efficacy. Information giving is pivotal in pain control, as fear of pain increases pain perception (see p. 583). An outline of some methods is provided.

It is vital that nurses understand the importance of simple (but by no means trivial) comfort measures that can be initiated as part of pain management, e.g. a carefully placed pillow (Box 23.21).

Reflective practice   Box 23.21

Comfort measures

Think about the comfort measures that you use to decrease pain and discomfort. For example, after a busy shift you may rest your aching legs on a chair or in a warm bath, or use a hot water bottle to relieve 'period pain'.

Student activities

- What simple comfort measures have you provided for people in pain?
- Discuss with your mentor how you might increase the use of comfort measures in pain management.

Pain type, severity and the patient's age are important factors to consider when planning the use of non-pharmacological approaches to pain management. It is also important to note that the patient's mental and emotional state are important in pain management and, as these are likely to vary over time, can affect the severity, tolerance and expression of pain.

Non-pharmacological methods (Box 23.22) can be classified into two groups: physical (counter-irritation) and psychological. However, some methods, such as massage, have both physical and psychological benefits. Many non-pharmacological methods are complementary and alternative medicine (CAM) therapies (Ch. 10). (See Further reading suggestions, e.g. Mantle & Tiran 2009).

Examples of non-pharmacological methods for pain control   Box 23.22

Psychological methods (central stimulation and enhanced pain modulation of the 'pain gate')

- Relaxation
- Distraction (cognitive strategy)
- Music therapy
- Humour
- Guided imagery
- Cognitive behaviour therapy – hypnosis, biofeedback.

Physical (counterirritation) methods (peripheral stimulation of the 'pain gate')

- Heat and cold
- Chemicals – topical applications causing skin irritation, e.g. products containing combinations of eucalyptus oil, menthol, methylsalicylate, etc.
- Massage
- Transcutaneous electrical nerve stimulation (TENS)
- Acupuncture.

Effective holistic pain management usually requires a combined pharmacological and non-pharmacological approach. In acute severe pain the dominant intervention is usually pharmacological along with explanation, anxiety reduction, emotional support and appropriate touch. Distraction and relaxation require patient participation as well as energy, which may limit their usefulness in severe pain. Relaxation is further limited in acute severe pain as there may be insufficient time to teach relaxation techniques. However, appropriate techniques can be taught in advance, e.g. prior to planned surgery.

Non-pharmacological methods of pain control (e.g. use of the hydrotherapy pool), which reduce pain perception by closing the 'pain gate', are probably most effective as coping strategies in chronic non-malignant pain rather than for reducing the intensity of pain (see Fig. 23.3 and Table 23.1). There are some exceptions to this, such as cold applications, but the most likely outcome of techniques such as relaxation and distraction is that the pain may become more bearable but not necessarily less severe in intensity. Specialized practitioners may be available via the pain specialist services for chronic pain or for cancer patients.

Despite the obvious benefits of pain relief achieved by using non-pharmacological methods, nurses must ensure that they possess the appropriate knowledge and skills to deliver such techniques (NMC 2008). It is also important to note that non-pharmacological methods may be overused in some circumstances and with certain people. For example, clients and patients who are cooperative and adapt to techniques such as distraction may suffer their pain in silence and not be provided with appropriate or adequate analgesia.

Simple comfort measures

These can improve the experience of the person in pain and include:

- Careful positioning and changes in position as required. Analgesia may be needed if the repositioning itself is painful

- Ensuring that people have sufficient rest and sleep (Ch. 10) can enhance coping strategies
- Pillows and footstools for support and a bed cage to keep heavy bedding off the legs
- Warmth with heated pads or warm baths, or cold applications/ice packs. Nurses must follow local safety guidelines when using heat or cold to prevent injury (Ch. 13)
- Attention to proper bed/cot making is important, e.g. ensuring that bedding is not creased (Ch. 18)
- Providing comfort for infants by swaddling or 'nesting', which means to snuggle, cuddle or cradle the infant.

These measures are also valuable for patient/clients and their carers who can become actively involved, especially in the management of chronic pain.

Information giving

Effective communication (Ch. 9) and the provision of high quality information are vital components of holistic pain management. Inadequate information leads to the fear of pain, especially when the cause is unknown, or fear of not coping and poor understanding of pain relief methods, which can all worsen pain (Box 23.23). RNs must ensure that all concerned have sufficient information about pain and pain relief. They should discuss options, give explanations and provide written information about methods of managing pain, all of which can help to minimize anxiety and fear. There are also expert patient programmes and self-help books designed to help patients cope with pain.

 Reflective practice Box 23.23

Information and coping with chronic pain information for patients

Access the pain toolkit devised to guide patients to manage their chronic pain independently (Moore 2007).

Student activity
- Reflect on the strategies recommended and the advice for those with chronic pain.

Relaxation

Relaxation may provide relief from pain and/or reduce anxiety. It may not lessen pain intensity but may decrease the distress associated with the pain. A patient/client cannot usually be relaxed and anxious at the same time. Relaxation aims to decrease skeletal muscle tension, as muscle pain can heighten painful stimuli, and the gate control theory predicts that decreasing muscle tension will reduce pain sensation. Relaxation is an effective coping mechanism for chronic or procedural pain. It can be initiated with music therapy, and relaxation techniques (Ch. 11) can be taught prior to, and in preparation for, painful procedures. A warm bath also aids relaxation. For infants, holding them in a well-supported comfortable position and/or rocking them rhythmically can facilitate relaxation.

Snoezelen multisensory rooms/environments, initially developed for people with a learning disability to create an environment for sensory stimulation, have recently been used to promote rest and relaxation for patients with chronic pain as a way to promote their coping strategies (Schofield 2002).

Hypnosis

Hypnosis is defined as focused attention, an altered state of consciousness or a trance that is followed by a period of relaxation. Hypnosis aids relaxation and is useful in relieving the distress of pain, depression, irritable bowel syndrome, in cancer, etc. Hypnosis is a valuable tool and its use by properly trained hypnotherapists in the NHS should be increased (Royal Society of Medicine's Hypnosis and Psychosomatic Medicine section 2011). It may not take the pain away but reduces or removes pain perception by stimulating the higher centres of the brain which inhibit opening of the 'gate'.

Distraction

Distraction is a means of putting the pain at the periphery of awareness (McCaffery 1990) and focusing attention on something else. The focus of attention is diverted to the 'distracter' rather than the pain. Distracters include:

- Company and conversation, especially when humour and laughter are involved
- Television, DVD, radio, personal music players, mobile phones
- Computers – social networks, games (valuable distracters for children, particularly if activity is limited)
- Hobbies
- Exercise, activity and sport (also linked to endorphin production)
- Pet animals
- Reading
- Play (see below).

Children in particular tend to be talented at using distracters as a means of pain relief. Additional distracters for children include:

- Having stories read to them
- Music, singing, and tapping to the rhythms of the song
- Talking books, especially via headphones (active listening is a strong distracter)
- Watching a favourite DVD or television programme
- Blowing bubbles
- Visits from role models such as the local football team
- Shouting or yelling.

The distracter can be increased or reduced according to the intensity of the pain (Box 23.24).

In children's wards, a play specialist may be available to support nurses with 'play as distraction'. This is beneficial, as boredom can be a factor that opens the 'pain gate'. Similarly, an activities coordinator working in a care home can arrange outings/social events that act as distracters for residents with pain.

Older people who live alone may find that social isolation is a negative influence on pain perception, as it is likely to open the 'pain gate'. Therefore, encouraging social interaction and hobbies, e.g. lunch clubs, reading groups, that stimulate and distract may be valuable strategies in pain management.

Imagery

Imagery is the use of imagination to modify pain responses and involves using sensory images to modify the pain, e.g. that the pain is a balloon and the person is trying to blow the balloon (pain) as far away as possible. In doing so, it makes the pain more bearable by providing a focus or substitution and organizes energies that facilitate the healing process. Imagery provides relief through relaxation, distraction and producing an image of the pain. Imagery can also empower patients/clients to take some control over their pain.

Imagery can be used in a guided way with children and is usually described as *guided therapeutic imagery*. The child imagines something about their pain that will help to reduce it, e.g. their pain flowing out of their bodies.

Massage

Massage may modify pain by stimulating the nerve fibres responsible for inhibiting pain perception by closing the gate and potentially stimulating endorphin production. The relief obtained by rubbing an area after a minor knock demonstrates this.

Where possible, the patient/client/parents should be involved in the decision-making process and appropriate permission should be sought. Using massage involves a level of physical contact that is an essential element of the therapy. Massage can provide carers with a useful role and make them feel that they are contributing something positive to the experience, e.g. the carer or relative can massage their loved one's back. Older adults especially may be deprived of physical contact and massage can have a dual effect of contact with another person and lead to relaxation.

Massage provides healing and relaxes tightly contracted muscles that may result from pain-induced stress. Therefore, massage can lead to relaxation and provide renewed energy needed for coping strategies.

Therapeutic touch

Touch is a means of communication (Ch. 9). It is normally a two-way process involving feelings and sensation, and indicates a caring or loving relationship; on the other hand, touch used therapeutically aims to aid healing.

Therapeutic touch is a non-invasive means by which the nurse can help to manage a person's pain. This is particularly important for certain groups such as children, people with mental distress or those with learning disabilities. Some patients in hospital are deprived of therapeutic touch, even though they are exposed to high levels of touch, especially in relation to observations and technical procedures (Box 23.25). In fact parents, especially those of children who are severely ill, touch their children more than the nursing staff.

Acupuncture

Acupuncture (see Ch. 10) aims to treat the person and not the disease or symptoms. After a systematic review Trigkilidas (2010) suggests that acupuncture can be better than standard care in people with chronic low back pain. There is also some evidence to suggest that acupuncture encourages the production of endorphins (see pp. 567–568).

Transcutaneous electrical nerve stimulation

Transcutaneous electrical nerve stimulation (TENS) is useful in localized pain and is thought to increase endorphin levels and act as a counterirritant. Ideally TENS should be used in combination with other treatments. The non-invasive device delivers controlled low-voltage electricity to the body via electrodes placed on the skin (Fig. 23.11). People using TENS often describe a tingling sensation when the device is active. It is useful for both acute and chronic pain and is used in labour (Box 23.26).

In chronic pain TENS provides a modality with fewer side-effects than other treatments and is attractive because it is controlled by the patient and does not limit mobility. However, some people may be unable to tolerate the electrodes on their skin.

Aromatherapy

Aromatherapy (see Ch. 10) involves the use of essential oils extracted from various plants. The oils can be used in massage, in the bath, compresses and inhalation. Aromatherapy massage

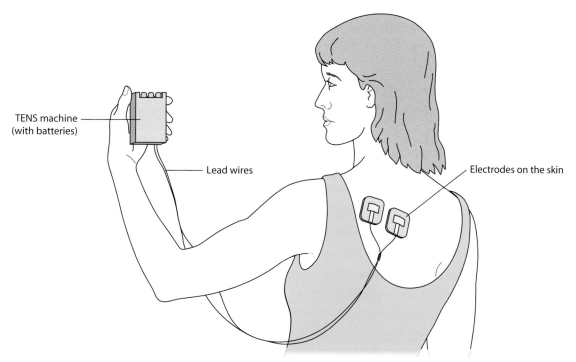

Fig. 23.11 • Transcutaneous electrical nerve stimulation (TENS).

 Critical thinking   Box 23.26

Non-pharmacological pain relief during labour

Women may choose to use TENS or other non-pharmacological methods as part of managing labour pain.

Student activities

- What non-pharmacological methods have you seen used during labour?
- How did these methods affect the woman's pain experience and the experience of her partner/supporter?
- Did women choose to combine the method with drug-based pain relief?

---

can offer several ways of reducing the pain experience, e.g. by acting on the 'pain gate', positively affecting the cognitive control mechanisms and by the release of endorphins. Aromatherapy is frequently used to reduce stress, promote relaxation, treat symptoms and relieve pain.

Aromatherapy must only be practised by trained practitioners, although once the oils have been made safely into an effective blend, patients/clients/parents can use them as prescribed by the therapist. Nurses must consult local guidelines and polices before using essential oils.

Surgical intervention

Sometimes necessary for intractable pain, surgical interventions include:

- Nerve ablation or destruction – temporary or permanent
- Spinal cord stimulation
- Brain stimulation using s.c. pulse generators.

These interventions are only used when other pain control methods have proved unsuccessful and usually fall within the remit of the specialist pain clinic.

SUMMARY

- Pain is a subjective, complex and multidimensional experience that has physical, psychosocial, emotional, cultural and spiritual elements.
- Accurate pain assessment is essential for effective management and requires good communication skills and an awareness of potential barriers to effective communication.
- Recognition of vulnerable people who cannot express pain easily is vital.
- Assessment tools improve the objectivity of pain assessment; the appropriate choice of tools requires the nurse to have an awareness of suitability for pain type and client group.
- The recognition that pain is multidimensional has encouraged holistic care, which recognizes the importance of pharmacological and non-pharmacological approaches.
- For people with chronic pain, empowerment to encourage independence and coping skills is important.
- Ineffective pain management seriously hampers rehabilitation following surgery and trauma and may lead to depression and disability if it becomes unrelieved chronic pain.
- Effective pain management is an important quality issue in nursing care across the lifespan and in all fields of nursing.
- Finally, remember that pain is 'whatever the experiencing person says it is, existing whenever he says it does' (McCaffery & Pasero 1999).

KEY WORDS AND PHRASES FOR LITERATURE SEARCHING

Acute pain

Analgesics

Chronic pain

Neuropathic pain

Nociceptive pain

Pain assessment

Pain clinics

Pain relief

 Useful websites

Bandolier – The Oxford Pain Internet Site http://www.medicine.ox.ac.uk/bandolier/booth/painpag/index2.html

British National Formulary and *British National Formulary for Children* www.bnf.org/bnf

British Pain Society www.britishpainsociety.org

Health Improvement Scotland www.healthscotland.com

National Institute for Health and Clinical Excellence www.nice.org.uk

Pain website www.pain-talk.co.uk

Scottish Intercollegiate Guidelines Network www.sign.ac.uk

All websites accessed September 2012.

References

Abbey, J., Piller, N., De Bellis, A., et al., 2004. The Abbey pain scale: a 1-minute numerical indicator for people with end-stage dementia. International Journal of Palliative Nursing 10 (1), 6–13.

Baker, C., Wong, D., 1987. QUESTT: a process of pain assessment in children. Orthopaedic Nurse 6 (1), 9–11.

Benesh, L., Szigrti, E., Ferraro, R., et al., 1997. Tools for assessing chronic pain in rural elderly women. Home Healthcare Nurse 15 (3), 207–211.

British National Formulary, 2012. Nurse independent prescribing. Online. Available: http://bnf.org/bnf/.

British Pain Society, 2006. Pain rating scale. Online. Available: www.britishpainsociety.org/pub_pain_scales.htm September 2012.

British Pain Society, 2007. Concise guidance to good practice, No. 8: assessment of pain in older adults. Online. Available: www.britishpainsociety.org/book_pain_older_people.pdf September 2012.

British Pain Society, 2010a. Opioids for persistent pain: good practice. Online. Available: www.britishpainsociety.org/book_opioid_main.pdf September 2012.

British Pain Society, 2010b. Opioids for persistent pain: information for patients. Online. Available: www.britishpainsociety.org/book_opioid_patient.pdf September 2012.

Chamley, C., 2011. Pain management. In: Brooker, C., Nicol, M. (Eds.), Alexander's nursing practice, fourth ed. Churchill Livingstone, Edinburgh.

Chronic Pain Policy Coalition, 2007. A new pain manifesto. Online. Available: www.policyconnect.org.uk/cppc/cppc/our-campaign September 2012.

Dalton, J., 1989. Nurses perceptions of their pain assessment skills pain management practices and attitudes towards pain. Oncology Nursing Forum 16, 225–231.

Davies, K., Taylor, A., 2003. Pain. In: Brooker, C., Nicol, M. (Eds.), Nursing adults. The practice of caring. Mosby, Edinburgh.

Department of Health, 2010. Essence of Care 2010 Benchmarks for the prevention and management of pain. Online. Available: www.dh.gov.uk/prod_consum_dh/groups/dh_digitalassets/@dh/@en/@ps/documents/digitalasset/dh_119977.pdf September 2012.

Field, B., Swarm, R., 2008. Chronic pain. Hogrefe & Huber, Cambridge, MA.

Fricker, J., 2003. Pain in Europe: a report. Online. Available: www.britishpainsociety.org/Pain%20in%20Europ%20survey%20report.pdf September 2012.

Greener, M., 2009. NSAIDS applied to the skin: A very topical subject. Nurse Prescribing 7 (70), 294–299.

Herr, K., Mobily, P., 1993. Comparison of selected pain assessment tools for use with the elderly. Applied Nursing Research 6 (1), 39–46.

Herr, K., Coyne, P., McCaffery, M., Manworren, R., Merkel, S., 2011. Pain assessment in the patient unable to self-report: position statement with clinical recommendations. Pain Managements Nurse 12 (4), 230–250.

Human Rights Act, 1998. TSO, London. Online. Available: www.legislation.gov.uk/ukpga/1998/42/contents September 2012.

James, G., 2011. Chronic pain: living with chronic pain. In: Randall, S., Ford, H. (Eds.), Long term conditions: A guide for nurses and health care professionals. Wiley-Blackwell, Chichester.

Kennedy, R.M., Luhmann, J., Zempsky, W.T., 2008. Clinical implications of unmanaged needle-insertion pain and distress in children. Pediatrics 122 (Supplement 3), S130–S133.

Lovering, S., 2006. Cultural attitudes and beliefs about pain. Journal of Transcultural Nursing 17, 389–395.

Mann, E., 2003. Chronic pain and opioids: dispelling myths and exploring the facts. Professional Nurse 18 (7), 408–411.

Mann, E., 2008. Neuropathic pain: could nurses become more involved. British Journal of Nursing 17 (19), 1208–1213.

Mann, E., Carr, E., 2009. Pain: creative approaches to effective management, second ed. Macmillan, Basingstoke.

McCaffery, M., 1990. Nursing approaches to nonpharmacological pain control. International Journal of Nursing Studies 27 (1), 1–5.

McCaffery, M., Pasero, C., 1999. Pain clinical manual, second ed. Mosby, St Louis.

Melzack, R., Katz, J., 1994. Measurement in persons in pain. In: Wall, P., Melzack, R. (Eds.), Textbook of pain, third ed. Churchill Livingstone, Edinburgh.

Melzack, R., Wall, P., 1965. Pain mechanisms: a new theory. Science 150, 971–979.

Merskey, H., Bogduk, N. (Eds.), 1994. Classification of chronic pain: descriptions of chronic pain syndromes and definitions of pain terms. Report by the International Association for the Study of Pain, second ed. IASP Press, Seattle.

Moore, A., Edwards, J., Barden, J., et al., 2003. League table of analgesia in acute pain. In: Bandoliers little book of pain. Oxford University Press, New York.

Moore, P., Cole, F., 2009 (Revised December 2012). The pain toolkit. Online. Available: www.paintoolkit.org/assets/downloads/Pain-Toolkit-Booklet-Nov-2012.pdf.

Nursing and Midwifery Council, 2008. The code: Standards for conduct, performance and ethics for nurses and midwives. Online. Available: www.nmc-uk.org September 2012.

Nursing and Midwifery Council, 2010. Standards for pre-registration nursing education. Online. Available: www.nmc-uk.org September 2012.

Parsons, G., Preece, W., 2010. Principles and practice of managing pain. A guide for nurses and allied health care professionals. Open University Press, Maidenhead.

Paz, S., Seymour, J., 2008. Pain theories, evaluation and management. In: Payne, S., Seymour, J., Ingleton, C. (Eds.), Palliative care nursing. Open University Press, New York.

Royal College of Nursing, 2009. The recognition and assessment of acute pain in children: update of full guidance. Online. Available: www.rcn.org.uk/__data/assets/pdf_file/0004/269185/003542.pdf September 2012.

Royal Society of Medicine (Hypnosis and psychosomatic medicine section), 2011. Take hypnosis out of the hands of "cowboys" – and bring it into the NHS. Press release

06.06.11. Online. Available: www.rsm.ac.uk/media/pr290.php.

Sarafino, E., 2008. Health psychology: Biopsychosocial interactions, sixth ed. Wiley, Hoboken.

Sepion, B., 2009. Communicating with children and young people. In: Childs, L., Coles, L., Marjoram, B. (Eds.), Essential skills clusters for nurses theory for practice. Wiley-Blackwell, Chichester.

Schofield, P., 2002. Evaluating Snoezelen for relaxation within chronic pain management. British Journal of Nursing 11 (12), 812–821.

Stebbings, J., 2010. Play. In: Trigg, E., Mohammed, T. (Eds.), 2010 Practices in children's nursing: guidelines for hospital and community, third ed. Churchill Livingstone, Edinburgh.

Trigkilidas, D., 2010. Acupuncture therapy for chronic lower back pain: a systematic review.

Annals of the Royal College of England 92 (7), 595–598.

Twycross, A., Dowden, S., Bruce, E., 2009. Managing pain in children. A clinical guide. Blackwell-Wiley, Chichester.

World Health Organization, 2005. Pain ladder. Online. Available: www.who.int/cancer/palliative/painladder/en September 2012.

Further reading

British Pain Society, 2010. Understanding and managing pain: information for patients. Online. Available: www.britishpainsociety.org/book_understanding_pain.pdf September 2012.

British Pain Society, 2010. Managing your pain effectively using 'Over the Counter' (OTC) Medicines. Online. Available: www.britishpainsociety.org/patient_pub_otc.pdf September 2012.

Department of Health, 2004. National Service Framework for children, young people and maternity services. Online. Available: www.dh.gov.uk/en/Publicationsandstatistics/Publications/PublicationsPolicyAndGuidance/DH_4089099 September 2012.

Glasper, A., Richardson, J., 2010. A textbook of children's and young people's nursing, second ed. Churchill Livingstone, Edinburgh.

Health Improvement Scotland, 2004. Post-operative pain management Best practice.

Online. Available: www.healthcareimprovementscotland.org/previous_resources/best_practice_statement/post-operative_pain_management.aspx September 2012.

Health Improvement Scotland, 2006. Management of chronic pain in adults. Online. Available: www.healthcareimprovementscotland.org/previous_resources/best_practice_statement/management_of_chronic_pain_in_.aspx September 2012.

Health Improvement Scotland, 2009. Best practice, management of pain in patients with cancer. Online. Available: www.healthcareimprovementscotland.org/previous_resources/best_practice_statement/the_management_of_pain_in_pati.aspx September 2012.

Hockenberry, M.J., Wilson, D. (Eds.), 2011. Wong's nursing care of infants and children, ninth ed. Mosby, St Louis.

NHS Choices, 2011. Alcohol and drugs during pregnancy. Online. Available: www.nhs.uk/planners/pregnancycareplanner/Pages/alcoholanddrugs.aspx.

National Institute for Health and Clinical Excellence, 2009. Low back pain: Early management of persistent non-specific low back pain. Clinical Guideline 88. Online. Available: http://guidance.nice.org.uk/CG88 September 2012.

National Institute for Health and Clinical Excellence, 2012. Opioids in palliative care: safe and effective prescription of strong opioids for pain in palliative care of adults. Clinical Guideline 140. Online. Available http://guidance.nice.org.uk/CG140 August 2012.

Mantle, F., Tiran, D., 2009. A-Z of Complementary and alternative medicine: A guide for health professionals. Churchill Livingstone, Edinburgh.

Caring for the person having surgery

24

Susan Watt

LEARNING OUTCOMES

This chapter will help you:

- Explain the differences between elective and emergency surgery
- Describe preoperative preparation of a patient
- Understand the nursing interventions needed to maintain the safety and dignity of people undergoing surgery
- Explain the principles of postoperative care
- Describe potential postoperative complications and their prevention
- Understand the principles of effective discharge planning.

Introduction

A person who has to undergo a surgical procedure or invasive investigation is likely to experience both psychological and physiological stress (see Ch. 11). Stressors can be reduced by careful planning and considered nursing intervention. This chapter will explore the care patients receive before (preoperative), during (intraoperative) and after (postoperative) surgery. Examples of invasive procedures, day surgery and in-patient stays are outlined, together with different reasons for and aims of surgery. The importance of the nurse's role in preoperative and postoperative care, in particular maintaining patient safety and dignity will be explored within this chapter. Discharge planning usually begins before admission for surgery and is explained in the final section. Surgical nursing care should be seamless, despite it being carried out in several different settings, and the factors that facilitate this are considered.

There is a wide range of terminology used to describe surgical procedures. By understanding the meaning of some commonly used prefixes and suffixes this becomes logical and much easier to understand (Table 24.1). It is good practice to look up the meanings of new terms encountered in practice.

Types of surgery

This section considers the different approaches to surgical interventions. There have been several advances in the way people can receive surgical treatment, including:

- Pre-assessment clinics prior to admission for surgery
- Combined investigation and surgical treatment, e.g. endoscopy (Box 24.1)
- Day surgery: the development of less, and minimally, invasive surgical procedures (including keyhole surgery, see Box 24.2) have reduced patients' stay in hospital from days to a few hours.

Table 24.1 Terminology used to describe surgical procedures

	Meaning	Example
Prefixes		
Angio~	Of a vessel	Angiography
Chol~	Bile	Cholecystectomy
Cysto~	Of the bladder	Cystectomy
Gastro~	Of the stomach	Gastrostomy
Laparo~	Abdominal	Laparotomy
Suffixes		
~ectomy	Removal of	Appendectomy
~oscopy	Viewing of	Laparoscopy
~ostomy	Opening of	Ileostomy
~otomy	Incision into	Osteotomy
~plasty	Reconstruction of	Angioplasty
~therm	Heat	Diathermy

Endoscopy   Box 24.1

Endoscopy is examination of internal structures using an endoscope. This instrument enables visualization of hollow organs and body cavities including the:

- Upper gastrointestinal tract – oesophagogastro-duodenoscopy (OGD), gastroscopy
- Lower gastrointestinal tract – colonoscopy, sigmoidoscopy
- Urinary tract – cystoscopy
- Bronchial tree – bronchoscopy
- Uterus – hysteroscopy
- Joints – arthroscopy.

Endoscopes are usually made from flexible fibreoptic material but are sometimes rigid metal devices. Endoscopy is used for:

- Diagnosis
- Taking tissue samples, known as biopsies, and/or fluid for diagnostic purposes
- Performing interventions such as sealing off bleeding points, e.g. peptic ulcers, removal of polyps from the large intestine, gallstones from the common bile duct or bone pieces from joints
- Photography of findings
- Surgery, e.g. laparoscopic cholecystectomy (removal of the gallbladder, see below).

Endoscopy may cause pain and discomfort and is usually carried out under light sedation or anaesthesia (general or local).

Keyhole surgery   Box 24.2

Laparoscopy

The laparoscope is an endoscope used for investigations or 'keyhole' surgery within the peritoneal cavity, e.g. laparoscopic cholecystectomy. Laparoscopic surgery is carried out under general anaesthesia and the immediate postoperative care is the same as that following conventional surgery (see pp. 598–605).

Advantages of laparoscopic surgery

- Small wound sites (around 12 mm)
- Less postoperative pain
- Early mobilization and discharge
- Fewer postoperative complications associated with immobility, e.g. chest infections, deep vein thrombosis (see p. 596).

Disadvantages of laparoscopic surgery

- Costly equipment required
- Training of practitioners is expensive.

Expected outcomes of surgery vary depending on the reason for intervention. This may be:

- A *curative* procedure that involves removal of diseased or damaged tissues that aims to restore health and may use radical methods, e.g. removal of an inflamed appendix or amputation of a limb following a crush injury
- A *conservative* procedure that involves the removal of diseased or damaged tissues using non-radical methods to improve health and preserve function, e.g. debulking/removal of a cancer
- A *palliative* procedure that is undertaken to relieve unpleasant or distressing symptoms when curative or

conservative procedures are not possible, e.g. insertion of a hollow tube into the oesophagus to relieve an obstruction caused by a cancer.

Surgical interventions may be classified as:

- *Elective* – this is planned beforehand and includes day surgery. It aims to improve a person's health and/or promote comfort and can be curative, conservative or palliative
- *Emergency* – this is unplanned and necessary for the person's survival and may be curative, conservative or, occasionally, palliative.

Elective surgery

People who undergo elective surgery are usually admitted on the day of surgery having already had pre-assessment and the necessary investigations (see below). Careful preparation ensures patients are in optimal health for their operation. This minimizes cancellation when further investigations are needed or unforeseen problems arise, thereby reducing the likelihood of postoperative complications. The type and extent of surgery, together with the individual's state of health before, during and after surgery, will determine the length of stay in hospital. When day surgery is undertaken, the patient goes home again the same day, whereas in-patient surgery usually requires a few days in hospital postoperatively. Some patients need a series of surgical interventions, e.g. reconstructive surgery following severe or disfiguring injuries.

Day surgery

Day surgery is becoming more common and accounts for approximately 80% of surgical procedures (British Association of Day Surgery 2011). This involves admission of selected patients for planned surgical interventions and discharge the same day. Many minor surgical procedures, such as cataract extraction, hernia repair, vasectomy or endoscopy, may be carried out as day cases.

There are many benefits of day surgery (Department of Health, DH 2002):

- Patients receive treatments tailored to their needs in dedicated day surgery units, which is associated with increased patient satisfaction
- Patients can recover in their own homes
- Short hospital stay with less risk of hospital acquired infections and least disruption to patient's lives
- Higher throughput of patients results in shorter waiting lists
- Fewer day surgery cases are cancelled at very short notice
- In-patient hospital beds can be kept for more serious cases.

Disadvantages:

- Not all procedures are suitable for day surgery
- Inadequate control of pain and nausea/vomiting after discharge
- Late complications may be missed

- Burden on relatives – all day surgery patients must have a responsible adult to care for them for 24–48 hours after discharge.

For some patients, day surgery is contraindicated, e.g. if the patient has a medical condition that may increase their chances of surgical complication, such as recent myocardial infarction or chronic obstructive pulmonary disease, psychological issues, e.g. unstable mental illness or social circumstances (patients may live too far away from the day surgery centre or have no-one to care for them afterwards).

Emergency surgery

This is sudden and unplanned. Patients may find this very stressful for many reasons, including fear of the unknown, fear of pain or dying and fear of hospitals. Bearing this in mind, the nurse must assess not only patients' physiological needs but also their psychological and emotional needs. In this situation, social needs are also very important, e.g. children may be waiting at the school gate or older adults or pet animals may depend on the person being at home at certain times. It is very important to establish a trusting nurse/patient relationship quickly. This relationship can be enhanced by the way the nurse informs and involves the patient during admission and preparation for urgent surgery. Effective communication skills (see Ch. 9) are therefore essential.

Preoperative care

The aim of preoperative care is to ensure that each patient receives holistic (physical and psychological) assessment and preparation for a safe and dignified surgical experience. For emergency admissions, this is accelerated and takes place very soon after admission; however, the principles are the same. Preparation usually begins with referral from the general practitioner (GP) for elective procedures. For patients in England, the 'Choose and Book' system provides the opportunity to decide which hospital they wish to use and the timing of their first out-patient appointment (NHS Connecting for Health 2011).

Preoperative assessment is carried out on most patients prior to elective surgery and this has been found to enhance the patient experience (NHS Institute for Innovation and Improvement 2008).

Pre-assessment clinics

Preoperative assessment enhances patients' surgical experience by:

- Ensuring patients are fully informed, which lessens stress and speeds up recovery
- Providing physical and psychological assessments which ensure patients are in good health preoperatively
- Involving patients and their carers in admission and discharge planning so they know what to expect
- Allowing patients to be admitted on the day of surgery

- Reducing the numbers of cancelled operations due to patient ill-health.

(NHS Institute for Innovation and Improvement 2008). A multidisciplinary approach is often used for pre-assessment; patients are seen not only by medical and nursing practitioners but also physiotherapists and occupational therapists.

Patients of all ages attending pre-assessment clinics are encouraged, if they wish, to bring a friend, partner or carer with them. Children should be accompanied by their parent or legal guardian during the pre-assessment process. However, there are some circumstances in which this may not be case, e.g. where an older child is deemed mature enough to understand the procedure and its implications and is competent to make their own decisions about their care, e.g. a girl of 15 years with sufficient maturity having a termination of pregnancy without her parents' knowledge. At pre-assessment clinics patients have the opportunity to:

- Discuss their treatment options with members of the care team
- Identify whether day surgery or in-patient surgery is more appropriate
- Undergo all, or some, of the investigations required on the same day
- Discuss lifestyle changes that will improve postoperative recovery, e.g. weight reduction, smoking cessation (see below)
- Receive information about what to expect before, during and after surgery e.g. options for pain management postoperatively (NHS Quality Improvement Scotland, NHS QIS 2004)
- Learn preoperative exercises which can reduce postoperative complications (Valkenet et al 2011)
- Discuss the local fasting policy so that they understand what is required
- Discuss personal and domestic circumstances e.g. who will help care for them after discharge. If the patient is a main carer for a child or elderly person, who will help with this role while the patient is in hospital or recovering at home? Members of the care team, e.g. social worker, home help or the community health team, may be included to provide specialist advice and help
- Discuss the local policy regarding routine medicines, e.g. a patient may be advised to cease taking warfarin (medication which thins the blood) a few days prior to admission.

It is important that everyone, including both children and parents, is provided with information in a way that is understood (see below).

Investigations

Preoperative investigations are performed for different reasons including confirmation of the diagnosis to ensure the correct course of treatment is offered, to provide information regarding the risks of surgery and to predict potential postoperative complications (National Institute for Health and Clinical Excellence (NICE) 2003). Some investigations are carried out routinely on all patients; others are specific to the type of intervention being considered. Routine investigations include:

- Blood samples – full blood count, urea and electrolyte levels, blood glucose, liver function tests, coagulation studies, and blood grouping and cross-matching if a transfusion (see Ch. 17) may be required
- Chest X-ray
- Electrocardiogram (ECG)
- Urinalysis.

Depending on the type of surgery, some of the following may also be carried out:

- Respiratory function tests (see Ch. 17)
- Microbiology tests, e.g. sputum, urine to exclude infection
- Other X-rays
- Computed tomography (CT) scan
- Magnetic resonance imaging (MRI) scan
- Ultrasound scanning
- Barium studies
- Angiography.

A simple explanation of some of these investigations that will help you provide patient information can be found on the Patient.co.uk website (see Useful websites, p. 606). More detailed information can be found in Brooker and Nicol (2011).

Smoking cessation

Patients who smoke should be advised to give up, as smoking is a risk factor for many postoperative complications, e.g. chest infections, deep vein thrombosis (DVT, p. 595), poor wound healing and pressure ulcers (see Ch. 25). Ideally, interventions to promote smoking cessation should start between four and eight weeks before surgery and include weekly counselling and the use of nicotine replacement therapy (Thomsen et al 2010). It should be recognized that stopping smoking may be difficult for patients and withdrawal of nicotine can increase stress levels. Nurses must not be judgemental or critical if a patient cannot heed this advice; however, information about potential postoperative complications related to smoking should always be provided.

Psychological preparation for surgery

Effective psychological preparation of patients prior to surgery is essential. The pre-assessment clinic provides an opportunity for patients and their relatives to have information clarified and questions answered using language that they understand. Lack of information can increase patients' anxiety.

At the pre-assessment clinic, the care team can explain to the patient what will happen, before, during and after surgery. Advice can also be given regarding recovery after discharge. Healthcare practitioners involved in the care of children undergoing surgery must recognize the importance of a providing a family friendly environment (Royal College of Surgeons of England 2007).

Even when patients appear to be fully informed, they often find the preoperative waiting period stressful. Some surgery may not have a favourable outcome and this may add to people's fears and impair their ability to cope with bad news (see Ch. 9).

As patients are unlikely to remember everything discussed at a pre-assessment clinic, published material, e.g. pamphlets and DVDs, can be provided to reinforce what was discussed and provide further information which should reduce misunderstanding. This gives the opportunity for people to read or watch when they feel able to concentrate and is a useful reminder of what to expect. For those for whom English is not their first language, material in their own language should be provided whenever possible; sometimes an interpreter may be needed (see Ch. 9).

When faced with an impending operation, some people seek information from other sources including the Internet. It should be recognized however, that information found on the Internet may not always be correct or accurate.

Preoperative considerations for children

Preoperative preparation of children depends on the age of the child. Older children will cope with full explanations whereas younger children should be given simple and straightforward information in a language they can understand, and may benefit from books about what to expect in hospital. Reading together will make the surgery seem less threatening. Play may also be helpful in alleviating the anxiety of smaller children, e.g. the 'temperature' and 'pulse' can be taken on a doll or teddy to show them what to expect. A visit to the hospital and ward before the surgery allows children to become familiar with the environment and gives them the opportunity to meet some of the staff.

It is important to be honest with children, e.g. if they will experience pain postoperatively they should be told that they will be given medicine to help, not simply told that they will not have pain.

Some children think that going into hospital or having an operation is some form of punishment, so reassurance should be given that this is not the case. Others will fear separation from their parents, therefore parents should be allowed to stay with children until they are anaesthetized.

Benefits of providing preoperative information

A study by Wong et al (2010) found that providing information and education preoperatively significantly reduced the pain patients experienced postoperatively. Several seminal research studies identified other postoperative benefits of providing preoperative information, including fewer postoperative complications and reduced patient anxiety (Hayward 1975; Boore 1978; Wilson-Barnett 1979).

Common sources of preoperative anxiety

It is important to recognize that apprehension can build up while waiting for an operation, despite effective planning (Box 24.3). Fear of the unknown and loss of independence are common anxieties, other patients may be fearful of needles,

Reflective practice   Box 24.3

Preoperative anxiety and coping strategies

Some patients undergoing surgery report anxiety about having an anaesthetic, the possibility of waking up during the operation and being unable to tell anyone, not recovering from the anaesthetic or that they may behave inappropriately under the anaesthetic. Anxiety may also be increased when the potential prognosis is poor.

Normal coping strategies may be inadequate in patients having surgery. Franklin (1974) found that anxious patients needed more reassurance as well as more information about their treatment, prognosis and surroundings.

Student activities

- What would be your greatest anxiety if you needed to have (or have had) an anaesthetic?
- Consider what coping strategies you could use to reduce your anxiety.
- Observe your mentor speaking to a patient preoperatively to identify potential sources of anxiety and think about the communication skills used.
- Consider how you could help reduce patients' anxiety.
- Identify the communication skills that you might use to reduce patients' anxieties.

being anaesthetized or the consequences of surgery (Pritchard 2009).

Surgery that changes body appearance will affect people's body image (see Ch. 11), e.g. removal of a breast due to cancer is a common source of preoperative anxiety. However, to other people the same surgery may bring positive outcomes despite postoperative discomfort, e.g. breast reduction or amputation of a painful gangrenous extremity.

Anxiety can cause a person to develop either introverted or extroverted behaviour. In children, this may manifest itself by a change in behaviour, e.g. withdrawal, regression, overactivity or increased parent dependence.

Efforts should be made to minimize patients' anxiety preoperatively. The care team at the pre-assessment clinic can discuss people's fears about the anaesthetic or clarify any other concerns, e.g. relating to fear of needles or the wearing of dentures and hearing aids until induction of anaesthesia. Patients who need initial postoperative care in a high dependency or intensive care unit may find visiting the area useful but this should not be imposed as it may increase their anxiety. A meeting with an ex-patient, or the parent of a child, who has undergone the same surgery may also be beneficial.

When a patient is admitted for surgery, recovery room nurses can visit them on the ward preoperatively, which can facilitate seamless care from the ward to theatre and back again, reducing their anxiety.

Some patients use their spirituality to help them cope. Coping strategies can be observed and discussed at the pre-assessment clinic and also at the time of admission (see Box 24.3). Identifying postoperative coping strategies beforehand may help patients to work through postoperative problems using their own stress-reducing mechanisms, e.g. yoga exercises that reduce tension may assist postoperative pain management (see Ch. 23).

Obtaining consent

Prior to any operation or invasive investigation people must sign a consent form for both legal and ethical reasons (see Chs 6, 7). For consent to be valid, it is essential that three criteria are satisfied: that it is voluntary, that it is informed and that there is mental capacity to make the decision (see Ch. 6). The options, risks and benefits of the surgery should be discussed with the patient prior to obtaining consent. A qualified interpreter must be provided when obtaining consent from non-English speaking patients. Young people aged 16 and 17 are deemed to be competent to provide consent themselves. Children younger than this who fully understand what is involved in the surgery can give consent, although ideally their parents would also be involved. The Department of Health published a useful guide to consent for children and young people (DH 2001a).

It is essential that people are able to understand information given to them about an operation or investigation beforehand. This allows them to weigh up the benefits or implications of it before they provide consent. Some people however, may not be able to provide consent, e.g. those with learning disabilities or dementia and unconscious patients. In cases where patients lack 'capacity' to provide consent, treatment can be given if it is deemed as being in the person's 'best interests'. The healthcare professional responsible for the patient's care would make that decision however, ideally, all of the healthcare team and the patient's family would also be involved in the process (DH 2001b,c).

While discussing impending surgery, if there is any doubt that a particular procedure may not be possible, e.g. when a more extensive procedure might be required, the patient should also sign for the proposed variation.

Critical thinking   Box 24.4

Obtaining consent

Mrs George signs a consent form for a laparoscopic cholecystectomy. During the operation, complications arise and a more invasive procedure (laparotomy) is carried out to complete the surgery safely. Mrs George had been well prepared for this eventuality. She had already agreed and signed the consent form indicating that she understood and was prepared to have the more invasive procedure if the need arose.

Student activities

- Negotiate an opportunity to observe a practitioner obtaining consent.
- Ask a patient how effectively the consent interview prepared them for their experience.

Sometimes consent may not be given, e.g. a patient may refuse a blood transfusion due to personal or religious beliefs or the fear of infection from blood-borne viruses. Student nurses should accept patients' religious or cultural beliefs and treat them in a non-discriminatory manner (NMC 2010).

- Find out which group of people may refuse a blood transfusion.
- Consider how you might support a patient who has refused a blood transfusion.

The surgeon undertaking the procedure must mark the site of operation when a limb or paired organ is involved. This is usually performed on the day of, or evening before, the operation to safeguard against later errors regarding the correct surgical site. A waterproof marker pen prevents removal of the marks during bathing or showering. The patient must be in agreement with the site marked.

Nurses must be aware that it is a patient's right to withdraw their consent at any time. If this occurs, the nurse in charge must be informed immediately. The Nursing and Midwifery Council (NMC 2008a) *The code: Standards of conduct, performance and ethics for nurses and midwives* points out that nurses must always respect patients' wishes to accept or decline treatment or care. Consent may also be withheld in relation to an aspect of treatment (Box 24.4).

In an emergency situation, a surgeon might operate on an unconscious patient without formal signed consent. In the absence of this, the intervention must be justifiable and carried out on the basis that it is in the patient's best interests.

Preoperative fasting

Usually, patients can eat and drink normally until 2–6 hours before surgery unless the surgery involves the gastrointestinal (GI) tract. The Royal College of Nursing (RCN 2005) suggests that:

- Clear fluids (water) can be taken up to 2 hours prior to surgery
- Breast milk can be given up to 4 hours prior to surgery
- Solids, cow's milk, formula milk and milky drinks can be given up to 6 hours prior to surgery.

The reason for fasting is to ensure safety during induction of general anaesthesia by preventing inhalation of acid stomach contents into the lungs when the gag reflex is lost. Sometimes, patients are still fasted overnight for surgery in the morning, however shorter fasting times, as outlined by the RCN (2005), increase patient comfort and hydration without adding risk.

Fasting (see Box 24.5) is also known as 'nil by mouth' or 'nil orally'. To enhance compliance, the local policy and the

rationale for fasting should be explained. Water jugs and other fluids are removed from the bedside and, in the case of children, sweets and biscuits should also be removed. A sign may be put above the bed or the side room door to remind those fasting and to inform others. Some patients may require an i.v. infusion during fasting to prevent or correct dehydration (see Ch. 19). Some patients are admitted to hospital so that their fasting regime can be monitored, e.g. people with diabetes.

If someone who is meant to be fasting is found to have taken anything orally, this must be reported promptly to the nurse in charge or anaesthetist who will decide whether it is safe for the intervention to go ahead.

Some patients who are having surgery under local anaesthesia, e.g. removal of a toenail, may not need to fast. However if sedation, e.g. midazolam, is required for a procedure, fasting may be necessary to avoid the risk of aspiration (inhalation of gastric contents into the respiratory tract).

In children and those who have communication problems, the nurse should also discuss effective ways of maintaining fasting with the parent or carer during pre-assessment and reinforce this on admission. Fasting should be implemented without causing undue stress, otherwise it may become an issue.

When a patient is admitted as an emergency, the last time they had food or fluids must be clearly established. In emergency situations, a tube may be passed into the patient's stomach to aspirate the contents, thereby reducing the risks from inhalation of gastric contents.

Skin preparation

Skin preparation is considered an important strategy in reducing surgical site infection. The evidence is largely inconclusive about best practice in relation to skin care, but the aim is to reduce not only the normal flora but also potentially harmful (pathogenic) microorganisms (see Ch. 15) that may be present on the skin or hair. Cleansing of the skin is important and best achieved by showering as running water rinses off loose hair and dead skin cells more readily. Showering is also a cultural requirement for many people. Care should be taken to avoid washing off any marks indicating the operation site.

Patients are encouraged to wash their hair, as some may be unable to wash their hair for several days postoperatively. People undergoing head and neck or eye (ophthalmic) surgery may be given specific instructions for hairwashing. Total bodywashing, where antiseptic solutions are used over a number of days, has been found to eradicate Meticillin-resistant *Staphylococcus aureus* (MRSA) in patients who are MRSA positive pre-admission.

Hair removal

There is inconclusive evidence regarding hair removal, the timing of this and where it should take place, e.g. ward or operating theatre, and so practice varies (Tanner et al 2007). Nurses must be sensitive to patients' dignity and recognize that body hair contributes to people's body image and cultural

---

Evidence-based practice   Box 24.5

Preoperative fasting

Preoperative fasting time is often based on ritual rather than evidenced-based practice. Recent evidence demonstrates that many patients still fast for longer than necessary (Baril and Portman 2007).

Prolonged fasting can lead to fluid and electrolyte imbalance, dehydration and malnutrition.

Student activities

Select a small group of postoperative patients or those who have undergone invasive investigations:

- Find out for how long they fasted.
- If the fasting time is longer than suggested, discuss the possible reasons for this with your mentor.

identity, and therefore hair removal may be distressing. The reasons for hair removal are explained and patients should be encouraged to do this themselves when possible, although the outcome should be checked before the final preparations for surgery (Box 24.6).

Evidence-based practice   Box 24.6

Preoperative hair removal

Hair is removed preoperatively to ensure the incision site can be viewed effectively and to allow adhesive drapes and wound dressings to be applied to the patient's skin. There is inconclusive evidence that hair removal reduces the risk of infection in the surgical site, in some studies it was shown to increase the risk (Tanner et al 2007).

There are three methods of hair removal: shaving, clipping and the use of depilatory creams. Shaving is the least expensive method, however, the risk of surgical site infection is highest with this approach to hair removal (Tanner et al 2007). Hair can be removed using clippers with disposable heads, thus reducing the incidence of cross-infection. Depilatory cream can be used but a small area (test patch) must be tested first to ensure there is no allergy.

Student activities

- Find out about skin preparation in your placement.
- Discuss the practices with your mentor.

Preventing potential postoperative complications

Many postoperative complications can be prevented or minimized by effective preoperative care. This section explains nursing interventions undertaken to achieve this.

Chest infection

This can be both life-threatening and debilitating, and people at increased risk include:

- Those who are overweight
- Cigarette smokers (see smoking cessation, p. 592)
- Those undergoing thoracic or major abdominal surgery
- Those with chronic respiratory disease, e.g. bronchitis (see Ch. 17)
- Older adults.

At the pre-assessment clinic, patients are given information about deep breathing exercises that minimize the risk of chest infection (see Ch. 17). Some people attend physiotherapy classes to learn these exercises and how to support their wounds when they need to cough postoperatively. Others are provided with written instructions to follow at home. People's knowledge is assessed on admission to ensure it is adequate and appropriate.

Deep vein thrombosis

A deep vein thrombosis (DVT) is the formation of a thrombus (clot) in the deep veins of the legs or pelvic veins (see Ch. 17).

Pulmonary embolism (blockage of a pulmonary artery by a detached thrombus that has travelled there in the bloodstream) is a potentially fatal consequence of DVT. All patients should be assessed for DVT risk preoperatively. Patients whose operations will last longer than 90 minutes (or 60 minutes if the pelvis or lower limbs are involved) and those who are expected to have reduced mobility postoperatively are at higher risk of DVT. Also obese patients, older patients (over 60 years old) and anyone with cancer or receiving treatment for cancer has a greater risk (NICE 2010).

For those having elective surgery, preoperative measures can be taken to reduce the risk of DVT, e.g. women can be advised to stop taking medicines containing oestrogen 4 weeks before or can be taught leg exercises to carry out postoperatively. Patients can be asked preoperatively to wear anti-embolism stockings to promote venous return in the legs (see Box 24.7). Mechanical devices can be used in some patients to stimulate the circulation in the legs and medicines used to prevent the development of the blood clots. Further information about the postoperative nursing and medical management of DVT can be found on page 595.

Nursing skills   Box 24.7

Anti-embolism stockings

- Establish whether knee, thigh or full-length stockings are needed. This depends on local policy, the operation and its aftercare
- Explain why the stockings are worn and for how long
- Using a tape measure, measure the widest circumference of the calf on both legs and the widest circumference of both thighs. (It may also be necessary to measure the patient's leg length if they are very tall or large, as the size may have to be adjusted to ensure the correct fit.)
- Select the correct size of stockings following the manufacturer's instructions
- Apply the stockings, ensuring that the toes are able to move freely and that the rest of the stocking fits the contours of the leg. It is important to ensure that stockings are not rolled over at the top; any excess should be eased back into the stocking to make a perfect fit
- The stockings are carefully removed prior to bathing or showering
- Written instructions about correct application, wearing and washing are provided when they are to be worn after discharge.

Bowel preparation

Bowel preparation prior to surgery aims to prevent:

- Defecation during anaesthesia
- Faecal contamination during surgery, particularly for surgery on the GI tract
- Postoperative stress on the wound
- Postoperative discomfort or constipation due to a full rectum.

Emptying of the bowel can be achieved by administration of oral or rectal laxatives (see Chs 21, 22) if necessary.

For procedures involving the lower GI tract, specific bowel cleansing laxatives, such as sodium picosulfate, may be prescribed, together with prophylactic antibiotic therapy. Patients may undertake some of their bowel preparation in relative comfort at home.

Any bowel preparation can cause distress, which can be reduced by effective nursing intervention. Good communication is essential to ensure that the patient receives the correct preparation and understands why it is necessary. The patient's ability to reach the lavatory promptly and safely is assessed (other nursing considerations are discussed in Ch. 21). Dehydration can occur during extensive bowel preparation, even when patients have achieved the recommended fluid intake. It is therefore important to be aware that headaches or changes in behaviour, such as loss of concentration, can be signs of dehydration. When extensive bowel preparation is carried out, it may be necessary to commence an i.v. infusion to:

- Prevent dehydration
- Restore fluid balance prior to surgery
- Reduce the incidence of postoperative nausea and vomiting.

Preparation for intravenous cannulation

Preparation for i.v. cannulation is especially important in children and those who have needle phobia. Topical anaesthetic cream such as EMLA (eutectic mixture of local anaesthetic) minimizes pain during i.v. cannulation and takes approximately an hour to act (Gilboy & Hollywood 2009, also see Ch. 23).

Final preoperative care

The nurse must implement local policies to prepare the patient safely for theatre. A checklist of specific measures is often used. Items included in such checklists and rationale for their inclusion are highlighted in Table 24.2.

After the patient is transferred to theatre, the bed space is prepared for their return from surgery (Box 24.8). Carrying out the activities in Box 24.9 will help you understand a patient's perioperative experience.

Transfer to theatre

Patients should be transferred to the operating theatre department with their documentation, including medical notes, their blood results and signed consent form, medicine prescription, fluid balance chart, observation chart, X-rays and the preoperative checklist. Adults are usually transferred there on their beds or theatre trolleys. In day surgery settings, patients may be able to walk to the operating theatre if they have not been given premedication. Children are usually accompanied by a parent and they may be transferred on child-friendly equipment, e.g. a Thomas the Tank Engine truck. They often take something personal and comforting with them such as their favourite teddy, doll, toy or comfort blanket. Small children may be carried by a parent or taken on a trolley depending on local policy.

Nursing skills — Box 24.8

Preparation of the bed space for postoperative care

This enables straightforward monitoring of postoperative progress and may involve moving the bed nearer to the nurses' station and assembling equipment, including:

- A sphygmomanometer (automated or manual) to record blood pressure
- A drip stand to suspend bags of i.v. fluids
- An observation chart to record temperature, pulse, respirations, blood pressure and oxygen saturation levels (see Chs 14, 17)
- A fluid balance chart to record fluid inputs and outputs (see Ch. 19)
- A vomit bowl and tissues
- A pulse oximeter to record oxygen saturation, if appropriate (see Ch. 17)
- Checking the oxygen supply and attaching clean tubing and mask (see Ch. 17)
- Checking and preparing suction equipment
- Additional equipment depending on the nature of the surgery.

Critical thinking — Box 24.9

Perioperative care

Student activities

Select a patient who is to undergo surgery and negotiate their permission to carry out the activities below. Ask your mentor if you can follow them from your placement to theatre, recovery and back to the ward.

1. Assist with their preoperative preparation
2. Accompany the patient to the anaesthetic room and observe:
   - The handover from the ward nurse
   - The patient's reactions to the experience
   - Who is involved in the anaesthetic room
3. In theatre, observe who does what during the operation
4. In the recovery room, observe:
   - The nursing care carried out
   - The handover to the ward nurse
5. Back on the ward, observe the immediate postoperative care.

Reflect on the extent to which preparation was effective in providing the patient with a realistic expectation of their perioperative experience.

Anaesthetic room

On arrival, the receiving nurse checks the name, hospital number, date of birth and the proposed surgery with the patient. The preoperative checklist is checked again and countersigned by the receiving nurse to ensure that all the safety measures have been carried out. The patient is transferred to the operating table in preparation for surgery, ready for their anaesthetic.

Table 24.2 Preoperative checklist

Check	Rationale
Correct patient?	To ensure the correct patient receives the surgery. Patients should be asked to verbalize their name and date of birth so this can be checked against the consent form and identity bracelets.
Correct procedure?	To ensure the correct patient receives the correct surgery. This can be checked from the consent form. Any discrepancies should be reported to the nurse in charge and surgeon.
Identity bracelets worn, showing name, date of birth, hospital number?	Patients should wear at least two identification bracelets, showing at a minimum, the information in column one. They should be checked for legibility and accuracy each time a patient is moved between clinical areas (e.g. between ward and operating theatre) and prior to medicine administration.
Consent form signed?	This is a legal requirement. It is also important that the patient understands what the procedure entails (NMC 2008b).
Operation site and side marked?	This ensures the patient undergoes the correct surgery. In the case of bowel surgery, the site where a stoma may be situated can be identified in advance and marked (Slater 2011).
Prescribed pre-medication administered?	The anaesthetist may prescribe preoperative medication (premedication), which will complement the anaesthetic, e.g. the sedative drug temazepam may be given to reduce anxiety. The patient should be instructed to remain in bed following administration of the premedication to ensure their safety. It is essential that the consent form is signed before premedication is administered.
Routine medicines taken?	Some medicines may be stopped in advance of surgery e.g. warfarin (anticoagulant). The anaesthetist will provide guidance on which drugs should be taken or if the patient is in hospital, prescribe them.
Make up and nail varnish removed (if required)?	Facial make up makes the patient's colour difficult to assess. Nail varnish prevents the colour of the nail beds from being observed and may also render oxygen saturation levels detected by a pulse oximeter inaccurate.
Jewellery, including body piercings, and hairclips removed, rings taped?	Metal jewellery may harm patients e.g. diathermy burns. Where possible, jewellery, including piercings, and hairclips should be removed and stored safely (consideration should be given to jewellery worn for cultural or religious reasons). Rings that cannot be removed should be taped to the patient's finger using hypoallergenic tape.
Removal of prosthesis, dentures, contact lenses	To ensure patient safety, e.g. loose dentures may cause airway obstruction. For dignity, some patients may not want to remove their dentures or wig until just before they are anaesthetized, this can be done in theatre and the dentures/wig given to the ward nurse for safe keeping. Contact lenses should not be worn as they may cause corneal abrasions.
Items to accompany patient to theatre (e.g. hearing aids)?	It is essential that theatre practitioners are able to communicate with patients before and after surgery. Ensuring deaf patients have their hearing aid will enable effective communication.
Dressed for theatre?	Clean gowns ensure the skin is exposed to the minimum possible number of bacteria after showering. These usually open down the back so that they can be easily removed during surgery if necessary. If anti-embolism stockings are required, the patients should be measured and have them fitted preoperatively. Children should be able to choose what to wear – arguing that theatre gowns are necessary and removing underwear can be distressing and bewildering.
Does the patient have any allergies?	This information is essential prior to any medicine administration or application of a wound dressing to prevent allergic reactions.
Has the patient passed urine?	An empty bladder prevents urinary incontinence during surgery and damage to the bladder during pelvic surgery. Ensure that any premedication is administered after the patient has passed urine to ensure safety after sedatives are given.
Urinalysis results recorded?	Any abnormalities should be reported to the nurse in charge, surgeon and anaesthetist.
Date of last menstrual period?	This should be documented in all women of child-bearing age to ensure there is no risk of pregnancy. Women who are menstruating should be instructed to use sanitary towels and not tampons to minimize the risk of infection

Continued

Table 24.2 Preoperative checklist—cont'd

Check	Rationale
Last food? Date: Time:	Food (including formula milk) can be taken up to 6 hours before surgery (RCN 2005). (Breast milk can be taken up to 4 hours before surgery). Fasting for longer may cause malnutrition. Ensuring no food has been eaten within 6 hours minimizes the risk of inhalation of gastric contents when the patient is anaesthetized. Special consideration should be given to diabetic patients who may become hypoglycaemic when fasting.
Last drink? Date: Time:	Clear fluids can be taken up to 2 hours before surgery (RCN 2005). Longer periods without fluids may cause dehydration.
Baseline observations BP: Pulse: Resp rate: Temp: Oxygen saturation:	Observation should be documented to provide a baseline for comparison in theatre and postoperatively.
Relevant information accompanying patient? Healthcare record X rays Drug chart Blood results Blood cross matched	The surgeon and anaesthetist need to have all the information they require in the operating theatre to prevent delays to the surgery.

Anaesthesia

Anaesthetics block sensation from the operative site so that surgery or investigations are not painful. There are three different types:

- *General anaesthesia:* Several drugs are used to induce unconsciousness, analgesia and muscle relaxation
- *Regional anaesthesia:* Techniques include spinal and epidural anaesthesia (see Ch. 23) where a local anaesthetic agent, e.g. lidocaine, is used to induce loss of sensation from a region of the body
- *Local anaesthesia:* A local anaesthetic agent, e.g. lidocaine, is used to induce loss of sensation from a small area around the site of administration.

Theatre

In theatre, all care is provided by experienced practitioners. (More information about what is involved can be found in Further reading, p. 606, e.g. Gibson & Magowan 2011.)

Recovery room

Patients recovering from an anaesthetic are cared for in a recovery room (a dedicated area within the operating department), where they are assessed, monitored and given individualized care during recovery from anaesthesia to allow the early detection of complications. Parents are encouraged to come to the recovery room to be with their child as they wake up after surgery. The length of time spent in recovery depends upon the patient's cardiovascular and respiratory stability and the time it takes them to waken up after anaesthetic.

Personal effects such as a hearing aid, wig and/or dentures, should be returned to the patient to in the recovery room to maintain their dignity.

Discharge from the recovery room

Certain criteria must be met (i.e. patient is fully conscious and able to maintain their own airway) to ensure they are fit enough to be discharged from the recovery room and transferred safely back to the ward (Scottish Intercollegiate Guidelines Network, SIGN 2004). It is essential that suitable analgesic and anti-emetic regimens are prescribed prior to the patient's return to the ward. The recovery room nurse gives the ward nurse a handover detailing the surgical procedure carried out, any complications identified and any specific postoperative care required.

Postoperative care

It is essential that the patient is reassured that the procedure/operation is over when they are back in the ward. Explanations of procedures being carried out on patients postoperatively, should be explained in a way that the patient understands. Patients who are well informed are more likely to have an uncomplicated and speedy recovery.

For patients who wear hearing aids, it is important to check that they have been reinserted and are working correctly. If a patient cannot hear adequately, it may heighten their anxiety. Hearing is the first of the senses to return after a period of unconsciousness and for this reason staff must avoid discussing patients' conditions near the bedside. At this stage, children often ask for their parents. The sound of the parent's voice gives reassurance and comfort that allows a child to rest and recover.

The principles of postoperative care are always the same, however specific nursing care may also be required depending on the surgery carried out. Postoperative care begins in the recovery room (see above) and continues through discharge from hospital until convalescence is complete. It aims to promote recovery and minimize postoperative complications. The principles and milestones after return to the ward are explored in this section. An overview of postoperative care can be found in Table 24.3.

Surgical patients can become acutely unwell postoperatively and therefore assessment and monitoring of patients is essential to detect complications (NICE 2007). Evidence shows that healthcare professionals may fail to recognize deteriorating patients and do not intervene promptly enough to prevent patients dying (SIGN 2004). Guidelines should always be followed and postoperative care should include:

- Clinical assessment and monitoring
- Cardiovascular management
- Respiratory management
- Fluid, electrolyte and renal management
- Nutrition
- Pain management
- Wound management.

Table 24.3 Care plan: the principles of postoperative care

Actual/potential problem	Aim	Nursing action	Rationale
1. Airway			
Airway obstruction	To prevent or detect, and report promptly	Nurse patient in the recovery position until conscious	Maintains airway patency and prevents the tongue occluding it
		Observe for stridor (Chs 14, 17)	Indicates partial airway obstruction
2. Breathing			
Inadequate breathing	To detect and report promptly	Observe oxygen saturation and rate, depth and effort of breathing	Changes may indicate inadequate respiratory function
		Observe skin for pallor or cyanosis	Indicates hypoxia
Hypoxia	To maintain normal oxygenation	Administer oxygen therapy as prescribed (Ch. 17)	Additional oxygen will increase level of oxygen available to tissues, thus preventing hypoxia
3. Circulation			
Haemorrhage or hypovolaemic shock	To detect early signs and report promptly	Record blood pressure, pulse	Falling blood pressure, increasing heart rate, pallor and cool peripheries may indicate shock
		Observe the patient's skin colour and temperature	
		Observe wound site for leakage	Increasing leakage can indicate haemorrhage. May require the application of pressure dressing or further attention from the surgeon
		Observe drain(s) for nature and volume of drainage	Increasing drainage can indicate haemorrhage
4. Fluid balance and renal management			
Dehydration or fluid overload	To maintain fluid balance	Maintain accurate record of fluid intake/output	Enables evaluation of fluid balance
		Monitor rate and flow of i.v. infusion if present	Important to ensure that the correct amount of fluid is administered
		Observe for presence of, and report increasing dyspnoea, cyanosis, tachycardia and expectorating frothy sputum (Ch. 17)	These indicate pulmonary oedema which can arise from fluid overload
		Offer patient sips of water when permitted	When fluids are well tolerated i.v. infusion can be discontinued
Urinary retention	To prevent or detect	Monitor and record urine output	To monitor fluid balance
			To ensure patient passes urine postoperatively
		Encourage patient to pass urine regularly	Reduces stasis time in bladder, which predisposes to urinary tract infection

Continued

Table 24.3 Care plan: the principles of postoperative care—cont'd

Actual/potential problem	Aim	Nursing action	Rationale
5. Nutrition			
Nausea	To minimize or alleviate	Administer antiemetics as prescribed Aspirate nasogastric tube if present	Recognize that opioid analgesia and anaesthetic drugs cause nausea Minimizes gastric contents
Malnutrition	To regain nutritional status	Introduce easily digested diet when tolerated	Re-establishes oral intake, providing energy and protein required for wound healing
6. Pain management			
Postoperative pain	To control pain by effective use of analgesia	Give analgesia as prescribed, particularly prior to painful events, e.g. physiotherapy Monitor effect of analgesia (Ch. 23)	Patient who is pain free will be able to cooperate with physiotherapy and move more easily in bed If analgesia not effective, medical staff should review prescription
7. Wound management			
Wound infection	To prevent infection occurring	Administer prophylactic antibiotics as prescribed Monitor patient's temperature 4-hourly. Note and report pyrexia, confusion and restlessness	Reduces the possibility of infection after major surgery Early identification of pyrexia allows prompt treatment
8. Mobilization			
Immobility	To prevent complications of immobility	*Prevent DVT by:* Providing passive leg exercises until patient is able to achieve this independently Encouraging deep breathing Applying antiembolism stockings Administering heparin if prescribed Observing calves for swelling, redness, temperature, pain. *Prevent pressure ulcers by:* Assessing patients risk Performing pressure area care/encourage early mobilization	Encourages venous return and prevents stasis of blood in leg veins Prevents DVT formation May indicate presence of DVT To highlight at-risk patients Prevents formation of pressure ulcers
9. Psychological care			
Anxiety	To alleviate patients' anxiety	*Lessen postoperative anxiety by:* Providing reassurance to patient Ensuring patient is well informed about postoperative care Ensuring patient receives adequate pain relief	Disorientation is common in the initial postoperative period Providing information reduces anxiety Providing information reduces postoperative pain (Hayward 1975)

Clinical assessment and monitoring

On immediate return to the ward, a registered nurse completes the initial assessment of the patient's condition, which forms the basis of their postoperative care. The observations should be documented accurately on the appropriate chart, e.g. Early Warning Scoring (EWS) chart (see Fig. 14.14, p. 333). A structured approach using airway, breathing and circulation should be followed (SIGN 2004). Observations are generally recorded every 15 minutes for the first hour postoperatively, gradually becoming less frequent thereafter depending on the patient's condition, e.g. every 30 minutes and then every hour. Any abnormalities in observations should be reported to the nurse in charge immediately.

Airway

Assessment begins with checking that the airway is clear. This can be confirmed if the patient is able to talk. Airway obstruction is an emergency and expert help is needed immediately.

Breathing

The following observations should be taken as part of a breathing assessment:

- Respiratory rate
- Oxygen saturation
- Symmetry of chest expansion during respiration
- Breathing sounds
- Effort of breathing/use of accessory muscles.

Circulation

The following observations should be taken as part of a circulation assessment:

- Pulse (rate, volume, regularity)
- Blood pressure
- Colour of patient's skin (normal for ethnicity)
- Temperature of peripheries (should be warm and well perfused with blood)
- Capillary refill time (should be less than 2 seconds)
- Drainage from wounds/drains
- Urine output and colour.

Cardiovascular management

Cardiovascular stability

It is essential that patients are cardiovascularly stable after surgery. Differences in heart rate and blood pressure, compared with baseline recordings may indicate that the patient is unwell and requires prompt investigation and treatment.

There are different causes of shock but postoperatively, the most common is due to hypovolaemia, which occurs when the circulating blood volume is reduced following excessive blood loss. Clinical features of hypovolaemic shock include tachycardia (pulse rate >100 b.p.m. in adults), tachypnoea, hypotension (systolic blood pressure <100 mmHg) and cold clammy skin. If these features are observed, they should be reported immediately to the nurse in charge.

Prevention of DVT

Preoperative preparation helps to reduce the incidence of DVT (see p. 595). Preventative postoperative measures include:

- Administration of prophylactic anticoagulants, e.g. heparin
- Mechanical DVT prophylaxis, e.g. wearing of anti-embolism stockings (see Fig. 24.7, p. 595), foot impulse devices, intermittent pneumatic compression devices (NICE 2010)
- Maintaining adequate hydration
- Effective pain management to assist mobilization
- Carrying out active or passive leg exercises (see Ch. 18)
- Early mobilization (see Ch. 18).

Not all patients who undergo surgery need these interventions as early mobilization and day surgery reduce the incidence of DVT. Specific guidance for different types of surgery can be found in the NICE (2010) Venous thromboembolism guideline.

The presence of pain, swelling or redness in the lower limbs is reported urgently, as these may be early signs of a DVT. It is important, however, to realize that the majority of DVTs cause no local signs and that some arise in the pelvic veins.

Respiratory management

There are many risk factors which increase patients' chances of developing postoperative respiratory complications, e.g. chronic lung disease, obesity, history of smoking, type of surgery. Recognition of complications and early treatment will improve patients' outcomes.

Preventing chest infections

Patients are encouraged to take deep breaths regularly postoperatively to aid lung expansion and to cough as necessary to expel anaesthetic gases and pooled respiratory tract secretions, which predispose to chest infections. The physiotherapist educates patients preoperatively (see p. 591) about these exercises. Chest physiotherapy and/or early mobilization reduce the incidence of chest infections and the need for antibiotics. In order to breathe deeply and cough, patients need adequate analgesia and support for chest or abdominal wounds. Placing a hand or pillow firmly over the wound will provide the support needed. Signs of chest infection include:

- Pyrexia
- Tachycardia
- Skin that is hot and damp to touch
- A productive cough with expectoration of purulent sputum (see Ch. 17).

A sputum specimen may be required for bacterial culture and testing of sensitivity to an appropriate antibiotic (see Ch. 17).

Fluid, electrolyte and renal management

The fluid and electrolytes the body requires every day are normally absorbed from the GI tract. It is essential that patients are adequately hydrated before, during and after surgery. One study found that many patients, particularly the elderly, are dehydrated preoperatively (National Confidential Enquiry into Patient Outcome and Death, NCEPOD 2010). Patients' fluid requirements can be further increased postoperatively due to fluid loss from wounds, stomas and nasogastric aspiration (Johnson & Monkhouse 2009). The principles of fluid balance in postoperative patients are to correct any pre-existing imbalance, to replace any unusual losses, e.g. wound drainage, and to ensure the body's requirements are met (SIGN 2004).

Fluid balance

All intakes (including i.v. medicines e.g. antibiotics) and outputs (including vomit) are recorded accurately on the fluid balance chart until urine output and oral fluids are re-established. Some patients may be catheterized postoperatively and hourly urine volumes are recorded. Fluid balance is reviewed regularly to ensure that patients are neither in negative balance nor fluid overloaded (see Ch. 19).

Fluid intake

Re-establishing oral fluids following surgical interventions depends on the type of procedure and local policy. Some patients may be able to drink almost immediately, e.g. after spinal or epidural anaesthesia. Those who have had anaesthetic throat spray administered, e.g. prior to upper endoscopic investigations, must remain 'nil by mouth' until the swallowing reflex returns (usually around 2 hours afterwards). When there has been handling of the intestines, the period of fasting is longer due to paralytic ileus (see p. 603).

For patients unable to drink, adequate hydration must be provided and an i.v. infusion may be required, often through an infusion pump. The volume of fluid administered should be individualized, e.g. children and those with cardiovascular problems will receive smaller volumes.

Appropriate volumes of i.v. fluids will ensure an adequate blood supply to the kidneys that maintains renal perfusion and urinary output (see below). This is essential to prevent kidney failure. Intravenous fluids are administered to replace fluid deficits due to:

* Preoperative or postoperative fasting
* Excess loss through a wound or fistula
* Pyrexia (excessively raised temperature) caused by inflammation or sepsis.

It should be noted that the presence of an i.v. infusion can reduce mobility and manual dexterity and so once an adequate oral intake is re-established without complications, the i.v. infusion can be discontinued.

Urine output

Adults, including those who have indwelling urinary catheters, should pass a minimum of 30 mL of urine per hour. Smaller volumes are normal in children (see Ch. 20). Well-hydrated patients should be able to void urine within 6–8 hours following a general anaesthetic. Inability to void postoperatively may be due to:

* The site of operation, especially when within the pelvic region, e.g. hysterectomy
* Spinal or epidural anaesthesia
* Muscle relaxant drugs administered during surgery – these can reduce the ability to void or cause voiding of small, frequent volumes
* Dehydration due to prolonged preoperative fasting, inadequate postoperative fluid intake or excessive loss, e.g. vomiting
* Poor pain control
* Embarrassment, lack of privacy or unusual position required for voiding.

When there is failure to pass urine following surgery or a significant drop in hourly urine output, this is reported to the nurse in charge. If there is difficulty in passing urine and the patient is in pain, analgesia should be administered as this may help them to relax and void. If all of these interventions fail, it may become necessary to insert a catheter to drain the bladder. This is retained until hydration is satisfactory and satisfactory urine volumes are sustained.

Nasogastric aspirate

Some surgical patients, e.g. after bowel surgery, will have a wide bore nasogastric tube *in situ* postoperatively to allow withdrawal (aspiration) of gastric secretions that accumulate when paralytic ileus (see p. 603) is present. The frequency of aspiration depends on the type of surgery and patient discomfort. Aspiration may be either continuous, using a low-pressure suction unit, or intermittent using a suction unit or syringe. The nasogastric tube may be attached to a collecting bag to allow the free passage of gas and drainage of gastric secretions. These may increase with abdominal pressure, e.g. when the patient coughs, breathes deeply or moves around to change position.

The colour and nature of each aspirate is noted and the volume recorded on the fluid balance chart. Sometimes the consistency is also recorded. The disadvantages of a nasogastric tube include:

* Restriction of the nasal passage reducing air entry
* Patient embarrassment and discomfort due to excessive nasal secretions if the tube irritates the mucous membrane lining
* Inability to blow the nose adequately
* Pressure and soreness around the nose or face
* Difficulty coughing.

The nursing care required by a patient with a nasogastric tube is shown in Box 24.10.

 Nursing skills   Box 24.10

~~Care of a patient with a nasogastric tube~~

* The nasogastric tube is firmly attached to the patient's nose using hypoallergenic tape to prevent it from sliding in and out of the nasal passage or becoming dislodged
* The tape is checked frequently to ensure that it remains adherent, as the nose can become moist and greasy, allowing the tape and/or the tube to move
* The nose, nostrils and face are checked for signs of pressure or soreness
* The skin around the nose and mouth is kept dry to prevent excoriation and infection
* Oral hygiene and/or mouthwashes keep the oral mucosa moist and prevent infections such as *Candida albicans* (thrush)
* Patients may be offered ice chips to moisten the oral mucosa if appropriate
* The nasogastric tube is aspirated continuously or intermittently as indicated on the care plan
* The colour, consistency and volumes of aspirate are observed and recorded on the fluid balance chart.

Nutrition

A recent survey found that 1 in 3 adults admitted to hospital are malnourished (British Association for Parenteral and Enteral Nutrition, BAPEN 2011). It is essential that surgical patients receive adequate nutrition as malnutrition causes complications postoperatively including:

- Delayed wound healing and potential infection
- Loss of muscle tone that may adversely affect mobilization
- Skin fragility, slow repair and development of pressure ulcers
- Impaired immune response
- Depression.

Patients who are undergoing minor surgery are usually able to eat normally again within 12 hours. Those who have been fasting for some time, may be reluctant to recommence solid food for fear that their preoperative symptoms will return. Patients may need assistance to select a diet that meets their nutritional needs in the postoperative period (Box 24.11). Meals and snacks should be served appropriately, taking people's medical and cultural needs into consideration (see Ch. 19).

 Reflective practice　　　　　　Box 24.11

Postoperative nutrition

Patients who are malnourished on admission to hospital have a higher risk of postoperative complications which can lead to a prolonged hospital stay (Drover et al 2010). Each nurse has a responsibility to ensure patients' nutritional status is assessed and managed appropriately (NMC 2010).

Student activities

- Consider the nutritional status of a patient that you have cared for before and after surgery
- How were the patient's nutritional needs assessed pre and postoperatively?
- How were the nutritional needs of this patient met before and after the surgery?
- In your opinion was this effective? Identify the possible reasons for your answer.

Sometimes, it will not be possible for patients to eat for several days or even weeks, such as after removal of large parts of the GI tract, and a preoperative referral to the dietitian should be made. Others cannot eat sufficient food to meet their energy requirements and food fortification or nutritional support may be used to prevent malnutrition (see Ch. 19). Factors, such as nausea, vomiting and constipation can affect nutritional status.

Nausea and vomiting

Nausea and vomiting sometimes occur following an anaesthetic or handling of the viscera during abdominal surgery, and also when people are in pain or anxious about the future. Children are twice as likely as adults to experience nausea and vomiting postoperatively (Association of Paediatric Anaesthetists of Great Britain and Ireland 2009). Postoperative nausea and

vomiting may be due to accumulation of gas within the GI tract or from hiccups due to the irritation of the diaphragm.

Postoperative nausea and vomiting can be reduced if patients are administered a prophylactic antiemetic, e.g. domperidone, before or during surgery. For those with ongoing nausea, nursing interventions that may help include:

- Positioning the patient upright, well supported by pillows, to assist drainage and reduce reflux of gastric secretions
- Reviewing analgesia as opioids, e.g. morphine, stimulate the vomiting centre in the brain
- Providing oral hygiene at least 3–4 hourly, or more often if necessary
- Giving ice chips to suck, if indicated on the care plan
- Reviewing the nasogastric drainage regime if present
- Other interventions shown in Box 19.9 (p. 469).

Preventing constipation

Patients may not pass faeces or flatus (gas) for several days postoperatively, especially when there is paralytic ileus or following preoperative bowel cleansing. Paralytic ileus occurs after surgery that involves extensive handling of the bowel when peristalsis (the muscular movements that normally move contents along the intestines) is temporarily lost. Flatus is passed when peristalsis returns. Before then many patients experience discomfort caused by trapped wind.

Opioid drugs predispose to firm stools, known as constipation. Postoperative passing of faeces is recorded in the nursing notes. The faeces may be watery at first as stools may take time to form normally again, even after a normal diet has been re-established. Laxatives (oral or rectal, see Ch. 21) are not normally necessary when patients are well hydrated, eating normally and ambulant again.

Pain management

Chapter 23 provides further information about all aspects of pain management. It is essential to assess patients regularly for pain postoperatively. Effective pain management reduces postoperative anxiety (Hayward 1975) and aids mobility. Benhamou et al (2008) found that pain management in surgical patients was often sub-optimal. Patients expect to encounter some pain following a surgical intervention but only to their degree of tolerance. Pain is not necessarily wound-related and can also be due to dehydration, a full bladder or the after-effects of being on the operating table. Pain may adversely affect postoperative recovery and is assessed and documented using a pain assessment chart (RCN 2009). Children and others who cannot verbalize their pain should be observed for other cues which indicate they are in pain, e.g. changes in behaviour (see Ch. 23).

Drugs used in pain management range from mild analgesics such as ibuprofen for mild pain to opioids, e.g. morphine, for moderate to severe pain. Several routes may also be used, including:

- Oral
- Subcutaneous

- Intravenous, including patient-controlled analgesia (PCA)
- Intramuscular
- Rectal.

PCA devices deliver preset doses of analgesic medication and allow patients to give themselves analgesia by pressing a button on the handset. Explaining how PCA works helps improve the effectiveness of this method of delivering analgesia (NHS QIS 2004). It can be used by people of all ages, provided they have sufficient understanding and the manual dexterity to push the delivery button. Some patients may use non-pharmacological methods of pain relief, such as visual imaging or yoga exercises (see Chs 10, 23), which may reduce the amount of analgesic medication needed. The activities in Box 24.12 will help you find out more about postoperative pain management.

 Critical thinking   Box 24.12

Postoperative pain management

Nurses play an essential role in the pain management of surgical patients (Badensten et al 2011). It is necessary for nurses to have a good understanding of medicines which can help to control patients' pain (NMC 2010).

Student activities

In your placement:

- Identify analgesic drugs used postoperatively and find out about their side-effects.
- Identify the routes used to administer them.
- Identify non-pharmacological methods of postoperative pain relief.
- Speak to a patient about their postoperative pain management.
- Discuss your findings with your mentor.

By anticipating the need for analgesia and speaking to patients about their pain levels well before increased activity is needed, e.g. chest physiotherapy, bed bathing/showering, getting out of bed and mobilizing, nurses can minimize pain experienced during these activities.

Wound management

The incision is usually covered with a dressing postoperatively. The purposes of wound dressings are to absorb exudate, ease pain and provide protection for the new tissue (NICE 2008). There is a large choice of dressings available. NICE (2008) guidance suggests 'an appropriate interactive dressing' should be chosen and this should be changed in accordance with local policy.

Surgical wounds normally heal by primary intention because skin closures, e.g. sutures, staples, glue or clips (see Fig. 24.2), are used to hold and support the skin edges together as healing takes place. The superficial layers close within 24–72 hours as epithelial cells migrate across the wound and initially the wound may appear inflamed, e.g. red and swollen. Wound healing is discussed in detail in Chapter 25.

Wound drainage

Some patients may have a wound drain (Fig. 24.1) to drain fluid away from surgical sites, especially vascular areas. This fluid may be:

- Sanguineous – heavily bloodstained
- Serosanguineous – blood and serum
- Serous – clear
- Purulent – cloudy.

A collection of fluid in a confined space causes pain, acts as a potential source of infection and impairs wound healing (see Ch. 25). The function of the drain is explained, as is the need to avoid pulling on it, especially when moving in bed or walking around.

The volume, consistency and type of drainage, as well as any fresh staining on the wound dressing, are noted and recorded during the initial postoperative assessment so that subsequent loss can be compared against this. Drains are checked for flow and patency if a vacuum system is used (Fig. 24.1). If patency is lost, leakage from the wound may increase. The type of drain and volumes draining dictate the frequency of checking. Drains can be:

- *Vacuum drains:* These draw fluid out from the drain tip, usually adjacent to the operation site, preventing accumulation of fluid and formation of a haematoma (blood clot). Drainage volumes are recorded on the fluid

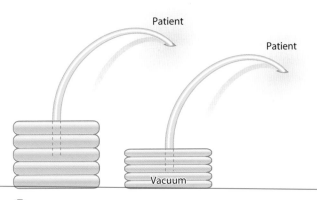

(A) Suction drain

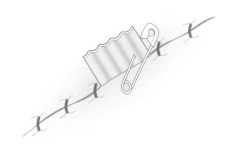

(B) Corrugated drain

Fig. 24.1 • Wound drains. (Reproduced with permission from Brooker, C., Nicol, M. (Eds.), 2003. Nursing adults. The practice of caring. Mosby, Edinburgh.)

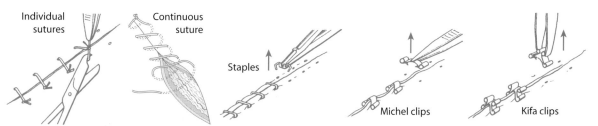

Individual sutures   Continuous suture   Staples   Michel clips   Kifa clips

Fig. 24.2 • Removal of skin closures.

balance chart and the characteristics entered in the nursing notes. Accurate records of the drainage will assist the decision about when to remove the drain. Prior to removal, the vacuum is released to prevent tissue damage and minimize patient discomfort. A small sterile dressing is applied over the drain site to absorb residual drainage and protect the area from infection.

• *Gravity drains:* These allow drainage of fluid into a collection bag, e.g. a corrugated drain (Fig. 24.1B).

Skin closure removal (Fig. 24.2)

Both adults and children may find the removal of skin closures frightening and the procedure is explained to reduce fear and anxiety. Distraction, e.g. talking to the patient while removing skin closures, often greatly reduces their anxiety.

Sutures are usually removed after 5–10 days unless they are absorbable; staples are normally removed after 2–5 days. More specifically, their removal depends on the reason for surgery, its location and the patient's age and general condition. If patients are discharged before skin closures are removed, then arrangements must be made for their removal by a community nurse.

Wound complications

• *Surgical site infection:* Around 5% of surgical patients develop a wound infection (NICE 2008). Early signs include pyrexia and/or pain in or around the wound. An inflamed area may appear red and swollen, and look quite different from a non-inflamed area. If an infection is superficial, sutures may be removed to allow pus to escape. A wound swab or sample of pus is sent for microscopy, culture and sensitivity testing (see Ch. 15)

• *Haematoma:* A small collection will gradually resolve spontaneously but larger collections cause pain, discomfort and predispose to infection. They may be evacuated by aspiration using a needle and syringe, or through a small incision

• *Dehiscence:* This is the splitting open of a wound exposing the underlying tissues that occurs only rarely (see Fig. 25.1). The causes include wound infection, poor nutrition, compromised immunity and increased tension on the wound by, e.g. abdominal distension or excessive coughing. The warning signs may be serosanguineous discharge from a previously dry wound and/or the patient saying that they 'felt something go'.

Regaining mobility

The type of surgery dictates the level of mobility and the timescale over which this can be achieved. Nurses must be aware of a patient's preoperative mobility when planning their postoperative mobility goals. Those having day surgery are mobilized soon after the procedure is completed. Patients who undergo major surgery without complications can usually walk to the bathroom the day after surgery; however, following some types of surgery, e.g. major vascular surgery (femoral popliteal bypass), bed rest for 24–48 hours may be required. Those confined to bed should have the call button nearby to summon assistance when needed.

Preoperatively, patients are given information about exercises that they can practise and implement soon after surgery (see p. 591). Patients are encouraged to carry out these exercises to reduce limb stiffness and aid venous return. When patients are unable to exercise by themselves physiotherapists or nurses carry out passive exercises (see Ch. 18).

Mobility is gradually increased postoperatively (Fig. 24.3). Initially, patients may be helped to sit out of bed in a chair. Walking distances and periods spent out of bed are thereafter increased gradually as the patient's condition allows until independence is regained. In the early stages, patients may experience dizziness (postural hypotension) therefore care should be taken to prevent slips or falls.

Patients who have had orthopaedic surgery may have specific mobilization programmes. The physiotherapist implements the planned activities with the nurse in a supporting role until the patient is confident and can mobilize safely.

Discharge planning

Discharge planning should begin at the pre-assessment clinic or on admission to hospital in emergency situations. Successful discharge planning provides a seamless transition between day or in-patient care and primary healthcare. Care required after discharge should be planned in partnership with the patient and their family or carers, the primary healthcare team and social services (Gibbens 2010). Some patients however feel insufficiently prepared for discharge (Boughton & Halliday 2009; Gilmartin 2007) and so many factors must be taken into account, including:

• Transport home
• Ascertaining who is at home and available to help with aftercare

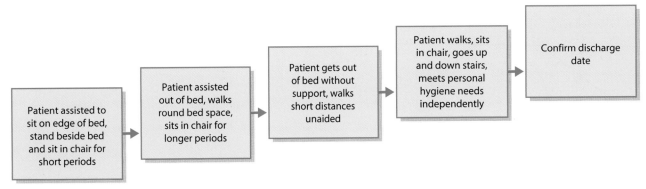

Fig. 24.3 • Steps of mobility.

- Removal of skin closures
- Availability of the patient's medicines, including analgesics, and instructions about taking them
- Date and time of follow-up appointments e.g. surgeon, specialist nurse, physiotherapist
- Specific advice about recovery and likely timescale, e.g. mobility, wound management, pain management, return to work/school, return to driving, resumption of sexual activity
- Support groups, counselling services
- Nutritional advice
- Need for aids or prosthesis
- Phone numbers or e-mail addresses for advice after discharge
- Information about when to seek help, e.g. chest pain, feeling hot
- Information booklets to reinforce verbal information
- Community services, e.g. meals on wheels.

Following surgery, including day surgery, people need at least a short period of convalescence. Planning an admission date helps patients to organize help at home during their convalescence. People with specific needs may have a home assessment arranged. Occupational therapists (OTs) can assess the patient's home environment and postoperative needs. They can then provide advice and supply aids, e.g. raised toilet seats or walking frames to assist following surgery such as hip replacement.

Other members of the MDT, e.g. social workers, may also be involved in discharge planning as some patients will be unable to care for themselves independently following surgery and will require a package of short- or long-term care. Sometimes a period of rehabilitation (see Ch. 11) or convalescence in a care home is arranged until patients can safely return home. Delayed discharge planning prolongs hospital admission until suitable arrangements can be completed and inadequate planning not infrequently results in readmission (Shepperd et al 2010). Hospitals usually have discharge policies that involve partnership working with other agencies such as primary healthcare and social services to provide a seamless return home from hospital.

Discharge planning is important for all patients, but especially following day surgery and for those who require arranged transport home and/or support from community services after discharge.

SUMMARY

- Pre-assessment clinics facilitate preoperative preparation and enable individual needs to be planned for.
- Preoperative anxiety is alleviated by effective communication and provision of information about the surgical experience.
- The aim of preoperative preparation is to ensure patient safety during the intraoperative and postoperative periods.
- Postoperative care aims to promote recovery and minimize postoperative complications.
- Effective discharge planning should start at the pre-assessment clinic and facilitates a seamless transition from home to hospital and home again.

KEY WORDS AND PHRASES FOR LITERATURE SEARCHING

Consent

Discharge planning

Patient communication

Perioperative care

Surgery

Surgical nursing

 Useful websites

Patient information

Patient.co.uk – Tests and investigations www.patient.co.uk/display/16777415

virtualmedicalcentre.com. Investigations http://www.virtualmedicalcentre.com/health-investigation/

Surgery

National Institute of Clinical Excellence – Surgical procedures http://www.nice.org.uk/guidance/index.jsp?action=bytreatment&TREATMENTS=Surgical+procedures#/search/?reload

British Association of Day Surgery www.daysurgeryuk.org/bads/joomla

All websites accessed September 2012.

CHAPTER 24

References

Association of Paediatric Anaesthetists of Great Britain and Ireland, 2009. Guidelines on the prevention of postoperative vomiting in children. Online. Available: www.apagbi.org.uk/sites/default/files/ APA_Guidelines_on_the_Prevention_of_Postoperative_Vomiting_in_Children.pdf September 2012.

Badensten, B., Frojd, C., Swenne, C., et al., 2011. Why pain is still not being assessed adequately? Journal of Clinical Nursing 20 (5–6), 624–634.

Baril, P., Portman, H., 2007. Preoperative fasting: knowledge and perceptions. AORN Journal 86 (4), 609–617.

Benhamou, D., Berti, M., Brodner, G., et al., 2008. Postoperative analgesia observation survey. Pain 136 (1), 134–141.

Boore, J.R.P., 1978. Prescription for recovery. RCN, London.

Boughton, M., Halliday, L., 2009. Home alone: patient and carer uncertainty surrounding discharge with continuing care needs. Contemporary Nurse 33 (1), 30–40.

British Association for Parenteral and Enteral Nutrition, 2011. Nutrition screening survey in the UK and Ireland in 2010. Online. Available: www.bapen.org.uk/pdfs/nsw/ nsw10/nsw10-report.pdf September 2012.

British Association of Day Surgery, 2011. Commissioning day surgery. Online. Available: www.bads.co.uk/bads/joomla/ images/stories/downloads/ CommissioningDaySurgery.pdf September 2012.

Brooker, C., Nicol, M. (Eds.), 2011. Alexander's nursing practice, fourth ed. Elsevier, Churchill Livingstone, Edinburgh.

Department of Health, 2001a. Consent – what you have a right to expect. A guide for children and young people. Department of Health, London.

Department of Health, 2001b. Seeking consent. Working with people with learning disabilities. Department of Health, London.

Department of Health, 2001c. Good practice in consent implementation guide: consent to examination or treatment. Department of Health, London.

Department of Health, 2002. Day Surgery: Operational guide. Department of Health, London.

Drover, J., Cahill, N., Kutsogiannis, J., et al., 2010. Nutrition therapy for the critically ill surgical patient: we need to do better. Journal of Enteral and Parenteral Nutrition 34, 644–652.

Franklin, B., 1974. Patient anxiety on admission to hospital. RCN, London.

Gibbens, C., 2010. Nurse facilitated discharge for children and their families. Paediatric Nursing 22 (1), 14–18.

Gibson, C.E., Magowan, R., 2011. Nursing the patient undergoing surgery. In: Brooker, C., Nicol, M. (Eds.), Alexander's nursing practice, fourth ed. Elsevier/Churchill Livingstone, Edinburgh.

Gilboy, S., Hollywood, E., 2009. Helping to alleviate pain for children having venepuncture. Paediatric Nursing 21 (8), 14–19.

Gilmartin, J., 2007. Contemporary day surgery. Journal of Clinical Nursing 16, 1109–1117.

Hayward, J., 1975. Information: a prescription against pain. RCN, London.

Johnson, R., Monkhouse, S., 2009. Postoperative fluid and electrolyte balance. Journal of Perioperative Practice 19 (9), 291–294.

National Confidential Enquiry into Patient Outcome and Death, 2010. An age old problem. A review of the care received by elderly patients undergoing surgery. Online. Available: www.ncepod.org.uk September 2012.

National Institute for Clinical Excellence, 2003. Preoperative tests: the use of routine preoperative tests for elective surgery. Online. Available: http://www.rcn.org.uk/ __data/assets/pdf_file/0020/109820/ 002778.pdf September 2012.

National Institute for Health and Clinical Excellence, 2007. Acutely ill patients in hospital. Clinical guideline 50. Online. Available: www.nice.org.uk/nicemedia/ live/11810/35950/35950.pdf September 2012.

National Institute for Health and Clinical Excellence, 2008. Surgical site infection. Online. Available: www.nice.org.uk/ nicemedia/live/11743/42378/42378.pdf September 2012.

National Institute for Health and Clinical Excellence, 2010. Venous thromboembolism: reducing the risk. Quick reference guide. Online. Available: www.nice.org.uk/ nicemedia/live/12695/47197/47197.pdf September 2012.

NHS Connecting for Health, 2011. Choose and book. Online. Available: www.chooseandbook.nhs.uk/ September 2012.

NHS Institute for Innovation and Improvement, 2008. Preoperative assessment and planning. Online. Available: www.institute.nhs.uk/ quality_and_service_improvement_tools/ quality_and_service_improvement_tools/ pre-operative_assessment_and_planning.html September 2012.

NHS Quality Improvement Scotland (NHS QIS), 2004. Postoperative pain management. NHS QIS, Edinburgh.

Nursing and Midwifery Council, 2008a. The Code: Standards of conduct, performance and ethics for nurses and midwives. NMC, London.

Nursing and Midwifery Council, 2008b. Consent. Online. Available: http://www.nmc-uk.org/Nurses-and-midwives/Advice-by-topic/A/Advice/ Consent/ October 2012.

Nursing and Midwifery Council, 2010. Essential Skills Clusters. Online. Available: http://standards.nmc-uk.org/Documents/ Annexe3_%20ESCs_16092010.pdf October 2012.

Pritchard, M., 2009. Identifying and assessing anxiety in pre-operative patients. Nursing Standard 23 (51), 35–40.

Royal College of Nursing, 2005. Perioperative fasting for adults and children. Online. Available: www.rcn.org.uk/__data/assets/ pdf_file/0020/109820/002778.pdf September 2011.

Royal College of Nursing, 2009. The recognition and assessment of acute pain in children. RCN, London.

Royal College of Surgeons of England, 2007. Surgery for children. Royal College of Surgeons of England, London.

Scottish Intercollegiate Guidelines Network, 2004. Postoperative management in adults. Guideline No. 77. SIGN, Edinburgh.

Shepperd, S., McClaran, J., Phillips, C. et al., 2010. Discharge planning from hospital to home. Cochrane Database. Online. Available: http://onlinelibrary.wiley.com/ doi/10.1002/14651858.CD000313.pub3/pdf September 2012.

Slater, R., 2011. Optimising patient adjustment to stoma formation. Gastrointestinal nursing 8 (10), 21–25.

Tanner, J., Moncaster, K., Woodings, D., 2007. Preoperative hair removal. Journal of Preoperative Practice 17 (3), 118–132.

Thomsen, T., Villebro, N., Moller, A., 2010. Interventions for preoperative smoking cessation. Cochrane Database. Online. Available: http://onlinelibrary.wiley.com/ doi/10.1002/14651858.CD002294.pub3/pdf September 2012.

Valkenet, K., van de Port, I., Dronkers, J., et al., 2011. The effects of preoperative exercise therapy on postoperative outcome. Clinical Rehabilitation 25, 99–111.

Wilson-Barnett, J., 1979. Stress in hospital: patients' psychological reactions to illness and healthcare. Churchill Livingstone, Edinburgh.

Wong, E., Chan, S., Chair, S., 2010. Effectiveness of an educational intervention on levels of pain, anxiety and self-efficacy for patients with musculoskeletal trauma. Journal of Advanced Nursing 66 (5), 1120–1131.

Further reading

Adam, S., Odell, M., Welch, J., 2009. Rapid assessment of the acutely ill patient. Wiley Blackwell, Chichester.

Greenstein, B., Gould, D., 2009. Trounce's clinical pharmacology for nurses, eighteenth ed. Churchill Livingstone, Edinburgh, E-book.

Jamieson, E.M., McCall, J.M., Whyte, L.A. (Eds.), 2007. Clinical nursing practices, fifth ed. Churchill Livingstone, Edinburgh.

Gibson, C.E., Magowan, R., 2011. Nursing the patient undergoing surgery. In: Brooker, C., Nicol, M. (Eds.), Alexander's nursing practice, fourth ed. Elsevier/Churchill Livingstone, Edinburgh.

Moore, T., Woodrow, P., 2009. High dependency nursing care, second ed. Routledge, Abingdon.

NHS Education for Scotland, 2006. A multi-faith resource for healthcare staff.

NES, Edinburgh. Online. Available: www.nes.scot.nhs.uk/media/3720/march07finalversions.pdf.pdf September 2012.

Nicol, M., Bavin, C., Cronin, P. et al., 2012. Essential nursing skills, fourth ed. Mosby, Edinburgh.

Wound management

Irene Anderson   Jacqui Fletcher

25

LEARNING OUTCOMES

This chapter will help you:

- Describe the various types of wound
- Describe the stages of wound healing
- Identify local and patient-related factors that delay healing
- Describe wound assessment, cleansing and débridement
- Identify treatment objectives when selecting wound dressings
- List the main dressing categories
- Identify risk factors for pressure ulceration
- Outline the prevention of pressure ulcers
- Describe the assessment and management of pressure ulcers
- Outline how venous leg ulceration occurs and the signs of venous insufficiency
- Outline the assessment and management of venous leg ulcers.

Introduction

Tissue viability encompasses a variety of clinical issues/problems. Although primarily related to the management of wounds, the term also includes preventing tissue damage and care of vulnerable skin. Skin can become damaged for many reasons, including trauma such as cuts, as a result of problems such as incontinence or during surgery, or may arise from an underlying disease, e.g. leg ulceration.

Although many aspects of wound care have been tradition-ally deemed a nursing role, good tissue viability care depends upon holistic assessment of the patient/client and involvement of the patient/carer and the relevant members of the multidis-ciplinary team (MDT).

In order to care for patients/clients with the potential for or compromised tissue viability, healthcare professionals must understand the normal structure and role of the skin and changes during the lifespan (see Ch. 16). This knowledge assists in determining deviations from the normal processes and helps to inform appropriate care plans and management.

Tissue viability includes the whole spectrum of patient/client care, including all age groups and all fields of nursing. Specific issues and problems may arise in particular settings, e.g. infants, wounds associated with childbirth (caesarean section, episiotomy and perineal tear), older people with dementia or people with limited mobility, but a broad under-standing of the fundamental principles gives a basis from which any nurse can begin to provide appropriate care.

Types of wound

The many different types of wound are classified in a variety of ways. This may relate to the aetiology (cause), the amount of tissue loss, whether they heal by primary or secondary inten-tion (see p. 611) or the length of time they usually take to heal. There are also many subcategories within the definitions which provide a more accurate description and assessment of the wound.

Wound classification and categories

Most commonly, wounds are described as being either acute or chronic (Table 25.1). Acute wounds are those where healing is straightforward and follows an orderly sequence, whereas chronic wounds are slow to heal with some delay in the healing process. Chronic wounds – pressure ulcers and venous leg ulcers – are covered later in the chapter (see pp. 620–628). This definition of what is acute or chronic is overly simplified and there are many examples where these definitions are inap-propriate. For example, a surgical wound that becomes infected, dehisces (bursts open) and fails to heal for many months does not fit the definition of an acute wound (Fig. 25.1); equally a laceration of the leg in an older woman with underlying venous disease is unlikely to heal in a straightforward way unless the underlying disease is also treated (Box 25.1).

Table 25.1 Common wound types

Type of wound	Acute or chronic	Primary or secondary healing
Surgical wound	Acute	Primary
Donor sites where skin has been removed for a skin graft	Acute	Secondary
Traumatic wound	Acute	Primary or secondary
Burn	Acute	Secondary
Fungating wound which occurs as cancer infiltrates the skin	Chronic	Secondary
Pressure ulcer (see pp. 620–625)	Chronic	Secondary
Leg ulcer (see pp. 624–628)	Chronic	Secondary
Diabetic foot ulcer	Chronic	Secondary

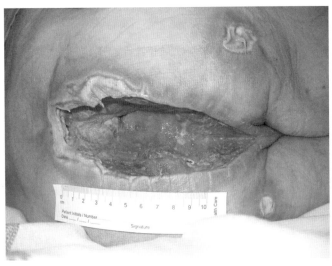

Fig. 25.1 • Wound dehiscence.

Acute wounds

Acute wounds may be categorized by type and cause of the injury. They include:

- *Incised wound* – caused by cutting with a sharp instrument. Examples include a surgical incision or trauma caused by glass
- *Laceration* – a wound where tissues are torn, usually with a blunt instrument or pressure or a tear such as a perineal tear during childbirth
- *Contusion* – caused by high-energy impact, usually with a blunt instrument (may also include bullet wounds). Contusions are usually more severe than lacerations; there is tissue layer separation and considerable tissue loss
- *Abrasion* – caused when the skin is forced against a resistant surface in a rubbing/scraping fashion. The

resulting wound may resemble a burn (abrasions are sometimes known as friction burns). Most commonly they are superficial and expose the nerve endings so they can be extremely painful. An abrasion is frequently contaminated by particles of the surface against which it was abraded, most commonly gravel/grit but often clothing fabric may be embedded in the wound

- *Shearing wounds* – occur when the skin is subjected to a twisting or tearing mechanism, the most severe example being a 'degloving' injury where the skin is peeled back, usually from a hand or foot, exposing the underlying structures
- *Puncture wounds* – such as a bite have a small opening, which penetrates to the underlying tissues, frequently driving microorganisms into the wound
- *Crush injuries* – occur when the tissues are trapped between an external surface and the underlying bone. Considerable internal damage may be present without a visible break in the skin.

Burn wounds are classified according to the depth and surface area of the skin affected (see Ch. 13).

Surgical wound categories (see Ch. 24)

The most common acute wounds result from surgical procedures that are frequently an elective (planned) event. Surgical wounds are further subdivided into categories based on the risk of wound infection occurring. Leaper and Harding (1998) describe four risk categories, which relate to the reason for surgery and the organs involved, as follows:

- *Clean*: Wounds are non-traumatic, i.e. elective surgery using aseptic technique (see Ch. 15) and without any septic focus or internal organ (viscus) being opened, e.g. a skin graft
- *Clean-contaminated*: Non-traumatic wounds, i.e. elective surgery with only a minor breach in aseptic technique or entry into a viscus without significant spillage, e.g. elective cholecystectomy (removal of gallbladder)
- *Contaminated*: Traumatic wounds from a relatively clean source, or with a major breach in aseptic technique or significant spillage from an open viscus, or when acute non-purulent infection (without pus) is encountered, e.g. surgery for appendicitis
- *Dirty*: Traumatic wounds from a dirty source, or following a delayed treatment, or when acute bacterial

contamination or release of pus (dead white cells and bacteria, cell debris and tissue fluid) occurs, e.g. surgery following trauma or where there is passage through the viscera such as following peritonitis (inflammation of the peritoneum).

Wound healing

In order to deliver appropriate care to patients/clients it is vital that nurses understand the processes by which wounds heal. The process involves a sequence of overlapping events or stages. It is important to link the theory to clinical practice so that recognition of the stage of wound healing informs treatment objectives. This is particularly important when documenting assessment findings and clinical decisions. It is logical to understand normal wound healing before considering abnormal and compromised healing.

Some injured tissue heals by regeneration and this can be seen in very superficial wounds affecting only the epidermal layer of the skin because these wounds heal without leaving any visible signs on the skin. Wounds affecting deeper layers of the skin are not able to do this and heal by a process of repair. New connective tissue is formed and healing occurs by fibrosis with scarring.

There are major differences in the healing process within fetal tissue. Wounds heal without scarring during the first 6 months of gestation; thereafter, healing resembles that occurring after birth. Fetal tissue heals by regeneration characterized by little inflammation, fibrosis or scarring.

Wounds can heal by primary or secondary intention. Primary intention healing occurs where there is minimal tissue loss and it is possible to draw the wound edges together with sutures (stitches), clips, staples or glue. Secondary intention healing occurs where there is tissue loss and it is not possible or desirable to draw the wound edges together. Wounds subject to extensive tissue loss usually heal by a process of granulation (formation of new capillaries and the growth of new healthy moist red tissue in the wound bed), contraction and epithelialization (epithelial cells move across the wound once it is filled with granulation tissue to resurface the wound).

Stages of wound healing

Wound healing is often described in four stages. These are:

- Vascular response
- Inflammation/inflammatory response
- Proliferation
- Maturation.

The four stages are considered separately but it is important to remember that the stages overlap, and progress and regress according to the circumstances of the patient's environment, lifestyle and underlying conditions (Fig. 25.2).

Stage 1 – Vascular response (0–3 days)

Stage 1 involves haemostasis and migration of cells that initiate healing. Blood vessels constrict initially and platelets

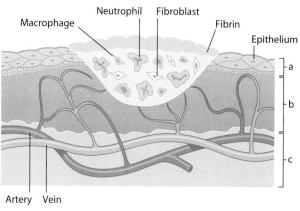

a = epidermis, b = dermis, c = subcutaneous tissue

(A)

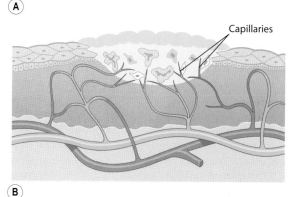

(B)

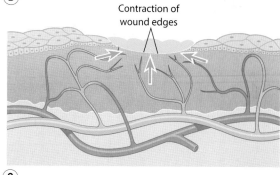

(C)

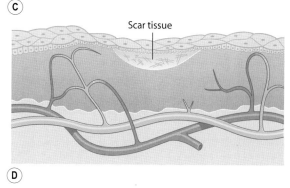

(D)

Fig. 25.2 • Stages of wound healing: (A) Inflammatory. (B) Proliferative. (C) Maturation. (D) Mature (early). (Reproduced with permission from Brooker, C., Nicol, M. (Eds.), 2003. Nursing adults. The practice of caring. Mosby, Edinburgh.)

accumulate at the breach in the vessel and stick together (aggregate), forming a plug to stop the bleeding temporarily. Coagulation factors cause the formation of a fibrin (insoluble substance formed from the soluble protein fibrinogen) clot.

Bleeding ceases as blood cells are trapped in the fibrin mesh to form the clot, which eventually dries to a scab.

Stage 2 – Inflammation/inflammatory response (1–6 days)

Blood vessels dilate due to the release of histamine by mast cells (tissue cells similar to basophils) that migrate to the wound. Gaps open up between the cells in the capillary walls and fluid leaks out into the tissues. The extra fluid and increased blood supply from the dilated capillaries result in redness, heat, swelling and pain, with some loss of function/movement in the area. This response can continue for some days. Therefore, it is important that wound assessment (see p. 614) includes wound history, otherwise these signs may lead to an assumption of wound infection.

The white blood cells (WBCs) neutrophils and monocytes (which become macrophages) are attracted to the area by protein growth factors, which stimulate specific cell division and proliferation. The WBCs move to the site by a process called chemotaxis to defend the body against bacteria and remove debris from the wound. The neutrophils and macrophages do this by engulfing bacteria and debris, a process known as phagocytosis.

WBCs stimulate fibroblasts (immature cells that form connective tissue) and the growth of new blood vessels (angiogenesis) in the wound. Fibroblasts begin to form collagen, a protein that provides the supportive framework in connective tissue. The wound contains fibrin debris known as slough (soft, creamy yellow tissue comprising cellular debris, which rises to the surface of the wound). Once enzymes in the wound fluid liquefy the slough, red granulation tissue is visible in the wound bed. Increased capillary permeability leads to fluid loss, or exudate (fluid containing serum, nutrients such as proteins, proteolytic enzymes and cell debris), from the wound.

An extracellular matrix (ECM) is formed in the wound, which serves as a platform over and through which cells can move and be supported as they act in the wound. The ECM constantly breaks down and reforms during healing and serves as a scaffold for new blood vessels.

Stage 3 – Proliferation (3–20 days)

Growth factors continue to stimulate fibroblasts and the ECM supports the new tissue. Other growth factors encourage angiogenesis and epithelial cell proliferation and migration. The deficit resulting from tissue loss is filled with new blood vessels and granulation tissue. At the same time, fibroblasts change shape, link with other fibroblasts and form a net-like structure. The changes result in fibres of collagen, which give the elasticity needed to retain shape and resist injury. The collagen fibres begin to contract, each cell pulling on others. The wound shrinks in size and now has a covering of new, paler epithelial tissue (epithelialization). The wound is healing by granulation, contraction and epithelialization.

Stage 4 – Maturation (21 days to >1 year)

In normal, healthy people this stage often begins at about 21 days. The wound appears 'healed' because it has a covering of epithelial tissue (new skin). The collagen matures, gains strength and has a more orderly structure, and the new blood vessels mature. Capillary dilatation reduces and the number of fibroblasts decreases. Because healing occurs by repair rather than regeneration, the healed wound leaves the skin looking different. This is scar tissue and, depending on the wound and the individual, takes a variety of forms. Scars are formed from fibrous tissue, which initially appears red and slightly raised, and are itchy. Eventually this will settle to an area commensurate with the original wound dimensions and flattens. Scar tissue takes a long time to mature, possibly up to 2 years, during which tissue is remodelling. Scars have little elasticity and are generally paler than surrounding skin once they have matured.

Factors influencing healing

The prerequisites for normal wound healing include:

- A diet containing sufficient protein, energy, vitamin C, iron, zinc and copper
- An adequate blood supply of oxygen and nutrients, and removal of waste
- The absence of contaminants, e.g. microorganisms, toxins, foreign bodies
- Freedom from wound trauma
- A healthy immune system
- Adequate rest and sleep.

Healing is influenced by a variety of factors and circumstances. Some factors that delay healing are local to the wound, including wound complications, whereas others are systemic or patient-related.

Local wound factors

A variety of local wound factors can impair or delay healing (Box 25.2), as follows:

- Poor surgical technique, e.g. rough handling, can damage tissues and delay healing
- Mechanical disruption caused by:
  - recurring trauma from scratching, deliberate self-harm (DSH) (see pp. 614–615), falls, inappropriate use of adherent dressings or careless dressing removal, all of which may damage delicate granulation tissue

 Critical thinking | Box 25.2

Amina

3-year-old Amina has had surgery and her mother asks why she needs a dressing over the wound.

Student activity
- What reasons do you think the registered nurse will give?

○ lack of protection during the maturation stage – patients/clients should be informed that the wound continues to heal and new tissue needs protection and should be kept moisturized and supple
- Foreign bodies, e.g. gravel, grit, sutures, etc., may set up a prolonged inflammatory response if not removed from the wound
- Toxic agents, e.g. inappropriate antiseptic use, can damage fragile tissue
- Reduced wound temperature caused by cold cleansing solutions or prolonged wound exposure reduces cellular activity
- Presence of excess slough and necrotic tissue (dead tissue caused by lack of oxygen to the local area) inhibits the cell migration required for healing and increases the risk of infection
- Proteolytic enzymes in exudate from chronic wounds can damage intact skin. Although the presence of exudate is vital for cellular activity, there needs to be management of the fluid if the wound and surrounding skin are not to suffer damage (World Union of Wound Healing Societies, WUWHS 2007)
- Local hypoxia (lack of oxygen in the tissues) caused by unrelieved pressure or prolonged oedema (abnormal collection of tissue fluid within the tissues) prevents cells from receiving sufficient oxygen for healing and delays granulation
- Dehydration of the wound bed caused by inappropriate dressings or exposure inhibits cellular activity.

Inappropriate wound management, poor assessment and clinical decision-making, and failure to set treatment objectives can all contribute to delayed and impaired wound healing.

Problems with wound healing may compromise scar formation. The scar, which remains proud of skin level, can be dry, flaky and itchy. In some skin types keloid scarring can occur. This is a hard, raised overgrowth of scar outside the proportions of the original wound, which can cause the person considerable emotional and physical problems.

Wound complications

Wound healing is seriously affected by complications that include:

- *Infection*: Bacteria compete with body cells for oxygen and nutrients. The wound is considered infected when increasing bacterial numbers induce a host reaction (normally heat, redness, pain and swelling) (see Ch. 15). Exudate and pain may increase and wound healing slows
- *Haematoma*: Bleeding and the collection of blood within a wound, which has been closed (by primary intention) or covered with a skin graft. This causes tension in the wound, leading to tissue damage and possibly infection
- *Dehiscence*: Partial or total breakdown of the wound. This can be due to increased tension on the wound edges or, more commonly, to infection (see Fig. 25.1, p. 610).

Systemic or patient-related factors

Many patient-related factors have an impact on healing, e.g. age and nutritional status. Patient-related factors that may affect healing should be considered during the holistic assessment (see pp. 614–618). Factors may impact directly on the healing process, e.g. severe malnutrition, or may impact on the planned objectives of care, e.g. for a patient/client with arterial disease it may not be possible to heal the wound and an alternative objective would be determined or the suggested time to healing modified (see pp. 618–620).

Age

The skin of older people often thins and becomes more vulnerable to damage (Norman 2004). When trauma occurs, healing may be delayed because of slower cell turnover, reduced collagen synthesis and age-related poor circulation (Box 25.3).

⚡ Reflective practice   Box 25.3

Wound healing rates

Think about the people with wounds you have met during placements.

Student activities

- What differences in healing rate did you observe between people of different ages?
- Discuss the observations with your mentor and consider other factors that influenced healing in the group you observed.

A newborn's skin is thin and fragile; 'The epidermis and dermis are loosely bound to each other and very thin …' (Kelsey & McEwing 2010, p 159). Infants and children have a greater body surface area than adults and this coupled with a thinner skin leads to a high rate of water loss through the skin, which has implications for fluid imbalance and a reduction in core temperature. The structure of the dermis continues to mature during infancy and childhood.

Nutritional status

Many individual nutrients (see Ch. 19) are vital in wound healing and a deficiency in any can affect healing. Protein-energy malnutrition (PEM), e.g. results in insufficient resource for the increased needs of a healing wound.

Dehydration

Dehydrated cells (see Ch. 19) are not able to function efficiently and cell replication will be impaired. All cells need a moist environment for survival and movement.

Systemic diseases

Many diseases impair or delay wound healing. These include:

- Clotting disorders, e.g. haemophilia, disrupt clotting and delay the arrest of bleeding
- Vascular, cardiac and respiratory conditions resulting in reduced oxygenation of tissues (see Ch. 17)
- Poor venous return causes congestion and collection of cellular debris within the wound area

- Cancer and its treatment with chemotherapy, e.g. methotrexate, or radiotherapy reduce the body's ability to heal. Chemotherapy, for example, adversely affects the inflammatory response and impedes cell proliferation. In addition, the reduction in WBCs affects immunity and increases the risk of infection
- Diabetes mellitus is associated with arterial disease, which impairs healing. Diabetes also damages peripheral nerves (neuropathy) and people may be unaware of tissue damage
- Impaired mobility and sensation can impact on wound healing. Reduced mobility, such as after a stroke, leads to reduced circulation and the associated problems.

Medication

Several commonly used drugs (see Ch. 22) have a negative impact on wound healing (Box 25.4). These include:

- Cancer chemotherapy, e.g. vincristine (see above)
- Non-steroidal anti-inflammatory drugs (NSAIDs), e.g. ibuprofen, affect the inflammatory response
- Corticosteroids, e.g. prednisolone, reduce the inflammatory and immune responses; reduced levels of immunity increase the risk of infection
- Anticoagulant drugs, e.g. warfarin, or long-term use of aspirin delay platelet aggregation, vasodilatation and attraction of cells. They affect the inflammatory response and healing is delayed.

 Reflective practice — Box 25.4

Drugs that affect wound healing

Think about the drugs commonly prescribed in your placement.

Student activities

- Are people asked if they are taking over-the-counter drugs, e.g. aspirin?
- Find out what people are told about the potential effects of their prescribed medication on healing.

Smoking

The adverse effects of smoking tobacco on wound healing include local hypoxia and altered platelet aggregation, which increase the risk of thrombus (clot) formation.

Stress

Psychological factors affecting patients/clients also influence wound healing. Stress and anxiety result in the production of glucocorticoid hormones, e.g. cortisol (see Ch. 11). Glucocorticoid hormones suppress inflammation and slow wound healing. They may also reduce blood supply. Everything possible should be done to relieve stress and anxiety, including ensuring adequate sleep and rest (see Ch. 10).

Wound management

This part of the chapter outlines wound assessment, cleansing, débridement and dressing products. Good wound management is dependent on a thorough holistic assessment of the patient/client and their wound. This is followed by the setting of appropriate patient/client-centred objectives and the use of evidence-based wound care to encourage healing or, where this is not possible, to manage the symptoms appropriately.

Wound assessment

Assessment of the wound is only one part of holistic assessment and should never be carried out in isolation. A full history is taken to identify any systemic patient-related factors which may influence healing, e.g. malnutrition, and also the causation and timescale of the wound.

Wound assessment is a multifaceted process and, in order to make best use of the information, it should be documented systematically and objectively. A variety of wound assessment charts exist but, whichever chart is selected, it should address all the elements of a holistic assessment outlined below. Re-assessments should be carried out at least weekly but may be more frequent depending on the individual wound characteristics (see Ch. 14).

Wound characteristics

When assessing a wound, several characteristics should be considered, including:

- Cause
- Location
- Condition of the surrounding skin
- Size
- Type of tissue present in the wound
- Exudate – type and amount
- Odour
- Wound pain.

Cause of the wound

The cause may impact on further assessment and care planning. The cause will also help determine the risk of complications. For example, if the knife causing the wound is contaminated with soil, the risk of infection is much higher than if it was a clean knife from a dishwasher. Sometimes, the cause is immediately obvious, but in other cases the cause may only be determined by careful and systematic history taking and in some instances sensitive questioning (see Ch. 9).

Particular consideration should be given to patients/clients whose wounds are self-inflicted, as their need for psychological support may be greater than an immediate need for wound care (Box 25.5). Frequently, an MDT approach to care is required, with involvement of mental health teams, psychologists and social services.

Deliberate self-harm (DSH) is very complex and can be a means of coping with deep psychological distress for some people (often young). There is concern that when self harmers are labelled as suicidal or mentally ill they become stigmatised which increases their vulnerability. A non-judgemental and compassionate approach is vital. Emerson (2010) suggests that

? Critical thinking   Box 25.5

Self-harm emergency care

A friend has told you that her daughter is cutting herself. On occasions, the injury has bled for some time but the girl was too frightened to go to the Emergency Department. Your friend asks you what will happen if they seek help.

Student activity

- Find out what treatment and help would be offered if they attend the Emergency Department.
- Discuss with your mentor why a young person may start to self-harm and which health professionals can provide psychological support.

Resources

National Institute for Health and Clinical Excellence (NICE), 2004. Self harm: short-term treatment and management: http://guidance.nice.org.uk/CG16 September 2012.

National Institute for Health and Clinical Excellence (NICE), 2011. Self harm (longer-term management): http://guidance.nice.org.uk/CG133 September 2012.

many nurses need additional information and training about self-harm.

The MDT is also important in managing patients with other types of wound and their individual input should always be considered. Many traumatic wounds require input from both physiotherapists and occupational therapists to maintain function and mobility; equally these team members help to manage chronic wounds such as venous leg ulcers where increased mobility may accelerate healing.

Location

Initially, wound location is considered in relation to its proximity to vital structures, as life-saving care takes priority. Location may provide clues to the cause of the wound. Buttock wounds tend to be automatically classified as pressure ulcers but this is often incorrect, as pressure ulcers usually (but not exclusively) occur over bony prominences (see pp. 623–624). Wounds appearing on or between the buttocks are more frequently caused by incontinence (see Chs 20, 21).

The position of the wound may also impact on the dressing choice (see pp. 619–620), e.g. keeping a dressing on the sacrum is notoriously difficult because it is subject to shear and friction forces. Equally, if the wound is easily visible, such as on the face or hand, the cosmetic impact of the dressing may be the overriding consideration. When managing wounds over or close to joints, consideration must be given to maintaining mobility and joint function.

Condition of the surrounding skin

The condition of the surrounding skin may indicate the patient's/client's general health or the presence of problems, e.g. eczema. This impacts on dressing choices; for example, if the surrounding skin is very fragile it may not be possible to use adhesive dressings. If there is gross oedema present there may be seepage of fluid onto the skin, which will lead to maceration (damage caused by excess moisture leading to

overhydration and increased susceptibility to trauma) if not adequately managed. Fluid is trapped on the skin surface when the dressing used does not manage the exudate adequately or is not changed frequently enough. Maceration also increases the risk of infection.

Size

The size of the wound is accurately measured and recorded in order to evaluate progress. Sometimes wounds appear to get bigger during healing; this may be because the full extent was previously masked by necrotic tissue or thick slough.

Measurement can be undertaken by using a disposable paper ruler to record the length and width. However, as most wounds are irregular in shape this does not record the overall size.

More frequently, a tracing is taken of the outline of the wound using a transparent overlay (Box 25.6). An overlay may be either a commercial wound tracing sheet (Fig. 25.3) or the clear part of a dressing packet. As the packet contained a sterile dressing the inside should be sterile and therefore safe to put in contact with the wound. This outline may then be traced onto paper and stored in the notes. If commercial tracing sheets are used, the backing film that had contact with the wound is removed and the initial tracing stored in the notes.

✋ Nursing skills   Box 25.6

Measuring wounds
Equipment

- Tracing grid
- Permanent marker pen.

Preparation

Ensure the patient/client understands what is happening and has given consent. If necessary, ensure that appropriate analgesia is administered. Ensure privacy. It may be necessary to clean the wound to remove any surface debris (see pp. 618–619). Mark the grid with head and foot, left and right.

Procedure

- Apply the grid lightly to the surface of the wound
- Ensure the patient is in the same position each time the wound is measured – this should be documented within the care plan
- Trace the outline of the wound, taking care not to apply too much pressure as this may cause pain. Mark on the proportion of different types of tissue present in the wound
- Carefully peel the grid away from the wound
- Remove the backing film that has been in contact with the wound and dispose of in a contaminated waste bag
- Place the tracing safely to one side until the dressing procedure is completed and the patient is comfortable
- Place the dated tracing in the patient's/client's nursing notes and record findings
- Compare the tracing to those done previously, noting any changes in the wound.

A tracing can also be used to record areas of different tissue types, e.g. slough or necrosis (Fig. 25.4 and pp. 616, 619). The change in percentages of these tissues may indicate wound progress as much as a change in overall size.

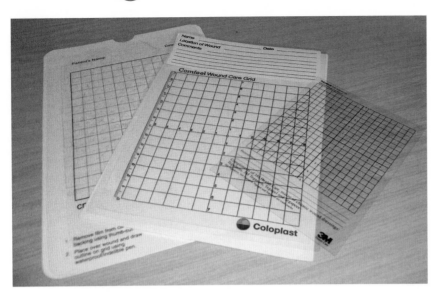

Fig. 25.3 • Wound tracing sheet.

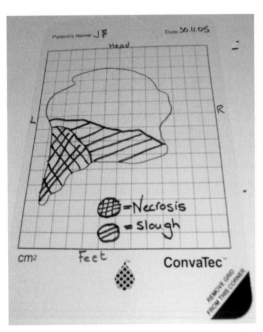

Fig. 25.4 • Wound trace of a sacral pressure ulcer showing different types of tissue.

- *Slough* is usually soft and stringy and may vary in colour from creamy yellow through brownish grey as the wound progresses. Despite removal of thick slough, a thin layer of creamy-coloured slough remains closely adherent to the wound surface, almost until healing is complete; this is not a cause for concern
- *Granulation tissue* contains many new capillaries and is bright red, moist and uneven in texture. Overgranulation occurs where the granulation tissue becomes overexuberant and grows above the surrounding tissue. This type of tissue is friable and may bleed easily. Unhealthy granulation tissue is a dull, deep red; it may be gelatinous and appear to be less well attached to the wound. Although its presence may indicate infection or poor blood supply, it is generally seen as an indicator of poor wound healing
- *Epithelial tissue* is pale pink or silvery white tissue, which denotes wound resurfacing. It develops from the wound margins and also as islands in partial thickness wounds where remnants of hair follicles and sebaceous glands remain.

If tracing materials are not available, a simple line drawing can be made with measurements marked on, as well as the areas of different tissues, e.g. slough, necrosis. Alternatively, a photographic record of wound size and condition can be obtained. If photography is used, written consent must be obtained from the person (see Chs 6, 7) and this must detail what the photograph may be used for, i.e. for use in the records or used for teaching purposes or for publication, when further written consent may be required by the publisher.

Types of tissue present in wounds

In addition to the size of the wound, it is important to record the type of tissue visible in the wound bed. For example:

- *Necrotic tissue* is black and hard or leathery; however, as it softens, it may become grey or brown

Exudate

All wounds produce protein-rich exudate throughout the healing process. Exudate bathes the wound, keeping it moist and supplying the substances needed for healing (see pp. 612, 613). In acute wounds, the level of exudate decreases as healing progresses; however, in chronic wounds exudate may persist or increase.

It is important to monitor the quantity of exudate but in practice this is not easy. Most wound assessment charts use subjective assessment of exudate quantity, e.g. low, moderate or high level, or symbols (+,++,+++). While most experienced nurses would claim to understand the meaning of these descriptions, they are not objective measurements and different nurses may have differing views of what constitutes a particular level. For this reason it is better to use an objective descriptor.

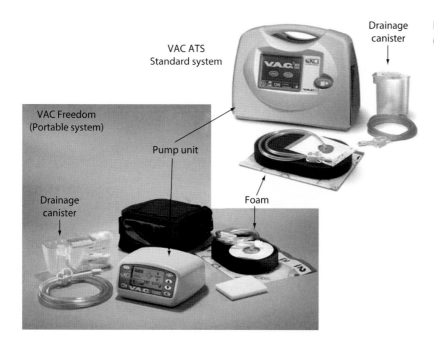

It is not usually possible to record the volume of exudate unless a wound drainage bag or topical negative pressure system is being used (Fig. 25.5). What can be recorded is the frequency with which the dressing becomes saturated and requires changing. For example, if initially the dressing requires changing twice daily and later progresses to once every 2 days, a clear reduction in exudate can be recorded or vice versa. This is dependent upon the same dressing type and size being used for consistency.

When observing for differences in exudate volume it is important to consider what else is happening to the wound. There may be an apparent increase in exudate but this may be due to the presence of other fluids, e.g. that produced by some dressings.

The type, colour and consistency of the exudate should also be recorded. Changes in the exudate are often the first signs of changes occurring within the wound. Exudate may be described as:

- *Serous* – clear, straw-coloured fluid
- *Serosanguineous* – usually clear but with streaks of blood. Becomes pink/pale red in colour as the fluids mix. May be observed prior to wound dehiscence
- *Sanguineous* – bloody fluid
- *Seropurulent* – serous fluid and pus
- *Purulent* – thick, pus-filled fluid of varying colour.

The consistency may vary from watery to thick and almost semi-solid.

Odour

Most wounds produce a typical smell, and odour within the wound is not necessarily abnormal. However, changes or increase in odour may suggest the presence of infection or progress within the wound. The odour normally becomes stronger and less pleasant as necrotic tissue is rehydrated and liquefies. Equally, some dressing products produce a typical odour. Assessment of odour is subjective and is often recorded as +, ++ or +++, but again this does not allow for comparison. One way of objectively describing the odour is to record when it is first detectable. For example:

- Very strong – odour obvious on entering the room with dressing intact
- Strong – odour obvious on entering the room when the dressing is leaking or removed
- Moderate – odour obvious within 2 metres with dressing intact
- Minimal – odour obvious within 2 metres when the dressing is leaking or removed
- Scant – odour obvious when standing next to the patient with dressing intact
- None – no odour obvious even when the dressing is removed.

Wound pain

It is only recently that pain has been widely acknowledged as being a problem in all wound types (see Ch. 23). A consensus document (WUWHS 2004) suggests that nurses:

- Assume that all wounds are painful
- Appreciate that they may become more painful
- Know that the surrounding skin can become sensitive and painful
- Realize that, for some patients, the lightest touch or even moving air over the wound can be intensely painful
- Know when to refer for appropriate specialist advice. The pain team may be helpful.

When assessing wound pain, the type, nature and intensity should be determined. The type of pain relates to what causes the pain: is it constant background pain, related to procedures such as dressing changes, or incident pain related to things such as coughing? This is important, as it influences the type of analgesic required. The patient should be encouraged to describe the nature of the pain; common words include dull or aching (e.g. with venous leg ulcers), burning, itching pain (with skin reactions) or sharp, stabbing pain. Pain should be assessed using an appropriate pain-rating scale (see Ch. 23).

Social factors

Wounds may impact on social aspects of life, and social factors may influence a person's wound and its management. For example, many older adults with leg ulcers become socially isolated, as they stay at home because of pain and embarrassment about the look and/or odour of the ulcer. Other groups have difficulty accessing services for wound care due to social circumstances, e.g. homeless people and people with wounds related to drug misuse where there is considerable stigma associated with the cause.

In children, older adults and other vulnerable groups such as people with a learning disability, the presence of traumatic wounds should alert the nurse to the possibility of non-accidental injury; however, it should be borne in mind that children, for example, frequently injure themselves (see Chs 3, 6).

Most dressing products and care from a tissue viability nurse are increasingly available in both hospital and community settings. However, some products remain non-prescribable in the community.

Environmental factors

The care environment may influence the management and also the risk factors such as infection. In hospital, the patient/client is vulnerable to cross-infection from contact with other patients and exposure to different microorganisms, which are more virulent/pathogenic than typical microorganisms found outside hospital (see Ch. 15). At home, the infection risk differs and there is less risk of cross-infection; however, the home environment is not always ideal. Many people have pet animals and both personal hygiene and general cleanliness vary considerably.

If the person is well and mobile, consideration must be given to where they go and what they do and what impact this will have on their wound. Children need a dressing that will withstand play and school activities. Work environments, e.g. where dressings are likely to become wet or contaminated, are considered in planning wound management. Caring for people with mental health problems presents particular difficulties and many usual nursing interventions cannot be used. For example, it may be judged unsafe to use a compression bandage for a patient with suicidal ideation or if other patients in close proximity are at similar risk.

Organizational factors

Nurses in both community and hospital usually deliver wound care. Care delivery should be at a time that meets the needs of both the patient/client and the need to provide appropriate care. Patients and families should be as fully involved as possible in the care provided. Involvement requires that they receive adequate and appropriate information, at an appropriate level and in a language they understand.

For children and those with ongoing care needs, the family and/or friends are frequently involved in providing wound care; this relies upon the carer being both willing and able to do this. For children, involvement of the family or their own participation in care of the wound can help to reduce pain and relieve anxiety. Family or patient participation in wound care, especially at home, means that the care can be provided at the most appropriate time and is not dependent on a nurse visiting. However, additional support is required to ensure that ongoing wound assessment is maintained and that the family feels fully supported and confident to call for nursing assistance when it is needed.

The need for input from other healthcare workers should be assessed. These include:

* Tissue viability nurse
* Doctor
* Healthcare assistant
* Dietitian
* Physiotherapist
* Occupational therapist
* Podiatrist
* Nurse specialists, e.g. diabetes, infection control, etc.
* Equipment/wound product suppliers
* Patients/clients and their carers, etc.

Input from most of these groups is equally important in caring for patients/clients with any type of wound. Other individuals whose participation may be needed include pharmacists, vascular surgeons and plastic surgeons, as well as domestic staff whose role in maintaining cleanliness is crucial.

Wound cleansing

Cleansing is important to clear loose debris from the wound. Frequently, this must be undertaken to facilitate wound assessment, particularly in acute traumatic wounds where the area may be obscured by blood or debris. However, 'sutured wounds rarely need cleansing unless leakage has occurred' (Fletcher & Anderson 2011, p 641). Wound healing occurs in a warm, moist environment and cleansing may cool the wound. The surrounding skin should always be cleansed to remove dressing material or exudate which has a detrimental effect on the skin. Wound cleansing is achieved by irrigating the wound with lukewarm fluid, either 0.9% sodium chloride solution or tap water to prevent cooling. Aseptic technique is used when there is an invasive component, such as in theatre, but otherwise a clean technique is used (see Ch. 15). The difference between clean and aseptic techniques is debated in the literature and is often poorly defined; however the key principles of rigorous hand cleansing, the use of protective clothing and clean surfaces for laying out dressing materials is essential for the protection of the patient and staff. Kingsley (2008) discusses the analysis of the evidence base and key differences between clean and aseptic techniques relative to wound care.

Many people cleanse their wounds in the shower where they flush the wound with the spray, or in the bath by splashing water on to the wound (Fletcher & Anderson 2011). Soaking is particularly suitable for leg wounds as the limb can be immersed in a bucket or bowl lined with a new plastic liner for each patient/client to reduce the risk of cross-infection.

Cotton wool/fibrous material must not be used to cleanse wounds as debris can become incorporated into the wound bed, causing inflammation. Slough or necrotic tissue may persist in the wound and this should be removed or débrided (see below). Dead tissue may act as a focus for infection, physically impede wound healing and cause, or increase, odour.

Wound débridement

Débridement is the removal of devitalized (dead) tissue which is adherent to the wound bed or the removal of foreign material from the wound. There are various methods that include:

- Surgical débridement in theatre
- Sharp débridement using scalpel and scissors. This is a highly skilled procedure and must only be undertaken by specially trained healthcare professionals who have been assessed as competent
- Chemical débridement using enzymes, e.g. streptokinase/streptodornase, to remove dead tissue. There may be discomfort and the potential for damaging the surrounding skin (Singhal et al 2001)
- Providing a moist wound environment by using appropriate dressings, e.g. hydrocolloids, to enhance natural débridement mechanisms whereby debris is liquefied by enzymes by autolysis. This is slower than sharp or surgical débridement but may be appropriate for some patients/clients
- Larval therapy (maggot therapy) may be used for wound débridement (Box 25.7). It is important the patient's skin is protected during therapy as the larvae produce enzymes that break down slough and necrotic material, and may damage peri-wound skin (Thomas et al 1996)
- Hydrosurgery, ultrasonic means and monofilament cloths.

◉ Reflective practice — Box 25.7

Larval therapy

Patients/clients, carers and nurses often have anxieties about having or using larval therapy.

Student activities

- How would you feel about a suggestion that 'maggots' could be used on your chronic wound?
- Ask the tissue viability nurse about patient preparation for larval therapy and what support is available during the treatment.
- Discuss with your mentor the measures needed to ensure that nurses feel confident in using larval therapy.

Wound dressings

Given the huge variety of wound dressings it is important to know how dressings work so that appropriate choices can be made. No single dressing will be appropriate for all wound types so nurses need know the wound circumstances for which each dressing is designed.

Aims of treatment

Following assessment, it is usual to develop a care plan to meet specific wound objectives. While it is tempting to set the overall aim of 'to heal the wound', this is too long term and lacks guidance for immediate wound management. More detailed objectives for specific wounds would typically include:

- For a *dry black necrotic wound* – débridement and rehydration. Dry, devitalized tissue is softened, liquefied and removed
- For a *yellow sloughy wound* – remove slough. Débridement and cleansing as above. If the wound bed is already wet, the treatment objective is to control fluid and encourage autolysis
- For a *red granulating wound* – protect the wound and maintain moisture balance
- For a *pink epithelializing wound* – protect and maintain moisture balance.

Additional objectives may be required for the prevention or management of infection. Specific objectives related to the wound aetiology should also be set, e.g. pressure reduction in the management of a pressure ulcer. These objectives must be considered together with other aspects of patient care and may have to be modified to meet more pressing objectives, e.g. increasing mobility.

Choosing an appropriate dressing

Essentially, the choice of dressing is determined by assessment findings, the aims of treatment and patient/client preferences. However, three key factors must be considered in dressing selection:

- Amount of exudate
- Condition of the surrounding skin
- Patient/client preference.

An estimation of exudate level (see pp. 616–617) can assist in dressing choice. Selecting a dressing designed for low levels of exudate, e.g. film dressing, may cause maceration and leakage on a wet wound, whereas choosing a dressing designed to cope with high exudate levels may allow drying of a wound with only minimal exudate.

The condition of the surrounding skin helps in determining the dressing type. Adhesive dressings may cause trauma on removal if applied to fragile skin, e.g. infants or older people. Where infection or copious exudate necessitates frequent dressing changes, it would be inappropriate to use adhesive dressings as these are designed to remain in place for a few days. The surrounding skin may be macerated or excoriated due to damage from excess fluid and for this reason the selected dressing should be designed to hold exudate within its structure away from the skin. It is important to read the manufacturer's instructions for use, as some dressings are cut to the shape of the wound and some cover the wound and surrounding skin.

Patient preference is an important consideration when assessing the patient, the wound and selecting dressings (Box 25.8). Before using any product there must be explanation for, and negotiation with, the patient who is to wear the dressing.

It is vital that the manufacturer's instructions for dressing use are read and understood before the final decision is made to apply any dressing. These instructions state at least:

- The structure of the dressing
- The wound types and circumstances for which it is designed
- The circumstances when it should not be used or when particular caution should be exercised.

Types of dressing

Depending on the type, dressings can be applied directly to the wound (primary) or applied over another dressing (secondary); for instance if a waterproof or bacteria proof covering is necessary or extra absorbency is required. Some primary dressings such as hydrogels, alginates and hydrofibre always require a secondary dressing and other dressings which can be primary or secondary such as hydrocolloid, foam and film dressings, would not have a secondary dressing. (Further information about the main dressing categories can be accessed in Fletcher & Anderson 2011, p 642–643; see also Further reading, e.g. British National Formulary 2012).

In addition to the main dressing categories, there are ancillary products used in wound management. These include:

- Tubular gauze – fix and retain dressings, particularly in awkward areas or where the skin is unsuitable for adhesive products
- Tape – there are many products available to suit different skin types and circumstances
- Paste bandages – cotton bandages coated with substances such as zinc oxide used to treat skin conditions.

Chronic wounds

Chronic wounds are those where healing is delayed or interrupted for some reason; most have persistent or recurrent inflammation and tend to have high levels of exudate. Most chronic wounds, including pressure ulcers and leg ulcers, will heal by secondary intention. Management of these wounds depends as much on management of the underlying cause as care of localized wound factors.

Pressure ulcers

Following a collaborative venture between the National Pressure Ulcer Advisory Panel (NPUAP) in the United States and the European Pressure Ulcer Advisory panel (EPUAP), new prevention and treatment guides were launched in 2009. Pressure ulcers are defined in the guides as:

> localized injury to the skin and/or underlying tissue usually over a bony prominence, as a result of pressure, or pressure in combination with shear. A number of contributing or confounding factors are also associated with pressure ulcers; the significance of these factors is yet to be elucidated.

(EPUAP 2009a, p 7)

All category 2 (partial loss of dermis with a red/pink wound bed or an open or intact blister) and above pressure ulcers should be documented as a clinical incident and the circumstances thoroughly investigated (NICE 2005). They occur in all age groups and across all specialities and care settings. They cause patients and carers distress, pain and embarrassment; they increase morbidity and increasingly are recorded as a cause of death (Fig. 25.6). In addition, they are costly, as management requires specialist equipment and dressings. Real costs are difficult to quantify, as costs also arise from the extra time that patients are hospitalized for what is a primarily preventable condition.

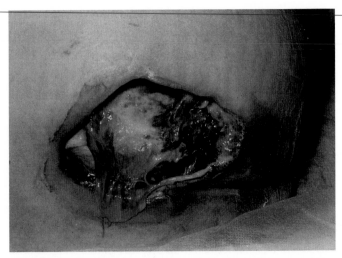

Fig. 25.6 • Pressure ulcer. (Reproduced with permission from Brooker, C., Nicol, M. (Eds.), 2003. Nursing adults. The practice of caring. Mosby, Edinburgh.)

It is becoming increasingly common for pressure ulcers to be investigated as causation is determined. However it must be remembered that not all pressure ulcers are preventable, these are usually termed as 'unavoidable'. Examples include: a patient who is acutely unwell and it is impossible to reposition them; the patient chooses to not have/refuses interventions; or if a patient has fallen at home and is on a hard surface for some time before they are discovered.

Risk factors for pressure ulcers

Several factors increase the risk of pressure ulcer development; these may be extrinsic (external to the patient, related to their environment) and intrinsic (directly about the patient).

Extrinsic factors

The extrinsic risk factors are (Fig. 25.7):

- *Pressure* – the direct application of force to the skin, usually the weight of the patient's body pressing down on a surface such as a bed or chair. The underlying blood vessels are compressed and blood supply to the area is reduced. This results in local tissue damage and, if the pressure is sustained, necrosis occurs
- *Friction* occurs when the skin is moved in a direction opposite to the surface with which it has contact. For example, if the patient/client slides down in bed, their skin drags along the sheet, which can result in removal of the superficial layer of the skin (epidermis)
- *Shear* is an internal force that occurs when the body slides down in bed or a chair. Before friction is overcome and the body moves, the bony skeleton moves inside the skin. Where the underlying blood supply is attached, it becomes stretched and twisted, eventually tearing or cutting off the local blood supply.

The role of moisture is less clear. However, when moisture is trapped against the skin, the skin becomes macerated, thus increasing susceptibility to trauma, e.g. from nurses'/carers' nails, rings, etc. and friction forces.

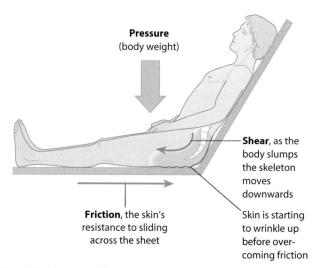

Fig. 25.7 • Relationship between pressure, shear and friction. (Reproduced with permission from Brooker, C., Nicol, M. (Eds.), 2003. Nursing adults. The practice of caring. Mosby, Edinburgh.)

Intrinsic factors

Intrinsic factors are numerous and individual to the patient:

- Increasing age is associated with changes in skin resilience and thinning, which increases susceptibility to trauma. Similar changes occur with some medications, e.g. long-term corticosteroids
- Concurrent disease that reduces blood flow or tissue oxygenation, e.g. arterial disease, chronic respiratory disease or anaemia
- Reduced mobility, such as after a stroke, or related to hospitalization, e.g. during surgery, or altered consciousness, physical disabilities or pain. Immobility may be associated with depression or caused by drugs, particularly night sedation, which reduces spontaneous movements
- Poor nutrition, particularly PEM (see Ch. 19), as nutrients are needed for cell replacement and to fuel activity. Recent weight loss is usually thought to be of greater importance than actual weight (EPUAP 2009b)
- Sensory loss impairs the response to pain normally associated with prolonged pressure. Without pain/discomfort the person is unaware of the need to move, thereby increasing their susceptibility to prolonged pressure
- Incontinence is a risk factor, both because of the effect of moisture on the skin and because urine and faeces may damage the skin, thereby reducing resistance to extrinsic factors
- Build/weight for height. Both extremes – being underweight or overweight – increase the risk of pressure ulceration. Underweight individuals have little subcutaneous tissue to buffer the impact of pressure. Overweight individuals, while they have additional padding over which to distribute the pressure, are sustaining much higher levels of pressure because of their additional weight.

Pressure ulcer risk assessment tools

In order to identify which patients/clients may be at risk of developing a pressure ulcer, a risk assessment tool is used (Table 25.2). Many such tools exist, e.g. Waterlow (see Fig. 14.2 and p. 622), Braden, etc. There are also tools specific to children (Anthony et al 2010).

The tools are based on a list of risk factors, each of which is allocated a numerical score which indicate risk; low, medium or high. In the Braden score, the lower the number, the higher the risk; however, in the majority of tools, the higher the score, the higher the risk of developing a pressure ulcer. Each tool and its risk factors were designed for a particular area of care, e.g. the Walsall tool for use in the community. Therefore the risk factors in each tool vary to take account of the particular issues associated with either a speciality such as intensive care or a particular care setting such as community (Table 25.2).

Although risk assessment tools cannot replace clinical assessment, they do provide a structure for recording the factors which together determine whether the patient/client is 'at risk' or not. Once a level of risk has been identified, appropriate preventative actions are implemented (see pp. 622–623). For example, if sections are scored indicating that

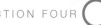
Table 25.2 Risk factors included in different pressure ulcer risk assessment tools

Risk factor	Risk assessment tool						
	Norton (Norton 1989)	Braden (Bergastrom et al 1987)	Waterlow (Waterlow 2005)	Gosnell (Gosnell 1982)	Maelor (Williams & Fonseca 1993)	Walsall (Chaloner & Franks 2000)	Andersen (McClemont et al 1992)
Physical condition	✓				✓	✓	
Mental condition	✓			✓			
Activity	✓	✓		✓	✓		
Mobility	✓	✓	✓	✓	✓	✓	✓
Continence	✓		✓	✓	✓	✓	✓
Nutrition		✓	✓	✓	✓	✓	✓
Build/weight for height			✓				
Skin condition			✓		✓	✓	✓
Age			✓				✓
Sex			✓				
Sensory perception		✓	✓				
Moisture		✓					
Friction and shear		✓					
Consciousness level					✓	✓	✓
Tissue malnutrition			✓				
Major surgery			✓				✓
Medication			✓				
Carer involvement						✓	
Dehydrated							✓
Pain					✓	✓	

the patient has discoloured skin, the care plan should include regular repositioning, skin assessment and skin care. Evaluation of risk should be carried out on a regular basis determined by the patient's overall condition; in acute care this will usually be at least weekly, but may be less frequent in a care home if the resident's condition is stable (Box 25.9). Assessment must be carried out if the patient's condition changes (deterioration/improvement) and on transfer to another care setting.

Pressure ulcer prevention

The prevention of pressure ulceration requires multidisciplinary working. The patient/client should, where necessary, have input from the appropriate health professional. These include:

- Nurses – assessment and evaluation of risk, positioning, holistic care, coordinating the MDT
- Tissue viability nurse – expert advice and education

 Reflective practice Box 25.9

Evaluating pressure ulcer risk

Which pressure ulcer risk assessment tool is used in your placement?

Student activities

- Is this tool appropriate for the patient/client group?
- Is pressure ulcer risk evaluated for all patients/clients on admission?
- Reflect with your mentor how frequently the risk is re-evaluated.

Resource

Department of Health, 2010. Essence of care 2010: Benchmarks for prevention and management of pressure ulcers. Online. Available: www.dh.gov.uk/en/Publicationsandstatistics/Publications/PublicationsPolicyAndGuidance/DH_119969 September 2012.

- Specialist nutrition nurse, dietitian – nutritional needs (see Ch. 19)
- Physiotherapist – improving mobility
- Moving and handling coordinator – expert advice and education about correct techniques (see Ch. 18)
- Occupational therapist – providing aids to independence and increasing mobility
- Specialist continence nurse – expert advice and education (see Chs 20, 21)
- Medical staff, nurse independent prescribers and pharmacists – review medication.

Repositioning

Where equipment is neither available nor suitable, it is still possible to prevent pressure damage by regular manual repositioning (see Ch. 18). Even when using specialist beds and mattresses, the patient should be regularly repositioned as this serves other functions, e.g. preventing sputum retention (see Ch. 17) and providing the patient with a changing view.

The skin should be examined at regular intervals and at every repositioning for the first signs of pressure damage (see below). Repositioning schedules should be tailored to the individual and should take account of when they may need to be in a particular position, e.g. sitting upright at mealtimes. While traditionally patients are repositioned from side to side and on their back, this increases the risk as they are being placed directly onto bony prominences. A more appropriate way of repositioning is to use the 30° tilt, where the patient's weight is supported on areas of large muscle bulk such as the buttocks. If the patient/client can tolerate the prone position it should be considered, as it gives full pressure relief to the back and increases the number of positions available and therefore the body surface area used to distribute pressure.

Pressure-redistributing equipment

This may include any type of equipment that enables the patient/client to maintain their independence, e.g. specialist seating, electric bed frames, etc., but more commonly includes a wide range of pressure area care mattresses and seating. Pressure-redistributing equipment is available to help reduce susceptibility to pressure ulcers and it is important that an appropriate product is chosen to meet individual patient's needs (Box 25.10). Particular problems may arise when supplying equipment for use at home, especially if the patient

---

sleeps in a double bed with their partner. Very few pieces of equipment are designed for this situation, with most mattresses taking up more than half the bed, leaving the carer with insufficient sleeping space; however, some do exist and must be considered. Equally, there are far fewer products for use with infants and children; most mattresses fit a standard hospital bed.

Equipment must be provided for both bed and chair. Pressure ulcer prevention is required throughout the 24 hours, as when seated there is increased risk of pressure damage as the body weight is supported on a much smaller area.

Skin assessment

Skin assessment is essential in preventing pressure damage. Key areas of the body are at greater risk of developing pressure damage because of an underlying bony prominence (Fig. 25.8). These include the:

- Sacrum
- Heels
- Ischial tuberosities (part of pelvis that supports the body when seated)
- Trochanters (at the hip)
- Between the knees
- Elbows
- Head
- Ears.

The most common place for pressure ulcers in the UK is the sacrum (approximately 29%), with the heels as the second most common location (EPUAP 2002). There is, however, some variation, e.g. in people who sit for long periods the ischial tuberosities are the most at-risk area. At-risk areas are different in infants whose head to bodyweight ratio differs from adults, making the head the most vulnerable area. Where pressure damage occurs over non-bony prominences it is usually caused by equipment, e.g. urinary catheter or oxygen mask/tubing (see Chs 17, 20).

Pressure ulcer grading

While it is estimated that 95% of all pressure ulcers are preventable, some people because of their poor general condition will develop one. Where a patient is admitted with existing pressure damage it is vital that this is clearly and comprehensively documented and, where possible, photographed.

The extent of damage is usually described as the depth of tissue damage using a grading/classification system. Several grading tools exist, the most common of which are the Stirling grading tool (Reid & Morison 1994) and the EPUAP grading tool (EPUAP 2009a) (Fig. 25.9).

Although the tools may appear straightforward, training is required to ensure reliability between users in describing the extent of damage. This is particularly so with the lesser degrees of damage where differentiating between blanching and non-blanching erythema (redness) may be difficult, and in people with darker skin. Blanching erythema is a patch of redness that resolves once the pressure is removed. Blanching refers to the test used to differentiate between this and persistent redness. Light finger pressure is applied to the reddened area. Where

---

Critical thinking   Box 25.10

Preventing pressure ulcers

Consider the following scenarios:
- Shami has a learning disability and limited mobility. She uses a wheelchair.
- Mick, who is fully mobile, has dementia. He sits by the TV all day and is reluctant to move around unless reminded.

Student activity
- Discuss with your mentor which pressure-reduction/relieving strategies would be appropriate for Shami and Mick?

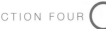

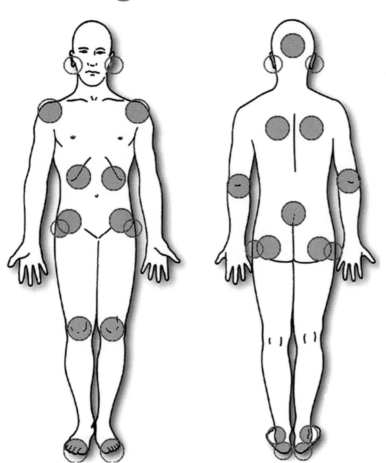

Fig. 25.8 • Areas of the body most at risk from pressure damage. (Reproduced with permission from the European Pressure Ulcer Advisory Panel, www.epuap.org)

the microcirculation is intact the area blanches (whitens). However, if the microcirculation is damaged, the colour does not change. Non-blanching erythema is a prime warning sign of imminent skin breakdown.

Another difficulty arises when the area is covered with necrotic tissue. It is not possible to see the full extent of damage and so the area is classified as probably EPUAP category 4. To assist with these difficulties, the EPUAP has proposed additional criteria for identifying the category of damage and also to exclude damage due primarily to moisture (Defloor et al 2005). As the pressure ulcer heals, it is usual practice to refer to its original grade but designated as healing, e.g. healing category 4.

The grading tools indicate the extent of the damage but provide little information about the appearance of the pressure ulcer and therefore cannot be used alone to set care objectives or to describe the wound. A thorough description should be supported by holistic wound assessment including a photograph (see pp. 614–618). Pressure ulcer management follows the wound care guidelines and dressing selection outlined above (see pp. 618–620) but with the additional objective of relieving pressure (Box 25.11).

Leg ulcers

Leg ulcers are a huge economic burden on NHS budgets. It is estimated that 1–2% of the UK population will experience a leg ulcer at some time, with the higher figure more likely in older people. Some 70% of leg ulcers have a venous aetiology, arterial disease accounts for 8–10%, some have a mixed venous and arterial cause (10–15%), and others are secondary to other diseases (2–5%), (Günnewicht & Dunford 2004). As nurses in the community usually manage venous leg ulcers, the emphasis here is on the principles of managing venous leg ulcers. The management of venous leg ulcers entails increasingly sophisticated care pathways involving the MDT, and improved wound care products and bandaging techniques. Importantly, the impact of leg ulceration on quality of life is well recognized.

Causation of venous leg ulceration

It is important to understand how venous leg ulceration occurs in order to carry out assessment and make safe and effective clinical decisions.

Blood returning to the heart in the leg veins is aided by the pressure changes occurring in the abdomen and thorax during respiration ('respiratory pump') and by muscle contraction in the lower limbs ('calf muscle pump'). The legs contain deep (high pressure) veins and superficial (low pressure) veins connected by perforating veins (Fig. 25.10A). Some blood returns to the heart through superficial veins but most drains from the superficial to the deep veins through the perforating veins and on to the heart. The calf and foot 'pumps' squeeze blood along the veins. The lining of the limb veins is modified to form

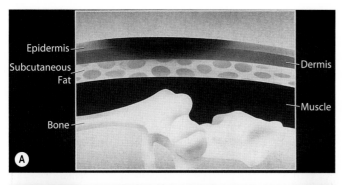

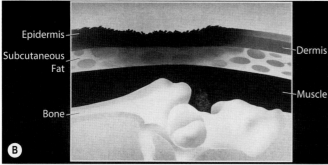

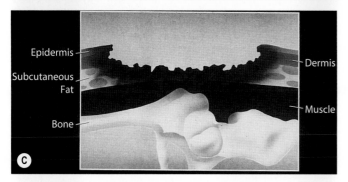

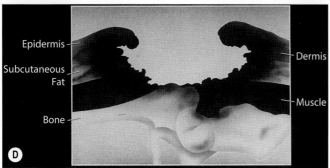

Fig. 25.9 • EPUAP four-grade classification tool: (A) Grade 1: non-blanchable erythema of intact skin. Discoloration of skin, warmth, oedema, and induration (hardness) may also be used as indicators, particularly in people with darker skin. (B) Grade 2: partial-thickness skin loss involving the epidermis or dermis, or both. The ulcer is superficial, which presents as an abrasion or blister. (C) Grade 3: full-thickness skin loss involving damage to, or necrosis of, subcutaneous tissue that may extend down to, but not through, the underlying fascia. (D) Grade 4: extensive destruction, tissue necrosis or damage to muscle, bone or supporting structures with or without full-thickness skin loss. (Reproduced with permission from Huntleigh Healthcare. In America, the NPUAP also recommend the use of two additional categories; Deep Tissue Injury (DTI) and Unstageable. Some clinical areas in Europe are also using these. *Note*: EPUAP (2009a) now use 'category' rather than 'grade' in the classification tool.)

 Evidence-based practice Box 25.11

Management of pressure ulcers

NICE (2005) has evidence-based guidelines which summarize the evidence supporting assessment and holistic management of pressure ulcers.

General findings and recommendations

1. Patients with category (grade) 1 pressure ulcers are at significant risk of developing more severe ulcers and should receive interventions to prevent deterioration.
2. The most benefit for patients with pressure ulcers is likely to be achieved with a multi-interventional interdisciplinary approach which includes:
   - Local wound management using modern or advanced dressings and other technologies
   - Pressure-relieving support surfaces such as beds, mattresses, overlays or cushions
   - Repositioning the person
   - Treatment of concurrent conditions, which may delay healing.
3. All category (grade) 2 and above pressure ulcers should be documented as a clinical incident and the circumstances thoroughly investigated.

Student activities

- How are pressure ulcers recorded in your placement?
- Does your clinical area have a guideline for pressure-relieving equipment selection?
- Do local guidelines include how to identify category (grade) 1 pressure ulceration?

valves which allow flow in one direction only and normally prevent backflow and pooling of blood in the legs.

The valves can be damaged by trauma or surgery, and by deep vein thrombosis (DVT) (see Chs 17, 24). Once the valve is damaged, it malfunctions and backflow occurs (Fig. 25.10B). Backflow between the high and low pressure veins results in increased blood volume in the leg and increased pressure in the thin-walled superficial veins; this is called venous hypertension. Further stretching of the vein and valve occurs, and if backflow continues, signs and symptoms of venous insufficiency and ulceration develop.

Characteristics of venous ulceration

The physical characteristics and symptoms of venous ulceration are outlined in Box 25.12; Figure 25.11 shows a 'typical' venous ulcer. However, it is very important to remember that ulcer appearance can vary significantly and it is impossible to determine ulcer aetiology on appearance alone.

Specific assessment

Assessment and documentation are vital in identifying the factors contributing to the ulcer; knowledge of underlying aetiology leads to safer management decisions.

The physical characteristics outlined in Box 25.12 are associated with venous disease and are important to consider

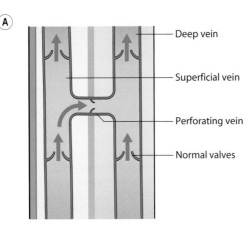 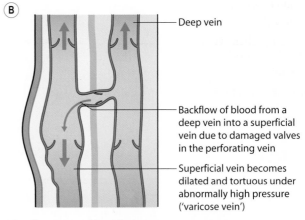

Fig. 25.10 • (A) Deep, superficial and perforating veins of the leg. (B) Valve damage and backflow. (Reproduced with permission from Bale S., Jones V., 1997. Wound care nursing. A patient-centred approach. Baillière Tindall, London.)

Physical characteristics of venous ulceration	Box 25.12

- Usual location – gaiter area of the leg (ankle/lower calf), commonly above the medial malleolus
- Appearance – shallow with ill-defined edges, often quite widespread
- High exudate level
- Oedema – excess fluid in the subcutaneous tissues around the foot and ankle. Caused by increased capillary pressure, stretching and increased permeability of the capillary walls
- Ankle flare – increased capillary pressure resulting from venous hypertension means that capillaries are visible through the skin as red, broken vessels (Morison et al 2007)
- Brown staining of the skin – red blood cells leak from the capillaries and staining results from a pigment (haemosiderin) released when the red cells disintegrate
- Varicose veins occur when the valves fail. There is backflow of blood from the deep veins and high-pressure blood enters the superficial veins, which are stretched and damaged. The vein becomes dilated and tortuous and is visible through the skin. The 'varicose' vein can be felt (palpated) and will often be tender or painful to touch, particularly after standing for a while
- Local skin change:
  - dry, flaky skin due to reduced cell turnover and lack of natural 'moisturization' as congestion reduces the nutrients reaching the cells
  - hypersensitivity and inflammation caused by exudate
  - itching caused by dryness and inflammation; scratching can then lead to breaks in the skin and increased risk of infection
  - skin hardening (lipodermatosclerosis) – the skin loses elasticity, taking on a hard 'woody' appearance and feel. It also leaves tissue very vulnerable to trauma (Morison et al 2007).

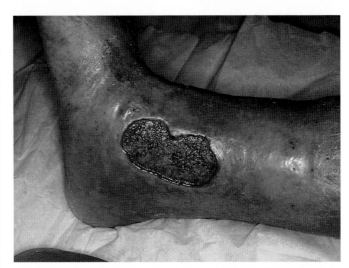

Fig. 25.11 • Venous leg ulcer. (Reproduced with permission from Brooker, C., Nicol, M. (Eds.), 2003. Nursing adults. The practice of caring. Mosby, Edinburgh.)

- History of venous or arterial disease
- Existing medical conditions and medication which may influence wound healing
- Family history of venous disease
- History of current ulcer, any previous ulceration and treatment(s)
- Members of the MDT involved in the care of the patient/client and the outcomes of any investigation or intervention
- Lifestyle factors, e.g. mobility, and activities such as standing for long periods or sleeping in a chair. This provides valuable information about action of the calf muscle pump and the likely pattern of oedema
- Nutritional assessment (see Ch. 19)
- Health beliefs – repeated episodes of leg ulceration are often associated with reduced quality of life. Understanding the patient's/client's perception of their ulcer is vital for partnership working. Involvement of the patient/client as a partner in care (concordance) is much

during assessment. Their presence indicates risk of ulceration through trauma, however trivial.

The assessment of a person with a leg ulcer must take account of factors influencing healing and general wound assessment, including description, wound measurement and photography, etc. (see pp. 614–618). In addition, specific factors include:

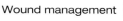

more likely where there are agreed goals and treatment strategies (Edwards 2003).

Once comprehensive knowledge is available, decisions can be made about further investigations that may be required. These include:

- Urinalysis to exclude undiagnosed diabetes and protein loss in the urine, etc.
- Blood tests – full blood count (FBC) used to detect anaemia or infection; a raised erythrocyte sedimentation rate (ESR) may indicate inflammation or infection and blood glucose testing will confirm diabetes
- Skin tests for hypersensitivity or allergy.

A vascular assessment including the use of Doppler ultrasound to assess the arterial blood supply to the lower limb is undertaken by an experienced nurse who has had specialist training to help determine the type of ulcer involved.

Doppler ultrasound is used to determine the arterial blood flow to the lower limb. The blood pressure (BP) is measured in the arms and compared to the BP at the ankles. The comparison between the arm and the ankle pressures gives a ratio, or index – the ankle brachial pressure index (ABPI):

$$\frac{\text{Ankle systolic BP}}{\text{Brachial systolic BP}} = \text{ABPI}$$

Management of venous leg ulcers

The aim of management is, where possible, to restore valve function in the veins to allow ulcer healing. It is also to protect the skin from further damage and manage venous hypertension. This will include:

- Holistic assessment and determination of ulcer type (see above)
- Measures to reduce the effects of high superficial venous pressure
- Improving venous return to the heart by encouraging ankle movement/calf muscle contraction
- Ensuring concordance with treatment by partnership between nurse and patient/client (Box 25.13)
- Preventing complications.

Compression therapy

Compression therapy is essential for uncomplicated venous ulcers. This can be applied by bandaging or compression hosiery (hosiery then needs to be continued once the ulcer is healed). A qualified nurse who has received additional training applies compression bandaging.

The veins are compressed to prevent/reduce backflow, thus reducing venous congestion in the leg and pressure in the superficial veins. Compression also enhances the action of the calf muscle pump, which squeezes the deep leg veins. The effects of this will be less oedema and increased comfort for the patient/client. Improvement in the circulation should allow the ulcer to heal and skin condition to improve. The precise pressures required to achieve these effects are unknown. Currently in the UK, there is an approximate value of 40 mmHg; however, this will vary according to the circumference of the

limb and the material used. The consensus is that some compression is better than none and it is what the patient/client will tolerate, the consistency in application and the wearing of compression bandaging/hosiery that really help healing. National leg ulcer guidelines should be followed to ensure evidence-based care for people with venous leg ulcers (See Further reading, below, e.g. Royal College of Nursing, RCN 2006; Scottish Intercollegiate Guidelines Network, SIGN 2010). Compression therapy includes:

- *Elastic systems*: These bandages apply pressure to the leg constantly and as the calf muscle changes shape the bandage resists this change to enhance the effect of the calf muscle pump. Elastic systems include long stretch, high compression bandages and multilayer systems ('4-layer')
- *Inelastic systems*: Short stretch bandages that form a rigid tube around the leg, applying low pressure when the leg is still. As the calf muscle changes shape it 'bounces' off the bandage, which redirects the force into the calf muscle. This system has a low resting pressure and a high working pressure. Some patients may find this more comfortable, particularly at night
- *Compression hosiery*: This is used after an ulcer is healed to treat venous hypertension and to reduce the risk of recurrence (Box 25.14). Sometimes it is possible to use hosiery for active ulceration if bulky dressings, which make application difficult, are not being used. Hosiery is available as below- or above-knee stockings and tights, but only stockings are provided on prescription in the UK. Hosiery must be properly fitted after careful measurement for the correct size. Measuring aids are available from hosiery manufacturers.

Hosiery items are classified by the pressure they deliver: Class I (14–17 mmHg), Class II (18–24 mmHg) and Class III (25–35 mmHg) (Morison et al 2007). Class III can be difficult to apply even for relatively young and able people. It can be helpful to apply two stockings of a lower class one on top of the other to reach the desired pressure to make application easier. There are aids available to help with application.

Health promotion   Box 25.14

Reducing recurrence of venous leg ulcers

Compression hosiery

- Wear hosiery as instructed
- Avoid damaging the skin when applying/removing hosiery
- Replace hosiery every 6 months.

Skin care (see Ch. 16)

- Wash legs in warm water
- Apply emollients after washing
- Pay special attention to toenails and foot care
- Visit the podiatrist as necessary.

Exercise

- Walk as much as possible and avoid standing
- Exercise toes/ankles several times an hour, even when resting
- Avoid sitting with legs crossed.

Elevation

- Position legs at heart level, e.g. lying on the bed with feet on a pillow.

Student activity

Access the article by Brooks et al (2004) and consider how the findings could be used to improve concordance with one of the aspects listed above.

Resource

Brooks, J., Ersser, S.J., Lloyd, A., et al., 2004. Nurse-led education sets out to improve patient concordance and prevent recurrence of leg ulcers. Journal of Wound Care 13 (3), 111–116.

SUMMARY

- While nurses have a pivotal role in the support and management of people with wounds, appropriate holistic care and management depend upon interdisciplinary working.
- Effective evidence-based care requires an understanding of wound type and aetiology.
- Knowledge of the physiology of wound healing underpins wound assessment.
- Management of the underlying condition, e.g. pressure relief, compression therapy, surgery and good nutrition are key aspects of wound management.

KEY WORDS AND PHRASES FOR LITERATURE SEARCHING

Dressing(s)

Healing

Leg ulcer

Pressure ulcer/sore

Tissue viability

Wound(s)

 Useful websites

European Pressure Ulcer Advisory Panel (EPUAP) www.epuap.org
European Wound Management Association www.ewma.org
Leg Ulcer Forum www.legulcerforum.org
Surgical Materials Testing Laboratory www.smtl.co.uk
Wounds International www.woundsinternational.com
All websites accessed September 2012.

References

Anthony, D., Willock, J., Baharestani, M., 2010. A comparison of Braden Q, Garvin and Glamorgan risk assessment scales in paediatrics. Journal of Tissue Viability 19, 98–105.

Bergastrom, N., Braden, B.J., Laguzza, A., et al., 1987. The Braden scale for predicting pressure sore risk. Nursing Research 36 (4), 205–210.

Chaloner, D.M., Franks, P.J., 2000. Validity of the Walsall community pressure sore risk calculator. British Journal of Community Nursing 5 (6), 266–276.

Defloor, T., Schoonhoven, L., Fletcher, J., et al., 2005. Statement of the European Pressure Ulcer Advisory Panel. Pressure ulcer classification: differentiating between pressure ulcers and moisture lesions. Journal of Wound, Ostomy and Continence Nursing 32 (5), 302–306.

Edwards, L.M., 2003. Why patients do not comply with compression bandaging. British Journal of Nursing 12 (11), S5–S16.

Emerson, A., 2010. A brief insight into how nurses perceive patients who self harm. British Journal of Nursing 19 (13), 840–843.

European Pressure Ulcer Advisory Panel, 2002. Summary report on the prevalence of pressure ulcers. EPUAP Review 4 (2). Online. Available: www.epuap.org/review4_2/index.html September 2012.

European Pressure Ulcer Advisory Panel and National Pressure Ulcer Advisory Panel, 2009a. Prevention and treatment of pressure ulcers: quick reference guide. National Pressure Ulcer Advisory Panel, Washington, DC.

European Pressure Ulcer Advisory Panel and National Pressure Ulcer Advisory Panel, 2009b. Pressure Ulcer Treatment. Online. Available: www.epuap.org/guidelines/Final_Quick_Treatment.pdf September 2012.

Fletcher, J., Anderson, I., 2011. Tissue viability and managing chronic wounds. In: Brooker, C., Nicol, M. (Eds.), Alexander's nursing practice, fourth ed. Churchill Livingstone, Edinburgh.

Gosnell, D., 1982. Pressure sore risk assessment: a critique. The Gosnell scale, Part 1. Decubitus 2 (3), 32–38.

Günnewicht, B., Dunford, C., 2004. Fundamental aspects of tissue viability nursing. Quay Books, London.

Kelsey, J., McEwing, G., 2010. Physical growth and development in children. In: Glasper, A., Richardson, J. (Eds.), A textbook of children's and young people's nursing, second edn. Churchill Livingstone, Edinburgh.

Kingsley, A., 2008. Aseptic technique: A review of the literature. Wound Essentials 3, 134–141.

Leaper, D.J., Harding, K.G. (Eds.), 1998. Wounds: biology and management. Oxford University Press, Oxford.

McClemont, E., Woodcock, N., Oliver, S., et al., 1992. The Lincoln experience – Part 1. Journal of Tissue Viability 2 (4), 114–118.

Morison, M.J., Moffatt, C.J., Franks, P.J., 2007. Leg ulcers: A problem based learning approach. Mosby, Edinburgh.

National Institute for Health and Clinical Excellence, 2005. Pressure ulcers: the management of pressure ulcers in primary and secondary care. Online. Available: http://guidance.nice.org.uk/CG29/Guidance September 2012.

Norman, D., 2004. The effects of age-related skin changes on wound healing rates. Journal of Wound Care 13 (5), 199–204.

Norton, D., 1989. Calculating the risk. Reflections on the Norton scale. Decubitus 2 (3), 24–31.

Reid, J., Morison, M., 1994. Towards a consensus: classification of pressure sores. Journal of Wound Care 3 (3), 157–160.

Singhal, A., Reis, E.D., Kerstein, M.D., 2001. Options for non-surgical débridement of necrotic wounds. Advances in Skin and Wound Care 14, 96–103.

Thomas, S., Jones, M., Shutler, S., et al., 1996. Using larvae in modern wound management. Journal of Wound Care 5 (2), 60–69.

Waterlow, J., 2005. Pressure ulcer prevention manual. Waterlow, Taunton.

Williams, C., Fonseca, J., 1993. Evaluation of the Medley Score. Part 1: the study plan. In: Proceedings of the 3rd European Conference on Advances in Wound Management, Harrogate, 19–22 October.

World Union of Wound Healing Societies, 2004. Principles of best practice: minimising pain at wound dressing – related procedures. MEP, London.

World Union of Wound Healing Societies, 2007. Principles of best practice: Wound exudate and the role of dressings. A consensus document. MEP Ltd, London. Online. Available: www.wuwhs.org/datas/2_1/4/consensus_exudate_ENG_FINAL.pdf September 2012.

Further reading

Anderson, I., 2006. Débridement methods in wound care. Nursing Standard 20 (24), 65–72.

Bale, S., Jones, V., 2006. Wound care nursing. A patient-centred approach, second ed. Mosby, Edinburgh.

British National Formulary, 2012. Appendix 5 Wound management products and elasticated garments. Online. Available: http://bnf.org/bnf/ September 2012.

Elliott, J., 2010. Strategies to improve the prevention of pressure ulcers. Nursing Older People 22 (9), 31–36.

Royal College of Nursing, 2006. The Nursing management of patients with venous leg ulcers. Recommendations. Online. Available: www.rcn.org.uk/development/practice/clinicalguidelines/venous_leg_ulcers September 2012.

Scottish Intercollegiate Guidelines Network, 2010. Management of chronic venous leg ulcers. Guideline 120. Online. Available: www.sign.ac.uk/guidelines/fulltext/120/index.html September 2012.

Glossary

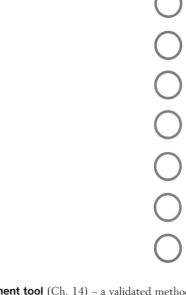

Accountability (Chs 2, 6, 7) – responsibility for something or to someone that applies when someone is answerable for what they do.

Active exercises (Ch. 18) – movements initiated by an individual that exercise their muscles and joints.

Acute pain (Ch. 23) – pain of brief duration commonly associated with tissue injury (nociceptive pain) which subsides as healing takes place.

Acute wound (Ch. 25) – one that heals in an uncomplicated way; usually a surgical incision or uncomplicated trauma.

Adaptation (Ch. 11) – alterations or adjustments in physiology, cognition and behaviour in response to changes in the environment. Adaptation implies that these changes improve the individual's condition in relation to the changed situation.

Adherence (Ch. 22) – an agreement between a patient/client and the healthcare professional that is negotiated in relation to the use of prescribed medication. *See* Concordance.

Adjuvant (Chs 12, 23) – additional treatment such as a drug that acts synergistically to increase the action of other drugs or therapy. Especially used to describe the use of drugs such as corticosteroids and antidepressant therapies in the management of pain.

Adverse drug reaction (ADR) (Ch. 22) – any unwanted effects of drugs.

Affect (Ch. 8) – overt emotional tone.

Allopathic (Ch. 10) – practice of conventional medicine.

Alternative medicine (Ch. 10) – any medical system based on a theory of disease or method of treatment other than the conventional/orthodox science of western medicine, e.g. complementary medicine.

Anaesthesia (Ch. 24) – loss of feeling or sensation.

Analgesics (Ch. 23) – drugs used to relieve pain.

Anuria (Ch. 20) – the absence of urinary output.

Apnoea (Chs 14, 17) – the absence of breathing.

Arousal (Ch. 11) – a state of heightened activity that includes cognitive, affective, physiological and behavioural changes.

Arrhythmia (Chs 14, 17) – an abnormal heart rhythm.

Aseptic technique (Chs 15, 25) – procedures that exclude pathogenic microorganisms from a particular environment, i.e. the use of sterile equipment and non-touch technique.

Asperger syndrome (Ch. 4) – a form of autism.

Assessment tool (Ch. 14) – a validated method of eliciting specific information that can minimize risk to individuals and augment holistic assessment.

Audit (Ch. 3) – the systematic, critical analysis of the quality of care including the procedures used for diagnosis and treatment; the use of resources and the resulting outcome and quality of life for the patient. When these are carried out against clinical standards it is referred to as clinical audit.

Auscultation (Ch. 14) – listening to sounds within the body using a stethoscope.

Autism (Ch. 4) – a lifelong condition that impinges on how an individual communicates and relates to others.

Autonomy (Chs 2, 7) – the ethical principle that individuals should make their own decisions about their lives.

Bacteriuria (Ch. 20) – bacteria in the urine. Bacteriuria can be symptomatic or asymptomatic.

Beneficence (Ch. 7) – the ethical principle that individuals should do good to others.

Bereavement (Ch. 12) – the loss of somebody or something of value, especially through death.

Bibliographic database (Ch. 5) – an electronic and searchable collection of information about articles within a specific subject area.

Biological body clock (Ch. 10) – an inherent timing mechanism that controls physiological processes and is not dependent on external factors.

Biopsy (Ch. 24) – tissue removed for laboratory examination.

Biorhythm (Ch. 10) – the cyclical patterns of biological functions unique to each individual, e.g. sleep–wake cycles.

Blood pressure (Chs 14, 17) – the force of blood against the arterial walls which varies during the cardiac cycle. Two pressures are measured: systolic, which represents the greatest pressure in the main arteries following contraction of the left ventricle, and diastolic, which is the lowest pressure in the main arteries and occurs at the end of ventricular relaxation while the heart is at rest, before the next cardiac contraction.

Body language (Ch. 9) – that part of communication which is not reliant on words.

Bradycardia (Chs 14, 17) – a heart rate slower than that expected for age. Less than 60 beats per minute (b.p.m.) in an adult at rest.

Breathing (Ch. 17) – the mechanical process by which air moves in and out of the lung.

Burnout (Ch. 11) – a state caused by work stress in which a person feels unmotivated, tired, less able to cope and low in mood.

Cachexia (Ch. 12) – emaciation resulting from rapid weight loss, often seen in patients with gastrointestinal or lung cancers as a result of complex metabolic changes.

Cardiac arrest (Ch. 17) – the total cessation of effective output of blood from heart function.

Catheterization (urinary) (Ch. 20) – insertion of a hollow tube into the bladder for the purpose of draining urine or instillation of medication into the bladder; catheterization can be urethral (via the urethra) or suprapubic (via the abdominal wall).

Chemotherapy (Ch. 12) – a term generally describing the use of anti-cancer (cytotoxic) drugs to destroy cancer cells.

Chronic pain (Ch. 23) – has a longer duration than acute pain – 3 months or more; it is further subdivided into malignant and non-malignant pain.

Chronic wound (Ch. 25) – one that has delayed healing for a variety of reasons, most commonly pressure ulcers, leg ulcers and diabetic foot ulcers.

Circadian rhythm (Ch. 10) – biological pattern based on a cycle approximately 24 hours in length.

Civil law (Ch. 6) – deals with the conduct and conflicts between people. A person (the claimant) who has suffered a perceived wrong can seek redress by bringing an action or claim in the civil courts. The claim may be settled with an award of financial compensation or damages, an order (injunction) banning an unlawful act or an order that requires some action.

Clinical governance (Ch. 3) – the system whereby NHS organizations are accountable for continuously improving the quality of services and safeguarding high standards of care by creating an environment in which clinical excellence will flourish.

Clinical nurse specialist (CNS) (Ch. 2) – a registered nurse who has acquired additional knowledge, skills and experience, who practises at an advanced level and who may have sole responsibility for a particular care episode or patient/client group.

Code of Conduct (Ch. 7) – the written expectations that The Nursing and Midwifery Council (NMC) has of registered nurses and midwives.

Colloid solution (Ch. 19) – a solution that contains particles (solutes) that stay in the bloodstream because they are too large to pass through the capillary membrane (e.g. gelatin solutions). Used intravenously to increase blood volume.

Colonization (Ch. 15) – a state where pathogenic microorganisms reside on or in the body without causing any disease symptoms.

Commensal (Ch. 15) – a microorganism that lives in close association with its host (*see* Normal flora). Commensals may become pathogenic if the host is immunocompromised.

Communication (Ch. 9) – the exchange of information between at least two people.

Competent (Ch. 2) – possessing the skills and abilities required for legal, safe and effective professional practice without direct supervision.

Complementary therapy (Ch. 10) – the use of skills and practice alongside conventional treatments to enhance patient welfare.

Compliance (Ch. 22) – the extent to which a patient/client uses their medication in relation to their prescription.

Compression therapy (Ch. 25) – the application of graduated pressure to the lower limb to reverse venous hypertension. Usually applied using compression bandages or hosiery.

Concordance (Ch. 22) *see* Adherence.

Confidentiality (Chs 6, 7) – information given on the understanding that it will not be divulged without the consent of the person who is giving the information, except under specified circumstances.

Consequentialist ethics (Ch. 7) – a theory in which the ethical focus is on the consequences of actions or inactions.

Constipation (Ch. 21) – an alteration in normal bowel movements, resulting in the less frequent and uncomfortable passage of hard stools.

Criminal law (Ch. 6) – deals with criminal offences relating to people and property and results in a prosecution, and, if the defendant is convicted, usually results in punishment (conditional discharge, fine, community penalty or a custodial sentence).

Crystalloid solution (Ch. 19) – a clear solution that moves between the bloodstream and the tissue fluid, e.g. 0.9% sodium chloride. Used intravenously to maintain hydration and electrolyte balance.

Culture (Ch. 8) – the way in which a society or group lives their lives together.

Cyanosis (Ch. 17) – bluish hue to the colour of the skin and mucous membranes.

Débridement (Ch. 25) – removal of devitalized (dead) tissue that is adherent to the wound bed or the removal of foreign material embedded in the wound.

Dehiscence (Ch. 25) – breakdown and bursting open of a wound, usually due to wound infection.

Dehydration (Ch. 19) – the loss of water and usually with varying degrees of electrolyte imbalance. It occurs when fluid intake fails to replace fluid loss.

Delusions (Ch. 8) – false beliefs, obstinate against reasoning and contrary evidence (e.g. persecutory thoughts).

Demography (Ch. 1) – the study of populations, e.g. the age, gender and size of subgroups and their vital statistics.

Deontological ethics (Ch. 7) – a theory in which the ethical focus is upon duties.

Diarrhoea (Ch. 21) – a loose, watery stool that occurs frequently.

Discharge planning (Ch. 14) – based on needs assessment, this aims to prevent readmission and provide seamless care to patients/clients and their families.

Disinfection (Ch. 15) – a process that reduces the number of viable microorganisms.

Dislocation (Ch. 18) – displacement of a body part, usually a bone, that affects joint movement.

Distress (Ch. 11) – bad stress (opposite of Eustress), which occurs when there is excessive adaptive demand. Health may suffer in response to this type of stress.

Diurnal rhythm (Ch. 10) – biological pattern based on a daily cycle; also called circadian rhythm.

Duty of care (Ch. 6) – the professional obligation and responsibility that nurses have to a patient/client, while caring for that patient or client.

Dyslexia (Ch. 4) – involves a variety of abilities or problems that affect several aspects of learning, including reading, spelling, writing and numbers.

Dysphagia (Ch. 19) – difficulty in swallowing.

Dyspnoea (Ch. 17) – difficult or laboured breathing.

Dysuria (Ch. 20) – usually taken to mean pain on passing urine, but can also mean difficulty and/or pain in passing urine.

Early Warning Score (EWS) (Ch. 14) – Early Warning Score (EWS) charts are assessment tools commonly used to monitor patient's vital signs in order to identify deterioration in condition.

Elective surgery (Ch. 24) – planned surgical treatment.

Electrolyte (Ch. 19) – any substance, such as sodium chloride, which when dissolved in water dissociates into electrically charged particles called ions and will conduct electricity.

Emollient (Ch. 16) – an oil-based substance applied to soften dry skin that acts by reducing water loss through the skin surface.

Empathy (Ch. 9) – the ability of a person to put him/herself in the other person's position and attempting to understand the world as they see it.

Encopresis (Ch. 21) – the repeated involuntary or voluntary faecal soiling of clothing by a child over 4 years of age.

End-of-life care (Ch. 12) – also known as terminal care, this is care given at the very end-of-life, e.g. last few hours, days or weeks.

Endoscopy (Ch. 24) – visualization of hollow structures and organs using an endoscope, e.g. the stomach (gastroscopy).

Enema (Ch. 21) – fluid introduced into the rectum or lower bowel to produce a bowel movement. Medication enemas for retention can also be given.

Enteral (Ch. 19) – within the gastrointestinal tract, such as enteral nutrition given orally or through a nasogastric, gastrostomy or jejunostomy tube.

Epidemiology (Ch. 1) – the study of the occurrence, patterns and spread of disease in the population.

Epithelialization (Ch. 25) – epithelial cells move across the wound, once it is filled with granulation tissue, to resurface the wound.

Ethics (Ch. 7) – a formal identification of values, attitudes, beliefs and behaviours that a society or culture considers necessary for its moral functioning.

Ethnography (Ch. 5) – originated within the field of anthropology and involves the research becoming 'immersed' within a culture in order to explain or explore particular phenomena. Data collection usually, but not exclusively, involves the use of observation, diaries and interviews.

Eustress (Ch. 11) – good stress (opposite of distress) and focuses on the optimal level of stress needed to promote growth and health. Eustress is often seen in action when stressful events enhance performance and feelings of pleasure or achievement.

Evidence-based practice (Ch. 5) – to base practice on the best available evidence in order to ensure the best quality care is delivered to patients and/or populations.

Exudate (Ch. 25) – fluid produced from the wound.

Faecal incontinence (Ch. 21) – the leaking of faecal matter or fluid from the bowel.

Family (Ch. 8) – a group of related individuals who live in close proximity and share resources.

First Aid (Ch. 13) – the initial treatment given in an emergency situation, with the aim of saving life, before the arrival of an appropriately qualified healthcare professional.

Flatus (Ch. 21) – an accumulation of gas in the bowel causing discomfort due to stretching of the bowel wall.

Flexibility (Ch. 18) – range of normal movements available at a joint.

Fomite (Ch. 15) – any non-living object that can spread infection.

Fracture (Ch. 18) – break in the continuity of bone.

Free-text term (Ch. 5) – words that describe an idea. These may include alternative spellings (including Americanisms), plurals, synonyms and abbreviations.

Frequency (Ch. 20) – the need to pass urine more often than is acceptable to the person. It can be a symptom of urinary tract infection.

Gate control theory (Ch. 23) – proposes that active processing occurs at the dorsal horn of the spinal cord, where the pain sensation first enters the central nervous system (CNS). The dorsal horn gate is opened or closed depending on the combination of sensory ascending inputs from the periphery or descending signals from the brain. Thus, pain will only be appreciated if the gate is open.

Glasgow Coma Scale (GCS) (Ch. 16) – a scale used to assess level of consciousness.

Granulation (Ch. 25) – the formation of new capillaries and the growth of new, healthy, moist, red tissue in the wound bed.

Grief (Ch. 12) – describes the emotional reaction to loss or death.

Grounded theory (Ch. 5) – originated in the late 1960s through the work of Barney Glaser & Anselm Strauss, who explored dying using a methodology that allowed the 'theory to emerge' from the data. 'An inductive qualitative research approach popular amongst sociologists and nurse researchers. Grounded theory provides a framework for collecting, coding and analysing data in order to develop concepts and hypotheses from the data by means of theoretical sampling of participants and settings to guide ongoing data collection. The ultimate goal of grounded theory is theory development' (Smith 1997, p 295.). Key data collection tools include interviews and observations.

Haematuria (Ch. 20) – blood in the urine.

Hallucinations (Ch. 8) – clear perceptions in the absence of relevant stimuli (e.g. imaginary 'voices').

Harm reduction (Ch. 13) – any intervention that reduces the likelihood of injury or impairment occurring to an individual.

Hazards of immobility (Ch. 18) – predictable problems that arise when mobility is restricted, e.g. pressure ulcers.

Health determinant (Ch. 1) – a factor that influences or determines health, e.g. poverty.

Health education (Ch. 1) – communication activity aimed at enhancing positive health and preventing or diminishing ill-health.

Health promotion (Ch. 1) – the process of enabling people to increase control over, and to improve, their health.

Healthcare (Ch. 3) – the systems and the professionals who help maintain, attain and regain good health and prevent illness.

Healthcare-associated infection (HCAI) (Ch. 15) – 'any infection that occurs as a result of the patient/client's care or treatment by healthcare staff, or an infection affecting healthcare staff in the course of their work' (Brooker 2010, p 343).

Hierarchy of evidence (Ch. 5) – a ranked structure of different types of evidence based on the ability of such evidence to predict effectiveness, remove bias and control confounders.

Holistic (Ch. 10) – a doctrine that considers the treatment of any subject as a whole integrated system, e.g. in treatment of disease, the complete person – physically and psychologically – is considered.

Holistic assessment (Ch. 14) – a comprehensive collection of information from primary and secondary sources to assist in decision-making for planning appropriate and individualized care.

Hospice (Ch. 12) – a place where people with palliative care needs may receive specialist care and attention.

Hospital-acquired infection (HAI) (Ch. 15) – 'one which occurs in a patient who has been in hospital for at least 72 h and did not have any signs or symptoms of such infection on admission...' (Brooker 2010, p 359).

Humanism (Ch. 2) – a system of beliefs concerned with the interests, achievements, capabilities, values and worth of human beings.

Hypertension (Chs 14, 17) – blood pressure that is greater than that expected for age.

Hypervolaemia (Ch. 17) – a high circulating blood volume.

Hypodermoclysis (Ch. 19) – the administration of fluids by subcutaneous infusion.

Hypotension (Chs 14, 17) – low blood pressure that is insufficient to maintain tissue blood flow and oxygenation.

Hypothermia (Ch. 14) – core body temperature below 35.0°C

Hypovolaemia (Ch. 17) – a low circulating blood volume.

Hypoxaemia (Ch. 17) – reduced oxygen in arterial blood.

Hypoxia (Ch. 17) – reduced oxygen level in the tissues.

Immobility (Ch. 18) – lack of movement in any muscle or group of muscles, caused by congenital disorders, trauma or disease. The loss of movement may be temporary or permanent.

Incontinence (Ch. 20) – involuntary or inappropriate passing of urine that has an impact on social functioning or hygiene.

Indexing term (Ch. 5) – a word assigned by a database producer to describe the content of an article. These words are arranged in a hierarchy from broad subject area to detailed specialism.

Infestation (Ch. 16) – invasion by a parasite that lives on a host, e.g. head lice.

Informed consent (Ch. 6) – information giving that is sensitive and informative over a period of time wherein the person may agree or disagree in making an informed decision.

Integrated care pathways (ICP) (Chs 2, 5, 12 and 14) – the multidisciplinary outline of anticipated care, placed in an appropriate timeframe, to help patients/clients with a specific condition, or set of symptoms, move progressively through a clinical experience to a positive outcome.

Integrated medicine (Ch. 10) – combining or adding parts to make a unified whole, e.g. the combination of conventional and complementary therapies.

Intermediate care (Ch. 3) – care given after traditional primary care and self-care, but before or instead of care that is available inside acute hospitals, such as preadmission assessment units, early and supported discharge schemes, community hospitals.

Interpersonal skills (Ch. 9) – the skills and capabilities to engage people in communication acts.

Interprofessional learning (IPL) (Ch. 4) – occasions when two or more different professionals learn with, from and about each other to improve collaboration and quality of care (CAIPE, 2011).

Interprofessional working (Ch. 3) – a group of professionals working together to plan care for specific patients/clients and may include social care workers, healthcare workers and voluntary or private healthcare workers.

Intertrigo (Ch. 16) – irritation that develops between two moist skin surfaces, e.g. under the breasts, between the buttocks.

Jet lag (Ch. 10) – fatigue and interruption of the sleep–wake cycle caused by disturbance of normal body biorhythms as a result of travelling across different time zones.

Justice (Ch. 7) – the ethical principle that individuals have rights, e.g. dignity, privacy, and that others have a duty to comply with these rights.

Language (Ch. 9) – the agreed sounds, symbols and expressions used to express information, ideas and feelings.

Lanugo (Ch. 8) – the soft, downy hair sometimes present on newborns, especially when they are pre-term. Usually replaced prior to birth with vellus hair. The development of lanugo on the back, cheeks and forearms may be a feature of anorexia nervosa.

Laxative (Ch. 21) – a medication used to stimulate or increase the frequency of bowel movements, or to aid formation of a softer, bulkier stool.

Learning (Ch. 4) – specific knowledge, skills and/or attitudes that someone has accomplished after participating in some form of instruction.

Learning outcomes (Ch. 4) – specific measurable results that are expected after participating in a learning experience. Outcomes may involve knowledge (cognitive), skills (behavioural) or attitudes (affective) that provide evidence that learning has occurred at the end of a specific learning experience.

Learning strategy (Ch. 4) – the way in which a person approaches a learning task.

Learning style (Ch. 4) – this reflects a person's typical way of thinking, remembering or problem-solving.

Learning theories (Ch. 4) – proposed explanations of how people learn.

Leg ulcer (Ch. 25) – wound of the lower leg related to a variety of underlying aetiologies (causes).

Listening (Ch. 9) – the visual, auditory and sometimes tactile process of perceiving language.

Literature review (Ch. 5) – the process of finding and appraising information, usually from a range of sources.

Maceration (Ch. 16) – softening of the skin caused by continual exposure to moisture.

Malnutrition (Ch. 19) – a disorder caused by dietary intake that is defective in either quantity or content, malabsorption or an inability to utilize nutrients.

Melaena (Ch. 21) – black tarry faeces, indicating the presence of partly digested blood from the upper gastrointestinal tract. It can also be due to disease such as cancer in the small intestine or upper colon.

Melatonin (Ch. 10) – hormone secreted by the pineal gland, considered to have a role in controlling daily biorhythms.

Milestone (Ch. 8) – competency usually attained at a given age, e.g. walking by 18 months of age.

Morals (Ch. 7) – behaviours considered to be ethically appropriate by a society or culture.

Morbidity (Ch. 1) – ill-health or disease.

Mortality (Ch. 1) – death, death rates and specialized mortality rates are explained in Chapter 1.

Motivation (Chs 4, 8) – what drives an individual and is closely related to their needs, emotions, beliefs, values and goals. The underlying causes of actions.

Moving and handling (Chs 13, 18) – the application of force to push, pull, lift, carry or support an inanimate object, or to support, roll, slide or move a person.

Multiagency team (Ch. 3) – practitioners from a range of different backgrounds or professions who work together with patients/clients to achieve results that could not be achieved by any one agency alone.

Multidisciplinary teams (MDTs) (Ch. 3) – groups of different healthcare professionals working together to plan and deliver care for patients/clients and may include nurses, doctors, physiotherapists, occupational therapists and social workers.

Nausea (Ch. 19) – a feeling of sickness that may be accompanied by sweating, pallor and excess amounts of watery saliva.

Necrosis (Ch. 25) – dead tissue caused by a lack of oxygen supply to the local area.

Negligence (Ch. 6) – an act with any element of carelessness or lack of regard resulting in injury, harm or loss. Any act or omission that falls short of a standard to be expected from 'the reasonable man.'

Neurological (Ch. 16) – of the nervous system.

Neuropathic pain (Ch. 23) – the experience of pain in the absence of any identifiable tissue damage due to abnormal processing of sensory input by the nervous system. Associated with chronic non-malignant pain.

Nociceptive pain (Ch. 23) – pain associated with tissue damage, which subsides as healing takes place.

Nocturia (Ch. 20) – waking up and needing to pass urine at night.

Non-maleficence (Ch. 7) – the ethical principle that individuals should not harm others.

Normal flora (Ch. 15) – microorganisms that colonize a host without causing disease.

Normalization (Ch. 8) – the process of becoming able to adopt the lifestyle usually expected of a member of society.

Nosocomial infection (Ch. 15) – *see* Healthcare-associated infection (HCAI); Hospital-acquired infection (HAI).

Nurse consultant (Ch. 2) – an expert practitioner who works with a specific group of patients or clients, influencing the quality of care through expert practice, professional leadership and consultancy, education, research and service development.

Nurse specialist (Ch. 12) – a nurse who works as part of a large multidisciplinary team, giving specialist advice, education and support to specific patients/clients and their carers, e.g. palliative care patients and carers, or patients/clients with a specific condition such as lung cancer or heart failure.

Nursing model (Ch. 14) – a framework to guide nurses, which is used with the nursing process to provide a unique perspective of nursing knowledge and practice.

Nursing process (Ch. 14) – a cyclical, problem-solving approach to providing nursing care that is based on the stages of assessment, planning, implementation and evaluation. Sometimes nursing diagnosis is made between assessment and planning.

Nutrition (Ch. 19) – the process of receiving and utilizing the materials needed for survival, growth and tissue repair. Alternatively, the science of food and its use by the body.

Oedema (Ch. 19) – an abnormal collection of tissue fluid within the tissues such as around the ankles and lower legs.

Oliguria (Ch. 20) – reduced urine output; includes very dilute/isotonic urine with a volume of less than 0.5 mL/kg per hour.

Opportunistic infection (Ch. 15) – caused by a microorganism that does not ordinarily cause disease but can become pathogenic under certain circumstances.

Orthopnoea (Ch. 17) – difficulty breathing when lying down.

Oxygen saturation (Ch. 17) – percentage of oxygenated haemoglobin present in the blood.

Pain modulation (Ch. 23) – inhibition of nociceptive impulses.

Pain threshold (Ch. 23) – the least or minimum experience of pain that an individual is able to recognize.

Pain tolerance (Ch. 23) – the intensity or duration of pain, and the maximum amount of pain that an individual is willing or capable of enduring.

Palliative care (Ch. 12) 'palliative care improves the quality of life of patients and families who face life-threatening illness, by providing pain and symptom relief, spiritual and psychosocial support from diagnosis to the end of life and bereavement' (WHO 2004).

Parenteral (Ch. 19) – outside or apart from the gastrointestinal (alimentary) tract such as parenteral nutrition given intravenously.

Passive exercises (Ch. 18) – movements of joints initiated by an external force, e.g. a physiotherapist, nurse or machinery to exercise muscles and joints.

Patient allocation (Ch. 2) – a system of workload allocation that enables nurses to be responsible for specific patients/clients rather than a series of tasks.

Peak expiratory flow rate (PEFR) (Ch. 17) – the greatest rate of airflow out of the lungs measured during a forced expiration.

Perioperative care (Ch. 24) – that given from arrival in the anaesthetic room, during a surgical intervention or operation and in the recovery area afterwards.

Person-centredness (Ch. 2) – respecting of the rights of each individual to make rational decisions and to determine their own ends, enabling them to reach their own decisions.

Pharmacology (Ch. 22) – the study of chemical substances, e.g. drugs, medications and other substances, that interact with the body.

Phenomenology (Ch. 5) – has its roots in philosophy and is a methodology, which explores the lived experience of the individual. It draws on a range of philosophers such as Hans George Gadamer, Martin Heidegger and Edmund Husserl, and has developed into a methodology which allows the researcher to explore in depth for meaning about experience. Key data collections tools include unstructured interviews.

Plaque (Ch. 16) – a sticky film of bacteria that continuously forms on the teeth and is removed by brushing.

Polypharmacy (Ch. 22) – the simultaneous prescribing of four or more different medicines, which increases the risk of adverse drug reactions and readmissions after hospital discharge, and reduces compliance.

Polyuria (Ch. 20) – excretion of large volumes of dilute urine.

Positive regard (Ch. 9) – the ability to hold and convey feelings for other people that are not based on negative beliefs about the person.

Postoperative care (Ch. 24) – that given following surgery.

Preoperative care (Ch. 24) – that given before surgery.

Pressure ulcer (Ch. 25) – a wound caused as a direct result of pressure, friction, shear or any combination of these.

Primary care (Ch. 3) – care provided in the community by GPs, the practice team and associated health professionals.

Primary intention healing (Ch. 25) – occurs where there is little tissue loss and it is possible to draw the wound edges together.

Primary nursing (Ch. 2) – a system of workload allocation, whereby patients/clients are allocated to the care of an individual registered nurse rather than a team of nurses. The focus is on individual, holistic care, where the participation of patients/clients and relatives is encouraged.

Professionalism (Ch. 2) – to guarantee and provide a consistently high standard of knowledge, skill and competence agreed between individuals, the professional body and society.

Prophylactic (Ch. 24) – an agent or treatment that can prevent or reduce the incidence of a disease.

Prosthesis (Chs 16, 24) – an artificial part that replaces a missing or dysfunctional body part, e.g. an artificial eye.

Proteinuria (Ch. 20) – the presence of protein in the urine.

Psychology (Ch. 8) – the study of mental processes and behaviour.

Public health (Ch. 1) – the science and art of preventing disease, prolonging life and promoting health through the organized efforts of society.

Pulse (Ch. 14) – rhythmic expansion and relaxation of an artery caused by ejection of blood from the left ventricle during systole.

Pyrexia (Ch. 14) – elevation of core body temperature above 37.5°C

Pyuria (Ch. 20) – the presence of white blood cells (WBCs) in the urine, indicating an inflammatory response of the urothelium (bladder lining) to bacterial invasion.

Qualitative research (Ch. 5) – an approach to research that explores experience, perceptions and subjective phenomena.

Quality assurance (Ch. 3) – planned system to provide service to an agreed standard within established resources and timescales.

Quantitative research (Ch. 5) – an approach to research that attempts to measure phenomena using objective, validated measures.

Radiotherapy (Ch. 12) – the use of high energy X-rays to destroy cancer cells, but which causes as little harm as possible to normal cells. May be used as curative or palliative treatment.

Reflection (Ch. 4) – a deliberate process of examining one's own and other people's behaviours, practices and effectiveness which leads to professional growth and greater understanding of oneself and others.

Relationships (Ch. 9) – the bond between people that maintains an effective connection.

Resident flora (Ch. 15) *see* Normal flora.

Respect for persons (Ch. 7) – the ethical principle that all individuals should be accorded respect, i.e. regard and consideration.

Rest (Ch. 10) – relaxation from exertion or labour, relief from worry or something troublesome.

Retention (Ch. 20) – inability to pass urine; can be caused by urethral obstruction or the inability to contract the bladder.

Risk assessment (Ch. 13) – the first stage of risk management that helps to identify the hazards to people's health.

Risk management (Ch. 13) – the whole process of identifying potential hazards and putting systems in place to decrease the likelihood of harm occurring.

Roles (Ch. 8) – behaviour expected of people in their varying social capacities.

Search strategy (Ch. 5) – the terms used to search a bibliographic database for a particular subject area.

Secondary care (Ch. 3) – hospital-based healthcare services: in-patient, out-patient and emergency care.

Secondary intention healing (Ch. 25) – occurs where there is loss of tissue and it is not possible or desirable to draw the wound edges together. The wound fills from the base with granulation tissue.

Self-awareness (Ch. 9) – exploration of thoughts, feelings and behaviours, including an understanding of how internal and external events influence people and how they behave.

Shift work (Ch. 10) – system of employment where an individual's normal hours of work are in part outside the period accepted as the normal working day, i.e. '9 to 5'.

Skin flora (Chs 15, 16) – the community of microorganisms that colonizes the skin.

Sleep (Ch. 10) – an altered state of consciousness occurring naturally in humans in a 24-hour biological rhythm.

Sleep disorder (Ch. 10) – change in normal sleep pattern or rhythm.

Slough (Ch. 25) – creamy yellow soft tissue comprising cellular debris, which rises to the surface of the wound.

Social care (Ch. 3) – a wide range of services provided by local authorities and the independent sector. Social care includes care at home for older people and for people with disabilities, care in day centres, residential or nursing homes as well as fostering services.

Social services (Ch. 3) – personal social services include social care and social work carried out through local authority social services departments and other statutory, private and voluntary agencies.

Socialization (Ch. 8) – the process by which a culture is transmitted from one generation to another, ensuring its continuity, e.g. the survival of its language, knowledge and way of life.

Sociology (Ch. 8) – the study of societies, their component groups and individual interactions.

Sprain (Ch. 18) – damage to the supporting ligaments surrounding a joint.

Sputum (Ch. 17) – mucus and other material coughed up (expectorated) from the lower respiratory tract.

Standard precautions (Chs 13, 15) – set of practice guidelines for infection control and precautions used to prevent contact with body fluids, secretions, non-intact skin and mucous membranes.

Statutory bodies (Ch. 1) – agencies duty-bound by law to undertake health work on behalf of government.

Sterilization (Ch. 15) – a process that renders an item sterile by eliminating all living microorganisms including bacterial spores.

Stoma (Ch. 21) – an artificial opening where the bowel is brought to the surface of the abdominal wall, e.g. a colostomy.

Stool (Ch. 21) – faeces which is passed from the anus.

Strain (Ch. 18) – overexertion of a muscle.

Stress (Ch. 11) – a reactive state to demands or potential demands made on the adaptive capacities of the mind and body.

Stressor (Ch. 11) – a physical or psychological event that produces stress (positive or negative).

Suppository (Ch. 21) – medication in a solid base that melts at body temperature. Inserted into the rectum to either produce a bowel movement or deliver medication, e.g. analgesics.

Symptom management (Ch. 12) – management of any physical, psychological or social occurrence or event that causes notable concern to a patient.

Tachycardia (Chs 14, 17) – a heart rate at rest that is greater than that expected for age. In an adult this is in excess of 100 beats per minute (b.p.m.).

Task allocation (Ch. 2) – also known as functional nursing, this is a mechanistic approach to the delivery of nursing care, where completing tasks and maintaining the ward routine takes precedence over the needs of individual patients/clients.

Team nursing (Ch. 2) – a group of registered and untrained nurses working together to provide individual care to a specific group of patients.

Terminal care (Ch. 12) *see* End-of-life care.

Tertiary care (Ch. 3) – hospital care for a patient with an unusual condition, or needing highly specialized treatments in a specialist centre such as a teaching hospital or regional centre.

Tissue viability (Ch. 25) – prevention of tissue damage and maintenance of tissue in a healthy state.

Transient flora (Ch. 15) – microorganisms that are present on a host for a short time without causing disease.

Trespass against the person (Ch. 6) – any interference with the person's bodily integrity and liberty, it includes assault and battery.

Values (Chs 1, 9) – those concepts that a person holds dear and are deeply important to them.

Vernix caseosa (Ch. 8) – fatty material, which covers and protects the skin of the fetus from maceration caused by fluid and friction. It is formed from 18 weeks of pregnancy, but increases during the last trimester.

Vicarious liability (Ch. 6) – describes an employer's liability for the wrongful acts and omissions of an employee during the course of their employment.

Violence and aggression (Ch. 13) – includes verbal and physical abuse towards an individual.

Virtue ethics (Ch. 7) – a theory in which the focus is upon promotion of intellectual and moral qualities that may enable individuals and communities to flourish.

Vital force (Ch. 10) – in early biological theory, a hypothetical force independent of physical and chemical forces regarded as being the causative factor of the evolution and development of living organisms.

Vital signs (Ch. 14) – indicators of body function such as blood pressure, temperature, pulse and respirations.

References

Brooker, C., 2010. Mosby's dictionary of medicine, nursing and health professions. First fully UK edition. Mosby, Edinburgh.

Centre for the Advancement of Interprofessional Education, 2011. Definition of Interprofessional learning.

CAIPE, London. Online. Available: www.caipe.org.uk September 2012.

Smith, P., 1997. Research mindedness for practice. Churchill Livingstone, Edinburgh.

World Health Organization, 2004. Palliative care. Online. Available: www.who.int/cancer/palliative/en September 2012.

Index

Index